D1064828

C. D. HAAGENSEN, M.D.

Professor Emeritus of Clinical Surgery,
The College of Physicians and Surgeons, Columbia University

DISEASES
OF
THE BREAST

Second Edition

W. B. SAUNDERS COMPANY Philadelphia · London · Toronto

W. B. Saunders Company: West Washington Square
Philadelphia, Pa.   19105

12 Dyott Street
London WC1A   1DB

833 Oxford Street
Toronto 18, Ontario

Diseases of the Breast   ISBN 0-7216-4440-6

Print No.:   9   8   7   6   5   4   3

To my wife,

Alice Munro Haagensen

Preface to the
Second Edition

During the 15 years that have elapsed since this book was published, my continuing experience with breast disease has confirmed, for me at least, the validity of the general point of view expressed in it. But as I reach the age at which my experience will begin to diminish, I realize more keenly than ever that nature is so infinitely varied in her manifestations — even in the limited domain of breast disease — that I cannot hope to achieve either a complete or an entirely accurate presentation of the subject. I am grateful to my colleagues and critics for the help they have given me in calling my attention to my omissions and errors.

During the 15 year period, there have been interesting developments in two aspects of breast disease. One is the use of newer methods of diagnosis such as radiography. The other is the significance of lobular neoplasia (the so-called lobular carcinoma), and multiple papilloma, as precancerous lesions.

It has given me great personal satisfaction in recent years to see a special Clinic for Breast Disease organized in our Columbia-Presbyterian Medical Center. In this clinic we achieve an adequate standard of recording the clinical and pathological features of breast disease, and of observing its natural history and evaluating the results of treatment. I am indebted to my associates in our Breast Clinic — Shivaji Bhonslay, David Habif, Sven Kister, Alfred Markowitz, Grant Sanger, and Philip Wiedel.

The statistical studies of our data, so important in a work of this kind, have been carried out by Dr. Edith Cooley and Dr. Andre Varma.

Robert Demarest, Lewis Koster, Rendal Von Muchow, and Edward Hajjar have prepared many new illustrations for this new edition.

Several generous friends, Mr. and Mrs. Emmanuel Cohen, Mr. and Mrs. Mike Levine, Mr. and Mrs. Morris Schapiro, and Mr. and Mrs. William R. Salomon, as well as another donor who wishes to remain anonymous, have made substantial contributions to the cost of preparing this new edition, and I am very grateful to them.

I am specially indebted to Dr. Raffaele Lattes, our Professor of Surgical Pathology, and to his associate, Dr. Nathan Lane, for help with pathology. During recent years I have come to rely for clinical and surgical help upon my associate, Dr. Sven Kister. Dr. Kister's knowledge of statistics has also been of great help to me. Finally, he has written Chapter 37 which deals with chemo-therapy. I am deeply indebted to him. Mrs. Kister has assisted with follow-up. Mrs. Grace MacQueen, long a member of the staff of the department, has helped in many ways.

I am deeply grateful to the late Lawrence Saunders, and to John Dusseau, Vice President and Editor-in-Chief, for their personal interest and encourage-ment, and to the Saunders staff for their expert assistance.

The preparation of this new edition has taken three years of intensive work. During all of this time my wife has patiently helped me by editing my manuscript and preparing the bibliography, sacrificing her own interests in the meanwhile. Her contribution has been a very great one.

I should particularly like to thank the many physicians who have referred patients with interesting problems in breast disease to us. I regret that I know most of them only through telephone conversations, but I have acquired a profound admiration for the sincerity with which they try to help their patients. As long as this spirit prevails, medicine will continue to be a rewarding profession.

C. D. HAAGENSEN

The Columbia-Presbyterian Medical Center
New York
March, 1971

Preface to the
First Edition

In this book I have tried to present a synthesis of what I have learned during twenty-five years of specialized concentration on diseases of the breast. I wish to emphasize at once that this knowledge is a product of the medical environment in which I have worked at the Columbia-Presbyterian Medical Center in New York. The book is based not only upon my personal experience, but upon all the data concerning diseases of the breast which have accumulated in our records during the forty year period 1915 to 1955.

When I came to Columbia in 1931 I had already acquired, from Dr. Ewing and his associates at the old Memorial Hospital, an abiding interest in neoplastic disease. At Columbia I found the environment of a modern medical center which permitted my specialized interest, particularly in diseases of the breast, to evolve. In these modern times, when the sum of knowledge concerning even a subject of limited scope has grown so that it is beyond the grasp of any one individual, I feel no need to justify specialization. More than 2000 years ago the Greeks first proved the value of specialization in the sciences. In modern medicine our specialization on an anatomical and disease basis merely carries this inevitable and desirable trend one step farther. A basic qualification, however, is that the specialist have ready access to the world of medical knowledge outside his own limited sphere. Otherwise he is hopelessly handicapped in dealing with the complex problems that sick patients usually present. The modern medical center— a family of specialized hospitals and services with closely integrated house and attending staffs—provides this kind of environment.

I should like to describe some of the basic facilities at the Columbia-Presbyterian Medical Center which have made this book possible. The first of these has been a Unit Record System. It was established in 1915 and has been organized with great efficiency by Miss Dorothy Kurtz. I am indebted to her for teaching me how to adapt the punch card method of statistical analysis to the problem of correlating the findings in our breast carcinoma cases.

In its establishment of a follow-up system for surgical patients the Presbyterian Hospital was preceded only by the Massachusetts General Hospital. Our follow-up system was organized in 1915 by Dr. James Corscaden and the late Dr. Hugh Auchincloss. One of the reasons why it has been so successful is that it has been a personal follow-up, each attending surgeon following his own ward patients just as if they were private patients. I have been able to trace every one of the ward and private patients in my personal series of radical mastectomies. In this task I have had the devoted assistance of Miss Florence Harvey, Miss Retta Pinney, and Miss Gertrude Taylor. A complete follow-up of this kind is, it seems to me, a fundamental obligation for us. Unless the fate of all our patients is known, their individual contributions to the knowledge of their disease—made at so great a cost—are entirely lost.

Dr. Arthur Purdy Stout, until his retirement three years ago the Director of our laboratory of Surgical Pathology, has contributed greatly, not only to this book, but to all the other aspects of our attack upon neoplastic disease at Columbia. Trained as a surgeon as well as a pathologist, Dr. Stout has been able to focus clinical as well as microscopical skill upon the special problem that tumors present. He has made the frozen section method of diagnosis a dependable, and therefore an invaluable, aid to our surgeons. His studies in the histogenesis of neoplasms are well known. Dr. Stout welcomed me into his laboratory when I first came to Columbia. He has been my inspiration ever since. This book is based upon the pathological material that he collected and studied over a period of forty years—1915 to 1955. We have worked together at interpreting it. The book is therefore his as much as it is mine.

All of us at Columbia who have worked at the special problems of neoplasia in the years gone by owe our opportunity to our beloved surgical chief, Dr. Allen O. Whipple. I am particularly indebted to him because he took me into his department and permitted me to specialize when specialization was not popular. He always supported and encouraged me in my clinical as well as my laboratory research.

There are a number of other individuals who have made important contributions to this book. Dr. Edith Cooley, our statistician, has worked tirelessly getting out the statistical data from our case records, analyzing them, and putting them into the form in which I have presented them. Mrs. Grace MacQueen, with her thorough familiarity with our records, and the subject matter itself, has been a great help in the preparation of the book. My wife has been my editorial mentor, correcting my manuscript with great patience, and verifying the entire bibliography.

In regard to the bibliography I should point out that it is a selected and not a complete one. I possess a substantially complete bibliography on diseases of the breast but it seemed wisest to select from it for inclusion in this book those items which not only contribute something but which are easily accessible to American and Western European readers.

I am deeply indebted to my surgical associates Dr. Joseph McDonald and Dr. David Habif for help with many of the surgical aspects of this work during the past years; to Dr. Stout's successor, Dr. Raffaele Lattes, for continuing assistance regarding matters of pathology; to Dr. John Pickren for certain pathological studies of his which I have included; to Dr. Virginia Apgar for help with the special problems of anesthesia; to Dr. Perry Hudson for assistance in regard to methods of hormone therapy; and to Dr. Maurice Lenz, until recently Director of Radiotherapy at the Francis Delafield Hospital, and to his successor, Dr. Ruth Guttmann, for help in all matters pertaining to radiotherapy.

For many years Dr. Stout, Dr. Lenz, Dr. John Hanford, and I conducted a Neoplasm Clinic in the Presbyterian Hospital. We learned to understand and value each other's point of view, and to integrate our surgical and radiotherapeutic attack upon breast carcinoma. Dr. Lenz taught us what intensive, highly fractionated irradiation, administered with meticulous care and great patience, can accomplish. In his hands radiotherapy is a precise weapon, and its use is

based upon principles which the surgeon can understand. The spirit of cooperation between surgeons and radiotherapeutists, both being guided by the facts
revealed by pathology, continues in our special cancer hospital, the Francis
Delafield Hospital, recently added to the Columbia-Presbyterian Medical Center.
The exceptional facilities for clinical cancer research provided in the Francis
Delafield Hospital have made possible a number of recent studies which I have
reported in this book.

Others who have helped with the preparation of the book have been Robert
Demarest and Leon Schlossberg, who made the drawings; Lewis Koster, who,
together with the late Walter O'Neil, made the photographs; Anton Samuel,
research technician; and the staff of the library of the College of Physicians and
Surgeons. The highly skilled staff of W. B. Saunders Company have made the
technical aspect of the preparation of the book easy for me.

C. D. HAAGENSEN

The Columbia-Presbyterian Medical Center
New York
September, 1956

Contents

Chapter One

Anatomy of the Mammary Gland

The mammary glands are a distinguishing feature of the zoological class which has been named after them — the mammals. The number of pairs of breasts varies greatly among different species of mammals, but has a general relationship to the number of young in each litter. For instance, the rodents have six or seven pairs of breasts and the lion but two. Man, the apes, and the monkeys (except for the marmosets) have but a single pair. The number of mammary glands has no relationship to the tendency of carcinoma to develop in them, for the disease is frequent in the mouse, in the dog, and in man, but is rare or unknown in other species.

FORM

The human female breast has a distinctive and unique protuberant conical form. In other primates the breasts are comparatively flat, even during pregnancy and lactation. The conical form of the human breasts is most marked in younger nulliparous women. With advancing age the breasts usually become somewhat flattened and pendulous and less firm. Popular opinion has it that these changes are aggravated by breast feeding, but there have been no scientific studies of this question. I have taken careful lactation histories in my patients and I have not been able to correlate my findings with the form of the breasts.

Although there appear to be some racial differences in the form of the breasts, the more pendulous type being more frequent in some primitive peoples, there can be no doubt that obesity is the most important factor concerned in variation in breast size and shape. As women gain weight, their breasts become more massive and pendulous.

It is important to point out that the two breasts are often unequal in size, although perfectly symmetrical in contour. This kind of breast inequality occurs in women who have no apparent endocrine abnormalities. The clinician alert for inequalities produced by neoplasms must not confuse differences in size which are developmental in origin with those due to pathologic changes.

These differences in the breasts may sometimes be marked. The following case illustrates the phenomenon.

C. G. came to the Presbyterian Hospital at the age of 13, complaining that her breasts were unequal in size. Menstruation had begun at the age of 11, and her breasts began to develop at about the same time. A year later it was noted that the left breast was smaller than the right. Both breasts slowly enlarged, but the left continued to be about one-half the size of the right. This discrepancy still persisted when the patient was last seen at the age of 19 (Fig. 1–1). At this time the right breast was entirely normal, but the left one continued to be smaller. There was no associated endocrine abnormality.

EXTENT

The protuberant breast extends from the second or third rib to the sixth or seventh

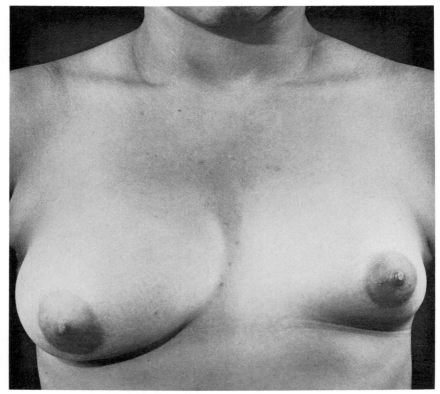

Figure 1–1.   Underdevelopment of the left breast.

costal cartilage, and from near the edge of the sternum to the anterior axillary line. The actual extent of the mammary tissue is considerably greater, however. It is spread out as a thin layer which often reaches the clavicle above, the midline medially, and the edge of the latissimus dorsi muscle laterally. This is a fact of importance to the surgeon attacking carcinoma of the breast, who should extend his dissection far enough to remove all of the breast. This wide superficial extent of the breast tissue is particularly evident in certain cases of acute postpartum engorgement of the breasts. We have also seen proof of it in studying microscopic sections from subcutaneous tissues from areas beyond the protuberant breast.

The upper outer sector of the breast is thicker than the remainder of the breast. The fact that this sector contains a greater bulk of mammary tissue than other sectors may account for the fact that both benign and malignant tumors are more frequent in it.

The breast also extends into the axilla to a variable degree. This axillary projection or "tail" is sometimes so large that it forms a visible axillary mass which enlarges premenstrually and during lactation. Such well-developed axillary projections of the mammary gland are commonly mistaken for axillary lipomas or enlarged axillary lymph nodes. Carcinoma may develop in the axillary projection and confuse the diagnostician.

Figure 1–2 shows a prominent left axillary projection of the mammary gland in a single woman, aged 32. She had noted the left axillary tumor for only one month. It was soft and measured about 5 cm. in diameter. Its lower pole merged with the upper outer part of the left breast, and there was no supernumerary nipple or areola to suggest that the axillary mass was a separate supernumerary mammary gland. There was a homologous but considerably smaller axillary projection on the right side. The left breast was considerably smaller than the right.

The left axillary mass was excised and proved to be mammary tissue. Microscopic

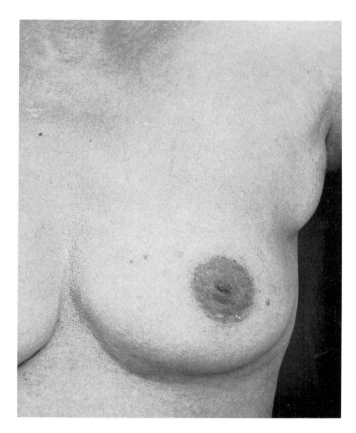

Figure 1–2. Axillary projection of the left mammary gland.

study showed that some of the ducts were dilated. There were papillary epithelial proliferations in others.

ANOMALIES

The extension of the breast into the axilla is so common that it can hardly be classed as an anomaly. True anomalies of the human breast include cases in which one or both breasts are absent or rudimentary, those in which there are accessory breasts or nipples, and those in which normally situated breasts have an abnormal structure. These anomalies are presumably genetic in origin, and are not due to disturbances in the neuroendocrine system that controls breast development and physiology. Such breast abnormalities will be discussed in Chapter 3.

The best discussion and documentation of these anomalies of the breast is to be found in Deaver and McFarland's book (1917) *The Breast: its Anomalies, its Diseases, and their Treatment.* To understand these anomalies it is necessary to keep in mind the embryology of the breasts. In the 4 mm. mammalian embryo, an epithelial ridge or "milk line" forms along each side of the body from the future axillary to the future inguinal region. It may extend onto the budding limbs. Somewhat later the ridge disappears and is represented by a number of minute points, each of which represents an epithelial anlage of a future breast. In some mammals all these anlagen develop into breasts; for example, the South American marsupial *Monodelphis henseli* has 25 pairs. In other mammals varying numbers of these pairs of breast anlagen are suppressed. In most of the primates and in man, only a single pair persists and develops into breasts in the pectoral region.

Absence of the breasts or nipples in human beings of either sex can be explained as the result of complete or imperfect suppression of these breast anlagen in the embryo. Accessory breasts, on the other hand, represent a reversion to a more primitive type of mammary arrangement in which more than a single pair of breast anlagen persist. Darwin himself, in his *Descent of Man* (1871), used polymastia as an example of atavism, or reversion to a more primitive ancestral type.

Amastia

Complete absence of one or both breasts is one of the rarest breast anomalies. Very small rudimentary breasts are less rare. Deaver and McFarland collected some 50-odd reports of this anomaly. During the last decade a few more such cases have been reported (Goldenring and Crelin; Jain, Sepaha, and Khandelwal; Kowlessar and Orti; Pierre and Bureau; Trier; Zilli and Stefani). Most of these subjects were females, although there were a few males in the series. The anomaly was usually unilateral, but in a few cases it was bilateral.

In a considerable proportion of cases of absent or rudimentary breasts there was associated underdevelopment or absence of structures of the shoulder girdle, chest, or arm. Several instances of mother and daughter with amastia are recorded, and in one family the anomaly was transmitted through three generations.

In our Presbyterian Hospital records we have one typical example of this rare anomaly. In this patient (R. P.) the right breast began to develop normally at the age of 11, but the left breast remained underdeveloped. Ten years later, when she was 21, her right breast was normal in size while the left breast was only about one-quarter the size of the right one (Fig. 1–3). The left pectoralis major muscle could not be demonstrated in physical examination. The left deltoid muscle was also underdeveloped. In this patient Dr. Jerome Webster performed a plastic operation to equalize the size of the two breasts, reducing the size of the right breast and transplanting part of it to augment the size of the left breast.

Accessory Breast Tissue

Accessory breasts or nipples are much more common than amastia. Deaver and McFarland tabulated 430 cases, and de Cholnoky, who has written more recently on this anomaly, refers to about 100 additional reports of such cases. None of the subjects of these reports can compete with the famous Diana of Ephesus, who displayed a total of 20 accessory pectoral breasts (Figure 1–4).

Accessory breasts or nipples occur in from 1 to 2 per cent of white subjects. This anomaly is apparently more frequent in Orientals. Iwai found it in 1.68 per cent of Japanese males and in 5.19 per cent of females. Takeya found it in 3.6 per cent of Chinese males.

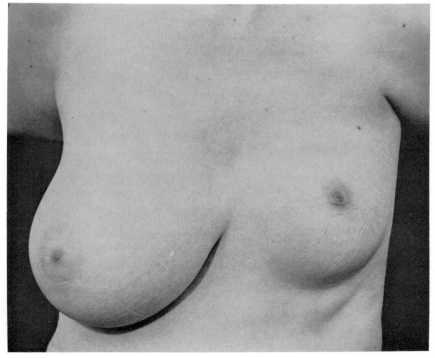

Figure 1–3.   Rudimentary left breast with absence of the pectoralis major muscle.

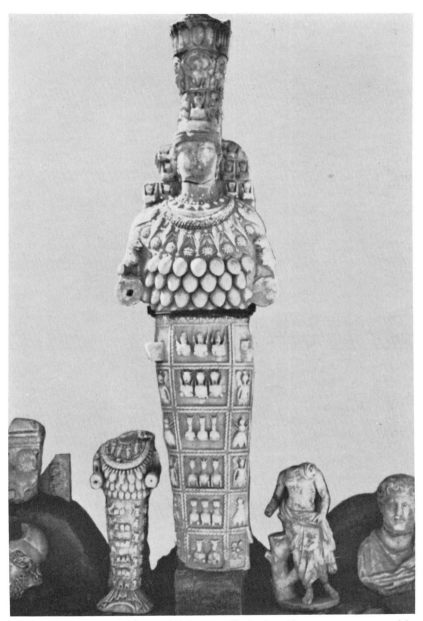

Figure 1–4. The statue of Diana of Ephesus, displaying 20 accessory pectoral breasts.

Accessory breast tissue appears to be about twice as frequent in females as in males.

This anomaly is clearly hereditary, for there are many reports of its transmission from parents to their children. Klinkerfuss has reported polymastia in four generations of a family.

Accessory breast tissue may occur as any combination, or as single elements, of the three components of the breast—its glandular parenchyma, the areola, or the nipple. The most frequent combination is a small areola and nipple. In many cases there is only a diminutive nipple.

These anomalous structures are usually situated along the embryologic milk line between the axillae and the groins. They are most frequent in the axilla. The next most frequent site is just below the normal breasts. In about one-half of the cases these anomalies are bilateral.

Figure 1–5 shows a woman, aged 35, with a well-developed supernumerary breast in the right axilla. She had noted its presence since she was 18 years old. During each of her three pregnancies it had enlarged, and during lactation it had secreted milk through the small protuberance in its center which resembled a small nipple. There was a similar but much smaller supernumerary breast, which did not possess a nipple, in the left axilla.

Because the large right axillary breast bothered her, the patient wanted it to be excised. This was done, and microscopic study showed abundant breast tissue with some cystic change, and a nipple of normal structure.

Figure 1–6 shows a 15 year old girl, otherwise normal, with a functioning supernumerary nipple about 10 cm. below the inframammary fold on the right side, and a supernumerary breast, complete with its own nipple, just below her normal left breast. This accessory left breast enlarged premenstrually. Both the right-sided extra nipple and the left-sided supernumerary breast were excised (service of Dr. J. P. Webster).

Figure 1–7 shows a man, aged 50, who had been aware since boyhood that he had

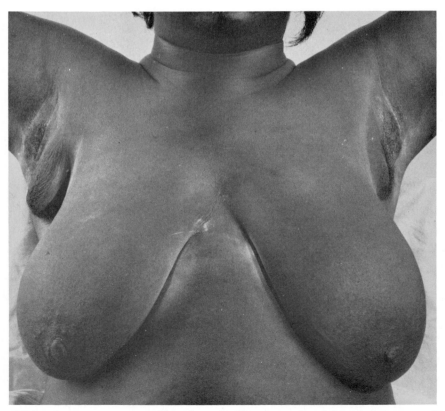

Figure 1–5.   Bilateral supernumerary axillary breasts. The one on the right side is larger and has a nipple.

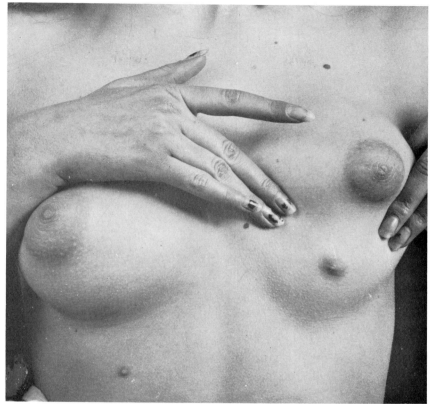

Figure 1–6. Supernumerary mammary development. Right supernumerary nipple. Left supernumerary breast.

accessory mammary structures. There were two on each side, extending along the mammary lines from a level about 8 cm. below the normal breasts down almost to the level of the umbilicus. The highest of these anomalous structures on the left side consisted of a small areola and a small nipple. The three others were only minute nipples.

More rarely, human anomalous breasts are found outside the embryonal mammary lines, corresponding to the location of the breasts in certain mammalian species. In one species of lemur (*Hapalemur griseus*) the breasts are situated in the acromial region, while in another lemur (*Chiromys Madagascariensis*) they are in the inguinal region. In the nutria (*Myopotamus*) the breasts are in the scapular region. The breasts of the *Cetacae* (whales and porpoises) are on the labia of the vulva. A South American rodent, the viscaccia (*Lagostomus*), has breasts on the dorsal aspects of its thighs, and the opossum (*Didelphys*) has breasts in the midline of the thorax and abdomen as well as along the mammary lines. There are reports of accessory breast tissue in man in all of these atypical locations outside the mammary lines. The most common are breasts in the inguinal region and vulva. Tow and Shanmugaratnam have recently collected reports of 15 such vulvar breasts.

Accessory breasts are of very little practical importance. Most of them consist only of a small areola and nipple, which have no physiologic function and are not subject to disease. Accessory breasts consisting only of glandular parenchyma but no areola or nipple are often wrongly diagnosed as lipomas or other benign neoplasms and are unnecessarily excised. Their mammary nature becomes apparent when they enlarge during pregnancy and lactation. When there is no normal duct system providing an outlet through a nipple, such accessory breast tissue usually involutes a few days or weeks after lactation begins. Complete accessory breasts of course lactate normally, and there are many reports of infants nursing from them.

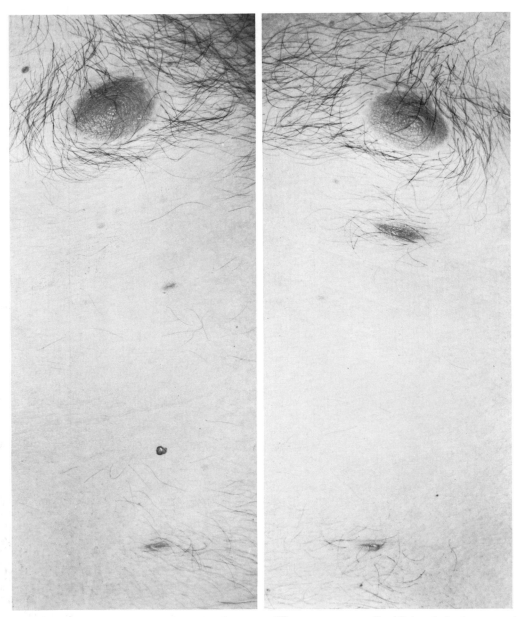

Figure 1–7. Accessory mammary structures in a man. There are two small additional nipples on each side along the mammary line below the normal breasts.

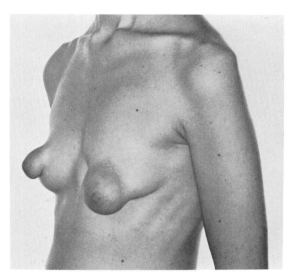

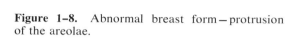

Figure 1–8. Abnormal breast form — protrusion of the areolae.

Accessory breasts containing glandular parenchyma are subject to all the diseases that afflict the normal breast. Adenofibromas, cysts, and carcinomas have all been reported as developing in them (Andreasen, Chiari, Cogswell and Czerny, de Cholnoky, Dickinson, Mornard, Noronha, Piccagli, Stringa, White).

Abnormal Breast Form

Absence of the nipple is apparently the rarest of all breast anomalies. Polythelia, in which a breast is provided with more than one nipple, has been observed in a small series of cases carefully tabulated and pictured by Deaver and McFarland. There may be two or more nipples within an otherwise normal areola, each nipple being connected with a portion of the duct system. Or there may be several separate and independent areolae, each with its own nipple, on the same breast. We have not observed this anomaly, but we have seen pedunculated neurofibromas of the areola simulating polythelia in a patient with neurofibromatosis.

Another abnormality of the breast which must be very rare, for we have not found a previous description of it, is protrusion of the areola to form a dependent sessile tumor. When the breasts begin to grow at puberty, the areolae sometimes appear to be disproportionately large and bulging. As the breasts enlarge and mature this disproportion corrects itself. In one of our patients, however, this protrusion of the areolae increased

with advancing age, forming true dependent tumors on each side. They are shown in Figure 1–8, when the patient was 25 years of age. The deformity was greater on the left side, but on both sides it was so disfiguring that correction by plastic surgery was performed by Dr. George Crikelair.

STRUCTURE

In addition to its epithelial parenchyma of acini and ducts and their supporting muscular and fascial elements, the breast consists of a varying amount of fat, blood vessels, nerves, and lymphatics. The connective tissue and epithelial elements are so inextricably intermingled that the surgeon can find no plane of dissection within the gland itself. He must always cut; attempts to use blunt dissection are futile.

The epithelial parenchyma is made up of 20 or more *lobes*, each emptying into a separate excretory duct terminating in the nipple. The lobes, in their turn, are divided into a multitude of lobules, or gland fields, each made up of from ten to 100 or more acini grouped around a collecting duct.

The *lobule* is thus the basic structural unit of the mammary gland, and as such deserves close study. The number and size of the lobules vary exceedingly, and not always according to the developmental stage of the subject. In general they are largest and most numerous during young womanhood (Figs. 1–9 and 1–10).

The *acini* in the resting mammary gland are lined by a single layer of cuboidal or cylin-

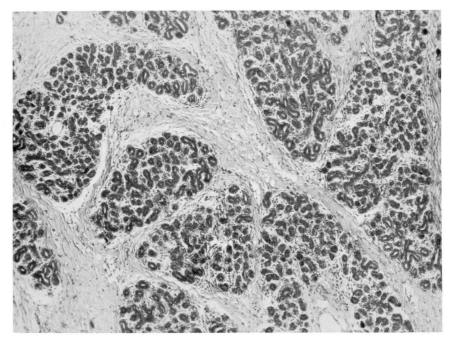

Figure 1–9.   Numerous and large lobules in the breast of a woman aged 22.

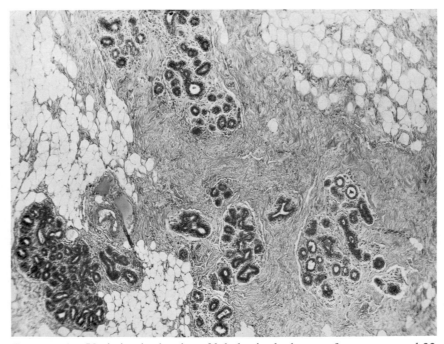

Figure 1–10.   Variation in the size of lobules in the breast of a woman aged 22.

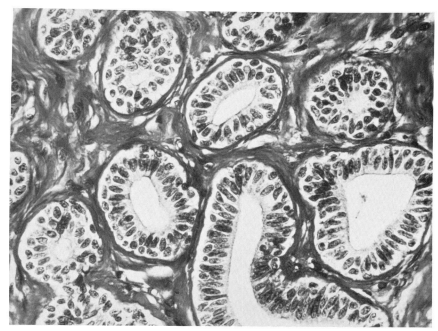

Figure 1–11. Normal epithelium of mammary gland acini.

drical epithelial cells (Fig. 1–11). Occasional additional cells around the base of the acinus suggest a second layer of epithelial cells. These basal cells are the so-called myoepithelial cells.

Each acinus is enveloped by a delicate but well-defined collagen sheath or basement membrane, which is best shown by a silver stain (Fig. 1–12). This sheath is prolonged to invest the collecting duct. The lobule as a whole is enclosed by a somewhat thicker collagen envelope.

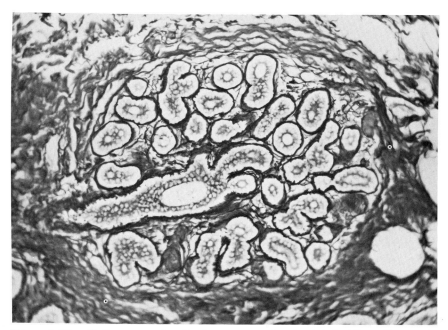

Figure 1–12. Collagenous sheath of mammary gland acini. Laidlaw silver stain.

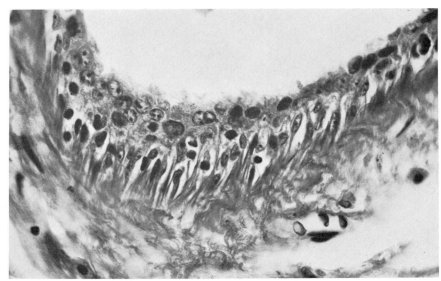

Figure 1–13.   Myoepithelial cells as seen in a transverse section through the wall of a small duct.

The *myoepithelial cells* of the breast have a special interest for the student of mammary neoplasms because they take part in certain benign proliferations which can be properly interpreted only in the light of the normal characteristics of the myoepithelial cells (Hamperl, Kuzma). These cells are best seen in the smaller ducts. They lie directly upon the basement membrane, beneath the inner layer of lining epithelium. They are elongated in shape, with dense oval nuclei and delicate cytoplasmic fibrils, closely resembling smooth muscle cells (Fig. 1–13). They have a spiral arrangement around the ducts, as shown in Figure 1–14 in which the duct wall has been sectioned eccentrically in its long axis. The

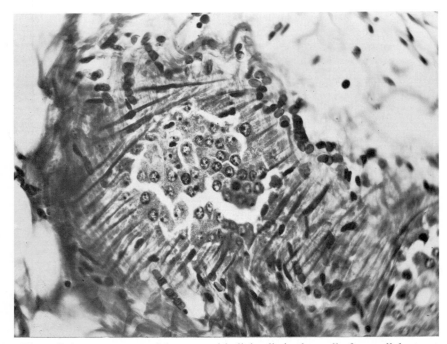

Figure 1–14.   The spiral arrangement of the myoepithelial cells in the wall of a small duct cut eccentrically in its long axis.

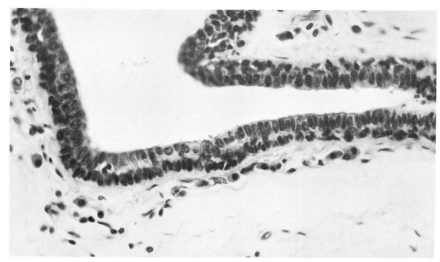

Figure 1–15. Main collecting duct of a mammary gland with two layers of epithelium.

myoepithelial cells provide a muscular mechanism for ejecting milk from acini and ducts (Richardson, Linzell), although this mechanism appears to be controlled by hormonal or metabolic factors; careful histologic studies have not demonstrated any innervation of the myoepithelial cells.

The details of the structure and arrangement of the myoepithelial cells can be seen only after proper fixation and staining. Masson's trichrome stain is the best means for demonstrating them. The myoepithelial layer of cells thins out as it approaches the acini, and is difficult or impossible to trace in normal acini. It is also lost to view in the larger collecting ducts. In these ducts there are two well-defined layers of cylindrical epithelial cells, as shown in Figure 1–15.

As the main collecting ducts enter the base of the nipple, they enlarge to form the milk sinuses which dilate and act as a reservoir for milk in nursing. They are about 20 in number. In cross-section, as seen in Figure 1–16, they have a characteristic accordion-pleated contour.

Just below the surface of the nipple the milk sinuses terminate in cone-shaped ampullae lined with stratified squamous epithelium. Figure 1–17 shows the milk sinuses and their ampullae in vertical section. In the resting breast these ampullae are filled with epithelial debris (Fig. 1–18) which effectively plugs the duct openings on the nipple surface.

The *nipple* and the *areola* contain several tissues which are of special interest in that they may give origin to neoplasms. Both the subareolar area and the nipple contain much smooth muscle. In the subareolar area its fibers are arranged in concentric rings, as well as radially. They insert into the base of the dermis, and function to contract the areola and to compress the base of the nipple.

The bulk of the nipple is made up of smooth muscle fibers arranged both circularly and longitudinally. When they contract they make the nipple erect, smaller, and firmer, and empty the milk sinuses.

The epithelium of the areolae and nipples is more deeply pigmented than normal skin. This pigmentation is more marked in brunettes than in blondes. It is also related to estrogen level, for the pigmentation is more marked in younger women, tends to fade somewhat at the menopause, and can be intensified at any age by the administration of estrogen.

The skin of the nipple is hairless and has well-developed dermal papillae. It contains large numbers of specialized sebaceous glands, which are often grouped around the openings of the milk sinuses. The skin of the areola has a few hair follicles around its periphery, and does not have well-developed dermal papillae. It contains three types of glands: sweat glands, specialized sebaceous glands, and not infrequently accessory mammary glands. The specialized sebaceous glands are large and superficially situated, and can often be seen as small nodules projecting above the areolar surface (Fig. 1–19). During pregnancy and lactation they enlarge, and they have come to be known as Montgomery's glands after the nineteenth century Irish obstetrician who de-

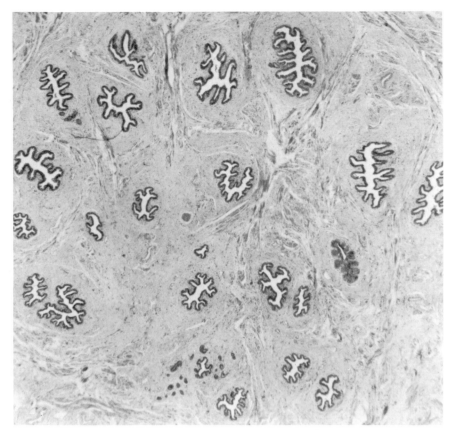

Figure 1–16. The milk sinuses seen in cross section of the nipple.

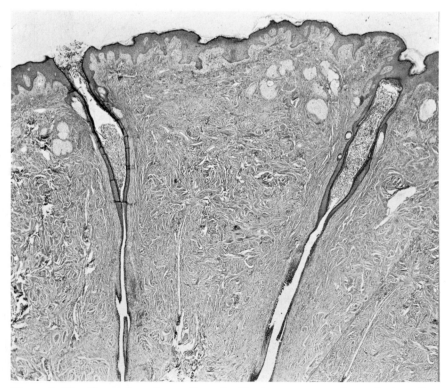

Figure 1–17. Cone-shaped ampullae of milk sinuses as seen in vertical section.

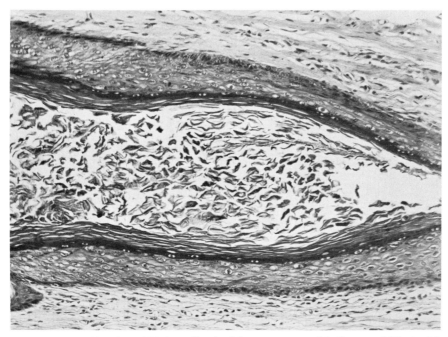

Figure 1–18. Ampulla of a milk sinus lined with squamous epithelium and filled with debris.

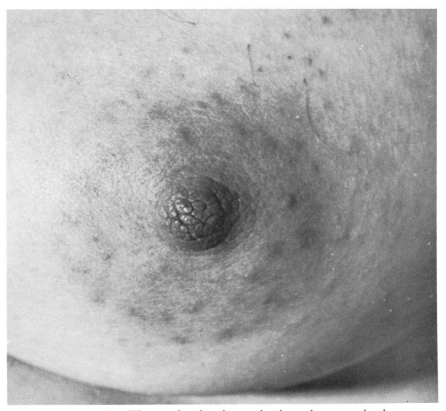

Figure 1–19. The areola, showing projecting sebaceous glands.

scribed them. The accessory mammary glands that are occasionally seen beneath the areola have the same structure as normal mammary gland acini. Their miniature ducts open into small sinuses in the areolar epithelium. The fact that they are indeed mammary glands is proved by their secretion of milk during lactation.

FASCIAL RELATIONSHIPS OF THE MAMMARY GLAND

Since the mammary gland is a modified cutaneous gland, an appendage of the skin, so to speak, it is enclosed between the superficial and deep layers of the superficial fascia. The superficial layer of this fascia is a very delicate but definite structure which will be seen only by the surgeon who looks sharply for it and who keeps the operative field dry enough to permit its identification. The anatomist in his dissecting room is usually unable to identify it. This fascial layer is important to the surgeon because it provides him with a good guide if he wishes to dissect up skin flaps through a relatively avascular plane and not include on them any mammary tissue. This is accomplished by dissecting just superficial to the superficial layer of the superficial fascia, and preferably by beginning at the caudad end of the radical mastectomy wound where the fascia is better developed. It becomes more and more delicate as the clavicle is approached. In thin individuals dissection through this plane leaves only 2 or 3 mm. of fat and areolar tissue on the skin flaps; in obese individuals several additional millimeters of fat may be found superficial to the fascia. Dissection in this plane passes deep to the network of small blood vessels in the corium, but is superficial to the larger vessels and lymphatics that lie beneath the superficial layer of the superficial fascia.

Cooper's "ligaments," which Sir Astley Cooper described and pictured so well a century ago, are peripheral tooth-like projections of the breast tissue in fibrous processes which reach and fuse with the superficial layer of the superficial fascia. "By these processes," Cooper wrote, "the breast is slung upon the forepart of the chest, for they form a movable but very firm connection with the skin so that the breast has sufficient motion. . . ." Figure 1–20 reproduces Cooper's original drawing of his dissection of the suspensory "ligaments." These fibrous processes are important clinically because the intimate connection between the breast and the skin which they provide results in skin retraction in carcinoma and in certain other breast lesions accompanied by fibrosis.

Stiles showed by means of his nitric acid method of fixation, which differentiates parenchyma and stroma in gross specimens, that the parenchyma of the breast is prolonged peripherally in these Cooper "ligaments" so that it "reaches almost up to the corium." Stiles quite properly concluded "that the surgeon who intends to excise the whole of such a gland (the breast) must either sacrifice a large amount of skin or keep so close to it in dissecting it off the mamma as to run some risk of sloughing."

Between the deep layer of the superficial fascia on the posterior aspect of the breast, and the deep fascia covering the pectoralis major and other muscles of the chest wall, there is a well-defined space, sometimes called the retromammary bursa. It contains loose areolar tissue which allows for a degree of mobility of the breast over the chest wall. The surgeon excising a portion of the mammary gland knows at once that he has reached the

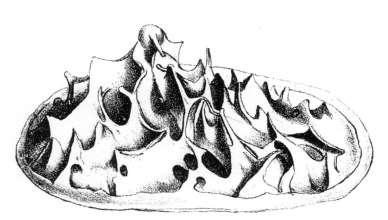

Figure 1–20. Cooper's ligaments of the breast. (*From* The Anatomy and Diseases of the Breast, by Sir Astley Cooper, Philadelphia, Lea and Blanchard, 1845.)

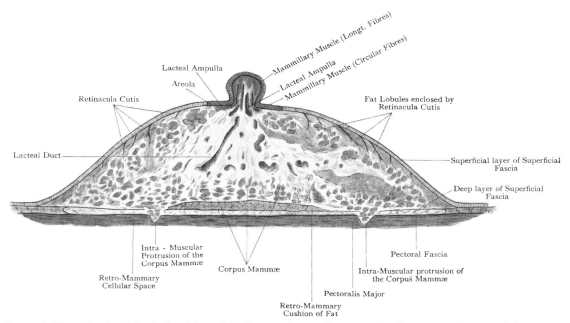

Figure 1–21. The fascial relationships of the breast shown diagrammatically. (*From* Cancer of the Breast: Clinically Considered, by Cecil H. Leaf, London, Constable and Company, Ltd., 1912.)

back of the breast when his knife falls into this loose areolar tissue.

Projections of the deep layer of the superficial fascia cross the retromammary space and fuse with the deep or pectoral fascia. These form the posterior suspensory ligaments of the breast. Stiles showed that small islands of breast parenchyma accompany these fibrous processes which are attached to the pectoral fascia. Deep projections of mammary parenchyma sometimes dip in between the muscle bundles of the pectoralis major muscle. In order to be certain of removing all breast tissue it is therefore necessary to excise not only the pectoral fascia which is intimately attached to the pectoralis muscle, but also a thin layer of the muscle itself. This is a difficult and bloody dissection.

These fascial relationships are well shown in Leaf's drawing (Fig. 1–21), which we have reproduced with his terminology.

Although it is customary to speak of the breast as lying upon the pectoral fascia, only a part of the gland, perhaps one half, in fact overlies the deep fascia of the pectoralis major. The remainder of the breast lies upon the other muscles clothing the chest wall lateral and caudad to the axillary border of the pectoralis major. When the arm is extended to shoulder level, the edge of the pectoralis major is elevated, exposing the fourth serra-

tion of the serratus magnus muscle. The breast then overlies the fourth, fifth, sixth, and seventh (in part) serrations of this muscle. More medially, it overlies the interdigitations of the external oblique with the serratus. Near the midline a small portion of the breast overlies the rectus abdominis. All of these muscles are of course covered by the same deep fascia which blends them together. Figure 1–22 shows these relationships.

THE AXILLARY FASCIAE

The fasciae of the axilla are of great practical importance to the surgeon, and he must know them thoroughly.

The deep layer of fascia which everywhere covers the muscle plane has a complex arrangement in the pectoral and axillary region. Here it not only forms septa which enclose and separate the two pectoral muscles, but in so doing it spans the axillary space and forms a bridge, so to speak, which stretches across the axilla from the deltoid muscle and the clavicle above to the chest wall muscles below. It has two strata, a superficial one called the *pectoral fascia* which invests the pectoralis major muscle, and a deeper one, the *costocoracoid fascia,* which invests the pectoralis minor muscle.

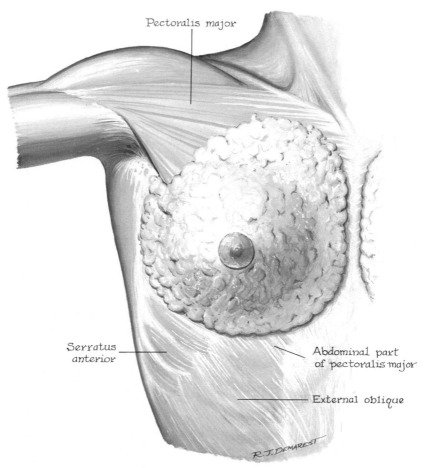

Figure 1–22.   Dissection of the breast to show anatomic relationships.

The *pectoral fascia* covers the external surface of the pectoralis major. Medially, it is continuous across the midline with the pectoral fascia of the opposite side. Laterally, it turns around the lateral border of the pectoralis major to cover its deep surface. Cephalad, it is continuous with the fascia of the deltoid and the fascia over the clavicle.

The *costocoracoid fascia* is a deeper and thicker layer of fascia spanning the axilla, revealed when the pectoralis major muscle is turned back or cut away, as in Eisler's drawing (Fig. 1–23). It has a special importance for the surgeon attempting to dissect the axilla, because it guards the nerves, vessels, and lymphatics that traverse the axilla. As Leaf said, this fascia gives coherence to the fat and lymph nodes of the axilla and makes their removal in one piece, together with all of the fascia, easier than would otherwise be the case. I have chosen to use the older English name, *costocoracoid* fascia, because it is the

most truly descriptive term. The German anatomists call it the "deep pectoral fascia." The French call it the "clavi-coraco-axillary aponeurosis," and some American anatomists prefer the term "clavipectoral fascia." Figure 1–24 shows these axillary fascial relationships in diagrammatic form as seen in a sagittal section through the pectoral region.

The portion of the costocoracoid fascia stretching across the inner portion of the axilla between the medial border of the pectoralis minor and the clavicle is irregularly four-sided. It contains an imperfectly rounded opening reminiscent of the fossa ovalis of the thigh, through which pass the cephalic vein, the thoracoacromial vessels, and anterior thoracic nerves. The crescentic medial edge of this opening is formed by a particularly thick and sometimes almost tendinous sheet of fascia which extends from the clavicle across the first intercostal space, to the second rib. The surgeon who wishes to expose the apex of

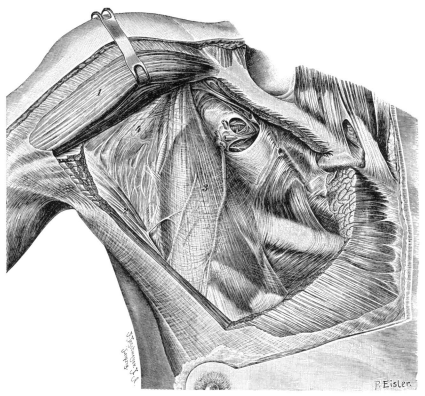

Figure 1–23. The costacoracoid fascia as shown after the pectoralis major has been removed to a large extent. *1*, deltoid; *2*, pectoralis major; *3*, pectoralis minor; *4*, coracobrachialis. (*From* Handbuch der Anatomie des Menschen, by Paul Eisler, Jena, Gustav Fischer, 1912.)

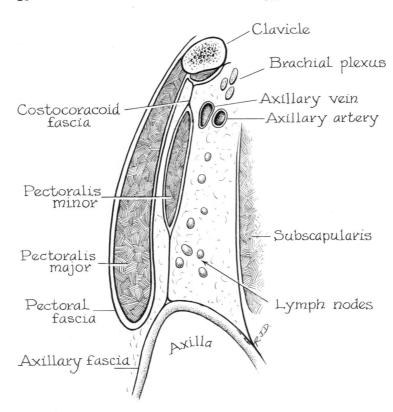

Figure 1-24. Relationships of the fasciae of the axilla as seen in a diagram of a sagittal section through the pectoral region.

the axilla must sever the attachment of this fascia to the clavicle, the adjacent portion of the first rib, and the deep fascia over the first intercostal space. This step reveals the axillary vein passing beneath the subclavius muscle, and parallel and just caudad to the vein, the collecting lymphatic trunks lying in areolar tissue and fat and also disappearing beneath the subclavius muscle.

The portion of the costocoracoid fascia stretching across the outer half of the axilla from the lateral edge of the pectoralis minor muscle to the coracobrachialis muscle is triangular in shape. At its base laterally it fuses with the so-called axillary fascia which forms the hollow of the axilla. This portion of the fascia is sometimes called, appropriately enough, the coracoaxillary fascia or the suspensory ligament of the axilla. From its apex at the coracoid process, band-like thickenings in the fascia stream laterally and caudad, reinforcing the fascia as it overlies the nerves and vessels of the lateral half of the axilla. The density of these reinforcing bands comes to the surgeon's attention as he severs this fascia cephalad and parallel to the axillary vein in the first step in axillary dissection.

THE BLOOD SUPPLY OF THE BREAST

Arteries

The chief blood supply of the breast is from the *perforating branches of the internal mammary artery*. The first, second, third, and fourth perforating branches perforate the chest wall near the sternal edge in the corresponding interspaces, and traverse the pectoralis major muscle to reach the mammary gland along its medial edge. The first perforating artery and its accompanying vein or veins usually emerge from the intercostal muscle plane near the caudad edge of the first interspace at the sternal border, and are closely applied to the surface of the second costal cartilage as they arch downward across it to enter the pectoral muscle. The second perforating artery is usually seen to emerge from the intercostal plane near the cephalad edge of the second interspace at the lower edge of the second costal cartilage. Thus the two largest vessels supplying the breast are encountered by the surgeon just above and just below the second costal cartilage. The lower perforators emerge at varying levels in their respective interspaces.

In the upper interspaces there is a series of much smaller perforating vessels which emerge from the intercostal muscle plane 2 or 3 cm. lateral to and parallel with the main perforators. These secondary perforators are large enough to justify the surgeon's taking care to identify and clamp and cut them after the main perforations have been clamped and cut.

Several branches of the axillary artery also share in providing blood for the breast (Fig. 1–25). The smallest and highest of these, *the highest thoracic artery,* is a variable and inconsequential vessel which crosses from the first part of the axillary artery to the chest wall above the upper border of the pectoralis minor muscle.

The *pectoral branch of the thoracoacromial artery* descends between the pectoralis minor and major muscles. It is the chief blood supply of the latter muscle. After traversing the pectoralis major, some of its branches reach the deep surface of the mammary gland.

A small artery, the *artery to the pectoralis minor,* arises from the second part of the axillary artery from 1 or 2 cm. lateral to the origin of the thoracoacromial trunk, or as a branch of the thoracoacromial trunk, and crosses the axillary vein, closely applied to its surface as it runs caudad to reach the deep surface of the pectoralis minor. The importance of this very small artery to the surgeon is out of all proportion to its size, for as we will point out in our description of the dissection of the axilla, cutting it and the medial anterior thoracic nerve which accompanies it, gives access to the axillary vein.

The *lateral thoracic artery* arises from the second part of the axillary artery, or as a branch of the thoracoacromial or subscapular arteries. Emerging from beneath the axillary vein, it crosses the axilla to the chest wall and the free outer edge of the pectoralis major to supply the lateral portion of the breast. It has been called the external mammary artery. It varies in size, and is not infrequently absent.

The *subscapular artery* is the largest branch of the axillary artery, arising from its third portion opposite the outer border of the subscapularis muscle. The subscapular gives off the scapular circumflex artery soon after it arises, and in its continuation across the surface of the subscapularis muscle to the lateral chest wall it is called the *thoracodorsal artery.*

It supplies the latissimus dorsi muscle and sends several large branches to the serratus magnus. Difficulty in controlling bleeding from these arterial branches and their accompanying veins during radical mastectomy has given the name "the bloody angle" to this region. The thoracodorsal artery is not an important supply for the breast, but in its course it is intimately associated with the central and scapular groups of lymph nodes which so often contain metastases from breast carcinoma; and the manner in which the surgeon deals with this artery in his axillary dissection is therefore very important.

Veins

The venous route is important to students of breast carcinoma not only because metastasis frequently occurs through veins, but also because veins are a key to the lymphatic pathways, which in general follow the course of the veins.

The superficial subcutaneous veins over the breast lie just below the superficial layer of the superficial fascia, and are large enough and close enough to the skin surface to be shown well by photographs taken in infrared light. Massopust and Gardner have made extensive photographic studies of this kind and have classified the anatomical patterns formed by these veins into two main types. In the transverse type of pattern the veins converge toward the sternal edge and then turn deeply to join the perforating vessels that pierce the chest wall and empty into the internal mammary veins. In the longitudinal type the veins converge toward the suprasternal notch and empty into the superficial veins of the lower neck that drain into the anterior jugulars. Infrared photographs from our own patients illustrate these two types of patterns (Figs. 1–26 and 1–27). Infrared photographs show that these superficial veins anastomose across the midline of the anterior chest wall in many patients.

Infrared photographs also demonstrate nicely the circumareolar veins, which are a relatively constant anatomic finding, and which surgeons who use circumareolar incisions know well.

The superficial veins over the breast are often dilated over an area of the breast that contains disease, and the dilatation is sometimes marked enough to be recognized by inspection in ordinary light. Tumors, whether

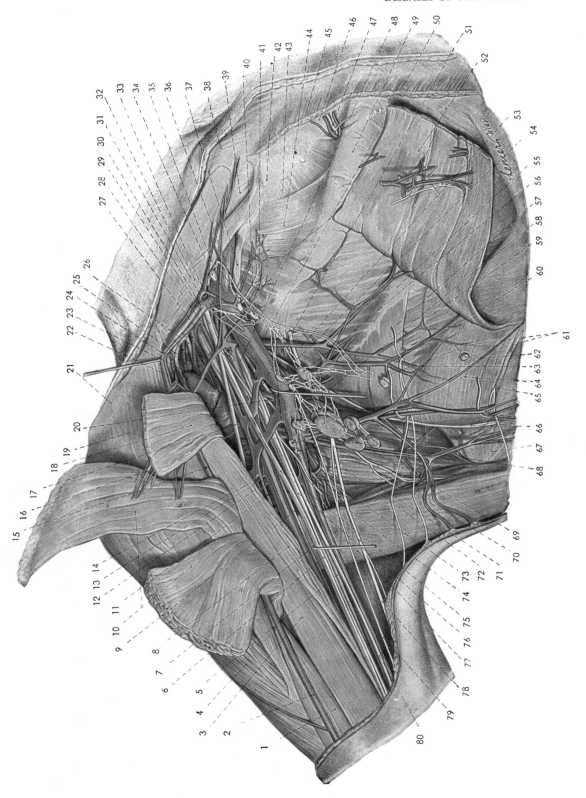

Figure 1–25. The anatomy of the axilla. (*From* Topographische Anatomie, by E. Pernkopf, Berlin and Vienna, Urban and Schwarzberg, 1937–1952.)

KEY TO DISSECTION OF AXILLA

1. Long head of the biceps muscle
2. Cephalic vein
3. Short head of the biceps muscle
4. Deltoid muscle
5. Ulnar nerve
6. Median nerve
7. Brachial artery
8. Coracobrachialis muscle
9. Radial nerve
10. Pectoralis major muscle
11. Brachial vein
12. Posterior humeral circumflex artery
13. Anterior humeral circumflex artery
14. Common head of the coracobrachialis and the short head of the biceps muscles
15. Cephalic vein
16. Anterior thoracic nerve and pectoral branch of thoraco-acromial artery
17. Musculocutaneous nerve
18. Pectoralis minor muscle
19. Deltoid muscle
20. Subscapular nerves
21. Acromial end of the clavicle
22. Acromial branch of thoraco-acromial artery
23. Thoraco-acromial artery
24. Coracoid process
25. Coracoclavicular fascia
26. Suprascapular artery, vein, and nerve
27. Posterior cord of brachial plexus
28. Medial anterior thoracic nerve, and a branch of the axillary artery to the pectoralis minor
29. Lateral cord of the brachial plexus
30. Terminal portion of the cephalic vein
31. Axillary artery
32. Subclavius muscle
33. Anterior thoracic nerves
34. Subclavicular group of axillary lymph nodes
35. Clavicular branch of thoraco-acromial artery
36. Axillary vein and subclavicular lymphatic trunk
37. Tendinous origin of the serratus anterior muscle from the first rib
38. Sternoclavicular joint
39. Costoclavicular ligament
40. Branch of the first intercostal nerve
41. Highest thoracic artery
42. Cartilage of first rib
43. Internal intercostal muscle (first intercostal space)
44. External intercostal muscle (first intercostal space)
45. Pectoralis major muscle (cut at its origin)
46. Sternum (manubrium)
47. Perforating vessels in first interspace
48. Medial cord of branchial plexus
49. Cartilage of second rib
50. Origin of serratus anterior muscle from second rib
51. Thoracodorsal nerve and artery
52. The pectoralis minor muscle reflected to show branches of the thoraco-acromial artery and the artery to the pectoralis minor, and branches of the anterior thoracic nerves, entering its deep surface
53. Lateral thoracic artery
54. Intercostobrachial nerve (lateral cutaneous branch of the second intercostal nerve)
55. Third rib
56. Central group of axillary lymph nodes
57. Origin of serratus anterior muscle from third rib
58. Long thoracic nerve
59. External intercostal muscle (third intercostal space)
60. Lateral cutaneous branch of the third intercostal nerve
61. External mammary group of axillary lymph nodes
62. Thoracodorsal vein
63. Costoaxillary vein
64. Origin of serratus anterior muscle from fourth rib
65. Lateral cutaneous branch of the fourth intercostal nerve
66. Long thoracic nerve
67. Insertion of serratus anterior muscle on inferior angle of scapula
68. Scapular group of axillary lymph nodes
69. Thoracodorsal nerve and artery
70. Axillary vein group of axillary lymph nodes
71. Teres major muscle
72. Subscapularis major muscle
73. Scapular circumflex artery and vein, and branch of subscapular nerve to teres major
74. Medial brachial cutaneous nerve (severed)
75. Lateral root of the medial nerve
76. Medial root of the medial nerve
77. Latissimus dorsi muscle
78. Intercostobrachial nerve
79. Medial branchial cutaneous nerve
80. Basilic vein and medial antibrachial cutaneous nerve

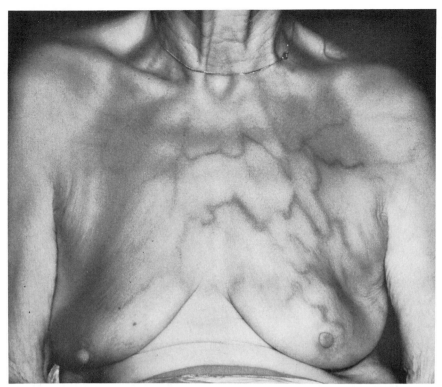

Figure 1–26. Superficial veins of the anterior chest wall as shown in an infrared photograph. Transverse type of pattern. The patient has a carcinoma of the upper central region of the left breast.

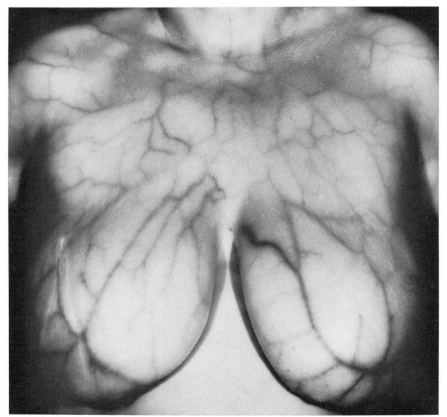

Figure 1–27. Superficial veins of the anterior chest wall as shown in an infrared photograph. Longitudinal type of pattern.

24

malignant or benign, that are growing vigorously demand an increased blood supply, and the prominent regional superficial veins are a manifestation of this increased blood supply.

There are three groups of deep veins carrying blood from the breast and chest wall which are of special interest to us:

1. The *perforating branches of the internal mammary vein* are the largest veins carrying blood from the breast. Those in the upper three interspaces are larger than those in the lower interspaces.

The internal mammary veins empty into the corresponding innominate veins. This venous pathway leads, of course, directly to the pulmonary capillary network, and provides a route for metastatic carcinoma emboli to the lungs.

2. The *axillary vein receives many tributaries* from the chest wall, the pectoral muscles, and the deep surface of the breast. In general they correspond to the branches of the axillary artery. They are, however, more variable in their arrangement. The tributaries entering the axillary vein are indeed so irregular that it is not worthwhile attempting to identify them, with the exception of the cephalic and thoracoacromial veins.

The axillary vein itself shows great variation. The junction of the basilic and brachial veins to form the axillary vein may take place at any point from the outer edge of the teres major up to the clavicle. When this junction occurs high up, the axillary vein is in effect double. Care must be exercised not to mistake, in such cases, the main venous trunk from the arm for a large branch of the axillary vein coming from the lateral chest wall. When, in the course of an axillary dissection, tension upon the specimen in a caudad direction bows the axillary vein downwards, its relationships may be distorted. Normally it lies medial (caudad when the arm is abducted as in an axillary dissection) to the axillary artery, overlapping it so thoroughly that the artery is not seen at all during the dissection.

A phenomenon which sometimes confuses the surgeon during his dissection of the axillary vein is the marked contractility of its lateral portion. When the vein is first exposed it has a large caliber throughout its whole extent, although tapering somewhat toward the arm. Dissection of the medial portion of the vein changes its caliber very little, but dissection of the lateral half produces such sharp contraction of that portion of the vein

that the surgeon may momentarily doubt that he is still dealing with the axillary trunk.

The venous pathway from the breast through the axillary vein leads, of course, directly to the pulmonary capillary network and provides a second route to the lungs for carcinoma emboli.

3. The third and one of the most important routes of venous drainage from the breast is directed posteriorly through the *intercostal veins*. These veins communicate with the vertebral veins and finally empty into the azygos vein. This route through the intercostal and azygos veins leads to the superior vena cava and to the lungs. It constitutes a third pathway by which carcinoma emboli produce pulmonary metastases.

These three venous routes for metastases from breast carcinoma to the capillary network of the lungs are shown especially in Figure 1–28.

The vertebral system of veins provides an entirely different route by which metastases reach the bones directly, without going through the caval veins and through the lungs.

The vertebral veins constitute a separate vertical system of veins, paralleling the caval system. They drain blood from the vertebral column, adjacent muscles, and the spinal cord. They form intricate venous plexuses both inside and outside the vertebral canal extending along its entire length. The so-called basivertebral veins form wide tortuous channels within the vertebral bodies, similar to those in the diploë of cranial bones, and empty into the anterior external vertebral plexus. The vertebral plexuses communicate at each vertebral segment with the intercostal veins. Figure 1–29 shows this communication as pictured in Gray's *Anatomy*.

Batson has proved with injection experiments in cadavers that the vertebral system of veins drains not only the vertebrae but also the bones of the pelvic girdle and the upper ends of the femurs, the bones of the shoulder girdle and the upper ends of the humeri, and the skull. This venous system is without valves, except in minor connecting channels. The pressure within it is low. Retrograde flow of blood occurs easily within it. Indeed, the blood surges back and forth from the vertebral to the caval system with slight changes in intra-abdominal pressure. The vertebral system can be readily injected through the tributaries of the caval system. Figure 1–30 shows the vertebral plexus well outlined in an injec-

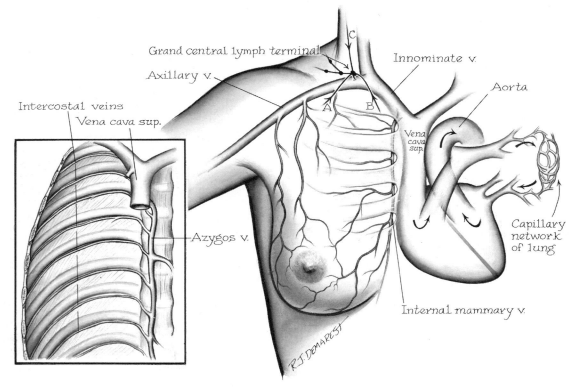

Figure 1–28.   The three venous routes of metastasis from carcinoma of the breast to the capillary network of the lungs, shown diagrammatically.

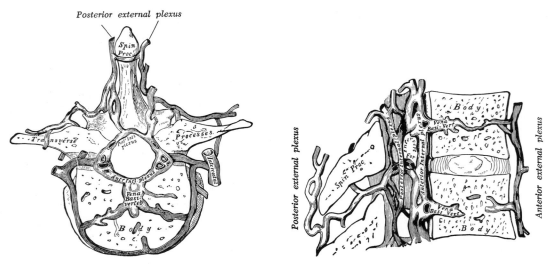

Figure 1–29.   Transverse and median sagittal sections of vertebrae showing the vertebral venous plexus and its communications with the intercostal veins. (*From* Gray's Anatomy, 26th ed., edited by Charles M. Goss, Philadelphia, Lea and Febiger, 1954.

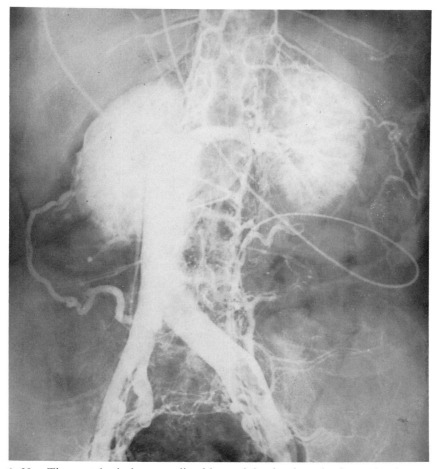

Figure 1–30. The vertebral plexus outlined by an injection into the femoral vein at autopsy.

tion made into the femoral vein, in an autopsy study.

Batson emphasizes that the vertebral system of veins provides a venous pathway in the long axis of the body along which metastases, escaping through the intercostal veins draining carcinoma of the breast, may spread to the skeleton without entering the caval venous system. The frequency with which metastases are seen in the vertebrae, in the pelvic bones, and in the skull, without evident parenchymal pulmonary metastases, strongly supports the argument that the vertebral system of veins is an important route along which breast carcinoma metastasizes.

Henriques has recently described and superbly illustrated the venous circulation of the vertebrae, corroborating the importance of the vertebral veins as a route for metastasis of breast cancer to the vertebrae.

THE NERVES OF THE MAMMARY REGION

The microscopic character of the innervation of the skin over the breast has been studied by Miller and Kasahara. They found an unusually large number of multi-branched free-fiber endings in the dermis of the nipple, and Ruffini-like endings and Krause end bulbs in the dermis of the areola and peripheral breast skin. They suggest that this special innervation is associated with the processes of erection of the nipple and milk flow, mediated through reflex stimulation of the pituitary.

The skin over the upper part of the breast is supplied by the third and fourth branches of the cervical plexus.

The skin of the lower part of the breast is supplied by the *thoracic intercostal nerves*. Their lateral cutaneous branches emerge between the digitations of the serrati muscles in the anterior axillary line and supply the lateral breast skin. Their anterior cutaneous branches emerge from the pectoralis major muscle with the perforating vessels close to the sternum and supply the medial breast skin.

The lateral cutaneous branch of the second intercostal nerve does not divide into an anterior and a posterior division, as do the lower lateral cutaneous nerves. Instead, the whole second lateral cutaneous nerve—and it is much the largest of this series of nerves—runs laterally across the axilla, forming a plexus with the medial brachial cutaneous nerve which lies cephalad to it (when the arm is abducted) and with the posterior division of the third lateral cutaneous nerve which lies caudad to it. This large second lateral cutaneous nerve has been named the intercostobrachial nerve. This nerve, and the plexus which it forms as it traverses the axilla to cross the white tendon of the latissimus muscle and run down the inner aspect of the arm, must of course be sacrificed in any axillary dissection. To attempt to save the intercostobrachial nerve and dissect it out from among the scapular vessels and lymph nodes, which often contain metastases, is bad cancer surgery. Sacrifice of the intercostobrachial nerve denervates the skin of the medial aspect of the upper half of the arm.

In the dissection of the axilla the medial brachial cutaneous nerve is often found lying caudad to the axillary vein, and it may have to be sacrificed to facilitate meticulous isolation and section of the numerous branches of the vein. When the medial brachial cutaneous nerve is also sacrificed, the area of anesthesia on the inner aspect of the arm extends down as far as the elbow.

In carrying out an axillary dissection the surgeon lays bare the cords of the brachial plexus by severing the fibers of the costocoracoid fascia and dissecting the delicate layer of fat and areolar tissue, which overlies the cords of the plexus and the axillary vein, downward across them. He has no need of disturbing the cords of the plexus by dissecting between them.

The only nerve sacrificed in this part of the dissection is the medial anterior thoracic nerve to the pectoralis minor. It crosses outward and downward over the axillary vein and must be cut if the vein is to be cleanly dissected.

At a later stage in the dissection of the axilla the surgeon has to deal with two important nerves, the thoracodorsal and the long thoracic.

The *thoracodorsal* or middle subscapular nerve emerges from beneath the axillary vein at the junction of its middle and inner thirds, and extends diagonally outward and downward in the fat and areolar tissue lying upon the subscapular muscle, usually closely applied to the thoracodorsal vessels, to enter the latissimus dorsi muscle which it supplies. In following this course the nerve traverses the central and scapular groups of axillary lymph nodes which often contain metastases. If the nerve is preserved, it has to be dissected out from among these nodes. This is a hazardous procedure if metastases are present, for the surgeon's knife or forceps may enter a carcinomatous node and smear carcinoma cells widely in the field of operation. It is therefore my custom to sacrifice the thoracodorsal nerve rather than to preserve it. I cut it as it emerges from beneath the axillary vein and dissect it downward with the thoracodorsal vessels, which are always sacrificed.

The *long thoracic nerve* emerges from beneath the medial third of the axillary vein and lies in the areolar tissue upon the digitations of the serratus anterior muscle as it descends along the chest wall. To expose this nerve, the surgeon reflects the costocoracoid fascia from the chest wall, forming as he does so a deep cleft, with the naked serratus digitations as its medial wall, and the axillary fat and areolar tissue to be removed in the dissection as its lateral wall. In the depths of this cleft the long thoracic nerve will be seen lying in the fat which the dissection has peeled off of the serratus digitations. This nerve should not be sacrificed, for lymph nodes are not ordinarily seen along or medial to it. It should be freed, displaced medially, and left intact.

THE LYMPHATICS OF THE BREAST

A knowledge of the lymphatic pathways from the breast is essential to an understanding of the natural course as well as the treatment of breast carcinoma. This knowledge has been gained in four epochs.

1. At the end of the eighteenth century both Cruikshank and Mascagni, with mercury injection studies of the lymphatics, independently discovered and described the two main lymphatic drainage routes from the breast.

Cruikshank (1786) identified ". . . two sets of absorbents, one accompanying the external thoracic artery and vein and the other the internal thoracic vein. The external absorbents arise from the nipple and from the external part of the mamma, from the integuments and the tubuli lactiferi. They run outwards towards the axilla and sometimes pass through small glands halfway between the nipple and the axilla. . . . Some of the external thoracic vessels pass over the pectoralis major and go to the glands under the middle of the clavicle. . . . The internal, or mammary absorbents arise from the posterior part of the mamma, perforate in many places the intercostal muscles and join the plexus . . . coming from the liver and diaphragm, and running on each side of the mammary artery and veins behind the cartilage of the true ribs."

Mascagni (1787) wrote: "From the superficial tissues of the thorax and epigastrium, besides the lymphatics which run to the axillary glands, other vessels of the same kind accompany the epigastric, intercostal, and internal mammary vessels."

2. A century later, Sappey, still using mercury injection, made a much more thorough study of breast lymphatics. He distinguished a superficial group of lymphatics originating in the skin over the breast, and a deep group draining the mammary gland itself. The two groups anastomosed extensively.

The superficial lymphatics of the breast are those of the skin overlying the gland. The breast is derived embryologically from the ectoderm, and is in this sense an organ of the skin. Breast tissue is found immediately beneath the dermis, and is therefore drained to some extent by dermal lymphatics. These consist of a narrow-meshed, superficial lymphatic network without valves, which sends branches up around the dermal papillae, and a wide-meshed, deeper lymphatic network made up of broader channels equipped with valves.

Sappey's well-known portrayal of a mercury injection of the lymphatics of the skin of the chest wall, including the mammary region (Fig. 1–31), shows the dermal lymphatics very well, but is not entirely correct for our purposes, since it shows a male subject. It is, however, worth reproducing to emphasize two points. The first point is the striking directional lymphatic flow to the axilla from the whole upper anterolateral chest. The second point is the watershed, at the umbilical level, between drainage from the chest wall and the upper abdominal wall to the axilla, and drainage from the lower abdominal wall to the groin. A carcinoma of even the most caudad portion of the breast involving the skin of the infra-

mammary region, therefore, drains into lymphatics which run to the axilla and not to the groin.

The deep lymphatics of the breast originate as a delicate network surrounding the mammary lobules. They constitute, in Sappey's words, "an inextricable network of prodigious richness." From this network, collecting lymphatic trunks follow the mammary ducts centripetally to the subareolar area of the breast, according to Sappey, where they empty into the subareolar lymphatic plexus. This plexus, which Sappey was the first to describe, is a dense network of lymphatics of large caliber, situated superficially beneath the areola. Sappey's drawing of the plexus has often been reproduced, and we include it here (Fig. 1–32). Out beyond the edge of the areola the plexus becomes less dense and its interstices widen. Sappey concluded that most of the lymph from the breast drains centripetally into the plexus.

3. The next step in our understanding of the lymphatic drainage of the breast was made in the last decade of the nineteenth century and the early years of the present century by anatomists (Grossman, Gerota, Oelsner, Mornard), using Gerota's improved method of postmortem injection, and surgeons (Heidenhain, Rotter, Stiles), studying the routes of spread of breast cancer in surgical specimens. These studies made it abundantly clear that Sappey's concept of the lymphatic drainage of the breast was an incomplete one, and that there are a number of additional lymphatic routes from the breast by which the disease spreads.

Lothar Heidenhain, working in Kuster's surgical clinic in Berlin, began in 1888 to study the breasts removed in that clinic, particularly with reference to the spread of carcinoma in the retromammary tissues, the pectoral fascia, and the pectoral muscles. It should be recalled that the deep surface of the breast is separated from the pectoralis major by loose connective tissue. The deeper fibers of this web of connective tissue coalesce with the pectoral fascia. The pectoral fascia is dense but thin, and gives off many delicate processes, which penetrate deeply in the interstices between the coarse fibers of the pectoral muscle. Heidenhain's microscopic studies showed that delicate extensions of breast parenchyma follow the pectoral fascia down into the muscle, and that foci of carcinoma are often found in this same deep plane.

Heidenhain showed that these retromam-

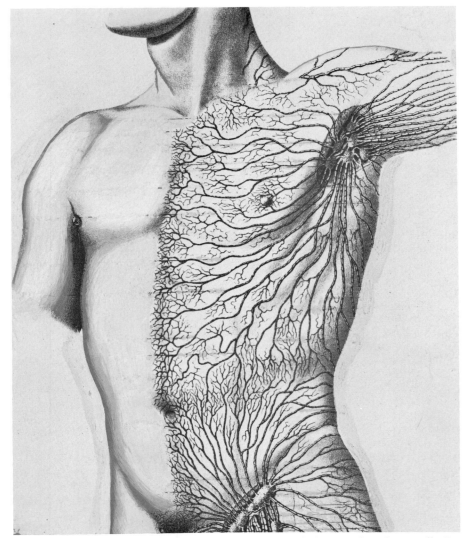

Figure 1–31.   Sappey's mercurial injection of the lymphatics of the anterior chest wall. *From* Sappey, P. C.: Anatomie, Physiologie, Pathologie des Vaisseaux Lymphatiques Considérés chez l'Homme et les Vertébrés. Paris, A. Delahaye and E. Lecrosnier, 18 [74] 85.

mary foci of carcinoma were in lymphatics. He traced them emerging from the posterior aspect of the breast, following the blood vessels to the pectoral fascia. He thought that these lymphatics ramified in the pectoral fascia and formed a plexus in it. Modern studies, however, have not confirmed the presence of a true lymphatic plexus in the pectoral fascia. Turner-Warwick found only a fine network of lymphatics in the pectoral fascia itself, and he believes that these very small lymphatics play no part in the early spread of breast cancer. He traced a few large lymphatics leaving the posterior surface of the

breast accompanying the larger blood vessels, passing across the retromammary space, and entering the pectoralis major muscle, with no suggestion of a plexiform arrangement.

Grossman, in 1896, carried out a special study of the lymph nodes in the axilla. Injecting adult cadavers with mercury, he found lymphatic trunks with several interspersed lymph nodes situated between the pectoralis major and minor muscles along the course of the highest thoracic artery in four of 25 subjects.

In 1899 Rotter, from the study of surgical specimens of breast carcinoma, extended

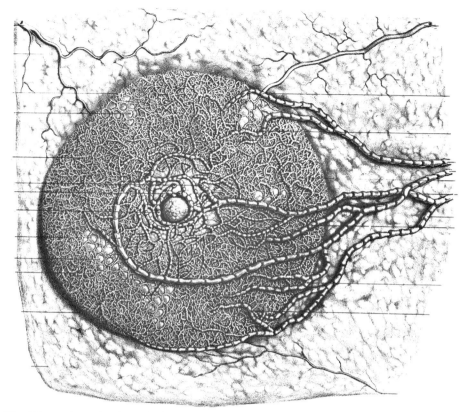

Figure 1–32. The subareolar lymphatic plexus according to Sappey. Sappey, P. C.: Anatomie, Physiologie, Pathologie des Vaisseaux Lymphatique Considérés chez l'Homme et les Vertébrés. Paris, A. Delahaye and E. Lecrosnier, 18 [74] 85.

Grossman's findings. He traced lymphatics from the posterior aspect of the breast penetrating the pectoralis major muscle to reach interpectoral nodes. In one-third of his cases, he found metastases along this lymphatic route between the pectoralis major and minor muscles. He emphasized that these metastases were often found in an early stage of breast carcinoma.

The lymph nodes that both Grossman and Rotter reported finding along this interpectoral lymphatic route, between the pectoralis major and minor muscles, were always found in close relation with the blood vessels, particularly where the blood vessels branched. Rotter found two or three such nodes in half the cases that he studied. They have since come to be known as Rotter's nodes.

During the same period, Harold Stiles in Edinburgh was carrying out similar and even more meticulous studies of surgical specimens of breast carcinoma. Between 1890 and 1895 he studied a total of 100 specimens. His description of the routes of lymphatic spread of

the disease confirmed and amplified those of Heidenhain, Grossman, and Rotter. Stiles' 1899 paper is worth reading today. He recommended removal of both pectoral muscles as part of the radical mastectomy. Halsted and Willy Meyer in the United States had already reached the same conclusion, and the modern era of breast surgery began.

Around the turn of the century, two German anatomists, Gerota of Berlin (1896) and Oelsner of Breslau (1901), carried out extensive injection studies of the lymphatics of the breast upon infant cadavers. Both confirmed the multiplicity of the routes of lymphatic drainage from the breast.

Regaud carried out a series of histologic studies of the lymphatics of the breast in the cat, cow, and guinea pig, between 1894 and 1900. He particularly studied the relationship of the lymphatics to the mammary lobules and the connective tissue stroma.

The last and the most thorough gross anatomic study of the lymphatics was Mornard's, reported in 1917 from Rouvière's Paris laboratory. He made bilateral injections in 50 fetuses. His work was the basis for Rouvière's description of the lymphatic routes from the breast, as well as for Rouvière's classification of axillary lymph nodes into six groups.

Rouvière's description of the main lymphatic route from the breast to the axilla can be summarized as follows: Two "enormous" collecting trunks originate from the periphery of the subareolar plexus, one medially and one laterally. The lateral collecting trunk emerges from the lateral edge of the subaoreolar plexus and is joined by a collateral trunk from the upper half of the breast. It runs laterally and upward to the axilla.

4. Recently our knowledge of the lymphatic system of the breast has been increased by the use of new techniques, such as lymphangiography and the injection of dyes and various isotopes into the breast, as well as more careful study of the lymph nodes in surgical specimens with the use of the clearing technique.

Radioactive colloidal gold has recently been used by Hultborn, Larsson, and Ragnhult, and also by Turner-Warwick, to study the lymphatic system of the breast. The Scandinavians measured the uptake of the isotope following radical mastectomy, in both the operative specimen and the patient, and concluded that the lymphatic flow from the breast is overwhelmingly toward the axilla. The axillary nodes took up 97 to 99 per cent of the isotope, while the internal mammary nodes took up only 1 to 3 per cent.

Turner-Warwick, in his studies, relied chiefly upon autoradiographs of surgical specimens. He found that "both the axilla and the internal mammary chain receive lymph from all quadrants of the breast; there is no striking tendency for any particular quadrant to drain in one direction. . . . The ipsilateral axillary nodes commonly receive more than 75 per cent of the total lymph from the breast. The remainder drains into the ipsilateral internal mammary chain. . . . The ipsilateral internal mammary chain undoubtedly represents an important pathway of lymph drainage from both the lateral and medial halves of the breast."

In contrast with Rouvière's concept, Turner-Warwick found that the subareolar plexus plays no essential part in the lymphatic drainage from the breast. His studies showed that the main lymphatics "run within the substance of the breast rather than on the superficial or deep surface, and as they run laterally they are joined by tributaries and pass through the axillary fascia within the thickness of the axillary tail." We believe that this description of the main lymphatic route is more accurate than Rouvière's, because Turner-Warwick's concept is based on the study of fully adult breasts, while Rouvière and the other anatomists who preceded him for the most part used infant cadavers, in which the breast was undeveloped.

Our own evidence, gained from studying the distribution of metastases in the axillary lymph node groups with the clearing technique in surgical specimens, leads us to believe that Rouvière also erred in concluding that the trunk lymphatics of the principal axillary route usually empty into the external mammary group of nodes. Table 22–11 (page 403), presenting our data, shows that the external mammary group of nodes contained metastases in only 14.6 per cent of our cases with involved nodes, whereas the central group of nodes was involved in 90 per cent, and the axillary vein group in 33.8 per cent. We believe that these facts gained from studying the actual distribution of metastases in the lymph node filter are more significant than information gained from the injection of lymphatics in infant cadavers.

Our own present concept of the lymphatic pathways from the breast to the axilla is shown diagrammatically in Figure 1–33.

Halsell and his associates studied the lymphatics within the breast by lymphangiography. The lymphatics in the areolar region were identified by vital dye staining and were injected with radiopaque material. They were visualized in 22 of 35 patients in which lymphangiography was attempted. They ran centrifugally from the areolar region, toward the axilla. Retrograde flow toward the areola was not demonstrated. Lewis and Beal also attempted lymphangiography of the breast, but not successfully.

Lymphangiography was used by Kendall, Arthur, and Patey to study the lymphatic drainage in patients with carcinoma of the breast. They compared their radiographic findings with the microscopic findings in the axillary lymph nodes after operation, and concluded that lymphangiography is not a reliable method of determining the presence of metastases.

Desprez-Curely and his associates have also studied the lymphatic drainage in carcinoma of the breast by means of lymphangiography. They claim to be able to distinguish

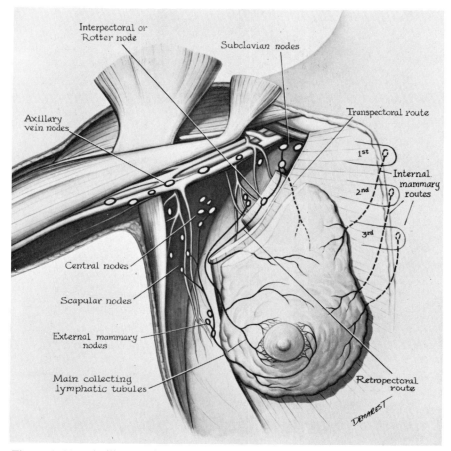

Figure 1–33.   Axillary and internal mammary lymphatic routes from the breast.

between chronic inflammation and metastases in axillary nodes with this method, but their evidence is not impressive.

The most extensive lymphangiographic studies of the axillary node filter are those recently carried out by Bobbio, Peracchia, and Pellegrino in Parma. They have obtained better visualization of the axillary nodes than anyone else, and have studied them in normal subjects, in patients with axillary metastases from breast carcinoma, and following radical mastectomy. They claim that they were able to correlate the radiographic images of lymph nodes with the microscopic findings.

This kind of evidence, however, is not yet, in my opinion, a reliable guide to the presence of metastases in lymph nodes. In our own clinic my associates Wolfgang Ackerman and Sven Kister have been working with lymphangiography but have found the method difficult and unreliable. We do not feel that it

is proper to carry out this procedure on patients with treatable breast carcinoma, for fear of pushing carcinoma emboli farther along the lymphatic pathway.

In our own experience the most helpful method of demonstrating the breast lymphatics and regional nodes has been the simple procedure of injecting Direct Sky Blue into the breast preoperatively. We usually inject 2 cc. into the subareolar area about 18 hours prior to operation. A central area of breast skin about 10 cm. in diameter is stained deep blue as shown in Figure 1–34. At operation, lymphatic trunks accompanying the blood vessels are easily identified. They resemble veins of small caliber, being similar in color because of the dye they contain. Some of the axillary nodes are usually stained blue by this dye. We have done radical mastectomies in many patients who have had these preoperative dye injections. The lymphatic trunks and lymph nodes demonstrated by this technique

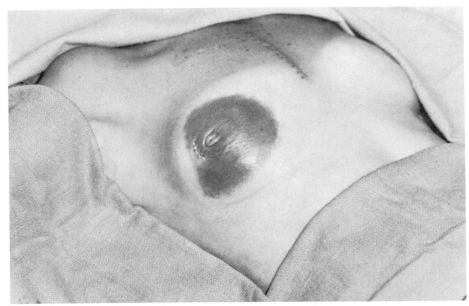

Figure 1–34. Preoperative subareolar injection of Direct Sky Blue. The skin over the central portion of the breast is stained blue.

are never quite the same. In most cases we see the lymphatic trunks running across the axilla from the tissues overlying the chest wall to the axillary vein nodes. In other cases the lymphatic trunks accompanying the medial perforating blood vessels or those following the blood vessels from the lower inner portion of the breast to the rectus fascia are seen. Sometimes the lymphatics that are seen best are those accompanying the many blood vessels from the serratus digitations to the operative specimen as it is dissected from the lateral chest wall. Our conviction from these preoperative injection studies with Direct Sky Blue is that lymphatics everywhere accompany blood vessels, and therefore that the lymphatics extend in all directions from the breast, although the main direction of lymphatic flow is toward the axilla.

We have recently had a convincing demonstration of the necessity for cutting the skin flaps thin in performing radical mastectomy. As we were dissecting back our lateral skin flap on a patient who had had preoperative dye injection, we came upon a minute blue nodule lying just beneath the skin in the subcutaneous fat over the upper outer sector of the breast. From this nodule a thin bluish line, representing a lymphatic trunk, extended toward the axilla, as shown in Figure 1–35. This was a very superficial lymph node, which happened to take up the dye. If our skin flap

had been thick, this node and its efferent lymphatic would certainly have been dissected up with the skin flap, and if there had been carcinoma in this node, prompt local recurrence in the skin flap would have resulted.

We recommend this method of preoperative injection of Direct Sky Blue for routine use in patients in whom radical mastectomy has been decided upon. When there is doubt as to the diagnosis or as to the indications for the radical operation, we do not use the dye, because the large blue discoloration of the skin is so disturbing to the patient, although it is, of course, harmless.

The Axillary Lymph Nodes

Grossman's study (1896) of axillary lymph nodes in adult cadavers was one of the first systematic attempts to define the number and position of the axillary nodes. He found 12 to 36 nodes in the axillae he studied, and he divided them into four groups. The later German students of the axillary lymph nodes, such as Gerota, Oelsner and Buschmakin, used a more complex grouping. Buschmakin, in his 1912 study based upon dissection of 60 adult subjects, found between 8 and 37 nodes which he classified in five different groups.

Bartels found the *Basle Nomina Anatomica* for these nodes unsatisfactory, and used his

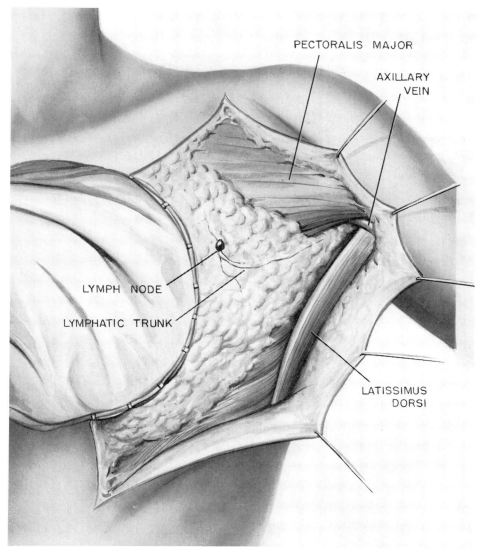

PECTORALIS MAJOR

AXILLARY
VEIN

LYMPH NODE

LYMPHATIC TRUNK

LATISSIMUS
DORSI

Figure 1–35.   Prepectoral lymph node and lymphatic trunk uncovered in dissection of the lateral skin flap in radical mastectomy.

own classification of seven node groups. The more recent *Nomina Anatomica* of Paris, listing five axillary lymph node groups, has the advantage of being simpler, but as a surgeon I do not find it altogether satisfactory.

Perhaps the best description and grouping of axillary lymph nodes is that of Poirier and Cunéo, which was adopted with modifications by Rouvière. I have chosen to follow it because the names for the different groups of nodes are simple and well chosen.

In Rouvière's classification, there are six different groups of axillary lymph nodes as follows:

1. The External Mammary Nodes.   This chain of nodes lies beneath the lateral edge of the pectoralis major, along the medial side of the axilla, following the course of the lateral thoracic artery on the chest wall from the sixth to the second rib. Rouvière stated that these nodes lie "upon, or within the thickness of, or beneath" the fascia covering the digitations of the serratus anterior muscle. This has not been my experience in dissecting the axilla hundreds of times. I make no attempt to dissect the fascia propria of the serratus digitations off the muscle fibers, but merely dissect the overlying mass of fat and areolar tissue containing the external mammary nodes away from the serratus digitations. These structures are very loosely attached to the serratus and are easily retracted laterally as the dissection proceeds. With this technique it has been only very rarely that I have seen any lymph nodes. I assume, therefore, that the external mammary nodes are few and small, and that they lie some little distance from, and *not within or beneath,* the fascia of the digitations of the serratus. Rouvière divides the external mammary nodes into two groups, a superior group at the level of the second and third intercostal spaces, and an inferior group at the level of the fourth, fifth, and sixth intercostal spaces. Nodes are infrequent at these lower levels. They were described by Kirmisson and also by Gerota, who called them paramammary nodes. When found, they may be comparatively superficial and very close to the lateral edge of the breast, or actually lying upon its surface.

2. The Scapular Nodes. Several lymph nodes lie closely applied to the subscapular vessels and their thoracodorsal branches, from the point of origin of the subscapular vein from the axillary trunk to the insertion of these vessels into the latissimus dorsi muscle and the lateral chest wall. As they cross the axilla toward the arm, the intercostobrachial nerves thread their way through the more cephalad of these scapular nodes. The thoracodorsal nerve, as it accompanies the thoracodorsal vessels, also runs through this scapular group of nodes. It is because these nerves are so intimately associated with the scapular nodes that these nerves should be sacrificed in any thorough axillary dissection for carcinoma. It is unreasonable to attempt to dissect them away from immediately adjacent lymph nodes, which may contain metastases, since sacrifice of these nerves does not produce any important disability.

3. The Central Nodes. These nodes lie embedded in fat in the center of the axilla. One or more of them may be situated surprisingly superficially beneath the skin and fascia of the center of the axilla, half way between the posterior and anterior axillary folds. They are therefore the nodes most easily palpated in the axilla, and the ones upon which our clinical estimate of the state of the axillary nodes is usually based. They are the largest and the most numerous of the axillary nodes. As our pathologic studies will show, they are also the group of nodes in which metastases most often are found. The central nodes are

therefore, from every point of view, the most important of the axillary nodes.

It is a very fortunate anatomic fact, from the point of view of the surgeon attempting to perform a thorough axillary dissection, that these nodes have a central position in the axilla. It makes it possible to carry the line of dissection at some distance on all sides from these central nodes, and therefore to get them out en bloc with the other axillary tissues without having to dissect too close to them.

4. The Interpectoral Nodes. The interpectoral lymph nodes, first described by Grossman but generally called Rotter's nodes, often are found lying between the pectoralis major and minor, along the pectoral branches of the thoracoacromial vessels. When found, they are small, and from one to four in number. Unless the pectoralis major muscle is removed in the operative attack on mammary carcinoma, these nodes will not be included in the excision.

5. The Axillary Vein Nodes. These nodes lie along the lateral portion of the axillary vein, on its caudad and ventral aspects, from the white tendon of the latissimus muscle where the most lateral nodes are found, to a point just medial to the origin of the thoracoacromial vein. It has been stated by some surgeons that it is necessary to excise the fascial sheath of the vein to get these nodes cleanly off of the vein. This is not true. If carcinoma has involved these nodes extensively, and has infiltrated the areolar tissue in which they lie and fixed them solidly to the vein, it is impossible to remove the disease and the nodes by any method. If the nodes are not fixed, they can be dissected out en bloc very easily following division of the delicate layer of fascia which covers the structures of the axilla. This fascia is divided along the cords of the brachial plexus cephalad to the vein and is dissected caudad across the axillary vein, taking with it the fat and areolar tissue and axillary vein nodes. The axillary vein is, of course, left cleanly denuded by this kind of dissection, even though the actual fascial sheath of the vein is not disturbed.

6. The Subclavicular Nodes. This is the highest, or most medial, group of axillary nodes. The nodes are situated along the ventral and caudad aspects of the axillary vein from a point just medial to the origin of the thoracoacromial vein to the very apex of the axilla, where the axillary vein disappears beneath the tendon of the subclavius muscle—

the highest point to which the surgeon can carry an axillary dissection. One or two of these subclavicular nodes are regularly seen lying on the axillary vein close to the point of origin of the thoracoacromial vein. The area is entirely inaccessible to the surgeon unless the pectoralis minor is divided.

There are usually several small nodes belonging to this subclavicular group lying in the areolar tissue in the crevice between the highest point of the axillary vein and the chest wall. These are the nodes we remove when we perform our *biopsy of the apex of the axilla*. In this procedure we do not disturb the more laterally placed nodes of the subclavicular node group.

The collecting trunks from all the other groups of axillary nodes empty into these subclavicular nodes; and from the plexus of lymphatic vessels which connects them one with another, one or more large lymphatic trunks arise and pass upward and medially beneath the tendon of the subclavius muscle and the clavicle to empty into the junction of the jugular and subclavian veins. These large trunks can be plainly seen at the apex of the axilla.

The subclavicular nodes have a great practical importance, because if they are involved I do not believe that surgical cure is possible. In order to be certain that the subclavicular nodes dissected out by the surgeon are always so classified by the pathologist, it has recently been my custom to sever this small group of nodes from the rest of the surgical specimen as soon as I have completed the dissection of the apex of the axilla. I place the small mass of fat and lymph nodes in a specimen bottle and set it aside for the pathologist. There is then no doubt as to the identification of the subclavicular nodes. I cannot see what harm can come from severing this small mass of apical tissue from the main surgical specimen. If metastases are present in these subclavicular nodes, surgery alone will not achieve cure, and if no metastases are present at this level, it is comforting to know it.

To summarize our concept of the remarkably efficient filter that the axillary lymphatic system provides, we can say that the main lymphatic trunks draining the breast run upward and laterally within its substance and emerge from its axillary prolongation and pierce the axillary fascia. They empty into the central group of axillary nodes. Other collecting lymphatic trunks emerge from the back of the breast, pierce the pectoralis major

muscle, and run cephalad between it and the pectoralis minor muscle to reach the axillary vein group of nodes or the subclavicular group of nodes. All the axillary nodes are connected by lymphatic trunks, through which the lymph flows to reach the subclavicular nodes at the apex of the axilla.

All these axillary nodes lie beneath the costocoracoid fascia, which encloses them, together with the blood vessels, nerves, connective tissue, and fat of the axilla, with a delicate but strong sheath. This fascia gives the structures that the surgeon needs to remove from the axilla a kind of coherence, and makes their removal in one piece, together with the fascia, easier than would otherwise be the case.

The fact is, of course, that the anatomists have been at a disadvantage, as compared with modern surgeons, in studying axillary nodes. With our modern methods of meticulous surgical dissection, and with study of the operative specimen with the clearing technique, we now remove and identify many more lymph nodes than the anatomists could possibly hope to find.

Monroe, in 1948, was one of the first to use the clearing technique for studying axillary lymph nodes. In a series of 87 radical mastectomy specimens he found an average of 30.4 lymph nodes per specimen.

Davis and Neis, in 1952, reported studying the distribution of axillary lymph nodes with the clearing technique in 77 mastectomy specimens. They found an average of 31.4 nodes per case. Unfortunately they used an anatomic grouping of lymph nodes which is different from that which I use, which makes comparison of our findings difficult.

Zeitlhofer, in Vienna, in 1952 reported the anatomic distribution of lymph node metastases in a series of 169 radical mastectomy specimens. Since he did not use the clearing method, his data are not as significant as they might otherwise have been.

In 1955 Berg published a similar study that had the same defect. Berg's method of identifying the position of the nodes in the specimens he studied was to divide them into three levels. He stated, "The assumption has been that metastases from breast carcinomas usually would first involve level I (nodes lateral and inferior to the pectoralis minor muscle), then level II (nodes behind the pectoralis minor), and only later level III (the few nodes medial and superior to the muscle)." In the light of the description of the axillary lymph node filter, which I present here, Berg's three-level classification is too simple. Two other omissions in his report should be noted. He did not state that the surgeons who did the dissections marked their specimens; without markings the pathologist *cannot* orient axillary specimens accurately. And Berg did not state the number of nodes he found per specimen. In view of these defects, Berg's data do not justify any conclusions as to the significance of metastases in the highest axillary nodes, the subclavicular nodes. He did not define these nodes with enough accuracy in his studies.

In our laboratory of surgical pathology, a much more thorough study of the lymph nodes of the axilla was carried out with the clearing technique, between 1951 and 1954. A total of 182 surgical specimens of axillary dissections were cleared. Most of the work was done by Dr. John Pickrin personally. He is an exceptionally assiduous and thorough pathologist, and I doubt that his study will be surpassed in accuracy for some time to come. That is why I have limited my interpretation of our cases to this 1951–1954 series. We have continued to clear all radical mastectomy specimens in our laboratory since 1954, but it has not been done as accurately as Pickrin did it. The pathologist can draw in, on a standard diagram, the lymph nodes he finds by clearing the specimen. The involved nodes are shown in solid black. Both the number of nodes and the anatomic group to which they belong are indicated, as in Figure 22–26. This kind of a record of the pathological findings is the most important information a clinician can have regarding the extent of metastasis in his patient's axillary lymphatic filter. It is of enormous value in deciding about subsequent therapy and prognosis.

The largest number of nodes found in an axilla in Pickrin's series of cases was 87, and the smallest was 8. An average finding of 35.3 nodes per specimen attests the value of the clearing method. Table 1–1 shows the numbers of nodes belonging to the six different axillary lymph node groups.

It will be seen that the central nodes are the most numerous, averaging 12.1 nodes. Although we have not systematically compared their size with that of the nodes in the other axillary node groups it has been our impression that the central nodes are much the largest. They are also, as I have already pointed out, easily palpated.

The axillary vein nodes are almost as numerous as the central nodes. They are not

Table 1–1. NUMBERS OF NODES IN THE AXILLARY NODE GROUPS

Node Group	Number of Nodes Found	Average Number of Nodes
External mammary nodes	311	1.7
Scapular nodes	1061	5.8
Central nodes	2199	12.1
Interpectoral nodes	262	1.4
Axillary vein nodes	1948	10.7
Subclavicular nodes	641	3.5
Total all groups	6422	35.3

palpable because they lie high up beneath the massive pectoral muscles.

The comparatively small number of nodes assigned in our studies to the external mammary group is possibly erroneous because of the fact that the surgical pathologist, in studying an axillary specimen, has more difficulty in orienting these nodes than the nodes in the other node groups.

The number of axillary lymph nodes found in relationship to the patient's age is shown in Table 1–2. There seems to be no significant diminution in the number of nodes with advancing age.

Prepectoral Lymph Nodes

We use the term *prepectoral* to describe a single lymph node which is occasionally found lying in the subcutaneous tissue or in the breast itself high up in its upper outer

Table 1–2. NUMBER OF AXILLARY NODES IN RELATIONSHIP TO AGE

Age of Patient	Number of Cases	Average Number of Nodes per Case
25–29	2	38
30–34	8	36
35–39	21	43
40–44	23	39
45–49	36	34
50–54	30	34
55–59	25	34
60–64	16	31
65–69	10	33
70–74	7	35
75–79	3	30
80–84	1	20
Total	*182*	*35*

sector. This node is not an axillary node, for it is not in the axilla at all. It is properly called a prepectoral node because it is superficial to the deep fascia covering the upper portion of the pectoralis major muscle. Its position is illustrated in Figure 1–35 which shows a very small prepectoral node which was too small to be palpable and was found during dissection of the lateral skin flap in a radical mastectomy after preliminary injection of Direct Sky Blue dye.

The prepectoral node is so infrequent that it is not known to the anatomists, and most surgeons are not familiar with it. In our laboratory of surgical pathology where we study several hundred mammary lesions yearly, we see only one or two of these prepectoral nodes each year. This node presents as a small, firm, well delimited, movable tumor in the upper outer sector of the breast. It is presumed to be a benign mammary tumor, and biopsy is performed or the node is removed locally. In the patients in whom we have removed a prepectoral node under these circumstances there has been no other regional lymph node adenopathy, with one exception. This was in a women who had lymphosarcoma involving axillary lymph nodes. She had, in addition, an enlarged prepectoral node that also contained lymphosarcoma.

Adventitious Mammary Lymph Nodes

Adventitious lymph nodes may be encountered almost anywhere in the body. A recent chance pathologic finding in studying a radical mastectomy surgical specimen suggests that this is true for the breast. The patient was 48 years old. She had a 3 cm. carcinoma of the right breast situated just caudad to the areola in the radius of six o'clock. There was a 1.5 cm. movable, clinically involved axillary lymph node. The axillary portion of the specimen was cleared and five lymph nodes of the central group were found to be involved. A block of tissue was cut through the deep aspect of the specimen immediately beneath the primary tumor. To our surprise this block showed two very small lymph nodes lying upon the deep fascia covering the pectoralis major muscle. The larger of these nodes, which measured about 5 mm. in diameter, was filled with metastatic carcinoma (Fig. 1–36). These lymph nodes were therefore situated beneath the breast slightly caudad to its center.

Termination of the Axillary Lymphatic Route in the Jugular-Subclavian Venous Confluence

From the highest subclavicular nodes at the apex of the axilla, two or three large lymphatic trunks pass medially through the small triangular space formed by the subclavian vein, the tendinous portion of the subclavius muscle, and the chest wall. These subclavian lymphatic trunks are large enough to be visible grossly if the surgeon keeps his operative field dry.

The subclavian lymphatic trunks are very short. In an autopsy study carried out at the Delafield Hospital, Ju found that the distance from the point where they pass beneath the tendinous portion of the subclavius muscle at the true apex of the axilla to their termination in the jugular-subclavian confluence, where they empty into the venous stream, averages only 3 cm. The subclavian lymphatic trunks terminate in several different ways: they may empty directly into the venous stream at the angle formed by the union of the subclavian and internal jugular veins; they may join other lymphatic trunks from the neck or mediastinum to form a common lymphatic duct, which on the right side of the neck then empties into the jugular-subclavian venous confluence, or on the left side of the neck into the thoracic duct or into the jugular-subclavian venous confluence; or finally, they may empty into so-called *sentinel* lymph nodes of the inferior deep cervical group situated close to the jugular-subclavian venous confluence.

These sentinel lymph nodes are often involved by breast carcinoma that has reached the subclavicular nodes situated only 3 cm. laterally at the apex of the axilla. Since the sentinel nodes lie deep beneath the lateral edge of the lower end of the sternocleidomastoid muscle behind the clavicle, they are not palpable unless they are considerably enlarged.

Lymphatic Route to the Supraclavicular Lymph Nodes

When the sentinel nodes around the lymphatic terminus in the jugular-subclavian venous confluence are involved by carcinoma and the lymphatic flow through them is to some degree blocked, the disease spreads in a retrograde direction along lymphatics con-

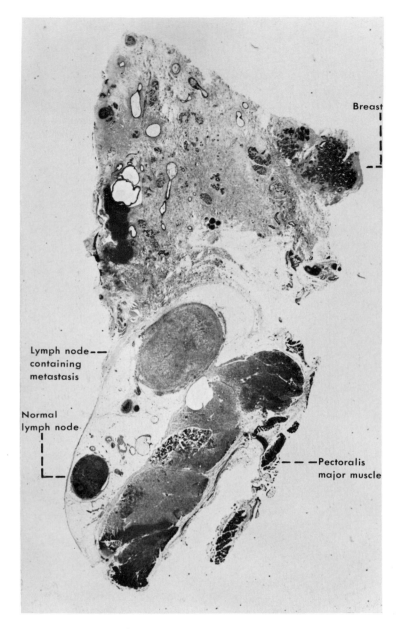

Lymph node——
containing
metastasis

Normal
lymph node

— —Pectoralis
major muscle

Breast

Figure 1–36. Adventitious lymph nodes lying on the fascia over the pectoralis major muscle deep to the lower portion of the breast.

necting the sentinel nodes with other lymph nodes of the transverse cervical group, which are situated more laterally and more superficially in the supraclavicular region. These are the nodes usually palpated when there are supraclavicular metastases. When they are involved it may be assumed that the deeper sentinel nodes contain metastases and that the disease has escaped into the venous circulation.

The lymphatic route from the axilla to the supraclavicular nodes via the sentinel nodes

at the jugular-subclavian confluence, which I have described, is properly called the *indirect* route to the supraclavicular nodes, although it is probably the usual route by which metastases from breast carcinoma reach them.

There is also, in some subjects, a *direct* lymphatic route from the axillary nodes, extending cephalad over the brachial plexus to reach the supraclavicular nodes. Both Bartels and Rouvière identified efferent lymphatics running from the subclavicular group of axillary nodes to nodes of the transverse

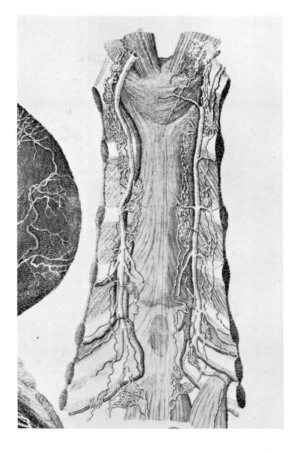

Figure 1–37. Mascagni's illustration of his injection of the internal mammary lymphatics. *From* Mascagni, P.: Lymphaticorum Corporis Humani Historia et Ichnographia. Siena, P. Carli, 1787.

cervical chain. In their recent lymphangiographic studies of the axillary lymph node filter, Bobbio, Peracchia, and Pellegrino demonstrated filling of supraclavicular nodes of the transverse cervical chain in half of their subjects, the contrast medium reaching these nodes through efferent lymphatics from nodes of the axillary vein and subclavicular node groups.

Although I have looked closely for lymphatic trunks extending directly upward over the cords of the brachial plexus toward the transverse cervical nodes, in patients in whom I have dissected the axilla after preoperative injection of Direct Sky Blue into the breast, I have not identified them. I suspect that this direct route from axilla to transverse cervical nodes is not a common one. We know that the main direction of lymphatic drainage is medially to the apex of the axilla, and then through the subclavian lymphatic trunks to the jugular-subclavian venous confluence. I have often seen these lymphatic trunks at the apex of the axilla dyed blue after injection of the dye.

There is a third possible route of breast carcinoma to the supraclavicular lymph nodes, namely, directly from the breast, bypassing the axillary lymph node filter. Mornard found such a route in 3 per cent of the subjects that he injected, but neither Oelsner nor Rouvière was able to demonstrate this pathway.

Internal Mammary Lymphatic Route

The most recent step in our understanding of the lymphatic drainage of the breast has been the realization of the importance of the internal mammary lymphatic route. The existence of this route was known to both Cruikshank and Mascagni. Mascagni's 1787 illustration of his injection of the internal mammary lymphatics (Fig. 1–37) is indeed so good that it can be studied with profit today. Yet 160 years were to pass before Richard Handley carried out biopsies in patients with breast cancer that proved how important the internal mammary route actually is.

Halsted had an inkling of the importance of the internal mammary route. In 1898 he wrote, "Dr. H. W. Cushing, my house surgeon, has in three instances cleared out the mediastinum on one side for recurrent cancer. It is likely, I think, that we shall in the near future remove the mediastinal contents at some of our primary operations." So far as I can determine, Halsted never mentioned this idea again.

In his excellent monograph on breast cancer published in 1912, Cecil Leaf described the internal mammary lymphatic route, and stated that cancers of the inner half of the breast more often metastasize to the internal mammary nodes than do cancers in other parts of the breast. But he did not describe these nodes and their anatomic relationships in detail, nor did he give any data as to the frequency with which they are involved, which suggests that he had very little actual knowledge of internal mammary metastases.

Sampson Handley, whose earlier studies of breast carcinoma were concentrated on the problem of whether it spread by embolism or by permeation of lymphatics, later became increasingly interested in the internal mammary lymphatic route. In the second edition (1922) of his important book on breast cancer, he reported exploring the anterior mediastinum and removing involved internal mammary nodes in six patients. In two of them, these nodes contained metastases. In 1927 he published reports of a series of cases of breast carcinoma with internal mammary metastases, and concluded that "by the time the axillary glands are enlarged, the disease has frequently, and perhaps usually, obtained access through the inner ends of the intercostal spaces to the internal mammary glands, and that in quite early and still operable cases these glands contain microscopic deposits of cancer cells." He reported excising the internal mammary routes in five cases, but he considered the operation impractical. Instead, he devised a method of inserting radium needles in the upper three intercostal spaces. By 1926 he had used this method prophylactically in a total of 56 patients. Although this technique did not gain acceptance, Sampson Handley was certainly the first to emphasize the importance of the internal mammary lymphatic route, and to devise a therapeutic attack on metastasis in these nodes.

One important result of Sampson Handley's emphasis on the internal mammary lymphatic route was the first anatomic study of this route. He encouraged the anatomist Stibbe to undertake such a study. This study, based on 60 autopsies, appeared in 1918. But surgeons gave it little attention.

The internal mammary lymphatic trunks originate from the anterior prepericardial lymph nodes lying anteriorly upon the upper surface of the diaphragm. These nodes receive collecting lymphatics from the anterior and superior portion of the liver via the falciform ligament, from the anterior portion of the diaphragm, and from the upper portion of the rectus abdominis muscle and the rectus sheath, as well as from the lower inner sector of the adjacent mammary gland.

The main efferent lymphatics from the breast to the internal mammary route emerge from the deep aspect and from the medial edge of the mammary gland. They lie upon the pectoral fascia, or pierce it to enter the pectoralis major muscle, and run medially, accompanying the branches of the perforating vessels, to reach the medial ends of the intercostal spaces. Here, usually at a point just above the costal cartilage of each rib, the vascular and lymphatic bundle turns inward at a sharp angle and penetrates the entire thickness of the pectoralis major as well as the intercostal muscles, to reach the internal mammary nodes and vessels. When the intercostal muscles over the inner ends of the interspaces have been removed, the internal mammary area is still roofed over by an exceedingly delicate but definite fascia. No name has been given to this fascia, but it might well be called the *internal mammary fascia*. Beneath it, the internal mammary lymphatics and blood vessels lie embedded in fat and areolar tissue. Sledziewski, who made careful studies in 1931 and 1937 of the internal mammary lymphatics, found that there are usually two or three delicate lymphatic trunks on each side. In the first, or the first and second intercostal spaces, the nodes lie upon and are separated from the parietal pleura only by a thin layer of fascia, which Stibbe named the costosternal fascia and which has also been called the endothoracic fascia. This fascia is so thin that the lung can be seen moving beneath it. In the lower interspaces this fascia is continuous with the transversus thoracis muscle, which constitutes another layer of tissue between the internal mammary vessels and the pleura. These relationships are shown in Figure 1–38.

The internal mammary lymphatic trunks eventually empty into the great veins by one of several routes. They may empty on the left side into the thoracic duct, and on the right

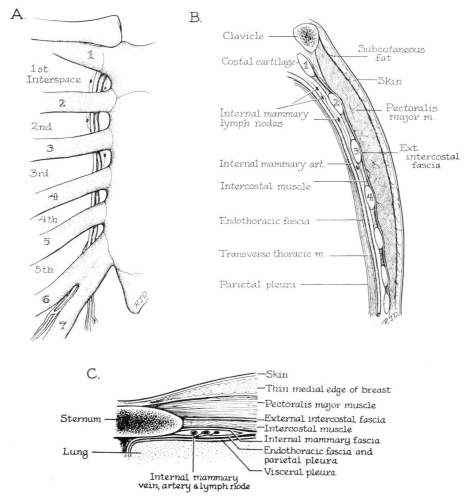

Figure 1–38. The internal mammary lymphatic route. *A*, Anterior view. *B*, Vertical cross section of the chest wall parallel to the internal mammary vessels. *C*, Horizontal cross section of the chest wall through the second interspace.

side into the right lymphatic duct. They may terminate on each side of the lowest lymph node of the inferior deep cervical group, which lies just behind the medial end of the clavicle, and thence into the great veins. Finally, they may empty directly into the jugular-subclavian vein confluence. The important point is that once a metastasis from breast carcinoma reaches a lymph node of the internal mammary chain in the first or second interspace, it is a very short distance from a point of entry into the venous circulation.

The Internal Mammary Lymph Nodes

The internal mammary lymph nodes are very small, usually measuring between 2 and 5 mm. in diameter. In addition to fully formed nodes, microscopic study of the fat and areolar tissue removed from the intercostal spaces along the course of the internal mammary vessels usually reveals minute foci of lymphocytes.

The internal mammary nodes are found interspersed along the course of the internal mammary trunk lymphatics. For the benefit of the radiotherapist who wishes to know the precise position of these nodes, it can be said that in almost all patients they are within 3 cm. of the sternal edge.

The nodes usually lie in the fat and areolar tissue upon the endothoracic fascia in the interspaces between the costal cartilages. The firm attachment of this fascia to the deep surface of the costal cartilages usually prevents

Table 1–3. Total number of internal mammary nodes on both sides in 60 subjects*

Space	Contained No Node	One Node	Two Nodes	More Than Two
First	4	91	19	6
Second	3	91	24	2
Third	21	75	19	5
Fourth	109	11	—	—
Fifth	105	15	—	—
Sixth (or behind sixth cartilage)	45	75	—	—

*From Stibbe, E. P.: J. Anat., 52:257, 1918.

the nodes from lying behind the cartilages, although a node sometimes may be partially in the groove under the edge of a cartilage.

Stibbe found the average total number of internal mammary lymph nodes per subject, including both sides, to be 8.5. The typical distribution was four on one side and five on the other, with one node in the upper three interspaces on each side, one in the sixth space on each side, and an extra node in one of the upper spaces. Stibbe's findings of grossly visible nodes are summarized in his table (Table 1–3).

Soerensen, at the suggestion of his surgical colleagues in Stockholm, studied the arrangement of the internal mammary nodes in 39 autopsies. He found an average total of 7 nodes per subject, or 3.5 on each side. Soerensen emphasized a fact that is of fundamental importance to surgeons searching for these nodes, namely their minute size. He pointed out that the great majority of the normal nodes are only 1 or 2 mm. in diameter, while a few measure as much as 5 or 6 mm. If the fat adjacent to the internal mammary vessels is removed when no node can be identified grossly by the surgeon, microscopic study will often reveal several small aggregations of lymphoid tissue.

At the Francis Delafield Hospital, my associate David Ju investigated the number and position of the internal mammary nodes in a series of 100 autopsies. The sternum and costal cartilages were removed in one piece, and the nodes subsequently were dissected out. He found an average total of 6.2 nodes per subject, or 3.1 on each side. Figure 1–39 shows the total numbers and arrangements of the nodes as Ju found them in 100 subjects. Stibbe reported a marked concentration of these nodes in the upper three interspaces and in the sixth interspace. Ju, on the other hand, noted the same concentration of nodes in the upper three interspaces, but found that the

lower three interspaces contained nodes infrequently but with about an equal incidence. Another point of difference in Stibbe's and Ju's findings was that according to Stibbe most of the nodes found in the first and second interspaces were situated to the medial side of the internal mammary artery. Ju found that they were about equally placed at each side of the artery.

In Rome, Putti (1953), at the suggestion of Margottini, studied the number and arrangement of internal mammary nodes in 47 cadavers. He found an average of 7.7 lymph nodes per subject, distributed as follows:

Site	Per cent
1st intercostal space	91
2nd intercostal space	89
3rd intercostal space	70
4th intercostal space	46
5th intercostal space	12
6th intercostal space	10
At the bifurcation of the internal mammary	23

Putti made a separate study, in 62 cadavers, of nodes lying behind the sternal extremity of the clavicle. In 21 of the cadavers he found a total of 31 lymph nodes lying behind the clavicle upon the innominate vein. The nodes were more frequently on the right than on the left, 26 per cent of the subjects having them on the right and only 6 per cent on the left.

Arão and Abrão presented still another study of the frequency and distribution of the internal mammary nodes in a series of 100 autopsies. Their findings are shown graphically in Figure 1–40, taken from their study. They found a larger number of nodes than previous investigators, an average of 8.9 on the right side and 7.3 on the left, that is, an average total of 16.2 per subject. In 56.6 per cent of their cases they found retromanubrial

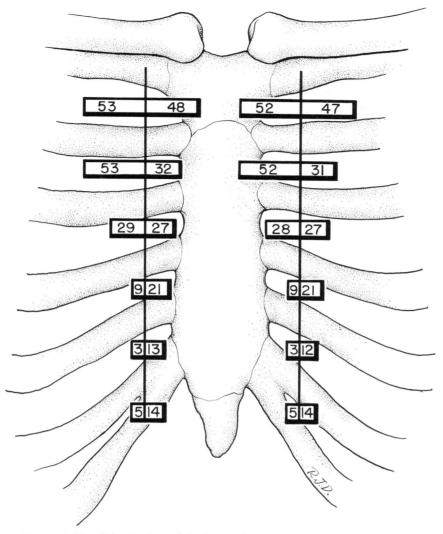

Figure 1–39. Distribution of the internal mammary nodes, according to Ju.

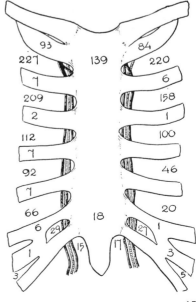

Figure 1–40. Distribution of the internal mammary nodes, according to Arão and Abrão. Arão, A., and Abrão, A.: Rev. paulista de med., *45*:317, 1954.

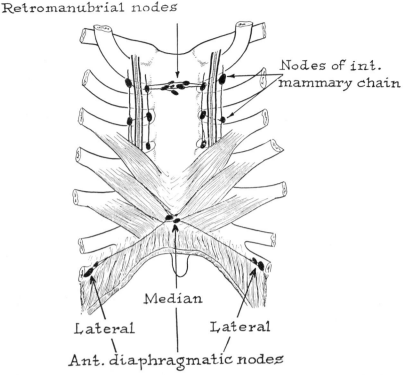

Retromanubrial nodes

Nodes of int. mammary chain

Median

Lateral   Lateral

Ant. diaphragmatic nodes

Figure 1–41. Retromanubrial nodes, according to Arão and Abrão. Arão, A., and Abrão, A.: Rev. paulista de med., *45*:317, 1954.

nodes situated in the path of connecting lymphatics between the left and right lymphatic trunks at the level of the first interspace (Fig. 1–41). In the subjects in whom such retromanubrial nodes existed, an average of 6.6 nodes were found. Rouvière was the first to point out this connection between the left and right internal mammary routes at the first interspace level. Sledziewski found it in 30 of 111 cases.

Lymphatic Route from Breast to Liver via the Rectus Abdominis Muscle

This lymphatic route was emphasized by Sampson Handley a half century ago. As Handley pointed out, the lower inner edge of the breast overlies the sixth costal cartilage, and is only two or three centimeters from the ensiform cartilage. Lymphatics accompanying the branches of the superior epigastric blood vessels, which run from this portion of the breast toward the epigastric notch, pierce the rectus fascia, and enter the rectus abdominis muscle. These lymphatics empty into the anterior prepericardial lymph nodes situated

upon the upper surface of the diaphragm over the falciform ligament. Other afferent lymphatics to these prepericardial nodes are from the diaphragm, the falciform ligament, and the anterior and superior portions of the liver. The internal mammary lymphatic trunks originate from these prepericardial lymph nodes. These relationships are shown diagrammatically in Figure 1–42.

The rectus muscle lymphatics thus provide a route by which metastases from breast carcinoma can reach the liver, although it is likely that this happens only when the internal mammary trunk is blocked higher up in the upper three interspaces where metastases to it are more frequent. When such blockage occurs, the direction of lymphatic flow may be reversed, and carcinoma emboli from the breast may reach the liver through the rectus muscle lymphatic route. Sampson Handley's examples of the process found at autopsy were from subjects with locally advanced breast carcinoma. Leaf published a good description with excellent illustrations of the rectus muscle lymphatic route. This route probably has no importance in early breast cancer unless the primary tumor happens to

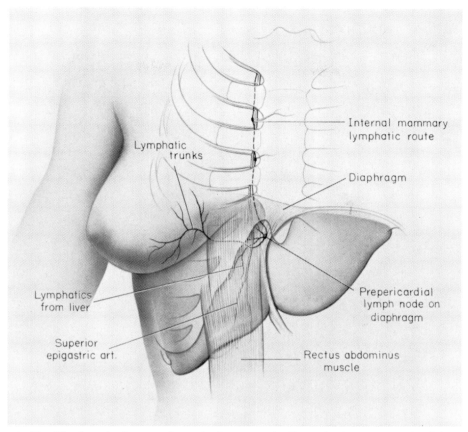

Figure 1–42. The lymphatic route from the breast to the liver via the rectus abdominis muscle.

be situated in the extreme lower inner portion of the breast. In our own data, carcinomas in this situation have a much poorer prognosis than those developing elsewhere in the breast. Metastasis via the rectus muscle route may be an explanation for this fact.

Lymphatic Drainage Across the Midline to the Opposite Breast and Axilla

The question of the likelihood of breast carcinoma spreading across the midline to involve the opposite breast and axilla is often raised. The anatomic evidence suggests that the lymphatics from one breast, or the skin over it, do not normally drain into the lymphatics of the opposite side. Oelsner long ago reported finding lymphatic trunks occasionally crossing the midline in his injection studies of infant cadavers, but modern studies of normal adults, such as that carried out by Turner-Warwick, do not confirm this finding. Turner-Warwick found "no significant drainage of lymph from the breast to the contralateral axilla or the contralateral internal mammary chain under normal conditions."

When breast carcinoma originating in one breast begins to spread in all directions, and the breast's normal principal routes of lymphatic drainage are to some degree blocked by metastases, it is to be expected that retrograde lymphatic spread to the skin of the opposite chest wall, the opposite breast, and the opposite axilla will occur.

Lymphatic Drainage of the Chest Wall Underlying the Breast

The lymphatics from the chest wall underlying the breast in general follow the course of the blood vessels that supply it. Those from the medial portion of the pectoralis major follow the perforating vessels into the internal mammary lymphatic route. The lymphatics from the remainder of this muscle as well as those from the pectoralis minor terminate in the lymph nodes of the axilla.

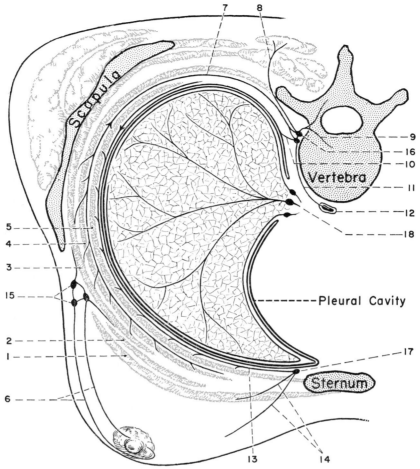

Figure 1–43.   Lymphatic drainage of the breast in cross section.

1. Pectoralis major m.
2. Pectoralis minor m.
3. Serratus magnus m.
4. External intercostal m.
5. Internal intercostal m.
6. Lymphatics from breast to axillary lymph nodes
7. External intercostal lymphatics
8. Lymphatics from spinal muscles
9. Lymphatics from vertebra
10. Lymphatics from parietal pleura
11. Lymphatics from posterior intercostal lymph nodes to thoracic duct
12. Thoracic duct
13. Internal intercostal lymphatics
14. Lymphatics from breast to internal mammary lymph nodes
15. Axillary lymph nodes
16. Posterior intercostal lymph nodes
17. Internal mammary lymph nodes
18. Lymph nodes of pulmonary pedicle

The lymphatics from the fascia overlying the serratus magnus and from its superficial surface follow the branches of the thoracodorsal vein and empty into the axillary lymph nodes. There is another set of lymphatics from the deep surface of this muscle which communicates with the lymphatics of the external intercostal muscles.

The external intercostal muscles are drained by collecting lymphatics, two or three in each intercostal space, which follow the intercostal vessels around posteriorly. These collecting lymphatics empty into the posterior intercostal lymph nodes, which lie in each interspace upon the inner aspect of the thoracic wall, close to the heads of the ribs. There are one to three of these nodes in each interspace. They are shown in Figure 1–43, a diagram of the lymphatic drainage of the breast as seen in cross section. In addition to the collecting lymphatics from the external intercostal route, these posterior intercostal nodes also receive

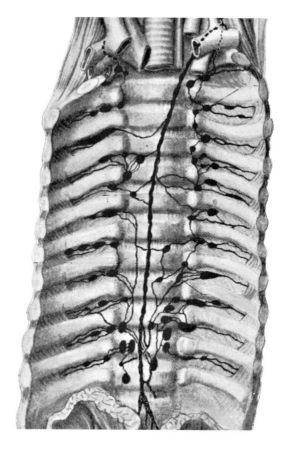

Figure 1–44. The posterior intercostal lymph node route. (*From* Rouvière, H.: Anatomie des lymphatiques de l'homme, Paris, 1932, p. 157.)

afferent lymphatics from the parietal pleura, the vertebrae, and the spinal muscles. These connections, of course, provide a route for carcinoma emboli from the breast to reach the pleura or the vertebrae by retrograde permeation.

The efferent lymphatic vessels from the posterior intercostal nodes in the lower five or six interspaces run downward and unite to form a common collecting lymphatic trunk on each side, which empties into the thoracic duct (Fig. 1–44).

The efferents from the posterior intercostal nodes of the first and second interspaces usually run upward, behind the subclavian artery, and either empty into a node of the inferior deep cervical (supraclavicular) group or join one of the other collecting lymphatic trunks and empty into the venous confluence. This connection provides another route by which a metastasis from breast carcinoma can reach the supraclavicular lymph nodes.

The efferents from the posterior intercostal nodes in the third, fourth, and fifth interspaces run transversely or obliquely and anastomose

to form an irregular plexus lying upon the vertebral bodies. In this prevertebral lymphatic plexus there are interposed a number of juxtavertebral lymph nodes. From these nodes efferent lymphatic trunks empty into the thoracic duct.

The internal intercostal muscles are provided by lymphatics that run anteriorly in the respective intercostal spaces and empty into the internal mammary lymphatic route. These internal intercostal lymphatics also receive lymphatics from the parietal pleura.

The Great Collecting Trunks of the Lymphatic System at the Base of the Neck

In our discussion of the pathways for metastases from breast carcinoma, we are particularly concerned with the lymphatic drainage of the breast and axilla, the anterior mediastinum, and the chest wall. The collecting lymphatic trunks from these areas all empty into the confluence of the internal

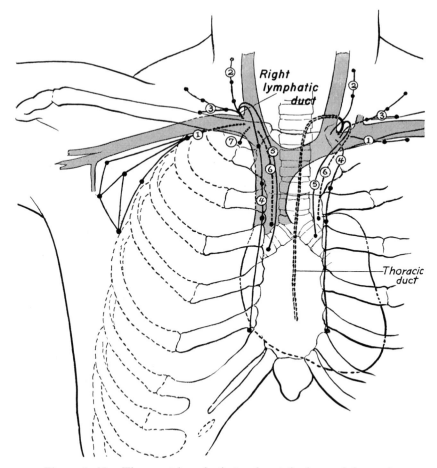

Figure 1–45. The great lymphatic trunks at the base of the neck.

jugular and subclavian veins at the base of the neck on each side, which may appropriately be called the *grand central lymphatic terminus* of the body (Fig. 1–45). The details of the anatomy of the terminal collecting lymphatic trunks in this region are of great practical importance for us.

There are essentially three groups of these terminal lymphatic trunks, the subclavian, the jugular, and the bronchomediastinal. Earlier anatomists pictured these as single collecting trunks, but the recent studies of Rodriguez and Pereira in Rouvière's Parisian laboratory and of Sledziewski in Warsaw have shown them to be very irregular both as to number and as to the manner in which they combine and empty in the venous confluence. Their findings can be summarized as follows, with reference to Figure 1–45:

1. The *subclavian trunks* (efferent from the axilla) are the most constant. There are usually two or three of them.

2 and 3. Instead of a single *jugular trunk* (efferent from the neck and supraclavicular areas) there are usually two or three collecting trunks from the internal jugular nodes, and one or two quite separate trunks from the transverse cervical chain of nodes (the supraclavicular nodes).

4. The *internal mammary trunks* run upward and terminate, quite independently of the other mediastinal trunks, in the venous confluence.

5. The right *anterior mediastinal trunk* originates in nodes situated along the phrenic nerve and the anterior portion of the root of the right lung. It runs upward anterior to the vena cava and empties separately into the right venous confluence. The left *anterior mediastinal trunk* is pre-aortic, ascending from the anterior portion of the root of the left lung. It empties into the terminal portion of the thoracic duct, or terminates separately in the left venous confluence.

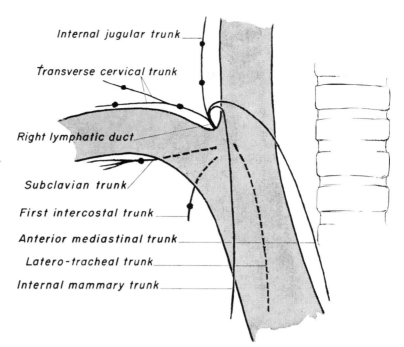

Internal jugular trunk

Transverse cervical trunk

Right lymphatic duct

Figure 1–46. The termination of the great lymphatic trunks at the base of the neck on the right side.

Subclavian trunk

First intercostal trunk

Anterior mediastinal trunk

Latero-tracheal trunk

Internal mammary trunk

6. There are usually several trunks on each side from the *posterior mediastinal* and *laterotracheal* groups of nodes. These trunks drain the roots of the lungs, ascend along the sides of the trachea, and empty into the venous confluence on each side.

7. Finally, there is sometimes a short collecting trunk from the posterior intercostal

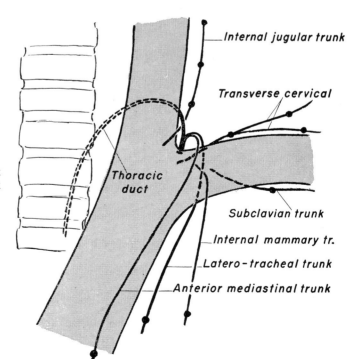

Internal jugular trunk

Transverse cervical

Thoracic duct

Figure 1–47. The termination of the great lymphatic trunks at the base of the neck on the left side.

Subclavian trunk

Internal mammary tr.

Latero-tracheal trunk

Anterior mediastinal trunk

lymph node of the first interspace which
ascends behind the great vessels and empties
into the venous confluence.

All seven of these groups of collecting
lymphatic trunks terminate finally in the confluence of the subclavian and internal jugular
veins on each side. In some subjects some of
these trunks combine in a variety of ways on
the right side to form a short common trunk
called the right lymphatic duct (Fig. 1–46).
The subclavian, internal jugular, and transverse cervical trunks are the ones which most
often unite to form the common duct. More
often, however, most of the trunks empty
separately into the venous confluence.

On the left side the various trunks empty
either into the internal jugular vein, into the
subclavian vein, or into the thoracic duct
(Fig. 1–47). The anterior mediastinal and the
laterotracheal trunks are the ones which most
often empty into the thoracic duct. The subclavian and the internal mammary trunks are
the ones which most often terminate independently in the great vein.

The lesson regarding carcinoma of the
breast which must be inferred from this
anatomy is that when emboli of carcinoma
cells filter through the defense zone of axillary
lymph nodes and reach the subclavian trunk,
their route of escape into the venous circulation is short and easy. Metastases into the
internal mammary nodes are almost as close
to this danger point.

REFERENCES

Anderson, R. E.: Two cases of axillary breast. Brit.
    Med. J., *1*:283, 1930.
Andreasen, A. T.: Medullary carcinoma in an axillary
    breast. Brit. J. Surg., *35*:322, 1948.
Arão, A., and Abrão, A.: Estudo anatómico da cadeia
    ganglionar mamária interna em 100 casos. Rev.
    paulista de med., *45*:317, 1954.
Bartels, P.: Das Lymphgefässsystem. *In* von Bardeleben,
    K.: Handbuch der Anatomie des Menschen. Jena,
    Gustav Fischer, 1909, Vol 3, Part 4.
Batson, O. V.: The function of the vertebral veins and
    their role in the spread of metastases. Ann. Surg.,
    112:138, 1940.
Batson, O. V.: The role of the vertebral veins in meta-
    static processes. Ann. Int. Med., *16*:38, 142.
Berg, J. W.: The significance of axillary node levels in the
    study of breast carcinoma. Cancer, *8*:776, 1955.
Bobbio, P., Peracchia, G., and Pellegrino, F.: Anatomia
    radiografica del sistema linfatico ascellare e sopra-
    claveare. Ateneo Parmense. *33* (supp.):5, 1962.
Bobbio, P., Peracchia, G., and Pellegrino, F.: Connes-
    sioni linfatiche presternali fra le regioni mammarie
    dei due lati. Ateneo Parmense, *33* (supp.):95, 1962.
Bonser, G. M., Dossett, J. A., and Jull, J. W.: Human and

Experimental Breast Cancer. London, Pitman Med.
    Pub. Co., 1961.
Bresslau, E. L.: The Mammary Apparatus of the Mam-
    malia. London, Methuen, 1920.
Buschmakin, N.: Die Lymphdrüsen der Achselhöhle,
    ihre Einteilung, und Blutversorgung. Anat. Anz.,
    41:3, 1912.
Chiari, H. H.: Zur Frage des Karzinoms in aberranten
    Brustdrüsengewebe. Brun's Beitr. Klin. Chir.,
    197:307, 1958.
de Cholnoky, T.: Accessory breast tissue in the axilla.
    N. Y. State J. Med., *51*:2245, 1951.
de Cholnoky, T.: Supernumerary breast. Arch. Surg.,
    39:926, 1939.
Cogswell, H. D., and Czerny, E. W.: Carcinoma of aber-
    rant breast of the axilla. Amer. Surg., *27*:388, 1961.
Cooper, Sir A. P.: The Anatomy and Diseases of the
    Breast. Philadelphia, Lea and Blanchard, 1845.
Cooper, W. A.: The history of the radical mastectomy.
    Ann. M. Hist., *3*:36, 1941.
Cruikshank, W. C.: The Anatomy of the Absorbing
    Vessels of the Human Body. London, G. Nicol,
    1786.
Dahl-Iversen, E.: Recherches sur les métastases micro-
    scopiques des ganglions lymphatiques parasternaux
    dans le cancer du sein. J. internat. chir., *11*:492,
    1951.
Davis, H. H., and Neis, D. D.: Distribution of axillary
    lymph node metastases in carcinoma of the breast.
    Ann. Surg., *136*:604, 1952.
Deaver, J. B., and McFarland, J.: The Breast: its Anom-
    alies, its Diseases, and their Treatment. Philadelphia,
    P. Blakiston's Son, 1917.
Delamere G., Poirier, P., and Cuneo, B.: The Lym-
    phatics. (Translated and edited by C. H. Leaf.)
    Chicago, W. T. Keener and Co., 1904.
Della Romana de Compte, L., and Radice, J. C.: Local-
    ización vulvar de una glándula mammaria aberrante.
    Obst. Gin. Lat. Amer., *15*:203, 1957.
Desprez-Curely, J. P., Bismuth, V., Fron, P., and
    Bourdon, R.: La Lymphographie du membre supéri-
    eur dans les affections tumorales malignes. Ann. de
    Radiol., *6*:437, 1963.
Dickinson, A. M.: Carcinoma of the axillary tail of the
    breast. Am. J. Surg., *49*:515, 1940.
von Eggeling, H.: Die Milchdrüse. *In* von Möllendorf,
    W.: Handbuch der Mikroskopischen Anatomie des
    Menschen. Berlin, Springer, 1927, Vol. 3, Part 1,
    p. 117.
Eisler, P.: Die Muskeln des Stammes. *In* von Bardeleben,
    K.: Handbuch der Anatomie des Menschen, Jena.
    Gustav Fischer, 1912, Vol. 2, Part 2, Section 1.
Fitzwilliams, D. C. L.: Lymphatic channels leading from
    the Breast. Brit. J. Surg., *12*:650, 1924-5.
Fraser, F. C.: Dominant inheritance of absent nipples
    and breasts. *In* Novant' anni delle leggi mendeliane.
    Roma, Istituto Gregorio Mendel, 1956, p. 360.
Fraser, J.: A study of the malignant breast by whole
    section and key block section methods. Surg., Gynec.
    & Obst., *45*:266, 1927.
Gerota, D.: Zur Technik der Lymphgefässinjektion.
    Anat. Anz., *12*:216, 1896.
Goldenring, H., and Crelin, E. S.: Mother and daughter
    with bilateral congenital amastia. Yale J. Biol. and
    Med., *33*:466, 1961.
Grant, R. N., Tabah, E. J., and Adair, F. E.: The surgical
    significance of the subareolar lymph plexus in cancer
    of the breast. Surgery, *33*:71, 1953.
Grossman, F.: Ueber die axillaren Lymphdrüsen. Inaug.
    Dissert., Berlin, C. Vogt, 1896.

Halsell, J. T., et al.: Lymphatic drainage of the breast demonstrated by vital dye staining and radiography. Ann. Surg., 162:221, 1965.

Halsted, W. S.: A clinical and histological study of certain adenocarcinomata of the breast. Ann. Surg., 28:557, 1898.

Halsted, W. S.: The results of radical operations for the cure of cancer of the breast. Ann. Surg., 46:1, 1907.

Hamperl, J.: Ueber die Myothelien (myo-epithelialen Elemente) der Brustdrüse. Virchows Arch. f. path. Anat., 305:171, 1939.

Handley, R. S., and Thackray, A. C.: The internal mammary lymph chain in carcinoma of the breast. Lancet, 2:276, 1949.

Handley, W. S.: Cancer of the Breast. London, John Murray, 1922, 2nd edition.

Handley, W. S.: Parasternal invasion of the thorax in breast cancer, and its suppression by the use of radium tubes as an operative precaution. Surg., Gynec., Obstet., 45:721, 1927.

Handley, W. S.: The radium treatment of sternal recurrences in cancer of the breast. Clin. J., 56:73, 1927.

Heidenhain, L.: Ueber die Ursachen der Lokalen Krebsrecidive nach Amputatio mammae. Arch. f. klin. Chir., 39:97, 1889.

Henriques, C.: The veins of the vertebral column and their role in the spread of cancer. Ann. Roy. Coll. Surg. Eng., 31:1, 1962.

Hitzrot, J. M.: A composite study of the axillary artery in man. Bull. Johns Hopkins Hosp., 12:136, 1901.

Hultborn, K. A., Larsson, L. G., and Ragnhult, I.: The lymph drainage from the breast to the axillary and parasternal lymph nodes, studied with the aid of colloidal AU[198]. Acta radiol., 43:52, 1955.

Iwai, T.: A statistical study on the polymastia of the Japanese. Lancet, 2:753, 1907.

Jain, S. R., Sepaha, G. C., and Khandelwal, G. D.: A case of unilateral amastia. J. Anat. Soc. India, 10:45, 1961.

Kendall, B. E., Arthur, J. F., and Patey, D. H.: Lymphangiography in carcinoma of the breast. Cancer, 16:1233, 1963.

Kirmisson, E.: Note sur la topographie des ganglions axillaires. Bull. et mém. Soc. anat. Paris, 7:453, 1882.

Klinkerfuss, G. H.: Four generations of polymastia. J.A.M.A., 82:1247, 1924.

Kowlessar, M., and Orti, E.: Complete breast absence in siblings. Amer. J. Dis. Child., 115:91, 1968.

Kuzma, J. F.: Myoepithelial proliferations in the human breast. Am. J. Path., 19:473, 1943.

Langer, E., and Huhn, S.: Der submikroskopische Bau der Myoepithelzelle. Zschr. Zellforsch., 47:507, 1958.

Leaf, C. H.: Cancer of the Breast: Clinically Considered. London, Constable, 1912.

Leborgne, F. E., Leborgne, R., Schaffner, E., and Leborgne, F. E., Jr.: Estudio de los linfáticos de la glándula mamaria con el radio oro 198. Torax, Montevideo, 4(4):233, 1955.

Lewis, R. J., and Beal, J. M.: Mammolymphangioadenography: direct radiographic visualization of the breast lymphatics. Surgical Forum, 14:112, 1963.

Linzell, J. L.: Flow and composition of mammary gland lymph. J. Physiol. Lond., 153:510, 1960.

Linzell, J. L.: The silver staining of myoepithelial cells particularly in the mammary gland, and their relation to the ejection of milk. J. Anat. Lond., 86:49, 1952.

Looney, C. M., Reichman, S. C., and Noel, O. F.:

Ectopic breast tissue: report of an unusual case. Amer. Surgeon, 25:219, 1959.

Mandl, F.: Versuche sur Klarlegung der Lymphverhaltnisse bei der Operation des Brustdrüsen Krebs. Wien. klin. Wchnschr., 37:1257, 1924.

Mascagni, P.: Vasorum Lymphaticorum Corporis Humani Historia et Ichnographia. Siena, P. Carli, 1787.

Masor, N.: An aberrant lactating breast of the axilla. New York State J. Med., 52:1674, 1952.

Massopust, L. C., and Gardner, W. D.: Infrared photographic studies of the superficial thoracic veins in the female. Surg., Gynec. & Obst., 91:717, 1950.

McGregor, A. L.: Accessory breast tissue. Med. Proc. Johannesberg, 7:440, 1961.

Miller, M. R., and Kasahara, M.: The cutaneous innervation of the human female breast. Anat., Rec., 135:153, 1959.

Monroe, C. W.: Lymphatic spread of carcinoma of the breast. Arch. Surg., 57:479, 1948.

Montagu, A.: Natural selection and the form of the breast in the female. J.A.M.A., 180:826, 1962.

Mornard, P.: Etude anatomique des lymphatiques de la mammelle, au point de vue de l'extension lymphatique des cancers. Rev. de chir., 51:462, 1916.

Mornard, P.: Sur deux cas de tumeurs malignes des mammelles axillaires aberrantes. Bull. et mém. Soc. nat. de chir. de Paris, 21:487, 1929.

Most, A.: Chirurgie der Lymphagefässe und der Lymphdrüsen. Stuttgart, F. Enke, 1917.

Most, A.: Zur Metastasenbildung und Chirurgie des Brustkrebses. Arch. f. klin. Chir., 183:209, 1935.

Most, A.: Die Glandula paramammaria in ihrer Bedeutung für die Diagnose des Brustkrebses. Arch. f. klin. Chir., 193:554, 1938.

Noronha, A. J.: Cystic disease in supernumerary breasts. Brit. J. Surg., 24:143, 1936.

Oelsner, L.: Anatomische Untersuchungen über die Lymphwege der Brust mit Bezug auf die Ausbreitung des Mammacarcinoms. Arch. f. klin. Chir., 64:134, 1901.

Pernkopf, E.: Topographische Anatomie. Berlin und Wien, Urban & Schwarzenberg, 1937-52.

Piccagli, G.: Carcinoma mammario aberrante. Ann. ital di chir., 17:241, 1938.

Pickren, J. W.: Significance of occult metastases. Cancer, 14:1266, 1961.

Pierre, M., and Bureau, H.: A propos de deux cas d'absence congénitale d'une glande mammaire. Ann. Chir. plast., 5:137, 1960.

Poirier, P., and Cunéo, B.: Les Lymphatiques. In Poirier, P., and Charpy, A.: Traité d'anatomie humaine., Paris, Masson, 1902, Vol. 2, Fasc. 4.

Putti, F.: Ricerche anatomiche sui linfonodi mammari interni. Chirurgia Italiana, 7:161, 1953.

Regaud, C.: Origine des vaisseaux lymphatiques de la glande mammaire. Bibliogr. Anat., 8:261, 1900.

Richardson, K. C.: Contractile tissues in the mammary gland with special reference to myoepithelium in the goat. Proc. Roy. Soc. Lond., Series B:136:30, 1945.

Rodriguez, A., and Pereira, S.: Sur les gros troncs lymphatiques de la base du cou. Ann. d'anat. path., 7:1019, 1930.

Rossi, R., Salvini, A., and Scortecci, V.: Il drenaggio linfatico mammario studiato per mezzo dell'oro colloidale radioattivo. Arch. Ital. Chir., 88:393, 1962.

Rotter, J.: Zur Topographie des Mammacarcinoms. Arch f. klin. Chir., 58:346, 1899.

Rouvière, H.: Anatomie des Lymphatiques de l'Homme. Paris, Masson, 1932.

Roux, J. P.: Lactation from axillary tail of breast. Brit. M. J., *1*:28, 1955.

Sappey, P. C.: Anatomie, Physiologie, Pathologie des Vaisseaux Lymphatiques Considérés chez l'Homme et les Vertébrés. Paris, A. Delahaye and E. Lecrosnier, 18 [74] 85.

Semba, V.: Anatomische Untersuchungen über die Lymphgefässsystem der Leber. Arch. f. klin. Chir., *149*:350, 1928.

Sledziewski, H. G.: Trajet des vaisseaux efférents des ganglions lymphatiques diaphragmatiques dans les médiastins. Compt. rend. de l'Assoc. d. anat., 26: 467, 1931.

Sledziewski, H. G.: Les métastases du cancer de l'estomac et les métastases "croisées" du cancer du sein aux ganglions lymphatiques de la base du cou, au point de vue de l'anatomie normale. Arch. d'anat., d'histol. et d'embryol., *24*:199, 1937.

Soerensen, B.: Recherches sur la localisation des ganglions lymphatiques parasternaux par rapport aux espaces intercostaux. Internat. j. de chir., *11*:501, 1951.

Speert, H.: Supernumerary mammae, with special reference to the Rhesus monkey. Quart. Rev. Biol., *17*:59, 1942.

Stibbe, E. P.: The internal mammary lymphatic glands. J. Anat., *52*:257, 1918.

Stiles, H. J.: Contributions to the surgical anatomy of the breast. Edinburgh M. J., *37*:1099, 1892.

Stringa, U.: Sui tumori delle ghiandole mammarie aberranti. Minerva chir., *6*:349, 1951.

Takeya, S.: Ueber die überzähligen Brustwarzen bei Chinesen. J. Orient. Med., *20*:32, 1934.

Taylor, G. W., and Nathanson, I. T.: Lymph Node Metastases. New York, Oxford Univ. Press, 1942.

Testut, L.: Traité d'Anatomie Humaine. Paris, Doin, 1905.

Tow, S. H., and Shanmugaratnam, K.: Supernumerary mammary gland in the vulva. Brit. Med. J., *2*:1234, 1962.

Trier, W. C.: Complete breast absence. Plast. Reconstr. Surg., *36*:430, 1965.

Turner-Warwick, R. T.: The lymphatics of the breast. Brit J. Surg., *46*:574, 1959.

Vogt-Hoerner, G., and Contesso, G.: Localisation anatomique de premier ganglion axillaire métastatique de cancer du sein. J. Chir., *86*:37, 1963.

Waugh, D., and Van Der Hoeven, E.: Fine structure of the human adult female breast. Lab. Invest., *11*:220, 1962.

Weinshel, L. R., and Demakopoulos, N.: Supernumerary breasts with special reference to the pseudomamma type. Am. J. Surg. (new series) *60*:76, 1943.

White, R. J.: Fibroadenoma in an accessory breast. Am. J. Surg., *8*:830, 1930.

Zaks, M. G.: The Motor Apparatus of the Mammary Gland. Springfield, Ill., Charles C Thomas, 1961.

Zeirhut, E.: Zur Röntgendiagnostik der Lymphabflusswege beim Mammakarzinom. Fortsch. Rontgenstrahl., *83*:702, 1955.

Zeitlhofer, J.: Ueber die axillare Lymphknotenmetastasierung des Brustdrüsenkrebses. Arch. f. klin. Chir., *272*:429, 1952.

Zilli, L., and Stefani, G.: Unilateral agenesis of the pectoralis muscles associated with mammary hypoplasia. Friuli Med., *15*:1522, 1960.

Chapter Two

The Normal Physiology of the Breasts

The mammary glands are an integral part of the reproductive system; and the physiologic changes in them are closely related to the physiology of the reproductive system as a whole and are under the same neuroendocrine control. Physicians must have a thorough understanding of the normal physiology of the breasts and the various aberrations in this physiology which are so common in modern women. Without this knowledge, physicians often mistake such physiologic phenomena for actual breast disease, and carry out needless and harmful diagnostic and surgical procedures.

There are three types of physiologic changes in the breasts: (1) growth and involution related to age; (2) changes associated with the menstrual cycle; and (3) changes due to pregnancy and lactation.

GROWTH AND INVOLUTION

The mammary glands develop in early embryonal life as a budding downgrowth from the ectoderm. By the time of birth the glands in the human being consist of a branching system of ducts emptying into a well-developed nipple. The gland fields are not yet apparent.

Within a few days after birth, in a considerable proportion of babies of both sexes, there is evidence of some slight degree of secretory function. The rudimentary breasts appear to enlarge, and there is slight secretion of a milky material from the nipples. After a week or so, this secretory activity subsides and the infantile mammary glands lapse into the inactive state which characterizes them during childhood. The epithelial elements consist merely of small ducts scattered throughout a fibrous stroma. Figure 2–1 shows such a breast from a 12 month old female child.

With the onset of puberty in the female, between the tenth and the fifteenth years, the areola enlarges and becomes more pigmented, and a discoid mass of breast tissue takes form beneath it. This grows to form the normal protuberant adolescent breast. As the breasts grow there is microscopic budding of the ducts to form gland fields. The breasts are often well developed by the time menstruation begins. Figure 2–2 shows the structure of the breast in a 14 year old girl. Occasionally breast development begins at an earlier age and may be mistaken for breast disease. This phenomenon is discussed in Chapter 4.

In adult women, breast character—that is, fullness, density, and nodularity—depends chiefly upon two factors. The first and most important is the corpulence of the individual. Since the breasts are in great part made up of fat, obese women usually have large and firm breasts. The second factor is whether or not the breasts have functioned. It is my impression that the breasts of women who have gone through pregnancy and nursed their

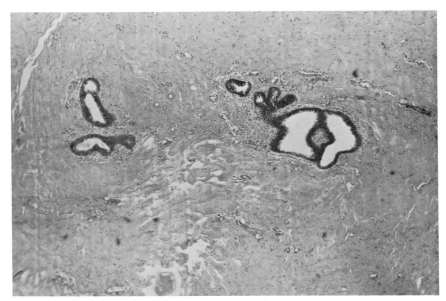

Figure 2–1.   Normal mammary gland in a 12 month old female child.

babies are softer and less nodular, that is, more normal. Increased density and nodularity are more characteristic of breasts that have never functioned. I must admit that I have not been able to correlate these differences in the physical characteristics of the breasts with any microscopic differences. There are marked differences in the number and size of the gland fields in breasts that are physically identical.

With the completion of the menopause the breasts commonly decrease somewhat in size and become less dense. If they have been abnormally nodular, the nodularity usually diminishes. With these postmenopausal physical changes in the breasts there is fre-

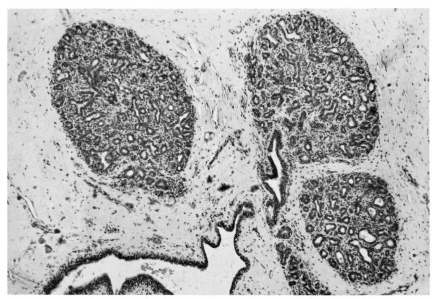

Figure 2–2.   Normal mammary gland in a 14 year old girl.

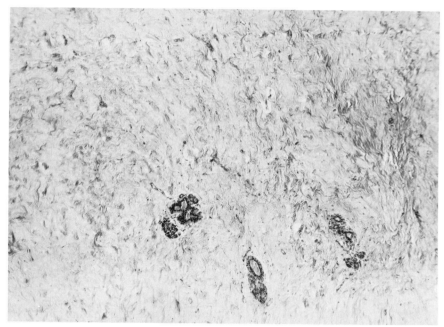

Figure 2–3. Atrophic lobules in the breast of a woman aged 61.

quently a decrease in the number and size of the gland fields. This is illustrated in Figure 2–3 which shows the breast of a 61 year old woman. Three atrophic lobules are seen lying in a dense fibrous matrix. Increase in the elastic tissue component of the breast stroma is a prominent feature of this aging process (Riedel).

It should be emphasized, however, that it is not unusual to find very little decrease in the epithelial elements in the breasts of postmenopausal women.

BREAST CHANGES ASSOCIATED WITH THE MENSTRUAL CYCLE

In the breasts the phenomen of *engorgement* is normally closely correlated with the menstrual cycle. Engorgement has several components—increase in the size, density, and nodularity of the breasts, as well as increase in sensitivity. Most women are conscious of some degree of breast engorgement during the three or four days preceding the onset of menstruation. Engorgement diminishes toward the end of menstruation and disappears with its completion.

The increase in size, density, and nodu-
larity of the breasts is usually not perceived in these terms by the patient; she complains only that her breasts are fuller. The great difficulty of measuring lesser variations in breast size makes it virtually impossible to prove that there is a cyclical increase in breast volume. But in many patients whom I have examined regularly there has been an obvious and marked increase in breast size premenstrually. In most women there is an increase in the density as well as the degree of nodularity of the breasts, usually beginning several days before menstruation and lasting throughout. It is such a regular phenomenon that it is my own custom not to examine the breasts during the week preceding menstruation, or during menstruation. I have very often seen patients in whom this increased cyclical nodularity has been mistaken for a dominant tumor caused by breast disease, and unnecessary biopsy has been advised. Indeed, it is fair to say that the decision clinicians are most frequently required to make regarding the breasts is that of distinguishing increased physiologic nodularity from real breast disease. Many unnecessary biopsies are performed because surgeons fail to make this differential diagnosis accurately. Whenever there is doubt, decision should be

reserved and the breasts re-examined at the midpoint of the succeeding menstrual cycle, when breast engorgement is minimal.

Unfortunately, in some women the increased physiologic nodularity does not have a cyclical pattern but persists for long periods of time more or less unchanged. It is in such patients that the examiner's diagnostic skill is most severely tested.

In this diagnostic dilemma the fact that the increased nodularity is bilateral and symmetrical, usually being most pronounced in the upper half of each breast, is a strong point in favor of the physiologic nature of the phenomenon. But in some patients simple increased physiologic nodularity is more marked in one breast than in the other, and may be concentrated in one sector of one breast, for example, in its upper outer sector.

Cystic disease is, of course, the lesion with which increased physiologic nodularity is most commonly confused. In both conditions the "tumors" are usually multiple and bilateral. Many clinicians do not really try to distinguish the two conditions and succumb to the temptation to call all increased nodularity of the breasts cystic disease. This is a bad practice. The two entities are entirely different. It is essential to try to distinguish them, and with careful and repeated examination it is usually possible to do so. I shall discuss the physical characteristics of both in Chapter 5.

Physicians do not realize what harm they do to their patients who have nothing more than increased physiologic nodularity when they tell them that they have cystic disease. This kind of inaccurate diagnosis makes patients worry and seek constant reassurance. Unnecessary mammograms are made. What such a patient needs in the first place is only careful examination of her breasts, explanation of the physiology of breast engorgement, and reassurance.

The increased sensitivity of the breasts that is a part of the cyclical physiologic phenomenon of engorgement deserves separate discussion. This sensitivity does not usually bother women enough to lead them to complain to a physician about it. In some women the sensitivity is so marked, however, that they call it pain. They try to find relief by supporting the breasts at all times with a brassiere. Exceptional patients complain that the pain is so severe that it cannot be endured. Search for relief comes to dominate their lives. They go from one physician to another, being given all sorts of combinations of hormones and other drugs, to no avail. Finally, some gullible surgeon may perform simple mastectomy. I have seen patients for whom this had been done, and ineffectually, for the patient still complained of pain. This is understandable, for it should be pointed out that women who complain of this degree of breast pain are in general unstable and hypochondriacal, although they are not frankly psychotic.

Breast engorgement is related to the patient's reproductive history, as well as to her age. It is my clinical impression that engorgement is more marked in nulliparous women, as well as in women who have not breast-fed their children—that is, in women whose breasts have not functioned normally. Breast engorgement is least apparent in the middle years of menstrual life. It often begins to increase in the 40's, and it is most severe just before the menopause. It normally disappears after the menopause, unless artificially prolonged by estrogen therapy.

Efforts to correlate these physical changes in the mammary glands during the cycle with histological changes in them have produced conflicting reports. Rosenberg, for instance, believed that he saw sprouting and budding of the duct epithelium in premenstrual breasts, and that following menstruation the newly formed acini disappeared. His evidence was based on autopsy material. In a similar study, however, Dieckmann found no evidence at all of budding of the ducts, or of other signs of epithelial proliferation during the premenstrual phase; but he did note that during this phase the intralobular stroma of the breast was loose, wide-meshed and edematous, and that the lumens of the acini were dilated and the basal layer of their epithelium vacuolated. In the interval phase of the cycle the intralobular stroma became compact, the vacuoles disappeared, and the lumens of the acini became smaller or disappeared.

In an effort to settle the controversy regarding cyclical epithelial proliferation in the breast. I carried out a histological study of breast tissues removed surgically in the Presbyterian Hospital, correlating the microscopic findings with the stage of the menstrual cycle. To determine whether or not there was actual budding of the ducts in the premenstrual phase of the cycle, I counted the numbers of lobules and acini in ten representative fields in each microscopic section. The result, shown in Table 2–1, revealed no statistically

Table 2–1. VARIATION IN NUMBER OF LOBULES AND ACINI ACCORDING TO PHASE OF MENSTRUAL CYCLE

Phase of Cycle	Number of Cases	Average Age	Average Number of Lobules per Low Power Field	Average Number of Acini per Lobule
Menstrual	23	39.3	5.8	32.0
Interval	59	37.3	6.7	36.2
Premenstrual	18	39.6	7.2	30.2
Total menstruating group	100	38.2	6.6	34.1
Menopause	10	54.8	2.3	11.2

significant difference in the different phases of the menstrual cycle. Epithelial proliferation, as evidenced by mitosis and apparent increase in the compactness of the acini, was seen as often in the interval phase of the cycle (Fig. 2–4) as at any other time. I therefore found no support for the claim that Rosenberg and others have made that there is an increased epithelial proliferation in the breast during the premenstrual phase of the menstrual cycle.

The phenomenon of vacuolization of the

basal layer of cells lining the mammary acini was described by Dieckmann as characteristic of the premenstrual phase of the menstrual cycle. I found it present in 33 per cent of the specimens removed during the premenstrual phase in my series of cases. It is illustrated in Figure 2–5. I also found such vacuolization in 12 per cent of my specimens from the interval phase. Its significance remains questionable.

Edema of the mammary lobule is another phenomenon which was thought by Dieck-

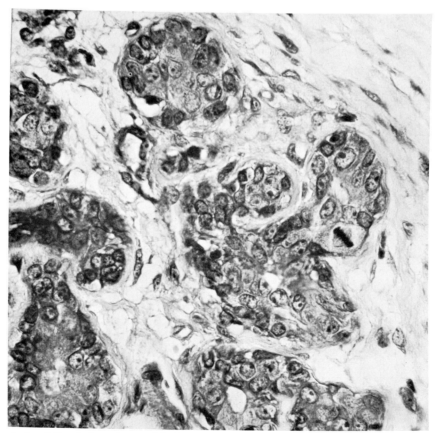

Figure 2–4. Mitosis in acinar epithelium during the interval phase of the menstrual cycle.

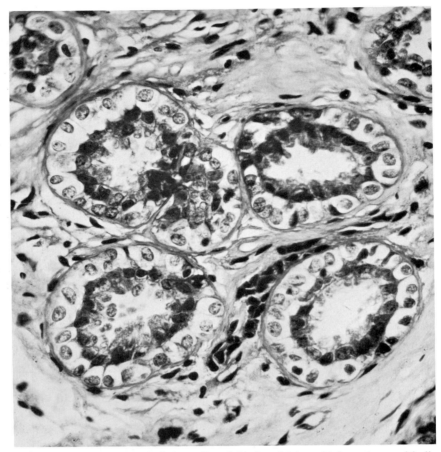

Figure 2–5.   Vacuolization of the cells of the basal layer of the acinar epithelium.

mann, by Moschowitz, and by others, to be characteristic of the premenstrual phase of the cycle. Such intralobular edema is shown in Figure 2–6, in a specimen from the menstrual phase of the cycle. By contrast, Figure 2–7 shows a large and active-appearing mammary lobule without edema in a specimen from the interval phase of the cycle. In my data, however, intralobular edema was found in only 28 per cent of the specimens from patients in the premenstrual phase of the cycle. It was also present to some degree in 22 per cent of the specimens from patients in the interval phase.

It has also been claimed that there is increased cellularity of the stroma of the breast and lymphocytic infiltration of the lobules during the premenstrual phase of the cycle. I was unable to confirm any of these claims.

It is, of course, obvious that the increase in the size and density of the breasts in the premenstrual phase must be the result of some physical change in them. Since no satisfactory evidence of epithelial proliferation, edema, or lymphocytic infiltration during the premenstruum has been found, it must be presumed that these changes are due to blood or lymph engorgement or to increase in the extracellular fluid tension. These are changes which we could not expect to demonstrate microscopically with ordinary microscopic techniques.

There is no reasonable treatment for breast engorgement except careful explanation of the nature of the phenomenon to the patient. She must be reassured that it is not disease, in the usual sense of the word, and that it does not predispose her to true breast disease. Estrogen and progesterone aggravate breast engorgement. Androgen has no apparent effect when given in doses short of those that will produce symptoms of masculinization, i.e., hirsutism, acne, voice changes, etc. A brassiere that supports the

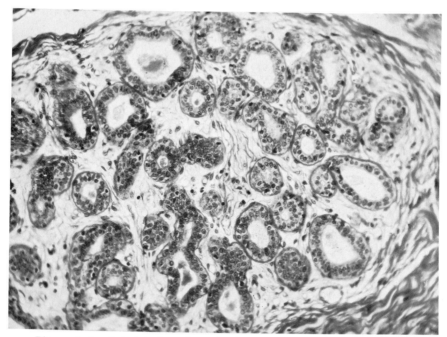

Figure 2–6. Intralobular edema in the menstrual phase of the cycle.

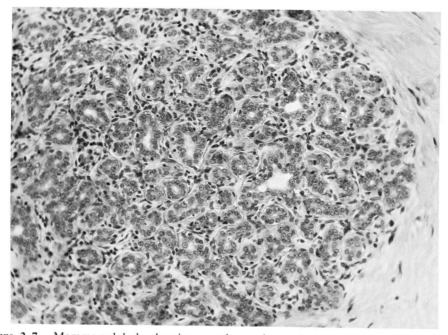

Figure 2–7. Mammary lobule showing no edema—interval phase of the menstrual cycle.

breasts well will help some patients. Obese patients with large dependent breasts are bothered more than thin patients by engorgement when they are so unfortunate as to have it in a severe form, even though their obesity has no causal relationship to their breast engorgement. Weight reduction is therefore advisable in these patients.

CHANGES IN THE BREASTS DUE TO PREGNANCY AND LACTATION

Within a few weeks after conception the effects of pregnancy are evident in the breasts. They become fuller and more firm. The areolar skin glands become more prominent, and the areolar skin darkens. The nipples enlarge and become more erect. The breasts enlarge steadily as the mammary lobules grow in size and number.

During the last half of pregnancy it is often possible to express a few drops of thin yellowish secretion from the nipples.

The first secretion from the breasts after delivery is the yellowish colostrum. If the baby is put to breast at once after delivery, and is permitted to nurse as long and as often thereafter as he wishes, the colostrum will usually give way to milk in 24 hours. If the baby is not put to breast until after the first 24 hours, however, and thereafter is permitted to nurse only on a fixed and limited schedule, it usually takes from three to five days for the milk to "come in." During this interval the breasts often become strikingly engorged—firmer, larger, and so distended with milk that they are painful. With nursing successfully established these symptoms soon subside.

When lactation terminates in the normal way after some months of nursing, with the baby taking only from one to three nursings a day and depending chiefly upon other food, the breasts soon return to approximately the same size and contour that they had before pregnancy. Lactation does not of course stop abruptly with the cessation of nursing. There is usually some leakage of milk from the nipples for some days afterwards. Occasionally this continues for a long time. Such abnormal and prolonged lactation will be discussed in Chapter 3.

Dawson described the histological changes in the postlactating breast very thoroughly. The retained secretion is gradually removed by phagocytosis. The epithelial cells lining the acini are shed into the centers of the acini and disintegrate. The process takes at least three months.

Pregnancy certainly changes the breasts. After pregnancy the breasts are less dense and nodular, and less protuberant than those of nulliparous women. But I do not believe that breast feeding has any great effect upon breast form and consistence. Women cannot justly claim that nursing harms their breasts.

WHY MOTHERS SHOULD NURSE THEIR BABIES

In a book such as this, which attempts to deal with diseases of the breast, I have only an indirect excuse for discussing the pros and cons of breast feeding. I can make the statement that it is my impression that certain diseases such as cystic disease and carcinoma are less frequent in breasts that have functioned naturally; but I cannot prove statistically that this is a fact in our patient population, because of a lack of a control group of women who have breast-fed their children. I have taken careful nursing histories of my patients for many years. These data confirm all too well the fact that in this country women have today largely abandoned nursing their babies. Among the women in my case series, the average total of breast feeding in a lifetime was only approximately four months. In a recent study by Salber and Feinleib it was shown that the breast feeding rate in the United States fell by almost one-half during a recent ten year period. In the New York area only 3.6 per cent of mothers today nurse their babies for as long as six months (Gerard). In Chapter 17, however, where I discuss the etiology of breast carcinoma, I will present what statistical evidence there is that tends to relate the origin of the disease to breast function.

Quite apart from the matter of statistical proof of the desirability of breast feeding as a preventive measure against breast disease, I wish to make a plea on a broader basis for mothers to nurse their babies. As a member of a family in which all the babies have always been nursed, and as a physician who has practiced medicine for 44 years, I feel strongly that breast feeding is an important part of normal life for both mother and baby. There is no question but that nursing gives much emotional satisfaction to the mother. It is not so easy to prove that it is just as emotionally rewarding to the baby, yet anyone with common sense who has observed the obvious love that a baby expresses for the mother who nurses him cannot doubt it. Nursing is one of the links in the chain of family love that stabilizes society.

A variety of reasons have been advanced for the recent decline of nursing in this country. My impression is that we physicians are mostly to blame. We are not only ignorant of the benefits of breast feeding, but most of us do not know enough about it to be of much help to the mothers who wish to nurse. In general the hospitals in which virtually all babies in this country are born provide an environment in which the mother who wishes to breast-feed her baby finds no expert help, and in which unreasonable rules and regulations make it very difficult for her to succeed if she tries. There are so few homes today in which there is a mother, a grandmother, or an aunt to help the young mother with the practical aspects of breast feeding that she is dependent on what advice her obstetrician or pediatrician can give her. If, as is often the case, the obstetrician is too busy to be bothered about the matter, and if the pediatrician is indifferent about it, the young mother has little chance of succeeding.

I was able to persuade one of my daughters, Mrs. Alice Gerard, to undertake a study of this question in the Columbia-Presbyterian Medical Center. Her findings have been published in book form.

Mrs. Gerard feels that the following are the basic requirements for increasing breast feeding:

1. The obstetrician and pediatrician should encourage breast feeding.
2. The nurses on obstetrical services should encourage breast feeding and assist in every way the mothers who wish to nurse their babies.
3. Hospital routines should be so flexible that the mother can nurse her baby soon after delivery, and keep it with her, nursing on demand and using both breasts at each feeding.
4. An ideal arrangement would be to appoint nursing counsellors to hospital obstetrical services, who could give the prospective mothers advice about breast feeding, instruct them in their initial efforts, and be available for advice after the mother leaves the hospital.
5. To avoid cracked nipples, one of the commonest difficulties in breast feeding, it is my impression that soap should not be used on the nipples, but that a special mildly acid cream should be applied to them after every nursing.

With this kind of help, we believe that almost all women who wish to nurse their babies can do so, and will have an adequate supply of milk. Nursing should be continued for a minimum of six months.

THE NEUROENDOCRINE CONTROL OF THE BREASTS

Breast development and function are controlled by the complex neuroendocrine system that governs reproduction. The ovaries, adrenals, pituitary, and hypothalamus are all essential components of this system. Our knowledge of the very complex mechanism of neuroendocrine control of the breast in some species, particularly in the rat and the mouse, has grown enormously during the last 25 years. But in human beings our knowledge of this mechanism is still rudimentary. The greatest handicap to progress is a lack of reliable chemical methods for determining the levels of the various hormones in the body fluids. Until chemists provide these assay methods, much of what we know continues to be based on clinical experience.

It seems reasonable to spare the reader a detailed account of our rapidly changing knowledge of the neuroendocrine mechanism of breast growth and function in laboratory and farm animals. I will merely try to summarize our present knowledge of this matter in human beings.

The growth and involution of the breasts appear to be largely dependent upon estrogen produced in the ovaries. At puberty a complex mechanism involving central nervous system receptors, the hypothalamus, and the pituitary initiates ovarian development and estrogen production. It should be kept in mind that estrogen in purified form did not become available until 1930. Shortly thereafter it was demonstrated that the hormone would make the breasts grow in castrated women (Werner and Collier), as well as in women with apparent ovarian deficiency (MacBryde). The relative decrease in breast size and density that occurs after the menopause is presumably due to decrease in estrogen production after the menopause.

Today, the therapeutic use of estrogens has become so common that examples of the effects of these hormones upon the breasts are of daily occurrence in the practice of medicine. The women who take oral contraceptives containing estrogen or progesterone usually develop breast enlargement comparable to that observed in early pregnancy. Women who are given estrogen at the menopause may obtain some relief from their hot flashes but they will usually experience some increase in breast engorgement. When estrogen is continued after the menopause the cyclical breast engorgement, which is often increasingly troublesome as the menopause approaches, persists. Relief from this breast engorgement is normally one of the benefits of the menopause, and those who take estrogen forego this advantage.

I have often been consulted for troublesome breast engorgement by women who were using enough estrogen-containing face cream to account for their breast symptoms. Speert long ago described the absorption of estrogen in an ointment or oily alcoholic vehicle through intact skin, and MacBryde reported breast growth obtained by this method.

In any department of surgical pathology breast tissue from women who have been given estrogen for considerable periods of time is often seen today. In such tissue a great variety of epithelial proliferation and cystic change is seen, attesting the fact that estrogen makes the breast epithelium grow. Figures 2–8 and 2–9 show an area of this kind of estrogen-induced epithelial proliferation from one of our cases. This tissue is from a 71 year old patient who had been given 15 mg. of stilbestrol daily for three months. Her breast tissue resembles that of a pregnant women, with a great increase in the number and size of the gland fields. The cells lining the acini show characteristic vacuolation. Huseby and Thomas published a good description of the microscopic changes produced by estrogen.

Such epithelial proliferation has also been observed in male mammary tissue, both in patients given stilbestrol for prostatic carcinoma and in workers handling stilbestrol (see Chapter 3).

There is very little precise information available concerning the effects upon the human breasts of the different components of the neuroendocrine mechanism that controls the menstrual cycle. Since progesterone has such an important role in the cycle we may assume that it has some effect upon the breast, but all that we really know is that progesterone, like estrogen, if given therapeutically will accentuate cyclical breast engorgement.

Although the precise neuroendocrine mechanisms that control the human breasts during pregnancy and lactation remain obscure, considerable progress has recently been made in understanding them. The placenta has been shown to produce comparatively large amounts of estrogen and progesterone, both of which stimulate the mammary lobules to multiply and to increase in size. In 1937 Turner and his associates identified a new anterior pituitary mammogenic hormone which, in many mammalian species, has a dual function of stimulating breast growth and milk secretion. This hormone has become known as *prolactin* or *mammotrophin*. Recently it has been shown that animal prolactin and the human anterior pituitary hormone *somatotrophin* have similar biological effects in animals (Cowie, Lyons and Dixon). Although final proof will not be available until reliable assay methods for the demonstration of mammotrophin-like activity in blood are developed, it is likely that this hormone has an important role in human breast physiology.

Recently an explanation has been found for another important aspect of breast function—milk ejection. The milk that collects in the subareolar milk sinuses can be withdrawn by suckling. But the ejection of milk from the mammary acini into the duct system—a process that has been commonly known as the "letting down" of the milk—is a much more complex mechanism, in which the mother's subjective response and the mechanical stimulation of suckling both play a part. During the last 30-odd years intensive study of this mechanism, carried on largely in cows, has revealed that it is a neurohumoral phenomenon in which the posterior pituitary has an essential role. Suckling produces nerve impulses that are carried by way of the lateral funiculus of the spinal cord to the hypothalamus. Via nervous pathways from the hypothalamus to the posterior pituitary, it is stimulated to release into the blood stream the specific hormone *oxytocin*. Oxytocin is carried to the breasts, where it causes the myoepithelial cells which surround the mammary acini to contract and eject the milk into the duct system. Oxytocin has been used

Fig. 2–8

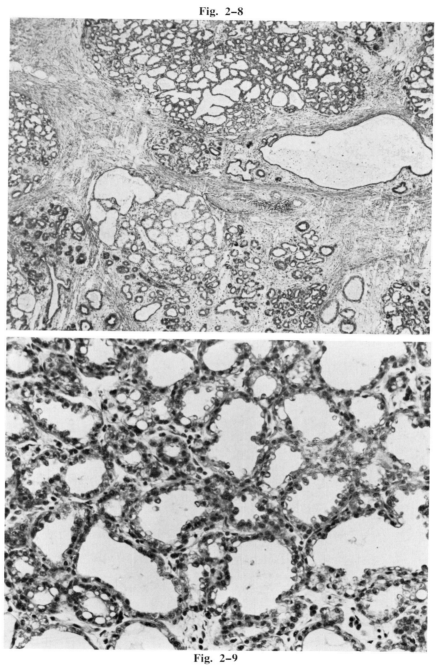

Fig. 2–9

Figure 2–8 and 2–9. Breast tissue from a 71 year old woman given stilbestrol for three months. Low and high power views.

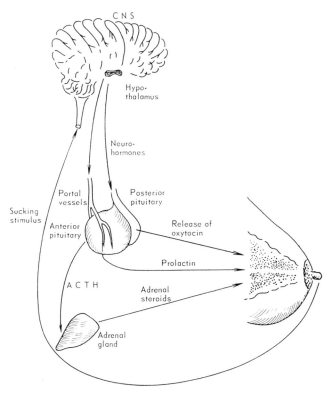

CNS

Hypo-
thalamus

Neuro-
hormones

Portal
vessels

Posterior
pituitary

Sucking
stimulus

Anterior
pituitary

Release of
oxytocin

Prolactin

ACTH

Adrenal
steroids

Adrenal
gland

Figure 2–10. The neuroendocrine factors concerned in lactation. (*From* World Health Org. Tech. Rep. Ser., 1965, 305.)

clinically with some success to help mothers let down their milk.

The complex neuroendocrine mechanism that controls breast function is shown diagrammatically in Figure 2–10.

REFERENCES

Auchincloss, H., and Haagensen, C. D.: Cancer of the breast possibly induced by estrogenic substance. J.A.M.A., *114*:1517, 1940.

Benson, G. K., and Fitzpatrick, R. J.: The neurohypophysis and the mammary gland. *In* Harris, G. W., and Donovan, B. T.: The Pituitary Gland. Berkeley, U. California Press, 1966, Vol. 3, p. 414.

Corner, G. W.: The hormonal control of lactation: positive action of extracts of the hypophysis. Am. J. Physiol., *95*:43, 1930.

Cowie, A. T.: Anterior pituitary function in lactation. *In* Harris, G. W., and Donovan, B. T.: The Pituitary Gland. Berkeley, U. California Press, 1966, Vol. 2, p. 412.

Dawson, E. K.: A histological study of the normal mammal in relation to tumour growth. II The mature gland in pregnancy and lactation. Edinburgh Med. J., *42*:633, 1935.

Dieckmann, H.: Ueber die Histologie der Brustdrüse bei gestörtem und ungestörtem Menstruationsablauf. Virchows Arch. f. path. Anat., *256*:321, 1925.

Gerard, A. H.: Please Nurse Your Baby. Hawthorn Books, 1970.

Haagensen, C. D., and Randall, H. T.: Production of mammary carcinoma in mice by estrogens. Arch. Path., *33*:411, 1942.

Huseby, R. A., and Thomas, L. B.: Histological and histochemical alterations in the normal breast tissues of patients with advanced breast cancer being treated with estrogenic hormones. Cancer, *7*:54, 1954.

Lyons, W. R., and Dixon, J. S.: The physiology and chemistry of the mammotrophic hormone. *In* Harris, G. W., and Donovan, B. T.: The Pituitary Gland. Berkeley, U. California Press, 1966, Vol. 1, p. 527.

MacBryde, C. M.: The production of breast growth in the human female. J.A.M.A., *112*:1045, 1939.

Meites, J., and Nicoll, C. S.: Adenohypophysis: Prolactin. Ann. Rev. Physiol., *28*:57, 1966.

Moschowitz, L.: Ueber den monatlichen Zyklus der Brustdrüse. Arch. f. klin. Chir., *142*:374, 1926.

Pickles, V. R.: Blood-flow estimations as indices of mammary activity. J. Obst. & Gynaec. Brit. Emp., *60*:301, 1953.

Riddle, O.: Lactogenic and mammogenic hormones. *In* Glandular Physiology and Therapy. Chicago, Amer. Med. Assoc., 1942, p. 67.

Riedel, G.: Die Entwicklung und Entartung des elastischen Gewebes in der senilen Mamma. Virchow's Arch. f. path. Anat., *256*:243, 1925.

Rosenberg, A.: Ueber menstruelle, durch das Corpus luteum bedingte Mammaveränderungen. Frankfurt. Ztschr. f. Path., *27*:466, 1922.

Salber, E. J., and Feinleib, M.: Breast-feeding in Boston. Pediatrics, *37*:299, 1966.

Speert, H.: The Normal and Experimental Development of the Mammary Gland of the Rhesus Monkey, with Some Pathological Correlations. Carnegie Institution of Washington Publication, No. 575, 1948.

Speert, H.: Local action of sex hormones. Physiol. Rev., *28*:23, 1948.

Trentin, J. J., and Turner, C. W.: The Experimental Development of the Mammary Gland with Special Reference to the Interaction of the Pituitary and Ovarian Hormones. Res. Bull. 418, Univ. Missouri College Agric., Mar. 1948.

Turner, C. W.: The mammary glands. *In* Allen, E., Danforth, C. H., and Doisy, E. A.: Sex and Internal Secretions. Baltimore, Williams and Wilkins Co., 1939, 2nd ed. p. 740.

Walchshofer, E.: Ueber Rückbildungsvorgänge in der alternden Mamma. Deut. Zeitschr. f. Chir., *224*:137, 1930.

Werner, A. A., and Collier, W. D.: The effect of theelin injections on the castrated woman. J.A.M.A., *100*:633, 1933.

Chapter Three

Abnormalities of Breast Growth, Secretion, and Lactation, of Physiologic Origin

THE FEMALE BREAST

In females the breasts, as a result of disturbances of the neuroendocrine system that controls them, may fail to develop normally at puberty, may enlarge prematurely, or may hypertrophy. These neuroendocrine breast abnormalities are symmetrical, and often occur in individuals who have other endocrine disturbances.

Failure of Development of the Female Breast

When the breasts fail entirely to develop at the normal age of puberty it may be due to ovarian agenesis. One of the features of the clinical syndrome originally described by Turner in which ovaries are absent is lack of breast development; the other characteristics are sexual infantilism, short stature, webbed neck, shield chest, and cubitus valgus. In these patients estrogen therapy will usually make the breasts develop. The breasts also fail to develop in patients with congenital adrenal hyperplasia (Jones and Scott).

A typical example of lack of breast development in Turner's syndrome is shown in Figure 3–1. This patient's breasts exist in a rudimentary form, but are undeveloped at the age of 18.

There is a larger group of young women in whom development of the breasts is delayed past the normal age of puberty, and then the breasts develop only to a limited extent. Such patients may begin to menstruate late, and have only a few periods before menstruation stops and they begin to have hot flashes. Their urinary gonadotrophin values are elevated. This syndrome is usually classified as premature menopause, and is due to a relative ovarian deficiency. A degree of breast development can usually be induced in these young women with estrogen therapy.

Precocious Development of the Female Breasts

In female children the breasts may begin to develop very early as part of the syndrome of precocious puberty. Most gynecologists consider puberty precocious when it begins before the age of eight or nine years. There are occasional children in whom the first signs of puberty appear within the first two or three years of life. These signs are, in most

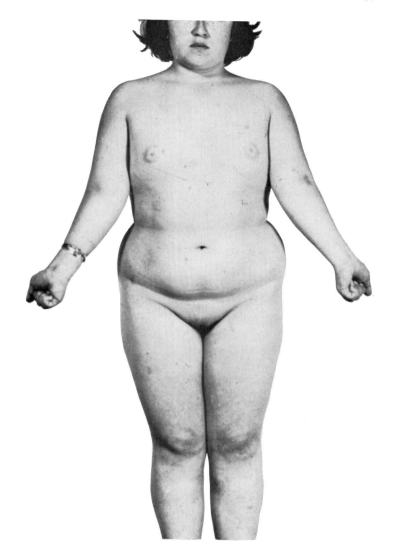

Figure 3–1. Turner's syndrome with lack of breast development at the age of 18 years.

instances, growth of the breasts and the appearance of pubic hair. Growth of the labia and menstruation develop later.

Because of our new knowledge of the dramatic endocrine effects of granulosa cell and other ovarian tumors, it has been the fashion to suspect the presence of an ovarian tumor in a child in whom puberty is precocious. Novak has quite properly emphasized, however, that in most cases of precocious puberty no demonstrable causative lesion is ever found. In this idiopathic or constitutional type of precocious puberty, as Novak calls it, the child develops perfectly normal puberal phenomena at an abnormally early age. During the subsequent life of these patients no etiologic factor explaining their pre-

cocity is ever found. Their adolescence, although premature, is normal.

Novak's designation, the *constitutional type,* for this type of precocious puberty, is an apt one, because not only the genital system but also the skeleton matures precociously. The children appear to grow with abnormal rapidity and are tall for their age. They not only menstruate unusually early but they also ovulate. It seems improbable that mere estrogen production, such as might be due to the presence of a granulosa cell ovarian tumor, could account for this complex precocious growth mechanism.

Studies of the excretion of sex hormones in these precocious children (Nathanson and Aub; Talbot et al.) have shown that there is an elevation of the excretion of gonadotrophins, estrogens, and 17-ketosteroids which approaches adult levels.

The hypertrophy of the breasts, which marks the onset of the genital development in the constitutional type of precocity, may be noted at an astonishingly early age. In Case No. 1 of Novak's series it was noted at 6 months of age. Menstruation began at 15 months. The child was normal, except for her precocity, at 10 years of age. In Novak's Case No. 5 breast enlargement began at 2 years, 3 months, and in his Case No. 8, at the age of 2 years.

The constitutional type of precocious puberty is much more frequent, according to Novak, than precocity due to granulosa cell ovarian tumor. He reported six examples of the former type occurring in his own practice, but of the three examples of the latter type which he described, none occurred in his own practice. This preponderance of the constitutional type has also been observed in the Babies' Hospital, from the records of which the following example of this condition has been chosen.

R.H. was admitted to the Babies' Hospital as a patient of Dr. Rustin McIntosh, on September 27, 1943. She was then 2 years and 7 months of age. Three months previously her mother had noted that she was growing abnormally fast and that her breasts were enlarging and some pubic hair had developed.

Examination showed the child to be within the range of normal for all body measurements except height, in which she was grossly above normal. There was noticeable growth of dark hair over her back and limbs. The breasts showed beginning development with definite palpable glandular tissue and well-defined areolae and nipples (Fig. 3–2A). A vaginal smear showed cells of the postpuberal type. The labia were enlarged but the clitoris was normal. Skeletal films showed the

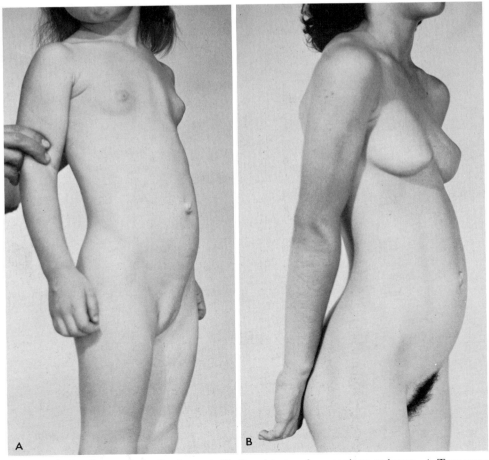

Figure 3–2. Breast hypertrophy in the constitutional type of precocious puberty. *A*, Two years, seven months. *B*, Seven years, four months.

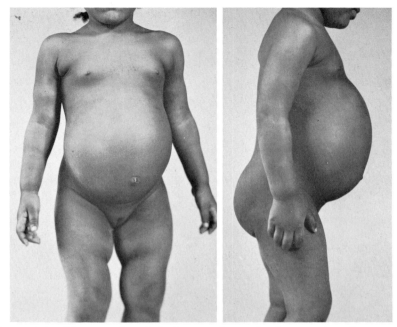

Figure 3–3. Hypertrophy of the breasts due to lutein cyst. Age three years.

skeletal age to be approximately 5 years. Urinary 17-ketosteroids totalled 0.9 mg. in 24 hours.

Her accelerated skeletal growth and her precocious sexual development continued during the following five years of observation. She menstruated first at the age of 6 years, 10 months. At the age of 7 she was found to have diabetes, which was controlled with insulin. At 7 years, 4 months, she weighed 74.5 lbs. and was 57.5 inches in height. Her breasts and external genitalia (Fig. 3–2B) resembled those of normal puberty.

At no time was there any evidence of ovarian, adrenal, or cerebral neoplasm.

Enlargement of the breasts in female children has in rare instances been associated with ovarian tumors. I have already referred to Novak's report of three cases in which such breast enlargement was part of a syndrome of precocious puberty caused by a granulosa cell tumor.

Lutein cysts of the ovary have also caused precocious development. The following is an example of this process, from the service of Dr. Edward J. Donovan in the Babies' Hospital.

C.C., aged 3 years, was admitted April 30, 1934. One month previously the mother noted that the child's abdomen was enlarging, and that her breasts were also abnormally prominent.

Examination showed the abdomen to be greatly enlarged owing to the presence of a soft, freely movable tumor. The breasts were enlarged, the mass of glandular tissue in each measuring 2 × 3 cm. (Fig. 3–3).

At laparotomy a cyst 14 cm. in diameter, arising from the left ovary, was found. It weighed 260 gm. It was filled with blood-stained fluid. The wall varied from 3 to 9 mm. in thickness, and from its thickest part a few low papillary ingrowths projected into the interior. Microscopic study showed it to be a lutein cyst. A wound infection developed and was followed by pneumonia and empyema, and the child finally died.

Microscopic study of the hypertrophied breast showed little evidence of epithelial proliferation. The number of ducts was somewhat increased but there was no acinar development.

Lesions of the third ventricle and tumors of the adrenal cortex are also rare causes of precocious hypertrophy of the female breast.

Early Development of the Female Breasts. Breast development beginning between 8 and 12 and a half years (the latter being the average age of puberty for girls of the North American continent) may be classified as early rather than precocious. This is not uncommon. The first indication is the discovery of a soft discoid mass of tissue, 2 or 3 cm. in diameter, beneath the nipple on one side.

Surgical Intervention in Precocious or Early Female Breast Development. When the mother of a little girl discovers a "tumor" beneath the child's nipple she is apt to overlook the possibility of precocious or early puberty and rush off to her local surgeon. He may be so inexperienced as to assume that the "tumor" represents disease, and proceed to excise it for biopsy. In so doing he removes in its entirety the breast in its early stage of growth, an irreparable surgical tragedy.

I have seen in consultation many of these children with beginning development of one breast, and have warned against any interference with this normal physiologic phenomenon. Curiously enough the tentative diagnosis of the referring physician has usually been "cyst" of the breast. Cystic disease does not occur in the breasts at this early age; 25 years is the earliest age at which I have seen it. Fibrous disease usually does not develop until later; our youngest patient with fibrous disease was 23. Adenosis is also a disease that occurs later; the youngest patient

with adenosis in our records was 19. The common breast tumor of youth is the adenofibroma. In our data the youngest patient with an adenofibroma was 13. Carcinoma of the breast below the age of 20 is so rare that it has no practical significance. I have discussed this question in detail in chapter 33. It is therefore safe to assume that a breast "tumor" in a child is not a neoplasm but merely the beginning of breast development.

I cannot condemn too strongly any kind of surgical procedure upon the breasts of children. The hazard of damage to an abnormally early developing breast is great. What is needed is patience and reassurance. Within a few months the opposite breast will usually show similar development.

Adolescent Hypertrophy of the Female Breast

The most frequent type of true hypertrophy of the female breast is that which oc-

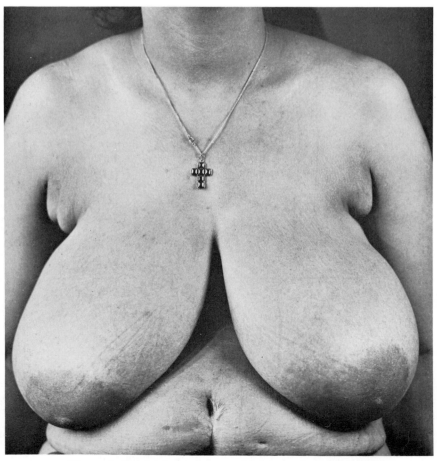

Figure 3–4. Adolescent type of hypertrophy of breasts.

curs during adolescence following normal puberty. The breasts, instead of ceasing to enlarge when they have reached normal limits, continue to grow. Over a period of a year or two of excessive growth the breasts may become so large that they are a great physical and psychological burden to the unfortunate girl. The abnormal drag of breast weight upon the shoulders in the erect position may cause so much distress that these patients are comfortable only when lying down.

The individuals thus affected may have a comparatively normal menstrual history, but in several of the patients whom we have studied, a degree of endocrine abnormality was suggested by low fertility.

When this adolescent type of breast hypertrophy develops, the breasts do not regress in size with maturing years. The patient has no hope of spontaneous relief from her burden.

The following is a typical example of the adolescent type of breast hypertrophy.

F.J. came to the Presbyterian Hospital at the age of 30 for relief of hypertrophy of her breasts, present since puberty. Her breasts had begun to develop at the age of 12, and efforts were first made to restrain their growth by applying a tight binder. They continued to grow rapidly, however, and soon reached an abnormally large size. This persisted up to the date of her admission (Fig. 3-4). Her breasts hung to below the level of her umbilicus, and dragged so heavily that she attempted to support them by means of a special bag-like brassiere.

The adolescent type of hypertrophy sometimes affects one breast much more than it does the other. This is difficult to explain on an endocrinological basis, for one would assume that the hormonal growth stimuli carried by the blood stream would reach both breasts in equal amounts.

The following is an example of asymmetrical adolescent breast hypertrophy.

H.S. came to the Presbyterian Hospital at the age of 19, complaining of hypertrophy of the left breast. At the age of 14 her left breast had begun to increase in size out of all proportion to her right breast, which developed normally with the onset of normal menses at the age of 14 and a half years. During the 18 months preceding her admission to the hospital, the rate of enlargement of the left breast had increased.

Examination showed a normally developed young woman, except for a greatly hypertrophied and dependent left breast (Fig. 3-5). The right

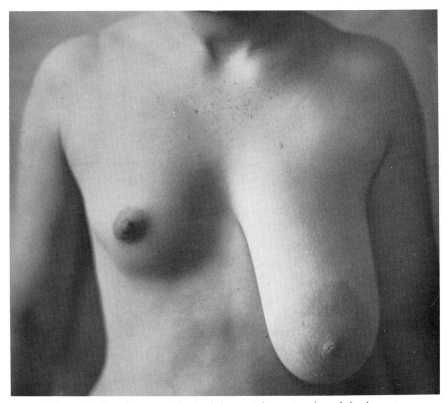

Figure 3–5. Asymmetrical adolescent hypertrophy of the breast.

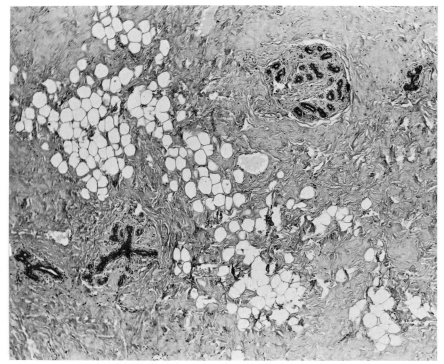

Figure 3–6.   Microscopic appearance of adolescent hypertrophy of the female breast.

breast was normal. A plastic resection of part of the hypertrophied breast was performed.

Microscopic study of this type of adolescent hypertrophy of the female breast shows surprisingly little that can be termed abnormal. The epithelial elements are not remarkable. The excessive growth appears to be on the part of the connective tissue and fat. The relative proportions of these elements in any particular example of breast tissue are difficult to assess from microscopic study. Figure 3–6 shows the microscopic appearance of adolescent hypertrophy.

Massive Breast Hypertrophy in Pregnancy

A few instances of massive breast hypertrophy during pregnancy have been reported (Burslem and Dewhurst; Luchsinger; Williams; Blaydes and Kinnebrew). In these cases the hypertrophy was so truly massive that in several amputation was performed, the breasts each weighing between 5 and 6 thousand grams. The hypertrophy began soon af-

ter the onset of pregnancy—usually a second pregnancy. We have no example of this phenomenon in the records of our medical center.

Nipple Discharge of Physiologic Origin in Females

Under this heading I wish to discuss nipple discharge resulting from systemic neuroendocrine causes, and not from disease within the breast.

1. Women who take oral contraceptives over a long period of time may develop a slight serous or milky nipple discharge. Gregg reported such a case. This kind of nipple discharge is bilateral, and is not bloody. It may be accompanied by the limited increase in the size of the breasts that oral contraceptives often produce. These facts serve to differentiate it from a nipple discharge due to intrinsic disease of the breast such as intraductal papilloma, in which the discharge is unilateral, more profuse, and occasionally blood-tinged.

2. Bilateral bloody discharge from the

nipples is a rare but definite phenomenon of pregnancy. In the patients in whom I have seen this type of discharge, the pregnancy has been a first or second one. The bloody discharge has begun during the middle or last trimester of the pregnancy, and has persisted as long as a month after delivery. I assume that this type of discharge is merely an expression of an exaggerated proliferation of the mammary epithelium accompanying the pregnancy. That it is not due to disease within the breast is apparent from the fact that in all the patients I have seen with the phenomenon it subsided spontaneously within a few months following completion of the pregnancy, although it continued for a while during lactation in several. None of the 12 patients with a bloody nipple discharge associated with pregnancy who consulted me between 1943 and 1967 has had subsequent evidence of breast disease. This phenomenon is so infrequent that all obstetricians are not familiar with it, and they and their surgical colleagues may be unjustifiably alarmed by it. Surgical exploration of the duct system in these patients should not, of course, be performed. All that is needed is reassurance of the patient.

The following is a good example of physiologic bloody nipple discharge during pregnancy.

Mrs. C.H., a 24 year old housewife, developed a spontaneous bilateral bloody nipple discharge during the seventh month of her first pregnancy. Her breasts were full. No tumor could be palpated in either one. During the first two weeks following delivery at term she attempted to nurse the baby and the bloody nipple discharge increased. She discontinued nursing because her supply of milk was inadequate. The bloody nipple discharge ceased spontaneously a month after delivery.

Kline and Lash carried out histological studies of the nipple secretion with the Papanicolaou technique in four pregnant women with frank bleeding from the nipple, such as I have described. In similar studies of nipple secretions in 53 other pregnant women they found occult red blood cells in 17. They concluded that such studies of nipple secretion are of no value in distinguishing physiologic bloody nipple discharge from that due to intraductal papilloma.

3. A still rarer type of physiologic nipple discharge is that which occurs in association with menstruation in young women with rapidly growing breasts. This consists of only a drop or two of serous discharge noted during the first days of the menstrual period. There is no accompanying evidence of breast disease, and the discharge disappears when the breasts have become more mature.

4. Women who are near the menopause sometimes discover that squeezing the breasts or nipples will produce a small amount of grayish, thick nipple discharge. This is a normal phenomenon in the inactive breast at this age.

Abnormal Lactation

Lactation not associated with pregnancy, or continuing long after breast feeding has been terminated, may be due to a variety of causes, as follows:

1. The stimulus of suckling, or manual manipulation of the breast and nipples, will induce lactation. Mead, writing of the Mundugumor women in New Guinea, states, "Even women who have never borne children are able in a few weeks, by placing the [adopted] child constantly at the breast and by drinking plenty of coconut-milk, to produce enough or nearly enough milk to rear the child, which is suckled by other women for the first few weeks after adoption."

Gilbert described the case of a woman aged 35 who sustained lactation for 15 years after she had weaned her first child, by daily breast manipulation.

2. Trauma to the chest wall, or any type of surgical procedure involving the chest wall such as thoracoplasty, pneumonectomy, or cardiac surgery, may be followed by lactation (Berger et al.; Salkin and Davis; Grossman et al.; White). The theoretical explanation of this kind of lactation would be that stimuli from thoracic nerves activate, as does sucking, the hypothalamic-pituitary mechanism that controls lactation.

3. Pituitary necrosis resulting from severe obstetrical hemorrhage (Sheehan's syndrome; the Chiari-Frommel syndrome) may cause persistent lactation (Levine et al.).

4. Pituitary adenomas, as well as other pituitary neoplasms, may disturb the hypothalamic-pituitary relationship and produce lactation (Russfield et al.; Krestin; Levin).

5. Section of the pituitary stalk performed for diabetic retinopathy produced lactation in one of 32 patients, according to Barnes.

6. Hypothyroidism, in both adolescent girls and adult women, has been reported by

Brown, Jenness, and Ulstrom to cause lactation.

7. The tranquilizing drugs—the phenothiazines, reserpine, and methyldopa—may induce lactation (Ayd; Hooper et al.; Sulman and Wennik; Johnson et al.; Pettinger et al.; Mendels).

8. Hormonal oral contraceptives occasionally produce galactorrhea (Gregg; Schachner; Yaffee).

Galactocele

In women in whom lactation has been established and is suppressed by terminating nursing more or less abruptly, the inspissated milk may produce a galactocele. This is a cyst containing thick creamy milk. The tumor thus formed has all the characteristics of a benign neoplasm, being rounded, well-delimited, and movable within the mammary tissue. It is usually situated near the central breast area. Whenever such a tumor develops in a woman who has lactated within six to 10 months it should be assumed that it may be a galactocele, and aspiration should be attempted. If the characteristic milky fluid is withdrawn, no further treatment is required. Since galactocele is a rather infrequent lesion, surgeons often fail to keep this possibility in mind, and operate unnecessarily.

THE MALE BREAST

Gynecomastia, as a transient hypertrophy of one or both breasts of limited extent, occurring at puberty or in older men, is fairly common. I have called the lesion in youth *puberal hypertrophy,* and that in old age *senescent hypertrophy.* In these forms of gynecomastia there are no recognizable endocrine abnormalities, and the etiology remains unknown.

Puberal Hypertrophy

A large proportion of boys between the ages of 13 and 17 show a slight degree of mammary gland enlargement which is transient and passes unnoticed. In occasional subjects the hypertrophy is more marked. It consists of a circumscribed discoid enlargement of the mammary gland directly beneath the areola, measuring 2 or 3 cm. in diameter. It is usually somewhat tender. Nydick and

his associates found this type of gynecomastia in 38.7 per cent of a series of 1855 adolescent boys. It was bilateral in three-fourths of them.

Microscopically, growth of ducts, without the development of gland fields, is seen. The lining epithelium of the ducts sometimes shows low papillary proliferation. The bulk of the lesion, however, is formed by an increase in the fibrous stroma. Karsner has described the histology of these lesions in detail.

The hormonal mechanism responsible for puberal hypertrophy of the breasts is not well understood. In studies of urinary gonadotrophins and steroids in these patients, Decourt and his associates found no definite abnormalities, but Jull and Dossett reported an increased concentration of the pituitary hormones. Collett-Solberg and Grumbach report that they are able to identify a greater estrogenic effect in urine cytograms in boys with puberal hypertrophy. They suggest that this is due to a delay in the reversal of the androstenedione-testosterone ratio that normally occurs at puberty.

Puberal hypertrophy is a self-limited phenomenon that usually disappears within four to six months. Occasionally it persists longer; in Nydick's large series of cases it persisted for as long as two years in 27 per cent and for three years in 7.7 per cent. Parents should be reassured that this is a normal physiologic phenomenon and that no treatment is required. Surgeons should not succumb to the temptation to operate upon this lesion.

In rare instances puberal hypertrophy progresses in one breast to a stage where the organ resembles, on a small scale, its female counterpart, and the expected regression does not occur. Surgical excision is then justified and should be done through a circumareolar incision in order to avoid a visible scar. The following case illustrates this condition.

M.K., aged 18, came to the Presbyterian Hospital complaining of enlargement of the right breast. The enlargement had developed four years previously, at the age of 14, and had persisted without undergoing any change. On examination the right breast resembled a small adolescent female breast with a well-defined areola and nipple (Fig. 3–7). The left breast was normal. In all other respects the boy was normal. His external genitalia were well developed, and he had more chest hair than most males.

On June 17, 1950, Dr. Jerome Webster, whose patient he was, excised the breast. Microscopic study showed the breast to consist for the most part of a dense fibrous stroma. The only epithelial elements were scattered ducts without accom-

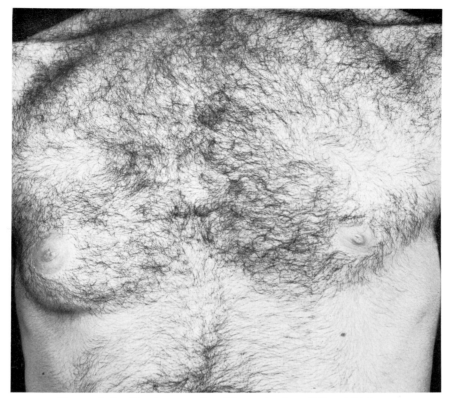

Figure 3–7. Persistent puberal hypertrophy of the right breast.

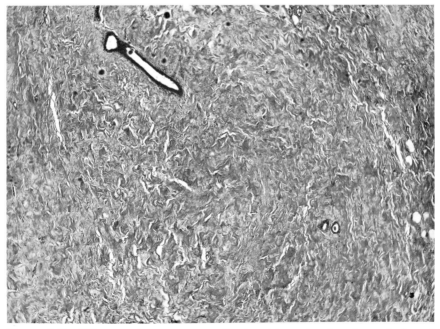

Figure 3–8. Microscopic appearance of puberal hypertrophy of a male breast.

panying acini (Fig. 3–8). This is the characteristic picture of puberal hypertrophy.

Senescent Hypertrophy

Older men, usually between the ages of 50 and 70, occasionally develop hypertrophy of the breasts which is similar to that occurring in boys at adolescence. The hypertrophy, which is not infrequently unilateral at first, with the opposite breast being affected later on or to a lesser degree, takes the form of a tender discoid tumor beneath the areola. It is usually from 2 to 4 cm. in diameter.

Microscopically this senescent hypertrophy resembles the puberal hypertrophy of youth. The bulk of the lesion is made up of fat and fibrous stroma. Scattered ducts, without acini, are seen.

This lesion, because it occurs in the cancer age, has to be differentiated from carcinoma. Its tenderness and the bilateral involvement, if present, are, of course, important points in favor of hypertrophy. But, in the great majority of cases, the lesion develops first on one side, or only on one side. The tumor that hypertrophy forms is usually situated centrally beneath the areola, although it may be large enough to extend beyond its border. Its edge is usually well defined and smooth. It is firm but not hard. Carcinoma, on the other hand, is not tender. It is usually eccentric to the nipple. Its edge is irregular, and not very well defined. It is hard, and it is usually fixed either to the underlying fascial plane or to the skin; and there may be nipple retraction. Senescent hypertrophy is much more common than carcinoma. But this differential diagnosis requires clinical experience. If doubt remains as to the nature of the lesion, biopsy should be done.

The senescent type of mammary hypertrophy usually regresses spontaneously within six to 12 months. If the diagnosis is reasonably certain, no treatment is required other than observation at monthly intervals until the hypertrophy regresses.

This transitory mammary hypertrophy of older men must be regarded as a kind of physiologic aberration, not associated with any recognizable endocrine abnormality. Nathanson (1947), in excretion studies of these patients, found the 17-ketosteroids and the gonadotrophic titer at normal levels for older males.

I suspect that there may be some associ-ation between senescent hypertrophy and carcinoma of the male breast, but carcinoma is so infrequent that I can not provide any statistical support for this thesis. I recall two striking cases. One was that of a man from a family with a high incidence of breast carcinoma. One of his grandfathers, and his own mother and one of her sisters, had the disease. In his own generation there were eight children, two of whom died in youth. Three of his four sisters, and his only living brother, had had it. At the age of 45 he developed characteristic unilateral mammary hypertrophy, which regressed spontaneously after six months. Ten years later he had had no further breast disease. The other case was one in which senescent hypertrophy was followed by carcinoma of the breast in the same patient. I first saw him when he was 51, when he came to me with a characteristic senescent hypertrophy of the right breast. He had noted the tenderness and enlargement six weeks previously. I reassured him, asking him to return if the hypertrophy had not disappeared in six months. He next consulted me seven years later, stating that although the breast enlargement had regressed after a few months, a small nodule situated to the outer side of the areola had remained. Examination showed that the hypertrophy had indeed disappeared. But in the radius of 9 o'clock beneath the areola, there was a firm 3 mm. nodule. There was no axillary adenopathy. I was puzzled by this finding, and I made the mistake of not performing biopsy. Instead I asked him to return for re-examination in three months. He did not return until 14 months later, when I found to my distress that the innocent-appearing nodule had grown to be a typical 5 cm. carcinoma, and that he had a 4 cm. clinically involved axillary node. He eventually succumbed to his carcinoma. This sequence of events strongly suggests that this carcinoma originated from senescent hypertrophy.

Hypertrophy Associated with Developmental Abnormalities of the Genitourinary Tract

Gynecomastia occurs with a variety of different types of developmental abnormality of the testes, with cryptorchism, and with hypospadias. Tillinger's study of testicular morphology was one of the earliest and most extensive. In addition to testicular biopsy there are now other methods of studying these cases, including the determination of urinary gonadotrophin and urinary steroids as well as study of the sex chromatin pattern in buccal epithelium, which are making it possible to classify them more accurately. From the general group of patients with hypogonadism several special syndromes have been identified.

Klinefelter's syndrome, described in 1942 by Klinefelter, Reifenstein, and Albright, is characterized by small testes which show atrophy and hyalinization of the seminiferous tubules, and aspermatogenesis. There is an XXY buccal epithelium chromatin pattern. Urinary pituitary gonadotrophin is increased, but 17-ketosteroids are approximately normal. Hypospadias is not present.

Reifenstein's syndrome, which he described in 1947, is a somewhat different form of hypogonadism, which is familial. The testicular atrophy is not as complete as in Klinefelter's syndrome, and the seminiferous

tubules contain both germinal cells and Sertoli cells. Buccal smears show a normal XY chromatin pattern. Hypospadias is always present.

Rosewater, Gwinup, and Hamwi have described another familial syndrome in which hypogonadism is associated with gynecomastia and a normal XY buccal epithelium chromatin pattern. But urinary pituitary gonadotrophin is low or absent, and there is no hypospadias.

The two following case reports of gynecomastia associated with genitourinary abnormalities from the records of the Presbyterian Hospital illustrate the degree of breast hypertrophy encountered in these cases, although data that would make it possible to classify them accurately are not available.

CASE 1

W.S. came to the Presbyterian Hospital at the age of 33 because of hypertrophy of the breasts.

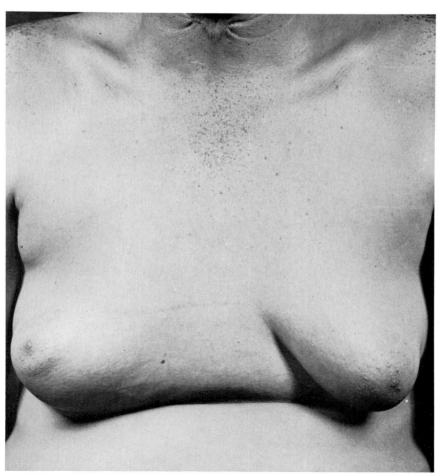

Figure 3–9. Hypertrophy of male breasts associated with eunuchism.

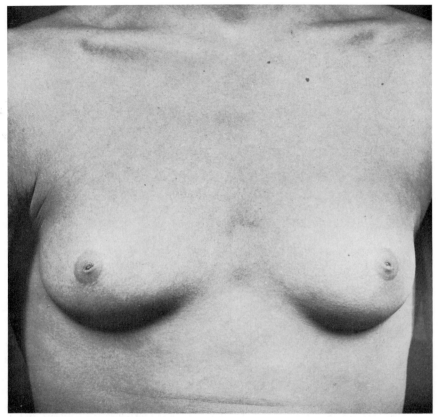

Figure 3–10.   Hypertrophy of male breasts occurring with hypospadias.

This had first been noted when he was 13 years of age, and had gradually increased during subsequent years. On admission he presented the typical picture of eunuchism. He weighed 260 lbs. His penis measured only 3 cm. in length, and no testes were palpable. The breasts were markedly enlarged, particularly the right one which was at least the size of a normal adult female breast. The left breast was about half as large. Both had well-developed areolae and nipples (Fig. 3–9).

On March 30, 1943, Dr. Jerome Webster, whose patient he was, performed bilateral mastectomy through circumareolar incisions. Microscopic study showed that the hypertrophic breast consisted largely of fat and fibrous tissue. No gland fields were seen, and there were only a few scattered ducts.

CASE 2

C.F., aged 12 years, came to the Presbyterian Hospital for the repair of a complete hypospadias, with which he had been born. The external genitalia were otherwise normal. The hypospadias was repaired in stages and was completed at the age of 15. At the age of 13 his breasts began to enlarge. They were not tender. The enlargement continued until at the age of 16 they resembled the breasts of a female of similar age (Fig. 3–10). They were quite symmetrical. The areolae and nipples were well developed.

When the boy was 17, Dr. Jerome Webster, whose patient he was, performed bilateral mastectomy through a semicircular intra-areolar incision. Microscopic study (Fig. 3–11) showed proliferation of ducts, with slight papillary heaping up of the lining epithelium in some. No acini were seen. The bulk of the hypertrophic tissue was fibrous stroma.

Idiopathic Hypertrophy

In contrast to these cases of hypertrophy of the male breast associated with developmental abnormalities of the genital tract, there are other cases in which hypertrophy develops at an early age and persists, without any evidence of associated abnormality of the genital tract, or organic disease elsewhere. The following case illustrates this type of lesion.

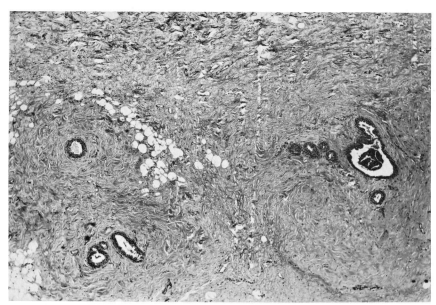

Figure 3-11. Microscopic appearance of hypertrophy of male breasts occurring with hypospadias.

R.R., aged 8, was brought to the Presbyterian Hospital because of swelling of the left breast. This had first been noted at the age of 6 and a half years and slowly increased over a period of a year and a half. Examination showed the left breast to be uniformly enlarged. It measured 6 by 4 by 3 cm., and resembled the breast of a female at the beginning of adolescence. The areola and nipple were well developed, in keeping with the breast hypertrophy. The right breast was undeveloped, as in a normal preadolescent boy (Fig. 3–12). There were no other signs of endocrine abnormality. The external genitalia were normal.

After following the boy for two years, during

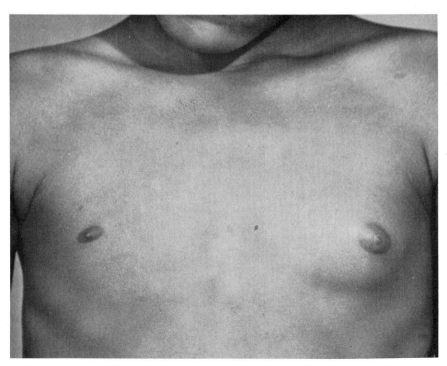

Figure 3-12. Idiopathic hypertrophy of the breast in a boy aged 8 years.

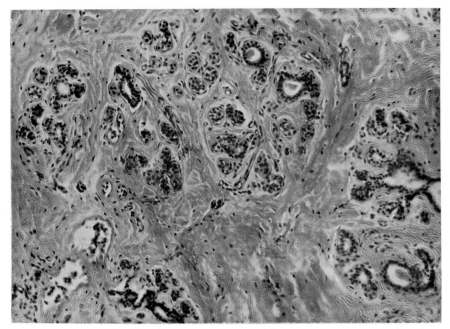

Figure 3–13.   Microsopic appearance of idiopathic hypertrophy of the breast in a boy aged 8.

which regression of the hypertrophied breast did not occur, Dr. Jerome Webster, whose patient he was, excised the left breast through a circumareolar incision, on August 8, 1951.

The microscopic sections showed extensive growth of acini around terminal ducts, to form small gland fields, giving the picture of active epithelial proliferation (Fig. 3–13). Snoga, Morgan, and Lundberg have described a similar case.

This form of gynecomastia differs from the others that I have described in that the breasts show proliferation of acinar as well as ductal elements. The stimulation to breast growth, whatever its origin, is therefore a complete one, resembling that in the pubescent female.

Hypertrophy Associated With Organic Disease

Hypertrophy of the male breast occurs, more often than is generally appreciated, in association with organic disease elsewhere in the body. Some of these forms of gynecomastia follow:
1. Lesions of the testis
   a. Orchitis due to mumps or leprosy (Rollier and Reboul; Job)
   b. Atrophy due to trauma (Apert and

Decléty) or pressure from varicocele or hydrocele
   c. Testicular neoplasms of all types may be accompanied by gynecomastia. In Treves' series of 525 of these neoplasms the incidence of gynecomastia was 10.3 per cent, and it was usually bilateral. Embryonal carcinoma was the type of neoplasm most commonly associated with gynecomastia in Treves' series of cases. Zondek made the original observation that there is a striking increase in urinary gonadotrophin in some testicular neoplasms. It has been found that other types of tumors of the testis produce estrogen (Twombly; Daly et al.)
2. Carcinoma of the adrenal cortex in the male, although a rare tumor, regularly produces gynecomastia (Wallach; Wilkins; Doerner et al., Stewart et al.; Bacon and Lowrey)
3. Pituitary adenomas have been reported to cause gynecomastia (Moehlig; McCullagh et al.)
4. Hyperthyroidism occasionally produces gynecomastia (Bauer and Goodwin; Berson and Schreiber; Larsson et al.)
5. Lesions of the Liver
   a. Infectious hepatitis has caused gynecomastia (Gilder and Hoagland)

b. Cirrhosis often produces gynecomastia (Lloyd and Williams; Bennett et al.)

c. Gynecomastia has been described as a symptom of hepatoma (Summerskill and Adson).

6. Starvation is a well-known cause of gynecomastia, and is presumed to be the result of liver damage. Weber and other German authors described its occurrence in men of all ages during the post-war years in Germany when severe malnutrition was widespread. Jacobs, as well as Klatskin and his associates, described it among Americans in Japanese prison camps. About 10 per cent of the prisoners developed it. This type of gynecomastia is usually bilateral.

7. Chronic thoracic diseases—such as empyema and tuberculosis—have been reported to produce gynecomastia occasionally. It is seen more frequently in lung cancer where it occurs in association with osteoarthropathy (Thibault; Hardy; Levi-Valensi et al.).

In these several types of disease that pro-duce gynecomastia, the mammary proliferation consists of stroma and ducts. Acini are not seen. The stimulus to breast growth is therefore an incomplete one.

Hypertrophy Induced by Androgen and Estrogen

Both estrogen and androgen given therapeutically will produce hypertrophy of the male breast. It may seem paradoxical that both of these hormones produce a similar effect, but it is a fact.

Breast hypertrophy is regularly seen in men who are given stilbestrol for carcinoma of the prostate. Figure 3–14 shows marked growth of the breasts in such a patient. Similar hypertrophy of the male breasts has been reported in workmen engaged in the manufacture of stilbestrol (Scarff and Smith; Finkler; Fitzsimons).

Moore and his associates were among the first to describe the microscopic character of

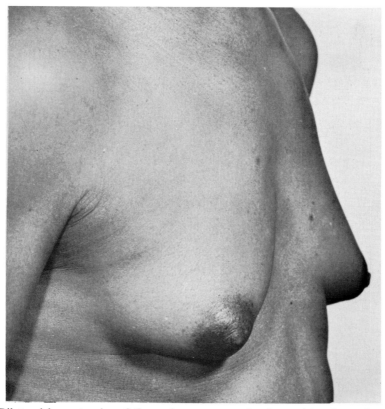

Figure 3–14. Bilateral hypertrophy of the male mammary glands resulting from the administration of 500 mg. of diethylstilbestrol daily for one year for carcinoma of the prostate.

this kind of breast hypertrophy induced by stilbestrol. There is marked increase in the mammary stroma with multiplication of ducts and proliferation of their lining epithelium. Moore, and most of those who have since described these lesions, have emphasized that although there may be some budding of the ducts, fully developed gland fields are not seen. Schwartz and Wilens have recently challenged this impression by reporting that they observed well-developed acini in eight of 25 subjects who had been treated with stilbestrol for prostatic carcinoma.

Hypertrophy Caused by Drugs

Digitalis has been reported to produce gynecomastia occasionally, irrespective of the preparation of digitalis used and the duration of the medication (Le Winn; Bloch; Rodstein). Isoniazid may cause gynecomastia, according to Molina and Aberkane. Spironolactone has recently been identified as the causative agent in some cases of gynecomastia (Mann; Clark).

Nipple Discharge of Physiologic Origin in Males

In males a nipple discharge may be produced by stimulation of the mammary epithelium by neuroendocrine mechanisms, without local disease of the breast.

Androgen, if given long enough and in sufficient dosage to males with breast hypertrophy, will produce a nipple discharge, as in the following case.

M.P., aged 34, came to the Presbyterian Hospital because of sterility. At the age of 4 he had had mumps. At the age of 18 it became apparent that he was undeveloped sexually, and during the following years he was given antuitrin S and testosterone in varying amounts without much change in his eunuchoid physique. He married at the age of 29 but remained sterile.

Examination on admission showed that the patient was still a typical eunuchoid. He was tall, slightly obese, with broad hips, smooth skin, and no facial hair. His pubic hair was scanty and had a female distribution. His testes were descended but small, and his penis normal in size. There was moderate hypertrophy of both breasts, including nipples and areolae.

The patient was given increased amounts of testosterone. Three years later, an occasional drop of bloody discharge was noted from the left nipple for the first time. By the following year a similar brownish discharge appeared from the right nipple. The breasts meanwhile had not changed in character.

Bilateral mastectomy was then carried out through circumareolar incisions. The terminal ducts beneath the nipples were grossly dilated and filled with brownish fluid. Microscopically the breasts showed dilated ducts with some papillary epithelial proliferation of the apocrine type, but no

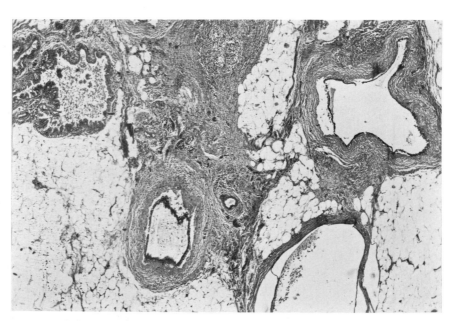

Figure 3–15. Dilated ducts in a hypertrophic male breast following treatment with androgen.

acini (Fig. 3–15). The dilated ducts had thickened walls and showed some periductal lymphocytic infiltration.

Chorioepithelioma of the testis produces colostrum-like secretion from hypertrophied breasts, according to Cooke.

The phenothiazines, reserpine, and methyldopa, will cause nipple discharge in males, just as they do in females. These drugs act upon the breast epithelium through the hypothalamus.

REFERENCES

Andreasen, A. T.: Medullary carcinoma in an axillary breast. Brit. J. Surg., 35:322, 1948.

Andrews, E., and Kampmeier, O. F.: Swellings of the male breast. Surg., Gynec. & Obst., 44:30, 1927.

Apert, E., and Decléty, J.: Gynécomastie unilatérale à la suite traumatisme des bourses. Bull. et mém. Soc. méd. d. hôp. Paris, 42:1091, 1918.

Arner, B., Ekwall, B., and Fürst, E.: Gynaecomastia factitia. Acta med. Scandinav., 168:105, 1960.

Ayd, F. J., Jr.: Thorazine and Serpasil treatment on private neuro-psychiatric patients. Am. J. Psychiat., 113:16, 1956.

Bacon, G. E., and Lowrey, G. H.: Feminizing adrenal tumor in a six-year-old boy. J. Clin. Endocrinol., 25:1403, 1965.

Barnes, A. B.: Diagnosis and treatment of abnormal breast secretions. New England J. Med., 275:1184, 1966.

Bauer, F. K., and Goodwin, W. E.: Acne and gynecomastia following I[131] therapy for hyperthyroidism. J. Clin. Endocrinol., 11:1574, 1951.

Bennett, H. S., Baggenstoss, A. H., and Butt, H. R.: The testis, breast, and prostate of men who die of cirrhosis of the liver. Am. J. Clin. Path., 20:814, 1950.

Berger, R. L., Joison, J., and Braverman, L. E.: Lactation after incision on the thoracic cage. New England J. Med., 274:1493, 1966.

Berson, S. A., and Schreiber, S. S.: Gynecomastia and hyperthyroidism. J. Clin. Endocrinol., 13:1126, 1953.

Blaydes, R. M., and Kinnebrew, C. A.: Massive breast hyperplasia complicating pregnancy. Obst. & Gynec. 12:601, 1958.

Bloch, K.: On the pathogenesis of breast hypertrophy from digitalis therapy. Ztschr. Kreislaufforsch., 50:591, 1961.

Bluestein, D. D., and Wall, G. H.: Persistent neonatal breast hypertrophy. Am. J. Dis. Child., 105:292, 1963.

Bowen, P., et al.: Hereditary male pseudohermaphroditism with hypogonadism, hypospadias, and gynecomastia (Reinfenstein's Syndrome). Ann. Int. Med., 62:252, 1965.

Brown, D. M., Jenness, R., and Ulstrom, R. A.: Study of composition of milk from patient with hypothyroidism and galactorrhea. J. Clin. Endocrinol., 25:1225, 1965.

Burslem, R. W., and Dewhurst, C. J.: Massive hypertrophy of the breasts in pregnancy. J. Obst. & Gynaec. Brit. Emp., 59:380, 1952.

Clark, E.: Spironolactone therapy and gynecomastia. J.A.M.A., 193:163, 1965.

Collett-Solberg, P. R., and Grumbach, M. M.: A simplified procedure for evaluating estrogenic effects and the sex chromatin pattern in exfoliated cells in urine. J. Pediat., 66:883, 1965.

Cooke, J. V.: Chorioepithelioma of testicle. Bull. Johns Hopkins Hosp., 24:215, 1915.

Curtis, E. M.: Oral-contraceptive feminization of a normal male infant. Obst. & Gynec., 23:295, 1964.

Daly, D. W., Dossett, J. A., and Jull, J. W.: An oestrogen-secreting sex-chromatin positive teratoma of the testis associated with gynaecomastia. Brit. J. Surg., 50:816, 1963.

Decourt, J., Jayle, M. F., and Massin, J. P.: Etude de 49 cas de gynécomasties apparemment isolées de l'adolescence. Semaine d. Hôp. Paris, 38:1266, 1962.

Doerner, G., Lisewski, G., and Wendt, F.: Feminisierendes Nebennierenrindenkarzinom. Endokrinologie, 41:297, 1961.

Dresch, C., Arnal, M., and Prader, A.: Premature development of breast: A study of 22 cases. Helv. Paediat. Acta., 15:585, 1960.

Edmondson, H. A., Glass, S. J., and Soll, S. N.: Gynecomastia associated with cirrhosis of the liver, Proc. Soc. Exper. Biol. & Med., 42:97, 1939.

Finkler, R. S.: Toxic effects of estrogens. Correspondence. J.A.M.A., 141:738, 1949.

Fitzsimons, M. P.: Gynaecomastia in stilboestrol workers. Brit. J. Indust. Med., 1:235, 1944.

Gilbert, B.: Persistent lactation. Brit. Med. J., 2:305, 1941.

Gilbert, J. B.: Studies in malignant testis tumors: Syndrome of choriogenic gynecomastia. J. Urol., 44:345, 1940.

Gilder, H., and Hoagland, C. L.: Urinary excretion of estrogens and 17-ketosteroids in young adult males with infectious hepatitis. Proc. Soc. Exp. Biol. & Med., 61:62, 1946.

Gregg, W. I.: Galactorrhea after contraceptive hormones. New England J. Med., 274:1432, 1966.

Grossman, S., Buchberg, A. S., Brecher, E., and Hallinger, L. M.: Idiopathic lactation following thoracoplasty. J. Clin. Endocrinol., 10:729, 1950.

Hamburger, C.: On the nature of gonadotrophin in cases of malignant tumors of the testis. Acta path. et microbiol. Scandinav., 18:457, 1941.

Hardy, J. D.: Gynecomastia associated with lung cancer. J.A.M.A., 173:1462, 1960.

Hertz, J.: Accidental ingestion of estrogens by children. Pediatrics, 21:203, 1958.

Hooper, J. H., Welch, B. C., and Shakelford, R. T.: Abnormal lactation associated with tranquilizing therapy. J.A.M.A., 178:506, 1961.

Hunt, V. C., and Budd, J. W.: Gynecomastia associated with interstitial cell tumor of the testicle. J. Urol., 42:1242, 1939.

Iwai, T.: A statistical study on the polymastia of the Japanese. Lancet, 2:753, 1907.

Jacobs, E. C.: Gynecomastia following severe starvation. Ann. Int. Med., 28:792, 1948.

Job, C. K.: Gynecomastia and leprous orchitis. Internat. J. Leprosy, 29:423, 1961.

Johnson, H. W., Poshyachinda, D., McCormick, G., and Hamblen, E. C.: Lactation with a phenothiazine derivative (Temaril). Am. J. Obst. & Gynec., 80:124, 1960.

Jones, H. W., and Scott, W. W.: Hermaphroditism, Genital Anomalies, and Related Endocrine Disorders. Baltimore, Williams and Wilkins Co., 1958.

Jull, J. W., and Dossett, J. A.: Hormone excretion studies of gynaecomastia of puberty. Brit. Med. J., 2:795, 1964.

Jung, F. T., and Shafton, A. L.: The mammary gland in the normal adolescent male. Proc. Soc. Exper. Biol. & Med., 33:455, 1935.

Karsner, H. T.: Gynecomastia. Am. J. Path., 22:235, 1946.

Keyser, L D.: Massive hypertrophy of the breast. Surg., Gynec. & Obst., 33:607, 1921.

Klatskin, G., Salter, W. T. and Humm, F. D.: Gynecomastia due to malnutrition. I. Clinical studies. Am. J. M. Sc., 213:19, 1947.

Kline, T. S., and Lash, S. R.: Bleeding nipple of pregnancy and post-partum period. Acta Cytologica, 8:336, 1964.

Klinefelter, H. F., Jr., Reifenstein, E. C., Jr. and Albright, F.: Syndrome characterized by gynecomastia, aspermatogenesis without A-leydigism, and increased excretion of follicle-stimulating hormone. J. Clin. Endocrinol., 2:615, 1942.

Krestin, D.: Spontaneous lactation associated with enlargement of the pituitary. Lancet, 1:928, 1932.

Larsson, O., Sundbom, C.-M., and Åstedt, B.: Gynaecomastia and diseases of the thyroid. Acta Endocrinol., 44:133, 1963.

Levin, M. E.: Persistent lactation associated with pituitary tumor and hyperadrenal corticism. Am. J. Med., 27:172, 1959.

Levine, H. J., Bergenstal, D. M., and Thomas, I. B.: Persistent lactation. Am. J. M. Sc., 243:118, 1962.

Levi-Valensi, P., et al.: Les gynécomasties en pratique pneumonologique. Semaine d. Hôp. Paris, 40:2882, 1964.

LeWinn, E. B.: Gynecomastia during digitalis therapy. New England J. Med., 248:316, 1953.

Ljungberg, T.: Hereditary gynaecomastia. Acta med. Scandinav., 168:371, 1960.

Lloyd, C. W., and Williams, R. H.: Endocrine changes associated with Laennec's cirrhosis of the liver. Am. J. Med., 4:315, 1948.

Luchsinger, J.: Pathological breast hypertrophy during pregnancy. Geburtsh. Frauenheilk., 20:1315, 1960.

Mandl, F.: Versuche zur Klarlegung der Lymphverhältnisse bei der Operation des Brustdrüsenkrebs. Wien. klin. Wchnschr., 37:1257, 1924.

Mann, N. M.: Gynecomastia during therapy with Spironolactone. J.A.M.A., 184:778, 1963.

McCullagh, E. P., Alivisatos, J. G., and Schaffenburg, C. A.: Pituitary tumor with gynecomastia and lactation. J. Clin. Endocrinol., 16:397, 1956.

Mead, M.: Sex and Temperament in Three Primitive Societies. New York, William Morrow and Co., 1963, p. 193.

Melikow, M. M.: Classification of tumors of testis. J. Urol., 73:547, 1955.

Mendels, J.: Thioproperazine induces lactation. Am. J. Psychiat., 121:109, 1964.

Moehlig, R. C.: Pituitary tumor associated with gynecomastia. Endocrinology, 13:529, 1929.

Molina, C., and Aberkane, B.: Les gynécomasties des tuberculeux pulmonaires. Semaine d. hôp. Paris, 36:834, 1960.

Moore, G. F., Wattenberg, C. A., and Rose, D. K.: Breast changes due to diethylstibestrol during treatment of prostate gland. J.A.M.A., 127:60, 1945.

Nathanson, I. T.: Studies on the etiology of human breast disease: Urinary excretion of follicle-stimulating hormone, estrogens, and 17-ketosteroids in adolescent mastitis of males. J. Clin. Endocrinol., 2:311, 1942.

Nathanson, I. T.: The Relationship of Hormones to Diseases of the Breast. In Endocrinology of Neoplastic Diseases. New York, Oxford Univ. Press, 1947, p. 156.

Nathanson, I. T., and Aub, J. C.: Excretion of sex hormones in abnormalities of puberty. J. Clin. Endocrinol., 3:321, 1943.

Novak, E.: The constitutional type of female precocious puberty with a report of 9 cases. Am. J. Obst. & Gynec., 47:20, 1944.

Nydick, M., Bustos, J., Dale, J. H., and Rawson, R. W.: Gynecomastia in adolescent boys. J.A.M.A., 178:449, 1961.

Peters, J. H., Sieber, W. K., and Davis, N.: Familial gynecomastia associated with genital abnormalities. J. Clin. Endocrinol., 15:182, 1955.

Pettinger, W. A., Horwitz, D., and Sjoersma, A.: Lactation due to methyldopa. Brit. M. J., 1:1460, 1963.

Rawson, R. W.: Gynecomastia in adolescents. J.A.M.A., 178:500, 1961.

Reifenstein, E. C., Jr.: Hereditary familial hypogonadism. Proc. Am. Federation Clin. Research, 3:86, 1947.

Richardson, K. C.: Contractile tissues in the mammary gland with special reference to myoepithelium in the goat. Proc. Roy. Soc., London, s.B., 136:30, 1949.

Rodstein, M.: Gynecomastia—an unusual manifestation of digitalis toxicity. G.P., 26:95, 1962.

Rollier, R., and Reboul, E.: La gynécomastie lepreuse. Internat. J. Leprosy, 27:221, 1959.

Rosewater, S., Gwinup, G., and Hamwi, S. J.: Familial gynecomastia. Ann. Int. Med., 63:377, 1965.

Rossi, R., Salvini, A., and Scortecci, V.: Il drenaggio linfatico mammario studiato per mezzo dell'oro colloidale radioattivo. Arch. ital. chir., 88:393, 1962.

Russfield, A. B., Reiner, L., and Klaus, H.: Endocrine significance of hypophyseal tumors in man. Am. J. Path., 32:1055, 1956.

Salkin, D., and Davis, E. W.: Lactation following thoracoplasty and pneumonectomy. J. Thoracic Surg., 18:580, 1949.

Scarff, R. W., and Smith, C. P.: Proliferative and other lesions of the male breast with notes on two cases of proliferative mastitis in stilboestrol workers. Brit. J. Surg., 29:393, 1942.

Schachner, S. H.: Galactorrhea subsequent to contraceptive hormones. New England, J. Med., 275:1138, 1966.

Schnurbusch, F.: Untersuchungen über die Morphologie der männlichen Brustdrüse während des Lebensablaufes als Grundlage für ein Studium der Gynäkomastie. Frankfurt. Ztschr. f. Path., 62:402, 1951.

Schwartz, I. S., and Wilens, S. L.: The formation of acinar tissue in gynecomastia. Am. J. Path., 43:797, 1963.

Shuster, S., and Brown, J. B.: Gynaecomastia and urinary oestrogen in patients with generalized skin disease. Lancet, 2:1358, 1962.

Sirtori, C., and Veronesi, U.: Gynecomastia. Cancer, 10:645, 1957.

Snoga, J. R., Morgan, R. L., and Lundberg, G. D.: Idiopathic prepuberal hypertrophy of the male breast. Am. J. Clin. Path., 44:458, 1965.

Starr, P.: Gynecomastia during hyperthyroidism. J.A.M.A., 104:1988, 1935.

Stewart, W. K., Fleming, L. W., and Wotiz, H. W.: The feminizing syndrome in male subjects with adrenocortical neoplasms. Am. J. Med., 37:455, 1964.

Sulman, P. G., and Wennik, H. Z.: Hormonal effect of chlorpromazine. Lancet, 1:161, 1956.

Summerskill, W. H., and Adson, M. A.: Gynecomastia

as a sign of hepatoma. Am. J. Digest. Dis., 7:250, 1962.

Takeya, S.: Ueber die überzähligen Brustwarzen bei Chinesen. J. Orient. Med., 20:32, 1934.

Talbot, N. B., et al.: Excretion of 17-ketosteroids by normal and by abnormal children. Am. J. Dis. Child., 65:364, 1943.

Thibault, P.: Gynécomastie et affections thoraciques. Presse méd., 67:1460, 1959.

Tillinger, K.-G.: Testicular morphology. Acta Endocrinol., 1957, Supp. 30, p. 95.

Treves, N.: Gynecomastia. Cancer, 11:1083, 1958.

Turner, H. H.: A syndrome of infantilism. Congenital webbed neck and cubitus valgus. Endocrinology, 23:566, 1938.

Twombly, G. H.: The Relationship of Hormones to Testicular Tumors. In Endocrinology of Neoplastic Diseases. New York, Oxford Univ. Press, 1947, p. 228.

Vague, J., et al.: Les gynécomasties familiales. Ann. d'endocrinol., 26:129, 1965.

Von Kessel, F., Pickrell, K. L., Huger, W. E., and Matton, G.: Surgical treatment of gynecomastia. An analysis of 275 cases. Ann. Surg., 157:142, 1963.

Wallach, S., Brown, H., Englert, E., Jr., and Eik-nes, K.: Adrenocortical carcinoma with gynecomastia; case report and review of literature. J. Clin. Endocrinol., 17:945, 1957.

Weber, H. W.: Ueber anatomische Befunde bei männlicher Brustdrüsenvergrösserung. Frankfurt. Ztschr. f. Path., 61:547, 1950.

Webster, J. P.: Mastectomy for gynecomastia through a semicircular intra-areolar incision. Ann. Surg., 124:557, 1946.

Wheeler, C. W., Cawley, E. P., Gray, H. T., and Curtis, A. C.: Gynecomastia. A review and analysis of 160 cases. Ann. Int. Med., 40:985, 1954.

White, A. E.: Nonpuerperal lactation. Ann. Int. Med., 52:1264, 1960.

Wilkins, L.: A feminizing adrenal tumor causing gynecomastia in a boy of five years contrasted with a virilizing tumor in a five-year-old girl. J. Clin. Endocrinol., 8:111, 1948.

Williams, M. J.: Gynecomastia. Its incidence, recognition, and host characteristics in 447 autopsy cases. Am. J. Med., 34:103, 1963.

Williams, P. C.: Massive hypertrophy of the breasts and axillary breasts in successive pregnancies. Am. J. Obst. & Gynec., 74:1326, 1957.

Yaffee, H. S.: Nonpuerperal galactorrhea. New England J. Med., 274:1446, 1966.

Zondek, B.: Ueber die Hormone des Hypophysenvorderlappens. Klin. Wchnschr., 9:245, 393, 964, 1207. 1930.

Chapter Four

Women's Role in the Detection of Breast Disease

Until very recently our attempt to control disease in the breast, particularly cancer, has concentrated upon diagnosis and treatment, even though it is obvious that refinements of methods of diagnosis and treatment can make only a limited gain in the control of cancer unless it is detected early in its evolution. Breast carcinoma is usually curable by good surgery when the primary lesion is small and only one or two axillary nodes are involved; but when axillary metastases of considerable extent are present, the rate of cure is greatly diminished; and when distant metastases have developed, no cures at all are obtained. For patients in this last category, improvement in surgical technique offers no hope whatever, because the disease is far beyond the surgeon's reach. It has been recognized too late. It is high time that we turn our attention to the problem of the early detection of breast disease.

In the detection of breast disease, both the patient herself and physicians have a role to play. I wish first to discuss the patient's share in the responsibility for the early detection of her disease, to analyze the reasons for her delay in its recognition and treatment, and to suggest methods of improving her ability to perceive breast disease and to act intelligently in securing medical help.

In the overwhelming majority of cases the initial symptom of breast disease is a tumor, which the patient herself discovers accidentally while bathing or dressing. Easily acces-

sible to palpation and inspection, the breasts offer a better opportunity for self-examination than almost any other organ in the body. The data from my personal series of cases of breast carcinoma presented in Chapter 23, in which I took the case histories myself, show that 85.3 per cent of my patients themselves noted the signs or symptoms of their disease. In only 14.7 per cent was the disease discovered by an examining physician.

Having discovered some symptom of breast disease, it is a tragic fact that women ordinarily wait a long time before consulting a physician. In my personal series of 495 cases of breast carcinoma studied between 1943 and 1955, the average delay was 7.5 months. In my more recent personal series of 938 cases studied between 1956 and 1967, this delay was reduced to an average of 4.9 months. This is an indication that our educational efforts are having some effect; but certainly women still delay far too long in consulting a physician.

My personal series of patients contained about equal proportions of private and ward patients. The private patients included a much higher proportion of individuals with good education and adequate financial means than the usual ward patients. Indeed, many of the ward patients with whom I have dealt in the Columbia-Presbyterian Medical Center have been so underprivileged and worn down by financial and social difficulties, so lacking in any basic education, sometimes even without an adequate knowledge of English, that it has often been impossible to find out with any reasonable accuracy when they first noted some sign of their breast carcinoma. Although I can not provide reliable data regarding the length of delay in our ward patients, I am convinced that it is considerably longer than in my private patients.

REASONS FOR DELAY

If we knew with more accuracy the reasons why women delay so long in seeking medical advice when they discover some sign of breast disease, we might be able to do something about getting them to consult us earlier. From my experience in questioning my patients regarding this delay, I have acquired the impression that the following factors are concerned, and that their importance is somewhat in the order that I discuss them.

1. Economic Factors. The excessive cost of medical care today is, I believe, an important factor in this matter of delay. Neither the voluntary insurance plans nor Medicare and Medicaid meet the entire cost of serious illness. Patients of limited means find that their hospital and doctor bills run into hundreds or thousands of dollars over and above what these systems provide; and when they are threatened with a new illness they delay doing anything about their symptoms.

Many of our patients are so poor that they have no resources beyond their needs for day to day existence; and when they face the threat of breast disease, which may involve hospitalization and surgical fees, they often put off doing anything, because they do not have the money for private care, and they have the illusion that ward patients get inferior care. The rarity of breast carcinoma in the ward services of the large municipal hospitals in our country is striking evidence of this prejudice.

Another important economic explanation for delay concerns the family obligations of a patient who is a mother of young children, or a wife of a handicapped or ill husband. She often sacrifices her own health for the good of her family. I have known many women who have made this kind of sacrifice.

One way of combating delay in the diagnosis and treatment of breast cancer as well as other major diseases would be for voluntary insurance companies, and Medicare as well,

to modify their provision that the patient pay the annual initial medical expense (in the case of Medicare, $50.00). This could be waived whenever consultation revealed a major disease.

2. Lack of Education. Many of our patients with breast cancer who delay a long time have had almost no education and have had only folklore upon which to rely. They naively assume that since they have no pain, and feel in general perfectly well, the breast lump that does not seem to change is innocuous. They so often say, "The lump hasn't bothered me and so I haven't bothered it."

This kind of ignorance is sometimes encountered even among high school and college graduates. As their level of education and sophistication rises, however, most modern women become aware of the threat of breast cancer. Magazine and newspaper articles have called their attention to it, and the disease is frequent enough so that some of their friends have had experiences with it.

Yet it is astonishing how poorly informed the average American woman continues to be regarding the basic facts of breast physiology and disease. Although we live in an age of science, almost nothing has been attempted in the way of including in our educational curricula the basic facts of health and disease that are so often of critical importance in the life of everyone. For example, it would not be at all difficult to include in the high school and college curriculum a basic health course in which cancer, among the other great diseases, would be discussed in a simplified way. The fundamental facts of how cancer develops as a single focus and extends and generalizes, the importance of early diagnosis and treatment, and the success achieved, could all be presented. The student would acquire a basic understanding of what cancer is and what can be done about it.

The University of Oregon requires all its students to take such a basic health course. In speaking to these students recently, I was impressed by their interest, and by the pertinent questions they asked.

One of the basic tasks of an educational program regarding breast cancer is to convince women that the disease is curable. Without any question, one of the most unfortunate reasons why women who suspect that they may have breast cancer delay for so long in doing anything about their symptoms is that they believe that the disease is incurable. Their scepticism is understandable, for many of them have not known anyone who has been cured of cancer. Surveys from Great Britain, Canada, and the United States (Table 4–1) indicate how widespread the disbelief in the curability of cancer is. These data do not suggest that we are making much progress in changing this prejudice.

Sensational journalism has done a good deal to harm women's confidence in the curability of breast cancer. For example, on December 16, 1963, across the top of the front page of the *New York Herald Tribune,* a bold headline announced—"Disturbing News About Breast Cancer," by Earl Ubell, Science Editor:

"There is dreadful news about breast cancer, compensated only by the promise of some progress against this most common single malignancy.

The news is this: a statistical review of all the known methods of surgery for breast cancer raises the ugly possibility that none increases the chances of survival of the female breast cancer victim. They all seem to be equally ineffective—a paradox of modern medicine."

Table 4–1. BELIEF IN THE CURABILITY OF CANCER

Can cancer be cured? (Paterson and Aitkin-Swan Survey, 1954)

Yes { Usually Sometimes Seldom	36 per cent
No, never	50 per cent
Do not know	14 per cent

Can cancer be cured or not? (Canadian Cancer Society Surveys)

	1954	1960
Usually or sometimes	63 per cent	71 per cent
Never	30 per cent	27 per cent
Do not know	7 per cent	2 per cent

Do you think cancer is curable? (American Institute of Public Opinion Surveys)

	1940	1950	1953
Yes	56 per cent	60 per cent	65 per cent
No	27 per cent	23 per cent	20 per cent
Do not know	17 per cent	17 per cent	15 per cent

Chances of recovering from cancer (American Cancer Society Study, Lieberman Research, 1966)

Very good chance	15 per cent
Fairly good chance	50 per cent
Not much chance	20 per cent
No chance at all	3 per cent
Depends, or don't know	12 per cent

It is difficult to believe that Mr. Ubell and the editors of the *Herald Tribune* did not realize that these statements were incorrect. The harm done by this kind of sensational journalism is very great. Our office telephone rang constantly after this article appeared, as anguished patients called, asking for reassurance.

3. Psychological Factors. In addition to economic and educational factors that cause women to delay consulting a physician for symptoms of breast disease, there is a whole series of psychological and emotional factors that may interfere with rational behavior. No one has studied this aspect of delay in disease of the breast as carefully as the late Dr. Mitchell A. Gold. Over a period of several years he interviewed our patients at the Francis Delafield Hospital, studying with keen insight and endless patience the reasons why they delayed seeking medical help. His conclusions are summarized in a paper published in 1964. He classified the chief psychologic reasons for delay as follows:

a. *Fear was a predominant deterrent.* The patients were not only afraid that they had cancer, and of the mutilation of mastectomy, but they feared that their emotional relationships with their husbands would be disturbed.

b. *False modesty and shyness.* Some women had led such sheltered lives that they hesitated to consult a physician regarding their breasts.

c. *Lack of breast tactilism.* Gold found that 47 per cent of the patients whom he studied had never experienced any emotional sensations associated with their breasts. Such women tend to ignore their breasts. They never palpate them, and are therefore not likely to find a breast tumor while it is still small.

d. *Negativism.* Women who grow up in a harsh and hostile environment may become introverted and negativistic, and often delay in seeking medical help until their symptoms are far advanced.

e. *Depression.* Some women, overwhelmed by the trials they have had, become depressed and neglect their health.

f. *Compulsion.* Women may develop a compulsive determination to achieve some goal in life. When symptoms of disease develop, they ignore them.

If we could overcome these financial and educational handicaps, and help women conquer their fear of breast cancer by persuading them that they have a chance of cure, we might substantially reduce the length of the time that women delay in consulting a physician after they discover some sign of breast disease. But this is not enough. We must also provide them with a method of detecting breast disease before it produces obvious signs and symptoms. Self-examination is, I believe, a partial answer to this challenge.

SELF-EXAMINATION

Having convinced women that it is of vital importance to find disease in the breast at an early stage of its evolution, our next duty must be to teach them how to do so. To those who object to women taking an active part in the detection of their own breast disease rather than leaving the problem to physicians, I can only point out that, even if all physicians were ideally trained and able to detect breast carcinoma in its earliest palpable stage, the proportion of breast carcinomas discovered in this way would be relatively small, because only a small proportion of all adult women present themselves for physical examination often enough to assure the diagnosis of breast carcinoma at an early stage. In order to be reasonably certain of detecting breast carcinoma at an early stage, the breast must, I believe, be examined at least every three months. There are not enough physicians, enough time, or enough money to achieve this, even if women could be persuaded of the desirability of consulting physicians this often for physical examination. Recent data collected by the American Institute of Public Opinion have shown that only about one-third of the women questioned in a survey of medical care had consulted a physician within two months. I see no escape from the simple fact that if breast disease is to be detected at an earlier stage in its development, it is the women themselves who must be taught to do it. When at first I realized the desirability of self-examination, I hesitated to recommend it, being doubtful of the ability of women to detect their own breast disease by self-examination, and fearful that the effort to do so would induce cancerphobia. As the years have gone by, my own experience has reassured me on both counts, and I am today firmly convinced that teaching women to examine their own breasts is an important means of improving the control of breast disease.

Breast disease in general indicates its presence by a tumor. In my series of personal cases (1942 to 1967), 1433 of a total of 1669 women with breast carcinoma themselves noted the signs and symptoms of their disease. In 70 per cent the primary symptom was a tumor. Retraction signs, while often present in breast carcinoma, are rarely perceived by the patient herself unless they are very marked. Retraction signs, therefore, are not of much importance in the problem of self-detection of breast disease. Breast disease does not in general produce pain, although physiologic disturbances in the breast often do so. The problem of self-detection of breast disease is therefore centered in the problem of training women to palpate their own breasts and find tumors in them.

Women ordinarily find their own breast tumors accidentally, while dressing or bathing. In passing a hand over the portion of the breast containing the tumor their attention is caught by the change in consistency of the breast tissue. Sometimes the tumor is very small when found. I have known many that were no more than 1 cm. in diameter, yet the woman herself found it. The following is such a case history.

Mrs. X, aged 60, was active in civic affairs, and one day was given a bundle of brochures concerning cancer to distribute to the members of her club. She had had no special interest in cancer, and the task had been thrust on her as a duty that a public-spirited woman ought to assume. As she lay in bed that evening thinking over the day's events, she recalled her promise to distribute the literature, and the fact that she had read none of it herself troubled her conscience. So she picked up one of the leaflets and read that a lump in the breast may be a sign of breast cancer. As she read, she instinctively put her right hand to the upper outer sector of her left breast. She was shocked to feel a very small firm lump. She slept badly and the next morning cancelled her plans for the day and consulted her internist. He confirmed her finding and sent her to me. Her tumor was hard, rather discrete, and measured 10 mm. in diameter. There was a suggestion of dimpling in the overlying skin. There were no palpable axillary lymph nodes. At the operation frozen section confirmed the clinical diagnosis of carcinoma. Radical mastectomy was done. The axillary lymph nodes were not involved. All this was 25 years ago, and she is still well. It is fair to say that this woman saved her own life by finding her carcinoma at this early stage.

If it is possible for women to discover small early carcinomas by fleeting casual palpation of this kind, it is certainly reasonable to expect women to discover tumors earlier if they have been taught to examine their breasts methodically. But neither folklore nor education have given the modern woman any idea of the possibility of purposeful self-examination of the breasts. The following case history illustrates this fact.

Mrs. Y, a woman aged 42, while undressing happened to pass her hand over her right breast and discovered a lump in it. A paternal aunt had had breast carcinoma. She came in for examination the following day. There was a firm, poorly circumscribed tumor 3.5 cm. in diameter in the upper central portion of the breast. It was a carcinoma. Metastases were already present in the internal mammary lymph node chain. She eventually succumbed to the disease. She had discovered it too late.

This tragedy occurred despite the fact that the patient was the daughter of a physician and the wife of a physician, and as such had a better access than most women to medical knowledge. She had had a college education, and following her marriage had taken a prominent part in the Parent Teacher Association work in her community. Nowhere in these experiences had she learned that she could guard against breast cancer by examining her breasts herself.

The great advantage of finding a breast lump while it is still small is apparent from our data of the natural history of breast carcinoma as presented in Chapter 22. Most breast carcinomas are easily palpable when they are a centimeter in diameter. At this stage the likelihood of metastasis is small. The average diameter of breast carcinomas in patients coming to the Presbyterian Hospital, however, has been 5.1 cm., and more than 60 per cent of the patients have had axillary metastases. The chance of cure is closely dependent upon the frequency of axillary metastasis. If we could teach women to find their own breast lumps while they are still small, it would be the greatest advance toward the control of breast carcinoma that has yet been made.

THE TECHNIQUE OF SELF-EXAMINATION

It is of great advantage to a woman in examining her own breasts, just as it is to a physician making such an examination, to use a correct and thorough technique. It seemed to me that self-examination could be taught best by a motion picture film. In 1949 I went to the officials of the National Cancer Institute of the United States Public Health Service and of the American Cancer Society and persuaded them to cooperate in such a teaching film. We made a 16 mm. sound film in color. I planned the script in cooperation with the technical staff of the American Cancer Society, and myself took the part of the examining physician teaching his patient how to examine her breasts. In the film we attempted to convince women that it is possible for them to feel tumors in their own breasts, and to demonstrate a precise technique of how to go about it.

The method of self-examination that I have taught my patients and which I presented in the film is based on my own method of examining the breast. In self-examination the technique is of course simplified.

The first step in self-examination should be careful inspection of the breast before a mirror. Women should be reassured about the inequality in the size of the breasts that many of them have, and which they may discover for the first time when they inspect their breasts carefully. They should look for asymmetry of the contours of the breasts and dimpling of the skin, as well as for flattening, broadening, and retraction of the nipples. They should be taught that any erosion of the nipple surface, no matter how minute, as well as any spontaneous serous or bloody discharge from the nipple (except that occurring during pregnancy) is an indubitable sign of breast disease requiring medical consultation.

The second step in self-examination should be to lie supine on a bed or couch. The arm on the side to be examined first should be raised above the head, and a small pillow, or if that is not available, a folded bath towel, placed under the shoulder (Fig. 4–1). This elevates the shoulder and shifts the breast somewhat medially, so that it is balanced and flattened out in as thin a layer as possible on the chest wall. If the shoulder is not elevated, the breast tends to fall laterally and fold upon itself, making palpation of the lateral half difficult (Fig. 4–2) because of its increased thickness.

In this supine position, palpation of the inner half of the breast is begun with the flat of the fingers of the opposite hand (Fig. 4–3). The palpation must be gentle, because tactile sensitivity is greatest with very gentle palpation. A little talcum power on the fingers of the examining hand makes the fingers glide

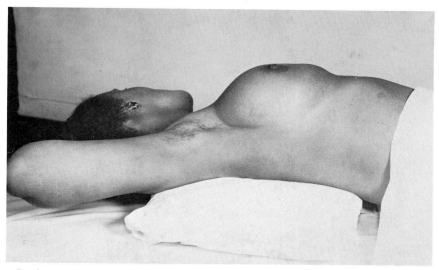

Figure 4–1.   Preferred position for beginning self-examination of the breast. The arm is raised. A pillow placed under the shoulder balances the breast upon the chest wall.

more easily over the skin of the breast and increases tactile sensitivity. The whole extent of the inner half of the breast is explored, the examining hand tracing a series of transverse lines from the nipple line to the sternal edge, beginning just below the clavicle and descending to the inframammary fold (Fig. 4–4). The mammary tissue may reach the clavicle above and the sternum medially as a thin layer, and small breast tumors arising near the breast periphery may seem to be so superficial that they are often mistaken for harmless cutaneous lesions. A dominant tumor anywhere in the breast area must be regarded as evidence of disease.

As a part of their instruction in self-examination women should be told of the existence of the inframammary ridge, and assured that it is not an indication of disease (see Chapter 5, page 110). Women often mistake this ridge for a tumor. Neoplasms do, of course, sometimes develop within it, and stand out as a lump within the ridge.

Having completed her palpation of the inner half of her breast, and of its lower edge, the woman is ready to examine the outer half of her breast. In this step it is preferable to have the arm down at the side; in this position the upper outer sector of the breast is more caudad, and therefore more accessible

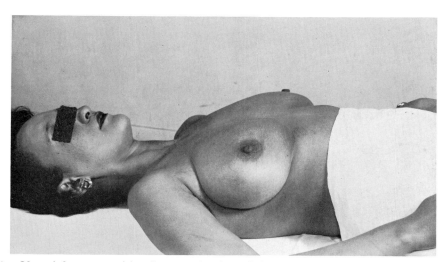

Figure 4–2.   Unsatisfactory position for examination of the breast. When the shoulders are flat on the table, the breasts fall laterally.

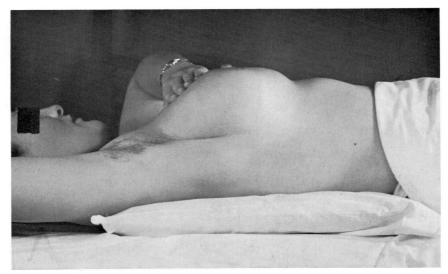

Figure 4–3.   Palpation of the inner half of the breast with the patient's opposite hand.

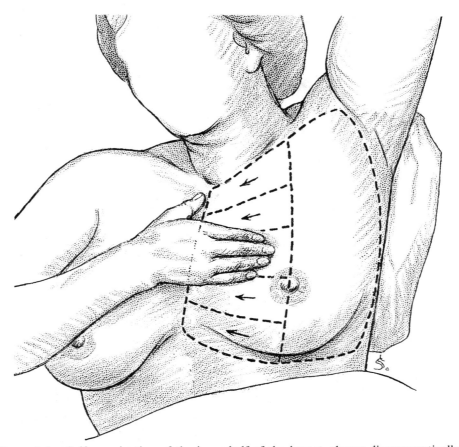

Figure 4–4.   Self-examination of the inner half of the breast, shown diagrammatically.

(Fig. 4–5). The examining hand explores the whole extent of the outer half of the breast, tracing a series of transverse lines from the nipple line outwards to the posterior axillary line, preferably beginning at the inframammary fold and ascending to the axilla (Fig. 4–6). The examination ends in the upper outer sector of the breast, which is the most difficult to examine because it is the thickest part of the breast. This sector, more often than any other part of the breast, shows nodularity that may be classified as within normal limits. It is also the sector in which dominant tumors representing disease are most often found. It is the sector of the breast, therefore, that should receive the greatest attention in any examination.

I believe that women should be discouraged from palpating their breasts while sitting up (Fig. 4–7). If the breast is of average or larger size, palpation is more difficult in the erect position than in the supine position. In the erect position the lower dependent half of the breast is folded upon itself, and a small tumor may be masked by this increased thickness.

When women adhere to the routine of this technique they become familiar with the physical characteristics of their breasts as revealed by repeated palpation with this one preferred method. They are then more likely to identify any small tumor that may develop.

In advising as to the frequency with which self-examination should be carried out, we face the dilemma of not wanting women to examine their breasts so often that they develop cancerphobia, but wanting them to carry out the examination often enough so that they have a reasonable chance of detecting carcinoma while it is yet in an early stage. My clinical experience with carcinoma of the breast has convinced me that the disease progresses more slowly than is generally thought. I believe that it takes at least from six to 12 months for a carcinoma to grow from a diameter of about 1 cm., at which it first becomes easily palpable, to 5.1 cm., the mean diameter of carcinomas in women coming for treatment in the Presbyterian Hospital. The aim with self-examination is, of course, to enable women to discover their breast tumors as soon as possible after they become palpable. We wish to push the moment at which the tumor is discovered backward in time into the six to 12 month period that now elapses between the time a tumor becomes palpable and the time it is actually found. It would be preferable, if it did not produce cancerphobia, to advise that self-examination of the breast be carried out at monthly intervals. In an effort to guard the patients whom I instruct in self-examination against cancerphobia, I appeal to them not to palpate their breasts at any other occasion than the monthly examination and not to think about breast disease except on this one occasion.

For women who have not reached the menopause it is important to choose the correct phase of the menstrual cycle for self-examination of the breasts. In a considerable proportion of women there is enough vascular

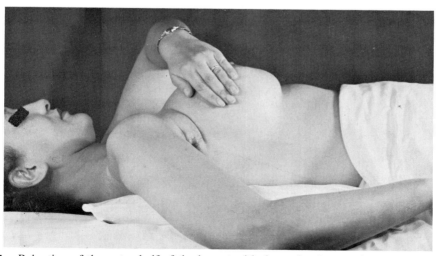

Figure 4–5. Palpation of the outer half of the breast with the patient's opposite hand. The arm is down at the side.

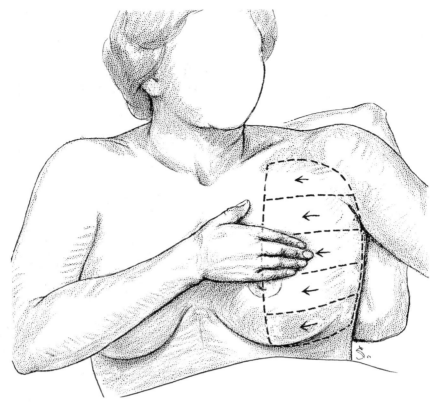

Figure 4–6. Self-examination of the outer half of the breast, shown diagrammatically.

engorgement of the breasts in the premenstrual phase of the cycle to produce slight enlargement and increased turgidity of the breasts, and some tenderness. In a smaller number of women the engorgement is sufficiently pronounced to produce a degree of nodular thickening that may deceive the examiner into thinking actual tumors are present. It is desirable to carry out self-examination at the time when these transitory physiologic changes are at a minimum, namely, in the immediate postmenstrual phase of the cycle.

The question of what age is the right one to introduce the subject of self-examination is a debatable one. It is ridiculous to attempt to teach it to girls in their teens. It is doubtful that even young women in their final college years are mature enough for this discipline. It seems reasonable to begin instruction when women are in their early 30's. This is the age at which breast carcinoma first begins to have a considerable frequency, and it is the earliest age, in my opinion, at which women are willing to give thought and attention to such a serious subject as the detection of breast carcinoma. At this age they have founded their own families, and the responsibility of parenthood has sobered them and lengthened the shadow of fate before them.

The concept of self-examination of the breast is so new that very few data are available as to what success there has been in teaching it. Gowen and his associates have reported that a follow-up study of 470 women 18 months after they had been taught my technique of self-examination revealed that 79 per cent of the 129 women who replied to the inquiry were practicing the method, and that as a result one had found a breast carcinoma, and eight had found benign tumors.

I know from my personal effort in teaching women to examine their own breasts that tumors, both benign and malignant, may, indeed, be found as a result of such teaching. Not all of the tumors thus discovered have been small, but some of those which proved to be malignant have not only been small but had not metastasized. The following is a case history.

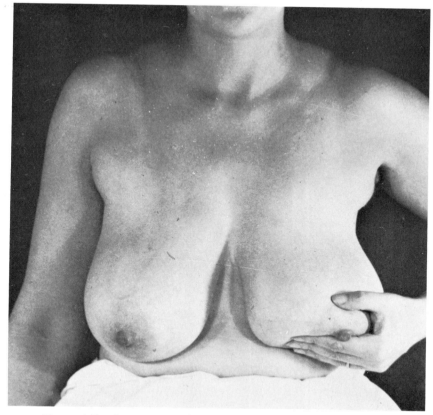

Figure 4–7. Improper method for self-examination of the breast.

Mrs. Z., aged 42, a physician's daughter, attended a showing of the film "Breast Self-Examination." That evening she examined her breasts according to the technique illustrated in the film, and found a tumor in the upper outer sector of the left breast. She came at once for consultation. The tumor was firm, poorly circumscribed, measured 2 cm. in diameter, and gave a definite retraction sign in the overlying skin on forward bending. Radical mastectomy was done. Fifty-four axillary lymph nodes were found, none of which contained metastases.

My own experience has convinced me that women can become comparatively expert at palpating tumors in their own breasts. They have advantages that an examining physician cannot possess. In the first place a women palpating her own breasts is concerned with the findings in two breasts only. As she examines them repeatedly she becomes thoroughly familiar with their special characteristics. An examining physician has to attempt to recall the comparative findings in a great many breasts, a difficult feat no matter how detailed his written records may be. A woman examining her own breasts has a sec-

ond important advantage: it is the proprioceptive tactile sense that helps her in palpating her own tissues.

To further emphasize that women may become expert at self-examination of their breasts, I must point out that in several instances women have come to me with small breast tumors which they discovered but which I was unable to find in my first palpation. As a result of such experiences I have learned, in all humility, to ask patients in whom I have not found a tumor whether or not they feel one, and if they do to show me its location.

Teaching women to examine their own breasts will, beyond question, produce cancerphobia in some women and do them more harm than good. There are some women so unstable mentally that fear of cancer, often focused by family tragedy due to the disease, makes any rational consideration of it impossible. Some cannot palpate their breasts at all without becoming terrified. Others palpate them daily and constantly torment themselves with thought of the disease. Physicians should therefore take care to teach self-examination only to those of their patients whom they know well enough to be certain that they will be able to think about the problem with the necessary degree of detachment. When the concept of breast self-examination is presented to women at large by means of the film, however, there can be no selection of subjects and some harm will certainly result.

The film "Breast Self-Examination" has now been shown to some millions of women but it is difficult to draw any conclusions concerning what effect it has had, if any, upon the early diagnosis of breast disease. Lewison reported that among 2358 women interviewed six months after they had seen the film, 80 per cent stated that they examined their breasts occasionally in the manner taught in the film, while 33 per cent examined them monthly.

In the last analysis the value of the concept of self-examination of the breasts will be determined only by teaching it widely over a long period of time and with the best modern educational techniques. Before this is done the idea should have the approval of physicians, for the public should and does look to physicians for judgment concerning a basic health concept of this kind. If physicians will but test out the concept of teaching self-examination of the breasts to their own patients, I am confident that they will eventually give the idea their approval. Some physicians will be tempted to condemn self-examination as a poor substitute for examination by a physician. They should face the fact that there are few women who can go to a physician for physical examination often enough to hope to have breast carcinoma discovered at an early and curable stage. To be reasonably safe a woman should be examined at least every three months. Self-examination is the only possible method of achieving this. It is a means of protection available to every women, no matter how remote she may be from her physician. It costs nothing.

Physicians must also face the fact that the practice of self-examination will add to their difficulties in the differential diagnosis of lesions of the breast. When women examine their own breasts they find a remarkable variety of tumors and tumor-like formations. Most of these are the nodular thickening due to physiologic changes in the breast and require no treatment, but some are small tumors due to disease that must be recognized as such and their pathological nature proved.

REFERENCES

Gold, M. A.: Causes of patients' delay in diseases of the breast. Cancer, 17:564, 1964.

Gowen, G. H., Hittle, E., Roe, N., and Crawford, I.: Is teaching breast self-examination for cancer effective? Illinois M. J., 102:179, 1952.

Haagensen, C. D.: Self-examination of the breasts. J.A.M.A., 149:356, 1952.

Hammerschlag, C. A., Fischer, S., DeCosse, J., and Kaplan, E.: Breast symptoms and patient delay: Psychological variables involved. Cancer, 17:1480, 1964.

Kaiser, R. F.: Experience with a special purpose program: breast self-examination for the detection of early cancer. Internat. Union against Cancer, 14:676, 1958.

Kelley, J. L., and Thieme, E. T.: Impact of public education about cancer on detection and treatment of cancer of the breast by surgery. Cancer, 20:260, 1967.

Lewison, E. F., et al.: Breast self-examination; educational and clinical effectiveness of the film. Maryland M. J., 3:123, 1954.

Lieberman Research, Inc.: A Study of Motivational, Attitudinal, and Environmental Deterrents to the Taking of Physical Examinations that Include Cancer Tests. New York, 1966.

Patterson, R., and Aitkin-Swan, J.: Public opinion on cancer. Lancet, 2:857, 1954.

Phillips, R. J., and Taylor, R. M.: Public opinion on cancer in Canada: A second survey. Canad. M.A.J., 84:142, 1961.

Chapter Five

Physicians' Role in the Detection and Diagnosis of Breast Disease

Physicians have the opportunity to look for disease every time they perform a physical examination in patients who consult them. Some members of the profession take a more active role and promote cancer detection clinics designed to find unsuspected cancers by periodic examination of apparently well individuals.

CANCER DETECTION CLINICS

The concept of the Cancer Detection Clinic originated about 25 years ago, and a number of such clinics were organized in larger cities in this country. Enough time has gone by to review their achievements critically. The final test of their value must, of course, be the number of unsuspected cancers that have been found in these clinics. The data so far available on this point as regards breast disease are not very impressive, although breast disease is certainly one of the types of disease most easily discovered by simple physical examination. Phillips and Miller report that among 7767 women examined once at the Cancer Prevention Center of Chicago between 1949 and 1951, a definite breast tumor was found in 129 or 1.7 per cent. Thirty-seven of these patients were proved to have benign breast disease, while ten had carcinoma. The incidence of unsuspected breast carcinoma in the series of 7767 patients was therefore 0.13 per cent. Axillary

metastases were found in only two of the ten patients with carcinoma—a strikingly low incidence. Walter and Atkinson found one carcinoma of the breast among 422 English women who volunteered to undergo an examination. Because it is a long-term study of the incidence of breast disease in symptomless women, the report by Macfarlane and her associates is the most important contribution to the subject that has yet appeared. In a group of 537 volunteer women without symptoms referable to the breast, a total of 11,203 semiannual breast examinations were made during the 11 year period—1942 to 1952. In the course of these examinations 11 breast carcinomas were found. But in every case the volunteer had found the carcinoma in her own breast before routine examination. It may perhaps be said that these 11 women found their carcinomas because their experience in having their breasts examined semiannually by a physician had taught them how to find breast tumors in their own breasts.

Several of the larger cancer detection clinics have reported their experience as regards breast cancer. From the Strang Cancer Prevention Clinic, Emerson Day reports that among 25,629 women, upon whom a total of 43,411 examinations were done during a three year period (1954 to 1956), 31 asymptomatic breast carcinomas were found. This amounts to one breast carcinoma for every 821 women. From the Cancer Detection

Center of the University of Minnesota, Gilbertsen reports that in a total of 6765 women at least 45 years of age and free of symptoms suggestive of cancer, 47 breast carcinomas were discovered at annual examinations conducted between 1948 and 1966. At operation only 19 per cent of these 47 women were found to have axillary metastases. During this same period of time, 19 of the 6765 women undergoing annual physical examination themselves discovered breast cancer as a result of self-examination. Gilbertsen's data must be viewed in terms of the expected attack rate for breast carcinoma in his 6765 patients over the period of time he followed them. He does not present such data.

From a practical point of view the number of breast carcinomas discovered each year in cancer detection clinics out of the total of approximately 70,000 new breast cancers diagnosed each year in our country remains very small. Further development of the cancer detection clinic concept faces several objections. The first and most important of these is that it is very doubtful that it is desirable, from the viewpoint of good medical practice, to establish special clinics for detecting only cancer, rather than all disease. Periodic medical check-ups, aiming at the detection of disease of all types, are certainly desirable. This concept is indeed a basic principle of modern medicine. Such periodic check-ups to find new disease should, of course, be carried on in every physician's office. I do not believe that the methods required to detect disease of the breast can be carried out any better in a cancer detection clinic than in the office of a well-trained modern physician.

A serious handicap of cancer detection clinics is the difficulty in staffing them with experienced examiners. The work is usually done by young physicians without much clinical experience, who are paid on a part-time basis.

METHODS OF DETECTION AND DIAGNOSIS OF BREAST DISEASE

Although the breasts are accessible organs situated on the surface of the body, and their examination is relatively easy, it must be admitted that physicians do not always take advantage of the opportunity they have to search for unsuspected breast disease every time that they carry out a regular physical examination. One might take it for granted that the breasts will certainly be examined as part of such an examination, but unfortunately this is by no means the case. A survey conducted in 1950 by the American Institute of Public Opinion revealed that when women went to physicians and asked specifically for a complete physical examination, in 30 per cent of the patients the breasts were not examined.

A more excusable kind of failure to examine the breasts is that which occurs in the routine care of patients being treated for other disease. This kind of oversight can be avoided by making it a rule to do a general physical examination upon all old patients every six months.

The methods that are useful in the detection and differential diagnosis of breast disease are relatively simple, and in the present chapter I shall describe the ones that I have come to rely upon.

The Medical History

A carefully taken medical history is as important in breast disease as in any other disease. The majority of patients who come for consultation regarding their breasts believe that they have discovered breast disease. A few are simply frightened because some friend or relative has developed breast cancer and their imagination has got out of hand. Careful questioning makes it possible to begin to sort out those who probably have no breast disease from those who may well have it. Chart 5–1 shows the relative frequency of the common breast conditions for which patients have consulted me. The largest group is made up of women with excessive and irregular engorgement of the breasts producing pain and tenderness, and increased nodularity and density. The relationship of these phenomena to the patient's menstrual cycle will at once become apparent on questioning.

Symptoms. In my history-taking I try to define the patient's initial breast symptom, when it was first noted, how it happened to be discovered, and how it evolved. I always ask how long the patient delayed before consulting a physician after she noted her first sign or symptom, and why she delayed. I inquire about secondary symptoms. I usually discuss symptoms in the following sequence.

TUMOR. The great majority of patients

BREAST CONDITIONS DURING LIFETIME—1000 ADULT WOMEN

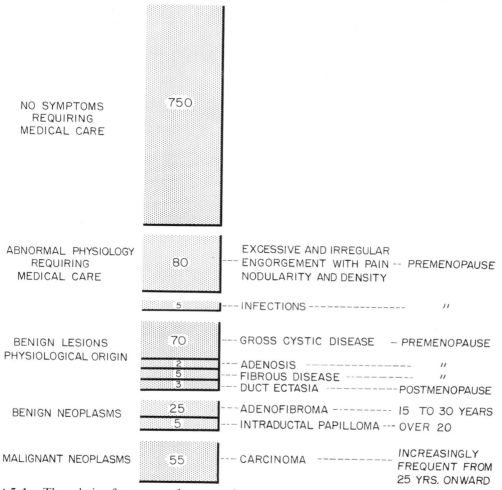

Chart 5–1. The relative frequency of common breast conditions for which patients have consulted me.

believe that they have a breast tumor, because they have found a "lump," a "thickening," or a "hardening" accidentally while dressing or bathing, or by self-examination. A minority have been told by a physician that they have a tumor and are convinced that they must have one even when they cannot feel it themselves. I always ask a patient who says she has a tumor whether or not it has changed since she first discovered it, and if it changes during her menstrual cycle. If she states that it is present only during the premenstrual and menstrual phases of her cycle it is likely that she has nothing more than increased physiological nodularity.

RETRACTION PHENOMENA. Women occasionally notice nipple retraction, but they regularly fail to see skin retraction and distortion of the contour of the breast even when it is pronounced. They are apt to exaggerate changes in the size of a breast.

PAIN. Cyclical pain and tenderness, usually affecting both breasts but more pronounced in one, are among the most frequent complaints. Even the most intelligent women often fail to realize that the cyclical character of these phenomena suggests that they are of physiologic rather than pathologic origin. Some unstable women magnify physiological discomfort to the point where they have to be reassured periodically. In a few women pain of physiologic origin is, apparently, so severe that it is a major handicap.

In addition to inquiring as to the relationship of pain to the menstrual cycle, if the patient is still menstruating, I try to define whether the pain is dull or sharp, constant or intermittent. Most cysts, as well as the benign neoplasms, are painless. Cysts that evolve rapidly to a considerable size, however, may be acutely painful and tender. Breast carcinomas, on the other hand, are usually painless, although in a few patients carcinoma produces occasional twinges of pain. Both River and Corry studied the frequency of pain in various lesions in the breast. My own impression is that, with the exceptions that I have mentioned, pain and tenderness are so inconstant that they play little part in the differential diagnosis of diseases of the breast.

NIPPLE DISCHARGE. Discharge from the nipple is not a frequent symptom. It occurs in only about 3 per cent of the patients with breast symptoms who consult me. Nipple discharge may be physiologic and harmless, or pathologic and an indication of inflammation or epithelial proliferation. Nipple discharge of pathologic significance escapes spontaneously from the nipple. Discharge that has to be elicited is usually not of pathologic significance. In many women of middle age, squeezing the nipple and subareolar area will produce a drop of thick grayish material from the nipple. If they discover this phenomenon they should be reassured and told that it is normal. It comes from terminal ectatic ducts. The examining physician has no need to attempt to express material from the nipple, and should not do so.

The character of a nipple discharge is an important distinguishing feature. There are two more common types of discharge — serous discharge and bloody discharge. Less frequently, nipple discharge may be thin and watery, thick and yellowish, grayish, greenish resembling pus, or milky.

A discharge that has the consistency and color of milk is usually just that. Occasionally women continue to secrete a small amount of milk for months, and in rare cases for years, after lactation would normally have ceased, as I have described in Chapter 3.

A *serous discharge* is thin, translucent, and faintly yellowish. It dries as a yellow stain upon the patient's brassiere or nightgown. Women who have taken oral contraceptives for a long time occasionally develop a slight bilateral serous discharge. In the great

majority of cases, however, a serous nipple discharge is due to an intraductal papilloma growing in one of the larger ducts in the subareolar region. Although the minute papillary processes of an intraductal papilloma are covered with epithelium, serum escapes from them, perhaps because they are easily traumatized. In a few instances a serous discharge occurs with carcinoma.

The presence of a sufficient number of red blood cells to color a discharge brown or red necessitates classifying it as a *bloody discharge*. This type of discharge is usually brownish in color. Sometimes it resembles frank blood. The bloody nature of the discharge has, however, no special significance; like a serous discharge, it is usually an indication of intraductal epithelial proliferation. In the majority of cases this epithelial proliferation is benign. It may be the papillary proliferation that is one of the components of cystic disease; it may be the papillary proliferation accompanying duct dilatation resulting from abnormal or excessive stimulation by hormonal therapy; but it is usually due to intraductal papilloma. In occasional patients with mammary duct ectasia a brownish or blood-tinged nipple discharge occurs. As I have pointed out in Chapter 3, there is sometimes a bloody discharge from the markedly engorged breasts of women in the last months of pregnancy. In rare instances a bloody nipple discharge accompanies the onset of menstruation in young women whose breasts are growing actively. Occasionally, a bloody discharge is due to malignant intraductal epithelial proliferation, as with intraductal papillary carcinoma.

Another type of nipple discharge is thin and watery, without any color. Lewison and Chambers present data suggesting that it signifies carcinoma. I agree with this interpretation, although I must point out that this type of nipple discharge is infrequent.

There is a surprising divergence in the reported frequency of nipple discharge in the various lesions occurring in the breasts. For example, Copeland and Higgins reported that 37 per cent of a series of 67 patients with nipple discharge had carcinoma, and McLaughlin and Coe found carcinoma in 25 per cent of a series of 46 patients with nipple discharge. On the other hand, Mercier and Redon reported finding carcinoma in only 11.6 per cent of a series of 120 patients with nipple discharge, and McPherson and MacKenzie found only 12.5 per cent of carcinomas in their series of 72 patients with a nipple discharge. Tailhefer and Pilleron operated upon 130 patients with a bloody nipple discharge but no palpable tumor, and found carcinoma in only two.

In studies of this kind the patients with induced nipple discharge should be excluded because this phenomenon does not represent disease. It is desirable to also exclude patients with prolonged and abnormal lactation, which is a physiologic aberration, as well as those in whom a discharge is produced by the use of oral contraceptives. The patients with erosion of the nipple surface due to Paget's disease should also be excluded, because the leakage of blood and serum from such erosions is not a true discharge from nipple ducts. In Table 5-1, which presents my experience with nipple discharge in 157 patients with this symptom consulting me between 1956 and 1967, such patients have been excluded.

My own experience as to the significance of spontaneous nipple discharge has therefore been very much like that of Mercier and Redon, and McPherson and MacKenzie. It is an important clinical sign, and except when it occurs during pregnancy, during menstruation in the growing breast, or in women taking oral contraceptives, it must not be ignored. If an accompanying tumor, or a pressure point producing the discharge, is not found at the initial examination, the patient must be carefully followed and re-examined until the probable site of the lesion in the breast is defined, and it is explored surgically and its nature proved.

Carcinoma is the cause of a nipple discharge in only a comparatively small percentage of the patients who have it. Whether the discharge is serous or bloody is not of diagnostic significance.

Past History of Breast Disease. An important part of the patient's history is, of course, inquiry about previous breast disease. The proportion of women who have had an earlier breast operation, or aspiration of a breast tumor, will be found to be surprisingly large. They usually are entirely ignorant as to the precise nature of the earlier lesion, unless it was carcinoma. I have learned not to accept the patient's version of her previous lesion, or indeed any pathological report of its nature. I insist upon obtaining the original microscopic sections and studying them myself. In this way I have occasionally uncovered errors in diagnosis that were of crucial importance in determining the status of the patient's breasts at the time she consulted me. It is not uncommon to find that the sections of the tissue removed at an earlier operation show only normal breast tissue.

Reproductive History. Since breast disease is closely related to the patient's reproductive history these data should be recorded. Included should be the age at onset of menses, their frequency, duration, and regularity, the marital state, age at first marriage, age at each pregnancy as well as its termination as an abortion or a viable birth, age of onset of menopause, and the facts regarding earlier gynecological procedures.

Hormones are so commonly administered today, in the form of oral contraceptives, for menstrual irregularity, or for the relief of menopausal symptoms, that it is important to inquire carefully regarding them. Such therapy often has definite effects upon the breasts. Many women are reluctant to admit that they have taken hormones. Many use face creams containing estrogen without being aware that the creams contain the hormone.

The patient's lactation history is, of course,

Table 5-1.   BREAST CONDITIONS PRODUCING SPONTANEOUS NIPPLE DISCHARGE
(Personal Series of Cases, 1956–1967)

| Condition | Type of Nipple Discharge | | | Total Number of Patients | Per Cent of Total Number of Patients |
	Serous	Bloody	Watery		
Pregnancy	—	10	—	10	6 per cent
Menstruation	—	1	—	1	—
Cystic Disease	3	—	—	3	—
Duct ectasia	3	2	—	5	3 per cent
Intraductal papilloma	53	55	—	108	69 per cent
Accessory subareolar gland papilloma	3	—	—	3	—
Papilloma of nipple ducts	9	—	—	9	5.8 per cent
Carcinoma of breast	7	10	1	18	11.5 per cent
Total				157	

part of her reproductive history. Whether or not she nursed her children, and how long she breast-fed each one, must be recorded.

From all these data it is possible to estimate the total number of years of menstrual life. I believe that it would be desirable to attempt to do this for every patient, because it is apparent from recent data concerning the etiology of breast cancer which I will discuss in Chapter 21, that the longer a woman's total duration of menstrual life, the greater the likelihood of her developing breast cancer.

I have also made it a practice to inquire whether or not the patient herself was breast-fed, but so few patients are certain about this that I doubt that these data are worth anything.

Family History Regarding Breast Disease. We know that breast carcinoma is a familial disease, and we may eventually discover that other breast diseases are familial. It is therefore of great practical importance to inquire as to the occurrence of breast disease in the patient's relatives, both male and female. If there is a history of breast carcinoma, the age at which it developed should be noted.

The Physical Examination of the Breast

A good deal of the success which a physician has in the differential diagnosis of breast disease depends upon the care that he takes in the examination of the breasts. If he merely passes his hand in a casual fashion over his patient's breasts as she sits erect, ready for an examination of heart and lungs, he will often miss lesions of the breast entirely. This kind of examination cannot give him any idea of the true status of the breasts. An adequate examination of the breasts should be a studied and methodical procedure, requiring several changes in the patient's position, and meticulous palpation of the entire extent of the breasts, which cover most of the anterior chest wall. This takes some time even when no abnormality is found. When the examiner finds something that arouses his suspicion of the presence of disease, still other maneuvers and more time are required.

Supraclavicular and Axillary Regions. The breast examination should be begun with palpation of the supraclavicular and axillary regions. The patient sits on a table facing the examiner, with her legs over the side. The supraclavicular and lower cervical areas are first carefully palpated (Fig. 5–1).

It is important for the examiner to understand that metastases in the so-called sentinel group of supraclavicular nodes, which lie upon the confluence of the internal jugular and subclavian veins hidden deep behind the inner end of the clavicle, are not palpable until they attain a large size. In supraclavicular biopsies metastases are occasionally found when no supraclavicular nodes are palpable. When nodes are palpated in this region they are usually the more laterally and more superficially situated nodes, involved by retrograde permeation from the sentinel nodes. Supraclavicular palpation is therefore useful only for the detection of advanced regional lymph node involvement.

In examining the axilla it is essential that the pectoral muscles be relaxed. To achieve this the examiner supports the patient's arm on one of his own. He palpates the axilla with the tips of the fingers of his other hand (Fig. 5–2). The more gentle his palpation, the better he will feel lymph nodes. Small nodes high in the axilla are difficult or impossible to feel. Nodes lying close behind the thick body of the pectoralis major muscle as it forms the ventral wall of the axillary space are also easily missed. In obese patients axillary palpation is particularly difficult.

Not only the number, but also the consistency and movability of the axillary nodes, should be noted. They may be fixed to the deep axillary structures or to the overlying skin. It is also important to estimate the transverse diameter in centimeters of the largest axillary node or mass of fused nodes.

We of course describe in the patient's unit record the clinical characteristics of all nodes that we palpate in the axilla, no matter how small and soft they may be, but we do not assume that all palpable nodes signify metastasis. A large proportion of women whose work involves sustaining small abrasions or cuts on their fingers or hands, as well as women who bite or pick their finger nails or push back the cuticle too much in manicuring, develop soft palpable axillary nodes up to 5 or 6 mm. in diameter. Such nodes are a sign of low-grade lymphadenitis. McNair and Dudley palpated axillary nodes of this kind in 37 per cent of a series of normal women. In our Columbia Clinical Classification we classify lymph nodes as "not clini-

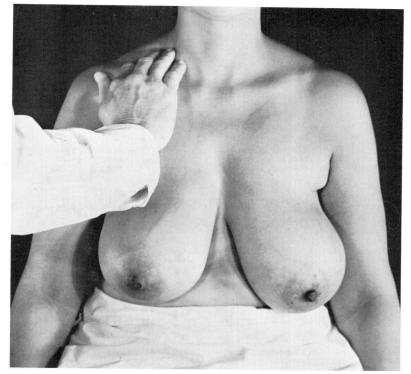

Figure 5–1. Palpation of the supraclavicular and cervical areas.

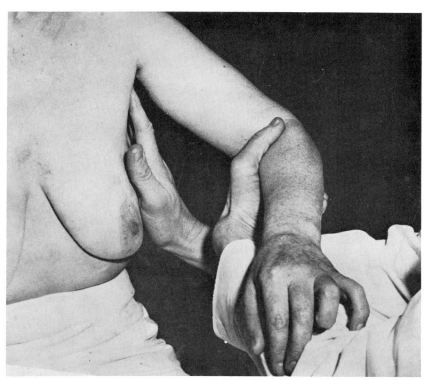

Figure 5–2. Palpation of the axilla.

cally involved" or "clinically involved." The axillae of patients with palpable small soft nodes that we regard as not being involved are classified as Stage A. Clinically involved nodes are, in general, harder and larger.

It is always, of course, essential to palpate both axillae, and to compare the findings in both before classifying nodes which are found in the axilla on the side of the diseased breast.

Occasionally very large axillary nodes may be visible on inspection of the axilla with the arms raised. Figure 5–3 shows such massive axillary metastases.

When the axilla is palpated with care, and in the manner that I have suggested, the findings, as verified by microscopic study of the surgical specimen, are surprisingly accurate. The data regarding the accuracy of clinical examination of the axilla are presented in Chapter 33 in my discussion of the clinical classification of the stage of advancement of breast carcinoma.

Inspection of the Breast. The next step in our routine of breast examination is a critical inspection of the breasts, first with the patient's arms at her sides and then with her arms raised high above her head (Fig. 5–4). The examination must be conducted in a good light if the examiner expects to see early retraction signs and slight changes in contour. The examiner compares the contour of the two breasts, following it from the anterior axillary fold to the midline on each side. An indentation or a bulge in the contour often betrays the site of the lesion.

The shrunken breast of advanced, slowly growing carcinoma, and the generally enlarged edematous breast of acute carcinoma are at once obvious, but slight retraction signs due to earlier lesions are not so evident.

It will occasionally be noted that one breast is slightly larger than the other, yet perfectly symmetrical with its mate. This mere disparity in size is often only a developmental defect and no cause for alarm.

The skin over the breast is carefully inspected for evidence of dilatation of subcutaneous veins, redness, and edema.

DILATED SUBCUTANEOUS VEINS. Rapidly growing neoplasms in the breast, both benign and malignant, induce an increased blood supply to the organ. Cystosarcomas seem to have a special tendency to cause enlargement of the regional veins. In occasional patients with carcinoma the subcutaneous veins over the upper part of the breast may be visibly dilated. Infrared photographs bring out this dilation in a striking manner.

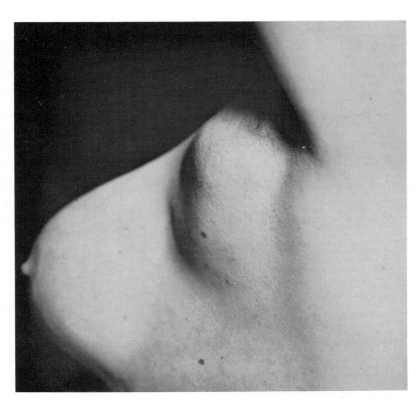

Figure 5–3. Carcinoma metastasis in a massively enlarged axillary lymph node.

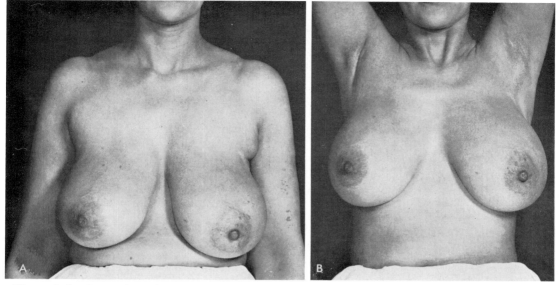

Figure 5–4. Inspection of the breasts (*A*) with the arms at the side and (*B*) with the arms raised.

REDNESS OF THE SKIN. Redness, and elevation of the skin temperature are of course seen with both acute and chronic infectious processes in the breast. These signs also occur, occasionally, with neoplasms.

The most striking example is the extensive redness of the skin in the so-called inflammatory type of carcinoma. I will discuss this disease subsequently in Chapter 31.

Redness of the skin of limited extent also occurs occasionally with the usual type of breast carcinoma, as the result of necrosis or infection within the lesion, or owing to impending ulceration.

With duct ectasia redness of the skin is to be expected when the irritating material within the ducts gets out into the breast stroma and sets up an inflammatory reaction.

Redness of the skin is also seen in rare cases of cystic disease in which a subacute inflammatory reaction within the cysts develops. Redness is therefore not pathognomonic of any special lesion in the breast.

EDEMA OF THE SKIN. Edema of the skin of the breast caused by blocking of the subdermal lymphatics develops in infections of the breast or axilla as well as in advanced carcinoma. Lymph accumulates within the skin until it is several times its normal thickness, and causes abnormal separation and deepening of the orifices of the cutaneous glands. Figure 5–5 shows extensive edema of the skin over the breast due to carcinoma. Figure 5–6 shows edema of the skin over the

breast in a patient with tuberculosis of the axillary lymph nodes.

When the area of edema is small, as in the patient with carcinoma shown in Figure 5–7, it easily escapes detection unless carefully looked for. It usually begins, as in this patient, in the skin within the areola, or just caudad to it, that is, in the most dependent part of the breast. This is regularly the site where edema appears when the carcinoma is situated deep in the center of the breast, but it may also be the earliest location of edema when the carcinoma is situated in the periphery of the breast. We have seen edema appear just below and medial to the nipple when the carcinoma was a small one located in the upper outer part of the breast.

There are, of course, other cases in which the edema first appears in the skin directly over a carcinoma situated more peripherally in the breast. In such cases the skin is usually somewhat adherent to the underlying tumor, and it seems probable that the lymphatics of the skin are obstructed by direct retrograde invasion from the surface of the growth outward.

CHANGES IN THE NIPPLES. While the patient is sitting erect it is important to look for changes in the nipples, such as deviation in the direction in which the nipples point, flattening, broadening, and retraction of the nipples, as well as nipple inversion.

The nipple epithelium must be carefully inspected in a good light. This is better done

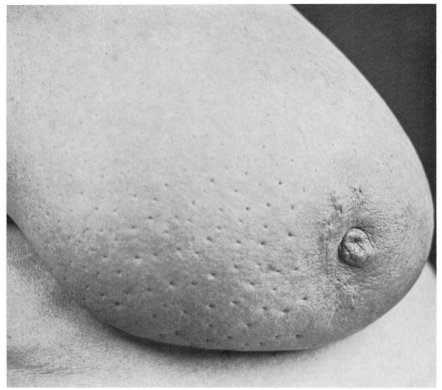

Figure 5–5. Extensive edema of the skin of the breast due to carcinoma.

with the patient lying down. At this point in my examination of the breasts, I therefore ask my patient to lie supine on the examining table. I inspect the nipple epithelium for thickening, reddening, or erosion. Any of these changes may signify Paget's carcinoma. I shall discuss them in detail in Chapter 29.

Palpation of the Breast. Having inspected the breasts, the examiner is ready to palpate them. This is best performed with the patient lying down, not sitting up. For adequate palpation, the breast should be balanced on the chest wall, so that it forms as even a layer as possible, flattened out upon the thoracic cage. To achieve this, I elevate the shoulder on the side being examined by placing a small pillow under it as for self-examination. This throws the breast medially, and tends to flatten it out upon the thorax. If the patient lies with her shoulders flat on the table, the breast falls to the side and palpation of its outer half is more difficult.

Palpation of the breast can and should be a gentle, precise, and orderly procedure. Palpation must never be so heavy-handed that it distresses the patient. Such an experience

may deter her from returning for subsequent vitally important re-examination. Gentle palpation is also more informative than rough examination. Indeed, it can be said that the more gentle the palpation, the more informative it will be. There is, moreover, a possible danger of causing metastasis by rough examination of a breast carcinoma. I have seen patients whose breasts showed ecchymosis caused by rough examination. Figure 5–8 shows such an area of ecchymosis in the lower outer sector of the breast which appeared following palpation by an enthusiastic surgeon. A good many examiners have a deplorable tendency to paw at the breast in examining it, using both hands to knead it like a batch of bread in their anxious search for a tumor. They are more likely to discover a tumor by precise and gentle palpation with the flat of the fingers of one hand.

The whole extent of the breast, as it lies relatively flattened out and balanced upon the chest wall, should be palpated systematically with the flat of the fingers of one hand. It is convenient to begin with the medial half of the breast. In palpating this area of the

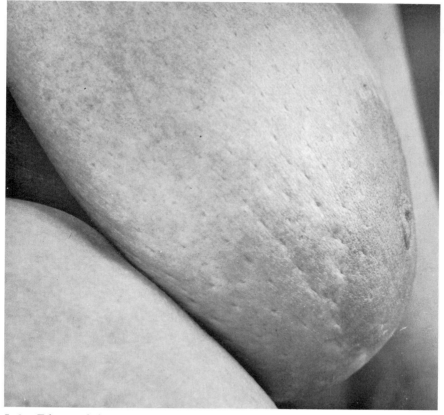

Figure 5–6.   Edema of the skin of the breast due to tuberculosis of the axillary lymph nodes.

Figure 5–7. Edema limited to the skin of the areolar region in carcinoma of the breast.

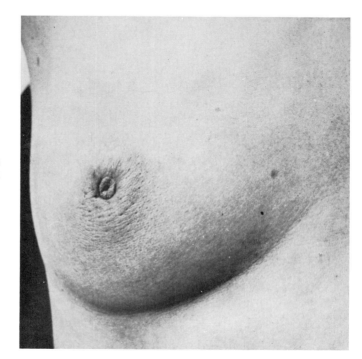

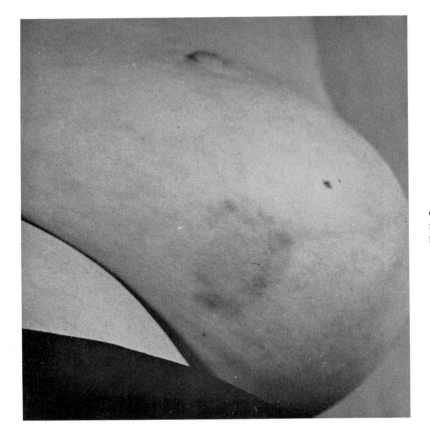

Figure 5-8. Ecchymosis of the skin of the lower outer sector of the breast following rough palpation.

breast, it is advantageous to have the patient's arm raised above the head (Fig. 5-9), a position that tenses the pectoral muscles so that it provides a flatter surface upon which the breast rests. The examiner's fingers trace a series of parallel transverse lines across the medial half of the breast from the nipple line to the sternum, beginning at the clavicle and ending at the inframammary fold.

One of the features of the normal anatomy of the breast which may confuse the examiner is the *inframammary fold*. In the more turgid breasts of adolescents and younger women who have not borne children no inframammary fold is found. But in the more flabby breasts of older women, and particularly in larger breasts, a prominent inframammary fold is often palpable. It forms a transverse ridge of denser nodular tissue at the caudad edge of the breast. Here the mammary tissue is bound down tightly to the deep fascia of the thoracic wall, compressed between the superficial and deep layers of the superficial fascia. The weight of the dependent bulky breast folds down over and presses upon it, and produces in it a degree of

congestion or fibrosis sufficient to make the lower edge of breast tissue palpable as a ridge. This ridge may be so prominent in some patients that it is mistaken for a tumor due to disease. It is not infrequently slightly tender. A tightly fitting brassiere may be a factor in accentuating the inframammary ridge.

Palpation of the lateral half of the breast is best carried out with the patient's arm at her side (Fig. 5-10). In this position the breast lies more caudad and its lateral half is more accessible to palpation. The examiner's fingers again trace a series of parallel transverse lines across this half of the breast from the posterior axillary line to the nipple line, beginning at the inframammary fold and ending in the infraclavicular region.

In examination of the breasts it should be kept in mind that the breast tissue often extends over a very wide area. A thin sheet of it may reach the lower edge of the clavicle above, the midline of the sternum medially, the lower edge of the inframmary fold caudad, and the edge of the latissimus dorsi muscle laterally. A small subcutaneous tumor

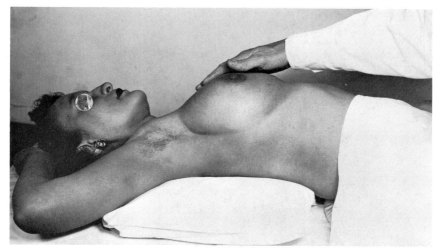

Figure 5-9. Palpation of the inner half of the breast; arm raised above the head.

near these outer limits of the breast may be mistaken for a benign subcutaneous lesion not associated with the breast when, in fact, it is a carcinoma of the breast. The axillary prolongation of the breast extends high into the axilla in some women, and a benign lesion or carcinoma arising in it is commonly mistaken for disease in the axillary lymph nodes.

Unless something is felt that arouses a suspicion of abnormality, each area of the breast need be palpated but once. The examiner should aim at minimizing his palpation, gentle though it may be. When the patient is referred to a surgeon, the surgeon must palpate both breasts once more to provide a complete case record, but repeated palpation

by other physicians and by students should not be permitted.

A little talcum powder on the examiner's fingers diminishes friction between them and the skin of the breast, and adds to the accuracy of palpation.

I have learned that palpation with the patient erect is an inaccurate method of examining the entire breast. The upper outer sector of the breast, where neoplasms are most frequent, is not conveniently accessible in this position. Unless the breast is small it hangs down and folds upon itself when the patient is erect, and in this dependent position it is thicker and more difficult to palpate than when it is flattened out upon the chest

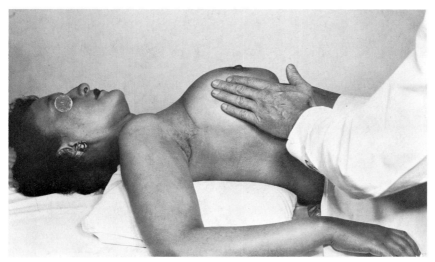

Figure 5-10. Palpation of the lateral half of the breast; arm at the side.

wall of the supine patient. Figure 5-11 shows how *not* to examine the upper outer sector of the breast.

The subareolar region and the portion of the breast just caudad to the areola, however, are areas which, in patients whose breasts are large, should be palpated with the patient sitting erect, as well as in the supine position. In the subareolar area, where the ducts converge to enter the base of the nipple, the breast structure is normally comparatively looser and less dense. In breasts that are thick and relatively firm in texture, the comparatively denser breast tissue of the upper half of the breast forms a sort of ledge above the softer subareolar region. This ledge is not infrequently mistaken for a tumor in such breasts. On the other hand, a real tumor of small size situated in the subareolar tissue or just caudad to the areola in such a thick, dense breast may be almost impalpable in the supine position, while it is readily felt when the breast is examined between the fingers with the patient in the sitting position.

In some patients the presence of a single, sharply defined dominant tumor in an otherwise unremarkable breast leaves no doubt in the examiner's mind as to the presence of disease. But in many other patients the findings of palpation are not as conclusive,

and the examiner has difficulty in interpreting what his fingers feel in the breast. In these patients he has to attempt to answer the question—*is the nodularity which he feels within the limits of the normal physiological variation in breast structure* or does it represent a *dominant tumor due to inflammatory or neoplastic disease?* If it is the former, no intervention is of course indicated, whereas if it is the latter, surgical investigation is imperative.

In keeping with its lobular structure the normal breast has a finely nodular character on palpation. With increased engorgement, and with perhaps other physiological changes which we do not understand, the coarseness of the nodules may be considerably increased. When such breast tissue is studied histologically nothing abnormal is seen and the conclusion is inescapable that the increased nodularity is a physiologic and not a pathologic change. Such increased nodularity may be generalized throughout the breast, but it is often more or less limited to one sector. The nodularity may be so marked that it becomes very difficult to decide whether or not it constitutes a dominant tumor representing disease.

In general it may be said that disease usually takes the form of a single dominant

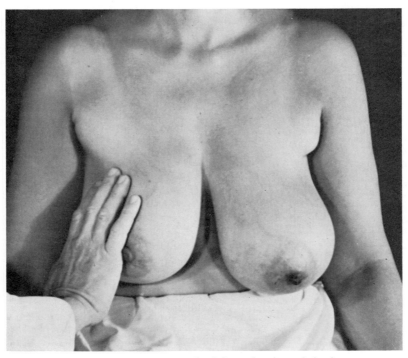

Figure 5-11.   Incorrect method for palpation of the breast.

tumor, whereas the increased nodularity due to physiologic change involves a considerable area in one breast or several sectors in both breasts. An exception must be made, of course, for cystic disease, which often produces multiple tumors. A localized area of increased nodularity representing nothing more than physiological change may give the impression of a dominant tumor. The differentiation of this kind of an area from a tumor representing real disease is the most difficult decision that an examiner has to make. It must be said that many surgeons tend to take refuge in the easy philosophy of operating when in doubt because this safeguards the patient. The result is that a large number of needless operations are performed upon the breast. The only hope that surgeons will improve their diagnostic accuracy lies in teaching them to examine the breasts with greater care, and to correlate their impressions from physical examination with the findings of their pathologists. I shall deal in detail with this matter of correlation of physical and pathological findings in the chapter on cystic disease.

The examiner needs not only a method for palpation such as I have outlined, but a system for expressing and for recording his tactile impressions of the lesion in terms of five physical qualities that tumors exhibit; namely, *size, shape, delimitation, consistence,* and *movability within the breast tissue.*

The *size* of the tumor should be determined and recorded in centimeters, by finding the tumor edges with two fingers and measuring the distance between them with a rule or tape. If the tumor is round, one diameter will suffice, but if it is discoid or elongated, two or more diameters should be recorded. The clinical measurements made in this way will be found to be about 1 cm. greater than the pathologist's measurements of the tumor in the operative specimen, because of the added thickness of the surrounding breast tissue. I can only deplore tumor size expressed in terms of fruits, nuts, or vegetables, but I have to admit that even present day medical students, who presumably have had a scientific education, continue to prefer these agricultural terms to the metric system.

The *shape* of tumors, whether rounded, discoid, elongated, nodular, or irregular, should be recorded. Most tumors when very small tend to be rounded, but when they become larger they often have more or less

characteristic shapes. For example, cysts are usually round, while carcinoma is often irregular in contour.

A very important quality is *delimitation.* By delimitation I mean the degree of sharpness with which the edges of the tumor are felt. This quality might be called demarcation, or circumscription, but delimitation is perhaps a more exact term. Cysts and adenofibromas are usually well delimited in the breast tissue. The edges of an area of adenosis, fibrous disease, or carcinoma, on the other hand, are not felt as sharply. They seem to fade out into the surrounding breast tissue. This lack of delimitation is due to the infiltrative character of these lesions.

There are, however, exceptions to these generalizations. An area of increased nodularity due to physiologic change, or a tumor formed by a multitude of minute cysts may be poorly delimited. In contrast, there are several types of carcinoma that are often remarkably well delimited—the type that we classify as the circumscribed form, papillary carcinoma, and well differentiated intraductal carcinoma.

The *consistency* of lesions in the breast is not always a reliable guide but it is certainly one of the most helpful indications of their nature. Most cysts have an elastic quality, some of the larger ones can be felt to fluctuate, and others are so soft that they can be felt only with the gentlest palpation. Very tense cysts may, however, be quite firm. Most carcinomas have a wooden hardness, but a calcified adenofibroma is equally hard. Papillary carcinoma may be soft. Adenosis may be almost as firm as carcinoma. An area of increased nodularity due to physiological change is usually not as firm as carcinoma. It is impossible to estimate accurately the consistence of very small tumors.

The degree of *movability* of a tumor in the breast tissue which surrounds it is perhaps the best guide to its nature. Fibroadenomas and cysts have the greatest degree of movability. Indeed, they often seem to be so freely movable, and slip about so readily under the fingers of the examiner, that he is at once convinced of their benignancy. Carcinoma, adenosis, and fibrous disease, on the other hand, are relatively fixed in the breast tissue in which they lie. They cannot be much moved about, as would be expected from their infiltrative nature. An area of increased nodularity due to physiologic change is often intermediate in its movability. It is not as freely movable as a cyst or adenofibroma but it is by no means as fixed as a carcinoma.

It is important for the examiner to be objective about his findings in palpation of the breast. In order to discipline myself in objectivity I make it a rule when I begin to take my patient's history to ask her *not* to tell me in which breast, and in what part of the breast, the tumor is situated. When I have finished my palpation, if I have found a tumor, I ask her if it is the one she or her previous examiner had found. If I have found no tumor, I tell her so and ask her to show me any tumor she or a previous examiner may have felt. It has been a humiliating experience for me on a number of occasions to have the patient demonstrate a definite tumor after I had missed it. This experience may humiliate the examiner but it may save the patient's life if the tumor is a carcinoma. It is, I am sure, a sound rule for the physician to check his findings with the patient's. As I have already pointed out, women can be very accurate indeed in palpating disease in their own breasts.

Another important safeguard in the diagnosis of breast lesions is to question the validity of conclusions based on palpation if the patient is examined during the premenstrual or menstrual phase of her cycle. Engorgement is so marked in some patients during these phases of the cycle that innocuous increased nodularity may give the impression of a dominant tumor due to disease. When there is any question as to the nature of the breast lesion in a patient examined during these unfavorable phases of her cycle, she should be asked to return for a reëxamination as soon as menstruation is over. Cysts not infrequently enlarge with striking rapidity in the premenstrual phase of the cycle and decrease sharply in size after menstruation. When an observing patient reports this phenomenon it is strong evidence in favor of cystic disease.

Palpation provides the most important evidence in the diagnosis of breast lesions but a search for retraction signs is also an essential part of an adequate examination of the breast in patients in whom there is any indication of breast disease. It is the next step in the examination of the breasts.

Retraction Phenomena in the Breast. Retraction signs constitute a whole series of clinical manifestations ranging from a small dimple in the skin over the tumor to shrinkage of the entire breast. They are due

to the fact that the growth of some neoplasms, or the evolution of inflammation from bacterial infection or fat necrosis, causes proliferation of fibroblasts not only within the lesion itself but into the surrounding breast tissue. This scar tissue, so to speak, contracts as it grows older, and since the breast is normally loose and fatty in structure, any or all of the tissue adjacent to the lesion may be pulled in toward it by the shortening strands of fibroblasts. This phenomenon is of fundamental importance in the interpretation of the clinical signs that disease produces.

This mechanism, by which carcinoma produces retraction phenomena, is illustrated by the accompanying drawing of a parasagittal section through the chest and the breast in the nipple plane (Fig. 5–12). I have already pointed out that the breast lies very close to the skin between the superficial and deep layers of the superficial fascia. The fascial septa of the breast, the so-called Cooper's ligaments, are intimately connected with this enveloping fascia. Superficially, this fascia is attached to the skin, and deeply, to the pectoral fascia. The fibrosis within the carcinoma, and radiating out around it, exerts an abnormal traction upon these fascial septa of the breast. They pull the skin inward to produce dimpling, and they fix the breast to a varying degree to the underlying pectoral fascia, limiting its movability and distorting its contour. If the pectoral muscles are contracted, carrying the pectoral fascia cephalad, the sector of the breast in which the carcinoma lies is pulled upward abnormally and its contour distorted. Contraction of the pectoral muscles may likewise bring out dimpling of the skin over the carcinoma, because of the abnormal fixation of the pectoral fascia to the carcinoma, and of the carcinoma to the overlying skin, by the fibrosis around it. When the fibrosis involves the larger mammary ducts, they are shortened, with the result that the axis in which the nipple points is changed, or the nipple is flattened, and finally retracted.

A good example of pronounced retraction is illustrated in Figure 5–13. Here, the carcinoma is situated in the upper central portion of the breast just above the areola. The skin over it has been drawn inward, forming a deep dimple. The areola has been pulled upward toward the carcinoma and, in its upper part, it is so narrowed that it is hardly discernible. The nipple is also pulled upward, and its axis is deviated so that instead of pointing

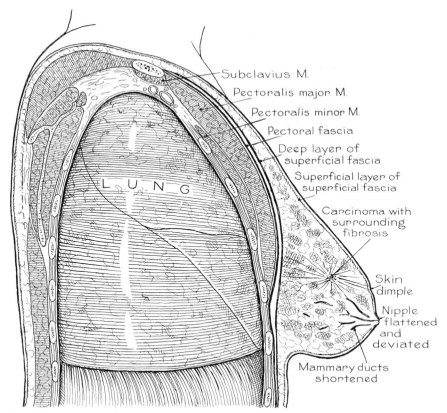

Subclavius M.
Pectoralis major M.
Pectoralis minor M.
Pectoral fascia
Deep layer of superficial fascia
Superficial layer of superficial fascia
Carcinoma with surrounding fibrosis
Skin dimple
Nipple flattened and deviated
Mammary ducts shortened

LUNG

Figure 5-12. Diagram of a parasagittal section through the breast and thorax to illustrate the mechanism of retraction in carcinoma of the breasts.

forward and somewhat laterally, it points upward toward the carcinoma.

Another example of a dimple in the skin over a carcinoma of the breast is shown in Figure 5–14. Here the dimple is a broad, shallow one. Again, the areola and the nipple are pulled upward toward the carcinoma.

These retraction signs are often less well developed. They may be so subtle that they can only be demonstrated by certain maneuvers.

The simple act of *raising the arms high above the head* will sometimes reveal asymmetry of the breasts, or retraction of the skin, which is of decisive diagnostic significance. Figure 5–15 shows a 30 year old patient in whom no asymmetry of the breasts is evident as she sits with her arms at her sides. In Figure 5–16, which shows her with her arms raised, a well-defined indentation is seen in the inner lower sector of the right breast adjacent to the small tumor indicated by the circle. As this fact suggests, the tumor was a

carcinoma. The fibrosis around the carcinoma has attached it abnormally closely to the underlying pectoral fascia and to the overlying skin. When the arms are raised, elevating the pectoral fascia, the carcinoma and the overlying skin are pulled upward and inward to a greater degree than the surrounding normal breast, producing the telltale asymmetry.

Another maneuver that is useful in revealing retraction of the skin is for the examiner to *lift the breast upward* with his hand. When the lesion is in the upper half of the breast, this maneuver will often bring out a dimple in the skin over it although none is seen when the breast hangs dependent. The mechanism of this phenomenon is a simple one. The skin over the lesion is tied down to it by fibrosis, while the skin over the normal surrounding breast lifts freely.

A variant of this same maneuver is *molding the breast* around the tumor. The examiner's fingers gently lift the breast up around the

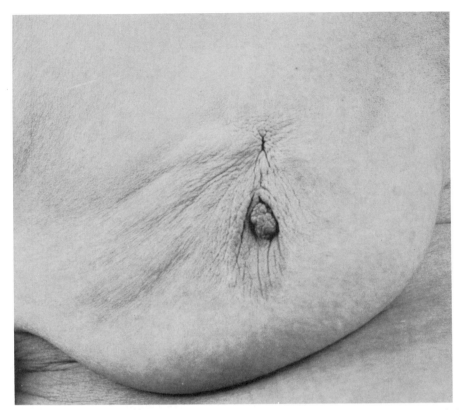

Figure 5–13.   Marked retraction produced by a carcinoma of the upper central portion of the breast.

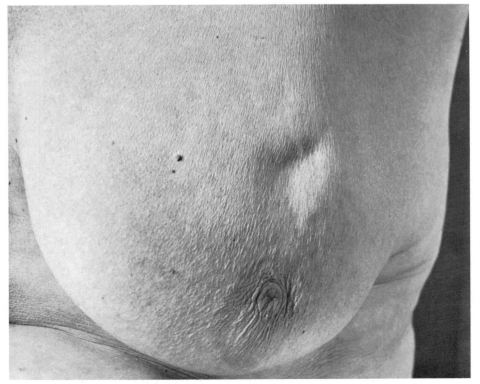

Figure 5–14.   Broad shallow dimple in the skin over a carcinoma of the upper outer sector of the breast.

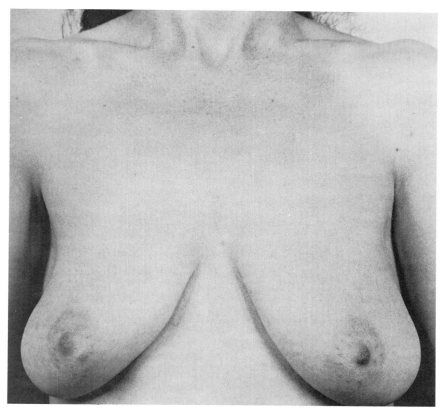

Figure 5–15.   Breasts symmetrical with the arms at the sides, in carcinoma of the inner lower sector of the right breast.

tumor, as shown in Figure 5–17. Here the carcinoma was situated in the upper outer sector of the breast. The dimple over it thus demonstrated is plainly seen. Dimpling occurs because the skin is tied down to the carcinoma by fibrosis, while the surrounding skin and breast tissue is elevated by the pressure of the examiner's fingers. Jackson and Severance have recently called this maneuver the "plateau test." When the tumor is in the lower half of the breast, this same maneuver, carried out with the patient lying down, will often bring out a dimple over the lesion, as shown in Figure 5–18.

Another maneuver that is often helpful in demonstrating retraction signs is that of *pectoral contraction.* While in the sitting position, the patient relaxes and rests her hands on her hips, giving the examiner an opportunity to compare the relative height of the lower edge of the breast and the level of the areola on each side, and to look for retraction signs over the tumor. The patient is then asked to press her hands against her hips, contracting her pectoral muscles, first on the

normal and then on the diseased side. The normal breast is pulled upward slightly by this motion, but the carcinomatous breast often rises sharply as compared with its mate. The breast as a whole may be abnormally elevated, or merely the sector of the breast in which the carcinoma is situated. This abnormal elevation occurs, of course, because the fibrosis in the carcinomatous area fixes it abnormally to the underlying pectoral fascia. When contraction of the pectoralis major elevates the pectoral fascia, the carcinomatous area in the breast is pulled up with it.

Pectoral contraction also brings out other retraction signs—deviation of the nipple toward the tumor, and furrows and dimples in the skin over it. Figures 5–19 and 5–20 demonstrate this pectoral contraction maneuver in a patient with a carcinoma in the outer upper part of the breast. Figure 5–19 shows the patient with her hand resting relaxed on her hip; no definite dimpling is seen in the skin adjacent to the carcinoma indicated by the circle. But in Figure 5–20 when her hand is pressed against her side, contracting the

(*Text continued on page 121.*)

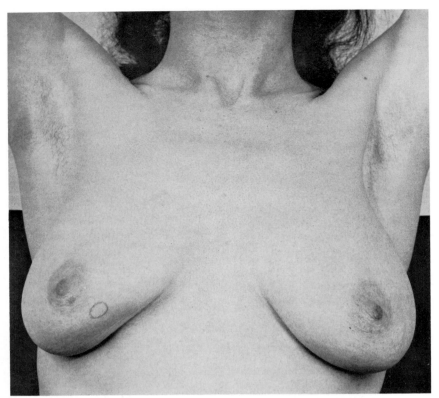

Figure 5-16. Indentation in the contour of the breast, with the arms raised, in carcinoma of the lower inner sector of the right breast, indicated by the circle marked on the skin.

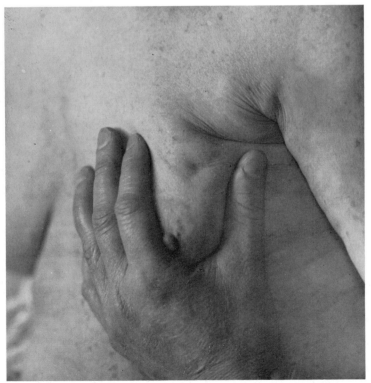

Figure 5-17. Dimple over a carcinoma in the upper outer sector of the breast, demonstrated by gentle molding of the breast tissue around the tumor.

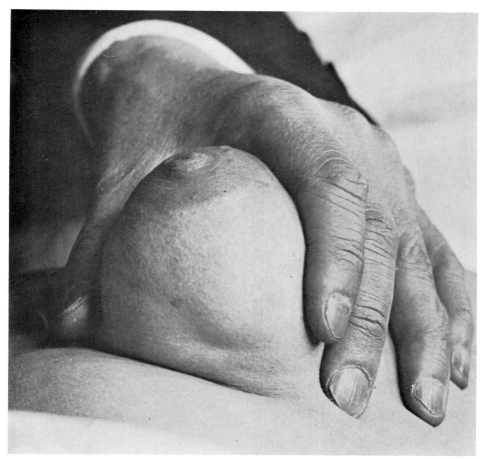

Figure 5-18. Dimple in the lower half of the breast, demonstrated by gentle molding of the breast tissue around the tumor.

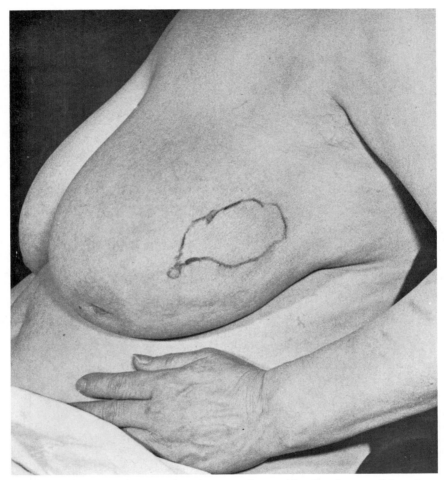

Figure 5–19. Pectoral contraction maneuver, arm resting on hip. Carcinoma of the upper outer sector of the breast.

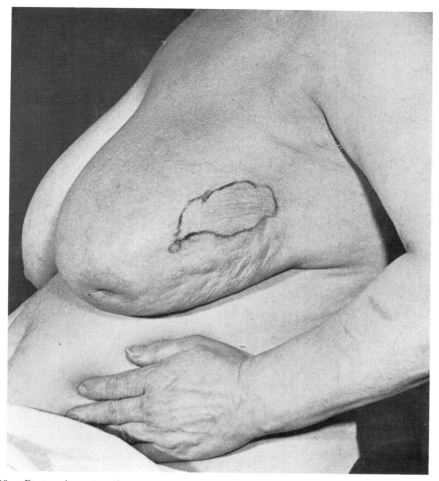

Figure 5–20.   Pectoral contraction maneuver, arm pressed against the hip, bringing out furrows in the skin over the carcinoma.

pectoral muscle, a whole series of furrows appear in the skin.

This is, of course, a rather marked example of skin dimpling brought out by pectoral contraction. Careful scrutiny should detect less well-developed dimpling, as in the patient shown in Figures 5–21 and 5–22. In Figure 5–21 where the hand is not pressed against the hip, no dimpling is seen over the carcinoma, which is situated in the outer middle sector of the breast. In Figure 5–22 in which the pectoral muscles are contracted, two small dimples are seen over the tumor.

Another procedure of great value in demonstrating retraction signs in the breast is the *forward-bending maneuver*. I learned of it from the late Hugh Auchincloss. The patient is asked to stand and bend far forward from the hips, keeping her chin up and extending her hands toward the examiner who supports

them on the tips of his own fingers as he sits before her (Fig. 5–23). In this position, normal breasts fall freely away from the chest wall and are perfectly symmetrical. But if a lesion producing retraction is present in one of them, even though it be small, the fibrosis that accompanies it will usually fix the diseased breast to the chest wall in some degree and produce an asymmetry that careful inspection from the side or from the front will detect. Over and over again, we have seen carcinoma in the breast betrayed by asymmetry demonstrated in this maneuver, although there were no other retraction signs. Figures 5–24 and 5–25 show a good example of the value of forward bending. There was a small carcinoma beneath the right areola, but no asymmetry was evident as the patient stood with her arms at her sides. When she bent forward, however, the

(*Text continued on page 125.*)

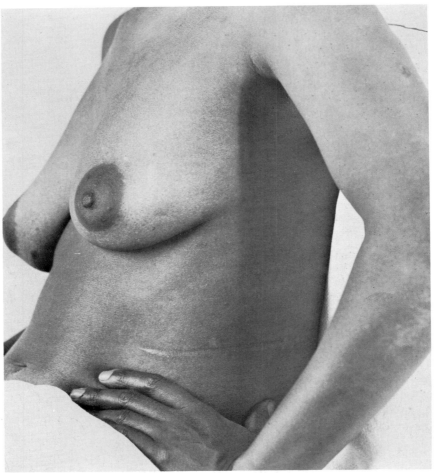

Figure 5–21. Pectoral contraction maneuver, arm resting on hip. Carcinoma of the middle outer sector of the breast.

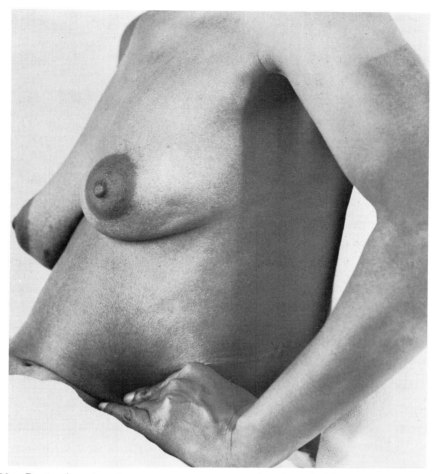

Figure 5–22. Pectoral contraction maneuver, arm pressed against the hip, bringing out small dimples in the skin over the carcinoma.

Figure 5–23. The forward-bending maneuver.

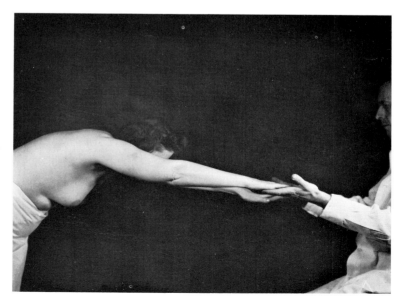

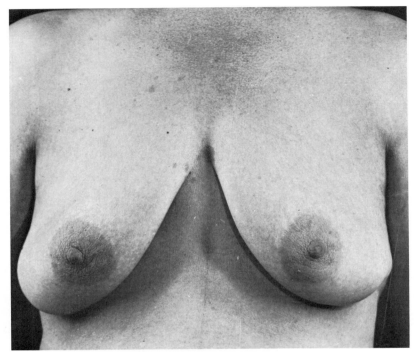

Figure 5–24.   Breasts symmetrical with patient in the erect position – carcinoma of the right subareolar region.

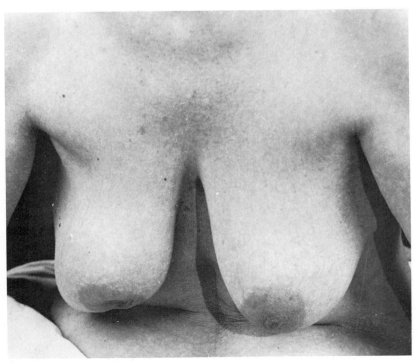

Figure 5–25.   Retraction of areola and nipple with patient in the forward-bending position. Carcinoma of the right subareolar region.

nipple and medial part of the right areola were pulled up deeply into the breast. No examiner could miss the distortion.

Figures 5–26 and 5–27 show another patient in the erect and forward-bending positions, and illustrate how forward bending accentuates the retraction signs produced by a carcinoma in the upper middle sector of the breast. Note how the right breast is held up against the chest wall, and its areola and nipple deviated laterally, in the forward-bending position.

The change that carcinoma produces in the contour of the breast in the forward-bending position is sometimes less obvious in patients with more dense, less atrophic breasts. In such breasts forward bending may reveal only a slight flattening of the contour of the breast adjacent to the carcinoma.

Fixation of the Breast. As carcinoma of the breast extends locally, the tumor itself, as well as the breast in which it lies, tends to become fixed to the underlying pectoral fascia and muscle, and finally to the thoracic cage. It is important to define this fixation in terms of degree. All surgeons are familiar with the advanced degree of fixation in which the breast is immovable upon the chest wall. But the early stages of the process often escape the examiner's attention, for they are brought out only by certain special maneuvers.

It has been my custom to classify fixation in three degrees. The first two degrees are somewhat different manifestations of abnormal attachment of the carcinoma to the underlying pectoral fascia and muscle. Third degree fixation is evidence of attachment of the tumor to the tissues of the chest wall beneath the pectoral muscle, or to the tissues of the chest wall lateral to the pectoral muscle.

First degree fixation is demonstrated with the patient sitting erect. She places her hands against her hips and contracts her pectoral muscles by pressing her hands against her hips. The breasts, if they are not too heavy, are normally pulled upward slightly by this action. But when carcinoma has produced abnormal fixation of the breast to the underlying pectoral fascia or muscle, the diseased breast is pulled upward to an abnormal degree, or in an asymmetrical manner. Figure 5–28 shows a marked example of first degree fixation. Pectoral contraction caused a 2 cm. elevation of the tumor and accentuated the skin dimpling. Such abnormal elevation may be apparent only along the lateral aspect of

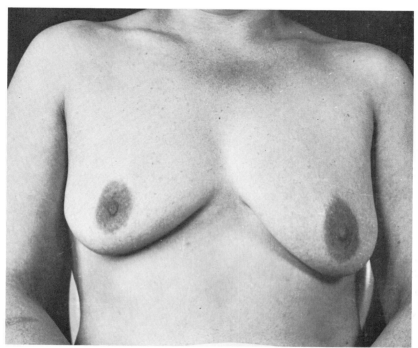

Figure 5–26.   Right breast slightly elevated but otherwise symmetrical with patient in the erect position—carcinoma of the upper central region of the right breast.

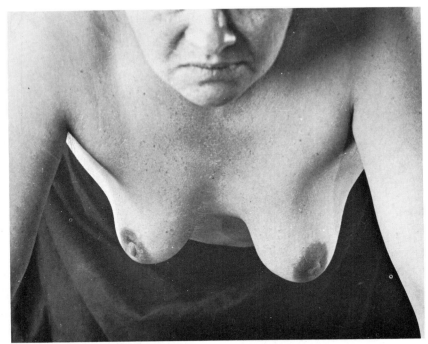

Figure 5–27.   Right breast held up against chest wall, its areola and nipple deviated laterally, with patient in forward-bending position—carcinoma of the upper central region of the right breast.

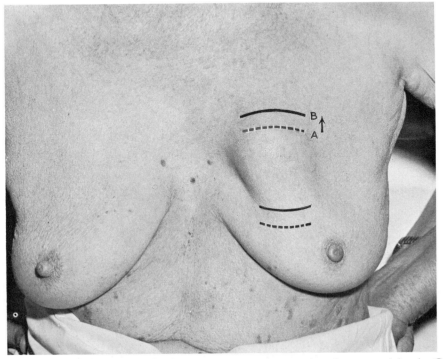

Figure 5–28.   A marked example of first degree fixation of a tumor to the pectoral fascia. Carcinoma of the upper inner sector of the breast. Contraction of the pectoral muscle elevated the tumor 2 cm. and accentuated the skin retraction.

the breast if the tumor is situated in its outer half. In these patients with only first degree fixation of the breast, the tumor within it can still be moved passively with freedom over the chest wall when the patient lies supine with the pectoral muscles contracted.

Second degree fixation is demonstrated with the patient lying supine with her hands placed upon her hips. With the pectoral muscles relaxed, the examiner gently tests the passive mobility of the tumor over the chest wall, as shown in Figure 5–29. The patient is then asked to press her hands against her hips to contract the pectoral muscles. In those patients with what I call second degree fixation, the movability of the tumor between the examiner's hands upon the chest wall will be sharply checked as the pectoral muscles are contracted. It is my impression that abnormal fixation of the tumor to the pectorals, as demonstrated by this maneuver, represents a more advanced stage of fixation than the phenomenon that I have described as first degree fixation.

Third degree fixation in my classification is the advanced stage when carcinoma is immovably fixed to the chest wall, even when the pectoral muscles are relaxed.

Retraction Signs in Nipple and Areola.

In his search for retraction signs, the examiner should pay special attention to changes in the areola and nipple. The horizontal levels of the areola and nipple are often elevated by a carcinoma in the upper half of the breast.

Deviation of the axis in which the nipple points is a subtle retraction sign. The fibrosis in and about the lesion pulls on the duct system and tilts the nipple so that it points toward the tumor. Figure 5–30 shows deviation of the axis of the right nipple upward and laterally toward a carcinoma of the upper outer sector of the breast.

When the lesion involves the area more or less directly beneath the nipple, the fibrosis shortens the whole duct system and pulls the nipple inward. In carcinoma this process may show itself merely as flattening and broadening of the nipple (Fig. 5–31) on the carcinomatous side as compared with its mate. As the fibrosis progresses, the nipple becomes flatter and broader until, in some instances, it is finally retracted beneath the surface of the surrounding areola (Fig. 5–32). Nipple retraction is also seen in benign lesions producing fibrosis in and about the collecting ducts, particularly in *ectasia of the ducts.*

Flattening or retraction of the nipple caused by these lesions should not be con-

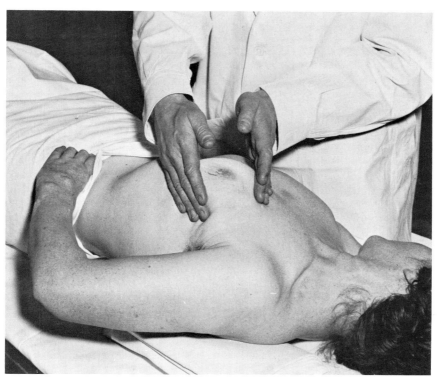

Figure 5–29. Testing the mobility of a carcinoma of the breast on the chest wall to determine second degree fixation.

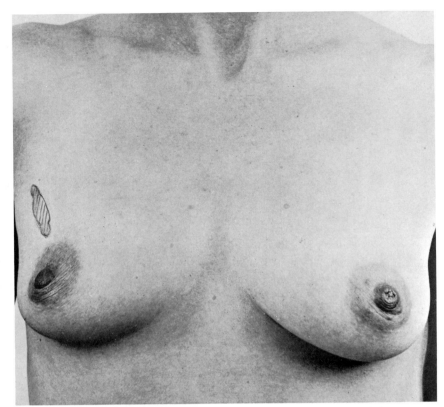

Figure 5–30. Upward and lateral deviation of the right nipple—carcinoma of the upper outer sector of the right breast.

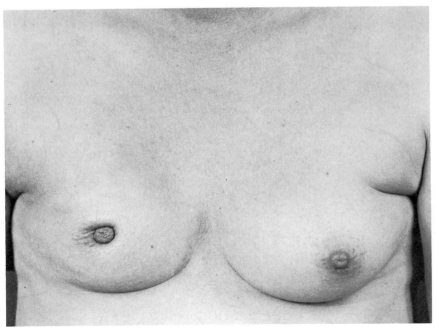

Figure 5–31. Flattening and broadening of the nipple produced by carcinoma of the central region of the right breast.

fused with mere *inversion of the nipple,* a condition seen in a good many women with no disease of the breast. Inversion of the nipple may be bilateral or unilateral. The patient will usually say that the inversion has been present for many years and that it interfered with nursing. Instead of protruding in the normal way, the nipple is hidden in a sulcus from which it can usually be pulled out. Figure 5–33 shows an inverted nipple, in a woman aged 67, that had been inverted since she was 30 years of age. There was no disease in her breast. The inverted nipple is not broadened and thickened and fixed, as is the nipple retracted by disease.

Carcinomas of the breast in which a careful examination fails to reveal any of the retraction signs described are few indeed. In my experience, these few have been either the papillary, the circumscribed, or the well-differentiated type. These varieties seem to produce less fibrosis in the surrounding breast than most carcinomas, and, therefore, less retraction.

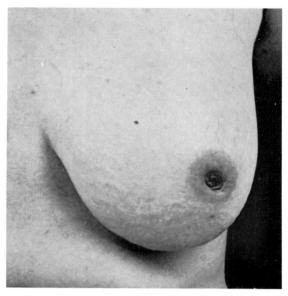

Figure 5–32. Retraction of the nipple below the surface of the areola in carcinoma of the central portion of the breast.

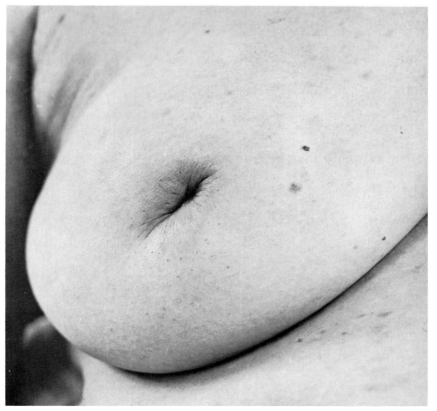

Figure 5–33. Simple inversion of the nipple—no disease of the breast.

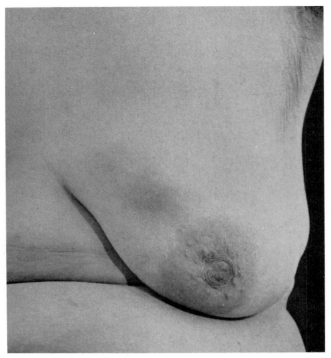

Figure 5–34. Pseudo-retraction of the skin caudad to a benign intraductal papilloma of the breast.

Although I have described retraction signs in general as being due to carcinoma it should never be forgotten that benign lesions also produce retraction. Duct ectasia, in particular, may produce very marked retraction signs that can deceive the most experienced clinician into thinking that he is dealing with carcinoma.

Pseudo-Retraction. Benign lesions of the breast which form a considerable mass, and sometimes protrude slightly above the level of the adjacent breast, not infrequently produce a sort of pseudo-retraction of the adjacent skin. This effect is merely the result of the contrast between the skin over the protruding tumor and the skin over the adjacent breast. Figure 5–34 shows such pseudo-retraction just caudad to a large benign intraductal papilloma.

Methods of Recording Physical Findings

There are four methods of recording the physical findings in breast disease. The first, a written description, is usually the only one available in the unit case history in most hospitals. It is the least accurate type of record.

Written by a junior intern who has very little knowledge of breast disease, often in an illegible hand, this kind of a record is often an insuperable handicap in classifying the clinical stage of the disease in subsequent studies.

A good photograph has the advantage of recording what can be seen more accurately than any other method. For many purposes photographs are indispensable. But they do not, of course, record what the examiner palpates.

A sketch is much the best kind of record of physical findings. I have made them in all the patients I have studied. These sketches are very simple and have no pretension of artistic merit. The effort to draw what I see and palpate, however, makes me look more sharply, and helps fix in my mind the characteristics of the lesion. I draw the outline of the thorax and breast in black ink, and put the pathologic findings in with red ink. If the tumor is well delimited, it is drawn in with a solid line, as shown in Figure 5–35.

Nodularity of the type commonly palpated with increased breast engorgement is shown in these sketches by coarse dots. Foci of more prominent nodules are shown by short

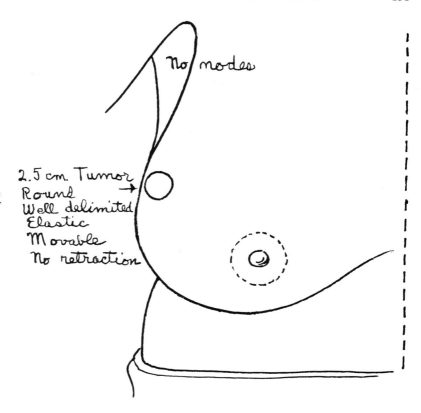

Figure 5–35. Sketch of the physical findings in a cyst of the breast.

curved lines within the dotted area, as indicated in Figure 5–36.

Poorly delimited lesions that form a dominant tumor are indicated by cross-hatching. Figure 5–37 shows my sketch of a carcinoma, indicated in this manner. Skin retraction is indicated by shading or lines. Distortion of the nipple and areola, or the contour of the breast, are drawn as seen.

I make a notation on the sketch as to the size of the tumor in centimeters, its shape, its delimitation, its consistence, its movability, and the accompanying retraction.

Any axillary nodes that are palpated are also shown in the sketch. Whether or not they are clinically involved, their size in centimeters, and their movability are all noted.

For those who cannot themselves make a reasonably accurate sketch, I have prepared printed stylized diagrams (Fig. 5–38) of the left and right thorax. They are bound up in pads from which they can be torn. On the reverse of each diagram our Columbia Clinical Classification is printed, so that it is readily available for reference. The physical findings can be drawn in on these diagrams, but the result is not as accurate as a sketch from life.

A statement as to the exact position of the tumor in the breast is an important part of the clinical record. If the lesion is a carcinoma its site has a relationship to the manner in which it may metastasize through the regional lymphatic filter. It is difficult to be exact regarding tumor sites in a written description. To facilitate accuracy in classifying breast tumors according to sites which appear to have some significance in terms of the lymphatic drainage, we have, in our printed stylized diagrams, divided the breast into seven zones, *A, B, C, D, E, F,* and *G,* as indicated in Figure 5–38. Any tumor lying beneath the areola, or any tumor whose edge reaches within 1 cm. of the edge of the areola, is classified as a central, or zone *G,* tumor and is presumed to be in contact with the rich subareolar lymphatic plexus. The upper and lower *parasternal* zones, zones *D* and *E,* are defined as zones limited medially by the midline of the sternum, and laterally by a vertical line drawn 3 cm. lateral to the sternal edge. The horizontal level of the nipple divides these two zones, as well as other zones, into upper and lower.

It is essential, for the accuracy of this method of classification, to chart the position

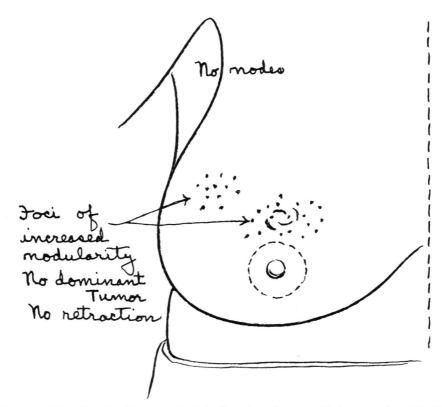

Figure 5–36. Sketch of the physical findings in a breast with increased nodularity.

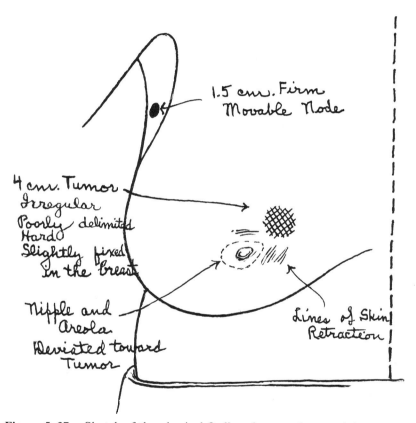

1.5 cm. Firm
Movable Node

4 cm. Tumor
Irregular
Poorly delimited
Hard
Slightly fixed
in the breast

Nipple and
Areola
Deviated toward
Tumor

Lines of Skin
Retraction

Figure 5–37.   Sketch of the physical findings in a carcinoma of the breast.

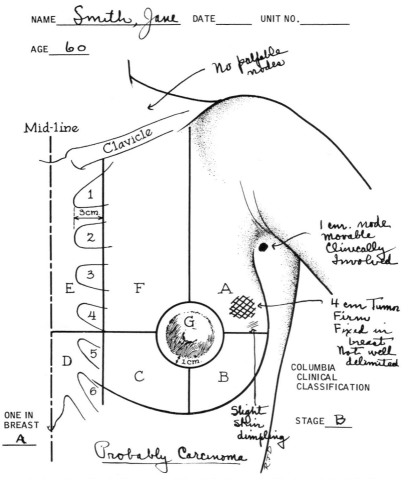

NAME *Smith, Jane* DATE_____ UNIT NO._____

AGE **60**

No palpable nodes

Mid-line

Clavicle

1

3cm

2

3

E   F   A

4

D   5   G   B
         1cm

6   C   B

ONE IN
BREAST
A

Slight skin dimpling

Probably Carcinoma

1 cm. node movable Clinically Involved

4 cm Tumor Firm Fixed in breast Not well delimited

COLUMBIA
CLINICAL
CLASSIFICATION

STAGE **B**

Figure 5–38.   Printed stylized diagram of the left thorax with the clinical findings drawn in.

of the tumor in the breast with the patient in the supine and *not* in the erect position. When the patient sits erect tumors of the lower portion of the breast are obscured by the dependent breast, and their exact site cannot be accurately depicted.

Other Techniques of Examination

Transillumination. Transillumination of the breast as a diagnostic aid was popularized by Cutler in the 1920's. Some clinicians, such as Huguenin, have found after a thorough trial that transillumination is a helpful aid in diagnosis. In my own experience, I have found it to be of such limited usefulness that I do not employ it. An intraductal papilloma in a dilated duct containing bloody fluid, situated in the subareolar area of a dependent breast, will show up well in transillumination as a sharply delimited, entirely opaque shadow. But even when it gives this picture, transillumination does not rule out carcinoma, and further diagnostic steps are necessary.

Roentgen-Ray Examination. There are two ways in which roentgen rays can be used to study the breasts: (1) the injection of an opaque medium into the duct system and roentgenographic study, and (2) soft tissue roentgen-ray studies of the breasts—the so-called mammograms.

INJECTION OF THE DUCTS WITH AN OPAQUE MEDIUM. This method of study was enthusiastically advocated by Hicken. He used colloidal thorium dioxide as a contrast medium. Romano and McFetridge, among others, later pointed out that the injection of iodized oil or thorium dioxide into the breast ducts not infrequently produced sharp foreign body reactions, and even abscess formation, sometimes necessitating mastectomy. This objection has of course now been overcome by the development of harmless contrast mediums.

The difficulty in injecting the mammary ducts, however, has kept most of the clinics in our country from taking up the method. It is much used in a number of South American clinics, where Leborgne has popularized it. He uses a concentrated iodine solution such as *Uroselectan B* as an injection medium and reports that he has observed no untoward reactions from it.

Sandblom and Löfgren, in Sweden, have refined the technique of injecting the nipple ducts with a contrast medium and studying them roentgenographically. They find the method indispensable for localizing the intraductal lesion in patients with a nipple discharge but no palpable tumor. Study of their reported results with the method reveals, however, that they failed to find a papilloma in 9 of the 20 patients without a palpable tumor in whom they used the method.

I hesitate to use the intraductal injection method of study in those patients with a nipple discharge. In those who have a tumor or a pressure point that localizes the lesion, intraductal injection is not necessary. Surgical exploration can be done at once. In the remaining smaller group of patients without localizing signs, repeated palpation over a limited period of time, searching for a pressure point, seems to me safer. In the infrequent carcinoma in this group of cases I would fear that injection of the ducts might produce metastasis. The disease is largely intraductal in these cases, and injecting the ducts under pressure might force carcinoma cells into blood or lymph vessels. Moreover, the information gained by roentgenography of injected ducts is not of decisive diagnostic significance. Biopsy, again, is the only sure guide to the nature of the lesion. The hazards of intraductal injection, to my mind, outweigh the value of what may be learned from it.

MAMMOGRAPHY. Although it had been known for half a century that roentgenograms of the breasts would reveal some forms of disease, interest in this form of examination has more recently been revived by Leborgne and by Egan. Mammography is now being extensively studied in many clinics with the support of the United States Public Health Service. Used as a screening method for detecting breast carcinoma, it has been reported that carcinomas have been found with it in from one to six women in every thousand examined.

Much the most extensive screening study, and one conducted with admirable care, is that directed by Strax. He has recently reported on his initial screening of a total of 20,211 women chosen at random from those enrolled in the Health Insurance Plan of Greater New York. They were screened both by mammography and by clinical examination carried out independently. With mammography alone carcinoma was found in 21 women whose breasts were normal on clinical examination. In a total of 24 other women carcinoma was detected by clinical examination alone; in 20 of these the initial mammograms were interpreted as negative. In 10 other women carcinoma was diagnosed on the basis of both mammograms and clinical examination.

In a control group of 29,694 women chosen in the same way as his study group, and who received only the usual medical care provided by the Health Insurance Plan, Strax reports that a total of 46 developed breast cancer during the first year of observation.

A similar screening study utilizing independent physical examination and mammography in a series of 12,245 women has been reported by Griesbach and Eads. With mammography alone carcinoma was detected in six women whose breasts were normal on palpation. In seven other patients carcinoma was found by palpation, the mammograms being reported as negative. In five other women both palpation and mammography indicated the presence of carcinoma.

Strax emphasizes several factors that limit the accuracy of mammography in the detection of breast cancer, some of which have been noted by other radiologists. The method is more accurate in older women; only three of the 21 cancers that Strax found with mammography alone occurred in women under the age of 50. Strax classified the breasts in his patients as "mainly glandular" or "mainly fatty" and reported that 18 of the 21 cancers found by mammography alone were in "fatty" breasts. He also found that mammography was comparatively inefficient in studying very small breasts.

The images of diagnostic significance in mammograms are of two general types — areas of increased density with characteristic shapes, and foci of calcification. The areas of increased density are numerous and of infinite variety. Only a very few of them, particularly those that are denser and have a stellate contour, are diagnostic of carcinoma. Figure 5–39 shows such a mammographic image of a carcinoma. This lesion was palpable, as are the overwhelming majority of carcinomas that produce this kind of an image.

A great variety of calcifications are also revealed in breasts by these soft tissue films. The most significant are the so-called microcalcifications that produce a very fine stippling effect. To be fully appreciated, they must be studied with an intensified light and a magnifying glass. They are an indubitable indication of disease in the breast and require biopsy. Many of these lesions are not palpable. When there was no palpable tumor in the breast, but mammograms revealed characteristic foci of microcalcification, we have found carcinoma in about half of our patients. The others had adenosis, cystic disease, or duct ectasia. There was no discernible difference in the appearance of the microcalcifications produced by these very different diseases. Hassler has recently tabulated the frequency of microcalcification in these various lesions.

The area of microcalcification produced by a carcinoma may be exceedingly small, as illustrated in Figure 5–40. Finding such a minute area of disease without removing a large sector of the breast and unnecessarily damaging it if the lesion is benign, presents a very real challenge to the surgeon. Crossed wires placed upon the breast (Fig. 5–41) sometimes help us localize these small areas of microcalcification. Very extensive microcalcification, such as that seen in Figure 5–42, is sometimes revealed by mammography, even when there is no palpable tumor in the breast.

As we today study microscopic sections of breast tissue we not infrequently see foci of calcification, which we have in the past overlooked. They are clearly the result of the deposition of calcium in old and dead masses of epithelial cells in ducts, or cysts or epithelial neoplasms of various types. They are often seen in the necrotic masses of cells filling up ducts in intraductal carcinoma of the so-called "comedo" type. This type of carcinoma is more slowly growing than other types, and has a more favorable prognosis. It is to be expected that in carcinoma detected by microcalcifications seen in mammography, without an accompanying palpable tumor in the breast, the incidence of axillary metastases will be low. Unfortunately this is not always true. My patient whose mammogram is shown in Figure 5–42 had no palpable breast tumor and no palpable axillary nodes, yet at operation 15 of 45 axillary nodes were

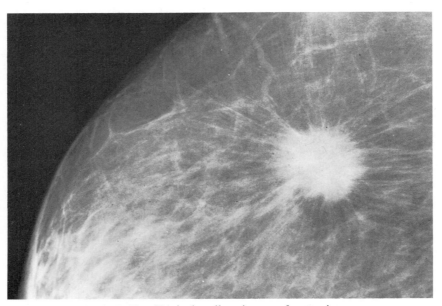

Figure 5–39.   Typical stellate image of a carcinoma.

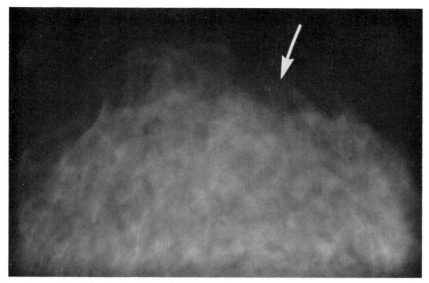

Figure 5–40.   A small area of stippling with five minute microcalcifications situated superficially in the breast to the right of center in the photograph (the reader should use a magnifying glass in studying them). This was the only indication of the patient's carcinoma. She did not have a palpable tumor.

found to contain metastases and she shortly succumbed to her disease.

The demonstration of these microcalcifications is not easy. The mammograms must be of very good quality. Artifacts in the processing of films simulate them. Figures 5–43 and 5–44 show two types of such artifacts.

Other forms of calcification revealed in the breast by mammography can be ignored.

Coarser small masses of calcium appearing in clumps or as isolated foci in the breast, as illustrated in Figure 5–45, presumably represent degenerative changes in ducts or small cysts and do not require biopsy. Old adenofibromas sometimes contain a great deal of calcium (Fig. 5–46). The walls of blood vessels in the breasts are occasionally calcified, and phleboliths are sometimes seen.

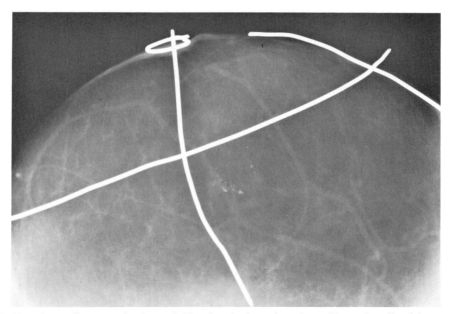

Figure 5–41.   A small area of microcalcification in intraductal papilloma localized by crossed wires placed upon the breast. There was no palpable tumor.

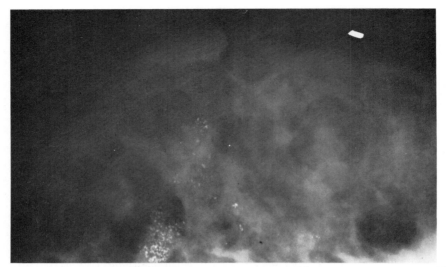

Figure 5-42. Extensive microcalcification produced by carcinoma. There was no palpable tumor.

Leborgne's book, published in 1953, is the classic work on mammography. Recently two excellent atlases of mammography have become available, one by Egan and the other by Baclesse and Willemin. The latter consists of reproductions of outstanding quality of a series of carefully selected mammograms.

While there is no doubt about the fact that mammography will detect a small proportion of carcinomas of the breast that cannot be found by clinical examination, it must be emphasized that the method has disadvantages. The most important of these is the fact that many carcinomas that are demonstrable by clinical examination are not detectable by mammography—as in 20 of 24 patients in Strax's series of cases. The exact proportion of these false negatives depends upon a

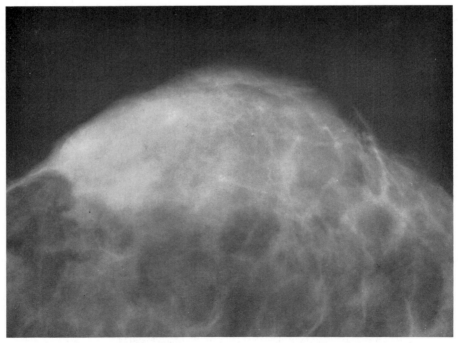

Figure 5-43. Artifacts consisting of groups of minute punctate densities with streaks of increased density radiating from them.

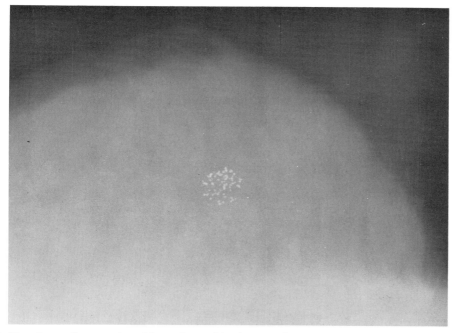

Figure 5–44. An artifact produced by a drop of barium on the cassette, simulating microcalcification.

Figure 5–45. Coarse small masses and clumps of calcium of no important significance.

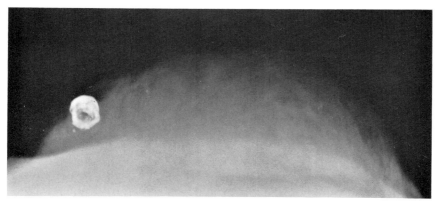

Figure 5–46. Calcified adenofibroma.

variety of factors, but it is so high that mammography cannot be relied upon as a method for detecting breast cancer. Physicians must learn that any patient in whom the physical findings suggest the reasonable possibility of carcinoma must have a biopsy, even though the mammogram is normal. It follows that physicians must not omit palpation of the breast and rely upon mammography alone, as some of them are now doing. We have seen a number of tragic cases in which a clinically obvious carcinoma was ignored for a long time because mammograms were reported as negative.

The opposite situation, namely over-diagnosis of mammograms when there is no clinical evidence of breast disease, is leading to a good many unnecessary biopsies. Although the finding of microcalcifications makes biopsy mandatory, the areas of increased density so often seen in mammograms are very difficult to interpret.

The question that we have to answer is how best to use mammography in helping us diagnose breast carcinoma in patients who consult us for presumed breast disease. The method has its greatest value in detecting small carcinomas in large fatty breasts in older women. Perhaps in such patients, particularly when they belong to the groups predisposed to have breast carcinoma that I have described in an earlier chapter, it is worthwhile to supplement the initial clinical examination of the breasts with mammography.

As a screening method for breast disease to be used in unselected women, or in the routine follow-up examination of patients who have no clinical evidence of breast carcinoma, mammography has not proved its value. I doubt that our society can afford $35,000 for mammography (mammograms today cost a minimum of $35 each) to detect one carcinoma of the breast in every thousand women examined, even though the disease is found at an earlier stage than if diagnosed later on by the usual clinical methods. More important is the fact that I do not believe that it is possible to persuade women to return for follow-up examination as often as they should if *both* mammography and clinical examination are required. All women over the age of 30 should have their breasts examined at least every six months as part of a general physical examination, and women who are predisposed to develop breast cancer should have a breast examination every three months.

XEROGRAPHY. Wolfe has claimed that xeroradiography of the breast, using a selenium plate, has several advantages over mammography with x-ray film. The method requires only 40 per cent of the radiation necessary for conventional mammograms, and provides an image of all breast structures, with a high degree of contrast.

THERMOGRAPHY. Lawson, in 1958, and the Williams', in 1960, were the first to attempt to identify disease in the breast by means of its infrared radiation. Dodd and his associates have recently reported their findings in studying the breasts of 4726 patients with this method. Their evidence as to the diagnostic value of thermography is not convincing.

ISOTOPE STUDIES. Studies of breast carcinoma have been made with several radioactive isotopes, with the hope of demonstrating their concentration in tumor tissue. McCorkle and Low-Beer studied the uptake of radioactive phosphorus in a variety of breast lesions, including carcinoma, but were unable to demonstrate differences of diagnostic significance.

The Tentative Diagnosis

When the clinical history and the examination of the breast have been completed, the physician must decide as best he can whether he is dealing with a harmless physiologic condition such as increased nodularity of the breast, or with real disease of the breast. For the former, nothing is required but reassurance. For the latter, steps must be taken to prove the presence and nature of the presumed disease. There are certain phenomena which are definite indications of disease in the breast, and which it is not safe to ignore. They are:

1. *A dominant tumor.* With certain infrequent exceptions which I will mention in dealing separately with cystic disease, adenosis, and so forth, a dominant tumor always requires investigation.

2. *Marked increase in the size and firmness* of one breast.

3. *Retraction signs*: dimpling of the skin, distortion of the contour of the breast, decrease in its mobility on the chest wall,

shrinkage of the breast, narrowing of the areola, deviation of the axis of the nipple, or retraction of the nipple.

4. *Redness or edema* of the skin over the breast.

5. *A spontaneous nipple discharge,* either serous, bloody, or watery, not accompanied by a palpable tumor, presents a special problem which I shall discuss later in chapters dealing with papilloma and with carcinoma.

6. *Change in the epithelium* of the surface of the nipple.

7. *Characteristic mammographic evidence* of breast disease.

Having tentatively determined that his patient has breast disease, the physician should next try to identify the disease. This is still more difficult. None of the symptoms and clinical signs that I have mentioned are pathognomonic. There are a number of benign lesions of the breast that simulate carcinoma more or less closely—a low-grade abscess, traumatic fat necrosis, duct ectasia, adenosis. Any of these may form a hard, poorly delimited tumor of the breast with skin dimpling. The circumscribed type of carcinoma, on the other hand, may seem as well delimited as a cyst. Nevertheless, it is a good intellectual discipline for the examiner to write down his tentative diagnosis when he has completed his history and examination. In this way he has a record of his mistake, if subsequent biopsy proves him wrong.

In the last analysis, experience is the only answer to the difficulties of the interpretation of clinical findings in the breast. This means experience in the clinical examination of the breast, strictly disciplined by accurate pathologic study of tissue removed for biopsy, and checked by follow-up reports of the patient's subsequent course. For every physician the accumulation of this kind of disciplined experience is an individual educational achievement. If he has a good pathologist and a good case record system to help him, and if he has the required intellectual honesty and humility, he will steadily improve his diagnostic skill.

Proving the Diagnosis

What the patient and surgeon both require, however, is not a tentative diagnosis, but a definitive one. The surgeon must have *proof* of the nature of the disease because his therapy is so different for different lesions. Benign lesions, in general, require only harmless limited local excision, whereas carcinoma requires a formidable and mutilating operation that must never be performed needlessly. There is no half-way therapeutic ground, such as partial or simple mastectomy, in which the surgeon can take refuge in his dilemma. *The truth is that the only kind of evidence upon which a surgeon can wholly rely today is pathologic.*

The form which this proof of the nature of breast disease takes depends upon the natural history and manifestations of the several common breast diseases. On the basis of my training and experience as both a clinician and a pathologist I have learned to proceed as follows in proving the diagnosis.

1. If the patient is under the age of 25, and her tumor has the rounded, well delimited character of an adenofibroma, and is very movable in the surrounding breast tissue, it is reasonably safe to assume that it is an adenofibroma. This means that the patient and her parents can be reassured, and the tumor removed at a convenient later date. Cysts, as well as carcinomas, are so rare in women under the age of 25 that this delay in obtaining pathologic proof of the nature of the lesion is reasonable. No harm would be done in the rare circumstance of the lesion being a cyst. The chance of missing a carcinoma, a lesion equally rare at this early age, is diminished by the fact that a carcinoma does not usually have the clinical characteristics of an adenofibroma.

2. If the patient is 25 or older and has not reached the menopause, and her tumor is rounded and well delimited, and movable in the surrounding breast tissue—thus presenting the clinical characteristics of a cyst— I anesthetize the skin with Novocain and insert a 20 gauge needle on a syringe into it. If I withdraw the characteristic cyst fluid, and no definite palpable evidence of disease remains, I am satisfied that I have reasonable proof that the lesion is a cyst. I do not examine the cyst fluid microscopically, because I have learned that it is a waste of time. I will discuss the validity of the aspiration method of diagnosing and treating cysts in Chapter 7.

3. Biopsy, and microscopic study of the lesion, is necessary to prove the diagnosis for all other lesions of the breast. The only question is what form the biopsy should take. A number of different methods of obtaining tissue are in use.

Aspiration Biopsy. Aspiration biopsy has been advocated by the Memorial Hospital group for some years and has gained some adherents. The procedure is ordinarily carried out in the surgeon's office before the patient has entered the hospital. After local anesthesia, a large-bore needle attached to a syringe is inserted into the tumor and, while suction is exerted, is withdrawn and advanced several times, sucking up a core of tumor cells into the bore of the needle. The material thus obtained is smeared on a glass slide and fixed and stained. In this manner, a fairly accurate impression of the cell types of the tumor is gained, although the details of cell structure are distorted by the crudity of the fixation and staining.

All such preparations give very little information, however, as to the cellular arrangement and the general architecture of the lesion. The pathologist is forced to rely solely on cytology, and usually upon poor cytology. This is a great handicap. For example, in distinguishing certain better differentiated types of carcinoma of the breast from benign epithelial proliferation, the arrangement of the cells within the ducts, as well as their invasive character, is just as important as the type of cells. Aspiration biopsy does not provide this crucial information. This is the main reason why Dr. Stout and I, working together at this problem over a period of years, came to believe that aspiration or trocar biopsy was not a reliable method of diagnosing lesions in the breast.

There is also a theoretical objection to needle biopsy on the ground of its roughness. A good deal of force is required to plunge a large-bore needle into the firm structure of mammary carcinoma—and this is exerted not once but several times. We fear that this trauma may squeeze carcinoma emboli into veins. If our emphasis on gentleness in manipulating carcinoma of the breast means anything, we should avoid a method as rough as aspiration biopsy.

A final objection to aspiration biopsy is that success with this method becomes more and more difficult as the carcinoma diminishes in size. It is difficult indeed to hit with the point of the aspirating needle a nodule located in the depths of the breast and measuring only 4 or 5 mm. in diameter. Yet, as the education of women in the detection of tumors of the breast improves, lesions of this size are seen more and more frequently. It is just in such difficult diagnoses, when one

must have a reliable method of proving the nature of the tumor, that the aspiration will most often fail. We have seen a number of patients in whom aspiration biopsy had been performed by an experienced aspirator, a specimen obtained which did not show carcinoma, and a reassuring opinion given; yet the subsequent course of events proved that carcinoma was present and had certainly been missed by the aspirating needle. In his defense of aspiration biopsy Robbins does not discuss the patients whose carcinomas were missed by aspiration biopsy and who subsequently went to other clinics where the correct diagnosis was made by incisional biopsy.

Trocar or Trephine Biopsy. Surgeons have devised a variety of trocars and trephines for boring out small cores of tissue from breast lesions. With them it is possible to obtain a somewhat better specimen that can be fixed, embedded, and cut in the usual way. In 1938, Silverman introduced the needle that bears his name and it has come to be widely used for biopsy. Christiansen, at the Copenhagen Radium Centre, began to use a similar instrument to biopsy breast tumors in 1939, and Kaae has reported that the use of this method has not had an unfavorable effect upon prognosis.

Ackermann, at our Delafield Hospital, has devised a good trocar with which a small core of tissue can be obtained.

All of these techniques have the disadvantage that they provide only a comparatively small specimen of the lesion, in which the architecture is not well shown, and such questions as invasion remain doubtful. The microscopic evidence is just not good enough.

Trocar and trephine biopsy also face the same objection as aspiration biopsy when the lesion is very small, namely, that they may miss it.

We use trocar biopsy only in special circumstances, as for example, in an aged and feeble patient, when the tumor is to be irradiated and the radiotherapist demands proof of its nature.

Intraductal Biopsy. Leborgne in Montevideo has devised a set of small instruments, dilators and loop curettes, which he inserts through the nipple ducts to reach the lesions and to secure small fragments of them. These fragments are sectioned and stained in the usual way.

I have already pointed out that *papillary*

lesions in the breast are among the most difficult to distinguish as benign or malignant, and that only a full-sized and carefully prepared histologic section is adequate.

Smears of Nipple Secretion. Sporadic attempts have been made to make diagnoses from smears of nipple secretion, but with indifferent success.

Saphir, in 1950, studied smears of nipple secretion in a series of 90 patients with spontaneous nipple discharge. He showed that the study of smears permits the diagnosis of papilloma as well as carcinoma in a considerable proportion of cases, but pointed out that he made some false positive as well as false negative reports.

Jackson and his associates in 1951 reported a study of nipple secretion obtained by *expression.* They attempted to express secretion from both breasts of every patient who came with a complaint referable to either breast. They make the point that they used only *gentle* pressure, yet they obtained secretion in 77 per cent of the breasts thus examined. Although they were able to demonstrate tumor cells in a considerable proportion of patients with intraductal papillomas and carcinomas, they could not differentiate these two lesions from each other by the study of smears.

Papanicolaou and his associates, in 1958, reported the most extensive study of nipple secretion *expressed* from the breasts of women who had no symptoms of breast disease as well as those who had such symptoms. Smears were studied from 726 breasts in 510 patients in the latter group. To obtain nipple secretion, the authors state, "the breast was subjected to gentle massage directed toward the areola. If secretion did not appear during palpation or massage, a hand breast pump was used to create mild suction over the areolar area." Only one carcinoma was discovered by the cytologic study of nipple secretions obtained in this manner from a total of 613 breasts in patients with no breast complaints. In this one patient, however, there was "minimal thickening under the areola" of the breast in which the carcinoma was found. In a series of 45 breasts with microscopically proved carcinoma the smear studies missed the disease in 31 per cent.

I have two objections to the use of smears of nipple secretion in the diagnosis of breast disease. The first is concerned with the *expression* of secretion for such smears. I have always emphasized that every kind of manipulation of a breast suspected of containing disease should be avoided, for fear of producing metastases from a possible carcinoma. I know enough about the heavy-handedness of many examiners not to trust them to attempt to express nipple secretion from the breasts of patients with disease.

Secondly, there is no doubt that the smear technique is not a reliable method of diagnosis. Smears often fail to reveal carcinoma when it is present in the breast, and they may give false positive diagnoses of carcinoma when it is not present. We have seen several errors of this kind. They are due to the fact that in the apocrine type of benign epithelial proliferation in the breast the epithelial cells sometimes enlarge and develop huge, atypical hyperchromatic nuclei. In smears they so closely resemble carcinoma cells that even the most skilled pathologist may be deceived. Figure 5–47 shows such abnormal carcinoma-like cells in an area of entirely benign intraductal papillary proliferation of the apocrine type. Figure 5–48 shows deceptively carcinoma-like cells in a smear of nipple secretion from the breast containing this lesion.

Incisional Biopsy. We prefer incisional biopsy and frozen section as the method of choice in proving the nature of tumors of the breast. Our procedure is as follows. The diagnostic problem is discussed fully with the patient, as gently and as hopefully as possible. Her consent is obtained for radical mastectomy, should it be required. She is admitted to the hospital and all preparations are made for the radical operation. The surgical pathologist often sees and examines the patient before operation. He is regularly present in the operating room when the biopsy is done. We use general anesthesia. Local anesthesia puts the patient on the rack of suspense while the diagnosis is being made.

If the tumor is presumed to be a carcinoma a small incision, 3 or 4 cm. in length, is made through the skin over it, and deepened to expose its surface. If the tumor is thought to be benign the incision is placed as indicated in Chapter 6. All vessels are meticulously caught with mosquito clamps and tied with fine silk, so that the wound is perfectly dry and the surgeon is able to see the cut surface of the lesion as he incises it. If the tumor is solid, a small wedge, measuring about 3 by 5 mm., is excised. This is ordinarily adequate for our frozen section. On infrequent occasions when the microscopic diagnosis is

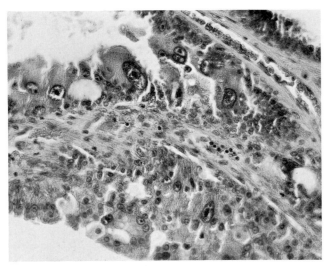

Figure 5–47. Atypical gigantic cells in the apocrine type of benign papillary epithelial proliferation of the breast.

difficult, the pathologist may ask for a second small wedge of tissue. We do not excise the whole tumor for diagnosis unless it is a very small one, measuring only a few millimeters in diameter, for we believe that the practice adds unnecessarily to the risk of producing metastasis. If the carcinoma is several centimeters in diameter, the line of local excision around its gross limits will cut across veins and lymphatics of considerable size which may carry off cancer emboli.

Excision of the entire tumor for biopsy is, however, the general practice throughout our country. Harrington, for example, stated "The tumor should be removed by wide excision, well away from the limits of the growth...." Saphir also recommended this

procedure. The usual argument in favor of this practice is that there is less chance of causing metastasis if the line of excision is around and not through the tumor. This reasoning does not have the support of pathology. We know that carcinoma frequently infiltrates far beyond the grossly visible limits of the disease and that no surgeon can hope that a local excision will get beyond it.

Since we cannot avoid cutting through carcinoma whether we incise the tumor and remove a tiny wedge, or excise the tumor as a whole, it seems reasonable to perform the smallest possible procedure which will yield a diagnosis. A tiny wedge almost always suffices. We have not had the experience that the structure of neoplasms of the breast is apt to differ much in different parts of the tumor. It is essential, of course, that the surgeon know enough gross pathology to be able to recognize disease in the breast when he exposes it, and that he have a meticulous enough surgical technique to enable him to keep the biopsy wound dry so that he can see the lesion.

A frozen section is made from a portion of the wedge biopsy. We cut a block of tissue of sufficient size to show the architecture of the tumor. We do *not* depend on a section so small that only a few cells are shown.

Although we believe that frozen sections made in this manner provide adequate microscopic evidence, we have learned that there is one type of neoplasm in the breast in which nothing except a good paraffin section

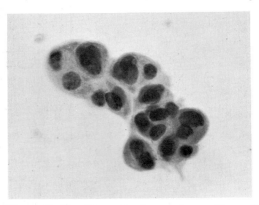

Figure 5–48. Deceptively carcinoma-like cells in a smear of nipple secretion from a breast containing benign intraductal papillary proliferation.

suffices. This is the papillary type of neoplasm. It is so difficult to distinguish papillary carcinoma from papilloma microscopically that all papillary lesions that are not grossly typical intraductal papillomas should be regarded as too difficult for frozen section diagnosis. Preliminary biopsy as a separate operative procedure, and careful study of paraffin sections, should precede any definite operative therapy.

There are rare occasions when the frozen-section method will fail to give an immediate diagnosis because the microscopic picture is confused by the presence of inflammation or by the variety and richness of the epithelial proliferation. The well-differentiated carcinomas, of course, give the most difficulty. On the rare occasions when the pathologist cannot be certain what the lesion is, the surgeon closes the wound and waits for paraffin section, available in 24 hours. *He does not proceed with mastectomy without being certain of his diagnosis.*

The surgeon who performs a radical mastectomy merely on the suspicion that he is dealing with a carcinoma, because he feels that it is not safe to wait until a definitive diagnosis is made, is using poor judgment and may mutilate his patient needlessly. A reasonable delay does not apparently prejudice the patient's chance of cure. We attempted to study this question in our clinic but found that the prognosis was better in patients in whom radical mastectomy was delayed. The explanation for this was apparently the fact that the well-differentiated carcinomas that have, of course, a better prognosis are the ones in which frozen sections are more often inadequate and definitive treatment must wait for permanent sections.

Siemens reported that in a series of 45 patients at Kiel, from 10 to 45 days elapsed between the biopsy and radical mastectomy, yet the cure rate was comparatively high. Jackson and Pitts, in Vancouver, had the same experience in a series of 51 patients in which the delay averaged 18.4 days. Scheel, in Oslo, found that biopsy performed several days before radical operation had no untoward effect upon the results in a series of 300 cases.

While we do not, of course, recommend delaying operation when it can be done at once, this evidence justifies delay that is unavoidable, as, for instance, when the frozen sections do not yield a definite diagnosis, or when a pathologist is not available to prepare frozen sections and the surgeon has no other course but to excise tissue for biopsy and send it to a pathologist in the community for a 24 hour paraffin section.

Simple mastectomy as an alternative procedure when the biopsy fails to yield an immediate microscopic diagnosis is, in our opinion, equally unwise. If the lesion finally proves to be benign, removal of the breast is unnecessary. If it proves to be a carcinoma, a simple mastectomy spoils the field, speaking in a technical sense, for a proper radical mastectomy, besides putting the patient through an additional major operation.

To return to the surgeon in the operating room who has just received word from the pathologist that the frozen section shows carcinoma, I recommend that he close his biopsy wound by suturing it tightly with a continuous running suture without disturbing the gauze packing that he left in the wound when he removed his biopsy. Since the danger of blood oozing from the biopsy wound and carrying cancer cells into the operative field of the subsequent radical mastectomy is very real, I seal the biopsy wound with a large patch of rubber dam cemented in place with a good cement.

Biopsies of breast tumors should not be performed in a physician's office, or in the out-patient department of a hospital, as has recently been recommended by Abramson. My objections are several, the most important being that when biopsy is done in this hasty and informal manner, usually by physicians without adequate training and experience, the lesion is not carefully described clinically, nor are proper records made, and the patient herself remains unaware of the possibility that she has serious disease, and has made no preparation for it. All patients who require biopsy of a breast tumor must have a full explanation of what they face, and should be admitted to a hospital bed within a reasonable time. There is such a shortage of hospital beds in many cities today that some delay is inevitable. For myself, I have set ten days as a reasonable limit to delay. If I cannot get my patient into my hospital within this period I send her to a colleague who can get her into his hospital.

Biopsy of Lesions of the Nipple. Lesions of the nipple epithelium—thickening, reddening, erosion—which are not accompanied by a palpable tumor in the breast may quite properly be biopsied in a physician's office or in the out-patient department. The extent of this kind of biopsy is so limited that it seems unreasonable to assume that there is any danger of producing metastases even if the lesion is Paget's carcinoma. Moreover, permanent sections are required for this type of biopsy and delay of a few days is inevitable. I inject a little novocaine at the base of a nipple, and with a small knife I excise a wedge of the abnormal epithelium about 3 mm. wide and deep. If this practice of immediate office biopsy of all suspicious changes in the nipple epithelium were followed, the long delay that usually occurs in the diagnosis of Paget's carcinoma would be eliminated.

Biopsy for Retraction Signs. I have stated previously that skin retraction and nipple retraction are signs of breast disease that must not be ignored. When they occur without any accompanying breast tumor they pose a special diagnostic problem. I have learned from experience that these retraction signs by themselves do not justify biopsy. In fear of missing carcinoma I have performed biopsy in several such cases, carefully excising the breast tissue beneath the area of retraction. I have found no evidence of disease in these cases. I have two other patients, both with marked localized skin retraction but no accompanying tumor, in whom I have not done a biopsy but have only re-examined them at appropriate intervals for more than ten years. No change has occurred. I assume that the retraction in these patients is due to fibrosis following fat necrosis in the distant past. My practice today is therefore to follow patients with retraction signs but no tumor very carefully, but not to perform biopsy.

THE FOLLOW-UP OF PATIENTS PREDISPOSED TO BREAST CARCINOMA

Physicians must not only be expert in diagnosing breast disease in patients who consult them with its symptoms. They should try to follow up all their patients systematically, with the aim of detecting breast carcinoma at an early stage should it develop in them. This is, of course, an almost impossible ideal because there are not enough physicians and not enough time to achieve it. Yet we can try as best we can.

For women in general who are not predisposed to breast carcinoma, we recommend that the breast be carefully palpated as part of a general physical examination to be carried out twice a year.

But for the women who are predisposed to develop breast carcinoma the problem is much more difficult. Elsewhere I have identified six different groups of women in whom the risk of breast cancer is significantly increased. They are:

1. The women whose breast physiology has been atypical. This includes women who have had no children, or if they have had children have had them comparatively late in life, and have had only a few. It also includes those who have not nursed their children for a considerable length of time. It is not possible to express in simple statistical terms the increased risk of breast cancer in these women, although Dunn has tried to do so; but there is no doubt about the fact that they are predisposed to develop the disease (see Chapter 21).

2. Familial breast carcinoma (sister, mother, or aunt), twice the expected incidence and 11 years earlier.

3. Previous carcinoma in one breast, seven times the expected incidence.

4. Gross cystic disease, four times the expected incidence.

5. Lobular neoplasia, (lobular carcinoma *in situ*), six (?) times the expected incidence within 25 years.

6. Multiple intraductal papilloma, seven times the expected incidence.

The women in these six different groups deserve special consideration in terms of follow-up. The women in group 1, who are in less peril than the others, must be kept track of, and without fail their breasts must be examined at least twice a year.

Ideally, the women in the other five groups should be examined every three months. If this were done most of their carcinomas would be detected in an early and curable stage.

When should these regular breast examinations begin for these women predisposed to breast cancer? For the women in groups 1 and 2, they should begin when they reach the age at which the disease has a considerable frequency—approximately 35 years. For the women in groups 3 to 6 these frequent breast examinations should begin when they first develop the breast disease which predisposes them to breast carcinoma. Since the disease is increasingly frequent with advancing age, this routine of frequent examination should be continued for life.

When the breasts must be examined as frequently as I have suggested, there is only one practical method — inspection and palpation. It takes only 15 minutes. It requires no equipment. It can therefore be done for a minimal fee, so that it is within the reach of almost all women. I myself have charged from $5 to $15 for this service. Mammography repeated three or four times a year will cost between $100 and $200 annually, which is more than most patients can afford for this purpose. Moreover, mammography should not be repeated very often because of the irradiation hazard involved. Repetition several times a year over a period of many years is out of the question. An equally important objection is the time and bother that mammography requires. Mammography requires perhaps an hour for the whole process of taking the films and checking their adequacy. It is not at all a simple process.

The physician's task of convincing his predisposed patients of the necessity of this routine of frequent breast examination, and of carrying it out expertly over a long period of years, is not an easy one. He must educate his patients and convince them of the importance of regular breast examination, without alarming them and making them hypochondriacs. Patients must not be frightened or bullied into returning for follow-up examination. As the physician wins the confidence, and often the friendship, of his patients the task becomes easier. Yet both parties are apt to be bored by these endless examinations. I find that no matter how hard I try to achieve the ideal of this kind of follow-up of patients predisposed to breast cancer, I eventually fail with many patients. They return faithfully for a few years and then I hear no more of them. When such a patient turns up with a well-advanced carcinoma I am conscience-stricken.

This sequence is so real to me that I try my best to persuade my patients to come for routine breast examinations as I have outlined here. My reward is that I occasionally find an early carcinoma which is easily cured.

REFERENCES

Abramson, D. J.: 857 Breast biopsies as an out-patient procedure: delayed mastectomy in 41 malignant cases. Ann. Surg., *163*:478, 1966.

Baclesse, F., and Willemin, A.: Atlas de Mammographie, Paris, Lib. de la faculté des Sciences, 1965.

Berg, J. W., and Robbins, G. F.: A late look at the safety of aspiration biopsy. Cancer, *15*:826, 1962.

Brill, R., and Koprowska, I: Diagnosis of early carcinoma of the breast by the Papanicolaou technic. Am. J. Surg., *90*:1016, 1955.

Christiansen, H.: An aspiration trepan for tissue biopsy. Acta radiol., *21*:348, 1940.

Copeland, M. M., and Higgins, T. G.: Significance of discharge from the nipple in nonpuerperal mammary conditions. Ann. Surg., *151*:638, 1960.

Corry, D. C.: Pain in carcinoma of the breast. Lancet, *1*:274, 1952.

Cutler, M.: Transillumination of the breast. Ann. Surg., *93*:223, 1931.

Day, E.: Personal communication.

Dodd, G. D., et al.: Thermography and cancer of the breast. Cancer, *23*:797, 1969.

Dunn, J. E.: Epidemiology and possible identification of high-risk groups that could develop cancer of the breast. Cancer, *23*:755, 1969.

Egan, R. L.: Fifty-three cases of carcinoma of the breast, occult until mammography. Am. J. Roentgen., *88*:1095, 1962.

Egan, R. L.: Mammography. Springfield, Ill., Charles C Thomas, 1964.

Gibson, A., and Smith, G.: Aspiration biopsy of breast tumours. Brit. J. Surg., *45*:236, 1957.

Gilbertsen, V. A.: Improving breast cancer prognoses. Geriatrics, *21*:128, 1966.

Goode, J. V., McNeill, J. P., and Gordon, C. E.: Routine aspiration of discrete breast cysts. Arch. Surg., *70*:686, 1955.

Griesbach, A. A., and Eads, W. S.: Experience with screening for breast carcinoma. Cancer, *19*:1548, 1966.

Harrington, S. W.: Diagnosis and treatment of lesions of the breast. Am. J. Cancer, *19*:56, 1933.

Harris, D. L., Greening, W. P., and Aichroth, P. M.: Infra-red in the diagnosis of a lump in the breast. Brit. J. Cancer, *20*:710, 1966.

Hassler, O.: Microradiographic investigations of calcifications of the female breast. Cancer, *23*:1103, 1969.

Hicken, N. F., Best, R. R., Hunt, H. B., and Harris, T. T.: The roentgen visualization and diagnosis of breast lesions by means of contrast media. Am. J. Roentgenol., *39*:321, 1938.

Hinchey, P. R.: Nipple discharge: Clinicopathologic study. Ann. Surg., *113*:341, 1941.

Holleb, A. I., Venet, L., and Hoyt, S.: Breast cancer detected by routine physical examination. Three year survey of the Strang Cancer Prevention Clinic. New York J. Med., *60*:823, 1960.

Holmquist, D. G., and Papanicolaou, G. N.: The exfoliative cytology of the mammary gland during pregnancy and lactation. Ann. New York Acad. Sc., *63*:1422, 1956.

Huguenin, R.: Intérêt et valeur de la transillumination dans le diagnostic des lésions de la mamelle. Bull. Assoc. franç. p. l'étude du cancer. *27*:496, 1938.

Jackson, D., and Severance, A. O.: Cytological study of nipple secretions. An aid in the diagnosis of breast lesions. Texas State J. Med., *41*:512, 1946.

Jackson, D., and Severance, A. O.: The plateau test in breast carcinoma. Texas State J. Med., *40*:328, 1944.

Jackson, D., Todd, D. A., and Gorsuch, P. L.: Study of breast secretion for detection of intramammary pathologic change and of silent papilloma. J. Internat. Coll. Surgeons, *15*:552, 1951.

Jackson, P. P., and Pitts, H. H.: Biopsy and delayed radical mastectomy for carcinoma of the breast. Amer. J. Surg., 98:184, 1959.

Kaae, S.: The risk involved by biopsy in breast cancer. Acta radiol., 37:469, 1952.

Lawson, R. N.: A new infrared imaging device. Canad. M.A.J., 79:402, 1958.

Leborgne, R. A.: The Breast in Roentgen Diagnosis. Montevideo, Imp. Uruguaya, S.A., 1953.

Leborgne, R.: Intraductal biopsy of certain pathologic processes of the breast. Surgery, 19:47, 1946.

Leborgne, R.: Diagnosis of tumors of the breast by simple roentgenography. Am. J. Roentgenol., 65:1, 1951.

Leborgne, R.: Estudio Anátomo-Radiológico de los Tumores Intracanaliculares de la Mama. Montevideo, Centenario-Augusta S. C., 1951.

Lewison, E. F., and Chambers, R. G.: Clinical significance of nipple discharge. J.A.M.A., 147:295, 1951.

Lydgate, W. A.: Does your family doctor give you adequate physical examinations? Today's Woman, Sept., 1951.

Macfarlane, C., Sturgis, M. C., and Fetterman, F. S.: Results of an experiment in the control of cancer of the female pelvic organs and report of a fifteen-year research. Am. J. Obst, & Gynec., 69:294, 1955.

McCorkle, H. J., Low-Beer, B. V. A., Bell, H. G., and Stone, R. S.: Clinical and laboratory studies on the uptake of radioactive phosphorus by lesions of the breast. Surgery, 24:409, 1948.

McLaughlin, C. W., Jr., and Coe, J. D.: A study of nipple discharge in the nonlactating breast. Ann. Surg., 157:810, 1963.

McNair, T. J., and Dudley, H. A. F.: Axillary lymph nodes in patients without breast carcinoma. Lancet, 1:713, 1960.

McPherson, V. A., and MacKenzie, W. C.: Lesions of the breast associated with nipple discharge. Canad. J. Surg., 5:6, 1962.

Mercier, J., and Redon, H.: La valeur diagnostique des écoulements par le mamelon. Semaine d. hôp. Paris, Ann. Chir., 13:745, 1959.

Mouriquand, J., and Dargent, M.: L'empreinte mammaire: étude cytopathologique. Bull. Assoc. franç. p. l'étude du cancer, 44:449, 1957.

Papanicolaou, G. N.: Atlas of Exfoliative Cytology. Cambridge, Harvard University Press, (for Commonwealth Fund) 1954.

Papanicolaou, G. N., Holmquist, D. G., Bader, G. M., and Falk, E. A.: Exfoliative cytology of the human mammary gland. Cancer, 11:377, 1958.

Phillips, M. A., and Miller, J.: Incidence of breast pathology in well women. Illinois M. J., 102:176, 1952.

River, L., et al.: Carcinoma of the breast: The diagnostic significance of pain. Am. J. Surg., 82:733, 1951.

Robbins, G. F., Brothers, J. H., III, Eberhart, W. F., and Quan, S.: Is aspiration biopsy of breast cancer dangerous to the patient? Cancer, 7:774, 1954.

Romano, S. A., and McFetridge, E. M.: Limitations and dangers of mammography by contrast mediums. J.A.M.A., 110:1905, 1938.

Rosemond, G. P., Burnett, W. E., and Caswell, H. T.: Aspiration of breast cysts as a diagnostic and therapeutic measure. Arch. Surg., 71:223, 1955.

Saltzstein, S. L.: Histologic diagnosis of breast carcinoma with the Silverman needle biopsy. Surgery, 48:366, 1960.

Sandblom, P., and Löfgren, F. O.: Diagnosis and treatment of the discharging nipple in the absence of a palpable tumour. Acta chir. Scandinav., 103:81, 1952.

Saphir, O.: Cytologic examination of breast secretions. Am. J. Clin. Path., 20:1001, 1950.

Saphir, O.: Early diagnosis of breast lesions. J.A.M.A., 150:859, 1952.

Scheel, A.: Some prognostic factors, particularly biopsy, in carcinoma of the breast. Acta radiol., 39:249, 1953.

Scheel, A.: The risk by excisional biopsy of cancer of the breast. Transactions of The Northern Surgical Association, Twenty-fifth meeting, Copenhagen, Ejnar Munksgaard, 1951.

Sicard, A., Flabeau, F., and Marsan, C.: Cyto-diagnostic des écoulements séro-sanglants par le mamelon. Presse méd., 63:111, 1955.

Siemens, W.: Der Einfluss der Probeexcision auf die Prognose des Mammacarcinoms. Arch. f. klin. Chir., 177:651, 1933.

Silverman, I.: A new biopsy needle. Am. J. Surg., 40:671, 1938.

Sparkman, R. S.: Reliability of frozen sections in the diagnosis of breast lesions. Ann. Surg., 155:924, 1962.

Stevens, G. M., and Weigen, J. F.: Mammography survey for breast cancer detection—a two year study of 1223 clinically negative asymptomatic women over forty. Cancer, 19:51, 1966.

Stout, A. P.: Observations on biopsy for diagnosis of tumors. Cancer, 10:912, 1957.

Strax, P., et al.: Mammography and clinical examination in mass screening. Cancer, 20:2184, 1967.

Tailhefer, A., and Pilleron, J. P.: 130 cas de 'mamelle saignante'. Mém. Acad. de chir., 82:612, 1956.

Walter, J., and Atkinson, E. C.: Early cancer detection and education: a pilot trial. Brit. M.J., 1:627, 1955.

Webster, A., et al.: Examination of the breasts and pelvic organs in apparently well women. Review of the findings in 1,600 women examined at the Cancer Prevention Clinic. Illinois M. J., 89:239, 1946.

Williams, K. L., Williams, F. J. L., and Handley, R. S.: Infra-red thermometry in the diagnosis of breast disease. Lancet, 2:1378, 1961.

Witten, D. M., and Thurber, D. L.: Mammography as a routine screening examination for detecting breast cancer. Am. J. Roentgenol., 92:14, 1964.

Wolfe, J. N.: Mammography as a screening examination in breast cancer. Radiology, 84:703, 1965.

Wolfe, J. N.: Mammography: errors in diagnosis. Radiology, 87:214, 1966.

Wolfe, J. N.: Xerography of the breast. Cancer, 23:791, 1969.

Chapter Six

The Technique of Excision of Benign Tumors of the Breast

A correct technique for the excision of benign tumors of the breast is a matter of great practical surgical importance, because these tumors are so common and because the results of the incorrect technique usually employed are so distressing cosmetically.

The surgeon's first duty is, of course, to expose, to diagnose, and usually to remove the lesion, doing as little harm as possible to the breast in the process. In keeping with this principle, it is the surgeon's duty to incise and suture the skin in a manner that will give the least visible scar. It is desirable to minimize the scar not only because a bad scar is ugly in itself, but because the modern patient, subjected to a good deal of propaganda regarding carcinoma of the breast, is reminded of this unpleasant possibility every time she notices her scar. If it is invisible, she avoids a good deal of mental anguish.

Unfortunately, a surgical tradition has developed, both in our country and abroad, of making radial incisions in operating upon the breast. Nothing could be worse. Radial incisions not only produce the worst possible scars, but they are entirely illogical. The reason for preferring them which is usually given is that they minimize damage to the ducts. In the first place, the ducts in the mature breast may be cut with impunity. I have severed all or part of the collecting ducts in many patients without any discernible late after-effects. In this regard Davis has reported a follow-up study of 24 patients in whom the ducts beneath the nipple were severed. There were no apparent after-effects. One patient subsequently bore three children and had no trouble in a breast in which the ducts had been severed. In the second place, the direction of the skin incision over the breast need have no relation to the direction of the incision in the breast parenchyma. A circular incision through the skin may give access to a radial incision into the breast if that is preferred. Personally, I am guided in incising the breast parenchyma only by my desire to find the most direct route through the breast tissue to the tumor.

In placing the skin incision, however, great care should be taken to follow the natural lines in the skin, which are the guides to the direction of the normal tension in the skin. Langer was the first to trace these lines in detail, and they are usually known as Langer's lines.

Incisions through the skin at right angles to these lines will gape, and the resultant scars will broaden and are apt to develop keloids. Incisions made parallel to or in these lines tend to fall together and give hair-line scars.

A good example of an ugly radial scar is shown in Figure 6–1. This young woman had

149

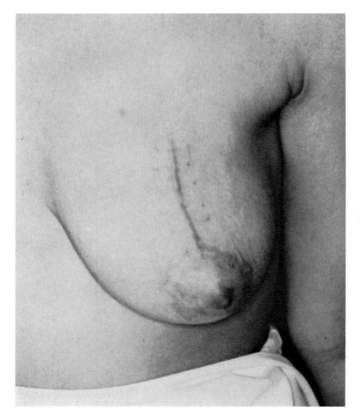

Figure 6–1. An ugly radial scar following excision of a breast cyst.

only a simple cyst which I would have treated by aspiration. But even if operation had been decided upon, biopsy of her tumor could perfectly well have been performed through a circumareolar incision that would have left virtually no scar. As it is her breast is badly disfigured for life. Since this operation she has become shy and introspective and has not married. What could have been a minor surgical procedure has become a personal tragedy for her.

I not infrequently see patients with several such radial scars subsequent to repeated operations for cystic disease. The appearance of their breasts has been ruined.

In contrast to radial scars, those resulting from incisions made in the skin lines and carefully approximated with fine suture material, are almost invisible. A circumareolar scar of this kind is shown in Figure 6–2.

Unfortunately, Langer did not work out the direction of the lines of skin tension over the female breast, nor have we found a satisfactory description of them from any other source. Figure 6–3 is a chart of these lines in the skin over the adult breast as I have determined them.

If a tumor is situated near the periphery of the upper part of the breast, far from the areola, at points *A, B,* or *C,* it is my custom to make curved incisions following Langer's lines, and to place them a little medial to the tumor. I prefer to place all incisions medial to the tumor, if it is at some distance from the center of the breast, as a precaution, should the lesion prove to be a carcinoma. It is advantageous to have the biopsy wound as near the center of the operative field as possible in planning the extent of a dissection for carcinoma.

For this same reason I rarely use a lateral paramammary incision, as at *H,* or an inframammary incision as at *I,* even though these incisions are very convenient for exposing tumors at the periphery of the breast, and even though they give good scars that are hidden from sight by the overlapping breast. If the tumor proves to be a carcinoma, the surgeon who has made a paramammary incision will have great difficulty in keeping his

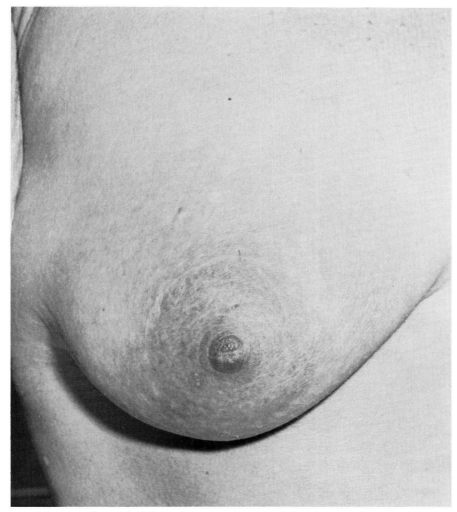

Figure 6–2.   An almost invisible circumareolar scar following excision of a breast cyst.

line of dissection sufficiently far away from the biopsy wound he must assume has been implanted with carcinoma cells. I make a paramammary incision only when I am certain the lesion is benign, and I cannot often have this degree of confidence in my clinical diagnosis.

If a tumor is situated midway between the periphery of the breast and the areola, as at points *D, E,* or *F,* and there is some suspicion that it is malignant, a curved incision directly over it or slightly medial to it is made. If, on the other hand, the clinical features of the tumor suggest that it is benign, a circumareolar incision is used.

The circumareolar incision is an exceedingly useful one. If it is correctly placed precisely at the edge of the areola, and if it is properly sutured, it eventually becomes

truly invisible, for the change in the color of the skin hides it. It is the preferred incision for all tumors near the edge of the areola, as at point *G,* and for tumors beneath the areola. In using it to expose presumably benign tumors situated some distance out from the edge of the areola, it is necessary to undercut a peripheral flap of skin and subcutaneous fat to reach and uncover the tumor.

The technique for using a circumareolar incision to expose a benign tumor at some distance from the areola is shown in Figures 6–4 to 6–6. The first step (Fig. 6–4) is to make a marking nick (*1*) in the edge of the areola at the center of the intended incision. This makes it possible to resuture the incision accurately. The circumareolar incision (*2, 3*) is then made through the skin around about half of the circumference of the areola. The cir-

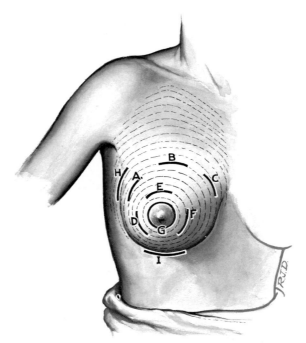

Figure 6–3. Langer's lines in the skin over the breast.

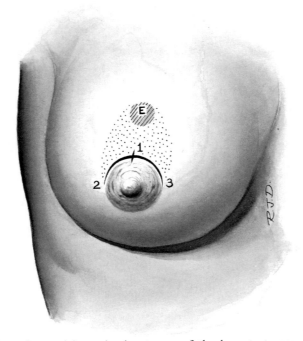

Figure 6–4. Technique for excising a benign tumor of the breast at some distance from the areola through a circumareolar incision. The incision has been made precisely at the edge of the areola.

cumareolar vein will be exposed, and its branches should be cut, clamped, and tied, as required. With the aid of skin hooks the peripheral edge of the incision is then elevated, and a flap, indicated by the dotted area, consisting of skin and the subcutaneous fat overlying the breast parenchyma, is dissected up to expose the tumor E (Fig. 6–5). This undercutting can be done with very little or no bleeding if the plane of dissection is kept just above the superficial fascia. When the flap has been undercut sufficiently, skin hooks are replaced with three small abdominal retractors to give satisfactory exposure of the breast parenchyma directly overlying the tumor (Fig. 6–6). This is then cut through to reach the tumor.

When the tumor has been exposed through an appropriate skin incision, and the wound has been got dry of blood so that it is possible to see the pathology as it is revealed, it is my practice to make a small incision into the lesion. If the cut surface seems characteristic of some benign type of tumor such as an adenofibroma, I proceed to excise the tumor, including a narrow rim of the surrounding normal breast parenchyma. If inspection of the cut surface leaves any doubt whatever in my mind about the nature of the tumor, I

excise only a small wedge, about 5 mm. wide and 10 mm. in length, to do a frozen section. I have had a long experience with the pathology of mammary lesions and am able to recognize some of them from their cut surface with a fair degree of accuracy. Surgeons who are less familiar with gross pathology will do well to excise a small wedge for frozen section from every tumor before going ahead with its excision.

In excising the various benign lesions of the breast I sacrifice as little of the normal surrounding breast tissue as possible. We do not believe that any of the benign lesions of the breast are precancerous in the sense that they are transformed into carcinoma. There is therefore no need to remove a wide margin of adjacent breast tissue in order to make certain that the benign lesion is excised in its entirety. It is better to leave some remnant of the lesion behind, since it is harmless, rather than to irreparably deform the breast. The primary reason for operating upon a benign lesion is to make certain that it is not malignant. A secondary purpose is to remove the gross tumor and to restore the breast to as normal a condition as possible — not to ruin it.

The lesion having been excised, I search the wound meticulously for bleeding vessels,

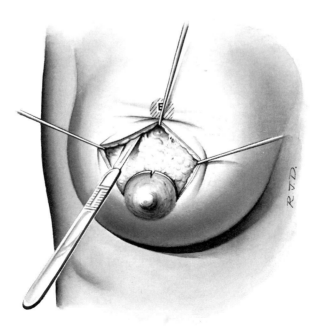

Figure 6–5. Technique for excising a benign tumor of the breast at some distance from the areola. The peripheral flap is being elevated with hooks, and undercut.

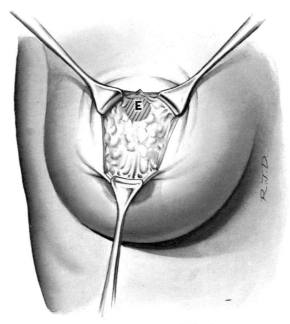

Figure 6–6. Technique for excising a benign tumor of the breast at some distance from the areola. The tumor at *E* is exposed and ready for excision.

and clamp and tie them with fine silk. I do not drain these wounds, preferring to devote a little extra time to achieving good hemostasis.

I have learned not to attempt to suture the breast parenchyma together in an effort to obliterate dead space after excising a tumor. No matter how carefully such deep sutures are placed, they deform the breast. This is because of its mobility. Sutures placed seemingly correctly in the breast flattened out on the chest wall as the patient lies supine on the operating table will prove to be wrongly placed and to cause distortion of the breast when the patient is erect and the breast is dependent.

All incisions through the skin over the breast should be closed with two layers of interrupted sutures. I use No. 00000 silk on small curved cutting needles (eye needles) for the deeper layer of sutures placed through the subcuticular tissue. When used for a circumareolar incision, these sutures also include the areolar muscle. The knots on these sutures must be tied precisely and tightly. Lying as they do just beneath the skin, the ends of the sutures must be cut flush upon the knots, and unless tied carefully, they will

loosen. This subcutaneous layer of sutures helps to keep the scar from widening after the superficial layer of interrupted sutures of No. 00000 nylon through the skin itself has been removed a week after operation.

I dress these wounds with a few gauze fluffs packed over the operative site, and a six-inch elastic bandage applied snugly but not tightly around the chest and fastened with small safety pins. No adhesive is used. A narrow cloth strap over the shoulder on the operative side holds this brassiere in place. I do not dress the wound for a week, at which time the supportive bandage is removed and the skin sutures are cut out.

Local excision of a breast tumor carried out according to this plan does not distort the breast. The skin incision is scarely visible. In occasional patients a postoperative hematoma will develop. It should be aspirated.

REFERENCE

Davis, H. H.: Effects on the breast of removal of the nipple or severing of the ducts. Arch. Surg., *58*:790, 1949.

Chapter Seven

Cystic Disease of the Breast

For more than a century, since the time that the English surgeons Sir Astley Cooper and Benjamin Brodie wrote of cystic disease of the breast, it has been recognized as the common benign lesion of the breast developing during middle age. The relationship of cystic disease to carcinoma has long been questioned, and it it still debated today. This makes cystic disease a subject worthy of thorough discussion.

The first comprehensive clinical and pathologic descriptions of cystic disease were written in France in the 1880's by Reclus and by Brissaud. Reclus' descriptions were so complete that in France, particularly, cystic disease has since borne his name. Reclus recognized the multiplicity of the cysts and the fact that both breasts are usually involved by the disease.

German surgeons turned their attention to cystic disease in the 1890's. Schimmelbusch discussed the disease in detail and it has since been called by his name in Germany. König wrote of the disease in 1893 and, believing it to be inflammatory in origin, called it *chronic cystic mastitis.* This name has been widely adopted, and remains one of the important handicaps to our understanding of the disease, for it leads to the false assumption that it is indeed inflammatory.

These French and German students of cystic disease not only gave it inexact names, but they failed to describe its pathological fea-

tures accurately. It must be admitted that this is not a simple task. Along with the cysts, which range from microscopic dilatations of ducts to large grossly evident thin-walled cavities, there are a great variety of forms of benign epithelial proliferation and fibrosis.

Definition

I prefer the simple term *cystic disease* for the lesion under discussion. The adjective *chronic,* while certainly expressing a truth regarding the natural history of the disease, makes the name unnecessarily complex. Cheatle's name, "cystiphorous desquamative epithelial hyperplasia," is the ultimate of prolixity. In the Scandinavian countries cystic disease is called "fibroadenomatosis." This is an unfortunate choice because it suggests to us the entirely different lesion, fibroadenoma.

In defining cystic disease it is first of all necessary to emphasize the fact that we are referring to a lesion characterized by *cysts*. If there are no cysts we do not classify the lesion as cystic disease. If the cysts are large enough to be easily visible, that is, 2 or 3 mm. or more in diameter, we refer to the lesion as "gross cystic disease;" if the cysts are seen only microscopically we use the term "microscopic cystic disease." There is no doubt that grossly evident cysts evolve from

155

microscopic cysts. The latter probably develop as the result of dilatation of ducts. From the point of view of their clinical significance, however, there is a fundamental difference between gross and microscopic cysts. Gross cysts often form a palpable tumor in the breast that can be detected clinically. We therefore have an approximate idea of the frequency of gross cysts. Their presence can be correlated with the subsequent development of carcinoma, and we are beginning to acquire some significant data on this question.

Microscopic cysts do not form a palpable tumor. They are discovered only by microscopic study of breast tissue that is excised when some other lesion is operated upon. We do not know how frequent they are in clinically normal breasts in living women. The result is that we do not know the significance of microscopic cysts in terms of the subsequent development of breast carcinoma. Autopsy studies do not help us answer this question.

A complex of microscopic changes usually accompanies cyst formation. Epithelial proliferation predominates, but fibrosis and atrophy also occur. The best description of these lesions is that which Foote and Stewart gave in connection with their study of the morphology of cancerous and noncancerous breasts. The most important of these benign lesions are: hyperplasia of duct epithelium, duct papillomatosis, blunt duct adenosis, apocrine metaplasia, and adenosis.

It must be emphasized that by themselves these microscopic lesions, like the microscopic cysts, which they often accompany, do not form a palpable tumor that can be detected clinically. They are diagnosed only microscopically. We therefore do not know their true frequency in normal breasts. Students of breast disease have not reported long term follow-up studies of women in which these microscopic lesions, not accompanied by gross cysts, were present. There is no solid evidence that the presence of these microscopic lesions by themselves predisposes to the development of breast carcinoma.

To return to my definition of cystic disease, it is, for the purposes of the present discussion, a lesion characterized by gross cysts with a characteristic natural history and morphology which I shall attempt to describe. By focusing upon the easily demonstrable gross cysts I hope to bring some order out of the confusion that surrounds cystic disease. Things have come to such a pass that most pathologists diagnose almost every specimen of breast tissue as showing "chronic cystic mastitis." The scrap basket that this diagnosis provides is an easy way of avoiding careful microscopic description and thoughtful classification of breast lesions.

There are several other types of breast cysts of quite different origin, that must be distinguished from those which are a manifestation of gross cystic disease as I have defined it. They are: (1) cysts containing inspissated milk—the so-called galactoceles; (2) cysts evolving in duct ectasia; (3) cysts resulting from traumatic fat necrosis; and (4) cysts associated with intraductal papilloma.

Frequency

Cystic disease is certainly the most frequent lesion of the breast. Even when only cysts large enough to be evident clinically are considered, cystic disease exceeds in frequency all other breast lesions. In my experience as a consultant, I certainly see more than twice as many women with proven cystic disease as with carcinoma. By proven cystic disease I mean that either palpable tumors were demonstrated to be cysts by aspiration, or grossly visible cysts were found at operation. This would suggest that at least one in every ten women in our contemporary society develops gross cystic disease as I have defined it.

Autopsy studies of the breast might be expected to help us determine more accurately the frequency of grossly visible cysts, but almost all fail to distinguish between microscopic proliferative changes, microscopic cysts, and grossly visible cysts. The study by Sandison (1962) of the breasts in 800 postmortem examinations is an example of this confusion. The only modern autopsy study providing data of sufficient accuracy and magnitude to justify quotation is that by Frantz and her associates. In 1951 they reported a study of the breasts in 225 autopsies of women without clinical evidence of mammary disease. Grossly evident cystic disease (cysts of 1 to 2 mm. or more) was found in 19 per cent. In one-half of these cases the grossly evident disease was bilateral. An additional 34 per cent of Frantz's cases showed microscopic evidence of cystic disease, i.e., microcysts, intraductal epithelial proliferation, or apocrine metaplasia of the duct epithelium.

The Natural History of Cystic Disease

Gross breast cysts are in general a phenomenon of middle life. They first begin to appear as isolated, unilateral lesions in young women in their middle twenties. The youngest patient with a gross cyst, in a series of 2017 women with the disease that I have been studying from several points of view, was 25 years old. The age distribution of the patients at the onset of their cystic disease in this series of cases is shown in Chart 7–1. It is seen from this chart that the disease attains its greatest frequency in the 15 year period between 35 and 50 years of age. It subsides and disappears with the menopause. It is remarkable how sharp the upper age limit for cystic disease actually is. In our total of 2017 patients with the disease there were only six in whom the age of onset was 55 years of age or older. Three were exactly 55; two of these had had their last menstrual period within three months, while the third had apparently entered the menopause three years previously. Two of the other patients were 57, and one was 59. The cysts in four of these patients were apparently induced by estrogen. The case histories of two of them are worth summarizing as examples of this phenomenon.

Mrs. H.E., aged 57, had had a hysterectomy at 43, but her ovaries were not removed. She had been using Revlon face cream (containing estrogen) generously for some months, when she discovered a tumor in her right breast. Clinically, it was a typical cyst, 4 cm. in diameter. It was

Table 7–1. LENGTH OF FOLLOW-UP IN 2017 PATIENTS WITH GROSS CYSTS

	Number of Patients
Less than 5 years	850
5 to 10 years	447
10 to 15 years	306
15 to 20 years	165
20 years or more	249
Total	2017

aspirated. She continued to use the face cream and 20 months later she developed another, 1 cm. cyst, in the same breast, which was also aspirated. She then stopped using the face cream and when last examined, three years later, her breasts were normal.

Mrs. D.P., aged 57, had entered the menopause at 53. Since then she had taken 1.25 mg. of prednisone daily for 20 days of every month. One week before consulting me she had found a tumor of her left breast. It was a 6 cm. group of cysts, which were aspirated. She stopped taking the prednisone and has developed no more cysts during the succeeding three years.

Realizing the need of more precise data regarding the natural history of gross cystic disease, I began many years ago to make a special effort to follow these patients in our medical center. The data that I am now able to present were accumulated by this personal effort.

The length of follow-up after the diagnosis of a gross breast cyst in the 2017 women in this series is shown in Table 7–1. The distribution of the initial gross cyst by location and

Chart 7–1. The age distribution of 2017 women with gross cystic disease.

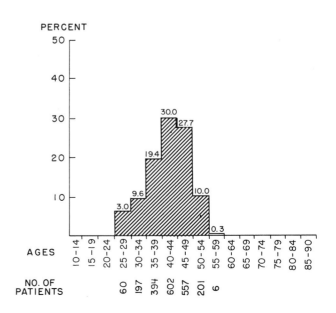

Table 7–2. Distribution of initial gross cysts in 2017 patients by age, location, and multiplicity of cysts

Age	Left Breast		Right Breast		Bilateral	Total
	Single	Multiple	Single	Multiple		
25–29	27	2	27	—	4	60
30–34	94	7	82	1	13	197
35–39	176	5	160	9	44	394
40–44	289	20	223	9	61	602
45–49	255	26	188	17	71	557
50–54	97	7	76	4	17	201
55–59	3	—	3	—	—	6
Total	941	67	759	40	210	2,017

age in our 2017 patients is shown in Table 7–2. Table 7–3 summarizes the data regarding the sites of the initial gross cysts.

These data show that more than 10 per cent of the women with gross cystic disease initially have palpable cysts in both breasts. They also reveal the interesting fact that the left breast is more often affected by the disease than the right breast. In 55.2 per cent of our patients the initial cyst developed in the left breast, and in 44.8 per cent, in the right breast. Breast carcinoma also has a predilection for the left breast. I have no explanation for this phenomenon.

Once cystic disease has begun, new cysts can be expected to develop at irregular intervals until the patient is through the menopause. Table 7–4 shows that approximately 40 per cent of our patients with gross cystic disease subsequently develop new cysts at intervals of from less than one year to 30 years after the initial cyst. Although these new cysts are sometimes situated in the vicinity of the initial cyst, they are usually widely scattered throughout one or both breasts.

Table 7–5 shows the average interval between the first and second gross cysts in the

893 patients who had subsequent gross cysts. In women who develop only a few cysts the interval between them may be long, whereas those who have many cysts are apt to have a continuous series of them. After the age of 40, women with gross cystic disease have more cysts, and the cysts develop at shorter intervals. Thus the disease reaches its most active phase in the premenopausal years and disappears after the completion of the menopause.

Table 7–6 shows the number of subsequent palpable cysts that developed in our 1167 patients followed for a minimum of five years. These data do not, of course, present a true picture of the actual numbers of cysts in this disease. We know from our inspection of these cystic breasts, at the operating table and in the pathology laboratory, that there are often countless gross cysts. We palpate only the larger ones, or those situated nearer the periphery of the breast where they are more easily felt.

Etiology

The fact that gross cystic disease does not become clinically evident until some years after ovarian function is fully evolved, that it subsides and disappears with the menopause, and that it frequently involves both breasts, suggests that it is in some way an expression of abnormal ovarian function. Whether this is an excess of estrogen, or some other type of hormonal dysfunction, we do not know. The induction of breast cysts well after the completion of the menopause by the administration of estrogen suggests that at least in these postmenopausal women an excess of estrogen is responsible. There is confirmatory

Table 7–3. Site of initial gross cysts in 2017 patients

	Number of Patients	Per cent of Total Number of Patients
Left breast		
Single cyst	941	46.7
Multiple cysts	67	3.3
Right breast		
Single cyst	759	37.6
Multiple cysts	40	2.0
Both breasts	210	10.4
Total	2,017	100

Table 7–4. INTERVAL BETWEEN FIRST DIAGNOSIS OF GROSS CYSTIC DISEASE AND THE FIRST SUBSEQUENT CYST IN 893 PATIENTS (EXCLUDING 23 PATIENTS WHO WERE OPERATED FOR A BREAST CANCER WHEN FIRST SEEN), BY AGE AT THE TIME OF FIRST CYST

Years After Entry	Age Groups							Total
	25–29	30–34	35–39	40–44	45–49	50–54	55–59	
less than 1	2	3	3	20	19	4		51
1	3	6	21	48	47	14		139
2	2	16	25	46	45	9	1	144
3	2	10	19	40	36	6		113
4	1	7	24	33	24	5		94
5		8	17	27	14			66
6	1	6	19	23	12			61
7	2	7	15	16	3	1		44
8		2	18	15	3			38
9	3	3	15	7	3	1		32
10	2	4	17	4				27
11	1	4	8	3		1		17
12	3	7	5	4	1			20
13	2	2	6	1	1			12
14	3	3	2					8
15		4	4	1	1			10
16	2							2
17		2						2
18	1				1			2
19	4	3						7
20			1					1
21					1			1
30			1		1			2
No subsequent cysts	26	100	170	310	335	155	5	1101
Total	60	197	390	598	547	196	6	1994

evidence from studies upon mice that estrogen produces breast cysts.

The French were pioneers in the experimental study of the effects of the ovarian hormones upon the breast in mice, and one of the earliest papers was that by Goormaghtigh and Amerlinck (1930) in which they reported that they had produced cystic disease by the injection of estrogen in ovariectomized mice.

As the knowledge of the effects of the ovarian hormones upon the mouse breast evolved from studies carried on in many laboratories, it became evident that estrogen not only stimulates the mammary epithelium to proliferate, but that it also causes dilatation of the mammary ducts and cyst formation. The latter process as seen in the mouse breast is similar in a general way to cystic disease in the human breast except that in mice the changes usually involve the whole extent of the mammary gland, while in a considerable proportion of women with cystic disease the changes are to some extent localized.

There are marked differences among different strains of mice in this tendency to develop cystic changes following estrogen administration. In a study carried out by Randall and myself (1942) in which we used three pure-bred strains of mice—the Paris R 3 strain, the Marsh strain, and the C 57 strain—this fact was well shown. The breasts of the Paris R 3 mice showed a great degree of epithelial proliferation accompanied by considerable cystic change. The breasts of the Marsh and C 57 mice showed little epithelial proliferation but very marked cystic change. In the C 57 mice, in particular, the breasts were transformed into masses of

Table 7–5. AVERAGE INTERVAL IN YEARS BETWEEN FIRST AND SECOND CYSTS BY AGE IN 893 PATIENTS WITH GROSS CYSTIC DISEASE

Age	Average Interval Between First and Second Cyst
25–29	9.86 years
30–34	6.90 years
35–39	6.13 years
40–44	3.95 years
45–49	3.15 years
50–54	2.41 years
55–59	2.00 years

Table 7–6. Number of subsequent cysts in 1167 patients followed for a minimum of 5 years

Number of Patients	Number of Subsequent Cysts
525	None
196	1
162	2
95	3
55	4
33	5
31	6
19	7
13	8
10	9
9	10
21	More than 10
Total 1,167	

cysts by long continued administration of estrogen in large dosage.

Engle, Krakower, and I treated a group of aged Rhesus monkeys with estrogen and produced cystic changes in the mammary gland but no epithelial proliferation.

Symptoms

Cystic disease of the breast often produces no symptoms and the patient is unaware of the disease until she discovers the tumor by palpation, either accidental or purposeful, of the breast. In other patients cysts produce pain and they may be tender to palpation. These symptoms may be present continuously, or may appear only in the premenstrual phase of the menstrual cycle. The pain and tenderness are more apt to be present when the cyst has enlarged rapidly. Perhaps the pain and tenderness have a relationship to the tension of the fluid within the cyst. Aspiration of the fluid certainly gives relief.

Another important clinical feature of cysts which helps to differentiate them from carcinoma and adenofibroma is that cysts are much more labile. They develop quickly, sometimes attaining a considerable size within a few days, and they may diminish in size just as rapidly. A rapid increase in size is not infrequently correlated with the premenstrual phase of the cycle, and diminution with the postmenstrual phase. When an intelligent and mentally stable patient gives a history of definite diminution in the size of her breast tumor, whether or not the diminution be correlated with the postmenstrual phase of her cycle, it is strong evidence that the lesion is a cyst and not a carcinoma. The only other breast lesion that regresses in this dramatic way is duct ectasia.

Discharge from the nipple occurs only rarely in cystic disease.

Physical Characteristics

Cysts of the breast are usually round and well delimited. When they lie deep in a thick breast, near its posterior aspect, their rounded form and circumscribed character are more difficult to appreciate.

Their consistency depends upon the pressure of the fluid within them. When it is low they are soft, and careful palpation may sometimes detect fluctuation. When they are tightly distended, however, they are firm. I have the impression that their tenseness may increase in the premenstrual phase of the cycle. When cysts are long-standing and have developed thick fibrous walls, they are also firm.

Cysts are usually relatively movable in the surrounding breast tissue. In this characteristic they resemble adenofibromas and are unlike carcinoma. When, instead of a single isolated cyst, the lesion consists of a group of cysts of varied size involving a segment of the breast, the tumor which they form lacks to a degree both circumscription and movability within the breast tissue.

Cysts are occasionally associated with signs of acute inflammation, pain, tenderness, and redness of the overlying skin. The fluid aspirated from such cysts is apt to be thicker and more opaque. It is usually sterile. Following aspiration, these signs of inflammation promptly subside. Perhaps this phenomenon is due to inflammation produced by the escape of some of the cyst fluid into the surrounding breast.

Pathology

The gross appearance of a typical breast cyst, with its round bulging contour and its bluish color, which have given it the name "blue-domed," are well known to surgeons and pathologists. Grossly visible cysts are of infinite variety in size and distribution. A single cyst with a thin wall and a smooth and glistening lining may be the only manifestation of the disease. Very large cysts sometimes have trabeculated walls (Fig. 7–1). Occasionally, the wall of a cyst is thick and fibrous and the lining is dull and granular; such cysts lack the characteristic bluish color.

At operation it is rather unusual to find a solitary cyst. The usual gross picture is that one large cyst, which formed the palpable tumor that led to operation, is surrounded by a number of small cysts in the immediately adjacent mammary tissue. However, the more extensively the surgeon operating on cystic disease explores the breast, the more cysts he will find. If he attempts to excise them all he will end up by removing a large sector of the breast and disfiguring it considerably.

A form of relatively localized cystic disease is that in which a limited area of the breast contains countless minute cysts that are only a few millimeters in diameter, intermingled with the microscopic epithelial proliferation and fibrosis that so often accompany cystic disease. There is no larger cyst to give such a lesion a rounded form and a circumscribed character. These lesions form a tumor that is firm and not very well delimited. It is, however, somewhat movable and not accompanied by retraction. The gross appearance of the cut surface of such a lesion is mottled brownish-gray, dotted with small

dark cysts (Fig. 7–2). An important feature differentiating it from carcinoma is a lack of the chalk streaks that are so often seen in carcinoma.

In some patients both breasts are riddled throughout with cysts, many of which are large enough to form palpable tumors. Figure 7–3 shows both breasts in this generalized form of the disease.

Microscopic study shows that the lining of larger cysts is a single layer of flattened epithelium. In many cysts, however, the epithelial lining has disappeared, leaving a bare connective tissue surface.

In cysts that are of recent origin the fluid that they contain is thin and straw-colored and resembles blood serum. In older cysts the fluid is darker in color, ranging from brown to greenish-gray to black, and slightly thicker. This color is due to the accumulation of hemosiderin which must originate from seepage of blood through breaks in the continuity of the lining epithelium. The fluid is almost always thin enough to be drawn easily through a 20-gauge needle. It contains formless debris. Nothing is to be gained by smearing it and studying it microscopically. Sometimes the cyst fluid is thicker and grayish, presumably as the result of an inflammatory reaction. Sometimes the aspirating needle hits a blood vessel and fresh blood is withdrawn. The fluid that is obtained by aspiration of a cyst into which a papilloma or papillary carcinoma is growing is quite

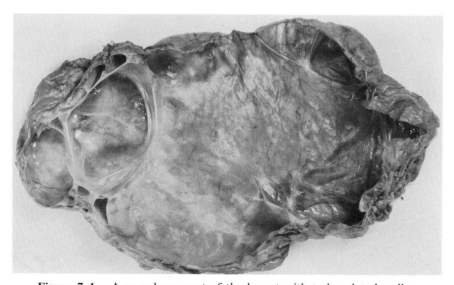

Figure 7–1. A very large cyst of the breast with trabeculated walls.

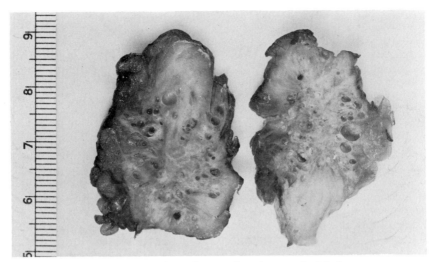

Figure 7-2.   A cluster of small cysts forming a palpable breast tumor.

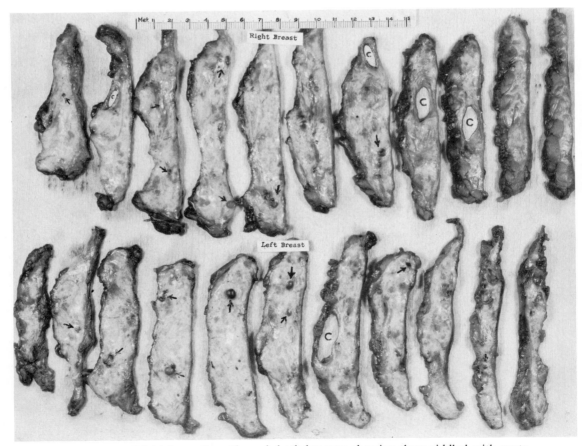

Figure 7-3.   Multiple sections through both breasts, showing them riddled with cysts.

different in character. It is thicker and resembles old blood. Moreover, aspiration of such a lesion does not get rid of the tumor, a residuum of which remains to remind the surgeon that he has not solved the diagnostic problem.

Although I have defined cystic disease for the purposes of our clinical studies as a lesion characterized by grossly visible cysts, because only visible cysts form a palpable tumor, the disease does have a microscopic component which warrants description, because some of its manifestations are usually found accompanying the grossly visible cysts. These microscopic features include the following:

1. Microcysts. I use the term to describe cysts that are so small that they are not visible to the naked eye. They are ubiquitous in the breasts of adult women, but tend to disappear after the menopause. They are usually lined by one or two layers of flattened epithelium without any evidence of proliferation. Figure 7–4 shows a group of these microscopic cysts. Whether these cysts develop merely as the result of the dilatation of ducts, or are the result of the process that Foote and Stewart have called "blunt duct adenosis," we can only guess. These minute cysts are not infrequently so numerous that it seems unlikely that they could have originated from ducts alone, since there could not

have been enough of these to form the multitude of cysts. Certainly there is no microscopic evidence that obstruction of ducts plays any role in the origin of these small cysts. Since there is every gradation in the size of these cysts it seems likely that the larger grossly visible cysts originate from the microscopic cysts.

2. Blunt Duct Adenosis. This term was devised by Foote and Stewart to designate a process in which ducts appear to divide and multiply, but instead of terminating in the normal manner in lobules of acini, end blindly as small rounded structures resembling microcysts. They therefore tend to have a lobular pattern. In the earlier phase of the process the epithelium lining of these structures is taller and their lumens smaller (Fig. 7–5); later on the epithelium becomes flattened (Fig. 7–6).

3. Proliferation of Duct Epithelium. The epithelium lining the small cysts and dilated ducts often shows a great variety of types of proliferation. The simplest form is heaping up of the duct epithelium as shown in Figure 7–7. In its extreme form this proliferation may be many layers thick, and may largely fill up the lumens of the dilated ducts (Fig. 7–8). Provided that the individual proliferating cells maintain the characteristics of benign cells, our follow-up experience has taught us that this kind of epithelial prolifera-

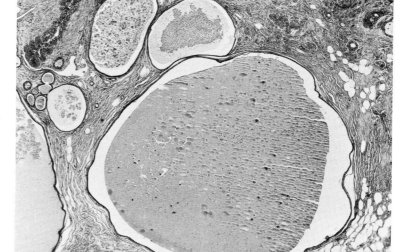

Figure 7–4. A group of microscopic cysts.

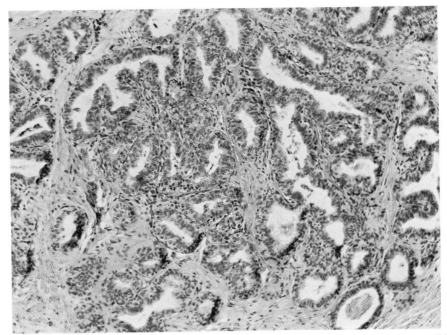

Figure 7–5. An area of blunt duct adenosis—early stage showing some papillary proliferation.

tion does not predispose to the development of carcinoma.

A good deal of the intraductal epithelial proliferation in cystic disease has a papillary pattern. This may consist merely of low, irregular projections of the epithelium into the duct lumen, which may coalesce to form a lace-like pattern partially filling the duct.

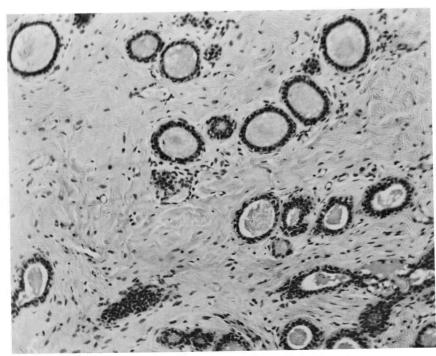

Figure 7–6. A later stage of blunt duct adenosis.

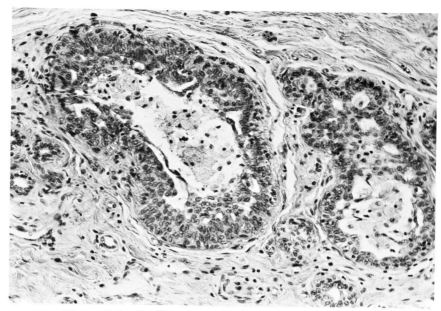

Figure 7–7. Proliferating epithelium heaping up in ducts.

Fully developed branching papillae with long stalks, as shown in Figure 7–9, are also seen. We classify these forms of benign microscopic papillary proliferation, so often seen as a component of cystic disease, as *papillomatosis*. We carefully distinguish it from intraductal papilloma which is a grossly visible organoid lesion, which I will discuss in Chapter 14.

4. Apocrine Metaplasia of Duct Epithelium. The normal cuboidal duct epithelium is transformed into columnar epithelium, with large cells with small regular nuclei and an abundant eosinophilic cytoplasm. This metaplasia can sometimes be traced from a duct with normal epithelium that divides in a lobular pattern, in which the newly formed branches all have apocrine

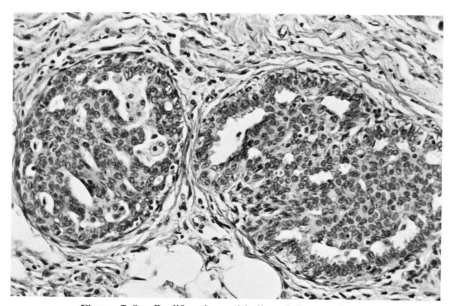

Figure 7–8. Proliferating epithelium filling up ducts.

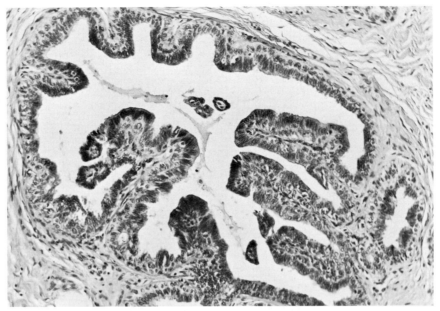

Figure 7-9.   Branching papillae growing in a duct.

epithelium, as shown in Figure 7-10. Small cysts are often associated with this process.

Speert produced apocrine metaplasia of the breast epithelium in the Rhesus monkey by the administration of very large doses of estrogen, but we have no evidence that this occurs in human beings.

5. Adenosis.   Adenosis is the name given by Ewing for the benign proliferation of acini and ducts in a lobular pattern which is one of the microscopic features of the cystic disease complex. Adenosis is usually seen in scattered small foci. The proliferating acini string out into the surrounding breast stroma, which is often sclerotic, and give the impression of infiltration. Although the individual proliferating cells are small and uniform, this fact is obscured by the fibrosis. Figure 7-11 shows such an area of adenosis. It is usually a minor component of the cystic disease

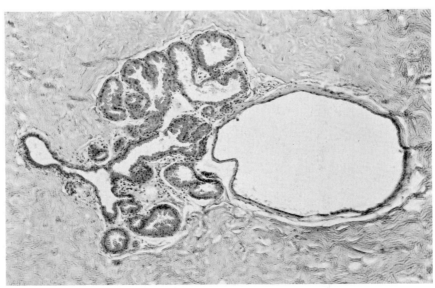

Figure 7-10.   Apocrine metaplasia of the epithelium of a duct that divides in a lobular pattern.

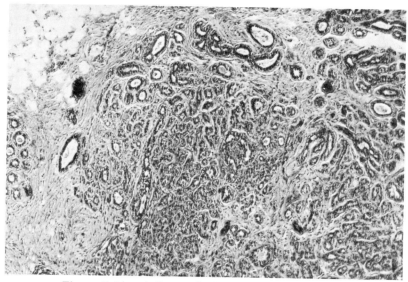

Figure 7–11. A focus of adenosis in cystic disease.

complex, but when it dominates the microscopic picture it becomes of great practical importance because its infiltrative character leads pathologists to mistake it for carcinoma. The most important features that distinguish adenosis from carcinoma are its lobular pattern and its patchy occurrence. There is no evidence that adenosis is a precursor of carcinoma of the breast.

Adenosis also occurs as a solid tumor without accompanying cyst formation which presents as a dominant tumor of the breast in younger women. Chapter 8 is devoted to this tumor-forming type of adenosis.

6. Fibrosis. An element of fibrosis often accompanies the microscopic features of cystic disease that I have been describing. It is as if the proliferation of epithelium stimulates a proliferation of the fibroblasts in the breast stroma. Figure 7–12 shows a typical focus of

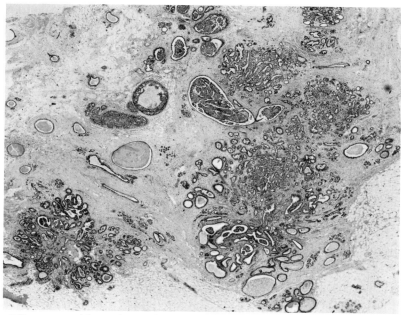

Figure 7–12. Microcysts, blunt duct adenosis, and papillary proliferation of duct epithelium in a fibrotic area in cystic disease.

the microscopic features of cystic disease, in which microcysts, blunt duct adenosis, papillary growth within ducts, and adenosis are surrounded by fibrosis.

The Importance, for the Education of the Surgeon, of Classifying Cystic Disease as Gross or Microscopic

I believe that it is important for pathologists to specify, in their diagnoses of cystic disease, whether they refer to the finding of grossly visible cysts, or only to the microscopic features of cystic disease. The diagnosis should read "cystic disease—gross" or "cystic disease—microscopic," or both.

This distinction has an important disciplinary value for the surgeon, who must, through correlation of his clinical findings with the pathologist's studies, learn to distinguish clinically recognizable disease in the breast from increased nodularity representing only physiological variation in the breast. This distinction is the fundamental one which a physician must learn to make correctly if he is to avoid missing disease on the one hand, or advising operation unnecessarily on the other hand. The latter error is, I believe, the more frequent one, at least among surgeons.

Grossly visible cysts in the breast often form a tumor which is palpable and therefore clinically recognizable. The breast lesions consisting solely of the microscopical features of cystic disease, without any grossly visible cysts, usually do not form a tumor and cannot be detected by clinical examination. When a surgeon biopsies a breast tumor and finds grossly visible cysts, his operation is justifiable in the sense that he found disease, although I would have dealt with it by aspiration. But when he biopsies what he regards as breast disease and finds only the microscopic features of the cystic disease complex, and no other breast disease, his biopsy is usually not justified. He should not have operated. What he thought to be a tumor was only increased nodularity within the limits of physiological variation. True enough, microscopic cystic disease is found, but it exists in the majority of all clinically normal breasts and, being undetectable, cannot be regarded as an indication for operation. If the pathologist does not distinguish between gross cystic disease and microscopic cystic disease in his report, the surgeon has no way of recognizing his error. When he gets the usual report of "chronic cystic mastitis" he will assume that his operation was justified, when in fact it may not have been.

THE RELATIONSHIP OF CYSTIC DISEASE TO CARCINOMA OF THE BREAST

No question is of more acute concern to the clinician dealing with breast disease than the relationship of grossly visible cysts to carcinoma. It is a problem which he must often face and for which the published evidence is confused and conflicting.

There are three main types of evidence bearing on this question:

1. The frequency with which breast carcinoma is preceded by a history of proven gross cystic disease.

2. The frequency with which carcinoma develops subsequent to gross cystic disease.

3. The frequency with which breasts removed for carcinoma show gross cystic disease.

I will discuss these three different types of evidence in order.

The Frequency with which Breast Carcinoma is Preceded by a History of Proven Gross Cystic Disease

Johnson (1924), studying a series of 444 cases of carcinoma of the breast, found only two in which there was a history of earlier proved breast cysts. In Foote and Stewart's study of 1200 patients with breast carcinoma at the Memorial Hospital they found that only 2.4 per cent had a past history of operatively proved benign breast disease. Patey reviewed the histories of 810 patients with breast carcinoma at the Middlesex Hospital and found that only 10, or 1.2 per cent, had previously had breast cysts.

I have studied this question in the case histories of our patients with breast carcinoma, and in new patients with the disease as I took their histories, and I have concluded that it is impossible to determine with a reasonable degree of accuracy, what proportion had proved gross cystic disease. Patients who have had previous operations for benign breast disease are almost always told that they have "fibrocystic disease," or simply "benign disease." I believe that the very low frequency of a history of previous cystic disease reported by Johnson, by Foote and Stewart, and by Patey merely reflects the inadequacy of case histories in answering this question.

The Frequency with which Breast Carcinoma Develops Subsequent to Proved Gross Cystic Disease

Clinicians have attempted to answer this question by long-term follow-up of their patients with proved cystic disease. Reviewing the numerous studies of this kind that have been published, I am forced to conclude that they all fail because they do not meet one or the other of the two basic requirements of this kind of research. The first requirement is a clear definition of what is meant by "chronic cystic mastitis." Most authors, exemplified by Lewison and Lyons in their 1953 presentation of the Johns Hopkins Hospital data, and by Veronesi in his 1968 report from the National Institute for the Study and Treatment of Tumors in Milan, make no attempt to describe their pathological criteria for what they call "chronic cystic mastitis." It is apparent, from the names used in the context and from accompanying illustrations, that some of these studies include every possible variant of benign microscopic change in the breast, as well as a number of well-defined benign lesions that have nothing whatever to do with cystic disease, such as adenofibroma, adenosis forming a solid dominant breast tumor, intraductal papilloma, duct ectasia, and lobular neoplasia (so-called lobular carcinoma *in situ*). These five lesions are quite separate and distinct lesions unrelated to cystic disease, which I have dealt with in separate chapters. When all these lesions are thrown together into a hodge-podge called "chronic cystic mastitis" nothing useful is learned from follow-up concerning the significance of gross cystic disease as I have defined it here, namely, a lesion characterized by the presence of grossly visible cysts.

A second basic defect in most studies of the frequency of carcinoma in patients who have had cystic disease is statistical. The numbers of patients studied are too few, the follow-up is not complete enough and long enough, and careful actuarial calculations of the exposure of the patients studied to the risk of developing carcinoma are not presented. Without this kind of evidence these studies are meaningless. Warren's much quoted 1940 study based on data from both Toronto and Boston, recommending mastectomy for recurrent "chronic mastitis," is an example of this kind of misleading study.

Perhaps the best study of the frequency with which carcinoma develops following cystic disease is that of Davis and his associates. A total of 284 patients with the disease were followed for an average of 13 years. Although it is not entirely clear from the data presented how many of them had gross cystic disease, mammary carcinoma developed in them 1.73 times as often as it does in the general female population according to Davis's calculations.

Many years ago I realized the great need for accurate data regarding the frequency with which carcinoma follows gross cystic disease of the breast, and I organized a special clinic in which I attempted to follow all of our ward patients with proved gross cystic disease. I have also made a special effort to get my private patients with the disease to come back for regular follow-up. In this manner I have accumulated data concerning a total of 2017 patients with documented gross cystic disease studied between the years 1930 and 1968.

The calendar years of entry, and the number of patients in each five year group, are given in Table 7–7. The ages and length of follow-up of the patients are shown in Table 7–8. Of the 2017 patients, 324 were followed for less than one year and have therefore been excluded. The remaining 1693 constitute the study group. Among the 324 patients who were excluded, 23 had gross cystic disease and carcinoma concomitantly during the year of entry.

In our 1693 patients followed for more

Table 7–7. CALENDAR YEARS OF ENTRY AND NUMBERS OF PATIENTS WITH GROSS CYSTIC DISEASE, 1930–1968

Calendar Year	Number of Patients
before 1930	3
1930–1934	52
1935–1939	86
1940–1944	132
1945–1949	211
1950–1954	282
1955–1959	450
1960–1964	518
1965–1968	283
Total	2017

Table 7–8. AGES AND LENGTH OF FOLLOW-UP OF
PATIENTS WITH GROSS CYSTIC DISEASE, 1930–1968

Age	Followed for Less than 1 Year	Followed for More than 1 Year	Total
25–29	6	54	60
30–34	22	175	197
35–39	39	355	394
40–44	96	506	602
45–49	108	449	557
50–54	51	150	201
55–59	2	4	6
Total	324	1693	2017

than one year breast carcinoma developed in
72. This incidence is compared in Table 7–9
to the incidence rates for the disease in wom-
en in the general population of the state of
New York. On the basis of these rates, adjusted for age, 17.35 breast carcinomas would
have been expected in our 1,693 women
exposed to the risk of the disease. In fact 72
developed it. This is more than four times the
expected incidence and is statistically highly
significant.

The age distribution of the 72 women who
developed breast carcinoma is shown in
Chart 7–2. Sixty-nine per cent of them were
older than 50 years. Thirty-two per cent were
in the 50 to 54 year age group. Their average

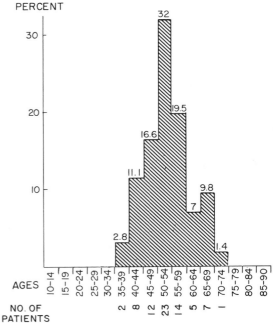

Chart 7–2. The age distribution of 72 women
with gross cysts of the breasts who developed
breast carcinoma.

age was 53.5 years. This is essentially the
same as the mean age of the breast cancer
patients in my personal series of cases—51.9
years. Carcinoma of the breast following
cysts therefore occurs in the same age range
as other breast carcinomas.

Carcinoma developed in 65 of the patients
with gross cystic disease followed for a mini-

Table 7–9. THE RELATIONSHIP OF GROSS
CYSTIC DISEASE IN 1693 PATIENTS TO THE
SUBSEQUENT DEVELOPMENT OF CARCINOMA
OF THE BREAST, 1930–1968

Age	Person Years	Observed Breast Carcinomas	Expected Breast Carcinomas
25–29	88.50		.004
30–34	586.75		.098
35–39	1552.50	2	.594
40–44	2999.50	8	2.138
45–49	3946.50	12	4.185
50–54	3377.00	23	3.963
55–59	2125.00	14	2.977
60–64	1107.25	5	1.835
65–69	492.25	7	.987
70 +	207.00	1	.569
Total	16482.25	72	17.35

Observed Incidence	72
Expected Incidence	17.35

The observed incidence is four times the expected incidence.

Note: 23 carcinomas were found concomitantly with
cysts and are excluded.

Table 7–10. THE RELATIONSHIP OF THE
DEVELOPMENT OF BREAST CARCINOMA TO THE
NUMBER OF GROSS CYSTS SUBSEQUENT TO THE
INITIAL CYST IN 1166 PATIENTS FOLLOWED
FOR A MINIMUM OF 5 YEARS, 1930–1968

Number of Patients with Gross Cysts	Number of Cysts Subsequent to Initial Cyst	Number of Carcinomas
522	0	32
197	1	14
161	2	9
93	3	4
54	4	2
33	5	0
31	6	2
19	7	1
14	8	0
12	9	0
30	10 or more	1
Total 1166		65

Table 7–11. THE RELATIONSHIP OF THE SITE OF THE INITIAL GROSS CYST TO THE SITE OF THE CARCINOMA IN 1166 PATIENTS FOLLOWED FOR A MINIMUM OF 5 YEARS, 1930–1968

Number of Patients with Gross Cysts	Number of Cysts Subsequent to Initial Cyst	Number of Patients who Developed Carcinoma		
		In the same breast as the initial cyst	In the opposite breast	Initial cysts in both breasts
522	0	13	14	5
197	1	6	7	1
161	2	3	4	2
93	3	3	0	1
54	4	0	0	2
33	5	0	0	0
31	6	1	0	1
19	7	1	0	0
14	8	0	0	0
12	9	0	0	0
30	10 or more	1	0	0
Total 1166		28	25	12

mum of 5 years. The relationship of the development of carcinoma to the number of cysts that occurred subsequent to the initial cyst in these women followed for at least 5 years is shown in Table 7–10. Forty-six carcinomas developed in a total of 719 women who had only one or two cysts—an incidence of 6.4 per cent. Among the 75 women who had more than eight cysts, only two developed carcinoma—an incidence of 2.6 per cent. Our data therefore do not indicate that the predisposition to carcinoma increases with the number of gross cysts.

The data bearing on the question of whether or not the carcinomas which develop in women who have had gross cysts occur in the same breast as that in which the initial cyst occurred is presented in Table 7–11. It will be seen that carcinoma developed just as often in the opposite breast as it did in the breast in which the initial cyst occurred. This fact should be considered by surgeons who propose removal of a breast containing gross cysts; they are only diminishing by one-half the predisposition to breast cancer.

The length of the interval between the initial gross cyst and the carcinoma which developed in 72 of our patients is an interesting and important aspect of this phenomenon. The pertinent data are presented in Table 7–12. For the younger women who had their initial breast cyst between the ages of 30 and 34 an average of 19.1 years elapsed before carcinoma developed, at the average age of 51.6 years. In the patients who developed their initial cyst beyond the age of 34 the interval until carcinoma developed was simi-

lar for the several quinquennial age groups: it averaged 9.7 years.

The data concerning the time relationship between the initial breast cyst and the subsequent carcinoma is shown in graphic form in Chart 7–3. About one-half of the carcinomas occurred within 10 years of the initial cyst. The mean age of the women who developed carcinoma between one and four years following their initial cyst was 47 years when carcinoma was diagnosed. In the women who developed carcinoma between five and nine years after their initial cyst the average age at which carcinoma occurred was 52. Those who had a 10 to 14 year interval between the initial cyst and carcinoma had a mean age of 51.7 years when their carcinoma was found. These ages are not significantly different.

Table 7–12. THE INTERVAL BETWEEN THE INITIAL GROSS CYST IN 1693 PATIENTS AND THE SUBSEQUENT DEVELOPMENT OF CARCINOMA, 1930–1968

Age of Patients with Initial Cyst	Average Number of Years Interval between Initial Cyst and Carcinoma	Average Age at which Carcinoma Developed
25–29	0	0
30–34	19.1	51.6
35–39	9.9	47.4
40–44	9.8	52.3
45–49	8.9	56.4
50–54	9.1	61.6
		53.5

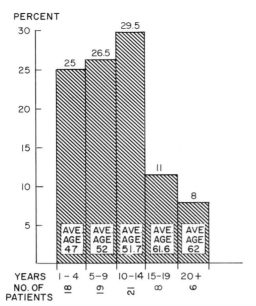

PERCENT

Chart 7–3. The interval between the initial gross cyst and carcinoma in the 72 patients in whom carcinoma developed.

The Frequency with which Breasts Removed for Carcinoma Show Gross Cystic Disease

It is surprising how difficult it is to find precise information as to the frequency of grossly visible cysts in breasts removed for carcinoma. There are numerous reports of the frequency of the hodge-podge of microscopic lesions referred to as "chronic mastitis" in carcinomatous breasts, but they do not help to answer the question.

Semb was one of the first to provide specific data on this point. In a series of 22 cancerous breasts he found grossly visible cysts (fibroadenomatosis cystica simplex) in 27 per cent.

Foote and Stewart carried out a similar but more detailed study. In their series of 300 cancerous breasts they found grossly visible cysts (1 mm. or more in diameter) in exactly the same proportion as Semb—27 per cent.

In our laboratory of surgical pathology the surgical specimens have been studied in a uniform and careful manner for many years. Written descriptions of the gross findings in all breasts removed for carcinoma are available. I went over the descriptions of 3000 breasts described between 1942 and 1967. I counted as gross cysts those which were recorded as being at least 2 mm. in

diameter, and at least several in number. On this basis 7.6 per cent of the specimens showed gross cystic disease. In 26 per cent of the specimens in which cysts were found, there were only a few, while in 74 per cent there were a great many cysts, usually scattered throughout the entire breast.

It is of interest that 90 per cent of the patients whose breasts showed gross cystic disease were under the age of 55 (for clinical purposes, premenopausal). Their average age was 45.6 years. This is, of course, in keeping with the fact that gross cysts are usually not found in the breasts after the menopause.

The fact that gross cystic disease is not often found in breasts amputated for carcinoma does not necessarily mean that the two diseases are unrelated. Both may have a common etiology going far back in the patients' life history, but the cystic disease disappeared in the older postmenopausal women, as we know it usually does.

THE DIAGNOSIS AND TREATMENT OF CYSTIC DISEASE

It is convenient to discuss the diagnosis and treatment of cysts of the breast together because both objects can be achieved in most instances by one procedure, namely aspiration. When I began my career as a surgeon, I accepted the dictum that still prevails in most surgical circles that a dominant tumor of the breast must always be explored surgically. As my experience in dealing with cystic disease grew I realized the folly of repeatedly operating upon this harmless disease when individual cysts can be diagnosed and treated perfectly well by aspiration. Thus I came more and more to attempt to aspirate tumors of the breasts which have the clinical character of cysts. For many years now this has been my standard practice and I recommend it strongly.

I am very cautious in my use of aspiration. I attempt it only for tumors that have the clinical characteristics of cysts. First of all, the patient must be within the usual age span for cystic disease, namely, between 30 and 55. Secondly, the tumor must feel like a cyst, that is, it must be rounded, well delimited, and movable in the surrounding breast tissue. It must not be hard or accompanied by retraction. The fact that the patient has previously had gross cysts proven by aspiration or operation of course suggests that the new tumor is also a cyst, but I do not permit this fact to persuade me to aspirate a tumor that does not feel like a cyst.

My procedure is first of all to explain to the patient that I believe that her tumor is probably a cyst, and that by putting a needle into it I can probably prove whether or not this is a fact, and at the same time cure it by withdrawing the fluid. I take care to emphasize that if I do not obtain the characteristic cyst fluid, and if the tumor is not entirely dissipated by withdrawing the fluid, I will have to recommend biopsy of the lesion in the hospital with all preparations made for whatever surgical procedure may be necessary. The patient almost always asks if the fluid in the cyst will not reaccumulate. I am able to assure her that it almost never does. I have no satisfactory explanation as to why this does not happen, but it is a fact that it does not.

In performing aspiration, I first anesthetize the skin with Novocain. I then gently insert a No. 20-gauge needle on a 20 cc. syringe into the tumor. I take great care not to plunge the needle through the tumor, and ordinarily insert it only once into the center of the lesion. I do not repeatedly insert my needle into the tumor in a stubborn attempt to get fluid. If the tumor is solid the resistance that the aspirating needle encounters is usually at once apparent.

If I withdraw the fluid characteristic of a cyst, and palpation reveals that the tumor is gone and no suspicious induration remains, I am content, and I dismiss the patient until her next examination, usually at an interval of three months. If I have not obtained fluid, and there is any suspicion of a different lesion, I tell the patient that my attempt at diagnosis has failed, and recommend admission to the hospital for biopsy.

Experience has taught me that lesions with the clinical characteristics of a cyst that I have attempted to aspirate unsuccessfully will, at subsequent operation, occasionally prove to be cysts with a thick wall. At operation for a presumed breast cyst the skin incision should be made as I have described in discussing the technique of excision of benign tumors of the breast in Chapter 6. It should be placed in the skin lines, and somewhat medial to the tumor if it lies near the periphery of the breast. A radial incision should never be made. When the cyst has been exposed, it is my practice, unless the cyst is very small, to open it and inspect its inner surface. In this way the mistake of locally excising a cystic papillary carcinoma or a circumscribed carcinoma with cystic change can be avoided. If a cyst is large, that is, some centimeters in diameter, I usually do not attempt to excise it in toto. I remove only a sector of its wall, together with a small amount of the immediately adjacent breast tissue. Such a partial excision of the wall of a cyst is just as efficacious as complete excision. Whatever a surgeon can do in minimizing the extent of the removal of breast tissue in operating for cystic disease is certainly worthwhile. If he is well informed as to the pathology of the disease he will know that he cannot hope to remove extensive cystic disease in its entirety.

In performing a limited local excision of cystic disease I try to maintain as good hemostasis as possible, carefully clamping small vessels as I cut them and keeping the wound from filling up with blood. The dissection should, of course, be done with the scalpel; blunt dissection with scissors is brutal, and indeed impossible, in mammary tissue, where there are no tissue planes. It is important to keep the wound dry so that the operator can see the extent to which the cystic disease involves the breast, and can see any other lesion that may be present. After completion of the excision, the extent of the wound and adjacent breast tissue should be carefully palpated to make certain that no lesion in the surrounding breast has been missed.

When a new tumor develops in a patient who has proved cystic disease, the question arises as to what to do. There are four possible courses of action. The radical one is to follow Warren's recommendation of mastectomy. Although Warren did not recognize the implication, this must be a bilateral mastectomy if the patient is to be entirely protected against further breast disease, because cystic disease is usually bilateral, and carcinoma, if it develops, appears just as often in the opposite breast as in the breast in which the first cyst occurred.

I have presented data that indicate that women who have had grossly evident breast cysts are more than four times as likely to develop breast carcinoma as women in the general population. The question that we must ask ourselves is whether or not this increased risk of carcinoma justifies prophylactic mastectomy. Every physician who serves his patients with understanding and compassion knows that mastectomy is a heavy penalty. It is, in my own opinion, entirely out of proportion to the hazard of developing carcinoma that cystic disease implies. I do not perform mastectomy for cystic disease even in the patients who have the disease in its extreme form, when both breasts are riddled with cysts. It is understandably more difficult to detect carcinoma in this type of the disease, but when these patients reach the menopause and their cysts regress it becomes easier to safeguard them.

A second alternative method of treatment for recurrent cysts is bilateral subcutaneous excision of the breasts and their replacement with implants of various plastic materials. I am even more strongly opposed to this operation than to mastectomy. As more surgeons are tempted to undertake this hazardous procedure, I see in consultation an increasing number of unfortunate patients who have undergone it with tragic consequences. Gurdin and Carlin have recently described the complications of breast implantations very well, with excellent illustrations of the bad results.

The worst complication of this operation is infection. With thin and long skin flaps that are prone to necrosis, and a large implant to which the tissues react as they do to a foreign body of any type, infection is very apt to occur. Once infection is established it is uncontrollable locally. Necrosis and wound disruption follow. The only solution for this situation is to remove the implant. The consequence is a badly scarred chest wall.

Even when the wounds heal well the cosmetic result is often poor. The implant may shift its position. Fibrosis of the tissues around the implant, with shrinkage and distortion, result in a breast which is too firm and does not look normal.

I cannot condemn these operations strongly enough. The anguish that often results from them is very great. They are never justified.

The third alternative course of action when a woman develops a new cyst is to excise it. This is the usual practice in most surgical circles. It is, I believe, an illogical one. It does not protect the patient against the development of carcinoma since she has much breast tissue remaining in which carcinoma may develop. It is not appreciably more efficient than aspiration in determining the nature of the individual tumor for which the surgical exploration is performed. Carcinoma is rarely found immediately adjacent to a cyst, because it does not evolve *from* cysts. It evolves anywhere in breasts in which there is some *common etiologic factor for both cystic disease and carcinoma*. The most important objection to repeated surgical excision of

cysts is that it is not a practical solution to the problem from the patient's point of view. Repeated excisions of areas of cystic disease are usually performed through radial incisions which leave ugly scars, and sensible women revolt against it. Repeated operations are, moreover, expensive and bothersome. Women who are given no other alternative than repeated operation will usually decide to ignore their cystic disease and avoid further medical consultation. This is the worst thing that any plan of therapy can lead to. If there is one thing that is imperative in cystic disease it is that the patient be persuaded to return regularly for follow-up examination for the remainder of her life.

The fourth alternative method of protecting women with cystic disease against carcinoma is frequent clinical examination of the breasts and aspiration of cysts as they develop. This is the method that I have come to depend upon. I tell my patients who have had a breast cyst that they must expect to have more cysts, probably in both breasts, and that the process will continue until the menopause. I assure them that the cysts themselves are harmless, that they do not transform into cancer, and that the problem which cysts present is a diagnostic one, namely, that the nature of every new breast tumor must be proven by aspiration, without delay. Otherwise a cancer may be missed. I warn them that the fact that they have cysts predisposes them somewhat to breast cancer, but I reassure them that this is not a very great hazard and that they can protect themselves by frequent breast examination.

If the patient is emotionally stable enough to be taught to examine her own breasts at monthly intervals she should be urged to do so. She must be impressed with the necessity of coming for consultation at once if she discovers a new tumor. In addition, her breasts should be examined by a physician every three months for the remainder of her life. I do not advise mammograms at these check-up examinations. Palpation is an overwhelmingly more accurate method of examination, and it is all that one can expect the patient to submit to every three months. With this kind of a program the patient with cystic disease can be reasonably confident that if she develops breast carcinoma it will be detected at an early and curable stage.

There has been a good deal of indiscriminate hormonal therapy for cystic disease. Both androgens and estrogens have been used. Since we do not know the nature of the underlying hormonal imbalance in cystic disease, hormonal therapy is necessarily empirical, and may well do harm instead of good. I have seen in consultation a good many patients with cystic disease who had been given one or another hormone, and I have not been able to find any evidence of benefit. Some women given androgen have developed the unpleasant side-effects that androgen regularly produces when it is given in sufficient doses. Other patients have been given estrogen and the disease has been aggravated. I have seen a number of patients whose cystic disease was prolonged by estrogen given for menopausal symptoms. Instead of regressing at the menopause in the expected manner, new cysts continued to form until the estrogen was stopped.

My critics will, of course, accuse me of running the risk of missing carcinoma of the breast or fatally delaying treatment, with my policy of relying upon aspiration in the diagnosis and treatment of cysts. I have indeed missed carcinomas in patients in whom I was following and aspirating cysts. What I am not certain about is whether I would have done any better if it had been my custom to operate upon cysts rather than to aspirate them. In most instances in which carcinoma has developed it has occurred in a different breast area from that in which the most recently aspirated cyst was situated.

I must also point out that if the patient is followed carefully enough all is not lost even when aspiration misses a carcinoma situated in the same sector of the breast. The following case history is illustrative.

Mrs. M. C. developed tumors with the characteristics of cysts in the upper outer sectors of both breasts when she was 47 years of age. I operated upon her and removed cysts from both sides. Fifteen months later she developed a new cyst in the lower outer sector of her right breast, which I aspirated. After eight months more, another cyst appeared in the middle outer sector of her left breast, and I aspirated it successfully. Four months later she came to me with a rounded but firm 2 cm. tumor close to the site of the cyst in her left breast that I had recently aspirated. I attempted aspiration of the new tumor and failed. I therefore admitted her to the hospital, made all preparations for a possible radical mastectomy, and did a biopsy of the new tumor. It proved to be an undifferentiated carcinoma. I performed radical mastectomy. Thirteen of 26 lymph nodes recovered from the axillary portion of the specimen were found to contain metastases. She was given postoperative prophylactic irradiation to the axilla. Twenty-three years later she was in good health. It can be fairly said, therefore, that I succeeded with my treatment despite the four months delay in the diagnosis of her carcinoma that my policy of aspiration of cysts was responsible for.

Looking back over my experience with the diagnosis and treatment of cysts I am convinced that aspiration is preferable to operation. I have successfully aspirated an enormous number of cysts—at least ten thousand—and have avoided an operation each time. This fact alone, I believe, justifies the method. The avoidance of the expense, anguish, morbidity, and also the possible mortality associated with this number of operations more than compensates for the harm done by the delay in the diagnosis of carcinoma that must be charged to aspiration in a small number of patients.

REFERENCES

Bloodgood, J. C.: The pathology of chronic cystic mastitis of the female breast. Arch. Surg., 3:445, 1921.

Bloodgood, J. C.: The blue-domed cyst in chronic cystic mastitis. J.A.M.A., 93:1056, 1929.

Bloodgood, J. C.: Borderline breast tumors. Ann. Surg., 93:235, 1931.

Böhmig, R.: Die Epithelproliferationen bei der Mastopathia fibrosa cystica. Zentralbl. f. allg. Path. u. path. Anat., 89:297, 1952.

Borchardt, M., and Jaffé, R.: Zur Kenntnis der Zystenmamma. Beitr. z. klin. Chir., 155:481, 1932.

Brissaud, E.: Anatomie pathologique de la maladie kystique des mamelles. Arch. de physiol. norm. et path., 3:98, 1884.

Brodie, B. C.: Lectures Illustrative of Various Subjects in Pathology and Surgery. London, Longman [and others], 1846.

Bull, W. T.: Notes on cyst of the breast. Medical Record, 55:557, 1899.

Campbell, O. J.: Relationship between cystic disease of the breast and carcinoma. Arch. Surg., 28:1001, 1934.

Clagett, O. T., Plimpton, N. C., and Root, G. T.: Lesions of the breast; the relationship of benign lesions to carcinoma. Surgery, 15:413, 1944.

Cooper, A. P.: Anatomy and Diseases of the Breast. Philadelphia, Lea and Blanchard, 1845.

Davis, H. H., Simons, M., and Davis, J. B.: Cystic disease of the breast: relationship to carcinoma. Cancer, 17:957, 1964.

Engle, E. T., Krakower, C., and Haagensen, C. D.: Estrogen administration to aged female monkeys with no resultant tumors. Cancer Research, 3:858, 1943.

Foote, F. W., and Stewart, F. W.: Comparative studies of cancerous versus non-cancerous breasts. II. Rôle of so-called chronic cystic mastitis in mammary carcinogenesis, influence of certain hormones on human breast structure. Ann. Surg., 121:197, 1945.

Frantz, V. K., Pickren, J. W., Melcher, G. W., and Auchincloss, H., Jr.: Incidence of chronic cystic disease in so-called "normal breasts". Cancer, 4:762, 1951.

Franzas, F.: Ueber die Mastopathia cystica latens und andere bemerkenswerte Veränderungen in klinisch symptomfreien weiblichen Brüsten. Arb. Path. Inst., Helsingfors, 9:401, 1935–36.

Goormaghtigh, N., et Amerlinck, A.: Réalisation expérimentale de la maladie de Reclus de la mamelle chez la souris. Bull. Assoc. franç. p. l'étude du cancer, 19:527, 1930.

Gurdin, M., and Carlin, G. A.: Complications of breast implantations. Plast. & Reconstruct. Surg., 40:530, 1967.

Haagensen, C. D., and Randall, H. T.: Production of mammary carcinoma in mice by estrogens. Arch. Path., 33:411, 1942.

Hendrick, J. W.: Results of treatment of cystic disease of the breast; Surgery, 44:457, 1958.

Hodge, J., Surver, J., and Aponte, G. G.: The relationship of fibrocystic disease to carcinoma of the breast. Arch. Surg., 79:670, 1959.

Humphrey, L. J., and Swerdlow, M.: Relationship of benign breast disease to carcinoma of the breast. Surgery, 52:841, 1962.

Johnson, R.: Some clinical aspects of carcinoma of the breast. Brit. J. Surg., 12:630, 1924–25.

Keynes, G.: Chronic mastitis. Brit. J. Surg., 11:89, 1923.

Kiaer, W.: Relation of Fibroadenomatosis ("Chronic Mastitis") to Cancer of the Breast. Copenhagen, Ejnar Munksgaard, 1954.

König, F.: Mastitis chronica cystica. Centralbl. f. Chir., 20:49, 1893.

Lewison, E. F., and Lyons, J. G., Jr.: Relationship between benign breast disease and cancer. Arch. Surg., 66:94, 1953.

Lindgren, S.: On mastopathia cystica. Acta chir. Scandinav., 79:119, 1936.

Logie, J. W.: Mastopathia cystica and mammary carcinoma. Cancer Research, 2:394, 1942.

Marcuse, P. M.: Fibrocystic disease of the breast; correlation of morphologic features with the clinical course. Am. J. Surg., 103:428, 1962.

Olch, I. Y.: On the treatment of gross cysts of the breast by aspiration. Int. Union Against Cancer, 15:1145, 1959.

Patey, D. H.: Chronic cystic mastitis and carcinoma; collective review. Internat. Abstr. Surg., 68:575, 1939.

Patey, D. H., and Nurick, A. W.: Natural history of cystic disease of breast treated conservatively. Brit. M. J., 1:15, 1953.

Pullinger, B. D.: Cystic disease of the breast: human and experimental. Lancet, 2:567, 1947.

Reclus, P.: La maladie kystique des mamelles. Rev. de chir., 3:761, 1883.

Sandison, A. T.: An autopsy study of the human breast. Nat. Cancer Inst. Monograph, No. 8, U.S. Dept. of Health, Education, and Welfare, 1962.

Schimmelbusch, C.: Das Cystadenom der Mamma. Arch. f. klin. Chir., 44:117, 1892.

Semb, C.: Pathologico-anatomical and clinical investigations of fibro-adenomatosis cystica mammae and its relation to other pathological conditions in the mamma, especially cancer. Acta chir. Scandinav. (supplement 10), 64:1, 1928.

Sloss, P. T., Bennett, W. A., and Clagett, O. T.: Incidence in normal breasts of features associated with chronic cystic mastitis. Am. J. Path., 33:1181, 1957.

Speert, H.: "Pale epithelium" in the mammary gland and its experimental production in the Rhesus monkey. Surg., Gynec. & Obst., 74:1098, 1942.

Veronesi, U., and Pizzocaro, G.: Breast cancer in women subsequent to cystic disease of the breast. Surg., Gynec. & Obst., 126:529, 1968.

Warren, S.: The relation of "chronic mastitis" to carcinoma of the breast. Surg., Gynec. & Obst., 71:257, 1940.

Chapter Eight

Adenosis Tumor

In describing, in the preceding chapter, the microscopic features of the complex lesion that we call cystic disease, I have already referred to the component that we call, for lack of a better name, "adenosis." The acini of the gland fields and, to a lesser extent, the small ducts proliferate, invade the breast stroma, and finally stimulate fibrosis, which has led to the name of sclerosing adenosis. As a common and relatively inconspicuous microscopic feature of cystic disease, adenosis is not a problem for the pathologist because he sees it so often. The clinician does not perceive it because it does not form a palpable tumor. But when adenosis grows as a pure type of epithelial proliferation, and produces a dominant tumor in the breast, it presents a special diagnostic problem of great importance. The surgeon perceives it as a tumor of unknown nature that he must subject to biopsy. The pathologist, unfortunately, is more likely to mistake it for carcinoma than most other lesions that develop in the breast. For this reason I wish to devote this chapter to tumor-forming adenosis.

Incidence

In defining this tumor-forming type of adenosis pathologically, I refer to the lesions in which the tumor is actually formed by the adenosis. No gross cysts, excepting in some instances a few minute ones measuring not more than a few millimeters in diameter, are seen.

Adenosis of this type, forming a tumor, has been relatively infrequent in my experience. Some pathologists and a good many surgeons are not familiar with this lesion, and it is often missed, being lost in the hodge-podge of conditions that are lumped together under the ambiguous term "cystic mastitis." I have had 70 patients with adenosis tumor operated upon between the years 1939 and 1967. I would estimate that one might encounter one case of adenosis tumor to every 25 or 30 cases of carcinoma. Heller and Fleming described a series of 15 cases of adenosis tumor, and stated that this lesion constituted 2 per cent of all breast lesions in their clinic.

Age Distribution

The mean age of my patients with adenosis forming a tumor was 37.3 years. The youngest was 19; the oldest 55. The latter had been using face cream containing estrogen and had not completed the menopause.

All the others were premenopausal. Their age distributions is shown in Chart 8–1. It can be said of adenosis, therefore, that like cyst formation, it is a phenomenon of the menstrual phase of life. The mean age of my patients with tumor-forming adenosis was

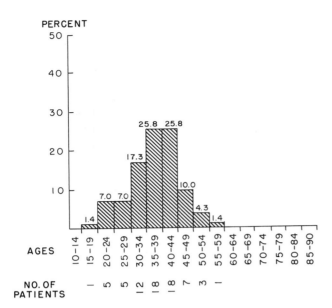

Chart 8–1. The age distribution of 70 patients with adenosis tumor.

somewhat younger than the mean age of our series of patients with cysts—37.3 as compared with 42 years.

Etiology

Seven of my 70 patients were single women. Among the married women 7 had never been pregnant. 52 others had produced 102 living children, and in the remaining four the information as to parity was lacking. These data do not suggest that the patients with adenosis tumor had anything abnormal in their reproductive history.

It has been suggested that the oral contraceptives, like other estrogens, stimulate the breast epithelium to proliferate, and thus predispose those who use them to develop adenosis and other epithelial tumors of the breast. Several of our younger patients with adenosis had indeed been using oral contraceptives, but their number is too small to have any statistical significance.

Our youngest patient with adenosis tumor, age 19, had been given estrogen intermittently for three years.

Clinical Features

Adenosis produces a tumor which may be clinically indistinguishable from carcinoma. It is firm and poorly delimited in the area of breast tissue in which it lies. It is also somewhat fixed in the breast tissue, like a carcinoma. Adenosis does not ordinarily produce retraction signs, although in a few cases where the lesion lay superficially in the breast, I have seen minimal retraction in the overlying skin. But this absence of retraction does not assist the clinician very much in his effort to distinguish between adenosis and carcinoma, because most of the tumors produced by adenosis are comparatively small, and the clinician should know that small carcinomas sometimes produce very little, if any, retraction.

The tumors produced by adenosis are in general small. Their mean diameter in my series of cases was only 2.4 cm. This is about one-half the average diameter of carcinomas coming to our clinic. In two of my patients with adenosis there was no palpable tumor; the lesion was identified by the fine stippling shown in mammograms by microcalcification in the lesions. In occasional cases of adenosis the lesion is much more extensive than the palpable tumor indicates.

Because the clinical characteristics of adenosis tumor do not distinguish it in any way from carcinoma, these tumors due to adenosis are often diagnosed clinically as carcinoma, and the surgeon comes to the operating table with this suspicion in his mind.

Pathology

There are certain gross features of adenosis tumor that should suggest to the critical pathologist that he is dealing with adenosis and not with carcinoma. Although adenosis is firm in consistence, it is not apt to be as hard as most carcinomas. The cut surface is slightly brownish, owing to the presence of small granular, brownish areas, which are in fact the foci of proliferating acini (Fig. 8–1).

The grayish-white streaks so typical of carcinoma are not seen. None of these gross features is, however, sufficiently characteristic to permit even the most experienced pathologist to distinguish surely between adenosis and carcinoma.

The microscopic features of adenosis may also superficially resemble carcinoma. The basic phenomenon is proliferation of the acinar epithelium. It grows without maintaining its usual acinar arrangement, and appears to infiltrate the surrounding mammary stroma, but the lobular pattern is to some degree preserved. An important distinguishing feature is the patchy character of this proliferation, as shown in Fig. 8–2. In the piece of tissue chosen for frozen section, however, the proliferation may be more solid and uniform, giving a deceptive impression of carcinoma.

Study of the lesion under higher magnification will show that the proliferating cells usually preserve to some degree an acinar arrangement (Fig. 8–3). The individual cells are small and rounded, and comparatively uniform (Fig. 8–4). Mitoses are infrequent. It has been suggested that they are myoepithelial cells, but this is certainly not proven.

As the lesion ages, fibrosis develops. The lobular pattern becomes less evident. The individual proliferating cells are compressed and distorted so that they increasingly appear to stream out into, and infiltrate, the mammary stroma, as shown in Figure 8–5. At this stage the proliferating cells appear to be smaller, with denser nuclei.

At a yet more advanced stage of fibrosis, adenosis may give a picture in which the effects of the fibrosis have so distorted the morphology of the original lobular proliferation that it can scarcely be recognized as such. Figure 8–6 is an example of this extreme degree of fibrosis. Such a microscopic field is strongly suggestive of carcinoma.

An area of adenosis jutting out into the mammary fat may simulate true invasion, as seen in Figure 8–7.

Taylor and Norris have pointed out that benign perineural invasion by normal mammary epithelium is occasionally seen in adenosis, and may lead the pathologist to the mistaken diagnosis of perineural carcinomatous invasion. They found 20 examples of this benign phenomenon in a series of 1000 consecutive breast specimens showing adenosis. Figure 8–8 shows it in one of our own cases. A group of three small epithelial structures resembling normal breast acini lie

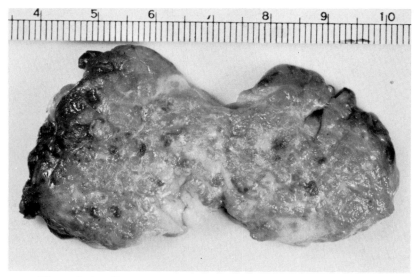

Figure 8–1.   Gross appearance of a tumor formed by adenosis.

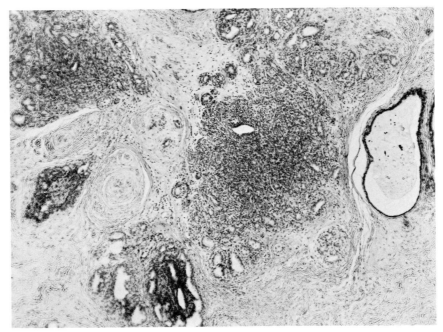

Figure 8–2. Adenosis, showing its patchy pattern.

beneath the epineurium of a nerve cut tangentially.

When the pathologist, already suspicious that he is dealing with carcinoma because of the clinical character of the lesion and its gross appearance, studies his frozen section and sees small epithelial cells indubitably infiltrating the breast stroma, he is very apt to mistake adenosis for carcinoma. He can save himself from the mistake only by always keeping adenosis in mind when he studies frozen sections of breast lesions, and by deferring his definitive diagnosis if he has the slightest doubt about the nature of the lesion.

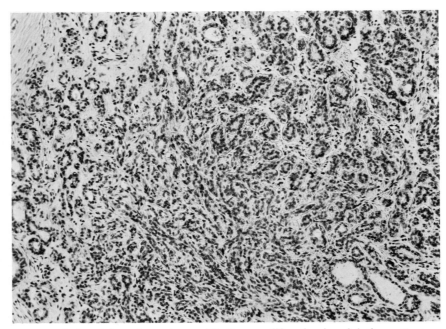

Figure 8–3. Adenosis—acinar epithelium proliferating in a lobular pattern.

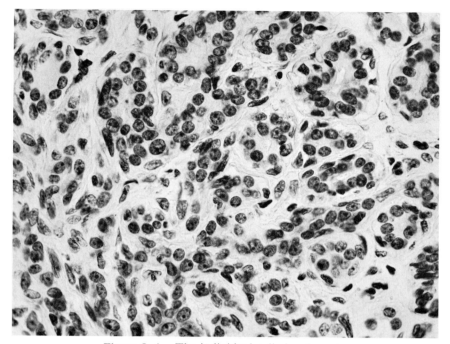

Figure 8-4.   The individual cells in adenosis.

He must cultivate a state of mind in which he takes no chances at all with this differential diagnosis. He must never gamble. If he will only wait, and prepare and study, with sufficient care, an adequate number of paraffin sections, he can distinguish correctly between adenosis and carcinoma every time.

Wellings and Roberts have reported that electron microscopy is useful in distinguishing adenosis from mammary carcinoma.

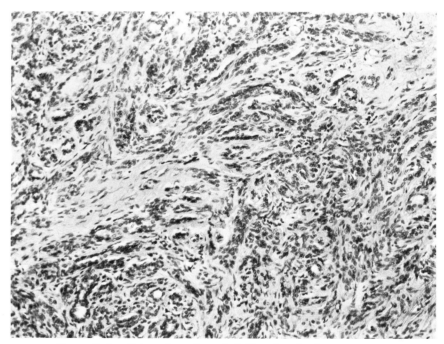

Figure 8-5.   Sclerosing adenosis infiltrating the breast stroma.

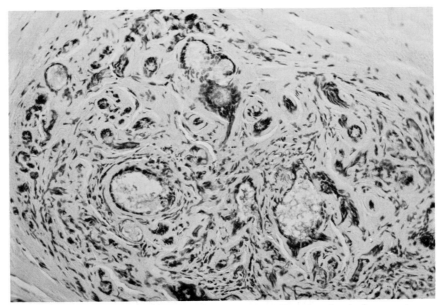

Figure 8–6.   Adenosis with an extreme degree of fibrosis, simulating carcinoma.

The surgeon on his part, when told that a reliable diagnosis is not possible from the frozen section, must not complain of his pathologist's uncertainty. He should be grateful that he has a pathologist who puts accuracy above everything else. He should close the wound after locally excising the small tumor from which he has excised a wedge for frozen section, and wait until the definitive diagnosis is made. We have no proof that waiting a few days for paraffin sections is a threat to the patient.

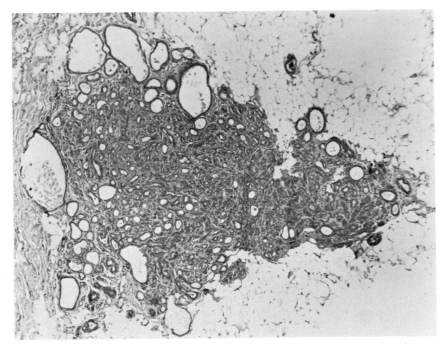

Figure 8–7.   An area of adenosis appearing to invade the mammary fat.

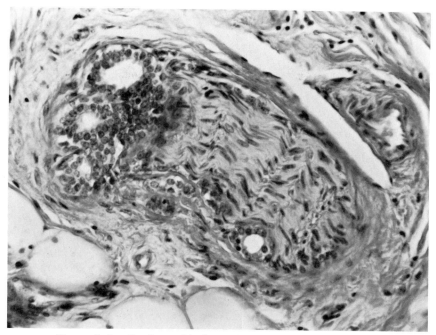

Figure 8–8.   Benign epithelium within a nerve in the breast.

Treatment

Adenosis tumor requires only local excision. The extensive removal of adjacent breast tissue, or mastectomy, is entirely unjustified.

This lesion apparently regresses after the menopause, like gross cystic disease. The following case history illustrates this fact.

Mrs. E.B., aged 45, consulted me because of a discharge from her right nipple. It had first appeared six months previously, when she noted a serous discharge over a three day period. She went to her family doctor who found no tumor in the breast and dismissed her. There was no further discharge for five months, when she noted a few drops of bloody discharge on her brassiere.

Palpation revealed only a poorly defined area of induration between the radii of 11 and 1 o'clock, just beyond the edge of the areola of the right breast. It was not well enough delimited to measure accurately. It was relatively fixed in the breast tissue. There was no retraction. Pressure over the induration produced a drop of serum from a nipple duct situated in the radius of 11 o'clock.

With all preparations for a radical mastectomy should it prove necessary, the area of induration was exposed through a circumareolar incision. The induration was seen to be due to the presence of a great many firm brownish nodules scattered throughout the softer whitish breast tissue. These nodules varied from a few millimeters to a centi-

meter or more in diameter. The entire upper outer sector of the breast was involved by the process. Several of the nodules were excised for frozen section, which revealed characteristic adenosis. To remove all of the lesion would have meant sacrificing almost half the breast. This seemed unjustified. Only the most prominent part of the lesion, that which had produced the area of induration, was excised.

When the patient reached the menopause, five years later, the residual induration had disappeared. Eleven years later her breast was normal.

This form of adenosis, which forms a dominant tumor in the breast, does not appear to predispose those who have it to subsequent breast carcinoma. Although the total number of patients in our series of cases is comparatively small, only one of them has as yet developed carcinoma. She was Mrs. D.S., who came to me when she was 43 with a firm 3 cm. tumor in the outer middle sector of her left breast. Biopsy was performed, and the tumor proved to be characteristic adenosis, and was excised locally. Five years later she discovered a tumor in her right breast. It grew rapidly, and when she consulted me a month later she had a typical carcinoma 5 cm. in diameter situated just medial to her right areola. There was a firm but movable 4 cm. node in the axilla. Internal mammary biopsy was done and a metastasis found in a node from the second interspace. She was treated by irradiation, and has no evidence of activity of her disease ten years and three months later.

REFERENCES

Cecconi, F.: Sulla adenosi sclerosante della mammella. Arch. ital. chir., *83*:501, 1958.

Ewing, J.: Neoplastic Diseases. Philadelphia, W. B. Saunders Co., 1942, 4th Ed., p. 541.

Heller, E. L., and Fleming, J. C.: Fibrosing adenomatosis of the breast. Am. J. Clin. Path., *20*:141, 1950.

Peremans, J.: Sclerosing adenosis. Belg. tijdschr. geneesk., *17*:1120, 1961.

Stewart, F. W.: Tumors of the Breast. Atlas of Tumor Pathology, Section IX, Fascicle 34, Washington, D.C., Armed Forces Institute of Pathology, 1950.

Urban, J. A.: Sclerosing adenosis. Cancer, *2*:625, 1949.

Taylor, H. B., and Norris, H. J.: Epithelial invasion of nerves in benign diseases of the breast. Cancer, *20*:2245, 1967.

Wellings, S. R., and Roberts, P.: Electron microscopy of sclerosing adenosis and infiltrating duct carcinoma of the human mammary gland. J. Nat. Cancer Inst., *30*:269, 1963.

Chapter Nine

Fibrous Disease of the Breast

The breast lesion that we call fibrous disease is not generally recognized as a disease entity. It is a benign, localized but not encapsulated, proliferation of the breast stroma that forms a definite dominant tumor. Because it is one of the less frequent benign lesions of the breast, its identity has usually been lost among the heterogeneous group of breast lesions that incurious pathologists and surgeons lump together as "fibrocystic" disease. Unless pathologist and surgeon really try to help each other identify fibrous disease, neither will succeed in doing so. It is worthwhile searching out and identifying this lesion however, because it has characteristics that are important clinically.

Incidence

Between the years 1939 and 1967 I have had 119 patients with fibrous disease of the breast. It is not, therefore, a frequent lesion of the breast. I have seen approximately one patient with fibrous disease for every 15 patients with breast carcinoma.

Age Distribution

The mean age of my patients with fibrous disease was 40.3 years. The youngest was 23; the oldest 56. The latter had had an estrogen pellet implanted 10 months previously and therefore had not completed the menopause despite her age. All these patients were thus properly classed as premenopausal. The age distribution of these patients is shown in Chart 9–1.

Etiology

The development of fibrous disease during the period of greatest ovarian activity suggests, of course, that it is caused by some form of hormonal dysfunction. This disease is the best example of selective stimulation of the fibroblastic element of the breast structure, because there is no associated epithelial proliferation.

In terms of their fertility, my patients with fibrous disease were normal enough. Fourteen of the 119 were not married. Twenty-five of the 105 married women had not been pregnant. The 80 parous women had produced a total of 150 children.

I have the impression that an unusually large proportion of these patients have heavy pendulous breasts. This is a difficult fact to document and I regret that I cannot be more precise. I can document another and perhaps associated fact, namely, that these fibrous disease tumors develop in the upper outer sector of the breasts much more often than is the case with other types of breast tumor.

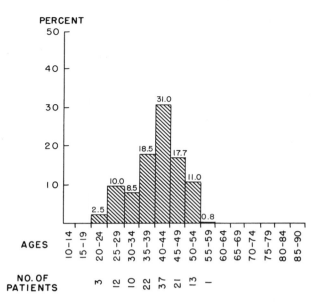

Chart 9–1. Age distribution of 119 patients with fibrous disease of the breast.

In my series of cases of fibrous disease 65 per cent of the tumors were in the upper outer sector of the breast, while in my series of carcinomas of the breast 44 per cent developed in the upper outer sector. One can theorize that in fibrous disease the weight of the breast transmitted through the fibrous stroma of its upper outer sector produces the localized tumor-forming hypertrophy of fibroblasts that characterizes this disease.

Clinical Features

Fibrous disease of the breast makes itself evident by the formation of a painless tumor. There are no other symptoms.

The tumor of fibrous disease is not well delimited like a cyst or an adenofibroma. Its edges merge into the surrounding breast tissue. This characteristic makes a skilled examiner fear that it is a carcinoma. Its shape is usually irregularly discoid, rather than rounded like a cyst or an adenofibroma.

It is firm in consistence, but not hard like a carcinoma. This is, however, a difficult distinction to make, particularly when the tumor is situated in a large dense breast.

The fibrous disease tumor lacks the easy movability of a cyst or an adenofibroma. It does not seem to slide around beneath the examiner's fingers. It is somewhat fixed in the bed of breast tissue in which it lies. This fixation is not as marked, however, as with

carcinoma. Again, this may be too finely drawn a distinction.

An important differentiating feature between fibrous disease and carcinoma is that fibrous disease does not produce retraction, while some manifestation of retraction can be demonstrated in almost every carcinoma.

The fibrous disease tumor rarely attains a large size. The largest one in my series of 119 cases was 5 cm. The mean diameter of the tumors was 2.3 cm. The smaller the tumors are, the greater is the difficulty of differentiating the various tumors of the breast from one another, and the small size of the fibrous disease tumor adds to the difficulty of distinguishing it from a small carcinoma in particular.

One feature of fibrous disease when it develops in the upper outer sector of the breast is the tendency for the lesion to be bilateral. One-fifth of my patients with a dominant tumor due to fibrous disease in this sector of the breast had a symmetrical tumor-like thickening on the other side. This contralateral thickening was not impressive enough to lead me to biopsy it, but it was a factor that led me to suspect that the dominant tumor on the other side was fibrous disease.

Pathology

The fibrous disease tumor is not encapsulated, and merges into the surrounding

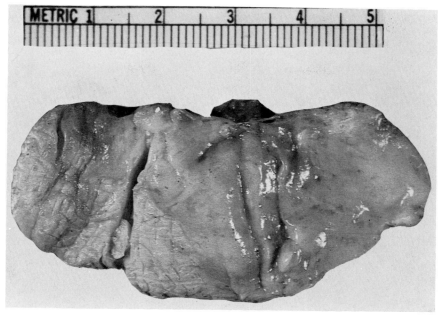

Figure 9–1. Gross appearance of fibrous disease.

breast tissue. Its cut surface is abnormally firm, with a dense, tough texture (Fig. 9–1). The knife does not grate going through, however, as it often does with carcinoma. Fibrous disease is more whitish in color, and more uniform in appearance, than normal breast tissue. It lacks the ominous chalky streaks of carcinoma. On the other hand no gross cysts are seen. While the pathologist cannot be entirely certain from the gross characteristics of the lesion that he is dealing with fibrous disease, he should strongly suspect it.

In the microscopic picture of fibrous disease two features predominate—proliferation of the fibrous stroma of the breast and atrophy of the mammary lobules. The stroma is dense, collagenous, and comparatively acellular (Fig. 9–2). The lobules are few in number, and

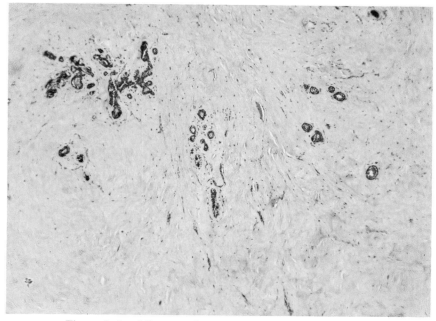

Figure 9–2. Microscopic appearance of fibrous disease.

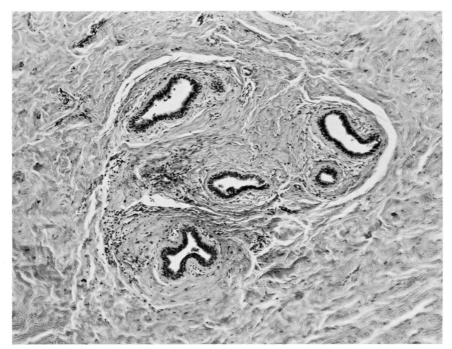

Figure 9–3.   A small fibrotic lobule in fibrous disease.

consist of only a few acini (Fig. 9–3). This kind of atrophy of the lobules is seen even in the youngest patients, in whom large and active lobules would be expected. Figure 9–4 shows this phenomenon in a patient aged 23.

In a minority of these lesions the element of lobular atrophy will be lacking. This makes the recognition of the lesion more difficult for the pathologist. Unless he is convinced that the patient indeed had a dominant tumor of

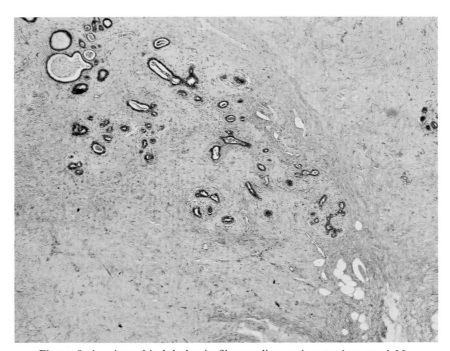

Figure 9–4.   Atrophic lobules in fibrous disease in a patient aged 23.

the breast and that his specimen came from it he is likely to classify it as normal breast tissue. Or if he finds a few dilated ducts and a little epithelial proliferation, insignificant changes that are present in the overwhelming majority of breasts of adult women and which do not produce a dominent tumor, he will blandly classify it as "fibrocystic disease." The way to convince the pathologist that fibrous disease is a genuine clinical and pathologic entity deserving of separate classification is to get him to palpate the tumor before operation. The surgeon, on the other hand, will be convinced when he sees the specimen cut by the pathologist who finds no gross cysts, but only dense fibrous tissue.

Stewart is one of the few pathologists who have recognized fibrous disease as a separate entity. He calls it "chronic indurative mastitis." Vassar and Culling have more recently published a good description of the disease, with a report of 20 cases.

Therapy

If the surgeon could be certain of the nature of a fibrous disease tumor he might reasonably leave it undisturbed. But he must perform a biopsy to prove its nature, and to rule out carcinoma. Having the lesion ex-posed and accessible, he had best excise it, after its nonmalignant nature has been proved, and in so doing relieve the patient of the worry that its continued presence would give her. This should be done in a manner that will leave a minimal scar, as I have described in my chapter on the excision of benign lesions of the breast.

Neither hormones nor irradiation therapy should be used for fibrous disease.

In two of my patients, fibrous disease recurred in the same region after I had excised it locally. I re-excised it and there has been no further recurrence.

I have no convincing evidence that fibrous disease has any relationship to carcinoma. Among a total of 57 patients whose fibrous disease was excised more than ten years ago, two have subsequently developed carcinoma. In both, the carcinoma appeared in the opposite breast, in one patient after an interval of three and one-half years and in the other after an interval of eight years.

REFERENCES

Stewart, F. W.: Tumors of the Breast. Atlas of Tumor Pathology, Section IX, Fascicle 34, Washington, D.C., Armed Forces Institute of Pathology, 1950.
Vassar, P. S., and Culling, C. F. A.: Fibrosis of the Breast A.M.A. Arch. Path., 67:128, 1959.

Chapter Ten

Mammary Duct Ectasia

For some years, surgeons and pathologists with extensive experience with breast disease have been aware that a benign condition in the aging breast characterized by dilatation of the collecting ducts in the subareolar region, and fibrosis and inflammation around them, is a separate clinical entity. It is important because its clinical picture may simulate carcinoma so closely that it has often been mistaken for it and needless mastectomy performed.

The lesion has been identified by a wide variety of names. Bloodgood, in 1923, wrote about it under the descriptive title of "the varicocele tumor — the clinical picture of dilated ducts beneath the nipple frequently to be palpated as a doughy worm-like mass." Adair called it "plasma cell mastitis." In so doing, he did not realize that he was describing merely the end stage of the process referred to by Bloodgood. In this end stage the irritative material within the dilated collecting ducts has passed through the duct walls and set up a low grade inflammatory reaction with many plasma cells. Dockerty called it "comedomastitis," and Payne and his associates labelled it "mastitis obliterans." Each of these names recalls some feature of the disease that I am describing, but none emphasizes its fundamental character as well as the term *mammary duct ectasia* which we prefer.

Sandison and Walker, as well as Asch and Frey, have recently adopted this name, but the disease is not well enough known to surgeons and pathologists to have won general recognition, and it is usually classified as an inflammatory process, or as one of the manifestations of that convenient catch-all, "chronic mastitis." I will describe its natural history and its pathological and clinical features in some detail, because it is important to establish it as a distinct and separate disease of the breast.

Incidence

Although occult duct ectasia is a comparatively common phenomenon, it evolves into clinically evident disease only infrequently. Between 1939 and 1967 I have had only 67 such patients: this amounts to only one patient with duct ectasia for every 25 or 30 patients with carcinoma.

Age Distribution

This is a disease of the aging breast. The overwhelming majority of those who develop it are near the menopause, or have passed it. The mean age of my patients with duct

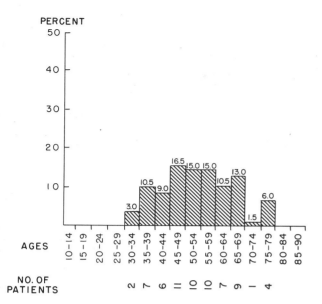

PERCENT

Chart 10-1. Age distribution of 67 patients with duct ectasia.

ectasia was 55 years. The youngest was 34 and the oldest 79. The age distribution of these patients is shown in Chart 10–1.

The Natural History of Mammary Duct Ectasia

Mammary duct ectasia begins with dilatation of the terminal collecting ducts beneath the nipple and areola. They become distended with cellular debris and lipid-containing material. The dilated ducts are bluish in color and from 3 to 5 mm. in diameter. At this initial stage there is no accompanying inflammation. There are no symptoms or clinical signs and the disease ordinarily escapes detection. Surgeons and pathologists with a broad experience in breast disease know of the existence of this kind of symptomless dilatation of the terminal ducts, having encountered it while exploring the breast for other lesions.

This initial symptomless form of mammary duct ectasia is more common than is generally appreciated. Frantz and her associates gave us for the first time an estimate of its true frequency. In their autopsy study of supposedly normal female breasts they found it in approximately 25 per cent of their subjects.

In a small proportion of these individuals with occult mammary duct ectasia, the lesion evolves to the stage of producing symptoms and clinical signs, as in the 67 cases in my personal series of cases. The earliest symptom is often a nipple discharge. It may be serous, bloodstained, or thicker and pus-like. The discharge is spontaneous and intermittent. Sixteen of our 65 patients had such a nipple discharge; in seven of the sixteen it was the only symptom of their disease. The discharge may be of long duration; in two of my patients it had been present for five years.

The development of a spontaneous nipple discharge of unknown etiology in a patient without a palpable breast tumor necessitates exploring the subareolar area surgically. I do this through a circumareolar incision centered over the axis of the subareolar area at which gentle pressure will produce the discharge. I dissect up the areolar flap and expose the terminal ducts at the base of the nipple. In duct ectasia several dilated ducts will be clearly seen. They are bluish in color and from 3 to 5 mm. in diameter. In some cases the majority of the terminal collecting ducts — normally some 20-odd in number — are involved. This finding is in contrast with the demonstration of a single dilated duct entering the base of the nipple in cases in which an intraductal papilloma is the cause of a nipple discharge. Papillomas are not found in mammary duct ectasia.

As the disease progresses, the duct dilatation extends peripherally. The distended ducts are strikingly defined in the as yet unchanged fatty breast stroma (Fig. 10–1). The duct walls are greatly thickened by fibrosis and by inflammatory infiltration of lymphocytes (Fig. 10–2). The fibrosis within the duct

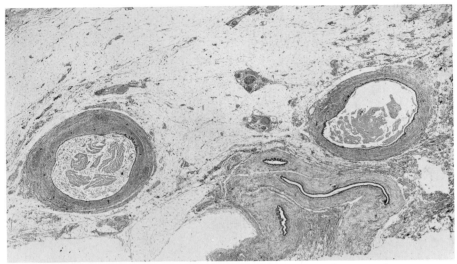

Figure 10–1. The dilated thick-walled ducts of duct ectasia.

walls not only thickens them but also shortens them, so that flattening and, eventually, retraction of the nipple, or deviation of the axis in which the nipple points, develops. These signs were present in 20 of our 67 patients, and in seven they were the first sign of disease. Figure 10–3 shows nipple retraction of six months' duration produced by mammary duct ectasia.

Strangely enough the duct epithelium is not stimulated to proliferate. In none of our cases was there any abnormal epithelial proliferation, either within the diseased ducts or in the ducts or acini of the adjacent uninvolved breast tissue. This absence of epithelial proliferation is one of the basic features of mammary duct ectasia. Atrophy, rather than proliferation, of the epithelium of the involved

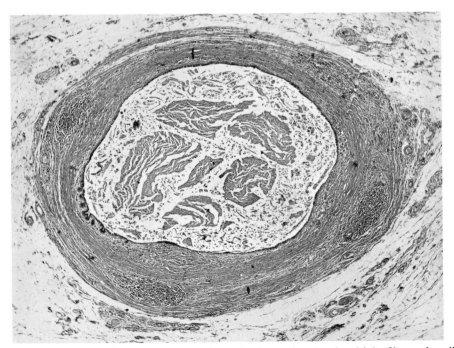

Figure 10–2. Higher power view of an ectatic duct, showing its thick, fibrosed wall.

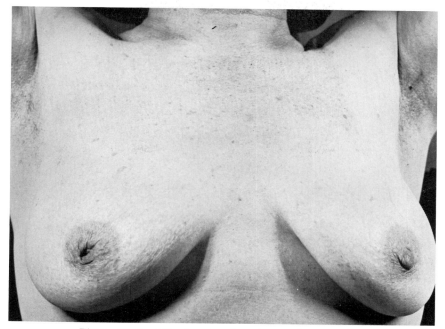

Figure 10–3.   Nipple retraction due to duct ectasia.

ducts is the rule. The epithelium is often so thinned out that it is barely visible in low-power magnification as a thin dark line lying upon the dense collar of fibrous tissue that forms the bulk of the much-thickened duct wall (Fig. 10–4). Outside the fibrous collar there is usually a zone of lymphocytic infiltration separating the duct from the surrounding fatty breast stroma.

The inflammatory changes in the duct walls

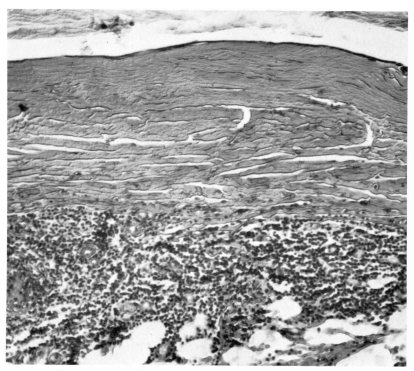

Figure 10–4.   High power view of wall of ectatic duct.

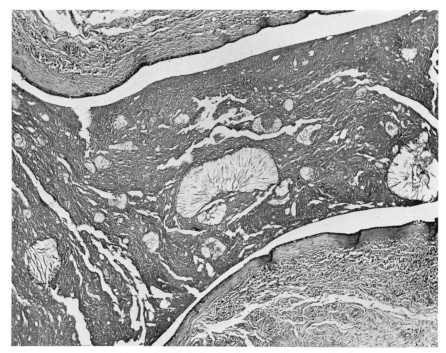

Figure 10–5.   Debris in the lumen of an ectatic duct.

apparently develop as a result of the irritative quality of the material with which they are distended. This material is amorphous debris with characteristic crystalline bodies scattered through it (Fig. 10–5). These crystalline bodies are round or oval, sometimes surprisingly large, and have a radial structure (Fig. 10–6). They have been identified in the dilated ducts in all our cases and are presumably another basic feature of mammary

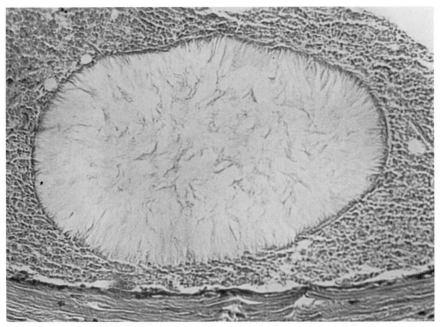

Figure 10–6.   Characteristic crystalline body in an ectatic duct.

duct ectasia that has evolved to the stage of producing symptoms and clinical signs.

We have made Scharlach-R stains of the material in the distended ducts and find that it stains intensely. The crystals themselves, however, do not stain. We assume from this evidence that the material is a lipid. We look forward to making analytical-chemical studies of the material when we have an opportunity to collect it in sufficient quantity. Lepper and Weaver have made such studies and report that "the material . . . consisted almost entirely of neutral fat."

When a surgeon explores duct ectasia at this stage of the evolution of the disease he cuts into firm tissue in which there are many dilated thick-walled ducts that ooze a surprising amount of pasty brownish material.

As mammary duct ectasia progresses, the continuity of the atrophic duct epithelium is broken in places. The irritating lipid material then sets up an inflammatory reaction in the thickened dense collagenous portion of the duct wall (Fig. 10–7). It eventually erodes through the whole thickness of the duct wall. Figure 10–8 shows a crystalline body, and an adjacent focus of lymphocytes, lying just outside the wall of a duct.

When the lipid material gets into the periductal tissues and the stroma of the breast, an intense inflammatory reaction, like that in fat necrosis following trauma, develops.

Phagocytic giant cells surround the lipid material (Fig. 10–9) and histiocytes, lymphocytes, and polymorphonuclear leucocytes form a zone of granulation tissue (Fig. 10–10). Its center may break down and form a small cavity filled with thick yellowish or brownish material. Such a lesion forms a palpable tumor that is firm, rounded, and relatively fixed in the breast tissue. Such a tumor was palpated in 54 of my 67 patients with duct ectasia. Since the tumor evolves from the terminal portion of the collecting ducts it is usually situated in the central sector of the breast, beneath or within a few centimeters of the areola. The great majority of these tumors are small, measuring from 1 to 3 cm. in diameter.

By the time duct ectasia has evolved to the stage at which there is a palpable tumor, reactive fibrosis around the lesion has often produced retraction signs in the form of dimpling of the adjacent skin and distortion of the contour of the breast. In 17 of our 67 patients, either there was obvious retraction, or it could be elicited by molding the breast, contracting the pectoral muscles, or by the forward-bending maneuver. Figure 10–11 shows a patient with duct ectasia in whom there was marked dimpling of the skin below the left areola. Her disease had produced a broad area of induration above the areola.

In some patients with duct ectasia the low grade inflammation produces a concentration

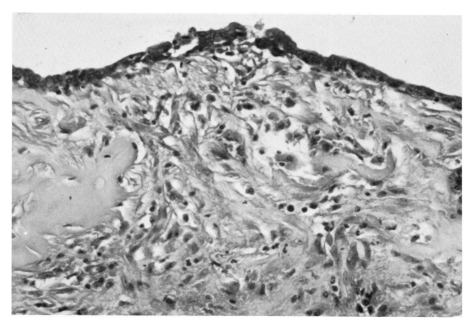

Figure 10–7.   Inflammatory reaction within the wall of an ectatic duct.

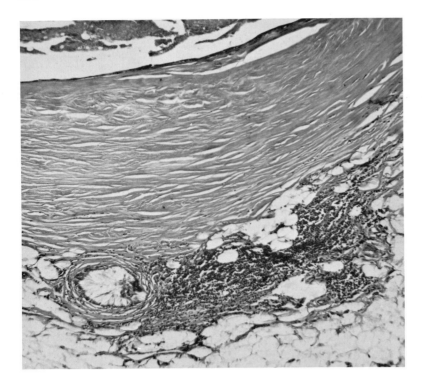

Figure 10–8. Crystalline body that has perforated the wall of an ectatic duct.

of plasma cells. This has so impressed some pathologists that they have called the lesion "plasma cell mastitis," thereby adding to the confusion regarding the nature of this disease.

The natural history of duct ectasia in the individual patient may be long. In two of our patients nipple retraction had been present for five and three years, respectively. In

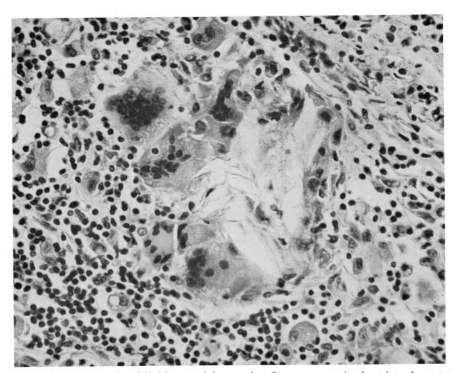

Figure 10–9.   Phagocystosis of lipid material escaping from an ectatic duct into breast tissue.

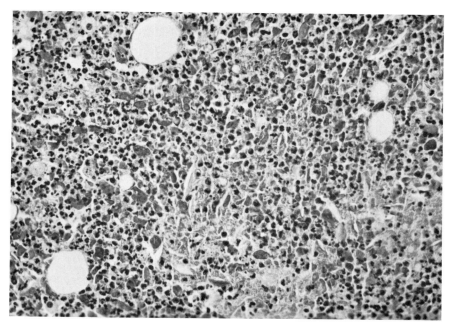

Figure 10–10. Granulation tissue resulting from the escape of lipid material from ectatic ducts into breast tissue.

another patient the small subareolar tumor had been present for eight years and had begun to enlarge a month before admission.

In a considerable proportion of patients with duct ectasia, episodes of acute inflam-

mation occur that suggest infection or abscess of the breast. These are heralded by acute pain and tenderness, redness and sometimes edema of the skin, and a tumor. The most remarkable thing about these

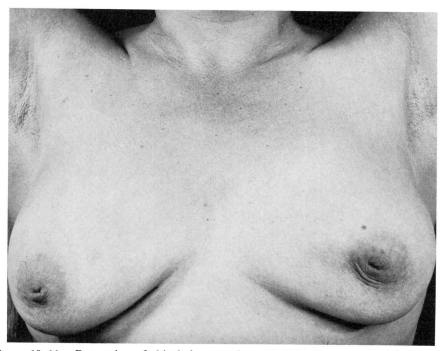

Figure 10–11. Retraction of skin below areola caused by duct ectasia of left breast.

episodes is the rapidity with which they develop, and, if left alone, the promptitude with which they subside. Within a week or ten days the breast may be almost normal again. Acute inflammation of this kind occurred in 12 of my 67 patients with duct ectasia. Pain and tenderness, not accompanied by changes in the skin, are more common: they were present in 23 of my 67 patients. They probably represent a less advanced stage of inflammation.

These episodes of inflammation in duct ectasia have a tendency to recur in the same breast, and to develop in both breasts. In five of our patients the disease was bilateral. One of these patients had had her right breast operated upon six and again two years previously with findings typical of duct ectasia, before she came to us with duct ectasia in her left breast. Another patient had had her left breast removed at another hospital, the presumed diagnosis being carcinoma, two years before she came to us with duct ectasia of the right breast. Review of the pathological findings in the left breast revealed that they were typical of duct ectasia, and that no carcinoma had been found. A third patient was found to have tumors due to ectasia in both breasts when she first came for consultation. The more advanced lesion in the left breast had given her symptoms for two months, and she was unaware of the small lesion in her right breast.

As might be expected in a disease in which inflammatory changes occur in the breast, the axillary lymph nodes are often enlarged. Such nodes were palpated in 13 of my 67 patients with duct ectasia.

Asch and Frey have recently pointed out that the ectatic ducts sometimes calcify, and that these tubular calcifications can be identified in mammograms, aiding in the diagnosis of the disease.

Etiology

Our studies of duct ectasia have given us no clue as to its etiology. The disease does not appear to have any relation to mammary function. Fifty-eight of my 67 patients were married. Fifty-two of those married had borne children, averaging 2.5 children each. The women with children had nursed for an average of 10 months. This is considerably longer than the total nursing time in all women consulting me regarding their breasts: they

nursed only for an average of 3.6 months. It cannot, therefore, be said that stasis in the mammary duct system as a result of not nursing was an etiologic factor in my series of patients with duct ectasia.

Illustrative Case Histories

Onset with Nipple Discharge. A. R., a 69 year old housewife, was admitted to the Presbyterian Hospital complaining of an intermittent brownish discharge from the left nipple of six months' duration. She had borne eight children, the last, 32 years previously, and had had her menopause at the age of 49. She had never previously had any trouble with her breasts. Examination revealed no asymmetry or tumor of the left breast. Pressure in the radius of 3 o'clock upon the areola produced a drop of brownish discharge from a duct in the center of the nipple. A presumptive diagnosis of intraductal papilloma was made.

At operation, a circumareolar incision was made between the radii of 2 and 8 o'clock. When the areolar flap was dissected back to the base of the nipple, several of the collecting ducts were seen to be dilated to a diameter of 5 mm. and were bluish in color. They were severed at the base of the nipple, allowing the escape of yellowish fluid. A pyramid-shaped sector of breast tissue surrounding the diseased ducts was then excised, the excision being carried out into the breast a distance of 10 cm.

Microscopic studies showed typical mammary duct ectasia. There was only minimal extraductal inflammation. No intraductal papilloma or other epithelial proliferation was found.

Onset with Nipple Retraction. M. H., a 51 year old housewife, was admitted to the Presbyterian Hospital with the complaint of retraction of the right nipple. She had first noticed flattening of the nipple five or six months previously. It had progressed until the nipple had recently become retracted beneath the surface of the areola. She had no other symptoms. She had borne two children, the last child twenty-one years previously, and had gone through the menopause at 49 years of age. She had never had any breast disease.

Examination showed the right nipple to be retracted to the level of the surrounding areola. It could not be everted. No tumor could be palpated. There was no asymmetry of the breast. With the possibility in mind that the nipple retraction might be an early sign of carcinoma, it was decided to explore the ducts at the base of the nipple.

At operation, a circumareolar incision was made around the cephalad half of the areola, and the areolar flap dissected up to expose the base of the nipple. The majority of the collecting ducts were seen to be bluish in color and dilated to as much as 5 mm. in diameter. When cut across at the base of the nipple, they oozed thick, grayish, creamy material. The ducts, together with a cone of surrounding breast tissue, were excised to a depth of about 5 cm. in the breast. At this level the ducts and the surrounding breast tissue appeared normal.

Microscopic study of the tissue showed typical mammary duct ectasia, with no intraductal epithelial proliferation and no extraductal inflammatory changes.

Onset with Tumor. M. R., a 46 year old housewife, was admitted to the Presbyterian Hospital complaining of tumor in the right breast of one month's duration. She had no other symptoms. She had had six pregnancies with three living children, the last child having been born 16 years previously, and she had nursed them all without difficulty, except for a caked breast on one occasion. Her periods had been regular.

Physical examination showed a hard 2 cm. tumor lying just beyond the edge of the areola of the right breast, in the radius of 10 o'clock. There was a definite shallow skin dimple over it. There were no enlarged axillary lymph nodes. A tentative diagnosis of carcinoma was made.

A circumareolar incision was made, exposing the tumor. When it was incised, it had the appearance of comedocarcinoma, being firm and mottled pinkish gray. Creamy material oozed from severed ducts. Frozen section did not show carcinoma, and the tumor was therefore excised locally.

Microscopic studies revealed typical mammary duct ectasia with a considerable amount of inflammatory infiltration and fat necrosis in the extraductal tissue.

Onset with Pain and Tenderness. A. F., a 39 year old housewife, was admitted to the Presbyterian Hospital with a complaint of pain and tenderness in the left breast of one week's duration. She had had one child 17 years previously and had nursed successfully. She had had no previous trouble with her breasts. The pain was in the left nipple region. The central portion of the breast was somewhat tender. There had been no nipple discharge.

Examination revealed a poorly defined, firm area of induration measuring about 4 cm. in diameter, lying beneath the upper half of the areola and extending cephalad from it. There was no redness of the overlying skin or elevation of skin temperature. On palpation there was definite tenderness over the area. In the forward-bending position there was slight flattening of the skin over the tumor. The white blood count was 8400. Her temperature on admission was 102° F. by rectum. It was decided to explore the lesion, with the presumption that it was inflammatory.

At operation, an incision was made around the upper half of the areola. When the lesion was cut into, dilated ducts oozed creamy material. At this point in the manipulations, creamy material also began to escape from the nipple. A small piece of tissue taken for frozen section showed only inflammation. The lesion was therefore excised locally.

Microscopic study showed typical mammary duct ectasia with acute inflammation of the extraductal tissues.

The Clinical Picture of Abscess. M. C., an unmarried 49 year old woman, came to the Presbyterian Hospital complaining of a tumor of the left breast. Five weeks previously she had discovered a lump in the lower part of her left breast. It was slightly tender, but she had thought nothing of it until four days previously, at which time the skin over it had become red.

Examination showed an elevated tumor measuring 3 cm. in diameter at the edge of the areola of the left breast between the radii of 3 and 5 o'clock. The skin over it was red and edematous. There was edema of the skin over the lower outer sector of the breast. There was a poorly defined area of induration deep in the breast in this sector. There was definite retraction of the skin just below the elevated tumor at the areolar edge. There were no enlarged axillary nodes. The white blood count was 9300, 58 per cent neutrophils. Body temperature was not elevated.

A diagnosis of abscess of the breast was made, and the elevated mass at the edge of the areola was incised. A cavity containing 3 cc. of thick pus was entered. Deep to the abscess the breast tissue was firm. Incision into this tissue revealed dilated ducts containing pasty material. Frozen section of this tissue revealed only inflammatory changes. The indurated area was therefore excised locally.

Microscopic study showed typical mammary duct ectasia, with acute inflammation and abscess formation.

The Clinical Picture of Carcinoma. N. G., a 42 year old housewife, came to the Presbyterian Hospital complaining of a tumor in the left breast, which she had first noted one week previously. The tumor had seemed to enlarge during the week that she had been aware of it. The entire breast, including the nipple, pained her. She described the pain as burning in character. There had been no redness of the skin. She had two children, now aged 11 and 5 years, respectively. She had not nursed them because of lack of milk. During the previous two years she had been troubled with painful engorgement of her breasts before and during menstruation.

Examination revealed a hard, poorly circumscribed tumor occupying a great part of the upper central part of the left breast. It measured about 6 cm. in diameter. The tumor was fixed in the surrounding breast tissue, and the breast as a whole was somewhat abnormally fixed to the chest wall, as evidenced by the fact that its mobility over the chest wall was lessened when the pectoral muscles were contracted. In the forward-bending position there was well-developed retraction in the skin over the tumor. The skin over the upper central portion of the breast was edematous but not reddened. The left nipple was flattened, and its axis deviated upward. In the left axilla there was a firm 2 cm. node. Skeletal and chest roentgenographic studies were negative.

I made a diagnosis of carcinoma, and radical mastectomy was performed without preliminary biopsy. When the breast was sectioned, the tumor was found to be made up of dense whitish tissue in which there were a multitude of dilated ducts filled with thick paste.

Microscopic studies showed typical mammary duct ectasia with accompanying infiltration. There was no carcinoma or, indeed, any form of epithelial proliferation anywhere in the breast.

Differentiation of Mammary Duct Ectasia from Carcinoma

The importance of duct ectasia depends upon the fact that it may present a clinical picture identical with carcinoma of the breast and betray the surgeon into doing an unnecessary radical mastectomy. The surgical literature, going back to the beginning of the modern pathologic classification of breast disease half a century ago, contains repeated instances of surgeons with extensive experience with breast lesions who performed mastectomy for mammary duct ectasia either because they did not understand and feared the lesion, or because they thought it to be carcinoma.

A series of eight cases in which mastectomy was unnecessarily performed for "plasma cell mastitis" simulating carcinoma was reported by Adair, in 1933. Lepper and Weaver, in 1937, described a group of eight cases with "generalized condition of distension of the ducts of the breast by fatty secretion," in which mastectomy had been done because of supposed carcinoma. In 1941, Cromar and Dockerty reported a series of 24 cases seen at the Mayo Clinic during the previous thirty years. A presumptive clinical diagnosis of cancer had been made in seventeen of the cases. Simple mastectomy had been carried out in fifteen cases, and radical mastectomy in nine. A subsequent study of the Mayo Clinic material, particularly of its pathological features, was reported by Tice, Dockerty, and Harrington.

In the present series of 67 cases of duct ectasia from the Presbyterian Hospital the presumptive diagnosis was carcinoma in 33. Radical mastectomy without preliminary biopsy was unfortunately performed in four. These mistakes were made many years ago, before we had learned never to trust the clinical diagnosis of breast carcinoma. I was personally responsible for the mistake in two of the patients. The last one occurred 26 years

ago. I have never since performed mastectomy without microscopic proof of the presence of carcinoma.

My own distressing experience of mistaking mammary duct ectasia for carcinoma, and study of the reports of other surgeons who have made the same error, convince me that it is impossible to distinguish the two diseases by clinical examination. When mammary duct ectasia has progressed to the stage in which inflammatory changes and consequent fibrosis have produced a tumor, the clinical picture may have all the features of carcinoma. The tumor is firm, poorly delimited, and, like a carcinoma, relatively fixed in the breast tissue that surrounds it. Retraction signs, including dimpling of the skin over the tumor, distortion of the contour of the breast, and retraction of the nipple, are regularly present. Axillary lymph nodes, enlarged as the result of inflammatory changes, are indistinguishable from lymph nodes containing metastases.

In order to emphasize the carcinoma-like clinical picture of mammary duct ectasia, I have summarized certain clinical features of the disease as reported by Cromar in the Mayo Clinic series of cases and from our own series of cases (Table 10-1).

A past history of the appearance and regression of signs of inflammation, such as pain and tenderness or redness of the overlying skin, or the presence of these signs, may suggest to the surgeon that the lesion with which he is dealing is due to mammary duct ectasia rather than to carcinoma, but I do not believe that we can safely exclude carcinoma on such a basis. Pain and tenderness, and slight redness of the overlying skin, are occasional features of mammary carcinoma.

Table 10-1. CLINICAL FEATURES OF MAMMARY DUCT ECTASIA

Clinical Features	Mayo Clinic (24 cases)	Haagensen, Presbyterian Hospital (67 cases)
Average age of patients in years	40	55
Per cent of patients with		
History of pain	79	35
Nipple discharge	21	24
Nipple retraction	42	30
Tumor	100	80
Skin retraction	83	26
Enlarged lymph nodes	72	12

My mistakes taught me that it is never safe to perform radical mastectomy without microscopic proof of the nature of the lesion. There are, of course, many advanced and inoperable cases of carcinoma in which the diagnosis can safely be made from the clinical picture, but all the clinical features of earlier and operable mammary carcinoma can be produced by mammary duct ectasia. Although this is a comparatively infrequent lesion, the hazard of mistaking it for carcinoma and performing a needless mastectomy is enough to justify making biopsy an absolute requirement preceding any mastectomy.

When a surgeon does a biopsy of a breast tumor caused by mammary duct ectasia, his impression may be that he is dealing with the comedo type of carcinoma. The cut surface of the lesion is mottled pinkish-gray and firm. As he cuts across it the dilated ducts ooze creamy or pasty material. A gross differentiation between carcinoma and mammary duct ectasia is impossible, but frozen section has enabled us to distinguish between the two diseases in every case in which we have resorted to it.

Treatment of Mammary Duct Ectasia

When the diagnosis of mammary duct ectasia has been made by surgical exploration and frozen section, the surgeon faces the problem of choosing the proper treatment. If the lesion is an early one, consisting only of dilatation and thickening of the collecting ducts, it has been our practice to sever all of these ducts at the base of the nipple, and to excise them together with a cone of surrounding breast tissue. We carry the excision deeply enough into the breast to reach a level at which the ducts and the surrounding breast tissue appear normal when cut across. This severance of the ducts at the base of the nipple, even though all were cut, has not had any apparent ill effects in the women in whom we have done it. None of the patients in whom we have severed the collecting ducts has subsequently become pregnant, so that we have no information as to what would happen if the breast were called upon to function.

In cases in which mammary duct ectasia has evolved to a more advanced stage in which periductal inflammation and fibrosis have produced a tumor, it has been our practice to excise the diseased area locally.

We have closed these wounds without drainage. The pus-like creamy material that oozes from the severed ducts in these lesions is not, in our experience, an indication for drainage.

Since mammary duct ectasia is a perfectly benign lesion, not associated with epithelial hyperplasia, there is no justification for the surgeon doing anything more than local excision.

The follow-up of these cases has not demonstrated any unexpected association with carcinoma.

REFERENCES

Adair, F. E.: Plasma cell mastitis—a lesion simulating mammary carcinoma; a clinical and pathologic study with a report of ten cases. Arch. Surg., 26:735, 1933.

Asch, T., and Frey, C.: Radiographic appearance of mammary-duct ectasia. New England J. Med., 266:86, 1962.

Bloodgood, J. C.: The pathology of chronic cystic mastitis of the female breast; with special consideration of the blue-domed cyst. Arch. Surg., 3:445, 1921.

Bloodgood, J. C.: The clinical picture of dilated ducts beneath the nipple frequently to be palpated as a doughy worm-like mass—the varicocele tumor of the breast. Surg., Gynec. & Obst., 36:486, 1923.

Bloodgood, J. C.: The changing clinical picture of lesions of the breast. Am. J. M. Sc., 179:27, 1930.

Cheatle, Sir G. L. and Cutler, M.: Tumours of the Breast. Philadelphia, J. B. Lippincott Co., 1931, p. 298.

Cromar, C. D. L., and Dockerty, M. B.: Plasma-cell mastitis. Proc. Staff Meet., Mayo Clin., 16:775; disc. 782, 1941.

Frantz, V. K., Pickren, J. W., Melcher, G. W., and Auchincloss, H., Jr.: Incidence of chronic cystic disease in so-called "normal breasts"; a study based on 225 postmortem examinations. Cancer, 4:762, 1951.

Lepper, E. H., and Weaver, M. O.: Generalized distension of the ducts of the breast by fatty secretion. J. Path. & Bact., 45:465, 1937.

Lübschitz, K.: A case of plasma cell mastitis. Acta Radiol., 24:403, 1943.

Manoil, L.: Plasma cell mastitis. Am. J. Surg., 83:711, 1952.

Payne, R. L., Strauss, A. F., and Glasser, R. D.: Mastitis obliterans. Surgery, 14:719, 1943.

Rodman, J. S., and Ingleby, H.: Plasma cell mastitis. Ann. Surg., 109:921, 1939.

Sandison, A. T., and Walker, J. C.: Inflammatory mastitis, mammary duct ectasia, and mammillary fistula. Brit. J. Surg., 50:57, 1962.

Seillé, G., and De Brux, J.: Une dystrophie mammaire peu connue: l'ectasie galactophorique secrétante. Presse méd., 66:2051, 1958.

Tice, G. I., Dockerty, M. B., and Harrington, S. W.: Comedomastitis. Surg., Gynec. & Obst., 87:525, 1948.

Chapter Eleven

Traumatic Fat Necrosis in the Breast

Fat necrosis is well known in those areas of superficial body fat that are exposed to trauma. The breasts, being composed largely of fat, and so situated that they are particularly vulnerable to trauma, are occasionally the site of fat necrosis. The importance of this lesion in the breast is that it simulates carcinoma in some patients, and obscures it in others.

The clinical importance of fat necrosis of the breast was first emphasized by Lee and Adair in 1920. They described two cases in which a firm tumor, adherent to the skin, was diagnosed clinically as carcinoma and the breast amputated. Pathologic study showed only fat necrosis. In one this was traced to a blow on the breast, and in the other to hypodermoclysis.

There are many examples in medical history in which the first good description of a comparatively infrequent disease stimulates valuable discussion of the disease. Lee and Adair's paper on fat necrosis of the breast had this result. During the next decade a number of case reports were published (Cohen; Stulz et al.; Cutler; Lecène and Moulonguet; Keynes; Gottesman and Zemansky; Moir; Hadfield; and Enzer). Lee and Adair, in two more papers on fat necrosis that appeared in 1922 and 1924, described a number of additional cases. Since then the most important contributions to the subject have been Harbitz's description of the pathology of the lesion, Adair and Munzer's report of their large series of 110 cases and Leborgne's description of its radiographic characteristics.

Incidence

Occult fat necrosis of the breast that produces no symptoms and goes undetected must be rather frequent. Leborgne, who has defined the radiographic appearance of old fat necrosis cysts with calcified walls, reports identifying them in 10 per cent of the subjects in whom he studied the breasts with mammograms.

Fat necrosis producing a breast tumor that is detected clinically is, however, not common. Between 1945 and 1967 I have had only 44 patients with such a lesion. Breast carcinoma has been more than 40 times as frequent in my experience.

Age Distribution

The mean age of the patients with fat necrosis in my series of cases was 51.9 years. The youngest was 27 and the oldest 80 years. Their age distribution is shown in Chart 11-1. The predominance of older women may be due to a greater tendency of older women to fall and injure their breasts.

Etiology

The earlier case reports of fat necrosis featured its traumatic origin. As experience with the lesion has accumulated it has become apparent that many of the patients who have

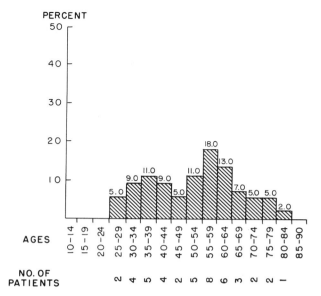

Chart 11-1. Age distribution of patients with traumatic fat necrosis.

typical fact necrosis are unable to recall any definite injury. In my series of 44 patients with proved fat necrosis only 32 per cent gave a definite history of trauma. Adair and Munzer reported that 44 per cent of their 110 patients gave a history of trauma. Yet it seems reasonable to assume that trauma is the cause of mammary fat necrosis in all cases except those secondary to infection, or to irritating material from the ducts getting into the breast stroma as in duct ectasia. Such cases of secondary fat necrosis, of course, have not been included in the present series of cases. The breasts, particularly in obese women, are certainly often traumatized, and it is not surprising that patients are unable to recall a specific injury. This supposition is borne out by the fact that occasional patients with fat necrosis have ecchymosis but nevertheless give no history of trauma. There were two such cases in the present series. Sixty per cent of the patients had neither a history of trauma nor ecchymosis. Fat necrosis occasionally develops from surgical trauma and forms a tumor that requires biopsy. In two of my patients the lesion originated in this way.

A strong point in favor of the traumatic origin of mammary fat necrosis is the frequency of gross or microscopic evidence of hemorrhage in these lesions. Harbitz found blood pigment in all but two of the 17 examples of fat necrosis that he studied.

There are several possible explanations for the manner in which trauma produces fat necrosis. The fat may be actually crushed and killed by the injury, or hemorrhage resulting from ruptured vessels may produce ischemia and necrosis.

Clinical Features of Fat Necrosis

The clinical features of fat necrosis are summarized in Table 11-1. In the patient in whom ecchymosis is present it is the most striking feature of the lesion. Figure 11-1 shows the ecchymosis over the central area of the breast in a nurse, aged 60, whom I saw twelve days after she had fallen and struck her breast. There was in addition a firm, poorly delimited tumor just beyond the areolar edge at 3 o'clock, as indicated in the photograph by the circle. It was relatively fixed in the breast tissue, and measured 2 cm. in diameter. The ecchymosis may be relatively limited, as in this patient, or it may extend over a great part of the skin of the breast.

In some patients in whom there is no ecchymosis the skin over the lesion is reddened. Eleven per cent of the patients in my series showed such reddening. It is due to the irritative effect upon the overlying skin of the area of necrosis situated close beneath it.

A characteristic feature of the majority of the fat necroses is that the lesion is situated very superficially in the breast, close to the skin. This, of course, is where trauma would be expected to be the most severe.

Fat necrosis may occur in any sector of the

Table 11–1. CLINICAL FEATURES OF FAT
NECROSIS

Clinical Features	Adair and Munzer	Presbyterian Hospital, Haagensen
Number of cases	110	44
Age range	14 to 80	27 to 80
History of trauma	44%	32%
History of pain or tenderness	34%	32%
Ecchymosis of skin	22%	27%
Redness of skin	9%	11%
Tumor	100%	100%
Retraction signs	58%	41%
Enlarged axillary nodes	29%	7%
Clinical diagnosis of carcinoma	27%	32%
Unnecessary radical mastectomy	2%	0

breast. The commonest site, however, is the areolar region. In 36 per cent of the cases in my series the lesion was in this region.

A tumor was present in all of my cases. It was usually small, the average diameter being 2 cm. These tumors are firm and they are often relatively fixed in the surrounding breast tissue. In these two features fat necrosis resembles carcinoma. The tumor of fat necrosis occasionally has one characteristic, however, that is unusual in carcinoma. This is its rounded, comparatively well delimited shape. A tumor due to fat necrosis often increases slowly in size for a period of days or weeks after it is discovered. This behavior of course suggests carcinoma. In most cases the tumor, if not removed, eventually regresses and disappears. In other patients it remains unchanged for years.

Fibrosis follows the initial necrosis, and produces retraction signs. In one form or another they were evident in 41 per cent of my series of cases. The commonest form is retraction of the skin over the tumor. Figure 11–2 shows marked dimpling of the skin over an area of fat necrosis just medial to the areola in an obese woman, aged 55, with large dependent breasts. Nipple retraction or axis deviation may also be produced by fat necrosis. These signs were present in five of the patients in our series of cases.

There is a type of clinical picture produced by fat necrosis that closely resembles abscess. In these patients there is no history of trauma or ecchymosis. The first sign of disease is pain or tenderness, localized over a small tumor situated usually beneath or near the areola. The skin over the lesion becomes red and warm. When the supposed abscess is

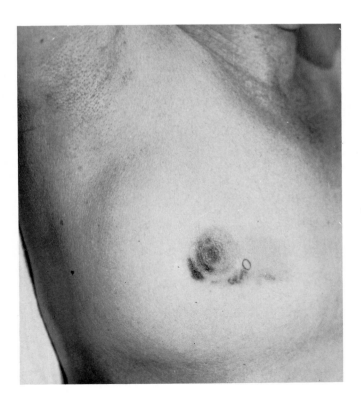

Figure 11–1. Ecchymosis associated with fat necrosis due to trauma.

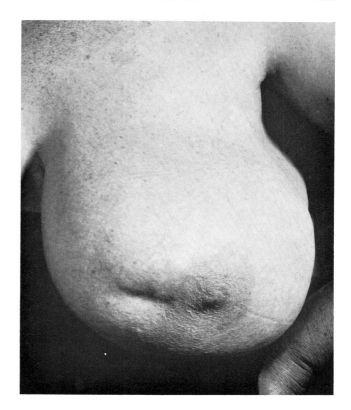

Figure 11–2. Skin retraction due to fat necrosis.

incised the process is found to be very superficial and comparatively localized. A cavity filled with old blood or thick grayish-yellow material is found. Microscopic study of the wall shows only fat necrosis. Such lesions usually occur in obese women with large breasts, and unlike the ordinary breast abscess, they are not associated with lactation.

Indeed, the great majority of patients with fat necrosis have large dependent breasts, as exemplified in Figure 11–2. It is understandable why this should be so.

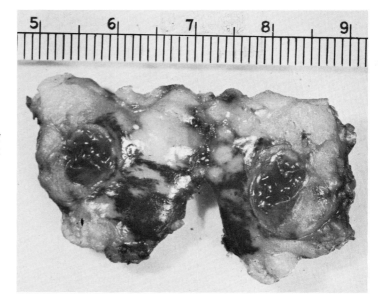

Figure 11–3. Gross appearance of the early hemorrhagic stage of fat necrosis.

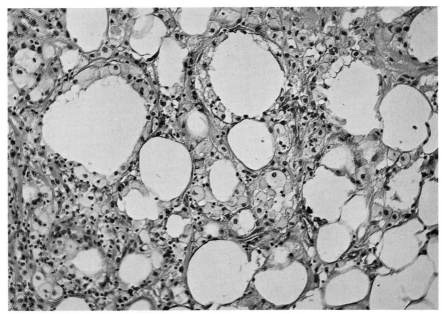

Figure 11-4. Microscopic appearance of early fat necrosis.

Pathology

The gross appearance of fat necrosis depends upon the stage of the lesion. The earliest picture is, of course, that of hemorrhage in an indurated area of fat. Figure 11-3 shows such a lesion.

After three or four weeks have elapsed the lesion forms a rounded firm tumor in the soft mammary fat. Its surface is yellowish-gray with scattered dark red zones. Incision into it may reveal a cavity filled with clear, oily liquefied fat, or old chocolate-colored sticky blood. In other cases the necrosis produces a cavity filled with thick grayish or yellowish

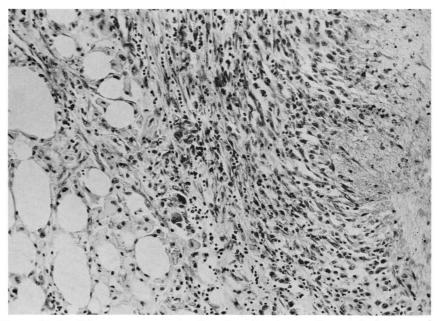

Figure 11-5. Fibrous zone surrounding the central necrotic area in fat necrosis.

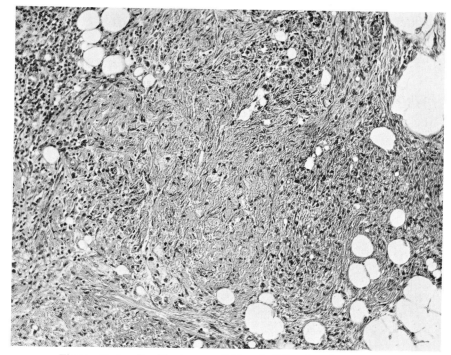

Figure 11-6. Residual area of fibrosis following fat necrosis.

necrotic material. Calcification of the walls of such cavities is common.

Microscopically the first step in the process of fat necrosis is the dissolution and fusion of the individual fat cells to form larger vacuoles. Between the vacuoles fibroblasts, lipoblasts, and large clear epithelioid cells proliferate. The epithelioid cells, which have also been called histiocytes, or clasmatocytes, or foam cells, engulf the fat debris. Their cytoplasms become reticulated. These epithelioid cells have a tendency to line the vacuoles as they carry on their function of fat absorption. Figure 11-4 shows these microscopic features.

At a later stage in the process the epitheli-

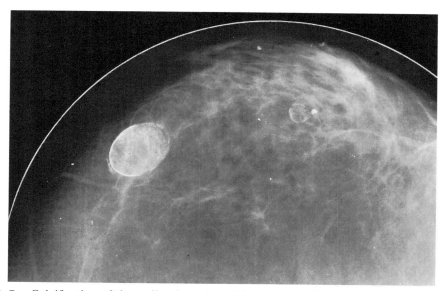

Figure 11-7. Calcification of the walls of cystic cavities resulting from fat necrosis, as seen in a mammogram. (Courtesy R. Leborgne.)

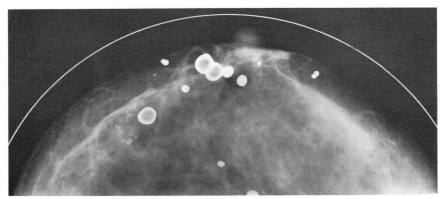

Figure 11–8. Calcification in the walls of small fat necrosis cysts producing small ring shadows seen in a mammogram. (Courtesy of R. Leborgne.)

oid cells are transformed into large multinucleated giant cells. These are most often seen in the vicinity of the fatty acid crystals, oil droplets, and blood pigment that result from the fat necrosis.

Fibrosis predominates at the periphery of the lesion, forming a zone of denser tissue around the central area of necrotic debris. Figure 11–5 shows this fibrous zone, with the necrotic debris at the right and the surrounding fat at the left.

Eventually the area of necrosis is entirely replaced by dense fibrous tissue, in which a few vacuoles filled with oil remain. Figure 11–6 shows such a lesion 18 months after the original traumatic fat necrosis.

Leborgne has called attention to the fact that the walls of the cysts filled with necrotic debris and lipid material that form in mammary fat necrosis often become calcified. He has illustrated this phenomenon with superb mammograms (Figure 11–7). He has also pointed out that the small calcified rings so often seen in mammograms represent calcification of very small fat necrosis cysts (Figure 11–8). In the past these rings have been variously interpreted, but on the basis of the pathology of fat necrosis I believe that Leborgne's explanation is the correct one.

Diagnosis

Because fat necrosis produces a firm tumor, often accompanied by skin dimpling, it suggests carcinoma. The preoperative diagnosis in 14 of the 44 patients in my Presbyterian Hospital series was carcinoma. Biopsy and frozen section were done in all our patients, and the nature of the lesion was correctly diagnosed.

A generation ago, when fat necrosis was first being recognized and discussed, it was often mistaken for carcinoma, no biopsy done, and mastectomy needlessly performed. When Hadfield, in 1929, collected a series of 45 cases of fat necrosis, he found that mastectomy has been mistakenly performed in 26 per cent. These were the cases, of course, in which there was no history of trauma and no ecchymosis to alert the surgeon to the possibility of fat necrosis. Such mistakes will only cease when the rule of biopsy for all breast lesions is generally adopted.

In patients who do give a history of definite trauma to the breast, and in whom ecchymosis and a tumor develop, there is danger that these signs may betray the surgeon into assuming that they are due to fat necrosis, and that it is safe not to perform a biopsy of the tumor and merely to watch it. I have seen several patients in whom trauma and subsequent ecchymosis called attention to a tumor which proved to be carcinoma. The carcinoma must have been present for some time in all these patients. It would have been missed if the rule of doing a biopsy on every breast tumor had not been followed.

Illustrative Case Histories

Fat Necrosis with a History of Trauma and Ecchymosis. Mrs. R. O., a woman aged 60 with large pendulous breasts, fell while carrying groceries. Her left breast was struck and severely bruised by a milk bottle. The skin over most of the breast became black and blue. Three weeks later she discovered a lump in the breast and came for consultation.

In the upper inner sector of her breast, 4 cm. from the areolar edge, there was a hard, poorly delimited 1 cm. tumor. There was slight skin retraction over it. At biopsy the tumor proved to be an area of fat necrosis with a central collection of old blood.

Fat Necrosis Without a History of Trauma but with Ecchymosis. Mrs. A. R., a 50 year old housewife, discovered a tender lump in her right breast while bathing. The following day the skin over it was ecchymotic. She could not recall any injury to her breast.

Examination showed a 6 cm. area of ecchymosis just above the areola. Beneath it there was a 3 cm. firm, but freely movable, well delimited, superficially situated tumor. At biopsy the tumor was found to be yellowish-red necrotic fat with a central area of hemorrhage.

Fat Necrosis Without a History of Trauma or Ecchymosis. Mrs. M. C., an obese housewife aged 44, came to the Presbyterian Hospital because of a tumor of her right breast that she had discovered three days previously. She could not recall any injury to her breast.

Examination showed a 2 cm. firm tumor situated superficially just medial to the areola. It was moderately well delimited, and fairly movable. The overlying skin was reddened, and showed slight retraction. There was three weeks delay in admission to the hospital for biopsy. During this period the redness of the skin disappeared and the tumor grew a little larger. At operation it was found to be a solid yellowish area of fat necrosis.

Fat Necrosis Following Surgery. Mrs. G. T., a housewife aged 45, with large dependent breasts, was struck on the left breast by the door of a subway train. Two days later she noticed that the breast was black and blue. Two weeks later, while bathing she found a lump in the region of the injury.

When she was examined the ecchymosis had disappeared. There was a 2 cm. firm, well delimited, movable tumor just medial to the areola of the left breast. There was skin attachment over it. At biopsy fat necrosis with a small cavity containing greenish-yellow, oily fluid was found and excised. Wound healing was uneventful.

Seven months later a 1.5 cm. firm, round, well delimited, movable tumor was found beneath the operative scar at follow-up examination. It had exactly the same clinical characteristics as the original tumor. We assumed that it was a new area of fat necrosis produced by the surgical trauma. Our supposition must have been correct, for the tumor persists unchanged, except for slight diminution in size, 15 years later.

Treatment of Fat Necrosis

The treatment of fat necrosis is local excision. The technique to be followed has been described in Chapter 6. In those cases of fat necrosis in which there is a cavity filled with necrotic material that looks like pus the surgeon need not fear to excise the lesion cleanly and to close the wound without drainage. Special care should be taken in these cases, however, to get the wound completely dry of blood, and to operate as gently as possible. These patients, who usually have large fatty breasts, are apt to develop fat necrosis anew from the trauma of operation unless these precautions are taken.

Paraffinoma

Mention should be made of the tumors of the breast that develop as a reaction to paraffin injection. The practice of injecting paraffin into the tissues for cosmetic purposes has now, fortunately, been thoroughly discredited, but it continues to be done occasionally by the unscrupulous.

Paraffin produces a low grade inflammatory reaction with fibrosis, and often abscess formation and the development of chronic fistulae. The paraffin, moreover, often migrates in the tissues, and has even penetrated the chest wall and gotten into the pleural cavity. Good descriptions of breast paraffinomas producing these complications have been presented by Krohn, by Schweitzer, by Bordet, by Delascio, and by Tinckler and Stock.

In our Presbyterian Hospital data we have a case in which Vaseline had been injected into the breast, not for cosmetic purposes, but for therapeutic purposes, with disastrous results.

A. B., a housewife aged 30, was admitted to the Presbyterian Hospital for draining sinuses of the left breast. Her first child had been born three years previously and she had nursed it successfully for three months. An abscess then developed in the left breast. Repeated incisions were required during the succeeding five months before the infection was brought under partial control. During this period of time several injections of "radioactive Vaseline" were made into the breast in an attempt to arrest the infection. (This therapy was not given at the Presbyterian Hospital.)

Subsequent to the Vaseline injections there had been repeated flare-ups of the breast infection, at intervals of three to six months. Several sinuses formed which drained pus and Vaseline. Pain had led the patient to drug addiction.

On examination the left breast was contracted and scarred by numerous incisions (Fig. 11-9). Beneath the scars were irregular firm areas of induration.

A simple mastectomy was done. When the breast was sectioned a number of greasy masses of Vaseline, surrounded by dense fibrous tissue, were

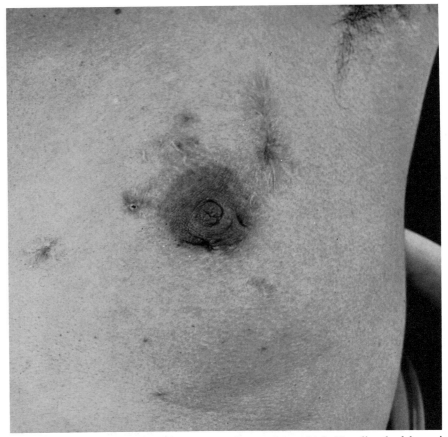

Figure 11–9.   Scarring and sinus formation in a breast into which Vaseline had been injected.

found. There were sinus tracts from the skin leading to several of these masses. Microscopic study showed chronic inflammation with necrosis and foreign body giant cell reaction about the injected Vaseline, and much fibrosis.

REFERENCES

Adair, F. E., and Munzer, J. T.: Fat necrosis of the female breast; report of 110 cases. Am. J. Surg., *74*:117, 1947.

Bordet, F.: Migration intra-pulmonaire d'un paraffinome mammaire. Arch. méd-chir. de l'app. respir., *13*:272, 1938.

Cohen, I.: Traumatic fat necrosis of the breast. J A.M.A., *80*:770, 1923.

Cutler, E. C.: Apoplexy of the breast. J.A.M.A., *82*:1763, 1924.

de Cholnoky, T.: Paraffinoma of male breast. Am. J. Surg., *44*:649, 1939.

Delascio, D., et al.: Parafinoma da mama. Rev. de ginec. e d'obst., *45*:419, 1951.

Dunphy, J. E.: Surgical importance of mammary and subcutaneous fat necrosis. Arch. Surg., *38*:1, 1939.

Enzer, N.: Traumatic fat necrosis of the breast. Am. J. Surg. n. s., *12*:102, 1931.

Gottesman, J., and Zemansky, A. P.: Fat necrosis of the breast. A study of twenty cases. Ann. Surg., *85*:438, 1927.

Hadfield, G.: Fat necrosis of the breast, with an account of a case. Brit. J. Surg., *13*:742, 1926.

Hadfield, G.: Fat necrosis of the breast. Brit. J. Surg., *17*:673, 1929.

Harbitz, H. F.: Lipogranuloma—a foreign body inflammation often suggesting a tumour. Acta chir. Scandinav., *76*:401, 1935.

Keynes, G.: A case of fat necrosis of the breast. Brit. J. Surg., *12*:663, 1925.

Krohn, K. H.: Ueber Paraffinome der Mamma. Zentralbl. f. Chir., *57*:2772, 1930.

Leborgne, R.: Esteatonecrosis quística calcificada de la mama. Torax, *16*:172, 1967.

Lecène, P., and Moulonguet, P.: La cytostéatonécrose ou saponification intracellulaire du tissu cellulo-adipeux sous-cutané. Ann. d'anat. path., *2*:193, 1925.

Lee, B. J., and Adair, F.: Traumatic fat necrosis of the female breast and its differentiation from carcinoma. Ann. Surg., *37*:189, 1920.

Lee, B. J., and Adair, F. E.: A further report on traumatic fat necrosis of the female breast and its differentiation from cancer. Surg., Gynec. & Obst., *34*:521, 1922.

Lee, B. J., and Adair, F. E.: Traumatic fat necrosis of the female breast and its differentiation from carcinoma. Ann. Surg., *80*:670, 1924.

Menville, J. G.: Fatty tissue tumors of the breast. Am. J. Cancer, 24:797, 1935.

Moir, P. J.: Traumatic fat necrosis of the breast. Brit. M. J., 1:640, 1929.

Sandison, A. T., and Walker, J. C.: Inflammatory mastitis, mammary duct ectasia, and mammillary fistula. Brit. J. Surg., 50:57, 1962.

Schweitzer, L.: Zur Kasuistik der Paraffinome. Zentralbl. f. Chir., 76:642, 1951.

Stulz, E., Diss, A., and Fontaine, R.: Granulome lipophagique du sein d'origine traumatique. Bull. et mém. Soc. anat. de Paris, 93:505, 1923.

Tinckler, L. F., and Stock, F. E.: Paraffinoma of the breast. Australian and New Zealand J. Surg., 25:142, 1955.

Zeitlhofer, J.: Ueber Fettgranulome der Brustdrüse. Arch. f. klin. Chir., 277:385, 1953.

Chapter Twelve

Adenofibroma of the Breast

The benign nature of the general class of fibroepithelial tumors of the breast was recognized a hundred years ago by such early pioneer students of breast disease as Sir Astley Cooper, who called them "chronic mammary tumours." But the varied microscopic pattern of this group of breast neoplasms, as it was revealed to the first few generations of pathologists who had the microscope to work with, led to a complex and confusing histologic classification which, even today, handicaps us. Depending upon whether the epithelial or the fibrous elements predominated, these tumors have been called adenofibroma or fibroma. When their stroma is myxomatous, they have been classed as myxoma. When it is highly cellular and cystic, they have been labelled cystosarcoma. When they appear to grow within ductlike spaces, they are called intracanalicular adenofibroma. Cheatle studied the histology of these tumors in great detail and classified them on the basis of the relationship of the new fibrous tissue proliferation to the elastica layer of the ducts and acini. McFarland reviewed a large number of them, deplored the confused nomenclature, and concluded that they are all varieties of a single well-characterized genus for which he preferred the name periductal fibroma. Güthert suggests that this whole group of breast tumors has an organoid character, and that they arise from embryonal rests. He considers the distinction of

intracanalicular and pericanalicular structure an artificial one, pointing out that almost every adenofibroma shows both types of structure.

We prefer to divide the fibroepithelial tumors of the breast into two groups on the basis of their microscopic structure—*adenofibroma* and *cystosarcoma phyllodes*. The two cannot be distinguished clinically. Adenofibroma is frequent and always benign. Cystosarcoma phyllodes is uncommon, and in rare instances malignant. In the present chapter I will deal with adenofibroma.

Etiology

Since adenofibromas develop most frequently during youth, it might be argued that their origin is in some way associated with the estrogenic stimulation of the breast tissues during this period of life. Soerensen reported histologic studies of several adenofibromas that were excised after the patient had been treated with estrogen. The tumors showed edema and hyperemia of the lobules, and lymphocytic infiltration.

Goldenberg and his associates have reported bizarre epithelial proliferation and secretory activity in adenofibromas excised from women who were taking hormonal oral contraceptives.

Adenofibromas also respond to the intense

212

growth stimulus to which the breast is subjected during pregnancy. Moran reported a series of ten patients in whom adenofibroma was excised during pregnancy. In nine there had been growth of the tumor during the pregnancy. Microscopic study of the excised adenofibromas revealed epithelial changes similar to those in the surrounding normal breast tissue.

While it is no doubt a fact that adenofibromas of the breast usually show some increase in size during pregnancy, I have not observed any harmful effects of this enlargement. In our patients the increase in the size of the tumor has not been great, and some of the tumors have regressed in size with involution of the breasts after completion of the pregnancy.

There has been a good deal of experimental work with adenofibroma of the breast in rats, a disease to which this species is especially prone (Heiman, Wright). It is doubtful, however, that any of the conclusions concerning the etiology and natural history of adenofibroma of the breast in the rat can be applied to this tumor as it occurs in human beings.

Incidence

Adenofibroma is the third most common tumor of the breast in present-day American females, being exceeded in frequency only by carcinoma and by cystic disease. During the 10 year period from 1951 to 1960 a total of 619 patients with adenofibromas were studied in the Presbyterian Hospital. During the same period 1428 patients with carcinoma of the breast were seen.

The group of 619 patients includes only those in whom the adenofibroma formed a tumor which was recognized clinically. Not included are a considerable number of cases in which minute adenofibromas were found in the course of gross and histologic study of breast tissue removed for other lesions. An accurate appraisal of the frequency of such very small adenofibromas requires the use of microscopic sections of the whole breast. Cheatle, who used this technique extensively, reported that unsuspected adenofibromas, often just visible to the naked eye, occur in about 25 per cent of all normal breasts.

In their study of the breasts in a series of 225 autopsies Frantz and her associates found adenofibroma in 21, or 9 per cent, of their cases. Only four of these tumors were large enough to be visible grossly; the other 17 were found microscopically.

Age Distribution

Adenofibroma is a disease of youth. This tumor may develop at any time after puberty and is overwhelmingly the most frequent breast tumor in young women under the age of 25 years. The youngest of our patients was a Negro girl in whom tumors were noted in both breasts when she was 12 years old, before she had menstruated. A year later two adenofibromas, measuring between 3 and 6 cm. in diameter, were removed from each breast. Our oldest patient was 76. But I have not seen a postmenopausal patient with an adenofibroma in whom I was convinced that the tumor had recently developed. In these postmenopausal patients it can be assumed that the lesion had originated before the menopause, and had only recently been detected. The mean age of our patients with adenofibroma who were under the age of 50 was 31 years. Chart 12–1 shows the age distribution of our 619 patients with the disease. In a series of 496 cases reported by Giacomelli the mean age of the patients was 21 years.

Racial Predisposition

It has been suggested that Negro women are predisposed to develop adenofibromas. In our hospitals at Columbia-Presbyterian Medical Center we have a large number of Negro patients, but their exact proportion is not known. We cannot, therefore, answer this question of racial predeliction from our data.

Natural History

The usual history of adenofibroma is that of a small, painless tumor discovered accidentally by a young woman in one breast in the course of bathing or dressing. Nipple discharge does not occur. The tumor grows so slowly in most patients that it takes six to 12 months for it to double in size. In a considerable proportion of patients, growth stops after the adenofibroma reaches 2 or 3 cm. in diameter. It is then likely to remain unchanged for the remainder of the patient's

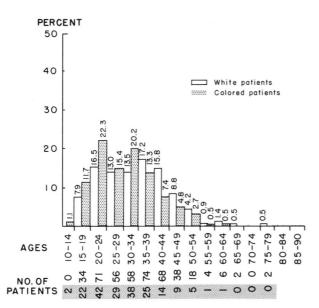

Chart 12-1. The age distribution of patients with adenofibroma of the breast.

life. Adenofibromas occasionally originate in the third or fourth decade, but they do not develop or grow after the menopause.

Some of these adenofibromas that develop during the later years of menstrual life show a surprising growth vigor, and continue to grow to a very large size. Although they have the gross and microscopic character of adenofibroma, they have often been called cystosarcoma merely because of their large size. We believe that this is incorrect. Cystosarcoma has a different natural history and requires somewhat different treatment.

The following is a typical case history of one of these large adenofibromas of middle life.

Mrs. C. P., a 34 year old housewife, had noted enlargement of her left breast six years previously. On admission her left breast was filled with a well-delimited nodular tumor, measuring 15 cm. in diameter. The skin over it was movable, and the tumor was not fixed to the underlying chest wall. At operation it was found to have a well-defined capsule, and after a frozen section of a biopsy specimen had confirmed its adenofibromatous character, it was easily dissected out of the surrounding breast tissue. Its microscopic structure was that of an adenofibroma, without any special features. The patient was well 11 years later.

Adenofibromas are not infrequently multiple, developing concurrently or successively, in one or both breasts. In our series of 619 patients with adenofibromas studied in our clinics between 1951 and 1960, more

than one adenofibroma was diagnosed or excised in 19.9 per cent. This is a minimal figure, because our patients with simple adenofibromas have not been systematically followed, and some may have subsequently developed additional adenofibromas without our knowledge.

Semb found adenofibroma to be multiple in 13.4 per cent of a series of 142 cases. Oliver and Major reported multiple adenofibromas in 15.7 per cent of a series of 352 patients with this lesion.

The following case history illustrates the multiple development of adenofibroma.

Mrs. N. G. first discovered bilateral breast tumors at the age of 28, and consulted me. She had three tumors in her left breast, a 1 cm. one in the upper outer sector, a 2 cm. one in the upper inner sector, and a 2 cm. one in the lower inner sector. In her right breast she had a 1 cm. tumor in the outer middle sector of the breast. All the tumors were very well delimited and movable within the surrounding breast tissue. I assumed that they were adenofibromas and advised their removal. She demurred. The tumors grew slowly and after four years were about twice the size they were when I first measured them. Thereafter they ceased to grow.

Fourteen years after she had first found these tumors she discovered a new one along the medial edge of her left breast. Although it was well delimited and movable like her other tumors, she was now 42 years old, and she consented to the removal of the new tumor as well as the largest of the old tumors in her breast. They all proved to be adenofibromas.

I last examined her when she was 52 years of age, 24 years after she had consulted me for the first time. Her adenofibromas had shown no change in many years. The largest was 2 cm. in diameter.

I have the impression that multiplicity of adenofibromas is more frequent in Negro women, but a review of this question in the 123 women with multiple adenofibromas in our series of cases suggests that there is no racial predilection (Table 12–1).

There are two special variants of the growth pattern of adenofibroma that merit special mention.

1. Massive Adenofibroma in Youth. The tumor is first noted at, or within a few years after, puberty. It may originate as a solitary lesion in one breast, and grow to a massive size, or there may be multiple tumors in both breasts, with one or two attaining a large size; these tumors are encapsulated grossly, and their microscopic structure is that of an adenofibroma. They do not recur if completely removed, and they do not metastasize. They have often been classified as cystosarcoma phyllodes, because they grow rapidly and attain a very large size. We have come to believe, in our department of surgical pathology, that this is incorrect. We make the diagnosis of cystosarcoma phyllodes not on clinical grounds but upon the characteristic

Table 12–1. MULTIPLICITY OF ADENOFIBROMA (Presbyterian Hospital, 1951–1960)

	Number of Patients	Number with Multiple Fibromas	Per cent with Multiple Fibromas
Caucasian	431	86	20%
Negro	188	37	19.7%
Total	619	123	19.9%

microscopic structure of these tumors, which I shall describe later.

Wulsin has written understandingly concerning these massive adenofibromas of adolesence, and there have been a few isolated case reports (Block and Zlatnik; Markowitz and Howell; Wulsin).

In our clinic we have had seven such cases. In these patients the age at which the tumor was first noted ranged from 12 to 16 years. Two of these patients were Caucasian and five were Negro. The size of the tumor in our patients varied from 10 cm. to 19 cm. Local excision sufficed to cure all our patients. In five of the patients there was a massive solitary tumor of one breast. The other two patients had multiple tumors in both breasts, some of which were very large.

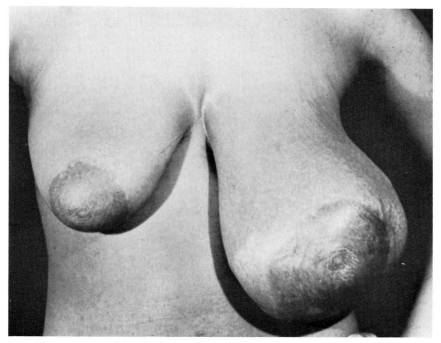

Figure 12–1. Massive adenofibroma of the breast in a girl aged 14.

The following is a characteristic example of a solitary adenofibroma of this type.

B. S., an unmarried Negro girl of 14, came to Presbyterian Hospital for treatment of a tumor of her left breast that she had discovered two years previously at about the time of her first menstrual period. It had grown steadily to reach a massive size (Fig. 12–1). At operation it was found to be well encapsulated and was excised locally. It measured 19 cm. in diameter and weighed 1070 grams. Its microscopic structure was that of an ordinary adenofibroma. Twelve years later there had been no recurrence.

The following is an example of multiple massive adenofibromas developing in youth.

G. C., a 12 year old Negro girl, came to the Presbyterian Hospital with tumors in both breasts. She had discovered the tumors three months previously. She had begun to menstruate a year previously. In her right breast she had a 3 cm. tumor just lateral to the areola. Her left breast was much larger than the right, and contained a lobular mass, which seemed to be made up of several separate components, measuring 20 by 15 cm. These tumors were all well circumscribed, and were freely movable within the surrounding breast tissue. They were excised locally. All

were characteristic adenofibromas. The mass on the left was made up of five separate adenofibromas, the largest 12 cm. and the smallest 2 cm. in diameter.

2. Multiple Successive Adenofibromas Developing Throughout the Entire Extent of the Breasts. This syndrome might be considered as the ultimate expression of the tendency of breast tissue to form massive yet benign adenofibromas beginning in adolescence. In this sense it is an exaggeration of the solitary massive adenofibroma of youth.

About the time of puberty in these patients, multiple adenofibromas begin to appear throughout both breasts. They grow steadily and often reach a very large size. At operation they are found to be well encapsulated, and microscopically they are ordinary benign adenofibromas. As they attain a substantial size and are removed, new ones develop. This process may continue as long as any remnant of mammary tissue exists. It cannot be described as malignant. Although some of the tumors attain a large size and are fixed to the thoracic wall because they develop in

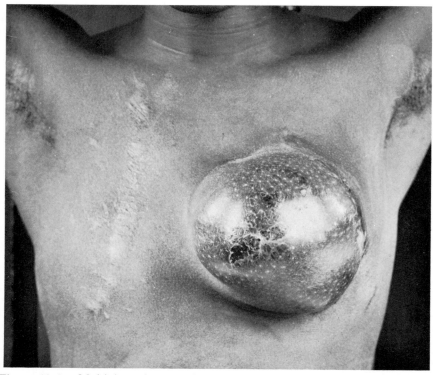

Figure 12–2. Multiple and successive adenofibromas beginning in adolescence.

scar tissue from previous operations, they do not invade adjacent tissues and do not metastasize.

The following is an example of this syndrome.

M. G., an unmarried Negro girl aged 18, came to the Presbyterian Hospital complaining of a recurrent tumor of the left breast. She had first noted tumors in both breasts five years previously when she was 13 years old. The tumors grew to approximately 10 cm. in diameter by the time she was 15. Bilateral partial mastectomy was then done at another hospital. Within a year after this operation a recurrent tumor developed on the left chest wall and grew steadily until her admission to the Presbyterian Hospital at the age of 18. Her condition at this time is shown in Figure 12-2.

There was a large, firm but not hard, well circumscribed lobular tumor measuring 12 cm. in diameter, solidly fixed to the left anterior chest wall. There were several small nodules situated both medial and lateral to the main tumor.

Biopsy of the main tumor showed a benign adenofibroma without any of the histologic characteristics of cystosarcoma phyllodes. Through a transverse incision across the whole anterior chest wall an attempt was made to excise all remaining breast tissue on both sides, together with the recurrent adenofibroma. Breast tissue was found to extend as a thin sheet laterally beyond the mid-axillary line on each side, however, and its complete removal was abandoned because it would have extended the scope of the operation unreasonably.

The patient moved to a southern state and was not seen until six years later. She was then 24 years of age and in good general health, but there were two recurrent adenofibromas, one measuring 3 cm. in diameter and situated at the lateral limits of the dissection on the right chest wall, presumably in residual breast tissue at this point, and another measuring 2 cm. in diameter near the left sternal edge. Nothing was done about these tumors.

The patient married and went through her first pregnancy when she was 27. In all she had seven pregnancies and uneventful deliveries, the last when she was 38. With each pregnancy her residual breast tissue and the two recurrent fibroadenomas enlarged somewhat, but subsequently regressed. The two adenofibromas finally began to grow slowly, and by 1967, when the patient was 46, the one on the left side measured 5 cm. and the one on the right side 8 cm. They were then excised locally by Dr. J. D. Ashmore, Jr. Microscopically, they were simple adenofibromas. The total duration of fibroadenomatosis in this patient was 33 years.

Dr. Ashmore has recently written me that this patient's 15 year old daughter has the same condition that her mother had. The daughter has eight large adenofibromas in her right breast, and five large ones in her left breast. I believe that this is the first report of the familial character of this disease.

Pathology

The gross appearance of adenofibroma is often characteristic. The tumor is so sharply delimited from the surrounding breast tissue that it seems to be encapsulated, although it does not have a capsule. The cut surface is whitish, resembling normal breast tissue in color. As the proportion of the epithelial component in the tumor is increased, the color appears more brownish. The cut surface often bulges. It frequently glistens with highlights owing to the mucoid content of the tissue. Figure 12-3 shows a characteristic adenofibroma. Clefts in the tumor are seen as dark lines, and are sometimes large enough to gap open.

Microscopically, adenofibromas are made up of two components, a proliferating connective tissue stroma and an atypical multiplication of ducts and acini (Fig. 12-4). These two components are present in varying amounts and provide a great variety of structure. Cheatle described and illustrated these variations in more detail than any other writer, and explained them in terms of the site of the connective tissue proliferation in relation to the duct structure; but this kind of exercise in classification has no practical value.

The clefts of the usual adenofibroma are lined by one or two layers of inactive-appearing epithelium. But the epithelial component of these tumors not infrequently shows a variety of proliferative processes, similar to those occurring in the ducts and acini of the mature breast. Piling up of the epithelium within the ducts, papillary proliferation, multiplication and atypical growth of ducts, and adenosis-like areas are often seen. Squamous metaplasia may occur in rare instances (Fig. 12-5).

In some adenofibromas the epithelial component is so dominant that they might almost be regarded as adenomas. Figure 12-6 shows such a tumor.

In our material we have no example which we were willing to classify as a pure adenoma of the breast. Such tumors must be exceedingly rare. It seems likely that the "adenomas" described by de Cholnoky and by Baker were adenofibromas in which the epithelial component predominated.

The fibroblasts which form the stroma of

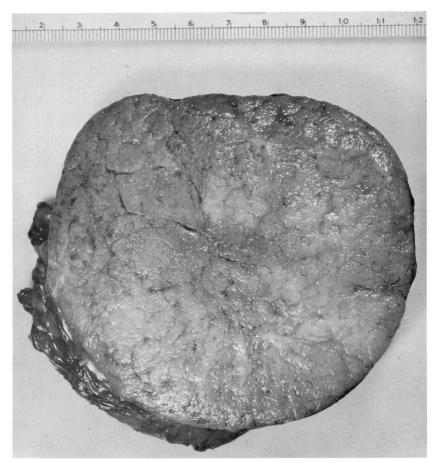

Figure 12–3. Gross appearance of adenofibroma of the breast.

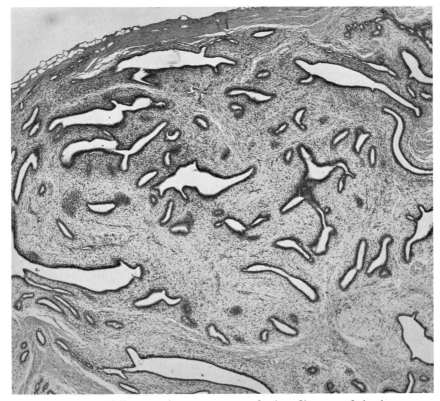

Figure 12–4. Microscopic appearance of adenofibroma of the breast.

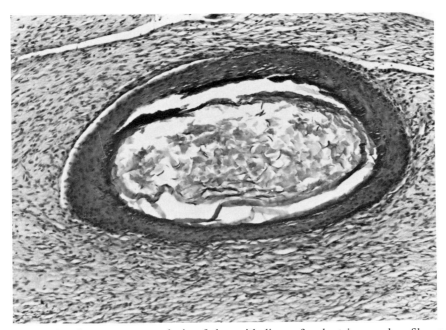

Figure 12–5. Squamous metaplasia of the epithelium of a duct in an adenofibroma.

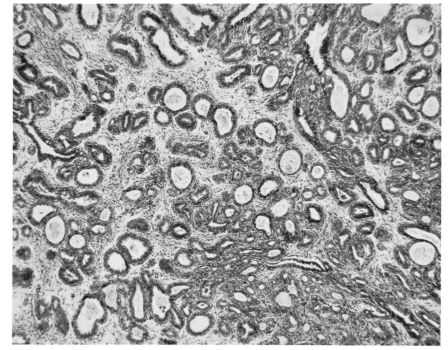

Figure 12–6. Adenofibroma in which the epithelial component predominates.

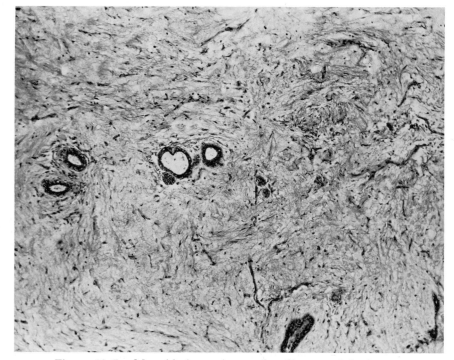

Figure 12–7. Myxoid change in an adenofibroma of the breast.

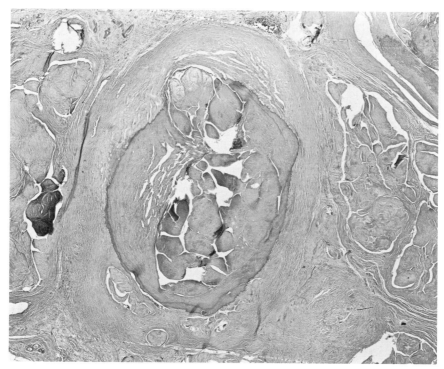

Figure 12–8. Calcification in an adenofibroma removed from a woman aged 62.

adenofibromas have the characteristics of benign cells, with small, elongated, regular nuclei. Mitoses are rarely seen. Some degree of myxoid change in the stroma is not uncommon. Figure 12–7 shows this variant.

Murad and his associates have studied the ultrastructure of adenofibromas with the electron microscope. They conclude that the stromal cells, and not the epithelial component, are the neoplastic elements in this tumor. They report that these stromal cells do not resemble the fibroblasts or any other stromal cells of the normal breast, but that they are similar to pericytes.

The stromal changes in adenofibroma that lead to the diagnosis of cystosarcoma phyllodes present a special challenge to the surgical pathologist. I will discuss them in Chapter 13.

The adenofibromas found in aged women occasionally show calcification. Figure 12–8 shows this phenomenon in an adenofibroma removed from a woman aged 62.

Diagnosis

Adenofibromas are usually well delimited. They are rounded, discoid, or lobulated. They may be soft, but more often have a rubbery firmness. They are not hard except when calcified. It is an occasional happy surprise for the surgeon to find that a stony hard tumor in an aged patient is not a carcinoma but instead a calcified adenofibroma.

The relative movability of the adenofibromas in the breast tissue in which they lie is one of their most distinctive characteristics. This is because of the fact that adenofibromas do not induce proliferation of fibroblasts in the breast tissue that surrounds them. Carcinoma and inflammatory lesions are immobilized by newly formed fibroblasts that fix them in the surrounding breast tissue as the guy ropes of a tent fix it to surrounding terrain.

For the same reason, adenofibromas do not produce true retraction signs. False retraction, the phenomenon whereby a relatively large, firm tumor in a flabby breast distorts the contour of the breast adjacent to the tumor, is sometimes seen with adenofibroma, but this phenomenon should not deceive a careful observer.

An adenofibroma cannot be distinguished by palpation from a dense gross cyst. Both lesions are circumscribed and slide around in the surrounding breast tissue. The age of the patient has diagnostic significance. Adenofibromas develop any time near puberty and are most frequent in youth. The youngest patient with a gross cyst in our series of some 2000 cases was 25, and the disease is most frequent in the decade before the menopause. Circumscribed and papillary carcinoma can mimic an adenofibroma, but they are infrequent lesions that occur in older patients.

My own practice has been to assume that a well-delimited movable tumor in a woman under 25 is an adenofibroma. If she is older I aspirate the lesion in an effort to determine whether it is a cyst or an adenofibroma. If it proves to be a cyst I have saved an unnecessary operation. If it is solid I have to perform a biopsy. Mammograms are of no help in this kind of differential diagnosis.

The pathologist should be asked to do an immediate frozen section upon a small wedge biopsy of every presumed adenofibroma, no matter how expert the surgeon and the pathologist may be at gross diagnosis. On several occasions surgeons in our hospital have excised a tumor that appeared grossly to be nothing more serious than a cellular adenofibroma, and not having asked for frozen section at the time of operation, have been shocked to learn later, when the routine microscopical sections came through, that the lesion was in fact a carcinoma. The distress that such errors cause to both the patient and the surgeon can be avoided by the simple rule of always doing an immediate frozen section.

Infarction of Adenofibroma

Adenofibromas occasionally undergo spontaneous infarction and necrosis, usually during pregnancy or lactation. This phenomenon was first noted by Delarue and Redon. Recently Hasson and Pope, and Wilkinson and Green, have again called attention to it. We have seen it in five of the last 1000-odd adenofibromas that we have studied in our laboratory. Table 12–2 shows the essential details in the five cases. There was nothing in the clinical history of any of these patients to indicate when the infarction had taken place. It had produced no symptoms. Figure 12–9 shows the gross appearance of one of these infarcted, necrotic adenofibromas. Figure 12–10 shows its microscopic appearance.

Localized infarction in the breast, occurring near to or at the termination of pregnancy, and forming a breast tumor simulating a neoplasm, has also been reported. The three cases of infarction that Hasson and Pope described were of this type. This phenomenon is apparently due to inadequate blood supply to physiologically hyperactive mammary tissue at term.

The Relationship of Adenofibroma to Carcinoma

Since the epithelial component of adenofibroma is presumably subject to the same biological stimuli as the breast epithelium in general, it might be expected that carcinoma might occasionally originate within an adenofibroma. This possibility was raised by reports such as that of Harrington and Miller. Although they did not present their evidence in any detail, they stated that carcinomatous transformation occurred in adenofibroma in 15 of their patients. Squartini and his associates at Perugia concluded from their

Table 12–2. Infarcted Adenofibromas of the Breast

Patient	Age	Duration of Tumor	Size of Tumor	Pregnant	Extent of Infarction
1. M.R.	14	2 months	3 cm.	No	Partial infarction and necrosis
2. H.M.	18	6 months	8 cm.	No	Partial infarction and necrosis
3. P.W.	27	5 weeks. Noted in 3rd month of lactation	3 cm.	Lactating	Almost complete infarction and necrosis
4. G.J.	23	5 months. Noted in 6th month of pregnancy		Had been pregnant	Total infarction and necrosis
5. D.B.	20	4 months. Noted in 7th month of pregnancy		Had been pregnant	Total infarction and necrosis

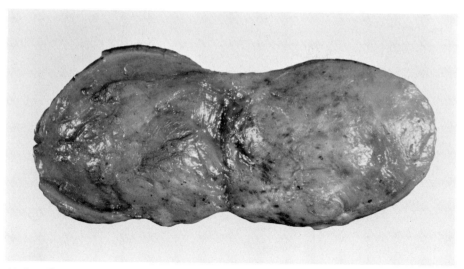

Figure 12–9. Gross appearance of an infarcted and largely necrotic adenofibroma of the breast.

microscopical studies of the growth pattern of carcinoma that some 15 per cent originate from adenofibromas, but they also failed to present any detailed evidence in support of this drastic statement.

Recent reports by McDivitt, Stewart, and Farrow, as well as by Goldman and Fried-

man, of "breast carcinoma" arising in fibroadenomas are in a different category because they present detailed evidence. Even so, both of these papers require careful reading because it then becomes apparent that the majority of the lesions were not carcinomas but lobular neoplasia (noninfiltrating lobular

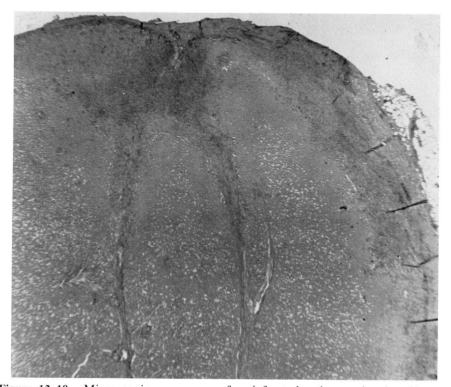

Figure 12–10. Microscopic appearance of an infarcted and necrotic adenofibroma.

carcinoma *in situ*). In Chapter 25 I have presented the reasons why this lesion must not be classified and treated as true carcinoma of the breast.

McDivitt and his associates, from their vast amount of pathologic material, described 13 cases, and Goldman and Friedman three cases, of lobular neoplasia occurring in adenofibromas. It is of basic importance, however, to know whether or not the lobular neoplasia exists *only* in the adenofibroma. There is nothing very remarkable about the epithelium of an adenofibroma being involved by this kind of proliferation if it exists elsewhere in the breast. This fact can be established only if mastectomy is performed and the entire breast studied microscopically. This kind of proof that the lobular neoplasia existed only in the adenofibroma was available in only four of the 16 cases that are described in these two reports.

In our clinic we have had two examples of lobular neoplasia occurring only within an adenofibroma which was excised locally. Figure 12–11 shows one of these lesions.

Both of the adenofibromas were otherwise not remarkable. Both were small, measuring 1.5 and 2 cm., respectively. Mastectomy was not done in either patient. One had had no recurrence of breast disease nine years later. The other had had two subsequent local excisions of lesions in the same breast. One was an adenofibroma removed six months after the original operation, and the other an area of cystic disease removed six years later. No lobular neoplasia was found in the breast tissue removed at these subsequent operations.

In the papers by McDivitt and his associates, and by Goldman and Friedman, a total of 17 adenofibromas containing true carcinoma were also described. Four of these were "infiltrating lobular carcinoma." In all four, radical mastectomy was performed. In three the lesion was not found outside of the adenofibroma.

The other 13 lesions were described as duct carcinomas. Mastectomy was done in eight of the 13. In five no carcinoma was found outside of the adenofibroma.

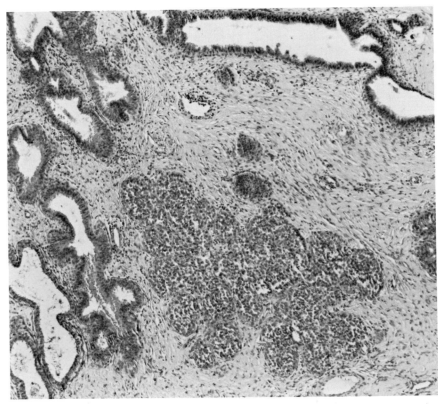

Figure 12–11. Lobular neoplasia within an adenofibroma removed from the breast of a 31 year old patient.

In our department of surgical pathology we do not have a single instance of carcinoma being found exclusively within an adenofibroma. In one case in which intraductal carcinoma was in close contact with the periphery of multiple adenofibromas, Dr. Stout concluded that the carcinoma developed from the breast tissue between the adenofibromas, and not from the adenofibromas themselves.

The fact remains, therefore, that carcinoma develops within adenofibroma only with great rarity, and that it is not a phenomenon of practical importance.

The question of the eventual development of carcinoma in the breasts of patients who had previously had adenofibromas removed is another matter. We do not have adequate follow-up data of patients with adenofibroma in our own clinic to provide a basis for an opinion.

Semb, however, did not find a single instance of the development of carcinoma among 142 patients with adenofibroma followed for from four to 27 years after operation.

Oliver and Major reported the follow-up of 175 patients with adenofibroma. After from four to 25 years, only one patient had developed carcinoma.

Treatment

When the presumptive clinical diagnosis of fibroadenoma has been made, excision is the only effective treatment. These lesions are entirely refractory to irradiation. Hormonal treatment has no influence upon them and may well do the patient's endocrine balance harm.

When the patient is under 25 years of age I take great care to reassure her, and I do not rush her to the operating room. The likelihood of her having a carcinoma at this age is so remote that there is no need for urgency. In our series of 6000 patients with carcinoma of the breast studied in our clinic between 1915 and 1966, only 9, or 0.2 per cent, were under the age of 25. Moreover, their tumors did not have the clinical characteristics of adenofibroma. When the patient is in her teens and the lesion is small—for example, not more than a centimeter or two in diameter—I often suggest that the patient return in three months for reëxamination. I have occasionally been pleasantly surprised to find

that the tumor has disappeared. It was only a prominent mammary lobule. This sequence of events is more frequent in young women who are taking oral contraceptives.

If the lesion persists, and if it grows, I advise excision. But in these younger women I defer the operation until a convenient time in relationship to their school schedule.

In women 25 years of age or older it is probably wise to proceed at once with biopsy and excision of the tumor.

In young patients in whom one adenofibroma has been excised and another tumor with the same characteristics develops, I have often been content to observe it. If it does not grow to such an extent that it deforms the breast, it seems reasonable not to put these young patients to the expense and trouble of another operation. Many such adenofibromas will remain stationary after reaching a moderate size. If a new tumor appears in a patient 25 years or older who has previously had an adenofibroma excised, it should, probably be removed, no matter how typical of an adenofibroma it may be. Beyond this age carcinoma has a significant frequency, and since clinical diagnosis is not entirely reliable, biopsy should be done unless there are special contraindications.

If the tumor is larger than 5 cm., or has a history of rapid growth, it is wise, after its surface is exposed, to excise a small wedge for frozen section study, in order to make certain that it is not a cystosarcoma. As I will describe in the following chapter, cystosarcoma requires a somewhat different technique of excision from adenofibroma.

At operation for a presumably benign lesion of this kind I take care to follow the technique for the excision of benign tumors that I described in Chapter 6. With this technique I leave an almost invisible scar.

REFERENCES

Austin, W. E., and Fidler, H. K.: Carcinoma developing in fibroadenoma of the breast. Am. J. Clin. Path., 23:688, 1953.

Baker, E. M.: Simple adenoma of the breast. Virginia M. Monthly, 74:505, 1947.

Block, G. E., and Zlatnik, P. A.: Giant fibroadenomata of the breast in a prepubertal girl. Arch. Surg., 80:665, 1960.

Botham, R. J., McDonald, J. R., and Clagett, O. T.: Fibroadenoma with sarcoma-like stroma: a benign tumor. Surgery, 43:510, 1958.

Cheatle, Sir G. L.: Hyperplasia of epithelial and connective tissues in the breast: its relation to fibro-adenoma and other pathological conditions. Brit. J. Surg., *10*:436, 1923.

de Cholnoky, T.: Benign tumors of the breast. Arch. Surg., *38*:79, 1939.

Clarke, J. C.: Giant intracanalicular fibro-adenoma of the breast. Ann. Surg., *127*:372, 1948.

Delarue, J., and Redon, H.: Les infarctus des fibro-adenomes mammaires. Semaine d. hôp. Paris, *25*:2991, 1949.

Frantz, V. K., Pickren, J. W., Melcher, G. W., and Auchincloss, H., Jr.: Incidence of chronic cystic disease in so-called 'normal breasts'. Cancer, *4*:762, 1951.

Geschickter, C. F., and Lewis, D.: Pregnancy and lactation changes in fibro-adenoma of the breast. Brit. M. J., *1*:499, 1938.

Giacomelli, V., and Re, A.: Studio statistico sulle affezioni displastiche della mammella in rapporto all'età. Tumori, *25*:213, 1951.

Goldenberg, V. E., Wiegenstein, L., and Mottet, N. K.: Florid breast fibroadenoma in patients taking hormonal oral contraceptives. Am. J. Clin. Path., *49*:52, 1968.

Goldman, R. L., and Friedman, N. B.: Carcinoma of the breast arising in fibroadenomas; with emphasis on lobular carcinoma. Cancer, *23*:544, 1969.

Güthert, H.: Der organoide Charakter des Fibroadenoms der Mamma. Arch. f. klin Chir., *194*:312, 1938.

Harrington, S. W., and Miller, J. M.: Malignant changes in fibro-adenoma of the mammary gland. Surg., Gynec. & Obst., *70*:615, 1940.

Hasson, J., and Pope, C. H.: Mammary infarcts associated with pregnancy presenting as breast tumors. Surgery, *49*:313, 1961.

Heiman, J.: The study of benign neoplasms of the rat's breast. Am. J. Cancer, *22*:497, 1934.

Heiman, J., and Krehbiel, O. F.: The influence of hormones on breast hyperplasia and tumor growths in white rats. Am. J. Cancer, *27*:450, 1936.

Llewellyn, H. D.: A giant adenosarcoma of the breast. Brit. J. Surg., *35*:214, 1947.

Markowitz, B., and Howell, H. L.: Rapid growth of a large breast fibroma in a young girl. J.A.M.A., *107*:1043, 1936.

McDivitt, R. W., Stewart, F. W., and Farrow, J. H.: Breast carcinoma arising in solitary fibroadenomas. Surg., Gynec. & Obst., *125*:572, 1967.

McFarland, J.: Adenofibroma and fibroadenoma of the female breast. Surg., Gynec. & Obst., *45*:729, 1927.

Moran, C. S.: Fibroadenoma of the breast during pregnancy and lactation. Arch. Surg., *31*:688, 1935.

Murad, T. M., Greider, M. H., and Scarpelli, D. G.: The ultrastructure of human mammary fibroadenoma. Am. J. Path., *51*:663, 1967.

Oliver, R. L., and Major, R. C.: Cyclomastopathy; a physio-pathological conception of some benign breast tumors, with an analysis of four hundred cases. Am. J. Cancer, *21*:1, 1934.

Owens, F. M., and Adams, W. E.: Giant intracanalicular fibroadenoma of the breast. Arch. Surg., *43*:588, 1941.

Salm, R.: Epidermoid metaplasia in mammary fibroadenoma with formation of keratin cysts. J. Path. Bact., *74*:221, 1957.

Semb, C.: Pathologico-anatomical and clinical investigations of fibroadenomatosis cystica mammae and its relation to other pathological conditions in the mamma, especially cancer. Acta chir. Scandinav. (supplement 10), *64*:1, 1928.

Smith, I. H.: Giant intracanalicular fibroadenomyxoma of the breast. Am. J. Surg., *30*:545, 1935.

Soerensen, F.: Histologische Untersuchungen einiger Oestrinbehandelter Fälle von Fibroadenomatosis Mammae. Acta path. et microbiol. Scandinav., *15*:333, 1938.

Squartini, F., Lotti, G., and Biancifiori, C.: Fibroadenoma e cancro della mamella. Lav. d. Ist. anat. e istol. pat., Perugia, *13*:201, 1953.

Vicari, F.: Contributo alla conoscenza della cisti di echinococco della mammella. Arch. ital. anat. pat., *31*:354, 1957.

Wilkinson, L., and Green, W. O., Jr.: Infarction of breast lesion during pregnancy and lactation. Cancer, *17*:1567, 1964.

Wright, A. W., Klinck, G. H., Jr., and Wolfe, J. M.: Pathology and pathogenesis of mammary tumors occurring spontaneously in Albany strain of rats. Am. J. Path., *16*:817, 1940.

Wulsin, J. H.: Large breast tumors in adolescent females. Ann. Surg., *152*:151, 1960.

Chapter Thirteen

Cystosarcoma Phyllodes

Cystosarcoma phyllodes is a tumor of the breast with frightening clinical and microscopic characteristics which have given it prominence beyond its due. For it is, in fact, not only common but usually benign. The great German pioneer student of neoplasms, Johannes Müller, named it cystic and "phyllodes," or leaf-like, because of the branching projections of tumor tissue into the cystic cavities within the tumor. He mistakenly called the lesion a sarcoma, although he knew that these tumors are in general benign.

Our first and most difficult task in discussing cystosarcoma is to define the lesion. It is of course a fibroepithelial tumor. It is also, without doubt, often derived from an adenofibroma. The evidence for this latter statement is both clinical and microscopic. The clinical evidence of an association with adenofibroma is that a significant number of the women with cystosarcoma have also at some time had an ordinary adenofibroma. The adenofibroma may have occurred in the opposite breast, in a different area of the breast in which the cystosarcoma developed, or in the same area in the same breast.

The following is an example of these two lesions occurring in separate breasts.

Mrs. D. F., a 54 year old housewife, came to the Presbyterian Hospital complaining of a tumor of her right breast which she had first noted 12 years previously. The tumor was "bean-sized." It had remained unchanged until 10 months previously, when it began to grow rapidly. When the patient was admitted, the tumor was lobulated, well-delimited, movable, and situated in the outer half of the breast. It measured 14 cm. in diameter and proved to be a characteristic cystosarcoma. There was also a circumscribed, movable 2 cm. tumor in her left breast. It was a simple adenofibroma.

An example of an adenofibroma developing in a different sector of the same breast in which a cystosarcoma later appeared follows.

Mrs. J., a 32 year old housewife, found a small tumor in her left breast. The tumor was situated in the upper outer sector of the breast near its periphery, and measured 1.5 cm. in diameter. It had the clinical characteristics of an adenofibroma, which was what it proved to be when excised locally. Twelve years later, when she was 49, this patient returned with a well-delimited, movable 5 cm. tumor in the upper central sector of the same breast. When excised it proved to be a typical cystosarcoma.

The most impressive kind of evidence that adenofibroma and cystosarcoma are in some way associated is the frequent microscopic finding of both lesions in the same tumor. The basic structure of the lesion is that of an adenofibroma, and within it, or adjacent to it, there are features that necessitate classifying it as a cystosarcoma. We have studied many such lesions and I will describe several of them in the course of the present discussion. Whether the adenofibroma and the cystosarcoma in a lesion of this kind have a common mesenchymal origin, or whether the cystosarcoma evolved from the adenofibroma, is a theoretical question. The practical point is that the two lesions are associated.

Our definition of cystosarcoma is, as I have emphasized in discussing adenofibroma, a pathologic rather than a clinical one. The first requisite is, of course, that the lesion be a fibroepithelial tumor, containing one or more components of mesenchymal origin as well as epithelial structures.

Many different types of sarcoma having no epithelial component occur in the breast, and if they are lumped together with the cystosarcomas, as Rogers and Flo, for example, have done, the malignancy of this group is high and the comparatively benign nature of cystosarcoma is obscured.

The second and most frequently invoked criterion of cystosarcoma is the character of the stroma. If the stroma is very cellular and made up of cells that vary considerably in size and shape, and have hyperchromatic nuclei with a significant number of mitoses—in short, a stroma that suggests a malignant character—the lesion is classified without question as a cystosarcoma. The fibroblasts that ordinarily form the stroma of adenofibromas have the characteristics of benign cells, with small elongated regular nuclei. Mitoses are usually not seen. Even though the stromal

cells of a tumor with the general architecture of an adenofibroma have this benign character, if they are too numerous our experience has taught us that we must classify the lesion as a cystosarcoma and treat it as such. Figure 13-1 shows such a cellular stroma in a tumor that recurred three times after local excision, leaving no doubt regarding its cystosarcomatous nature. Except for the cellularity of its stroma, this tumor had all the characteristics of a benign adenofibroma. In contrast, Figure 13-2 shows, at the same magnification, a typical adenofibroma with a stroma of normal cellularity.

Lester and Stout emphasized, in their important paper on cystosarcoma, that marked variation in the stromal pattern is often noted within a single tumor. In general the stroma may be relatively acellular, resembling that of an ordinary adenofibroma, but in some areas it may be anaplastic and sarcomatous. This patchy distribution of sarcoma-like change is illustrated by Figure 13-3, which shows a fibrosarcoma-like area in a tumor with a generally benign-appearing stroma. In some cystosarcomas the stromal overgrowth is so pronounced that no epithelial component is seen in broad areas of the lesion. Unless many blocks of tissue from different portions of the tumor are studied, the tumor can not be accurately classified.

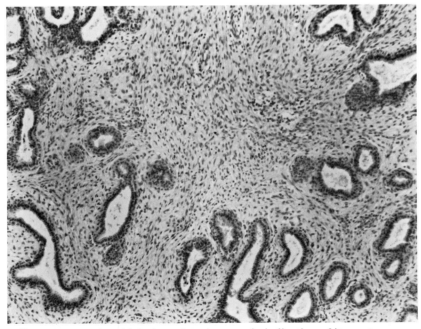

Figure 13-1. Cystosarcoma in which the only microscopic indication of its cystosarcomatous nature is a cellular stroma made up of benign-looking cells.

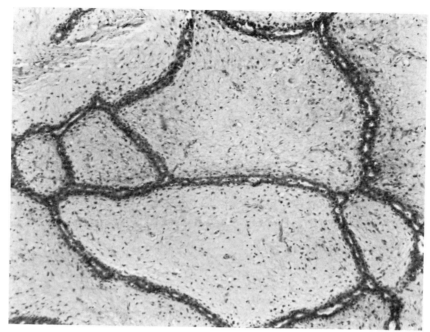

Figure 13–2. An adenofibroma in which the stroma has a normal degree of cellularity.

Admittedly, pathologists may differ in making the distinction between an adenofibroma with a somewhat more cellular stroma and a cystosarcoma that has the general architecture of an adenofibroma but has an unusually cellular sarcoma-like stroma. In making this distinction the pathologist unfortunately cannot depend upon the experience

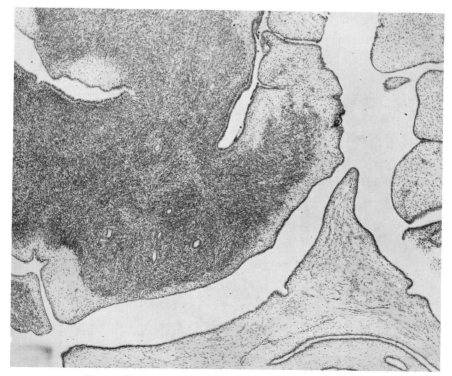

Figure 13–3. Sarcoma-like area in a cystosarcoma.

that follow-up ordinarily provides in other types of neoplasms. Cystosarcomas often look malignant, but they very rarely are. Although they recur locally unless completely excised, they rarely metastasize. The classification of cystosarcomas is therefore less rigid and more controversial than for almost any other type of breast neoplasm.

Another microscopic feature that is highly suggestive of a cystosarcomatous nature is the presence in a fibroepithelial tumor of remarkably elongated epithelial-lined clefts, such as those shown in Figure 13–4. The clefts in adenofibromas are usually shorter and narrower.

Myxoid change in the stroma does not in itself justify classifying one of these tumors as a cystosarcoma. However, if the myxoid change is so extensive that broken-down hemorrhagic and necrotic areas form within it, the tumor is properly called a cystosarcoma.

A gross pathologic feature that justifies the diagnosis of cystosarcoma is the presence of cysts within the tumor. The cysts vary greatly in size and number. They are often filled with polypoid masses projecting into them. These formations long ago suggested the term "phyllodes" or leaf-like to Müller. Figure 13–5 illustrates the gross appearance of one of these tumors.

These myxoid and degenerative changes in cystosarcomas, as well as the cysts usually seen in them, give them the gross pathologic character that suggests the diagnosis. They

are well delimited but have no true capsule. They are usually softer than adenofibromas. The cut surface of the solid portion of the tumor is moist, sticky, and gray, yellow, brown, or dark red in color.

A wide variety of types of sarcoma-like metaplasia are seen in the stroma of cystosarcomas. The most frequent type suggests fibrosarcoma. Figure 13–6 shows such a fibrosarcoma-like area in the stroma of a cystosarcoma.

Liposarcomatous change is the next most common. Most of the tumors reported as liposarcoma of the breast are not genuine primary liposarcomas but merely liposarcomatous metaplasia in cystosarcoma. The cases reported by Breckenridge, by Jackson, by Aronson, and by De Navasquez and Horton belong in this category. In the files of our department there were nine such cases sent to Stout and Lattes in consultation. In one of the cystosarcomas in our series of cases this liposarcomatous transformation was remarkable because it appeared to develop in countless independent foci around ducts. Figure 13–7 shows this tumor in a low power view. It had the general structure of an adenofibroma except that around every branching duct there was a separate zone of liposarcoma. Figure 13–8 shows the liposarcomatous component in higher magnification. This lesion developed in the left breast of a 33 year old woman, who had had an adenofibroma excised from the same breast nine

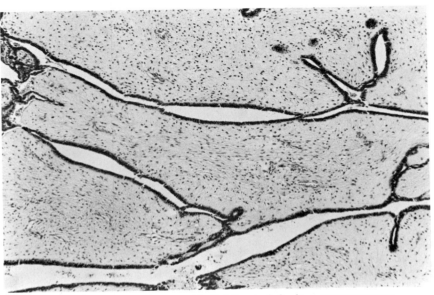

Figure 13–4.   Very long, epithelial-lined clefts in a cystosarcoma.

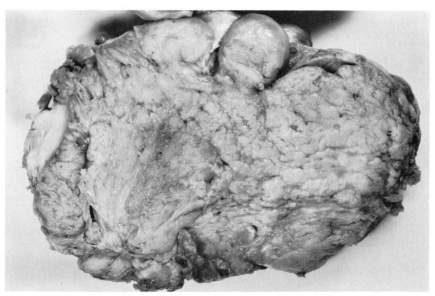

Figure 13–5. The gross appearance of cystosarcoma.

years previously. The new tumor was a large one, measuring 12 cm. in diameter. Mastectomy with removal of the underlying pectoralis major muscle was performed. One year later another tumor developed in the right breast. It was excised together with a rim of surrounding breast tissue and proved to be a cystosarcoma, quite different in character from the earlier left-sided lesion. This new right-sided lesion was predominantly myxoid. It recurred within a year. Partial mastectomy was then performed. Recurrence again developed and radical mastectomy was finally done. Eight years after the left mastec-

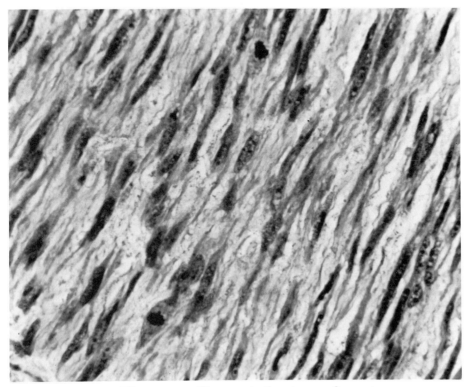

Figure 13–6. Fibrosarcoma-like area in the stroma of a cystosarcoma.

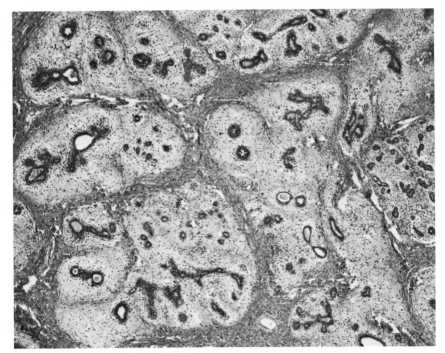

Figure 13–7. Foci of liposarcoma surrounding the ducts in a cystosarcoma — low power view.

tomy and five years after the right mastectomy the patient had had no further local recurrence and there was no evidence of metastases.

We have recently studied a cystosarcoma in which sarcoma-like metaplasia suggested fibrous histiocytoma. A storiform pattern as well as multinucleated histiocytes were well defined (Fig. 13–9). As in the cystosarcoma with liposarcomatous metaplasia already described, this histiocytic metaplasia was multi-focal, developing in seemingly independent foci around ducts (Fig. 13–10).

Fibroepithelial breast tumors that contain

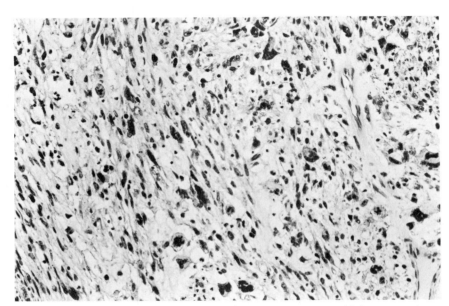

Figure 13–8. Liposarcomatous change in a cystosarcoma — high power view.

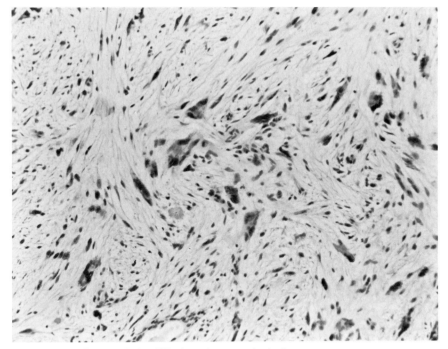

Figure 13–9.   Histiocytic metaplasia in cystosarcoma.

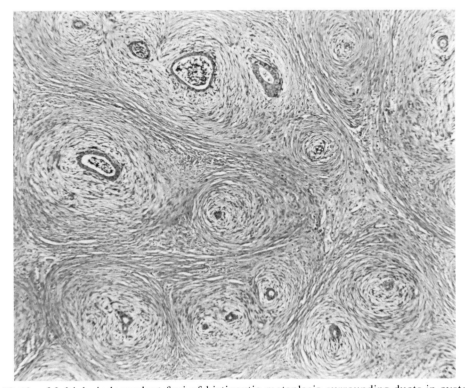

Figure 13–10.   Multiple independent foci of histiocytic metaplasia surrounding ducts in cystosarcoma.

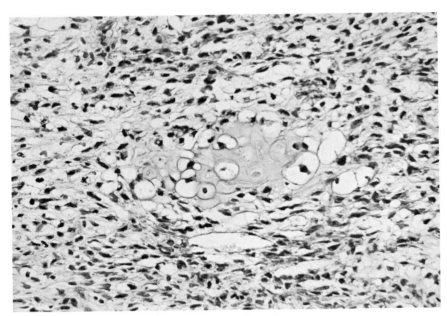

Figure 13–11.   An area of cartilage in a cystosarcoma.

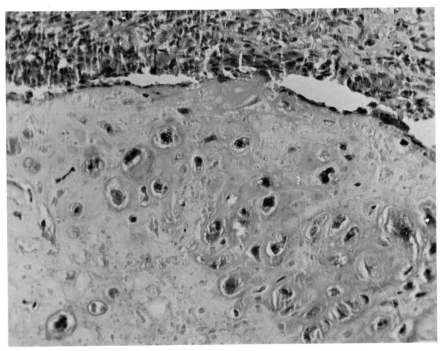

Figure 13–12.   An area of osteoid in a cystosarcoma.

cartilage (Fig. 13–11) or osteoid (Fig. 13–12) should be classified as cystosarcoma. Several of the tumors in the present series of cases showed these changes. They were not the tumors that metastasized. Smith and Taylor reported a similar experience.

Frequency

Cystosarcomas have constituted only 2 or 3 per cent of the fibroepithelial tumors of the breast in our clinics. Lester and Stout reviewed 36 of these tumors occurring in the Presbyterian Hospital over a 40 year period ending in 1952. Since then an additional 51 tumors have been studied in our breast clinics in the Presbyterian and Francis Delafield Hospitals. We have reclassified three of the tumors occurring in adolescent girls in Lester and Stout's series, and have grouped them with the massive adenofibromas of youth. The series of cystosarcomas here presented totals 84 cases.

Age Distribution

The age distribution (Chart 13–1) of our patients with cystosarcoma is quite different from that of our patients with adenofibroma. The cystosarcomas usually develop in older women, the mean age of our patients being 44.7 years as compared with a mean age of 31 years for our patients with adenofibroma. It should be kept in mind, however, that cystosarcoma sometimes occurs in younger women. Our series includes four under the age of 20. They were 14, 15, 16, and 18 years old.

As an example of the fact that cystosarcoma may develop at an early age, I can refer to our patient J. B., a 14 year old Negro girl. She had discovered a tumor in her right breast three weeks previously. It was well delimited, movable within the breast, and measured 8 cm. in diameter. It was excised locally. Its general architecture was that of an adenofibroma but its stroma was abnormally cellular (Fig. 13–13). The spindle-shaped stromal cells had hyperchromatic nuclei, which in some areas had a palisade arrangement. Mitoses were not seen. There was no recurrence 10 years later.

Bilaterality

In our Columbia series of patients there was only one in whom cystosarcoma developed, apparently independently, in both breasts. Norris and Taylor mention one case in which the disease was bilateral. Reich and Solomon, Bader and Isaacson, and Notley and Griffiths have each reported one such case. Cystosarcoma is, therefore, very much less likely to be bilateral than adenofibroma, which is not infrequently bilateral.

Chart 13–1. Age distribution among 84 patients with cystosarcoma of the breast.

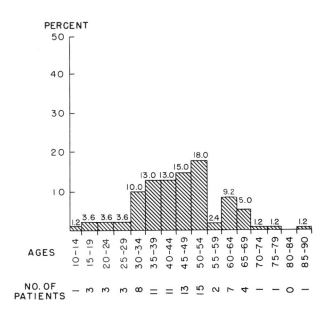

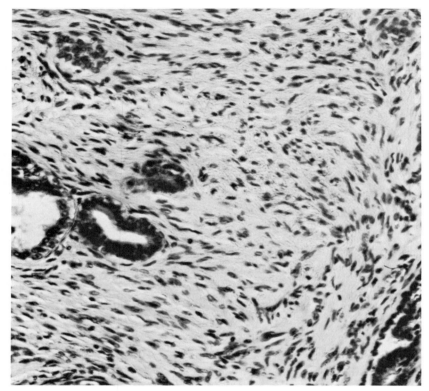

Figure 13–13. A cystosarcoma in a 14 year old patient.

Natural History

Most cystosarcomas grow rapidly and reach a large size before the patient comes for treatment. There is, however, great variation in the natural history of these lesions. The duration of the tumor in our series of 84 cases varied from one week to 42 years. The mean duration, which of course is not very significant when there are such extremes, was 24.4 months.

In one-sixth of our patients the tumor was very large, measuring 15 cm. or more in diameter. Figure 13–14 shows one of these large tumors in a 48 year old woman who had had her tumor for eight months.

Eleven of the 84 patients in our series had quite small tumors, measuring between 1 and 3 cm. in diameter. It is important for surgeons and pathologists to realize that all cystosarcomas are not large. They must be alert to the possibility of this lesion whenever a seemingly innocuous tumor of the breast is excised.

Cystosarcomas may exhibit great growth vigor in that they grow to be a very large size, but they have no great invasive tendency.

Although they have no true capsule, and microscopic study not infrequently shows invasion of the immediately adjacent breast tissue, this invasion is limited. The tumor does not grow along fascial planes and invade adjacent tissues aggressively, as carcinoma often does.

This is why cystosarcomas, as they grow in size and fill up the breast, remain well circumscribed, and movable on the chest wall. Their contour is often nodular. They do not adhere to and invade the overlying skin, although they sometimes distend it to such an extent that pressure on it produces ulceration. Two of the largest tumors in our series of cases were accompanied by this kind of skin ulceration.

The important and much debated question regarding cystosarcomas is how often they metastasize, and whether or not it is possible to predict from their microscopic structure that metastasis is likely. One of the most comprehensive studies of this problem was that of Treves and Sunderland, who reviewed 77 cases seen at the Memorial Hospital, New York, over a 20 year period. They classified 18 as malignant. Nine (13 per cent) metastasized. Treves and Sunderland concluded that the best criterion of malignancy in these tumors is not their gross size but rather the presence of microscopic areas of focal sub-epithelial stromal cellularity and anaplasia. The presence of bizarre giant cells in an otherwise benign-appearing stroma was not, in their experience, an indication of malignancy.

Lester and Stout attempted to apply the Treves and Sunderland criteria of malignancy in the 58 cases available to them for study. They found, however, that only two of their five metastasizing tumors could be classed as malignant by these criteria. They concluded that it is unsafe to rely for therapeutic guidance upon these criteria as applied to biopsy specimens. The malignant-appearing area in one of these rare truly malignant cystosarcomas may be so small that only meticulous study of many sections from the entire tumor will find it. On the other hand, many cystosarcomas will be found to contain highly malignant-appearing stromal areas, yet their clinical course is entirely benign. They have been cured by local excision. The following case is an example.

L. S., a 61 year old white housewife, came to the Presbyterian Hospital, complaining that a tumor which had remained unchanged in her right breast for 42 years had begun to enlarge one month previously. Examination showed a well circumscribed, lobulated, movable tumor 9 cm. in diameter in the outer half of the right breast. There was no retraction. Biopsy was performed, and the tumor proved to be a cystosarcoma and was excised locally through a curved lateral incision. Microscopically it had the pattern of an adeno-fibroma, except for several areas in which there were foci of anaplastic spindle-shaped cells varying considerably in size and shape, and containing frequent mitoses, that suggested fibrosarcoma (Fig. 13–15). There had been no recurrence or metastasis from this lesion eight years later.

Oberman reported a small series of cystosarcomas. Four of the eight lesions metastasized. This is surely an abnormal experience.

Norris and Taylor have recently studied a series of 94 cystosarcomas from the Armed Forces Institute of Pathology. They had follow-up data regarding 88 of their cases. In 15, i.e., 17 per cent, metastasis and death occurred.

In their series of cases, Norris and Taylor studied the correlation of three microscopic

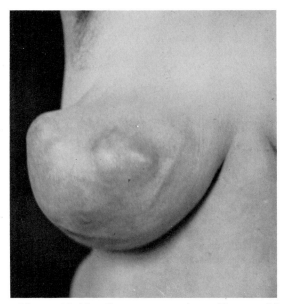

Figure 13–14. Cystosarcoma in a 48 year old woman.

features with the results of treatment—namely, the presence of an infiltrating tumor margin, the degree of stromal cellular atypism, and the number of mitoses. Some degree of correlation was found for each of these prognostic features, but the correlation was most striking as regards mitotic activity. None of the 23 patients whose tumors showed from none to two mitoses per high power field died, whereas 15 of the 64 patients whose tumors showed a greater degree of mitotic activity died. None of the tumors less than 4 cm. in diameter metastasized, but except for this fact the size of the tumor was not related to its malignancy. The metastases that developed in 15 of Norris and Taylor's series of patients were usually to lungs, to other viscera in a few instances, to bones in one case, to an axillary lymph node in one case, and to a periaortic lymph node in another case.

Minkowitz and his associates have recently described another case in which cystosarcoma metastasized to an axillary lymph node. This is, however, a very rare phenomenon.

Ariel reported one case in which cystosarcoma had metastasized to bone. He could find reports of only four other cases in which skeletal metastases occurred.

In our series of 84 cystosarcomas from our clinics in the Presbyterian and Francis Dela-

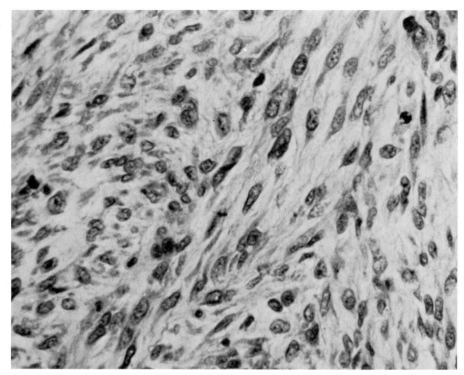

Figure 13–15.   Fibrosarcoma-like area in the stroma of a cystosarcoma.

field Hospitals there were only four that are known to have metastasized. In determining the proportion of metastasizing tumors we might follow the same procedure that Norris and Taylor used. They deducted the number of patients lost to follow-up and dying from other disease before five years. On this basis, 15 of their total of 87 patients (17.2 per cent) developed metastasis. In our Columbia series of 84 cystosarcomas, eight patients were lost to follow-up before five years, four patients died within five years from other causes, and eight had been treated less than five years previously. Among the remaining total of 64 patients with cystosarcoma only four developed metastases and succumbed. The incidence of metastasizing lesions in our series was therefore only 6.2 per cent.

I believe that this figure is closer to the truth than either the Treves and Sunderland Memorial Hospital data or Norris and Taylor's data from the Armed Forces Institute of Pathology. Because of their reputation as institutions dealing with difficult diagnostic problems, unusual malignant lesions are referred to them and are included in their case series. Indeed, Treves and Sunderland themselves admitted that their series of cystosarcomas may have been overweighted with referred malignant tumors.

Studying referred cases is not entirely satisfactory, because the initial clinical facts and the details of treatment are usually not accurately known. Stout, and his successor Lattes, in our Department of Surgical Pathology, have been referred many such cystosarcomas, but I have chosen not to include them in the present series of cases. In all of our cases the clinical studies and treatment were carried out in our own clinics.

The details of the four cases in our series of cystosarcoma in which metastases occurred follow.

CASE 1

S. H., a 50 year old nulliparous Negress, was admitted because of a rapidly enlarging breast tumor present for four months, with ulceration noted two weeks previously. The left breast was enormous, and showed a small area of ulceration over its most protuberant portion (Fig. 13–16). Simple mastectomy with removal of low axillary nodes was performed. The specimen weighed 8 pounds. The tumor was lobulated and circumscribed. The cut surface presented a mixture of firm, white, whorled tissue with multiple cysts, large gelatinous areas, and foci of hemorrhage and necrosis.

About two months later she returned with partial intestinal obstruction due to intussusception produced by multiple polypoid tumors in the small intestine. At this time a laryngeal tumor and large cervical nodes were noted, and specimens were taken for biopsy. Segments of gangrenous bowel were removed. She died seven months after the discovery of her breast tumor, with generalized peritonitis, a sequel of the intestinal gangrene.

Multiple sections of the original breast tumor showed the pattern of an intracanalicular fibroma with many compressed and distorted ducts lined by uniform epithelial cells in a moderately cellular stroma, portions of which were dense while other portions were myxomatous. Occasional mitoses were encountered but there was no significant degree of pleomorphism. There were large foci of hemorrhage and necrosis. A single section among numerous additional ones made from the original tumor after its malignant clinical course had become evident, contained an unusually cellular focus composed of large spindle-shaped and polygonal cells with variation in nuclear size and staining (Fig. 13–17). Occasional giant forms and numerous mitotic figures were seen.

Many of the multiple small intestinal tumors were polypoid (Fig. 13–18) and one such tumor formed the head of the intussuscepted segment. These tumors, one of which is shown in Figure 13–19, as well as biopsies of the laryngeal tumor and a cervical mass, presented a similar microscopic picture. They were vascular, cellular tumors with large spindle-shaped cells containing ovoid, vesicular nuclei which varied considerably in size and shape. In some areas the cells tended to be rounded or polygonal, resembling those seen in the cellular focus in the primary breast tumor.

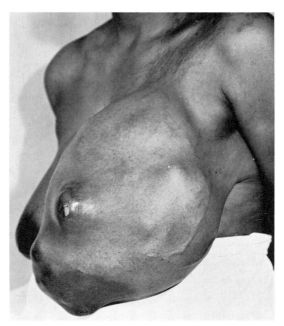

Figure 13–16. Malignant cystosarcoma phyllodes. Case 1.

At postmortem examination similar metastatic lesions were found in the heart, lungs, stomach, intestinal tract and cervical region. Tumor was not found in any lymph nodes. Tissue from the cervical region removed operatively and at autopsy could not be identified as nodal in origin. Epithelial

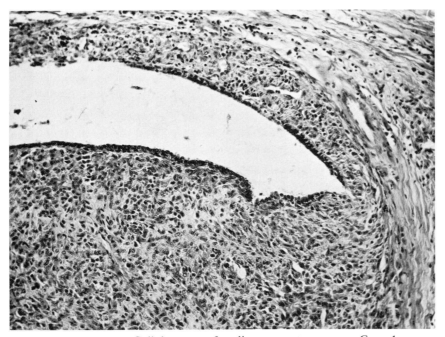

Figure 13–17.   Cellular area of malignant cystosarcoma. Case 1.

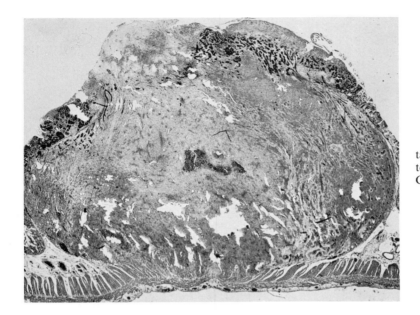

Figure 13–18. Polypoid metastasis to the ileum from cystosarcoma—low power view. Case 1.

elements were not found in any of the metastatic deposits.

This huge, rapidly growing, fibroepithelial breast tumor produced widespread visceral metastases and killed the patient within a year. Histologically the major portion of the tumor had the structure of a fibroadenoma with a moderately cellular stroma. Only the connective tissue elements were represented in the metastases as an anaplastic sarcoma similar to that seen in one small portion of the original breast tumor.

CASE 2

R. H., a 36 year old Negro housewife, had first noted a tumor of her left breast 20 years previously, at the time of her first pregnancy. She delivered normally but did not nurse the baby. The tumor was not treated and slowly increased in size during subsequent years. Meanwhile she completed two more pregnancies. Three months prior to admission the tumor began to enlarge rapidly, and became painful.

On her admission to Presbyterian Hospital two separate tumors were palpated in her left breast.

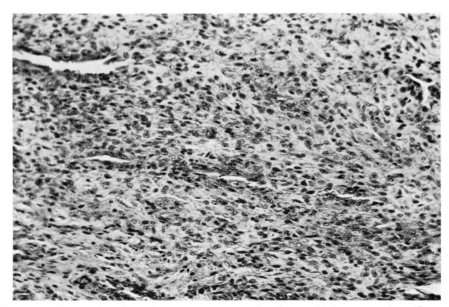

Figure 13–19.   Metastasis of cystosarcoma to the ileum—high power view. Case 1.

The larger one distended the center of her left breast. It was firm and irregularly nodular in contour, and well delimited from surrounding breast tissue. It measured 12 by 14 cm. Cephalad to but in contact with the large tumor, there was a separate small 2 cm. tumor with similar clinical characteristics. There were no clinically involved axillary nodes.

The tumors, thought to be adenofibromas, were exposed through a circumareolar incision and dissected out by blunt dissection. Only then was a frozen section of the larger tumor done, and its cystosarcomatous nature discovered. An attempt was then made to excise a rim of mammary tissue surrounding the site of the tumors.

The smaller of the two tumors was grossly and microscopically a typical adenofibroma.

Most of the larger tumor had the gross character of an adenofibroma, but about one-third of its bulk was made up of soft brownish tissue in which there were hemorrhagic areas as well as small cysts. The firmer portion of the tumor had the microscopic structure of an adenofibroma (Fig. 13-20), but the softer areas were highly cellular and resembled fibrosarcoma (Fig. 13-21).

Three months postoperatively, local recurrence was evident. The entire left breast was indurated and was twice the normal size. A chest film now revealed right-sided pulmonary metastases.

Irradiation of the rapidly enlarging local disease in the left breast failed to check it. The tumor ulcerated, and in a final attempt to control the local disease the breast and pectoral muscles were excised.

The patient succumbed to pulmonary metastases 16 months after her original operation. The tumor grew through the apex of the right thorax into the right supraclavicular region. There were also metastases to the adrenals, the colon, and the wall of the aorta. The character of the tumor in these metastases remained unchanged.

CASE 3

Mrs. H. B., a 53 year old housewife, developed a tumor in the upper portion of her right breast. The tumor grew rapidly, attaining a diameter of 15 cm. within a year. It was then excised locally in another hospital and diagnosed as a cystosarcoma. Microscopically, part of the tumor had the structure of an adenofibroma without any special features (Fig. 13-22), but its bulk was made up of highly anaplastic spindle-shaped cells and osteoid, suggesting osteosarcoma (Fig. 13-23). The patient was referred to us. On admission her wound was not entirely healed. It was decided to do no further surgery for the time being.

Six weeks later a 3 cm. local recurrence in the operated area of the right breast was apparent. At this time a small firm 2 cm. subareolar tumor was noted in the left breast. At operation this left breast tumor was excised and proved to be a calcified adenofibroma. The recurrent tumor in the right breast was excised and proved to be recurrent cystosarcoma.

Within two months local recurrence in the right breast was again apparent. Radical mastectomy was performed. No metastases of her cystosarcoma were found in 54 lymph nodes. However, a small node contained a minute focus of metastatic adenocarcinoma in a peripheral sinus. We found no carcinoma in the amputated breast, and the finding remains unexplained.

Eight months later the patient was found to have pulmonary metastases. She died three months

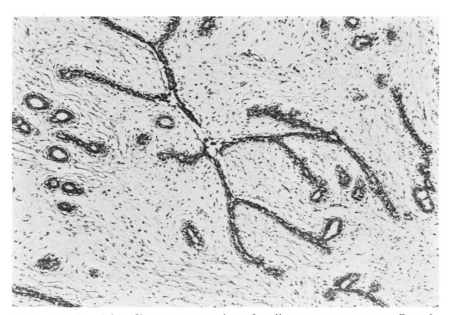

Figure 13–20.   Adenofibromatous portion of malignant cystosarcoma. Case 2.

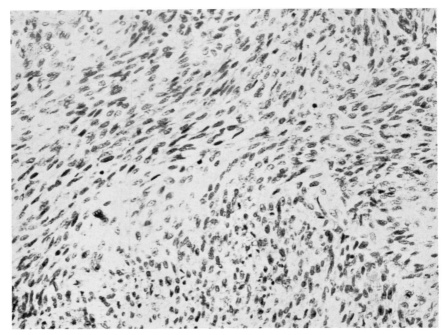

Figure 13–21. Fibrosarcoma-like portion of malignant cystosarcoma. Case 2.

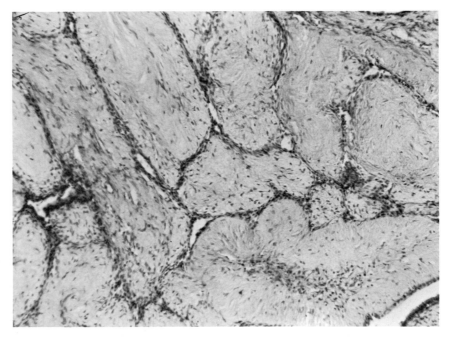

Figure 13–22. Adenofibromatous portion of malignant cystosarcoma. Case 3.

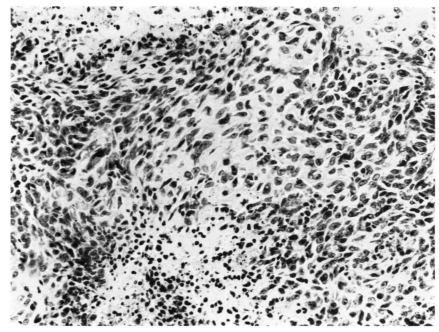

Figure 13–23. Osteosarcoma-like portion of malignant cystosarcoma. Case 3.

later, 29 months after she first discovered her breast tumor and 17 months after the first surgical attempt to remove it.

CASE 4

A 64 year old Negro housewife came to the Presbyterian Hospital in February, 1961, because she had a tumor of her right breast which she said had been present for two months. Ten years previously she had had an intraductal papilloma excised from the subareolar region of the same breast.

Examination revealed a firm, irregular, but movable 8 cm. tumor in the upper outer sector of

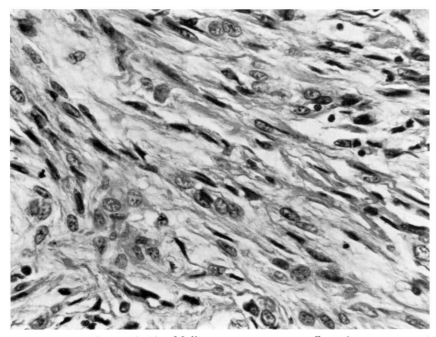

Figure 13–24. Malignant cystosarcoma. Case 4.

the breast, adjacent to the radial scar of the previous breast operation. There was no skin retraction.

Biopsy was done, and the frozen section was interpreted as showing carcinoma. Radical mastectomy was performed. The gross appearance of the lesion, however, was more suggestive of cystosarcoma, being well circumscribed and containing soft mucinous and cystic areas. Microscopic study showed that the bulk of the lesion was made up of fibrosarcomatous tissue with a loose myxoid stroma. In many areas the spindle-shaped cells varied considerably in size and shape and appeared to be malignant (Fig. 13–24). Slit-like spaces and cysts lined with epithelium were scattered throughout the tumor. There were extensive areas of squamous metaplasia. There were no metastases in 41 axillary lymph nodes.

Within six months the patient developed local recurrence on the chest wall, and pulmonary metastases. She died one year after operation.

Epithelial Proliferation in Cystosarcoma

We have seen five types of proliferation of the epithelial component of the cystosarcomas in our series.

1. It is not uncommon to find, in cystosarcomas, small scattered areas in which the epithelium grows in a benign papillary manner, partly filling up dilated ducts. Figure 13–25 shows this phenomenon.

2. Proliferation of epithelium in a pattern resembling adenosis is also seen.

3. Squamous metaplasia is occasionally seen in the lining epithelium of the ducts of cystosarcomas. Norris and Taylor referred to this phenomenon in eight of their 94 cases. We have seen it in several of our cases. It was especially prominent in one of our malignant cystosarcomas (Case 4). It is shown in Figure 13–26.

4. Lobular neoplasia (lobular carcinoma *in situ*). In close association with four of the cystosarcomas in our series we found typical lobular neoplasia. (The reader will understand, after referring to Chapter 25 dealing with this interesting precancerous lesion, why we prefer the term lobular neoplasia.) In two of our cystosarcomas the lobular neoplasia was entirely within the lesion, in one being found only in a single microscopic field. In the second case the lobular neoplasia was seen in several different areas within the tumor and had a striking arborescent pattern in low power magnification (Fig. 13–27). Figure 13–28 shows it in somewhat

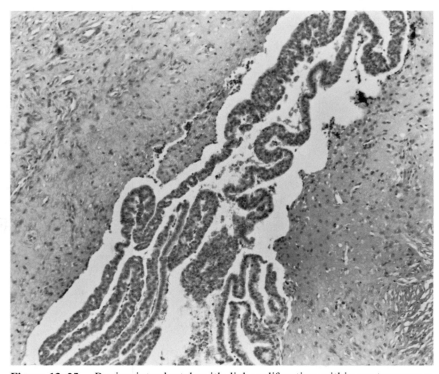

Figure 13–25. Benign intraductal epithelial proliferation within cystosarcoma.

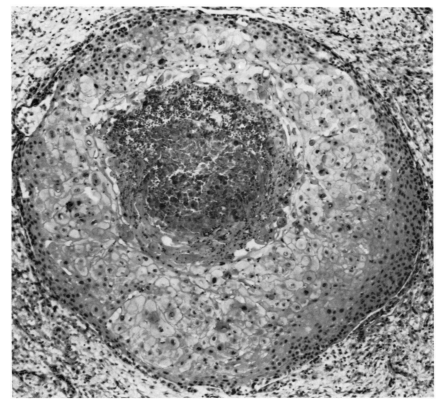

Figure 13-26. Squamous metaplasia in a cystosarcoma.

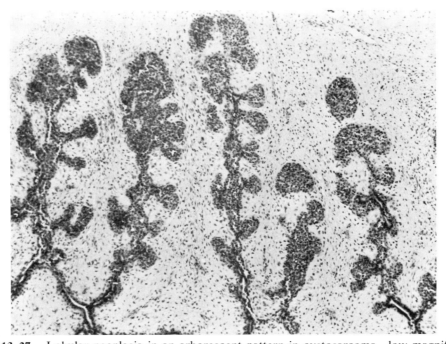

Figure 13-27. Lobular neoplasia in an arborescent pattern in cystosarcoma—low magnification.

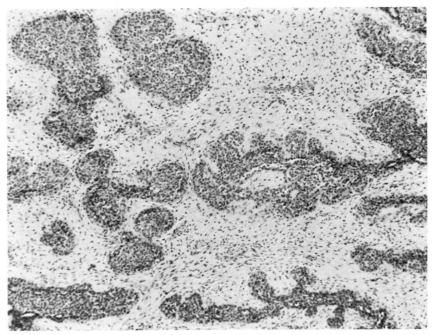

Figure 13–28.   Lobular neoplasia in cystosarcoma—higher magnification.

higher magnification. In a third cystosarcoma in our series, the lobular neoplasia was found not only within the lesion but in the adjacent breast tissue. In a fourth cystosarcoma the lobular neoplasia was seen only in breast tissue adjacent to the tumor. A remarkable feature of this fourth case was that a minute focus of papillary carcinoma was also found in the breast tissue removed with the cystosarcoma.

5. Carcinoma. Within the substance of two of their 94 cystosarcomas, Norris and Taylor found microscopic foci of infiltrating carcinoma. In one other patient intraductal carcinoma was found in breast tissue outside the cystosarcoma. Norris and Taylor did not report breast carcinoma occurring subsequent to the treatment of cystosarcoma in any of their patients; but they unfortunately do not report fully the extent and length of the follow-up in their series of cases.

In our Columbia series of 84 cystosarcomas, concurrent carcinoma was found in three. In one patient aged 40, a small infiltrating carcinoma was found in the breast removed because of the presence of a cystosarcoma. Eight years later, a new and independent carcinoma developed in her opposite breast and was treated by radical mastectomy.

In a second patient, aged 66, a 3 cm. tumor was excised locally, and on frozen section a diagnosis of cystosarcoma made. A margin of breast tissue surrounding the cystosarcoma was then excised. Study of permanent sections of breast tissue adjacent to the cystosarcoma showed a minute carcinoma limited to a single microscopic field. Radical mastectomy was then carried out. The patient succumbed postoperatively.

The third patient, aged 51, was the one referred to previously as having both lobular neoplasia and a minute focus of papillary carcinoma in the breast tissue adjacent to her cystosarcoma. Radical mastectomy was performed and the patient was well 10 years later.

In addition to these three concurrent carcinomas in our series of patients with cystosarcoma, two of our 64 patients followed for five years or more developed carcinoma subsequent to their cystosarcoma. In one of them it occurred four years later in the same breast as the cystosarcoma. In the other it was found one year later in the opposite breast.

While these data are not statistically significant because the numbers of cases are too small, they suggest the possibility of an etiologic association between cystosarcoma and carcinoma. Certainly patients who have had cystosarcoma should be followed with special care for the remainder of their lives.

Treatment

There has been wide divergence in the recommendations for treatment of cystosarcoma. Treves and Sunderland recommended radical mastectomy for all of these tumors containing histologically malignant-appearing cells. This category would include many of the tumors we classify as cystosarcoma. Norris and Taylor, who are not clinicians, advise mastectomy with low axillary dissection for cystosarcomas over 4 cm. in diameter, if axillary lymph nodes are enlarged, and if biopsy shows a histologically aggressive type of tumor. In Norris and Taylor's recent series of cases, mastectomy was carried out in 59 per cent of the patients.

Our practice at Columbia has been to excise these lesions locally together with a zone of the surrounding breast tissue. We have been led to adopt this conservative point of view by the following facts.

1. Local excision was successful—even though it occasionally had to be repeated—in all of our benign cystosarcomas in which it was tried. In our four malignant cystosarcomas—constituting only 6 per cent of all our cases—all methods failed to control the disease locally. In one of the four patients in whom radical mastectomy was done there was prompt local recurrence.

2. When they do metastasize, cystosarcomas, like other sarcomas of mesenchymal origin, almost always metastasize through the blood stream, usually to the pulmonary capillary bed, and only with great rarity to the axillary nodes. Axillary dissection is therefore unreasonable.

3. If it were possible to predict, from the clinical or the microscopic features of these tumors, which ones will metastasize, it might be justifiable to treat selected patients by mastectomy in the hope of avoiding metastasis. Lester and Stout, however, found no reliable criteria for distinguishing the cystosarcomas that metastasized. Our more recent experience in the same laboratory supports this point of view. We continue to see cystosarcomas that look very malignant indeed, but do not metastasize.

There is, of course, another way in which a neoplasm manifests a malignant character, that is, by local recurrence. I have reserved a discussion of the local recurrence of cystosarcoma until last because it is a very complex problem.

The first point I must make is that local recurrence of cystosarcoma following local excision as it is ordinarily carried out is very frequent. Among our 64 patients followed for a minimal period of 5 years (those dying from intercurrent disease excluded) 43 had been treated initially by local excision, 14 by simple mastectomy, and 7 by radical mastectomy. Twelve, or 28 per cent, of the 43 patients treated by local excision developed local recurrence, after an interval of from two months to 17 years. In 11 of the 12 patients the local recurrence appeared within six years. The local recurrence after 17 years in the 12th patient was remarkable, but beyond question genuine local recurrence. The recurrent tumor developed at the exact site of the original cystosarcoma, and was identical in structure.

None of the 14 patients treated by simple mastectomy in our series of cystosarcomas developed local recurrence.

Six of the seven cystosarcomas treated by radical mastectomy in our series of cases were benign. In three of the six the radical mastectomy was not done because of the cystosarcoma, but because of the finding of a coincidental carcinoma. Two of these six patients died post-operatively. None of the remaining four developed local recurrence. The seventh patient treated by radical mastectomy had a malignant cystosarcoma, and she promptly developed local recurrence and pulmonary metastases.

While 28 per cent is, of course, a high local recurrence rate following the treatment of cystosarcoma by local excision, it is perfectly understandable in terms of the facts of pathology, and the manner in which the local excision is often performed by surgeons who do not fully understand the problem they are facing. Although cystosarcomas may appear in gross inspection to be encapsulated, they are not. Microscopic study will show the surrounding breast tissue to be compressed, but it is often infiltrated for a short distance by the cystosarcoma. The cystosarcoma cells, unlike those of an adenofibroma, possess sufficient autonomy and growth vigor so that if they are left in the wound they will form a recurrent tumor. The average surgeon, thinking that he is dealing with an adenofibroma because the tumor is so well delimited and movable in the surrounding breast tissue, dissects the tumor out so closely that he leaves foci of it behind, from which recurrence develops.

The obvious way to avoid this result is to recognize that the tumor is a cystosarcoma before any attempt is made to excise it, and then to secure ample surgical exposure, and carefully excise it with a rim of a couple of centimeters of surrounding breast tissue. This means cutting into every tumor of the breast and excising a small wedge for frozen section before any further surgery is carried out.

A good example of how to attack a cystosarcoma in such a way that local recurrence is assured is exemplified by the following case history. The operator was one of our resident surgeons. The patient had a large 12 by 14 cm. lobulated, well delimited tumor of the central and lateral sectors of the breast. The operator assumed that it was an adenofibroma and elected to remove it through a circumareolar incision without preliminary biopsy and frozen section. The reader can imagine the brutality of the dissection required to excise a tumor of this size with the very limited access of a circumareolar incision. In the process of removal the tumor was broken into, and its obvious cystosarcomatous nature was revealed and confirmed—but too late—by a frozen section. Although a rim of surrounding breast tissue was excised, this could not be adequately done through the inadequate incision. Local recurrence was apparent three months later.

It is of course a considerable chore to perform a biopsy on every seemingly benign tumor of the breast and remove a small wedge of the lesion for frozen section, yet this is the only way in which cystosarcoma, as well as other types of breast lesions, can be detected and the appropriate treatment selected. I admit that I myself have violated this rule, my excuse being that as a pathologist of long experience, I may be more expert in recognizing special types of breast lesions on the basis of their clinical and gross characteristics. I at once confess that this has not prevented me from making mistakes in diagnoses, and I realize all too well as I approach the end of my active surgical career, that it is impossible to recognize the nature of all breast tumors without frozen section. If I had my surgical life to live over again, I would follow the rule I have suggested, and I am sure that I would have had fewer local recurrences of cystosarcomas.

The following case is one in which I myself operated and failed to cure the patient with my first local excision, but succeeded with my second local excision.

Mrs. J. R., a woman of 45, had had a slowly growing tumor of her left breast for 15 years when she consulted me. The tumor filled the upper and central sectors of her left breast. It was rather soft, well delimited, and irregularly lobular. It was freely movable over the chest wall. I assumed that it was a cystosarcoma and exposed it through a generous lateral paramammary incision. I excised it with a narrow margin of surrounding breast tissue, taking care not to break into the lesion at any point.

At follow-up four years later, a recurrent tumor mass was noted in the central portion of the breast. It had the same character as the original tumor. Using the original paramammary incision, I exposed and excised the recurrence, again removing a rim of breast tissue around the lesion. Microscopically the original tumor and the recurrence were cystosarcomas with a good deal of pleomorphism of the stroma and mitotic activity. Five years later there had been no further recurrence.

I must point out, however, in defense of local excision as the method of choice for the treatment of cystosarcoma, that in our Columbia series of 43 cases treated by local excision, this method was successful in terms of eventual cure. Even though there was a local recurrence in 28 per cent (and I believe that there would have been many fewer recurrences if the local excision had been done as I have described above) re-excision succeeded in all the nonmetastasizing cystosarcomas in which it was done; and the women did not lose their breasts.

Two patients who were originally treated by local excision and developed local recurrence were treated by simple mastectomy; in both, the second more extensive operation was successful. In two other patients with metastasizing tumors that were originally treated by local excision, local recurrence developed. It seems very unlikely that more aggressive initial local treatment would have saved these patients because in both pulmonary metastases appeared within a few months.

It is this experience that leads us to advise local excision of the tumor together with a rim of surrounding tissue as the most reasonable primary treatment for cystosarcoma.

When recurrent cystosarcoma has the same microscopical character as the original lesion, with a benign epithelial component and a stroma consisting entirely of benign looking cells or predominantly of benign looking cells with a few scattered more cellular fibrosarcoma-like areas, I believe that local excision is still the right treatment.

But we have learned that in rare instances the stroma of the cystosarcoma progressively changes its microscopical character with repeated recurrence, in each recurrence becoming more malignant looking. The character of the epithelial component, however, does not change. A stage is finally reached in which the stroma is entirely made up of malignant looking hyperchromatic spindle shaped cells with many mitoses, and resembles fibrosarcoma. This kind of a lesion infiltrates the surrounding mammary tissue and fat. For this type of recurrent cystosarcoma Lattes and I advise mastectomy, without an axillary dissection since these lesions do not metastasize to regional lymph nodes. Such malignant evolution of the stroma of a cystosarcoma is rare, but we have recently seen two examples. They occurred in women aged 22 and 34, respectively, at the time the original tumor appeared. In both it was a rather benign looking cystosarcoma. The lesion recurred three times within 20 months in the younger patient. In the older patient there were five recurrences within 5 years, the last three developing within the last year. In both patients the stroma finally resembled highly malignant fibrosarcoma. Complete mastectomy was done, but too recently to provide meaningful follow-up.

REFERENCES

Ariel, L.: Skeletal metastases in cystosarcoma phylloides. Arch. Surg., 82:275, 1961.

Aronson, W.: Malignant cystosarcoma phyllodes with liposarcoma. Wisconsin M. J., 65:184, 1966.

Bader, E., and Isaacson, C.: Bilateral malignant cystosarcoma phyllodes. Brit. J. Surg., 48:519, 1961.

Breckenridge, R. L.: Liposarcoma of the breast. Am. J. Clin. Path., 24:954, 1954.

Cooper, W. G., and Ackerman, L. V.: Cystosarcoma phylloides. Surg., Gynec. & Obst., 77:279, 1943.

DeNavasquez, S., and Horton, R. E.: Liposarcoma of the breast. Guy's Hosp. Rep., 96:57, 1947.

Dyer, N. H., Bridger, J. E., and Taylor, R. S.: Cystosarcoma phylloides. Brit. J. Surg., 53:450, 1966.

Dyke, S. C.: A bony tumor of the breast. Brit. J. Surg., 14:323, 1926.

Engelbreth-Holm, J.: Giant-cell tumors of the breast. Acta path. et microbiol. Scandinav., 17:506, 1940.

Estrade, J.: Tumeurs phyllodes ou adénofibromes géants du sein. Bull. Assoc. franç. p. l'étude du cancer, 40:29, 1953.

Hafner, C. D., Mezger, E., and Wylie, J. H.: Cystosarcoma phyllodes of the breast. Surg. Gynec. & Obst., 115:29, 1962.

Jackson, A. V.: Metastasising liposarcoma of the breast arising in a fibroadenoma. J. Path. Bact., 83:582, 1962.

Lester, J., and Stout, A. P.: Cystosarcoma phyllodes. Cancer, 7:335, 1954.

McDivitt, R. W., Stewart, F. W., and Berg, J. W.: Tumors of the Breast, Atlas of Tumor Pathology, Washington, D.C., Armed Forces Institute of Pathology, 1967, Second Series, Fascicle 2.

McDonald, J. R., and Harrington, S. W.: Giant fibroadenoma of the breast—"cystosarcoma phyllodes." Ann. Surg., 131:243, 1950.

Minkowitz, S., Zeichner, M., DiMaio, V., and Nicastri, A. D.: Cystosarcoma phyllodes: a unique case with multiple unilateral lesions and ipsilateral axillary metastases. J. Path. Bact., 96:514, 1968.

Müller, J., Uber den feinern Bau und die Formen der krankhaften Geschwülste. Berlin, G. Reimer, 1838.

Norris, H. J., and Taylor, H. B.: Relationship of histologic features to behavior of cystosarcoma phyllodes. Cancer, 20:2090, 1967.

Notley, R. G., and Griffiths, H. J. L.: Bilateral malignant cystosarcoma phyllodes. Brit. J. Surg., 52:360, 1965.

Oberman, H. A.: Cystosarcoma phyllodes. Cancer, 18:697, 1965.

Oberman, H. A.: Sarcomas of the breast. Cancer, 18:1233, 1965.

Reich, T., and Solomon, C.: Bilateral cystosarcoma phyllodes, malignant variant, with 14 year follow up. Ann. Surg., 147:39, 1958.

Rogers, R., and Flo, S.: Sarcoma of the breast. New England J. Med., 226:841, 1942.

Ross, D. E.: Cystosarcoma phyllodes (giant intracanalicular myxoma). Am. J. Surg., 84:728, 1952.

Rottino, A., and Willson, K.: Osseous, cartilaginous and mixed tumors of the human breast. Arch. Surg., 51:184, 1945.

Smith, B. H., and Taylor, H. B.: The occurrence of bone and cartilage in mammary tumors. Am. J. Clin. Path., 51:610, 1969.

Stephenson, H. E., Gross, S., Gumport, S. L., and Meyer, H. W.: Cystosarcoma phyllodes of the breast. Ann. Surg., 136:856, 1952.

Treves, N.: A study of cystosarcoma phyllodes. Ann. New York Acad. Sc., 114:922, 1964.

Treves, N., and Sunderland, D. A.: Cystosarcoma phyllodes of the breast: a malignant and benign tumor; a clinicopathological study of seventy-seven cases. Cancer, 4:1286, 1951.

White, J. W.: Malignant variant of cystosarcoma phyllodes. Am. J. Cancer, 40:458, 1940.

Chapter Fourteen

Intraductal Papilloma

The papillary neoplasms of the breast continue to present one of the most difficult diagnostic and therapeutic problems that surgeons face. There are two main types of papillary lesions—the benign intraductal papillomas, which are relatively frequent, and the malignant papillary carcinomas, which are rare. Both give rise to a serous or bloody nipple discharge. These two lesions, so different in their prognosis, have often been confused. The key to this confusion is the same as for most other breast neoplasms: namely, close correlation of the clinical features of these tumors with their pathological characteristics.

In the present chapter I shall deal with the benign intraductal papillomas. The malignant papillary carcinomas will be discussed in Chapter 28.

J. Collins Warren, in a paper which he wrote in 1905, presenting a new classification for benign tumors of the breast and emphasizing the necessity for closer cooperation between pathologist and surgeon, was one of the first to recognize the benign character of "papillary cyst-adenoma," and to recommend that the surgical attack on these lesions be limited to local excision. Earlier observers had often regarded these lesions as malignant, and had used a variety of terms to describe them—adenocystoma papilliferum mammae, villous papilloma, papillary fibroma, duct papilloma, cysto-adenoma intracanaliculare,

proliferous cysts, or carcinome villeux. Warren reported nine cases of intraductal papillary cysto-adenoma from the Massachusetts General Hospital, six of which were treated successfully by local excision.

Greenough and Simmons in 1907 made another study of the Massachusetts General Hospital data and reported 20 cases of papillary cysto-adenoma. In 17 patients the lesion was benign. Seven of these patients had simple mastectomy, and the remaining ten had local excision. The follow-up of this group of patients was not complete, only one of them being followed for as long as four years. Nevertheless, Greenough and Simmons believed that they had sufficient evidence to conclude that papillary cysto-adenoma ordinarily requires only local excision.

In 1916 Dean Lewis, of Chicago, in a discussion of bleeding nipple, emphasized that a discharge of serum or blood from the nipple was usually indicative of benign intraductal papilloma, and not of carcinoma. He advised operative search for and excision of the papilloma, even when no tumor could be palpated. He pointed out that in these cases the situation of the papilloma could be determined by the appearance of the discharge when pressure is made over it. Lewis believed that local excision sufficed for intraductal papilloma, and that in the occasional case in which malignant transformation occurred this change could be detected from the gross appearance of the lesion.

Miller and Lewis, in 1923, reviewed their experience with 40 patients with a serous or bloody discharge from the nipple and found that the discharge was due to benign intraductal papilloma in 32 per cent, and to carcinoma in 68 per cent. This predominance of cases of carcinoma led Lewis to take a more grave view of nipple discharge than he had presented in his earlier paper. He emphasized that a serous or bloody nipple discharge is evidence of a pathological lesion which should be searched for and identified.

In 1917 Judd reviewed the Mayo Clinic records of 100 patients with serous or bloody nipple discharge, and reported that 57 per cent were proved to have carcinoma. All the patients with carcinoma had a palpable breast tumor, a fact which led Judd to use the presence of a tumor as a distinguishing feature between nipple discharge due to carcinoma and nipple discharge due to intraductal papilloma. None of Judd's intraductal papillomas formed a palpable tumor. He therefore advocated mastectomy for all patients with nipple discharge and a palpable tumor, but conservative treatment for those in whom no tumor could be detected.

Joseph C. Bloodgood was another contemporary student of breast neoplasms who discussed intraductal papilloma in a series of papers (Bloodgood, 1921, 1922, 1932). He regarded it as a relatively innocuous lesion. He did not think it precancerous. In his opinion a serous or bloody discharge was ordinarily due to intraductal papilloma—not to carcinoma. In his series of cases of carcinoma of the breast a discharge from the nipple was noted in only 1 per cent prior to the palpation of a breast tumor.

In 1927 Deryl Hart reviewed the Johns Hopkins' data concerning "intracystic papillomatous tumors of the breast, benign and malignant," and wrote one of the best available papers on the subject. He studied 95 cases with benign papillary lesions and 24 with malignant ones. Forty-eight per cent of the benign lesions had a nipple discharge, which in a relatively large number had been present for many years. In 20 per cent no tumor was palpable. Local excision sufficed for cure of these benign papillomas.

A nipple discharge occurred in only 12.5 per cent of Hart's cases with malignant papillary lesions. The duration of symptoms was usually short. A tumor was present in every malignant lesion, and in most cases the clinical picture suggested malignant disease. Hart emphasized the necessity of carrying out radical mastectomy for these malignant lesions.

In Hart's series there was only one case in which the clinical history suggested that a benign papillary lesion had transformed into a malignant one.

Adair (1930) presented a very different point of view. He reviewed 108 cases of sanguineous discharge from the nipple, and reported that in 47.2 per cent the symptom was due to malignant and in 52.8 per cent to benign lesions. Forty-nine out of 57 benign lesions were classified as intraductal papillomas or papillary cysto-adenoma, and 17 out of 49 carcinomas were classified as papillary adenocarcinoma. Adair concluded that a serosanguineous or bloody discharge signified the presence of a carcinoma about as often as it did a benign lesion, and that benign papillary cysto-adenomas eventually developed into papillary adenocarcinomas.

In their book, published in 1931, Cheatle and Cutler presented elaborate histologic evidence in support of their belief that benign papillomas may evolve into carcinoma. They did not include any convincing clinical evidence in support of this belief. Nevertheless they advocated simple mastectomy as the proper treatment for papilloma.

Saphir and Parker in 1940 made an interesting study of the papillary lesions of the breast. They studied 58 intraductal papillomas and divided them into three groups. Forty-two were placed in Group I, and designated as the fibrous type, nine were placed in Group II and called the glandular type, and seven were placed in Group III and termed the transitional type. They regarded the first two groups as well differentiated tumors, and benign, but felt that the latter group, which was not glandular in structure, being made up of more or less solid masses of cells without connective tissue stalks, was potentially malignant.

In 1941 Gray and Wood again reviewed the experience at the Mayo Clinic regarding discharge from the nipple. Eighty-eight patients with a serous or bloody nipple discharge proved to have benign papilloma. Simple mastectomy was carried out in almost all of these cases. In 87 other patients with a serous or bloody nipple discharge a diagnosis of malignant papilloma was made. The details of the clinical signs in these patients with presumed malignant lesions are not given beyond the fact that 52, or 60 per cent, had no palpable tumor. The diagnosis of carcinoma was based upon the microscopic findings. It is of interest to note that the Mayo Clinic pathologists classified the lesions in 44 of these 52 patients as Grade I adenocarcinoma. This fact, and the photomicrograph which Gray and Wood include of one of these tumors, leads us to believe that they were only benign papillomas.

Estes and Phillips in 1949 studied a series of 87 cases of intraductal papilloma seen in their clinic, and concluded that simple mastectomy is the proper treatment, although none of their patients treated by local excision subsequently developed carcinoma.

It is the tendency to employ a comparatively radical method of treatment for what is in our opinion a benign breast lesion that stimulated Dr. Stout and me to review our experience with intraductal papilloma in the Presbyterian Hospital and to present it in a paper in 1951.

In the 1951 study we concerned ourselves with the papillomas growing in ducts as characteristic neoplasms, generally stalked, and usually large enough to be grossly visible in careful inspection. These intraductal papillomas are autonomous neoplasms. They usually produce a nipple discharge. They grow slowly and eventually produce a palpable tumor. We did not include in our study the ubiquitous microscopic papillary proliferation of duct epithelium, in which the epithelium of slightly enlarged ducts is heaped up or forms low papillary processes. This microscopic low-grade papillary proliferation is seen to some degree in the majority of breasts. It produces no signs or symptoms, and has, so far as we know, no special prognostic significance. It has commonly been regarded as a manifestation of cystic disease. True intraductal papilloma is not common in the breast, but when it does occur it presents a diagnostic problem, and requires treatment.

The intraductal papillomas are of two broad classes—the *solitary papillomas* that usually develop in the terminal portion of a duct, and the *multiple papillomas* that develop throughout the duct system of a sector of the breast. The overwhelming majority of papillomas are of the solitary type. Multiple papillomas are infrequent.

There is a third group of papillomas—those within the nipple itself. They are the most infrequent of all.

SOLITARY INTRADUCTAL PAPILLOMA

The solitary type of grossly visible intraductal papilloma of the terminal ducts is certainly a disease *sui generis*. In the Presbyterian Hospital between the years 1916 and 1941 inclusive, Stout and Phillips and I found case histories of 81 such papillomas. Our study of these cases confirmed our conviction that this lesion can be accurately diagnosed and localized by simple clinical methods, that it is benign, and that local excision is all that is required to cure it. Our study also showed that solitary intraductal papilloma does not transform into carcinoma, and is not associated with carcinoma in a significant proportion of cases.

Since our 1951 study of intraductal papilloma a number of interesting papers dealing with this disease have appeared.

In 1957 Hendrick reported his experience in dealing with 208 patients with intraductal papilloma. He confirmed our Columbia point of view that it is a benign lesion that can be treated by local excision. He followed 92 per cent of his patients for from 5 to 18 years. Only two of them developed carcinoma, and in them it was in the opposite breast.

Madalin and his associates from the Mayo Clinic, also in 1957, described their findings in a series of 100 breasts amputated in 100 patients who had a nipple discharge. In 58 a centrally situated intraductal papilloma was found. In the others duct ectasia and cystic disease were the most frequent lesions. Carcinoma was found in only one breast.

Two important studies of the significance of a nipple discharge soon followed. In 1959 Mercier and Redon reported that only 12 per cent of a series of 120 patients with a nipple discharge proved to have carcinoma. In 1962 McPherson and MacKenzie reported that in their series of 72 patients with a nipple discharge 12.5 per cent had carcinoma.

In contrast to these several reports in which there was agreement that a nipple discharge usually signifies a benign papilloma, Copeland and Higgins in 1960 reported that in a series of 67 patients with a nipple discharge 37 per cent proved to have carcinoma.

Buhl-Jorgensen and his associates from the Radium Center in Copenhagen have recently presented a study of 183 patients with intraductal papilloma or papillomatosis in which they suggest that both of these lesions are associated with an abnormally high incidence of mammary carcinoma. Unfortunately, they fail to describe adequately the lesions that they write about. Without careful clinical and pathological description and classification of the various papillary lesions occurring in the breast any discussion of the subject is meaningless.

In the present discussion of intraductal papilloma I will use the data from my personal series of cases studied between the years 1943 and 1967. These data are more precise than those from our hospital service in general of a generation ago that Stout, Phillips, and I referred to in our 1951 paper. My personal series of cases includes a total of 160 patients with proven solitary intraductal papilloma (excluding those developing in the nipple). I shall also refer to 23 additional patients of mine with a nipple discharge but no palpable tumor, in whom the site of the presumed papilloma could not be defined. These 23 patients were not operated upon because while they were being followed and re-examined in an effort to localize the presumed papilloma, the discharge ceased spontaneously. After an interval of from five to 14 years they had had no further sign of breast disease.

Incidence

The solitary type of intraductal papilloma, while it is the only form of intraductal papilloma that has a considerable frequency, is nevertheless not a very common breast lesion. During the 25 year period in which I have dealt with a total of 160 solitary intraductal papillomas in my personal practice, I was consulted by 1669 patients with carcinoma—more than ten times the number of my patients with intraductal papilloma.

Age Distribution

Patients with solitary intraductal papilloma tend to be older than any other group of patients with benign breast lesions, excepting those with duct ectasia. The ages of patients with intraductal papilloma (including those with solitary papilloma of the breast as well as those with papilloma of the nipple) in my personal series of cases ranged between 18 and 85 (Chart 14–1). The mean age of these 179 patients was 48 years.

Clinical Features of Solitary Intraductal Papilloma

Nipple Discharge. The predominant symptom of solitary intraductal papilloma is, of course, a nipple discharge. In Chapter 5, I have discussed the various types of nipple discharge and their significance in the different diseases of the breast in which the symptom occurs. Reference to Table 5–1 (p.

Chart 14–1. The age distribution of 179 patients with solitary intraductal papilloma.

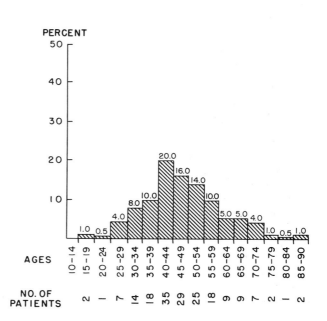

103) will show that among a total of 157 patients consulting me between the years 1956 and 1967 with a spontaneous nipple discharge, 108, or 69 per cent, had a proven intraductal papilloma. Only 18, or 11.5 per cent, had carcinoma.

My conclusion is that the patient who comes with a spontaneous nipple discharge will usually prove to have an intraductal papilloma, although the possibility of carcinoma must, of course, be kept in mind.

In my personal series of 160 patients with proven solitary intraductal papilloma a nipple discharge was the presenting symptom in 129, or 81 per cent, of the patients. It was the only symptom of the disease in 79, or 49 per cent.

The discharge was serous in 64, or 49.6 per cent. It was bloody in 65, or 50.4 per cent. Each of the delicate finger-like processes in a papilloma must have a blood supply, and very slight trauma would be expected to break some of them off and fill up the duct with serum or blood.

The character of the nipple discharge—whether serous or bloody—does not in my experience distinguish intraductal papilloma from carcinoma. In the 17 patients with breast carcinoma and a nipple discharge who consulted me between 1956 and 1967, the discharge was serous in seven, colorless in one, and bloody in nine. This is not a significantly different ratio of serous to bloody discharge from that in my patients with intraductal papilloma noted above.

The nipple discharge in solitary intraductal papilloma is usually noted only intermittently, as evidenced by an occasional yellowish or brownish stain on the brassiere or nightgown. Long intervals may go by without any discharge in some patients. In other patients the discharge is more constant and abundant, slight pressure on the breast being sufficient to produce a flow of several drops of serum or blood.

Several of my patients have pointed out that their nipple discharge was increased with the onset of menstruation, but this is not the usual experience.

The location on the surface of the nipple of the duct from which the discharge escapes is an important indication of the radial situation of the papilloma in the breast. Approximately 20 ducts open into the nipple surface, and the arrangement of these orifices has a close relationship to the radial course of ducts out into the breast. For example, when a discharge is noted from a duct orifice at 9 o'clock on the nipple surface, the lesion, be it an intraductal papilloma or some other disease, will almost always be found in the corresponding 9 o'clock radius of the breast.

In patients with a nipple discharge in whom no tumor can be found, palpation of the circumareolar region will often reveal a pressure point over some radius of its circumference. Gentle pressure over this point produces a discharge from a duct orifice situated in a corresponding radius in the nipple surface. Figure 14-1 shows this maneuver producing a drop of discharge from the nipple. Moistening the nipple surface will sometimes assist in eliciting the discharge. In this manner the site of the papilloma can often be localized.

Tumor. A generation ago we occasionally saw a patient with a large breast tumor produced by intraductal papilloma. For example, Figure 14-2 shows a 59 year old housewife who came to the Presbyterian Hospital in 1939 with a tumor of the left breast, which she said she had had for a year. She had no nipple discharge. The tumor was well delimited and freely movable and measured 13 cm. in diameter. It was a benign intraductal papilloma.

Today, if a tumor exists in a patient with intraductal papilloma, it is almost always small. In my personal series of 160 patients there have been 31 who consulted me only because of a tumor that they or a physician had discovered. Fifty others with intraductal papilloma came to me because they had both a tumor and a nipple discharge, and 79 consulted me because they had only nipple discharge. Nevertheless, in 45 of the 79 with careful palpation I found a tumor, the presence of which was unknown to the patient. In all but two of the 126 patients with a tumor it was situated in the subareolar area, or close to the edge of the areola. In one patient the tumor was in the upper outer sector of her breast, and in the other it was in its upper inner sector. The tumors in my personal series of cases were all small, varying between 3 mm. and 2 cm., except for one measuring 3 cm. in diameter. The mean diameter of the tumors was 1 cm.

There were two types of tumors. One type was subareolar in position, and linear in form, representing the dilated terminal duct distended with serum or blood and the papilloma growing within it. These linear tumors were minute in size, usually measuring only 2 or 3

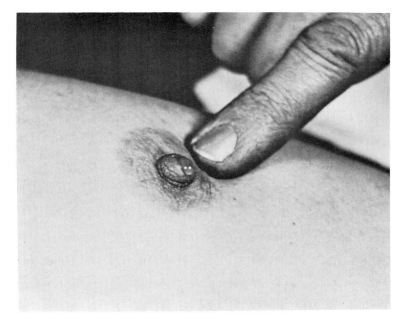

Figure 14-1. The expression of a drop of discharge from the nipple in a patient with intraductal papilloma, by gentle pressure over the site of the papilloma in the subareolar region.

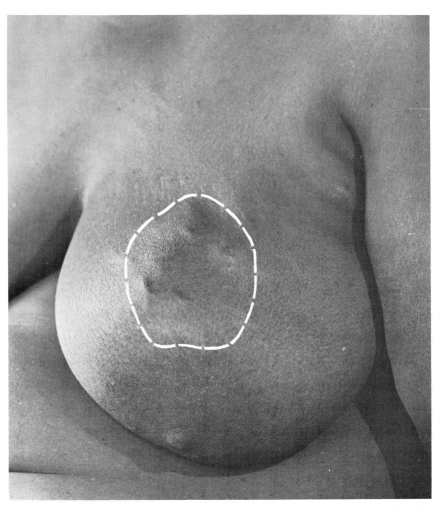

Figure 14-2. A solitary papilloma within a cyst forming a 13 cm. tumor of the breast.

mm. in width and 10 or 12 mm. in length. They were often very difficult indeed to detect, requiring exceedingly gentle and thorough palpation. The other type of tumor was round and well delimited, a little larger in size, and representing the papilloma growing to form a cyst-like structure in a duct that was blocked off.

In a few patients there is a relationship between tumor formation and the discharge. A tumor will develop slowly over a period during which there will be no nipple discharge. A profuse discharge will then occur and the tumor will disappear as the distended duct or cyst empties. This cycle may be repeated over and over again.

Retraction Signs. Intraductal papillomas do not ordinarily produce retraction, but occasionally skin dimpling, retraction of the nipple, or distortion of the contour of the breast develops. A good example of retraction was seen in the case of Mrs. E. F. whose history can be summarized as follows.

She was a 72 year old housewife who came to the hospital complaining of a bloody discharge

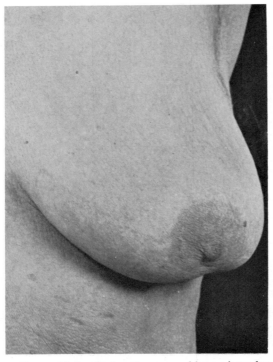

Figure 14–3. Retraction caused by an intraductal papilloma, evidenced by a notch in the contour of the lower edge of the breast.

from the left nipple which she had noted for the previous four months. The discharge consisted of a drop of very black blood noted every other day. She went to her local physician, who discovered a tumor in the breast, and referred her to the hospital.

Examination showed a firm, 3 cm. tumor lying beneath the edge of the areola of the left breast in the radius of 4 o'clock. The mass was relatively fixed in the surrounding breast tissue and there was marked dimpling of the overlying skin. When the arms were raised, a deep notch became evident in the contour of the breast at the site of the tumor, as shown in Figure 14-3. The breast and the tumor within it were freely movable over the chest wall.

The surgeon mistakenly chose to do a radical mastectomy without frozen section. Pathologic examination of the breast showed that the tumor mass consisted of an intraductal papilloma solidly filling a cystic structure. On microscopic examination the lesion proved to be a benign intraductal papilloma.

Signs of Inflammation. In one of our patients the clinical picture suggested an abscess. The patient, a woman of 41 years who had not been pregnant for some years, developed swelling and tenderness of the left breast, accompanied by throbbing pain and the escape of a few drops of blood from the nipple. A week later, when she came into the hospital, there was a 4 cm. indurated area in the outer middle section of the breast. The skin over the outer half of the breast was reddened and abnormally warm. Pressure upon the area of induration produced a flow of "dark reddish pus" from the nipple. Culture of this material showed hemolytic *Staphylococcus aureus*.

The lesion was excised and proved to be a small intraductal papilloma filling a distended duct, accompanied by acute inflammation in the surrounding breast tissue.

Duration of Symptoms

The solitary intraductal papillomas have very little growth vigor, and enlarge so slowly that in some patients the symptoms have been of long duration. The duration of symptoms in my series of 160 patients is shown in Table 14-1. It will be seen that 15 patients had had symptoms for more than three years. Three had had a nipple discharge, for 16, 17, and 18 years respectively.

A typical case history of an intraductal papil-

Table 14–1. DURATION OF SYMPTOMS IN 160 PATIENTS WITH SOLITARY INTRADUCTAL PAPILLOMA

Duration	Number of Patients
3 months or less	85
4 to 6 months	17
7 to 12 months	19
13 to 36 months	17
37 to 60 months	10
61 to 120 months	2
121 months or more	·3 (16 years, 17 years, and 18 years)
Not stated	3
Discovered by examining physician	4

loma of long duration was that of S. K., a housewife 38 years old. Seventeen years previously, after weaning her first child, she had developed a discharge from the left nipple. It consisted of a few drops of a brownish fluid which she noted only at intervals of from one to three months. She learned that by squeezing the breast she could express a small quantity of the discharge. This seemed to relieve her of a feeling of discomfort in the breast which she had from time to time. During two subsequent pregnancies, 12 and eight years previously, the discharge had disappeared, and did not reappear until after the babies were weaned.

Two years previously she had noted a small lump beneath the areola of the left breast. This seemed to decrease somewhat in size when she squeezed her breast to express the discharge. Examination showed a freely movable 2.5 cm. tumor beneath the areola. There were no retraction signs.

At operation a thin-walled cystic structure filled with brown fluid and containing a papilloma growing from a broad base was found. The lesion was excised locally, together with a small amount of adjacent breast tissue. Twelve years later there had been no recurrence of either tumor or discharge.

Long intervals of freedom from the discharge are not uncommon, as in the case of A. L., a nursemaid aged 62.

She had first noted a serosanguineous nipple discharge ten years previously. After a few weeks the discharge ceased and never reappeared. Five years previously she had first discovered a tumor beneath the nipple. This had not changed in size, but it had recently become tender.

Examination showed a firm 3 x 3 cm. mass beneath the areola of the right breast. The mass was attached to the skin of the overlying areola, and to the nipple, which was somewhat flattened. At operation the tumor was found to be a cyst containing brownish fluid and partly filled by a papilloma. The cyst was excised. The patient had had no recurrence when last seen 11 years later.

Pathology

Most solitary intraductal papillomas are so small that some surgical pathologists and many surgeons have never seen one, not knowing how to find and demonstrate them.

When the surgeon has correctly diagnosed the presence of an intraductal papilloma, identified the duct in which it is situated, and removed the duct containing it together with a small cone of surrounding breast tissue, the surgical specimen should be laid out flat, with the central end of the diseased duct, which was severed from the base of the nipple, marked with black silk. Beginning at this point the duct is slit open with fine scissors. As the duct is opened, extending peripherally, the papilloma will be found filling and distending it. The papilloma is brownish in color, and very soft and friable. It is usually only 2 or 3 mm. in diameter. It is usually attached to the duct wall only by a delicate pedicle, and is very easily torn loose. Otherwise it lies free within the duct, along which it usually extends for a distance of 1 or 2 cm. Figure 14–4 shows such a papilloma.

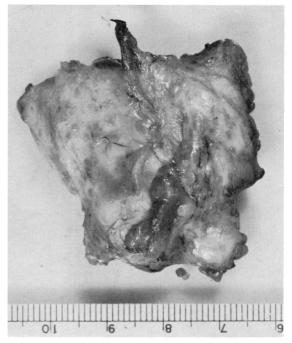

Figure 14–4. Gross appearance of a solitary intraductal papilloma lying in a duct which has been opened. The proximal end of the duct, severed at the base of the nipple, projects from the top of the specimen.

Occasionally it extends for 4 or 5 cm. along the duct in which it arose, and may grow into its branches. Solitary intraductal papillomas are usually situated in a major collecting duct in the subareolar area within a few centimeters of its termination. As I have mentioned above in discussing the site of the tumor formed by intraductal papilloma, in rare instances this same type of solitary intraductal papilloma occurs in a duct farther out in the breast.

If a surgical pathologist is presented with a mass of breast tissue, with no information as to its orientation, which was excised by a surgeon blindly removing a portion of the breast in the hope of finding disease responsible for a nipple discharge, and the surgical pathologist slices through the specimen at random he is very apt to miss one of these small papillomas even when the surgeon was lucky enough to remove it.

When solitary intraductal papillomas grow to a larger size they form a friable, soft, hemorrhagic mass within a cystic cavity formed by the greatly dilated duct, as shown in Figure 14-5. We have seen lesions of this kind as large as 10 or 12 cm. in diameter.

Microscopically, intraductal papillomas are simply proliferations of duct epithelium

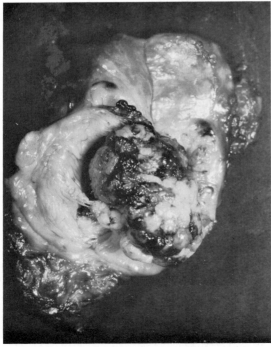

Figure 14-5. Gross appearance of an intraductal papilloma forming a soft, friable, hemorrhagic mass within a cyst.

which project outward into a dilated lumen from one or more focal points. The proliferated epithelial cells are supported upon vascular stalks which may be thin and delicate (Fig. 14-6) or broad and heavy (Fig. 14-7). The proliferation may be obviously papillary, or so completely anastomosing as to seem to form gland-like spaces. The individual proliferating epithelial cells in these lesions are small and quite regular in size and shape. Mitoses are rare. The proliferating cells give the impression of being benign.

We have occasionally seen a solitary papilloma that has become completely necrotic, presumably because its blood supply has been cut off. The sharpest study is required to identify the ghost-like outlines of its structure. Figure 14-8 shows such a necrotic papilloma.

One of the important ancillary aspects of the pathology of intraductal papilloma is the fact that sclerosed papillomas may be mistaken for carcinoma. This is perhaps the lesion most frequently mistaken for carcinoma of the breast according to Lattes, the Director of our Laboratory of Surgical Pathology at Columbia.

Presumably as the result of repeated trauma, hemorrhage and fibrosis occur in the lesion. The proliferating papillary epithelium is caught in this process and distorted. The fibrosis obliterates to a degree the general architecture of the papilloma, and the boundaries between the papilloma, the wall of the duct in which it lies, and the surrounding breast tissue, are lost. A false impression of carcinoma is given by this process. Figure 14-9 shows such a lesion. Here the outlines of the duct wall have been lost, and the epithelial cells of the papilloma have been forced into an abnormal pattern. Pathologists and surgeons should beware of this diagnostic trap.

The microscopic criteria that make it possible to distinguish between a sclerosed intraductal papilloma and a carcinoma are not only the general architecture of the lesion, but the cytology of the tumor cells themselves. The epithelial cells of a papilloma resemble the cells of normal duct epithelium, whether of the usual type, or of the so-called apocrine type with small nuclei and large acidophilic granular cytoplasms. It must be remembered, however, that normal duct cells vary considerably. Not only are they capable of enlargement when engaged in secretory activity, but they undergo degenerative changes

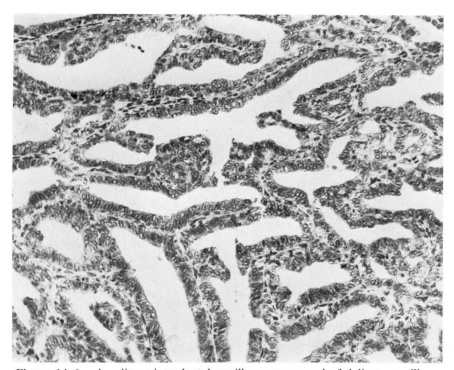

Figure 14–6. A solitary intraductal papilloma composed of delicate papillae.

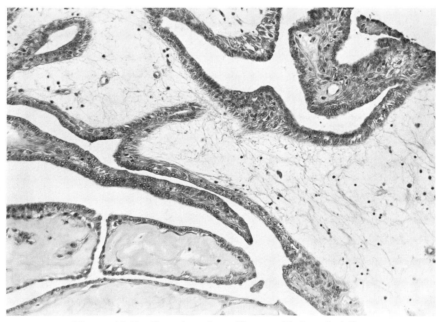

Figure 14–7. Intraductal papilloma with broad stalks.

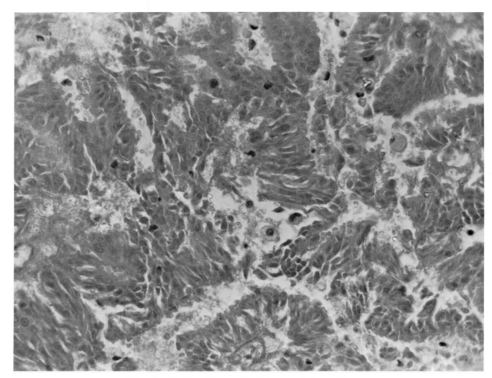

Figure 14–8. Necrotic intraductal papilloma.

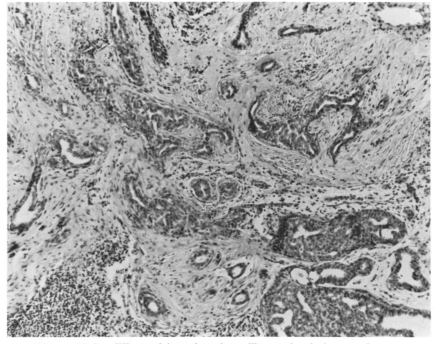

Figure 14–9. Fibrosed intraductal papilloma simulating carcinoma.

with swelling and fatty infiltration. In order to judge whether or not such abnormal-appearing cells are cancerous, one must be familiar with these various changes which can take place in noncancerous cells. In doubtful cases, the decision generally rests upon the character of the nuclei; if they have the appearance of anaplasia with hyperchromatism, accentuation of the chromatin network, or large nucleoli, and particularly if there are more than rare, widely separated mitoses, the lesion must be considered carcinoma. I will discuss the question of the microscopic differentiation between intraductal papilloma and papillary carcinoma in more detail in Chapter 28 in which I deal with papillary carcinoma.

I must emphasize that these difficult differential pathologic diagnoses should not be attempted on the basis of frozen sections. We have a rule in our laboratory of Surgical Pathology, which Dr. Stout laid down many years ago, that the definitive diagnosis of papillary lesions in the breast must not be attempted from frozen sections. We still adhere to this rule and it has saved us many times from mistaken diagnosis.

The Clinical Diagnosis of Solitary Intraductal Papilloma

I have emphasized the fact that the majority of patients with intraductal papilloma consult a physician because they have a serous or bloody nipple discharge. If there is an accompanying tumor one can go ahead with the appropriate surgical exploration. But if careful palpation does not reveal a tumor, and a pressure point in the areolar region producing the discharge cannot be found, the reasonable thing to do is to explain this dilemma to the patient and re-examine her at intervals of every couple of weeks. The risk to the patient of this sort of delay is exceedingly small. Carcinoma producing a nipple discharge not accompanied by a palpable tumor is rare. On the other hand, if the surgeon explores the duct system of one of these patients without any idea as to the radial postion of the papilloma in the subareolar region he is greatly handicapped. He may make his circumareolar incision on the wrong side of the areola and do a good deal of unnecessary damage to the breast before he finds the lesion.

Sandblom has made a great point of solving this dilemma by cannulating the nipple duct from which the discharge escapes and injecting it with contrast medium. I have not used this method because I have usually succeeded with simple palpation in localizing the radial position of the lesion in patients in whom the nipple discharge continued.

This brings me to the interesting question of what the explanation is when the nipple discharge ceases and does not recur. I have a series of 23 such patients followed for from five to 14 years. Seventeen of these patients came to me with a nipple discharge but no breast tumor, and I could not find a pressure point that would elicit the discharge and enable me to localize the radial position of the papilloma. Repeated examination did not solve the dilemma. Finally the discharge ceased. No operation was done and there has been no further evidence of disease in the breast. The explanation in this group of patients may, of course, be that they did not have intraductal papilloma, but had duct ectasia or cystic disease that resolved spontaneously.

But in six other women with all the classic signs of intraductal papilloma, including a small subareolar tumor, operation was refused or delayed for one reason or another, and the discharge ceased. No operation was performed and there has been no further evidence of breast disease after a mean follow-up period of six and one-half years. In these patients I believe that the papilloma must have undergone spontaneous necrosis. That this may occur I have already mentioned in discussing the pathology of this lesion. The following case is an example.

Mrs. D. W., aged 70, consulted me because she had had an intermittent serous discharge from her right nipple for five years. Beneath the edge of the areola there was a 5 x 10 mm. elongated tumor. Pressure on it produced serous discharge from a central nipple duct. Surgery was refused, the discharge disappeared, and eight years later her breast was normal.

Bilateral Occurrence of Solitary Intraductal Papilloma

Solitary intraductal papilloma is only rarely a bilateral disease. In my personal series of 160 patients with solitary papillomas only three have developed solitary papillomas in both breasts. The interval between the bilateral lesions averaged 11 years.

Association of Solitary Intraductal Papilloma with Gross Cystic Disease

Nine of the 160 patients in my personal series of patients with solitary intraductal papilloma have also had proven gross cystic disease. In one of the patients the cystic disease was bilateral, in four it developed in the same breast as the papilloma, and in four others it occurred in the opposite breast. These data are not statistically significant because the numbers of cases are too small, but they do not suggest that there is any association between solitary intraductal papilloma and gross cystic disease.

Association of Solitary Intraductal Papilloma with Carcinoma

The question of whether or not solitary intraductal papillomas transform into papillary carcinoma, or are an indication of a predisposition to breast carcinoma, is an interesting and important one. In my personal series of 160 patients with solitary intraductal papilloma, 118 were treated more than 10 years ago. Eight of the 118 have developed breast carcinoma. Four died of intercurrent disease before 10 years. Eighteen were lost track of before 10 years. Of the 42 patients with intraductal papilloma whom I have treated during the past 10 years two have to date developed mammary carcinoma.

This may appear to be a suspiciously high frequency of carcinoma. But from the point of view of statistical proof of any relationship beween the two diseases the numbers of cases are too small to permit valid conclusions. There are, however, features of these cases that argue against an association between solitary intraductal papilloma and carcinoma.

In the first place the carcinoma and the solitary intraductal papilloma occurred in opposite breasts in eight of my 10 patients. In three of the 10 the carcinoma preceded the papilloma, whereas in seven it followed the papilloma. The interval between the first symptom of solitary papilloma and the development of carcinoma in these seven patients was long. It varied from three to 18 years, averaging 9.3 years.

Another argument against the evolution of solitary intraductal papilloma into carcinoma is the fact that among the 10 patients who developed carcinoma in my personal series of 160 patients with solitary papilloma, only three had carcinoma of the apocrine papillary or cribriform intraductal type—the type we should expect if transition from papilloma to carcinoma occurs. It is interesting to present the details of these three cases.

CASE 1

Mrs. J. S. was 35 when she consulted me for a serous discharge from her right nipple which she had had for four years. I found a 1 cm. rounded tumor at the edge of the right areola. At operation a solitary intraductal papilloma was identified and excised.

Eighteen years later I found an area of induration in the periphery of the upper outer portion of her right breast. Biopsy revealed a carcinoma of the apocrine type, which was treated by radical mastectomy.

She is well six years after her radical mastectomy.

CASE 2

Mrs. G. S. began to have a serous discharge from her left nipple when she was 59, and came at once to consult me. She had no palpable tumor, but a subareolar pressure point at 11 o'clock produced a discharge from a corresponding duct. With my usual technique a small solitary papilloma was found in a terminal duct and excised. Fourteen years later she developed a bloody discharge from her right nipple. A cord-like thickening was palpable beneath the areola. At operation a solitary papilloma in one of the terminal ducts was identified and resected.

Two years later a poorly defined area of induration was palpated in the inner portion of her left breast over the 3rd costal cartilage. At operation this proved to be a carcinoma and was treated by radical mastectomy. This was 16 years after I had excised the solitary intraductal papilloma from the subareolar region of this breast.

Mrs. S's carcinoma was also of the apocrine papillary and cribriform type, which suggests an evolution from papilloma.

She is well three years after her radical mastectomy.

CASE 3

Miss B. H. was 48 when she discovered a small tumor in her left breast. She consulted me a month later. She had no nipple discharge. Her tumor was round and well delimited, 1.5 cm. in diameter, and was situated beneath the edge of the areola. With my usual operative technique it was identified as a solitary papilloma in the terminal portion of a duct, and was excised.

Three years later she found a small tumor in the upper outer portion of her right breast. It was only 1 cm. in diameter but had the clinical characteristics of a carcinoma, which it proved to be on biopsy. Radical mastectomy was performed.

Her carcinoma was intraductal, and in part apocrine with papillary and cribriform areas. In the adjacent breast tissue there was a striking amount of benign intraductal papillary proliferation of the apocrine type.

She has no evidence of breast disease 11 years later.

In two of these three patients the microscopic evidence is suggestive that the carcinoma may have evolved from pre-existing papilloma. In the third patient the carcinoma developed in the opposite breast. If carcinoma does evolve from solitary intraductal papilloma it does so so rarely that it is not greatly to be feared. In multiple papillomatosis of the breast, which I will subsequently discuss, the facts are quite different.

My conclusion from these data is that with rare exceptions solitary intraductal papillomas are not precancerous lesions. They should be treated conservatively. Patients who have had this disease should be followed for at least a 20 year period, and I suggest at intervals of six months.

Treatment of Solitary Intraductal Papilloma

The disagreement regarding the correct treatment of intraductal papilloma, and the mistakes that are made in treatment, result chiefly from a lack of knowledge of the pathology of the disease on the part of the surgeons. Many are not familiar enough with the gross appearance of a duct containing a papilloma to be able to find it at operation. The dissection must, moreover, be a meticulous one in which bleeding is carefully controlled, or it will not be possible to see the lesion. Handicapped by these difficulties, the average surgeon who attempts local excision of an intraductal papilloma has been content merely to excise blindly the area of breast tissue which he presumes contains the lesion, without dissecting out the lesion and identifying it. When local excision is done in this manner, it is not surprising that recurrence occasionally develops from papilloma left behind. Such recurrences are mistakenly interpreted as a malignant transformation of the papilloma, and needless mastectomy is performed.

Another cause for confusion regarding the treatment of intraductal papilloma is the difficulty that some pathologists have in distinguishing benign papilloma from papillary carcinoma. The less courageous pathologists tend to classify a good many entirely benign lesions as malignant. I know that this distinction is not an easy one, but I believe that with adequate experience it can be made with certainty in almost every case. When the pathologist is in doubt, he had better delay and seek more expert diagnostic help before deciding that the lesion is malignant. He should remember that papillary carcinomas are infrequent, and that even if the lesion in question proves to be a carcinoma, a reasonable delay will not impair the chance of cure by radical surgery, because the growth vigor of papillary carcinoma, like the other well-differentiated carcinomas of the breast, is decidedly less than that of the ordinary breast carcinoma.

My own experience convinced me long ago that solitary intraductal papillomas can be accurately diagnosed and localized, and that local excision of the involved duct or ducts is all that is required to cure the disease. Nevertheless, a number of patients with solitary intraductal papilloma have been treated in our hospital by radical mastectomy or by simple mastectomy. In some of these cases the surgeon was responsible for this drastic treatment. For example, some years ago before the necessity of biopsy to establish the diagnosis of all breast lesions was generally accepted by all members of our staff, radical mastectomy was done in two patients who proved to have only intraductal papilloma. Simple mastectomy was done in several cases by surgeons who tried to find a small papilloma and failed, and solved their dilemma by removing the breast.

In other instances our pathologist was responsible for the drastic surgery, having mistaken intraductal papilloma for carcinoma. This happened in five instances prior to 1945 when the rule was adopted in our department of surgical pathology that if a surgeon finds a papillary lesion, a definitive microscopic diagnosis must not ordinarily be attempted from frozen section. We wait for permanent sections, and study them with great care.

This limitation does not handicap the surgeon or endanger the patient. When a patient has the classic clinical signs of a centrally located solitary intraductal papilloma, and its radial position has been defined, and the duct containing it identified at operation, the duct and a cone of surrounding breast tissue are excised, the duct is opened, and the papilloma is usually identified grossly at once. No frozen section is attempted.

When the patient has a tumor situated peripherally in the breast, biopsy is of course done through an incision directly over the tumor, and a small wedge is removed for frozen section. If this reveals that the lesion is papillary and well differentiated the wound is closed and no further surgery carried out until a definitive microscopic diagnosis is made from permanent sections.

My technique for the surgical excision of solitary centrally situated intraductal papilloma is as follows. The problem and procedure have of course been fully explained to the patient, and the unlikely possibility of carcinoma discussed.

In the operating room, under general anesthesia, an incision through the skin is made about halfway around the circumference of the areola (Fig. 14-10A). The incision is centered at the radius in which the lesion is presumably situated, as indicated by the position of the tumor, or by other localizing signs. The incision is placed pre-

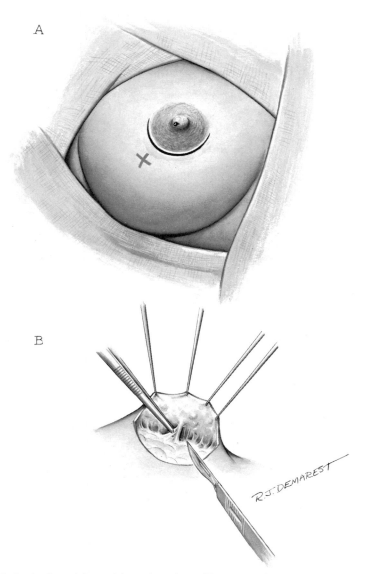

Figure 14-10. Method of excision of intraductal papilloma. *A,* Circumareolar incision; X marks the site of the papilloma. *B,* Dissection to the base of the nipple of the dilated duct containing the papilloma.
Illustration continues on opposite page.

cisely at the areolar edge. This minimizes the scar. The incision should not extend more than halfway around the areola, for fear of causing necrosis of the areolar flap.

Traction of the areolar flap is made with four skin hooks of the type described in Chapter 6. I then dissect up the areolar flap to the base of the nipple and dissect out the ducts which radiate from it. The dissection must be performed with delicacy, and meticulous hemostasis achieved with mosquito hemostats, otherwise the pathology will be obscured. The duct containing the papilloma can usually be identified by its size and color. It will be dilated to a diameter of something like 3 or 4 mm., and the serum or blood which it contains gives it a bluish appearance (Fig. 14–10B). Having identified and isolated the duct containing the papilloma, I clamp it and cut across it at the base of the nipple. Unless the involved duct is dissected out to the very base of the nipple, there is danger of not removing the papilloma in its entirety, for the branching processes sometimes grow along the duct very close to the nipple base. I often cut across all the ducts at the base of the nipple

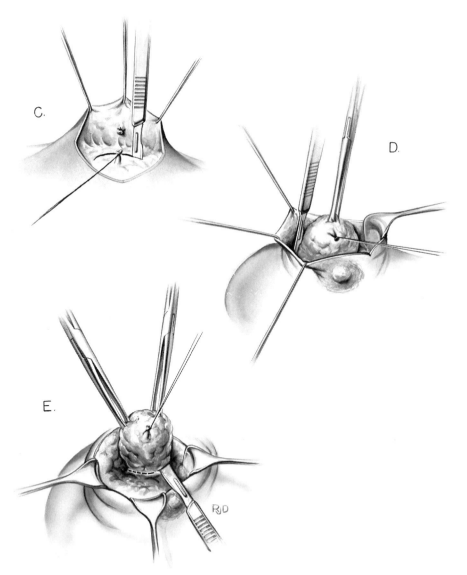

Figure 14–10. *Continued. C*, Beginning excision of cone of breast tissue surrounding the duct containing the papilloma. *D*, Dissecting up a flap of skin and subcutaneous tissue from the underlying breast tissue on the side of the wound opposite the nipple. *E*, Cutting across the base of the cone of the breast tissue containing the papilloma.

in making certain that I have found the duct containing the papilloma. No harm results.

Without further effort to trace the diseased duct out into the breast, I then excise a cone-shaped sector of mammary tissue surrounding the diseased duct. To accomplish this the first step is to incise the breast tissue centrally to the diseased duct to form the central edge of the area of breast tissue to be excised (Fig. 14–10C).

The next step is to elevate a flap of skin and subcutaneous tissue from the peripheral edge of the wound, uncovering the peripheral portion of the cone of breast tissue to be excised. This is done by retracting the peripheral edge of the wound with skin hooks and undercutting the skin for a distance of 3 or 4 cm. (Fig. 14–10D). This done, the skin hooks are exchanged for four small abdominal retractors, and the area of breast tissue to be excised is exposed. The size of the sector excised varies somewhat with the size of the breast, but it is my practice to carry the excision about 5 cm. out toward the periphery of the breast. With the diseased duct at its center, the cone of breast tissue to be removed is then elevated and excised, beginning at its central edge and encircling it peripherally (Fig. 14–10E). As the base of the cone of breast tissue is being cut across, great care is taken to keep the operative field dry, so that if any ducts are seen to contain extensions of the papilloma as they are cut across, a wider excision can be carried out.

It is very unusual to find the central type of intraductal papilloma originating in more than one of the main terminal ducts. The lesion is solitary in the sense that it originates in one duct, and extends a variable distance along it, usually not more than 1 or 2 cm. I have, however, seen one of these papillomas extend along a duct for 5 or 6 cm., and even grow into its branches. In cutting across the base of the cone of breast tissue that is resected with the diseased duct, a number of dilated branches of the main duct, all containing serum, will be encountered. The fact that they are dilated and filled with serum does not mean that they contain papilloma. It indicates that the main duct into which they drain is blocked by papilloma nearer its termination, and that the serum produced by the papilloma has backed up into its branches.

When the specimen is out, I ask the pathologist to open the duct that presumably contains the papilloma while I watch him. I wish to make certain myself that I have found and removed the lesion producing the nipple discharge.

After careful hemostasis the wound is closed without drainage. The circumareolar incision is closed with subcuticular sutures of silk and skin sutures of nylon. I dress the wound with gauze fluffs held in place by an Ace bandage to give gentle compression. The wound is left undisturbed for a week, when the sutures are removed. Some blood or serum not infrequently collects in these wounds, and requires aspiration when the wound is dressed. This is preferable, in my opinion, to placing a drain in the wound.

This procedure hardly distorts the breast at all, and leaves a scar that is almost invisible.

With this technique I have rarely failed to find and remove intraductal papillomas when they are the cause of nipple discharge. Occasionally cystic disease or duct ectasia will be found, and of course excised. When I encounter papillary proliferation in many ducts, and involving an extensive area of the breast, I at once suspect that the lesion is a papillary carcinoma. With this finding I do not proceed with either wide local excision or mastectomy. Instead, I remove a small biopsy from a representative portion of the lesion and close the wound. As I have already pointed out, frozen section differentiation between the benign intraductal papilloma and intraductal carcinoma is too difficult to be reliable. We depend only upon good paraffin sections. In this manner we safely and surely identify benign papilloma and avoid needless sacrifice of the breast.

The results of this conservative surgical attack on solitary centrally situated intraductal papillomas have been very satisfactory when properly carried out. In the 1951 study that Stout, Phillips, and I made of our Presbyterian Hospital data there were 56 patients in whom the lesion was excised locally. Only three of these 56 patients were lost track of. Three others died of intercurrent disease. Forty-eight were well after five years or more. In two patients there was local recurrence, which was to be expected in view of the lack of understanding of the problem on the part of the surgeons who performed the operations. The details of these two cases follows.

CASE 1

Mrs. O. R., a 38 year old woman, was first seen in 1930, complaining of a bloody discharge from the left nipple of seven years' duration. She had

had a lump in her breast for six weeks. On examination she had a 4 x 5 cm. freely movable mass at the areolar margin. Local excision was attempted, but the surgeon failed to recognize that the lesion was a papilloma. He cut directly down on the tumor and excised it without tracing the diseased duct to the nipple, or identifying its peripheral extension. With this kind of limited excision it is very likely that part of the duct or ducts containing papilloma were left *in situ*. Microscopically the original lesion was a benign intraductal papilloma.

Approximately four years later there was a recurrence in the scar of the previous operation. Biopsy of the new tumor was done, a frozen section diagnosis of carcinoma made, and radical mastectomy carried out. Fixed sections, however, proved the recurrent lesion to be identical with the original benign intraductal papilloma. The mastectomy was clearly unnecessary.

CASE 2

Mrs. D. B. was first seen in 1937, when she was 34 years of age. She complained of a bloody discharge from the left nipple of three years' duration, a lump in the breast of one year's duration. Examination revealed a 2 x 3 cm. shotty mass at the upper inner areolar margin. A partial mastectomy was done. In this patient also, the tumor was cut down upon and broken into several pieces, and shelled out bluntly, without any attempt to trace the diseased duct, either centrally or peripherally. Microscopically it was a benign intraductal papilloma.

In 1941 there was a 0.5 cm. recurrent tumor in the scar of the previous operation. A second partial mastectomy was done. At this time a pyramidal sector of breast tissue, including the diseased duct system centrally and peripherally and down to the pectoral fascia, was removed. Five years later, she was free of disease in both breasts.

In my personal series of 160 patients with solitary intraductal papilloma, 118 were treated with my method of local excision more than 10 years ago. Four died of intercurrent disease less than 10 years after operation. Eighteen have been lost track of. Ninety-five patients have had no further evidence of papilloma in the breast in which it had occurred, during a follow-up period of from 10 to 24 years. I have had only one patient develop a local recurrence of her papilloma. My failure in this case was presumably because I failed to remove an exceptionally long extension of the papilloma along the involved duct. The details of the case follow.

Mrs. J. K., aged 42, discovered a very small tumor beneath her right areola. Three months later she consulted me. The tumor was only 5 mm. in diameter and round and movable. At operation I found a dilated duct, and after transecting it at the base of the nipple I excised it and a cone of breast tissue surrounding it for a distance of about 4 cm. into the breast. But as I cut across the base of this cone I encountered the diseased duct filled with papilloma even at this depth. In an effort to make certain I got the papilloma all out I excised an additional 2 cm. of breast tissue extending down into the breast.

Seven years later the patient discovered a small new tumor beneath her right areola adjacent to the scar of my earlier operation. It was very similar to, and in almost the same site as her earlier tumor. I excised this new tumor, together with a 2 cm. margin of surrounding tissue. It proved to be an intraductal papilloma situated within a duct. Whether this was a new papilloma developing in a new duct, or a remnant of the original papilloma which I had failed to remove in its entirety, I do not know. But the patient's breast is normal five years later.

PAPILLOMA OF THE NIPPLE

When a disease is so infrequent that even an experienced clinician will see it only a few times in a lifetime it is apt to go unrecognized and be mistreated except in clinics in which there is close cooperation between clinicians and pathologists. This is particularly well illustrated by papilloma of the nipple, a rare but distinctive lesion, in which papilloma develops within the nipple.

In our clinic we recognized this form of papilloma 30 years ago and treated it successfully by locally excising the involved sector of the nipple, as detailed in the following case report.

Mrs. M. R., aged 30, came to the Presbyterian Hospital in 1938. She had noticed a small crusted area on her left nipple for over a year. There was a small amount of yellowish discharge from it from time to time. Palpation of the breast failed to reveal any tumor. Close inspection of the nipple showed that the orifice of one of the nipple ducts was dilated, and that projecting from it was a soft, reddish, papillary mass about 3 mm. in diameter. This was assumed to be a papilloma of the terminal portion of the duct. At operation a sector of the nipple, including the diseased duct, was excised. The excision was carried to the base of the nipple and a little way down into the breast. Microscopic examination showed that the lesion was indeed an intraductal papilloma. It projected from the orifice of the duct and extended down along its branches to the base of the specimen. It was not certain from the study of the microscopic sections that the papilloma had been excised in its entirety.

The follow-up of this patient showed, however, that the excision was adequate, for she had no further trouble with the left breast. But nine years later, in 1947, she entered another hospital for bleeding from the right nipple. A local excision of the subareolar area was done and benign intraductal papilloma found.

Stout and Phillips and I described and illustrated one of these papillomas of the nipple in our 1951 paper, and in the first edition of this book, published in 1956, I described the lesion, emphasizing its benign character.

In 1955 Jones presented the first paper devoted to this special lesion, and gave it the name "florid papillomatosis." He described five cases. Three of them had been mistaken for carcinoma.

Nichols, Dockerty, and Judd at the Mayo Clinic were impressed by Jones' description. They adopted the name he had given the lesion, and found 16 of these tumors in their case records. Thirteen had been diagnosed as carcinoma, and radical mastectomy had been done in 15.

Le Gal and his associates, at Strasbourg, in 1959, described 5 cases. Four had been initially diagnosed as epithelioma. These authors emphasized the adenomatous character of the lesion and suggested the name "erosive adenomatosis."

The following year Moulonguet described one of these lesions, which was clearly papillary, and expressed a preference for the name "extruding papillomatosis" of the nipple.

In 1962 Handley and Thackray published a careful description of eight cases observed at the Middlesex Hospital. In five of the earlier cases the lesion had been mistaken for carcinoma and mastectomy performed. The more recent lesions had been recognized as benign and treated successfully by removal of the nipple or local excision. Handley and Thackray emphasized the adenomatous character of the lesion and suggested that it may originate from sweat glands.

Robert and his associates reported five more cases in 1963.

A description of 10 cases published in 1965 by Miller and Bernier was remarkable because of the fact that one of the patients was a child aged nine, and another a man aged 66.

Taylor and Robertson at the Armed Forces Institute of Pathology have recently described 29 cases that they have collected. Ten were treated by mastectomy.

This, then, is a lesion that has recently had enough publicity to acquaint most pathologists with the fact that it is entirely benign. Surgeons, however, still do not know how to recognize the disease in its early stage, and they remain confused as to how best to deal with it. Most of the clinical descriptions hitherto published have described an advanced stage of the disease with a granulomatous tumor of considerable size fungating out onto the surface of the nipple. It is quite possible to recognize this lesion at a much earlier stage, before it has appeared on the surface of the nipple.

The first sign may be a drop of blood appearing from the opening of a duct on the nipple surface when the nipple is compressed. The opening of the duct may be dilated, and a minute granuloma-like lesion 2 or 3 mm. in diameter be visible in it. In other cases there will be no visible break in the nipple epithelium but it will appear reddened over a sector of the nipple surface. This redness is due to the papilloma within the substance of the nipple near its surface with consequent thinning of the overlying nipple epithelium. Paget's disease due to carcinoma growing beneath and in the nipple epithelium also has a pre-erosive stage that gives the same appearance. Another early manifestation of papilloma of the nipple may be a minute mound-like tumor elevated above the nipple surface and covered with intact epithelium.

It is so difficult to photograph these early stages of the lesion that I am unable to illustrate them.

As the disease progresses within the nipple, the nipple becomes thickened, and even enlarged.

The final stage, which is the one usually featured, is that of a soft granuloma-like tumor growing out on the nipple surface. It may occupy a considerable part of the nipple surface as shown in Fig. 14–11. The lesions bleed easily. It is worthy of note that the discharge from papilloma of the nipple, when there is a discharge, is almost always bloody, rather than serous. One of the reasons why "florid papillomatosis" is not a good name for this lesion is that it describes only the advanced stage of the disease. The most appropriate name is papilloma of the nipple.

I am able to report experience with 19 of these papillomas of the nipple. In all, the lesion was recognized as a benign papilloma. Mastectomy was not done in any of the patients.

The duration of these nipple papillomas

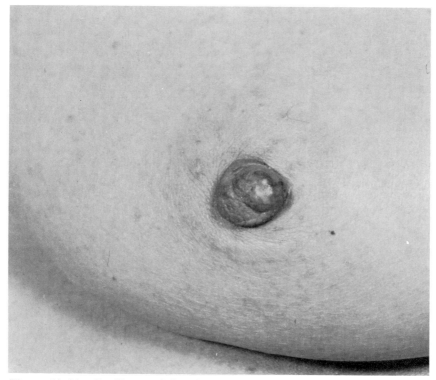

Figure 14–11. Papilloma of the nipple fungating out onto the nipple surface.

may be as long as that of the other forms of duct papilloma. Indeed, the patient with the longest duration in my series of patients with papillomas of all types was a woman aged 78 with a papilloma of the nipple. She had had a serous nipple discharge for 48 years. Another of my patients with a nipple papilloma had had an intermittent bloody nipple discharge for 19 years. The mean duration of symptoms in my series of cases, if the patient with a duration of 48 years is excluded, was 34 months.

None of the 19 patients in my series has had bilateral nipple papilloma. Two of the 19, however, have also had solitary intraductal papilloma in the subareolar region of the contralateral breast. Two others, among the 19, also had gross cystic disease; in one it was bilateral, while in the other it occurred in the same breast as the nipple papilloma.

One of the 19 patients had carcinoma in addition to nipple papilloma. The details of her disease are worth describing.

Mrs. L. W., aged 78, had had a serous discharge from her left nipple for 48 years when she came to the Presbyterian Hospital because of a hard tumor which she had discovered a month previously in the same breast. The nipple was flattened. On its surface there was a central dilated duct in which a papilloma presented. Within the substance of the nipple a 1 cm. tumor was palpable.

In the lower outer sector of the same breast there was a 5 cm. hard tumor fixed in the breast tissue. Its central edge was immediately adjacent to the base of the nipple. There was marked skin dimpling over the lower sector tumor. Radical mastectomy was done.

The pathologic study revealed the nipple tumor to be a sclerosed solitary papilloma contained in a dilated nipple duct. The epithelium of the papilloma was almost entirely of the apocrine type, but benign in character. The tumor in the lower outer sector of the breast was a carcinoma which was in part intraductal, with a comedone structure. A few of the intraductal cell masses had a papillary arrangement. In several dilated nipple ducts filled with carcinoma immediately adjacent to the nipple papilloma, the carcinoma cells not only were apocrine in type but were growing in papillary formation. These facts suggest that in this case the carcinoma may in fact have evolved from the long existing adjacent papilloma.

The patient succumbed to a cerebral hemorrhage four years later, without further evidence of breast disease.

The Pathology of Papilloma of the Nipple

Although they have similar clinical manifestations, there are two quite distinct pathologic forms of nipple papilloma. The less frequent is the *solitary papilloma* growing within a dilated milk sinus in the nipple. It is wholly contained within the well-defined wall of the milk sinus. Figure 14–12 shows a solitary papilloma of this type. This lesion may grow upwards from a terminal duct at the base of the nipple, extend along a milk sinus, and finally present through the opening of the duct on the nipple surface; but it does not originate near the surface of the nipple. Five of the 19 nipple papillomas in my series of cases were of this solitary type. It does not present any special difficulty in diagnosis for the pathologist.

The more frequent type of nipple papilloma consists of a diffuse adenomatous and papillary epithelial proliferation, that usually develops in the superficial portion of the nipple, and at a comparatively early stage erodes the nipple epithelium and presents on its surface as a granulating area. Figure 14–13 shows a very small lesion of this type. Figure 14–14 shows one that has progressed to involve most of the nipple. We prefer the name *papillary adenoma* for this nipple lesion. Fourteen of my 19 nipple papillomas were of this type. This lesion presents diagnostic difficulties for the pathologist who is not familiar with it. The proliferating epithelial cells are comparatively small, and regular in size and shape, and do not suggest malignancy. But they grow in an irregular glandular and papillary arrangement, and are not enclosed by a limiting duct wall. Figure 14–15 shows the advancing edge of one of these lesions.

The temptation to call this type of lesion a

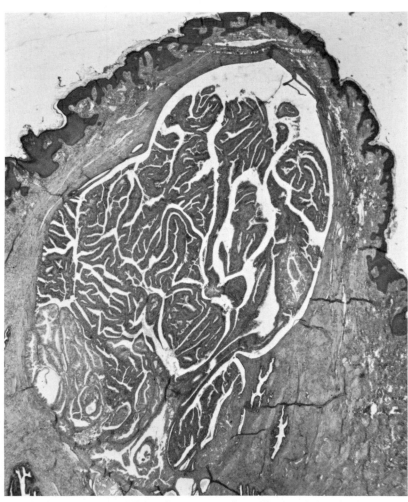

Figure 14–12.   The solitary type of papilloma of the nipple.

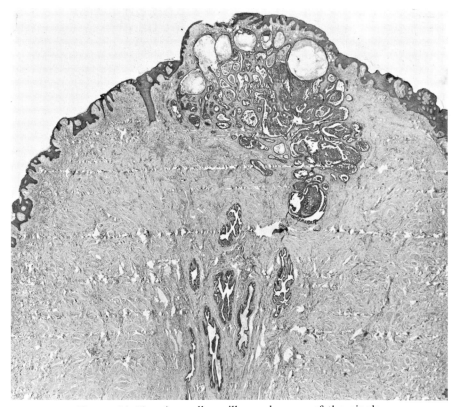

Figure 14–13.   A small papillary adenoma of the nipple.

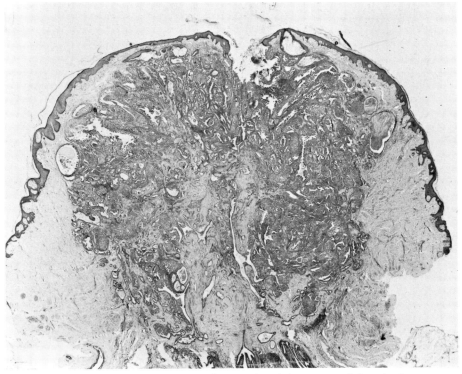

Figure 14–14.   A papillary adenoma involving most of the nipple.

carcinoma is accentuated when fibrosis develops within it, perhaps as the result of infection following erosion of the nipple epithelium. Caught in the fibrosis, the proliferating epithelium loses its papillary arrangement and appears to invade the nipple stroma in the form of tubules and strands of cells (Fig. 14–16). This distortion has often led pathologists to mistake papillary adenoma of the nipple for carcinoma and to recommend radical mastectomy. The truth is that these lesions are entirely benign. Not a single one has, to our knowledge, behaved like a carcinoma.

I believe that papillary adenoma of the nipple develops from the epithelium of the milk sinuses. The accordion-pleated contour of the milk sinuses makes it easy to identify them. In two of these papillary adenomas of the nipple that we have studied in serial section, and in other examples of this lesion, I have been able to trace its origin from the epithelium of a milk sinus. Figure 14–17 shows the very earliest stage of this process where there is a minute papillary outgrowth of the milk sinus epithelium. Figure 14–18 shows an advanced stage in which the papillary adenoma is filling up the upper end of a milk sinus.

There are two diseases of the nipple that have to be differentiated from nipple papilloma that has involved the nipple epithelium: (1) chronic inflammation of the nipple epithelium—sometimes due to fungus infection—called eczema for want of a more specific term; and (2) the Paget's form of mammary carcinoma growing up along ducts into the nipple epithelium and eroding it.

(Text continues on page 275.)

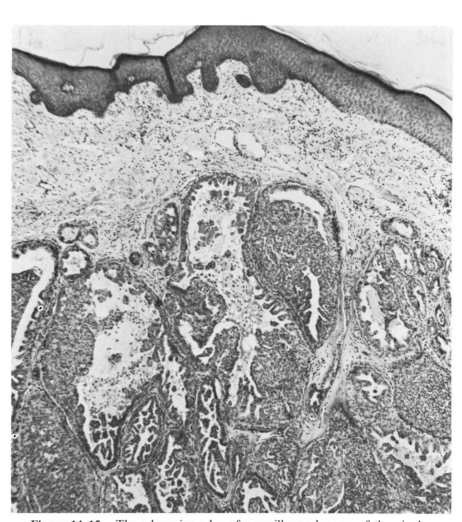

Figure 14–15.   The advancing edge of a papillary adenoma of the nipple.

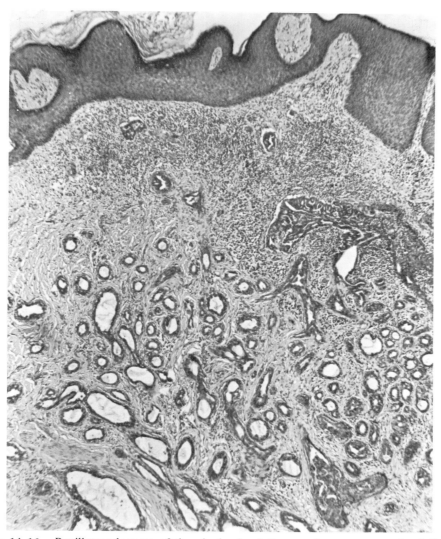

Figure 14–16. Papillary adenoma of the nipple simulating carcinoma as a result of fibrosis.

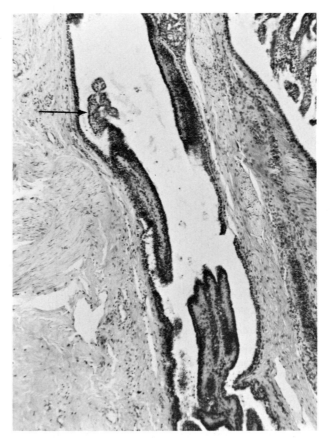

Figure 14–17. Minute papillary adenoma (*arrow*) originating from the epithelium of a milk sinus.

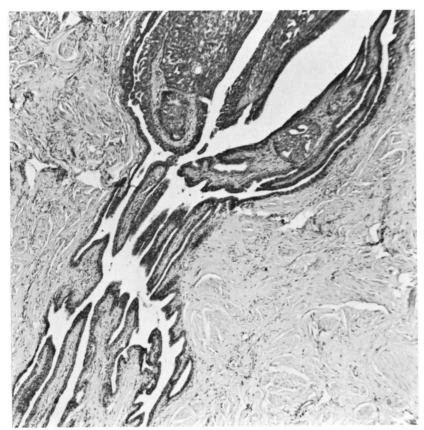

Figure 14–18. Papillary adenoma originating from and distending the upper end of a milk sinus.

The Treatment of Papilloma of the Nipple

The first step in treatment is to establish the diagnosis by excising a minute wedge of the abnormal nipple epithelium, or of the lesion protruding from its surface, and studying it microscopically. This is done with local anesthesia as an office procedure.

The great majority of these nipple papillomas can be cured by excision of the diseased portion of the nipple, preserving enough of the nipple to retain a semblance of it. In a small proportion of these cases in which the entire nipple is involved by the lesion it is necessary to remove the nipple. Mastectomy is never justified for this lesion.

In the 19 patients in my series of papilloma of the nipple, I was responsible for the treatment in all but two. In these two I made the diagnosis but the treatment was carried out by colleagues; it consisted of partial excision of the nipple in one patient and removal of the nipple in the other patient.

In 13 patients the papilloma involved only a part of the nipple, and I was able to remove it by partially excising the nipple. In three other patients the papilloma involved so much of the nipple that I had to excise it. For my patient whose history has been detailed above, who had a solitary papilloma of the nipple and an accompanying adjacent carcinoma of the breast, I of course performed a radical mastectomy.

My method of local excision that conserves the nipple is as follows. With radial incisions on each side of the lesion I split the nipple, retract its two halves, and carefully excise the papilloma. It can be recognized as a dense grayish lesion. I excise a narrow shell of the surrounding nipple tissue with it. I trace the lesion down to the base of the nipple where the wall of the duct in which the papilloma arises can sometimes be identified.

With this technique, carried out in 13 patients, I have had no recurrence after from one to 24 years. In eight of these patients the operation was done more than five years ago.

Both of the two patients in whom I excised the entire nipple have been recent ones. In them there has been no recurrence after two years.

MULTIPLE INTRADUCTAL PAPILLOMA

Our experience with papillary epithelial lesions of the breast has taught us the basic fact that *multiple papilloma* should be carefully distinguished from *solitary papilloma*, which I have been describing. Multiple papilloma has clinical and microscopic characteristics that are very different from those of solitary papilloma. Most important of all, multiple papilloma seems to be associated with carcinoma, whereas solitary papilloma is not. Multiple papilloma is, therefore, in our opinion, a separate disease that is important for clinicians and pathologists to recognize.

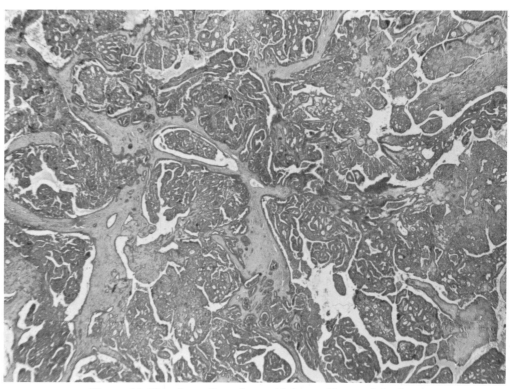

Figure 14–19. A portion of a multiple papilloma of the breast.

The basic feature distinguishing multiple from solitary papilloma is, of course, pathologic. Solitary papilloma is, as its name implies, a single papilloma, usually growing in the terminal portion of a main duct. It may extend several centimeters along the duct in which it originates, and grow into its branches, but it is easy enough to see that it is one papilloma. Infrequently such a single papilloma fills a cyst situated far out in the breast; it is still a solitary papilloma.

Multiple papilloma, on the other hand, consists of a great many grossly visible papillomas seemingly originating independently in many ducts in a portion or sector of the breast. The fact of the multiplicity of the papillomas is at once obvious to the pathologist. Figure 14–19 shows a small portion of an extensive lesion of this kind.

Pathologists have usually grouped all multiple papillary lesions together under the general term "papillomatosis." In so doing they fail to distinguish between the ubiquitous epithelial proliferation of minor degree in small ducts and microcysts, often papillary, that is seen in most adult breasts, and the infrequent papillary neoplasm for which we reserve the name multiple papilloma. The former phenomenon, illustrated in Figure 14–20,

does not produce a palpable tumor, is not grossly visible, and has no proved prognostic significance. Papillomatosis is an appropriate name for it and should be retained.

Multiple papilloma, on the other hand, is a disease *sui generis* that forms a palpable tumor in the breast, is grossly visible to the surgeon and the pathologist, and is a precancerous lesion.

Incidence

Multiple papilloma is a very infrequent disease. During the period in which I dealt personally with 160 patients with solitary papilloma, I had only 15 with multiple papilloma. In order to get a large enough series of cases of multiple papilloma for an adequate study of the disease, I have had to review all the cases in our hospital files between 1940 and 1967. They totalled only 39.

Age Distribution

Multiple papilloma develops at a younger age than solitary papilloma. The ages of patients with multiple papilloma in this series of cases ranged from 16 to 73, and the mean age

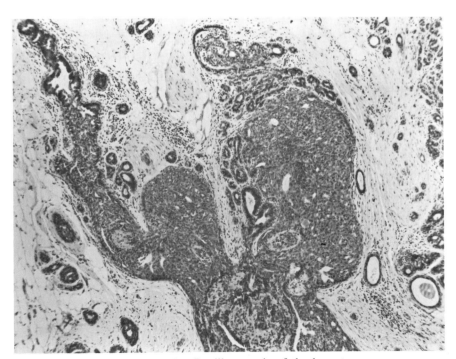

Figure 14–20. Papillomatosis of the breast.

was 39.6 years. The mean age of my patients with solitary papilloma was 48 years. Four of our patients with multiple papilloma were under 20 years of age—being 16, 17, 18, and 19 years old, respectively.

Clinical Features of Multiple Papilloma

A nipple discharge is not as frequently seen with multiple papilloma as with solitary papilloma. Only 14 of our 39 patients with multiple papilloma had a nipple discharge; in eight it was bloody, and in six serous.

In all but one of the patients with multiple papilloma a tumor was palpated. This was often small, and sometimes consisted of a group of nodules.

In 10 of the 38 patients with a tumor it was situated beneath the areola or close to its edge. In the other patients the disease was situated well out in the breast, sometimes involving an entire sector and extending down to the deep surface of the breast.

Multiple papilloma was bilateral in nine of the 39 patients of our series. This is an impressive proportion of bilateral involvement. Only 1.5 per cent of my patients with solitary papilloma had bilateral lesions.

These clinical features of solitary and multiple intraductal papillomas are compared in the following table:

Clinical Feature	Solitary Papilloma	Multiple Papilloma
Mean age of patients	48 years	39.6 years
Nipple discharge	81%	36%
Situated in subareolar zone of breast	95%	26%
Bilateral occurrence	1.5%	26%

One of the most remarkable clinical features of multiple papilloma as exhibited in our series of cases is the exceedingly slow course and tenacious nature of the disease. One of our patients died of cardiovascular disease only three years after local excision of her multiple papilloma. Nine others have been treated within the past 10 years, too recently to permit an accurate assessment of the course of their disease. One other patient was treated by bilateral simple mastectomy and, as would be expected, had no further evidence of the disease.

Among 13 other patients with multiple papilloma followed for 10 years or more after the onset of the disease, four were apparently cured by local excision, because they had no further evidence of their disease after 10, 11, 13, and 17 years respectively. Nine of the 13 patients had local recurrence following local excision of the multiple papilloma. Three of them had one local recurrence, two had two local recurrences, two had three local recurrences, one had four local recurrences, and one had five local recurrences. These local recurrences developed over a period of from five to 16 years. Thereafter, these nine patients had no further evidence of multiple papilloma. The mean total follow-up period in these nine patients was 16 years.

The following case history illustrates the natural history of multiple papilloma.

Mrs. L. J., aged 40, had had an intermittent bloody discharge from her left nipple for two years when she came to the Presbyterian Hospital in September, 1957. She was found to have a right subareolar tumor. It was well delimited and 4 cm. in diameter. At operation the tumor was found to be a cyst containing a papilloma. In the surrounding breast tissue there were many small intraductal papillomas. The area of disease was excised locally.

Within six months there was obvious local recurrence, as a lobulated 3 cm. tumor, in the region of the previous operation. A second local excision was performed.

Four and one-half years later, in September, 1962, a second recurrence was apparent farther out in the breast. It was situated halfway between the areola and the lower inner edge of the breast and measured 2.5 cm. in diameter. Again, local excision was performed.

Twenty-one months later, in June, 1964, a third local recurrence of the disease in the same sector of the breast was detected. It measured 2.5 cm. in diameter. Again, it was excised locally.

During the seven years of microscopic observation the character of the multiple papilloma remained unchanged. Its chief features were the ones usually seen in this disease—benign-appearing intraductal papillary epithelial proliferation, marked apocrine metaplasia of duct epithelium, and adenosis. I will illustrate each of these features of multiple papilloma in a subsequent description of the pathology of the disease.

At the present writing, 15 years after the symptoms of her disease first appeared, Mrs. L. J. has no clinical evidence of further recurrence.

Relationship of Multiple Papilloma to Cystic Disease

Gross cystic disease has developed in only three of our 39 patients who have had multiple papilloma. Two of these patients had bilateral multiple papilloma, which was diagnosed in one at the age of 23 and in the other at the age of 33. The younger patient developed cysts in one breast when she was 42, and the older got a cyst in one breast when she was 43.

Relationship of Multiple Papilloma to Carcinoma

Fifteen of our 39 patients with multiple papilloma have also had carcinoma. In all, the carcinoma was of the special intraductal apocrine papillary and cribriform type that we have come to associate with multiple papilloma.

In two of the 15 patients the carcinoma was bilateral.

In six of the 15 patients the carcinoma apparently evolved from multiple papilloma during the period following local excision of the disease. The interval between the initial symptom of papilloma and the diagnosis of carcinoma in these 6 patients was 4, 5, 8, 8½, 9, and 9½ years, respectively. There is in these case histories, therefore, evidence that when carcinoma evolves from multiple papilloma the process takes some years.

In the nine other patients, multiple papilloma and carcinoma were found to co-exist. In these patients we have, of course, no proof that the carcinoma evolved from multiple papilloma. We can theorize that the two diseases may have evolved independently in breast tissue predisposed to develop neoplastic processes.

Whatever the true relationship of multiple papilloma to intraductal apocrine papillary cribriform carcinoma may be, the fact remains that in our data, this special form of carcinoma has been found in 38 per cent of our patients with multiple papilloma. This fact alone is of sufficient importance to distinguish multiple papilloma from solitary papilloma in terms of treatment and follow-up.

The clinical course of this special type of breast carcinoma associated with multiple papilloma is often unusually slow. The history of one of our patients illustrates this fact.

Mrs. L. G., in 1942 when she was 38, developed a discharge from her right nipple. She was operated upon at another hospital and a "papilloma" was reported to have been excised.

Two years later the nipple discharge began again. A right-sided breast tumor also developed. In 1945 a second operation was performed, again with excision of a "papilloma."

In 1947 a new tumor appeared in the upper outer sector of the same breast. This tumor was excised locally in 1951, and was reported to be a papilloma. We later studied the microscopic sections of this lesion. Multiple papilloma, marked apocrine metaplasia of the duct epithelium, and intraductal carcinoma of the papillary cribriform type were seen. The carcinoma had been missed.

In 1956 a fourth local excision was performed for a "cyst" in the same sector of the right breast. We later studied the sections of this tissue and found the same multiple papilloma and the same type of carcinoma that had been missed in 1951.

In 1964 there was again local recurrence in the same area of the right breast. A fifth local excision was done in 1966. On this occasion the correct diagnosis of carcinoma was made and a radical mastectomy was done. The type of carcinoma was the same as when it was first apparent in 1951. There were no axillary metastases.

In this case the special type of intraductal apocrine papillary and cribriform carcinoma associated with multiple papilloma existed for 15 years without metastasizing to regional lymph nodes. The multiple papilloma with which it was associated had been present for at least 19 years.

The Pathology of Multiple Papilloma and the Carcinoma that may Evolve from it

The disease multiple papilloma has three basic pathologic features: papillomas growing in many ducts, adenosis, and widespread apocrine metaplasia of the proliferating duct epithelium. I will try to describe each of these features.

1. The papillomas vary greatly in structure. Some have broad stalks clothed with small regular epithelial cells (Fig. 14–21). In others a good deal of the intraductal proliferation has a glandular arrangement, and the epithelial cells may have cytoplasmic snouts projecting into the gland lumens (Fig. 14–22). Occasionally the papillomas are almost solid (Fig. 14–23). Spindle-cell metaplasia of the epithelium is seen in some of these more solid papillomas (Fig. 14–24). None of these variations appears to have any special significance. It is exceedingly difficult, if not impossible, to discriminate, by means of cytologic differences alone, between some benign multiple papillomas, and papillary carcinoma in which the hyperchromatism and variation in nuclear size and shape are not marked. The distinction has to be based on more obvious characteristics such as growth pattern.

Text continues on page 282.

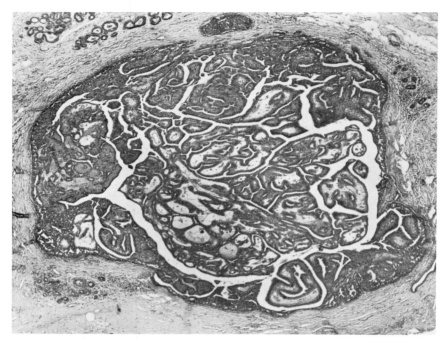

Figure 14–21. Multiple papilloma with broad stalks.

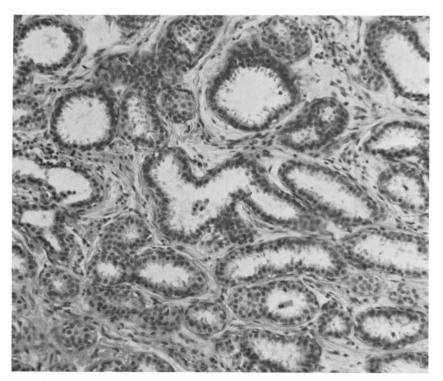

Figure 14–22. Multiple papilloma in which the intraductal proliferation has a glandular arrangement in some areas and the epithelial cells have cytoplasmic snouts projecting into the gland lumens.

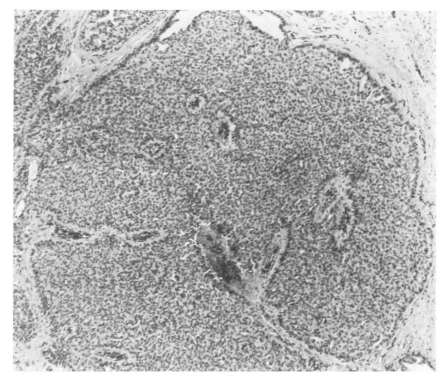

Figure 14–23. Multiple papilloma with a solid structure.

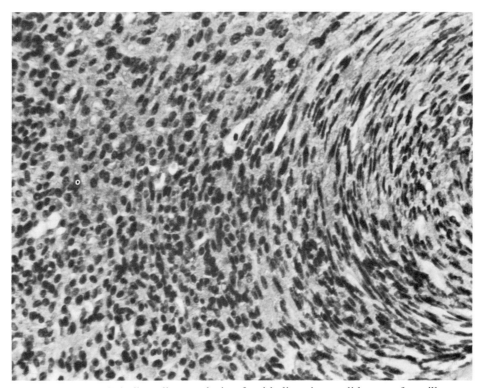

Figure 14–24. Spindle cell metaplasia of epithelium in a solid type of papilloma.

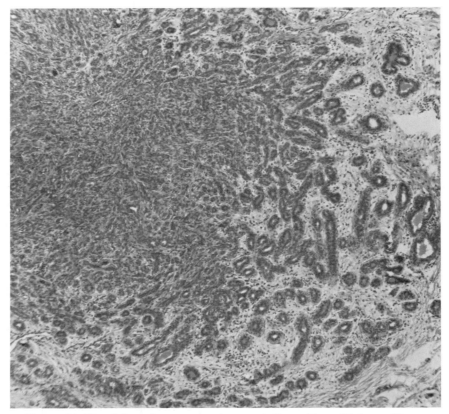

Figure 14–25.   Adenosis occurring in association with multiple papilloma.

2. Adenosis is not uncommon in the otherwise normal breast. But in breasts with multiple papilloma, adenosis of marked degree is so often seen that it must be regarded as one of the basic microscopic features of the disease. In several of our cases the adenosis dominated the microscopic picture. Figure 14–25 shows a portion of a large and active-looking area of adenosis associated with multiple papilloma. The intraductal papillary proliferation in this disease sometimes has a growth pattern like that of adenosis, as illustrated in Figure 14–26.

3. Apocrine metaplasia is a phenomenon commonly observed in the duct epithelium in the otherwise normal breast. The duct epithelium normally consists of two layers of small regular cells. It is transformed into a single layer of larger so-called apocrine cells. These apocrine cells have large, pale, acidophilic cytoplasms with regular nuclei situated near the basement membrane and luminal apocrine snouts. With this kind of apocrine metaplasia there is usually dilatation of the ducts. Groups of small cysts lined with apocrine epithelium, as seen in Figure 14–27, are found. This phenomenon, occurring to a limited degree, has no significance.

In breasts with multiple papilloma, however, apocrine metaplasia of a very marked degree is seen so often that I believe that it is an integral part of the disease. Figure 14–28 shows a portion of a multiple papilloma with areas of apocrine metaplasia. Figure 14–29 shows a small papilloma composed exclusively of the apocrine type of cells. Figure 14–30 shows another multiple papilloma in which long finger-like processes are made up of the apocrine type of cells.

The proliferating apocrine-type cells assume a great variety of forms, and in some cases a basic cellular pattern associated with carcinoma evolves. The first step is illustrated in Figure 14–31. Here, the tips of the finger-like papillary processes have begun to coalesce, suggesting the cribriform pattern of the special apocrine papillary type of carcinoma. Figure 14–32 shows a small focus of this type of carcinoma in which low papillary processes have fused to form the characteris-

Text continues on page 290.

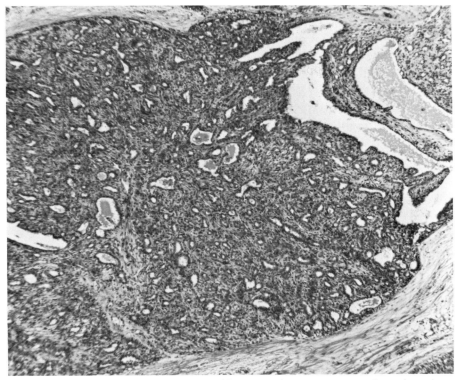

Figure 14–26. Multiple papilloma with a growth pattern suggesting adenosis.

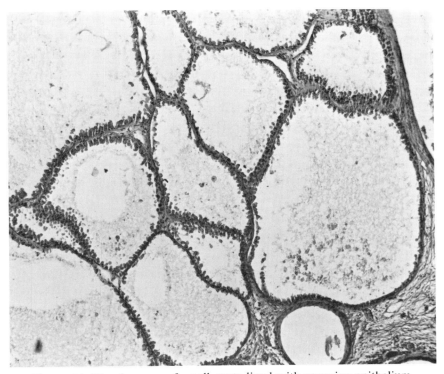

Figure 14–27. A group of small cysts lined with apocrine epithelium.

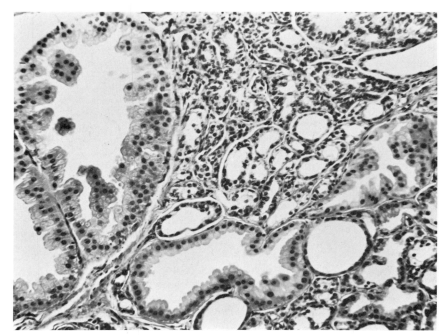

Figure 14–28. An area of apocrine metaplasia within a multiple papilloma.

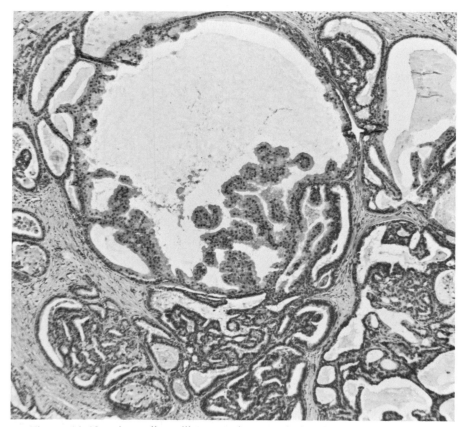

Figure 14–29. A small papilloma made up entirely of apocrine-type cells.

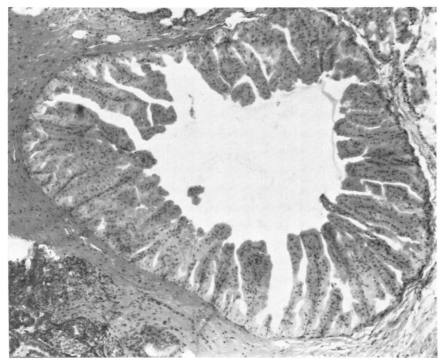

Figure 14–30. A multiple papilloma with long finger-like processes of the apocrine-type cells.

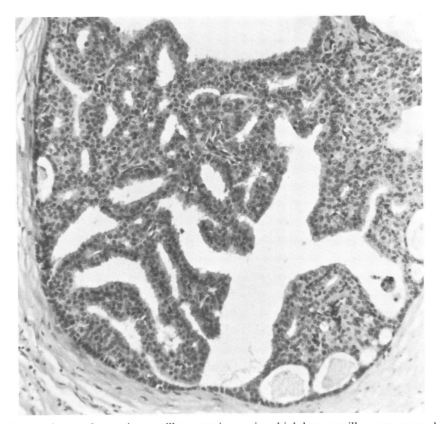

Figure 14–31. A focus of apocrine papillary carcinoma in which long papillary processes begin to form a cribriform pattern.

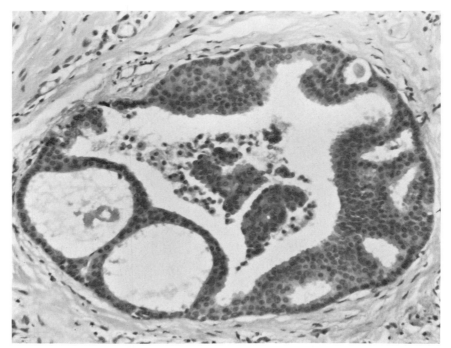

Figure 14–32. A small focus of apocrine papillary carcinoma in which low papillary processes have coalesced to form a cartwheel pattern.

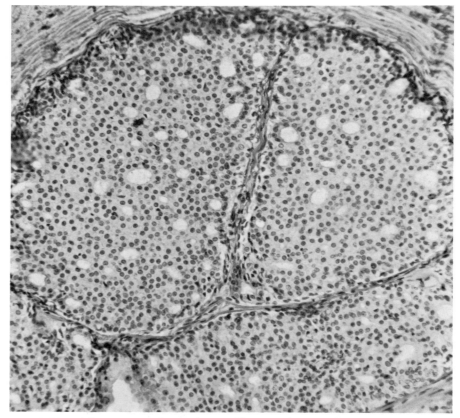

Figure 14–33. A larger area of apocrine papillary carcinoma with the cribriform pattern.

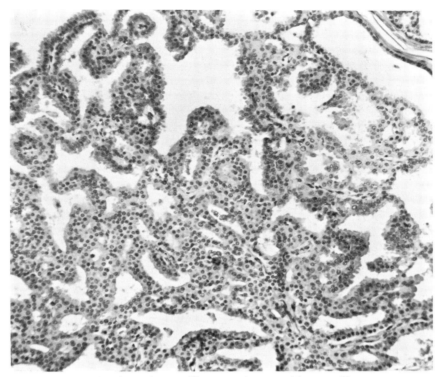

Figure 14–34. Apocrine papillary carcinoma with a papillary pattern.

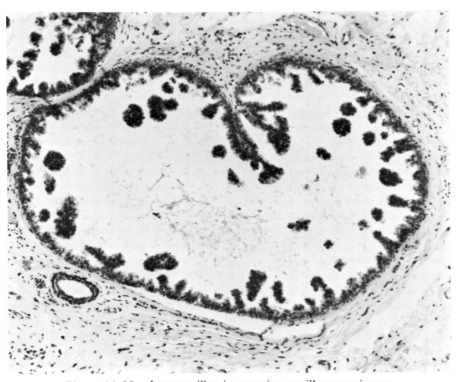

Figure 14–35. Low papillae in apocrine papillary carcinoma.

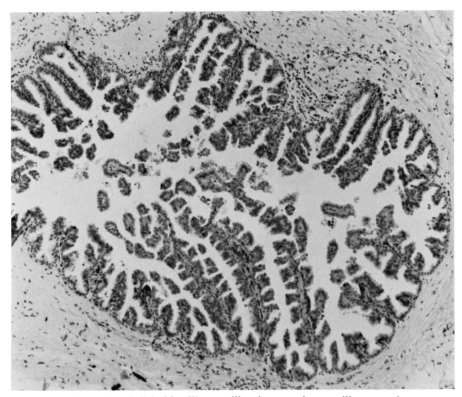

Figure 14–36. High ladder-like papillae in apocrine papillary carcinoma.

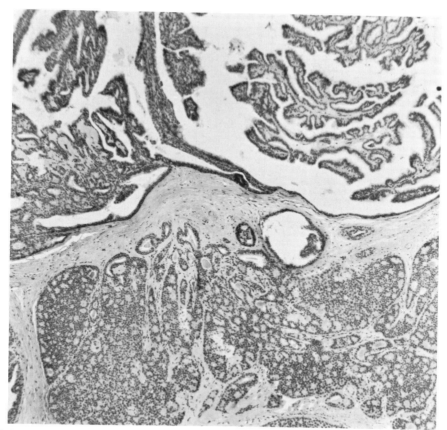

Figure 14–37. An area of apocrine carcinoma with the cribriform pattern adjacent to benign multiple papillomas.

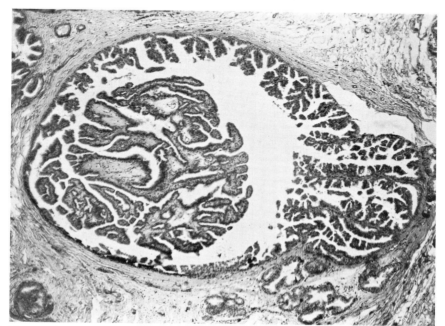

Figure 14–38. Benign-appearing multiple papilloma growing within a cystic structure lined by apocrine papillary carcinoma.

tic cartwheel pattern. Figure 14–33 shows the edge of a larger area of apocrine papillary carcinoma with the cribriform pattern. In Figure 14–34 the papillary pattern of this same type of carcinoma is shown. The cribriform and papillary patterns are usually both present in varying proportions in this special type of carcinoma. It can be seen from these microphotographs that the cell type is the same in both growth patterns. In the papillary pattern the papillae may be very low, as shown in Figure 14–35, or they may be long and ladder-like, as in Figure 14–36.

The intimate association of benign appearing multiple papilloma and apocrine papillary carcinoma is illustrated in the two following microphotographs. Figure 14–37 shows an area of carcinoma of the cribriform pattern with adjacent entirely benign-appearing multiple papilloma. Figure 14–38 shows an entirely benign-appearing papilloma growing *within* a cystic structure lined by apocrine papillary carcinoma.

The Treatment of Multiple Papilloma

I have emphasized my belief that multiple papilloma should be distinguished from solitary papilloma. The latter is not associated with carcinoma and is easily dealt with by local excision. Multiple papilloma is, on the other hand, a tenacious disease which usually recurs after local excision, and is apt to evolve into, or be associated with, the apocrine-type of carcinoma. The treatment of multiple papilloma therefore presents a more difficult problem.

In the light of our experience with this disease, I do not believe, however, that mastectomy is justified. Even though recurrence after local excision is to be expected, we have, in the majority of cases, succeeded in controlling the disease by repeated local excision. When the apocrine type of carcinoma is found in association with multiple papilloma, radical mastectomy should, of course, be done. This type of carcinoma is exceptionally favorable, and a good radical mastectomy will in all likelihood be successful.

There are four kinds of errors that must be guarded against in the treatment of multiple papilloma.

1. The diagnosis must be established by an initial biopsy and the study of permanent par-

affin sections. Frozen sections are in general not a dependable method of distinguishing between multiple papilloma and papillary carcinoma.

2. When local excision of the lesion is carried out, the surgeon must take great care to try to remove all of the grossly evident disease. The brownish papillomas growing in ducts and cysts are not easy to define unless the surgeon's exposure is adequate and the operative field is kept very dry. I use a curved incision in the skin lines to obtain exposure. I usually have to excise a sector of the breast, but I do not needlessly sacrifice normal-appearing breast tissue.

3. Patients with multiple papilloma should be carefully followed and examined every three months for the remainder of their lives.

4. A meticulous microscopic study of all the tissue excised at operation for the disease should be carried out. We know from our experience in our own laboratory of surgical pathology that it is easy to miss minute foci of the apocrine type of carcinoma which is likely to occur in this disease.

REFERENCES

Adair, F. E.: Sanguineous discharge from the nipple and its significance in relation to cancer of the breast. Ann. Surg., 91:197, 1930.
Bloodgood, J. C.: The pathology of chronic cystic mastitis of the female breast; with special consideration of the blue-domed cyst. Arch. Surg., 3:445, 1921.
Bloodgood, J. C.: Benign lesions of the female breast for which operation is not indicated. J.A.M.A., 78:859, 1922.
Bloodgood, J. C.: Borderline breast tumors. Am. J. Cancer, 16:103, 1932.
Buhl-Jorgensen, S. E., Fischermann, K., Johansen, H. and Petersen, B.: Cancer risk in intraductal papilloma and papillomatosis. Surg., Gynec. & Obst., 127:1307, 1968.
Cheatle, Sir G. L., and Cutler, M.: Tumours of the Breast. Philadelphia, J. B. Lippincott Co., 1931.
Chester, S. T., and Bell, H. G.: Intraductal and intracystic papillomas of the breast. West, J. Surg., 59:603, 1951.
Copeland, M. M., and Higgins, T. G.: Significance of discharge fron nipple in nonpuerperal mammary conditions. Ann. Surg., 151:638, 1960.
Estes, A. C., and Phillips, C.: Papilloma of lacteal duct. Surg., Gynec. & Obst., 89:345, 1949.
Goldenstein, A.: Mama sangrante. Diagnóstico e tratamento pela exérese dos ductos afetados. Rev. paulista de med., 41:246, 1952.
Gray, H. K., and Wood, G. A.: Significance of mammary discharge in cases of papilloma of the breast. Arch. Surg., 42:203, 1941.
Greenough, R. B., and Simmons, C. C.: Papillary-cystadenomata of the breast. Ann. Surg., 45:188, 1907.
Greenough, R. B., and Simmons, C. C.: Results of con-

servative treatment of cystic disease of the breast. Ann. Surg., *60*:42, 1914.

Haagensen, C. D., Stout, A. P., and Phillips, J. S.: The papillary neoplasms of the breast. I. Benign intraductal papilloma. Ann. Surg., *133*:18, 1951.

Handley, R. S., and Thackray, A. C.: Adenoma of nipple. Brit. J. Cancer, *16*:187, 1962.

Hart, D.: Intracystic papillomatous tumors of the breast, benign and malignant. Arch. Surg., *14*:793, 1927.

Hendrick, J. W.: Intraductal papilloma of the breast. Surg., Gynec. & Obst., *105*:215, 1957.

Hicken, N. F.: Intracystic papilloma of the breast. Surgery, *7*:724, 1940.

Hollenberg, H. G.: Bleeding from the nipple. Arch. Surg., *64*:159, 1952.

Jones, D. B.: Florid papillomatosis of the nipple ducts. Cancer, *8*:315, 1955.

Judd, E. S.: Intracanalicular papilloma of the breast. Journal Lancet, *37*:141, 1917.

Kaump, D. H., and Mendes Ferreira, A. E.: Papillomas of the breast: study of 273 specimens. J. Lab. & Clin. Med., *22*:681, 1937.

Kilgore, A. R., Fleming, R. and Ramos, M. M.: The incidence of cancer with nipple discharge and the risk of cancer in the presence of papillary disease of the breast. Surg., Gynec. & Obst., *96*:649, 1953.

Kraus, F. T., and Neubecker, R. D.: The differential diagnosis of papillary tumors of the breast. Cancer, *15*:444, 1962.

LeGal, Y., Gros, C. M., and Bader, P.: L'adénomatose érosive du mamelon. Ann. d'anat. path., *4*:292, 1959.

Lewis, D.: Bleeding nipples. Surg., Gynec. & Obst., *22*:666, 1916.

Lewison, E. F., and Chambers, R. G.: Clinical significance of nipple discharge. J.A.M.A., *147*:295, 1951.

Madalin, H. E., Clagett, O. T., and McDonald, J. R.: Lesions of the breast associated with discharge from the nipple. Ann. Surg., *146*:751, 1957.

McLaughlin, C. W., and Coe, J. D.: A study of nipple discharge in the non-lactating breast. Ann. Surg., *157*:810, 1963.

McPherson, V. A., and MacKenzie, W. C.: Lesions of the breast associated with nipple discharge; prognosis after local excision of benign lesions. Canad. J. Surg., *5*:6, 1962.

Mercier, J., and Redon, H. Le valeur diagnostique des écoulements par le mamelon. Semaine d. hôp. Paris, Ann. chir., *13*:745, 1959.

Miller, E. M., and Lewis, D.: The significance of a serohemorrhagic or hemorrhagic discharge from the nipple. J.A.M.A., *81*:1651, 1923.

Miller, G., and Bernier, L.: Adénomatose érosive du mamelon. Canad. J. Surg., *8*:261, 1965.

Moore, S. W., Pearce, J., and Ring, E.: Intraductal papilloma of the breast. Surg., Gynec. & Obst., *112*:153, 1961.

Moulonguet, P.: Papillomatose bourgeonnante du mamelon. Mém. Acad. Chir., *86*:458, 1960.

Moulonguet, P., and Merot, Y.: Les écoulements sérosanglants par le mamelon causés par un adénome du sein. Gynéc. et obst., *51*:209, 1952.

Nichols, F. C., Dockerty, M. B., and Judd, E. S.: Florid papillomatosis of nipple. Surg., Gynec. & Obst., *197*:474, 1958.

Robert, H., DeBrux, J., and Winaver, D.: La papillomatose bénigne du mamelon. Presse Méd., *71*:2713, 1963.

Saltzstein, H. C., and Pollack, R. S.: Localization and treatment of papillomas of the breast. Cancer, *1*:625, 1948.

Sandblom, P., and Löfgren, F. O.: Diagnosis and treatment of the discharging nipple in the absence of a palpable tumor. Acta. chir. Scandinav., *103*:81, 1952.

Saphir, O., and Parker, M. L.: Intracystic papilloma of the breast. Am. J. Path., *16*:189, 1940.

Stowers, J. E.: The significance of bleeding or discharge from the nipple. Surg., Gynec. & Obst., *61*:537, 1935.

Taylor, H. B., and Robertson, A. G.: Adenomas of the nipple. Cancer, *18*:995, 1965.

Wakeley, Sir C.: Duct papillomata of the breast. Lancet, *252*:62, 1947.

Warren, J. C.: The surgeon and the pathologist. J.A.M.A., *45*:149, 1905.

Warren, S.: The prognosis of benign lesions of the female breast. Surgery, *19*:32, 1946.

Chapter Fifteen

Nonepithelial Neoplasms of the Breast

In grouping together in one long chapter a number of different types of neoplasms of the breast that are of mesenchymal origin, I have the excuse that they are all comparatively infrequent, and for this reason scarcely deserve discussion in separate chapters.

I have included in this chapter both benign and malignant nonepithelial neoplasms of the breast, grouped according to their histogenesis. Virchow long ago said "Die Mamma ist die Amme der Geschwülste Lehre,"* because so many different types of neoplasms develop in it.

The various types of true soft tissue sarcoma of the breast are distinguished from the cystosarcomas by the fact that the cystosarcomas, at least in their primary manifestation, have an epithelial component. When they recur or metastasize, this epithelial component is often lost. Unless the pathologist has carefully studied the primary lesion he may wrongly classify the recurrence as a true breast sarcoma. This kind of mistake accounts for many so-called breast sarcomas. There are also occasional breast carcinomas that contain areas of spindle cell, cartilaginous, or osseous metaplasia. They should not be classified as carcinosarcoma, or as fibrosarcoma, chondrosarcoma, or osteogenic sarcoma. They are merely carcinomas showing metaplasia.

A general review of sarcomas and related mesenchymal tumors of the breast such as that recently presented by Norris and Taylor, which puts such very dissimilar lesions as benign fibrous histiocytoma (dermatofibrosarcoma protuberans) and highly malignant fibrosarcoma and malignant hemangioendothelioma (angiosarcoma) in one general category, is not helpful. Even though these mesenchymal tumors of the breast are infrequent it is useful to classify them as to their histogenesis as accurately as possible, and to correlate each microscopic type with its natural history.

Berg and his associates report that "stromal sarcomas" of the breast form a homogeneous group. Our experience with mesenchymal sarcomas of the breast is quite the reverse. These tumors differ greatly in character, and it is certainly useful to classify them as to their histogenesis, although this is sometimes not easy to do. In his 1965 paper, Oberman reported 13 of these lesions and made a commendable attempt to classify them. Lattes has also written briefly and understandingly regarding the classification of these breast sarcomas.

In classifying these breast neoplasms of mesenchymal origin I will follow the classification Stout and Lattes use in their new fascicle, "Tumors of the Soft Tissues," in the *Atlas of Tumor Pathology* (Second Series), published by the Armed Forces Institute of Pathology. Stout and Lattes based their study upon a total of 8686 soft part tumors studied in the Laboratory of Surgical Pathology of

---

*"The breast is the wet nurse of the student of tumors."

Columbia University. I have studied the same case material, and I will describe and illustrate the types of breast tumors of mesenchymal origin included in it.

FIBROUS HISTIOCYTOMA (DERMATOFIBROSARCOMA PROTUBERANS)

These lesions may develop in the skin over the breast and infiltrate the underlying breast. They have the whorled storiform pattern that characterizes this lesion. Stout and Lattes believe that they are made up of facultative fibroblasts derived from histiocytes.

Most of these lesions are benign, but a few are malignant. In our clinic we have seen examples of both types of lesions in the breast.

Benign Fibrous Histiocytoma. Although these fibrous histiocytomas with benign histologic characteristics infiltrate the skin and sometimes grow down into deeper tissues, and although they may grow to a comparatively large size, they do not metastasize and are not truly malignant.

Oberman described two of these lesions occurring in the mammary region. In our clinic we have had three. These are not true breast tumors but fibrous histiocytomas developing in the skin and subcutaneous tissues of the mammary region. They oc-

curred in women aged 27, 33, and 64. In two of the three patients the lesion developed in the scar of a previous operation. In the 33 year old patient the scar resulted from the removal of an adenofibroma four years previously. In the 64 year old patient the scar resulted from the excision of a tumor of unknown nature 30 years previously. This patient's story is characteristic for this lesion. Eight months before consulting me in October, 1960, she had noticed several small nodules in the lateral portion of the scar, which was transverse and extended from the sternal edge across the inner half of her left breast. The nodules had grown slowly. On admission, examination showed three firm nodules in the old scar, each about 1 cm. in diameter, projecting about 5 mm. above the skin level, and covered by thin, shiny, pink epithelium.

The lesion was excised locally, along with an ellipse of skin about 5 cm. in width on each side of the nodules, and including underlying breast tissue to a depth of 5 cm. Figure 15–1 shows the operative specimen.

Microscopic study showed the lesion to be a characteristic fibrous histiocytoma made up of spindle-shaped cells arranged in a storiform pattern (Fig. 15–2). Mitoses were rare. The tumor grew up to the epidermis and infiltrated the underlying mammary parenchyma (Fig. 15–3).

The patient had had no recurrence when she died of another disease seven years later.

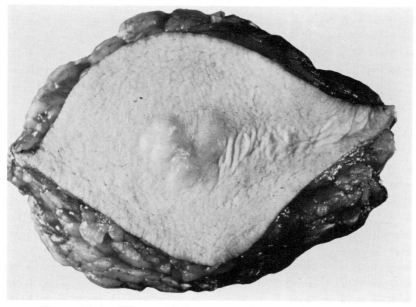

Figure 15–1. Fibrous histiocytoma—the operative specimen.

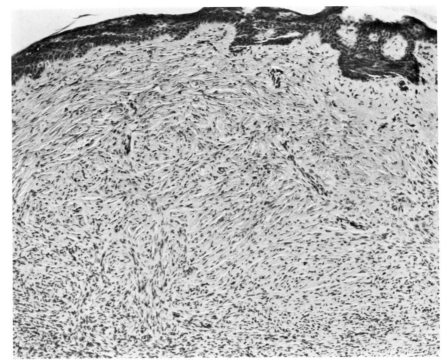

Figure 15–2. Microscopic appearance of a fibrous histiocytoma of the breast.

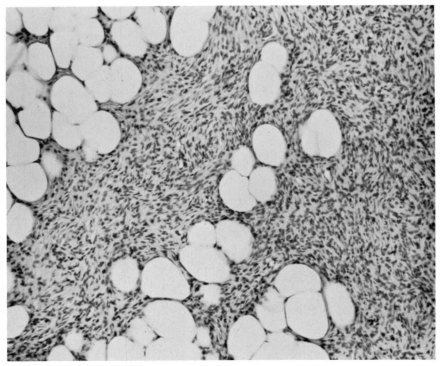

Figure 15–3. Fibrous histiocytoma invading the underlying mammary fat.

Our other two patients with benign fibrous histiocytoma were also cured by local excision of their tumor. The 27 year old patient had had no recurrence 21 years after operation. The 33 year old patient developed a local recurrence of her lesion three years after I first excised it. I re-excised it more extensively, and she had had no further recurrence when she died of a primary carcinoma of the lung 14 years after her breast lesion was first diagnosed.

Malignant Fibrous Histiocytoma. O'Brien and Stout reviewed a total of 1516 fibrous histiocytomas and classified 15 as malignant because of high mitotic rate, active infiltrative growth, or known metastases.

One of these malignant lesions occurred in the breast. It is described below. Judging from the ease with which it has been controlled, it was not very malignant.

Mrs. A. O., aged 49, developed a 2 cm. tumor of the inner sector of her breast. It was excised together with a narrow margin of surrounding breast tissue, the surgical specimen measuring 3 cm. in diameter. The lesion was 12 mm. in diameter, firm, and grayish white. It was a fibrous histiocytoma that did not have any features that suggested a malignant character.

Ten months later the patient returned with a hard recurrent tumor at the site of the original excision. It was adjacent to the edge of the sternum and was fixed to the underlying thorax. There was retraction of the skin over the tumor. It was excised together with the underlying pectoral muscle. The tumor was 5 cm. in diameter and infiltrated the overlying skin, and extended down into, but not through, the underlying muscle.

The histologic character of this recurrent lesion was strikingly different from that of the original tumor. The storiform pattern characteristic of the lesion was preserved, but the tumor was much more cellular, there was more variation in cell size, and mitoses were much more frequent (Fig. 15–4). Altogether, the recurrent tumor gave the impression of being malignant.

Nevertheless the patient had no evidence of further recurrence seven years later, although the re-excision had not been particularly wide. (This case was submitted to Dr. Stout by Dr. Homer Kesten, and we are indebted to him for permission to include it here.)

Treatment of Fibrous Histiocytoma

These lesions, whether classified histologically as benign or malignant, are not much to be feared, and are usually controlled by reasonably extensive local excision. When they occur in the mammary area, mastectomy is not necessary.

Of the 1516 examples of this lesion that O'Brien and Stout reviewed, only 13 metastasized.

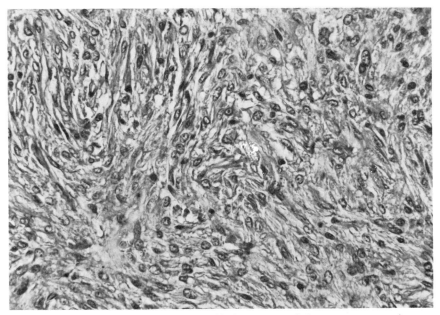

Figure 15–4. A malignant fibrous histiocytoma of the mammary region.

FIBROSARCOMA

When the strict criteria for fibrosarcoma that Stout worked out during the later years of his life are followed, the number of true malignant fibrosarcomas is markedly reduced. The majority occur in the superficial soft tissues of males.

Oberman, in his study of 13 sarcomas of the breast, classified seven as fibrosarcoma. In our own case material we have only two tumors that we are willing to classify as fibrosarcoma. The details of these cases follow.

CASE 1.

Mrs. C. M., a 48 year old housewife, was admitted in June, 1934, to the Presbyterian Hospital complaining of a tumor of the breast that she had noted five days previously.

Examination revealed a hard, rounded tumor in the right breast, situated caudad to the areola. It measured about 5 cm. in diameter. It was movable within the breast tissue. The overlying skin was not involved. There was no retraction.

At operation the tumor was excised locally, together with a 2 or 3 cm. margin of surrounding breast tissue. No lymph node dissection was done.

Grossly, the tumor was well circumscribed and measured 3.5 cm. in diameter. Its cut surface was fibrous and trabeculated. Microscopically it was a characteristic malignant fibrosarcoma without any apparent relationship to the breast tissue except for invasion at the margins. Its spindle-shaped cells varied considerably in size and shape, and showed an average of two mitoses per high power field. There were several areas of typical osteoid in the tumor. Dr. Stout classified it as a poorly differentiated malignant fibrosarcoma with osseous metaplasia.

When she was last seen 34 years later the patient had had no recurrence or metastasis from her breast tumor.

CASE 2

Mrs. L. L. G., a 48 year old housewife, came to the Presbyterian Hospital in April, 1965, with the complaint that she had found a tumor in her right breast two weeks previously. She had had a solitary intraductal papilloma excised from the subareolar region of her left breast eight years earlier.

Examination of the right breast revealed a 1.5 cm., firm, poorly delimited tumor situated in the upper outer sector, 2 cm. from the areolar edge. The left breast was normal.

At operation a circumareolar incision was used to expose the lesion. Several small cysts were first encountered. But beneath them, and deep in the breast, there was a firm, grayish, poorly delimited tumor which was excised. Frozen section revealed that it was an unusual lesion and the wound was closed.

Microscopic studies showed a highly cellular tumor composed of spindle-shaped cells, varying considerably in size, and with an average of two mitoses per high power field (Fig. 15–5). The

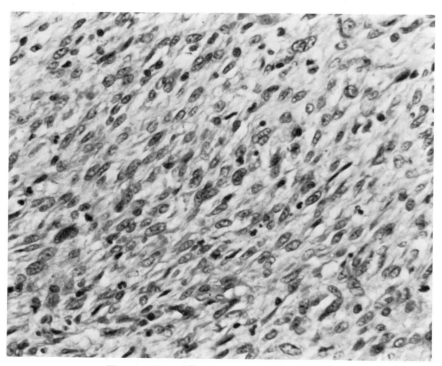

Figure 15–5   Fibrosarcoma of the breast.

lesion invaded the surrounding breast tissue and had the appearance of being fully malignant. It was classified as a fibrosarcoma. There was no evidence that it was a cystosarcoma. A simple mastectomy was performed 10 days after the local excision. Eighteen months later a cough developed. A chest film showed right-sided pulmonary metastases. Irradiation was ineffective. Skin metastases and metastases to lumbar vertebrae developed, and she died in February, 1967, 22 months after the onset of her disease.

The number of cases reported is too small and their treatment has been too varied to permit any statistically based conclusions as to treatment of fibrosarcoma of the breast.

In the less highly malignant lesions wide local excision appears to succeed. For the very malignant lesions more radical surgical attack fails, as it did in our Case 2, because of blood-borne metastases. I therefore favor wide local excision for fibrosarcoma of the breast.

LEIOMYOMA

Outside the uterus and gastrointestinal tract leiomyomas are uncommon. They develop in the deeper tissues from the smooth muscle of blood vessels and can be classed as *vascular leiomyomas,* or they develop from the smooth muscle of the skin, and are called *superficial leiomyomas.*

In the breast superficial leiomyomas have occasionally been observed arising in the skin of the areolar region. Melnick collected reports of 10 such tumors. There is, of course, a well-developed layer of smooth muscle in the corium of the areolar region, from which leiomyoma might arise. Contraction of this smooth muscle is readily observed upon stimulation of the nipple or areola.

At the Presbyterian Hospital we have had three examples of this superficial type of leiomyoma. Two were in the skin of the areola, and the third was in the skin of the upper inner sector of the breast, several centimeters from the areola.

Our patients were 25, 50, and 57 years of age. In two of them the lesions were of long duration, two and four years, respectively. In all three patients the lesion was a small, slightly elevated, reddish tumor, obviously developing in the skin, and movable over the deeper mammary tissue. It was mistaken for a sebaceous cyst in two cases.

The following case illustrates this unusual lesion.

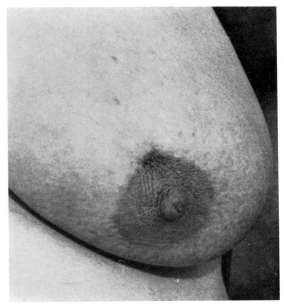

Figure 15–6. Superficial leiomyoma of the areolar region.

F. J., a housewife aged 57, came to the Presbyterian Hospital complaining of a tumor of the breast of two years' duration. The patient stated that the tumor varied in size and that at times it was painful and reddened "and stood up like a nipple." Figure 15–6 shows the tumor in the radius of 11 o'clock, at the edge of the areola of the left breast. It was a 1.5 cm., poorly circumscribed, firm lesion of the skin. It was slightly elevated above the skin surface, and its surface was somewhat reddened. It was excised locally and proved to be a characteristic leiomyoma (Fig. 15–7).

All three of our patients were cured by simple local excision.

The vascular type of leiomyoma developing in deeper tissues is rarer in the breast. Striking examples of such tumors in the breast have been described, however, by Strong, by Stein, by Melnick, by Libcke, and by Craig. In these cases the tumors grew slowly over a period of years to reach a large size. They were encapsulated and freely movable within the breast. At the Presbyterian Hospital we had two of these leiomyomas developing within the breast parenchyma, and perhaps of vascular origin. Since the two lesions were rather different I include brief descriptions of both.

CASE 1

Mrs. S. P., a housewife aged 52, came to the Presbyterian Hospital in September, 1967, with a right breast tumor of two weeks' duration. It was

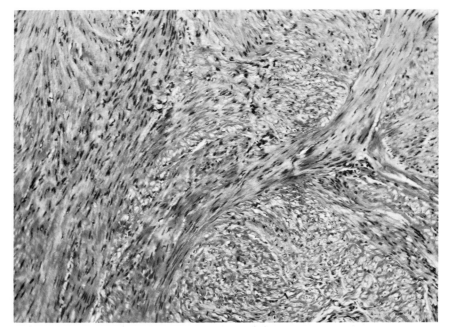

Figure 15–7. Microscopic appearance of a superficial leiomyoma of the areolar region.

situated deeply in the breast beneath the areola, was well delimited, and measured 2.5 cm. The lesion was exposed through a circumareolar incision. A cyst was first encountered. In the deeper portion of its wall there was an indurated area which was excised. This proved to be a characteristic leiomyoma made up of elongated cells with blunt-ended nuclei, accompanied by reticular

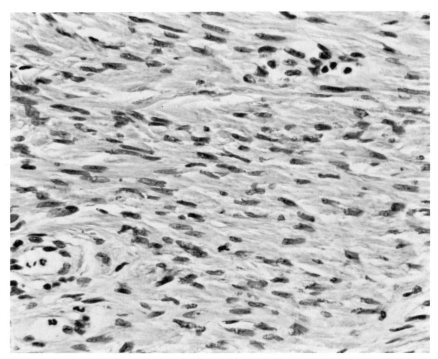

Figure 15–8. Leiomyoma of the mammary parenchyma.

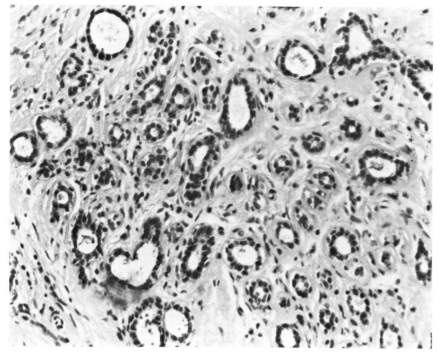

Figure 15–9.   Epithelial component of a leiomyoma of the mammary parenchyma.

fibrils paralleling their long axes. The lesion was not demarcated from the surrounding breast parenchyma.

There had been no recurrence of the lesion one year later.

CASE 2

Mrs. E. K., a housewife aged 40, came to the Presbyterian Hospital in April, 1962, with a tumor of her left breast. She had discovered the tumor a month previously. It was situated in the upper outer sector of the breast, 2 cm. from the edge of the areola. It was lobulated and well delimited, and was 3 cm. in diameter.

At operation it was found to be situated at some depth in the mammary parenchyma and was excised. Grossly it had the appearance of an adenofibroma, but microscopically it was a leiomyoma (Fig. 15–8). However, it contained a feature that we have not seen before, namely, an epithelial component. This took the form of groups of small ducts or mammary acini, lined by benign-looking epithelial cells, as shown in Figure 15–9. These epithelial structures were clearly a part of the tumor. They were not mammary lobules or ducts infiltrated and distorted by the leiomyoma. This lesion might therefore be called an adenoleiomyoma. It is unique in our experience.

The patient remains well six years after operation.

LEIOMYOSARCOMA

Leiomyosarcoma is most frequently seen in the viscera and in the retroperitoneal region, but it occasionally develops in the soft tissues elsewhere.

I do not find any reports of this lesion in the breast, but we have one breast tumor that is probably a leiomyosarcoma.. It occurred in a 77 year old woman who consulted one of our surgeons in January, 1939, for a tumor of her left breast. She had first noted the tumor two weeks previously. It was well delimited, movable, and soft, and measured 8 cm. in diameter. It occupied most of the upper part of the breast.

After biopsy and frozen section revealed that it was some type of sarcoma, a complete mastectomy was performed.

The lesion was very cellular and looked highly malignant. It was made up of elongated, blunt-ended cells that varied greatly in size and shape and were arranged in interlacing bundles. Mitoses were very frequent. Occasional small giant cells and elongated strap-shaped cells were seen (Fig. 15–10). On reviewing this lesion recently, Lattes classifies it as a probable leiomyosarcoma.

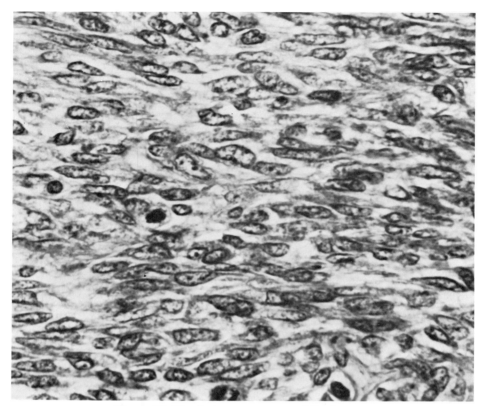

Figure 15–10.   Leiomyosarcoma of the breast.

The patient was last reported to have reached the age of 91 without recurrence of her breast tumor.

RHABDOMYOSARCOMA

This infrequent and vicious tumor ordinarily develops from skeletal muscle, but is occasionally found in tissues where striated muscle is not expected. It is often difficult to distinguish microscopically between fibrosarcoma, rhabdomyosarcoma, and liposarcoma. The final proof of origin from striated muscle rests upon the demonstration of cross-striations. Sailer, Oberman, and Toni have all published good microphotographs of cross-striations in breast tumors that they classified as rhabdomyosarcoma. Evans and Botham and his associates have also reported breast lesions that they regarded as rhabdomyosarcomas.

In our own clinic we have had no unquestionable example of this rare breast tumor. Two, however, which have been sent to Stout in consultations, may be accepted as rhabdomyosarcoma. The patients were 73 and 84 years old, respectively. Both were treated by radical mastectomy. In the younger patient metastases were found in four of 17 axillary lymph nodes (it is of interest to note that rhabdomyosarcoma developing in other parts of the body has been known to metastasize to regional lymph nodes). In this patient there was no local recurrence, but she developed pulmonary metastases and died five years after her operation. In the older patient there was local recurrence in the axilla and metastasis to the lungs, pleura, and pericardium.

In both of these patients the lesion had the classical microscopic features of rhabdomyosarcoma. They were exceedingly anaplastic. The cells varied greatly in size and shape, and many had racquet-shaped or strap-like cytoplasms. The nuclei were often bizarre and multiple. Mitoses were numerous. In both tumors longitudinal and cross-striations were seen. Figure 15–11 shows one of these lesions.

To judge from the course of the disease in the acceptable rhabdomyosarcomas, no form of treatment has much value. The disease grows locally out of control, metastasizes widely, and is fatal in a short time.

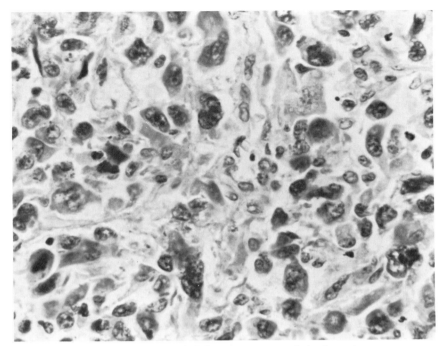

Figure 15–11. Rhabdomyosarcoma of the breast.

MALIGNANT HEMANGIOENDOTHELIOMA (ANGIOSARCOMA)

This highly malignant tumor, in which endothelial cells forming atypical capillaries dominate, was originally named hemangioendothelioma by F. B. Mallory. It has been recognized with increasing frequency in recent years, partly as the result of the studies of Stout and his associates. In their recent fascicle on "Tumors of the Soft Tissues," Stout and Lattes reported on 165 of these tumors studied in our laboratory at Columbia. Although this lesion is most often seen in viscera and bones, a rather surprising number have been reported occurring in the breast. In 1965, Steingaszner and his associates collected reports of 28 of these breast tumors and added 10 examples. In addition to these cases Robinson and Castleman, Gulesserian and Lawton, and Khanna and his associates have reported examples of this lesion. In our clinic we have seen four patients with malignant hemangioendothelioma of the breast.

This lesion develops in women of all ages, but the patients are younger than women with carcinoma. Our patients were 18, 51, 54, and 60 years of age, respectively. Twenty-nine of the 38 patients whose histories Steingaszner collected were under 40 years of age.

The usual clinical history is that the lesion grows rapidly to form a bulky breast tumor. Its vascular character is suggested by bluish-red discoloration of the overlying skin. Both breasts were involved by the disease in eight of the cases collected by Steingaszner. This lesion does not metastasize to the regional lymph nodes, but metastasizes widely to viscera, and is rapidly fatal. In our four patients the total duration of disease was 20 months, 13 months, 9 months and 9 months. In Steingaszner's series of 30 patients with follow-up information the mean survival time from onset to death was approximately two years.

The following is an abstract of the history of one of our Presbyterian Hospital cases. It is typical of the history of malignant hemangioendothelioma.

J. M., an 18 year old girl, came to the Presbyterian Hospital complaining that two months previously she had noted a "blue mark" in the areola of the right breast. For one week there had been a tumor beneath the blue mark.

The right breast was slightly enlarged and the nipple inverted. There was bluish discoloration of the upper half of the areola. Beneath this discoloration there was a firm, rounded, freely movable tumor 6 x 3 cm. in diameter.

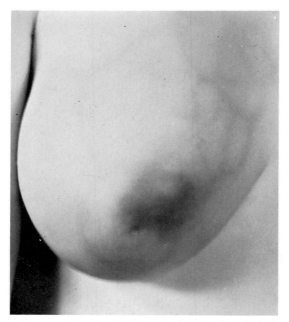

Figure 15–12. Malignant hemangioendothelioma of the areolar region at an early stage, as seen in an infrared photograph.

Under the direction of a gynecological consultant the patient was treated with estrogen under the illusion that the breast lesion represented a functional condition.

The tumor continued to enlarge. An infrared photograph taken nine months after her first admission (Fig. 15-12) showed its vascular character. It appeared as a dark area visible through the skin of the areolar region. Its vascular character was further confirmed by the fact that upon pressure with the patient supine the volume of the tumor markedly diminished.

During the succeeding six months the tumor grew rapidly to the massive size shown in another infrared photograph (Fig. 15-13). A simple mastectomy was then done. Pathological study showed the lesion to be a malignant hemangioendothelioma. Figure 15-14 is a high power view of its microscopic appearance, and shows anaplastic endothelioblasts filling atypical capillaries.

A metastatic tumor nodule in the abdominal wall, and widespread bone metastases developed shortly after operation, and the patient died 20 months after the onset of her disease. There was never any clinical evidence of involvement of regional lymph nodes.

Treatment of this highly malignant neo-

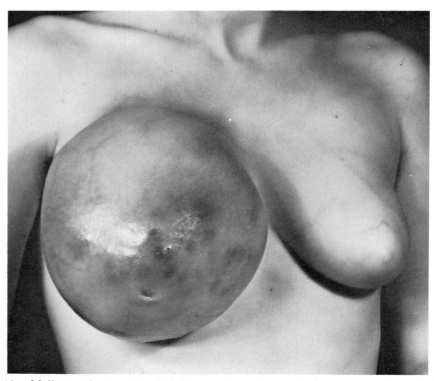

Figure 15–13.   Malignant hemangioendothelioma at an advanced stage, as seen in an infrared photograph.

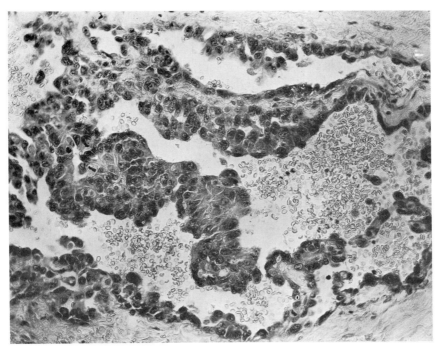

Figure 15–14. Malignant hemangioendothelioma of the breast.

plasm has in general been futile. It grows so fast and metastasizes so widely that attempts at surgical excision regularly fail, and it is so radioresistant that only slight regression is obtained by irradiation. Steingaszner was able to find reports of only two long-term survivors — one patient treated by radical mastectomy who survived 14 years, and another patient whose tumor was excised locally who survived seven years. In both the primary tumor was of short duration and small size. Radical mastectomy is certainly unjustified for this lesion because it does not metastasize to regional lymph nodes. When the tumor is large, as it usually is, palliative wide local excision of the primary tumor is all that is indicated.

LYMPHANGIOSARCOMA

A special type of sarcoma which is appropriately called lymphangiosarcoma, develops in the arms of patients with severe and prolonged arm edema following radical mastectomy. Stewart and Treves in 1948 were the first to identify this lesion. By 1963 Chu and Treves were able to collect reports of more than 50 cases, and by 1965 Herr-mann found reports of 83 cases. Since then reports by René and his associates, by Fisher, by Re and his associates, by Eby and his associates, by Krückmeyer and his associates, by Mackh, by Malik and Samter, by Kappey, by Bachulis and his associates, by Ende, and by Nemoto and his associates, have brought the total number of cases to approximately 100. Thus it can be said that although this lesion is uncommon, it is not rare.

There have been a few pathologists like Salm who have suggested that these arm lesions are metastases from the original breast carcinoma. More than a dozen cases, such as that reported by Baes of lymphangio-sarcoma developing in an extremity that was edematous for some reason other than carcinoma, have been reported, however, and the fact that severe chronic edema of a limb predisposes to this disease can not be seriously challenged.

Among my own patients upon whom I have performed radical mastectomy, not one has developed lymphangiosarcoma. This is probably because arm edema is infrequent following the type of radical mastectomy I perform, and when it does develop it is usually mild in degree. Perfect wound healing, and avoidance of postoperative irradiation to the axilla, are of basic importance in avoiding arm edema.

Two patients who had radical mastectomy elsewhere and who had developed edematous arms in which lymphangiosarcoma developed have consulted me. Both had had postoperative irradiation to the axilla, and had developed massive arm edema. The arm lymphangiosarcoma developed nine years later in one, and 11 years later in the other.

Stout and Lattes have been consulted regarding this diagnosis in 10 additional cases. The mean duration of the arm edema before the lymphangiosarcoma appeared was 9.1 years in this group of cases.

The interval between the onset of the arm edema and the development of the lymphangiosarcoma has varied in the reported cases, between one and 24 years. The mean interval was 10.5 years as tabulated by Herrmann.

The clinical picture of this lesion is a striking one. Faint reddish macules develop in the brawny skin of the edematous arm. The inner and anterior aspects of the upper arm are the sites first involved in most patients. The macules coalesce, their color deepens, and induration develops. At this stage the lesion is apt to be mistaken for ecchymosis. Raised purple nodules soon develop in the affected skin, and ulceration follows. The lesion metastasizes very widely throughout the body.

The mean survival from onset to death in this disease was tabulated by Herrmann as 18.8 months in the treated patients, and 5.7 months in the untreated patients.

The history of one of my patients illustrates these features very well.

M. C., aged 55, an Irish housewife, had a left radical mastectomy in another hospital, in September, 1937. She was given prophylactic postoperative irradiation from October, 1937 to April, 1938.

In May, 1938, local recurrence was noted and additional irradiation was given to the recurrence. In August, 1938, local excision of part of the irradiated area was done in another hospital with slow wound healing.

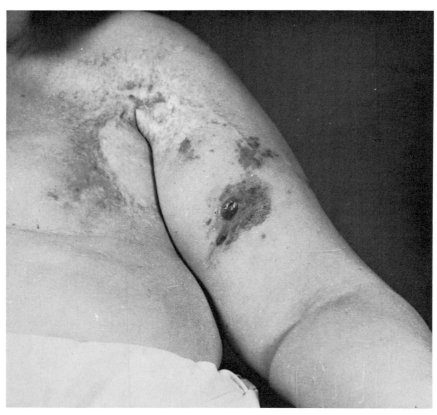

Figure 15-15. Lymphangiosarcoma developing in an edematous arm 13 years after radical mastectomy.

The arm had become markedly edematous by this time, and the edema persisted and increased.

She consulted me in April, 1950, because of "purple spots" which had developed in the skin of the upper part of the edematous arm. They had first appeared a year previously and had recently progressed.

Her condition when I examined her is shown in Figure 15-15. There was an old mastectomy scar, of the type that is carried out onto the anterior aspect of the upper arm. There were marked irradiation changes in the skin along the whole length of the scar, but these changes were most marked over the upper portion of the scar on the anterior aspect of the shoulder.

The whole arm was markedly edematous, the tissues being firm and the skin thickened. On the anterior aspect of the upper arm, beginning just distal to the outer limits of irradiation changes in the skin, there were isolated and confluent groups of purplish, slightly elevated macules. In the center of the largest group of macules there was an elevated, soft, purplish tumor nodule measuring 2 cm. in diameter. Biopsy of the nodule showed the characteristic microscopic picture of lymphangiosarcoma (Fig. 15-16). Interscapula-thoracic amputation was advised but the patient refused and went elsewhere.

The treatment of lymphangiosarcoma presents a formidable problem. Herrmann in his review of the results of treatment found only three patients who had survived apparently cured for over five years — Bowers' patient who had a forequarter amputation, Dembrow and Adair's patient who had the same operation followed by excision of local recurrence a year later, and Southwick and Slaughter's patient treated by external irradiation alone. Herrmann and Ariel have recently reported the five year survival of one additional patient who was treated by the intra-arterial injection of yttrium.

The mean duration of life from onset of the disease to death in a total of 25 patients treated by amputation of the arm was 16.8 months according to Herrmann. On the other hand, he found that the mean duration of life in 22 patients treated only by irradiation was 18.5 months.

In the face of these facts concerning the results of surgery and irradiation in this almost invariably fatal disease, it seems reasonable to attempt to control it with irradiation.

LIPOMA

Since the lipoma is one of the commonest benign neoplasms and is found in all parts of the body, it is not surprising that it is not rare in the breast. In our clinic we have seen several of these tumors yearly. Over a 40 year

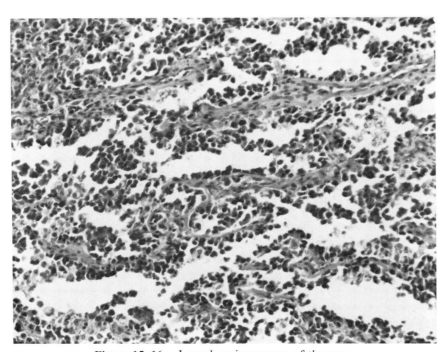

Figure 15-16.   Lymphangiosarcoma of the arm.

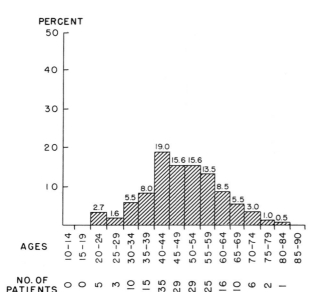

Chart 15-1. The percentage distribution of ages of 186 patients with lipoma of the breast.

period (1927 to 1968) a total of 186 were recorded in our laboratory of surgical pathology.

Lipomas develop in the breasts of older, rather than younger, women. The mean age of our group of patients was 45. Their age distribution is shown in Chart 15-1.

Breast lipomas are usually solitary lesions. We have seen only six patients in whom the breast lipoma was associated with multiple subcutaneous lipomas in other parts of the body.

These tumors produce no symptoms. They grow slowly. Twenty of our 186 patients had had their tumors for more than two years. In four the duration was 15 years or more.

The average diameter of the lipomas in our series of cases was about 2 cm. But with a long duration they may grow to a large size. In one-sixth of our patients the tumor

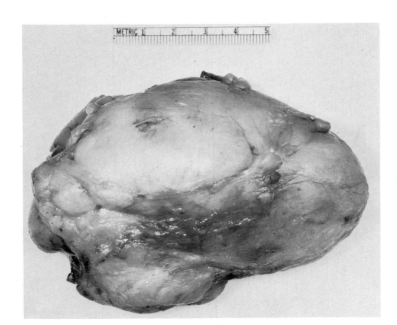

Figure 15-17. Gross appearance of lipoma of the breast.

measured more than 5 cm. in diameter, and 10 of these tumors were 10 cm. or more in diameter.

Breast lipomas are soft, movable, and fairly well delimited, although their outline tends to be lost in the soft texture of the breast. They do not, of course, produce retraction.

The lesions that lipomas of the breast are most apt to be confused with clinically are mesenchymoma and cystosarcoma. The latter tumor is apt to grow more rapidly, but this is a small point in differentiation.

The gross pathologic appearance of lipoma of the breast is so similar to that of normal fat in a fatty breast that close inspection is sometimes necessary to identify it. The lipoma has of course a delicate capsule (Fig. 15-17) and its color is usually slightly different from the normal fat of the breast, being more yellow.

Cystosarcoma sometimes has a pale yellowish color that suggests lipoma at first glance. It is important to distinguish the two lesions, and a frozen section should always be made if there is any doubt. A lipoma may be shelled out, whereas cystosarcoma, as I have already pointed out, should be excised with a margin of the surrounding breast tissue.

The following case history is typical of lipoma of the breast.

Miss M. W., a 58 year old woman, came to the Presbyterian Hospital with the complaint that her breast tumor had reached a size that inconvenienced her. She had had it for fifteen years, and it had slowly increased in size during the last few years. It was situated in the lower inner sector of the left breast, and measured 10 cm. in diameter. It was soft, well delimited, and movable. It was exposed and excised through an inframammary incision, chosen because I was convinced it was benign; and it proved to be a simple lipoma.

ADENOLIPOMA

A special type of fatty tumor, peculiar to the breast, has been called adenolipoma. It is indeed a lipoma, but one in which fat is intermingled with epithelial lobules.

Spalding published a good description of one of these tumors seen at Guy's Hospital. At the Presbyterian Hospital we have studied 22 adenolipomas during the 25 year period 1943 – 1968. Although this group is too small for the age distribution to be of any significance, the patients were a little younger than those with simple lipomas. Their mean age was 42 years. In several of our patients the lesion had been present for a number of years. In size the tumors were not dissimilar from our series of simple lipomas.

A rather striking example of adenolipoma in our group of cases follows.

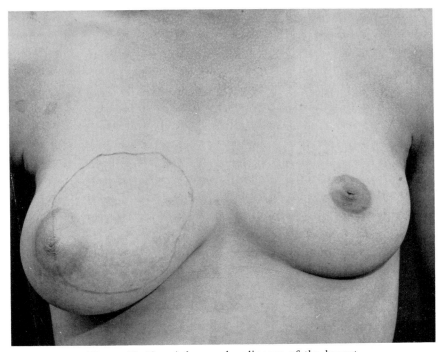

Figure 15-18. A large adenolipoma of the breast.

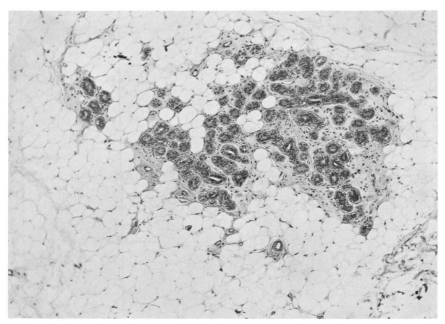

Figure 15-19.   Microscopic appearance of an adenolipoma of the breast.

M. L., an unmarried girl aged 18, was admitted to the Presbyterian Hospital complaining of a tumor of the right breast of six months' duration.

The inner half of the right breast was distended by a soft, well circumscribed, movable tumor measuring 12 cm. in diameter (Fig. 15-18).

It was excised and found to be a typical encapsulated adenolipoma. The gross appearance of its cut surface was characteristic of these tumors. It showed yellowish fat with small, brick red, slightly raised lobules of more firm epithelial tissue dispersed throughout.

The moot question regarding adenolipoma is whether the epithelial elements, as well as the fat, are neoplastic, or whether the neoplastic fat merely infiltrates the normal mammary epithelial elements. The frequency with which lipomas diffusely infiltrate other tissues such as skeletal muscles is of course well known. The fact that in adenolipomas the mammary acini are seen lying naked, so to speak, in immediate contact with the neoplastic fat, as shown in Figure 15-19, suggests that the second explanation is the best one.

The tumors are, of course, entirely benign, and local excision suffices.

LIPOSARCOMA

Primary liposarcoma is one of the rarest of all breast tumors. We have had none in pa-

tients coming to our clinic, but Stout and Lattes have been consulted regarding six tumors that they classified as genuine primary breast liposarcoma. One of these was reported by Stout and Bernanke. I have found reports of two additional apparently genuine cases. These eight cases are summarized in Table 15-1.

It will be seen from this tabulation that these tumors are in general comparatively small, and do not appear to have a high degree of malignancy, although the number of cases is too small to permit any firm conclusions.

I have carefully excluded from this tabulation the cystosarcomas that show liposarcomatous metaplasia. I have discussed them in Chapter 13. These tumors are much more frequent than primary liposarcoma of the breast.

The case reported by Stout and Bernanke remains probably the best example of primary liposarcoma of the breast. A summary of it follows.

A married woman, aged 43, noted a tumor in her left breast. Examination showed a freely movable 2.5 x 1.7 cm. tumor of the upper outer sector of the breast. It was not attached to the skin. There were no enlarged axillary nodes.

At operation the tumor was excised locally with a wide margin of surrounding breast tissue. Gross examination revealed that it was well circumscribed, soft, light brown in color, and 1 to 2 cm.

Table 15–1. PRIMARY LIPOSARCOMA OF THE BREAST

Source	Age of Patient	Duration of Tumor	Size of Tumor	Treatment	Follow-up
Laboratory of Surgical Pathology, Columbia					
Case 42472	42	2 weeks	4 × 2 cm.	Local excision	Well 12 yrs. when killed in a tornado
Case 69657	43	7 years	1 cm.	Local excision and axillary dissection	Well 6 years
Case 69012	18	Unknown	5 × 3 cm.	Local excision	Well 7 years
Case 79018	29	5 years	2.5 cm.	Local excision	Lost track of
Case 84463	44	Unknown	2 cm.	Local excision and simple mastectomy	Recent case (1968)
Millo*	51	6 months	Lower half of breast	Radical mastectomy	Pulmonary metastases, died in 2 months
Stout and Bernanke†	43	2 weeks	2.5 cm.	Local excision	Well 7 years
MacFarlane‡	68	Several months	2.5 cm.	Local excision	Lost track of

*Millo, L.: Arch. ital. di patolog. e clin. dei tumori, 2:610, 1958.
†Stout, A. P., and Bernanke, M.: Surg., Gynec. & Obst., 83:216, 1946.
‡MacFarlane, A.: Brit. J. Surg., 45:106, 1957.

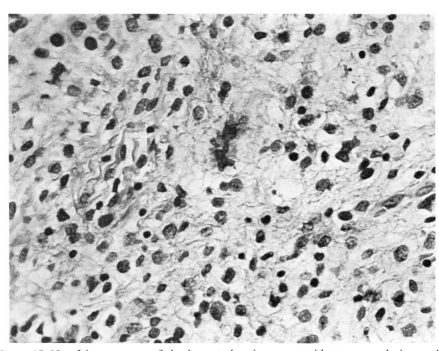

Figure 15–20. Liposarcoma of the breast showing a myxoid stroma and giant cells.

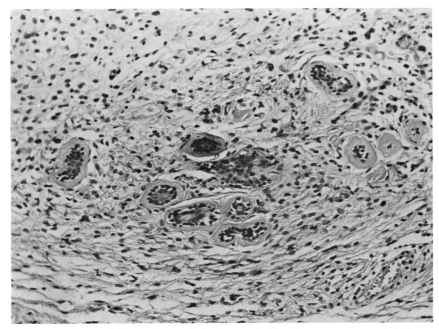

Figure 15–21. Liposarcoma of the breast infiltrating a mammary lobule.

in diameter. Microscopically it was a partially differentiated liposarcoma. Figure 15–20 shows its myxoid stroma and bizarre giant cells. The infiltrating character of the tumor is shown in Figure 15–21, where it is seen infiltrating a mammary lobule. The patient was well seven years later.

GRANULAR CELL TUMOR

In 1926 Abrikossoff described a neoplasm characterized by cells with a granular cytoplasm and small nuclei. He believed that the neoplasm originated from myoblasts. It was subsequently realized that this view was incorrect, and this lesion is now known as the "granular cell tumor." It is seen in numerous organs of the body, most commonly in the tongue. The next most frequent sites are striated muscle and skin.

In 1946 Stout and I described five of these tumors that we had seen in the breast. Since then, sporadic reports and reviews have appeared from many clinics. In such papers, lesions of the skin and subcutaneous tissues overlying the breast are usually included with lesions of the mammary gland. This has tended to dilute and confuse the true incidence and clinical picture of granular cell tumor in the mammary gland. While this interesting tumor presents little difficulty in

diagnosis and treatment when it occurs in most situations, when located within the breast it presents a more important problem for accurate differential diagnosis. Mulcare has recently discussed this subject, collecting reports of 15 of these breast lesions, and reporting the cases from our own clinic.

At Columbia we have observed 15 of these granular cell tumors of the breast. One tumor was an incidental finding in the surgical specimen. Fourteen patients came to the surgical services of the Presbyterian Hospital or the Francis Delafield Hospital for signs and symptoms directly related to granular cell tumor.

Of our 15 patients, 14 were female and one was male. That patient represents the only reported case of the disease in the male breast.

The average diameter of the tumor was 1.75 cm., with a range from 0.5 cm. to 4 cm. Eleven of the 14 lesions were located in the upper inner quadrant of the breast (Zones F and E of the Columbia classification nomenclature, Figure 15–22). The three other lesions were situated in Zones A, B, and C, respectively. In two patients there was retraction of the skin overlying the tumor. The lesion was usually described as firm or hard, and fairly well circumscribed.

Only one of our patients had a granular cell

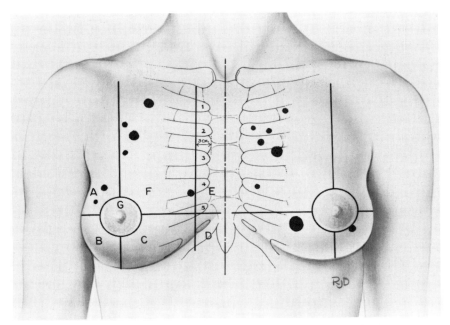

Figure 15–22. The location of 15 granular cell tumors of the breast.

tumor elsewhere. It had been excised from the skin of the right groin, adjacent to the labia, five years prior to the discovery of her breast mass.

The preoperative diagnoses were stated in 13 of the 14 cases. In seven, the leading impression, based on the clinical findings, was carcinoma, while in six, it was fibroadenoma. Although the average age of our patients was nearly 20 years younger than that of patients with carcinoma of the breast, our diagnostic errors are an indication of how often granular cell tumor can mimic carcinoma.

When biopsy was done or the lesion was locally excised, a frozen section diagnosis was attempted in nine of the 14 cases. Six of the nine were correctly diagnosed. In one case, in 1931, when granular cell tumor was less well known, the frozen section diagnosis rendered was only that the lesion was benign. In two patients, the initial frozen section diagnosis was carcinoma. In one of these two, this impression was immediately corrected to granular cell tumor while the patient was still under anesthesia, and local excision was performed. In the other case the initial diagnosis of carcinoma was not revised until the permanent sections of the biopsy were studied. Then there was a failure of communication between the pathologist and the surgeon and a radical mastectomy was mistak-

enly performed. The initially incorrect diagnosis of carcinoma by frozen section in two of our nine cases emphasizes that granular cell myoblastoma can represent a difficult differential diagnostic problem to the pathologist as well as the surgeon.

The history of one of our cases might be taken as typical of this lesion.

Mrs. N. B., a Russian-born Jewess, first came to the Presbyterian Hospital in 1928 when she was 47 years of age. She was found to have hypertensive cardiovascular disease and mild diabetes. She failed to follow her diet and gained a good deal of weight as the years went by. In 1935 she was put on insulin.

In February, 1944, at the age of 63, she discovered a tumor in her left breast. It presented on the inferior aspect of the large dependent breast just cephalad to the inframammary fold. It was, therefore, concealed when the patient sat erect and in this position the only evident abnormality was slight elevation of the breast. It was very evident with the patient in the supine position, however, as a projecting tumor situated over the fifth interspace half way between the sternal edge and the nipple line. It was hard, and measured 4 cm. in diameter. The tumor and the breast tissue in which it lay were relatively fixed to the underlying chest wall. When the breast was pushed medially toward the tumor a definite dimple appeared in the skin over it. No enlarged axillary nodes were detected.

A presumptive diagnosis of carcinoma of the breast was made, and all preparations were completed for a radical mastectomy. Fortunately, a biopsy was done, a small wedge being removed from the surface of the lesion for frozen section. The only feature of the gross appearance that suggested something unusual was the fact that the cut surface of the tumor was whiter than most carcinomas (Fig. 15-23). When the frozen section revealed that the lesion was a granular cell tumor it was excised locally and the wound closed. Healing was uneventful. There had been no recurrence when the patient was last seen ten years later.

The tumor was made up of cells with small oval nuclei and large finely granular cytoplasms (Fig. 15-24). The cells lay in solid masses and strands, often in immediate contact with one another without any intervening collagenous reticulum. The Scharlach R stain failed to show any lipoid in the cells. The edge of the lesion was sharply defined against the adjacent mammary tissue, but there was no true capsule.

The granular cell tumors developing as primary breast lesions have all been benign. There is, therefore, no need for anything more drastic than local excision. Thirteen of our 14 patients who came to our clinic because of their breast tumor were treated by local excision, and recurrence has not developed in a single one of them after an interval of from one to 36 years. One of our patients was unfortunately treated by radical mastectomy, because of a misunderstanding on the part of the surgeon as to the correct diagnosis.

The clinical importance of granular cell tumor of the breast lies in the fact that it can produce all the clinical signs of early carcinoma. The tumor is hard. It is relatively fixed in the breast tissue surrounding it. It may be abnormally attached to the underlying pectoral fascia. It may cause dimpling of the overlying skin. The gross appearance of the lesion is enough like carcinoma to betray most pathologists into making this diagnosis if they depend upon the gross appearance alone, without taking the precaution of making a frozen section. The closest scrutiny will show that this lesion is more sharply circumscribed than most carcinomas, and that its cut surface is whiter and more uniform than the grayish, chalk-streaked surface of the typical carcinoma. These differences, however, are slight and easily missed. This

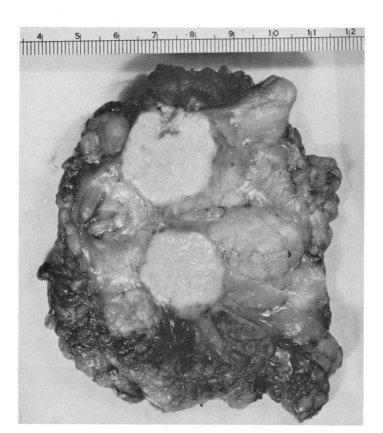

Figure 15-23. Gross appearance of a granular cell tumor of the breast.

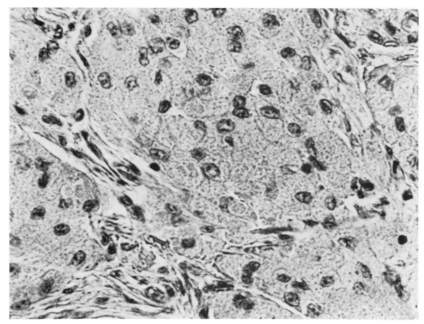

Figure 15–24. Granular cell tumor of the breast.

fact is yet another reason why we do a biopsy of every breast tumor and do a frozen section before deciding how to treat the tumor.

BENIGN MESENCHYMOMA OF THE BREAST

There are a number of benign tumors made up of mixtures of mesenchymal tissues. They have been called by many names, such as hamartoma, angiomyolipoma, and so forth. Stout, in 1948, described a number of these tumors and urged the use of the term "mesenchymoma" for them, and it has been widely adopted. The tumors of this type that occur in the subcutaneous tissues are largely composed of fat but contain angiomatous foci. Howard and Helwig wrote a good description of this lesion and called it angiolipoma.

Tumors of this type occasionally occur in the breast, and we classify them as benign mesenchymomas. Their true nature has usually been missed and they have been called lipomas, which they very much resemble both clinically and grossly. During the last 10 years, during which we have been alert to the occurrence of this lesion in the breast, we have seen six examples of it.

The clinical details of these cases are shown in Table 15–2. In all these patients the

Table 15–2. BENIGN MESENCHYMOMA OF THE BREAST

Age of Patient	Duration of Tumor	Size of Tumor	Site in Breast	Treatment	Follow-up
56	2 weeks	3 cm.	Upper inner sector	Local excision	Well 11 years
57	1 week	8 mm.	Subareolar	Local excision	Well 6 years
43	6 months	4 cm.	Lower inner sector	Local excision	Well 4 years
26	3 weeks	3 cm.	Lower inner sector	Local excision	Well 5 years
52	2 weeks	2 cm.	Upper inner sector	Local excision	Well 6 months
51	Found at follow-up examination	2 cm.	Sternal edge, 4th interspace	Local excision	Well 5 months

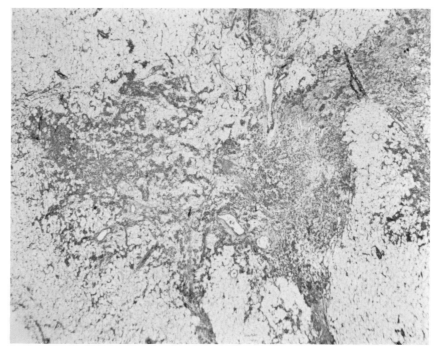

Figure 15–25. Mesenchymoma of the breast—low power view.

tumor was soft, well delimited and movable within the breast. The largest was 4 cm. in diameter. Clinically, this lesion cannot be differentiated from a lipoma.

This lesion, like a lipoma, has a delicate capsule. The only gross feature that suggests that this tumor is a mesenchymoma rather than a lipoma, is that it is more grayish in color.

Microscopically, this tumor is composed of

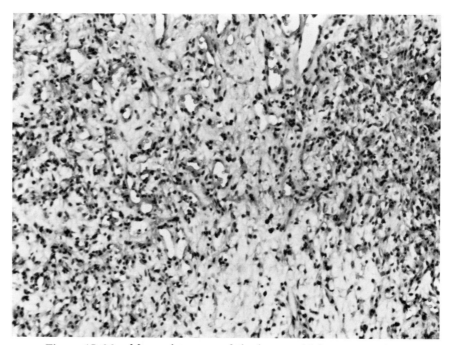

Figure 15–26. Mesenchymoma of the breast—higher power view.

adult fat in which there are angiomatous areas. These are seen in a low power view in Figure 15–25. These areas are composed of a fibrous reticulum enclosing a meshwork of capillary-like structures. The predominant cell type is small, ovoid, and quite regular. Mitoses are infrequent. The capillary-like spaces sometimes contain red blood cells but often do not (Fig. 15–26). There is great variation in the amount of the angiomatous elements in these tumors.

Simple excision is of course all that is required for these lesions.

NEUROFIBROMATOSIS OF THE BREAST

Neurofibromatosis may involve the skin and subcutaneous tissues over the breast. There seems to be a special tendency for the papillary fibromas, which are one of the features of neurofibromatosis, to develop in the areolar and nipple area. Striking cases of this kind have been described by Schilling, and by Ottow. We have had a good example in the Presbyterian Hospital.

Miss D. H. came to the Presbyterian Hospital at the age of 29, complaining of a tumor of her tongue. She had the fully developed syndrome of neurofibromatosis, with typical café-au-lait spots on her skin (Fig. 15–27), numerous small pedunculated cutaneous neurofibromas, and several subcutaneous neurofibromas. She had in addition two typical neurofibromatous lesions: (1) Along the left side of her tongue there was a thick, submucous mass of neurofibromatous tissue. (2) There was a cluster of elevated and pedunculated neurofibromas projecting from the areolas and nipples bilaterally.

During the 10 years following her admission the patient's nipple lesions slowly increased in size. Individually some of the papillomas became as large as 2 cm. in length. Figure 15–28 shows their appearance. They were so disfiguring and troublesome that excision of the papillomas and plastic reconstruction of the nipples was performed. Pathologically the lesions were characteristic neurofibromas.

LYMPHOSARCOMA

All types of lymphosarcoma have appeared initially in the breast, without concurrent manifestations of the disease elsewhere. In such cases the disease usually soon appears in other areas of the body, in lymph nodes, or in the chest, and follows its characteristic course. The primary mammary manifestation in the breast is often mistaken for carcinoma. In other cases lymphosarcoma apparently originates in the breast, is successfully treated, and does not develop elsewhere.

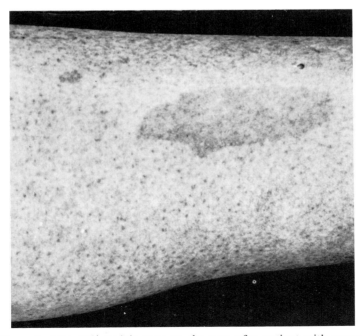

Figure 15–27. Characteristic café-au-lait spot on the arm of a patient with neurofibromatosis of the breasts.

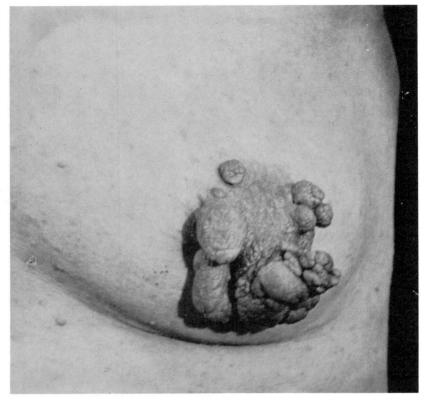

Figure 15–28. Pedunculated neurofibroma of the nipple region.

There are, of course, other patients in whom lymphosarcoma has generalized, and as the disease evolves, a focus appears in the breast. I have not included such cases in the present discussion.

Case reports of lymphosarcoma developing initially in the breast include those made by Thür, by Harrington and Miller, by Pohl, by Kreitner and Ulm, by Stringer, by Kay, by Bellini, by du Roy and Sawyer, and by Jernstrom and Sether. De Crosse and his associates have reported a series of 14 cases. In all, approximately 75 of these cases have been reported.

From our own clinic we have nine cases in which lymphosarcoma appeared initially in the breast. They were all of the reticulum cell type. All have been followed. The details of these cases are shown in Table 15–3.

In the files of our Department of Surgical Pathology there are a total of 24 additional cases of lymphosarcoma appearing initially in the breast, that were sent to Stout or to Lattes for consultation. These cases are not as fully documented clinically as our own, so that I have not included them in Table 15–3.

All histologic types of lymphosarcoma are included in the combined group of 33 lymphosarcomas of the breast studied in our Department of Surgical Pathology. There were 27 cases of the reticulum cell type, three of the lymphocytic type, two of the mixed type, and one of the follicular type.

There is a tendency for the disease to involve both breasts. This occurred in eight of the 33 cases that we studied.

While the lymphosarcomatous breast tumor in some of our patients formed a well-delimited movable mass, in other patients the clinical picture was indistinguishable from that of carcinoma, the tumor being poorly delimited and fixed in the surrounding breast tissue, with retraction of the overlying skin. This clinical picture, and the fact that it is easy to mistake lymphosarcoma for undifferentiated small cell carcinoma in frozen section, has often led to radical mastectomy. This happened in seven of the 33 cases that we have studied. In two of our own group of nine cases the frozen section was misread as carcinoma, but radical mastectomy was carried out in only one of them.

Table 15–3. LYMPHOSARCOMA OF THE BREAST (Columbia-Presbyterian Medical Center)

Age of Patient	Duration	Size of Breast Tumor	Axillary Nodes	Treatment	Follow-Up
Case 1 55	2 months	12 cm.	2.5 cm.	Biopsy and irradiation	Breast tumor did not respond to irradiation. Patient died of cerebral metastases in 3 months
Case 2 71	3 weeks	2 cm.	2 cm. bilateral	Biopsy and irradiation	Well 3 years
Case 3 50	1 week	2 cm.	0	Biopsy, radical mastectomy	Died of generalized lymphosarcoma in 6 years
Case 4 46	6 weeks	5 cm.	0	Simple mastectomy, irradiation	Died of generalized lymphosarcoma in 4 months
Case 5 65	1 year	14 cm. Ulcerated	8 cm. Fixed	Biopsy and irradiation	Died of cardiovascular disease 14 years later. Persisting microscopic breast lymphosarcoma
Case 6 60	3 months	8 cm.	1 cm.	Biopsy and irradiation	Well 4½ years
Case 7 74	5 weeks	3 cm.	1 cm.	Biopsy and irradiation	Died of generalized lymphosarcoma 3 years later.
Case 8 25	1 month	Movable upper outer 3 cm.	0	Local excision, irradiation	Died of generalized lymphosarcoma 11½ years later
Case 9 48	8 months	4 cm.	6 cm.	Biopsy, irradiation	Died of generalized lymphosarcoma 8 years, 2 months later

A typical case history of lymphosarcoma appearing initially in the breast follows.

Mrs. G., a 25 year old housewife, discovered a lump in her right breast and came for consultation a month later. Her tumor was situated in the upper outer sector of her right breast and measured 3 cm. in diameter. There were no clinically involved axillary nodes. The breast tumor was excised locally and proved to be reticulum cell lymphosarcoma.

The breast, axilla, and supraclavicular regions were irradiated. There was never any reappearance of her disease in these areas, and she was in apparent good health until 11 years later when she developed generalized lymphosarcoma and died within six months.

In another of our patients the disease had atypical clinical features.

Mrs. I. B., a 65 year old Scottish widow, came to the Presbyterian Hospital because of a tumor in her right breast. She had discovered it one year previously. At that time it was a small, firm tumor situated just lateral to the areola. It steadily enlarged. Six months previously the skin over it had ulcerated. Three months previously she had first noticed a tumor in her right axilla.

Examination showed a large ulcerated tumor in the right breast, situated in the upper half of the breast (Fig. 15-29). The edges of the ulcer were raised and crenelated. Its base was necrotic. The lesion was situated superficially in the breast and did not extend down in the breast substance more than 2 or 3 cm. Its edges were remarkably well

defined in the breast tissue. The breast as a whole was freely movable over the chest wall.

In the axilla there was a massive group of enlarged nodes, 8 cm. in diameter, fixed in the deeper structures of the axilla. Palpation of the infraclavicular region gave a sensation of fullness in the upper axilla. There were no palpable supraclavicular nodes. No enlarged lymph nodes could be palpated anywhere else in the patient. The chest film was negative. Skeletal films showed no definite evidence of metastasis.

Biopsy of the ulcerated tumor of the breast showed reticulum cell lymphosarcoma (Fig. 15-30).

Both the breast and the axilla were treated with irradiation. A tumor dose of 2740 R. was delivered within a period of three weeks. Within a month the ulcer healed and both the axillary nodes and the breast tumor disappeared. A scarred indurated area remained beneath the site of the ulceration. The patient never developed any signs of generalized lymphosarcoma.

She died suddenly 14 years after treatment. At autopsy the cause of death was shown to be acute congestive heart failure. Sections through the indurated area in the breast showed an exceedingly dense, almost avascular, collagenous tissue in which there were a few scattered foci of atrophic cells with dense hyperchromatic nuclei. Although the nature of these cells remained uncertain, it was my own opinion that they represented the sclerotic remnant of her lymphosarcoma.

The treatment of lymphosarcoma appearing initially in the breast must be predicated on the fact that lymphosarcoma is usually an

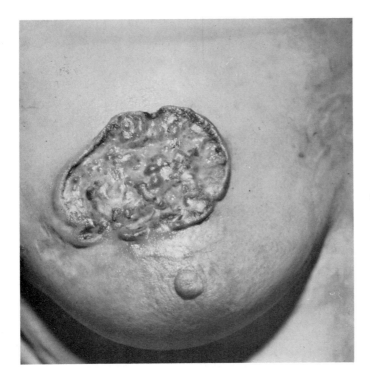

Figure 15-29. Ulcerated reticulum cell lymphosarcoma of the breast.

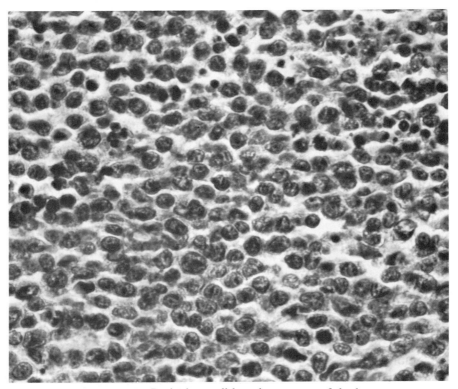

Figure 15-30. Reticulum cell lymphosarcoma of the breast.

incurable disease that finally becomes generalized. Although some authors, such as De Crosse, recommend radical mastectomy supplemented with irradiation, we prefer to rely upon irradiation exclusively, not only because mastectomy is usually futile, but because lymphosarcoma is highly sensitive to irradiation.

In the group of 33 cases that we have studied, 12 were treated by simple or radical mastectomy followed by irradiation. Ten have been followed for more than three years, and all developed generalized lymphosarcoma and succumbed to it. Their mean survival time from the beginning of treatment was 39 months.

On the other hand, among the nine patients from our own clinic, six were treated by irradiation alone. One survived symptom-free for 14 years, and two others have no evidence of their disease four and a half and three years, respectively, after irradiation was begun. The three others who have succumbed had a mean survival of 44 months after irradiation was begun.

Cerebral involvement occurred at an early stage in several of the patients in our series. These are the most fulminating cases in which no form of treatment is effective.

In connection with this discussion of lymphosarcoma of the breast, I cannot forego describing an unusual case in which the final classification of the disease remains uncertain.

CASE 1

Mrs. A. v. de E., aged 51, a woman of German origin, was admitted to the hospital in April, 1952, because of a lesion of the skin of the left breast. It had been first noted two years prior to admission. It began as an eczema-like manifestation involving a small area of the skin above the nipple. It itched and she scratched it a good deal. It responded temporarily to topical applications but after a period of quiescence the lesion extended until it involved the skin over the entire breast.

Examination on admission revealed no abnormalities other than the lesion of the breast. The skin over the entire left breast was thickened, indurated, roughened, and reddened. There were scattered areas of shallow ulceration covered with foul smelling exudate and crusts. The areola and nipple were intact. Figure 15–31 shows the appear-

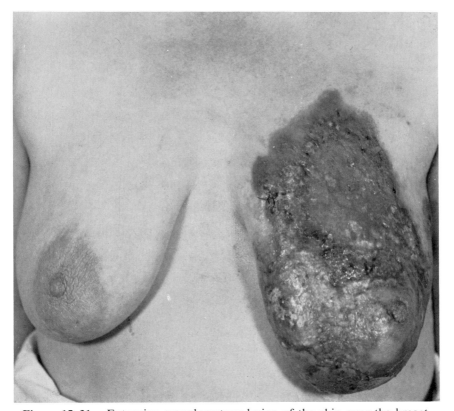

Figure 15–31. Extensive granulomatous lesion of the skin over the breast.

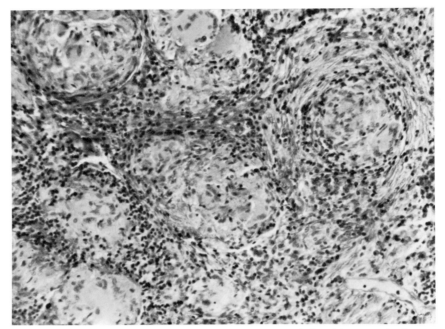

Figure 15–32. Microscopic appearance of a lesion of the skin over the breast.

ance of the lesion. No mass could be palpated in the breast. A single enlarged but movable lymph node was felt in the mid-axilla on the side of the lesion.

The laboratory data were within normal limits. A chest roentgenogram was negative. Cultures from the lesion revealed various organisms, including *Pseudomonas aeruginosa, nonhemolytic Streptococcus, B. pyocyaneus, Staphylococcus aureus* and *diphtheroids*. At no time were acid-fast bacilli demonstrated.

Several biopsies of different portions of the

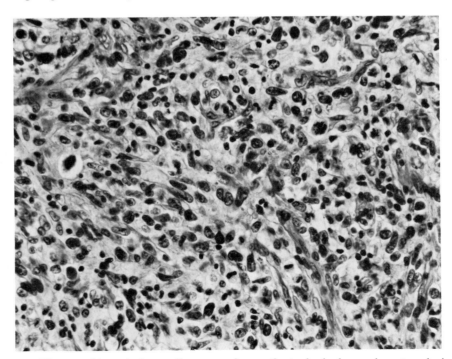

Figure 15–33. Pleomorphic reticulum cell sarcoma in a patient who had granulomatous lesion of skin of the breast.

lesion were taken. Microscopic study revealed a striking granulomatous inflammation characterized by tubercles containing giant cells, but without caseation or necrosis. No acid-fast bacilli could be demonstrated. The diagnosis of sarcoid was suggested. Figure 15-32 shows the microscopic appearance of the lesion.

The lesions proved to be refractory to parenteral antibiotic therapy but were somewhat improved by topical applications of neomycin. The ulcerations finally healed. The residual lesion consisted of a patchy induration and discoloration of the skin. On follow-up examination it became obvious that the lesions were showing spontaneous improvement as time went by. No specific therapy was prescribed.

When she was last seen in our clinic, five years after her initial admission, the breast lesion had to a great extent regressed.

Three years later a skin lesion, similar to the one she had had on her left breast, developed in her left axilla and spread to her left scapular region. She went to another clinic where the new lesion was described as necrotic. It involved an area of skin 11 cm. in diameter. A biopsy revealed a malignant neoplasm, which in our laboratory of surgical pathology has been classified as a pleomorphic reticulum cell sarcoma (Fig. 15-33). The dominant cells were large and pleomorphic, with many atypical mitoses. Some were multinucleated. They were clearly not epithelial in origin.

Chest films showed a patchy infiltrate at the right base and fluid in the left thorax. The patient died five weeks after admission and an autopsy was not obtained.

HODGKIN'S DISEASE

Hodgkin's disease manifests itself initially in the breasts with great rarity. We have no example of this breast lesion in Presbyterian Hospital data. Kückens was the first to report such a lesion. It occurred in a 16 year old girl. A tumor removed from the upper portion of her breast proved to be typical Hodgkin's disease. In 1945, Adair and his associates described four cases, among a total of 406 with Hodgkin's disease, in which tumors of the breast were presumed to be Hodgkin's disease. Microscopic proof that the breast lesion was indeed Hodgkin's disease was available in only two of these cases. More recently, well-documented additional cases have been described by Bertrand and Lataix. A very interesting case has been described by Randall and Spalding. The patient, aged 28, had had a breast tumor for 10 years which grew during pregnancy and lactation. The clinical picture was that of carcinoma, and radical mastectomy was done. Both the primary lesion in the breast and its axillary metastasis proved to be typical Hodgkin's

disease. McGregor has reported another example of this disease in which the breast tumor developed after five and one-half months of lactation. The affected breast enlarged rapidly, and redness and edema of the overlying skin, accompanied by a temperature elevated at 102°, suggested an inflammatory process. The lesion eventually proved to be Hodgkin's disease, which was fatal in six months.

LEUKEMIA

Leukemia manifests itself as an infiltration of the breast in occasional cases. McWilliams and Hanes reported such a case from our hospital in which bilateral radical mastectomy was done. Gelin et al. described one in which the breast lesion simulated an abscess. Blackwell has recently reported a very instructive case in which a 42-year-old patient who had a 10 cm. movable tumor of the breast was operated upon without preliminary blood studies, with the assumption that she had a carcinoma. A simple mastectomy was done. There was profuse postoperative bleeding, the wound became infected, and death followed after 14 days.

In a patient of mine, whose history follows, I could not differentiate clinically between the inflammatory type of carcinoma and leukemia.

L. C., an unmarried nurse aged 49, began to have chills, anorexia, nausea, and some vomiting, night sweats and general malaise, in April, 1942. She had intermittent fever of between 100° and 103°. Erythematous nodules appeared on her lower legs. Blood studies were at first not remarkable, but by the middle of May a few immature white cells resembling blasts began to be seen.

At this time a lesion developed in her right breast. The breast was considerably enlarged by a diffuse induration involving its lower portion. The skin was red, abnormally warm, and showed early edema. The lesion was tender. There were no enlarged lymph nodes. The clinical picture resembled that of the inflammatory type of carcinoma, or a low grade inflammatory process of some sort. The blood picture, however, suggested leukemia. While the diagnosis was being debated the lesion on the right side extended to involve most of the right breast, and a similar lesion appeared in the upper central part of the left breast. A biopsy was then done upon the right breast, and myelogenous leukemia found (Fig. 15-34). The appearance of the breasts at this time is shown in Figure 15-35.

Irradiation was given to the breast lesions without much response. The patient failed rapidly,

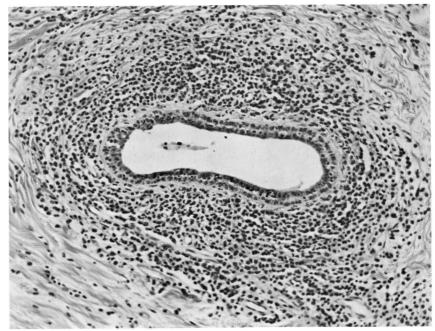

Figure 15–34.   Myelogenous leukemic infiltration around a mammary duct.

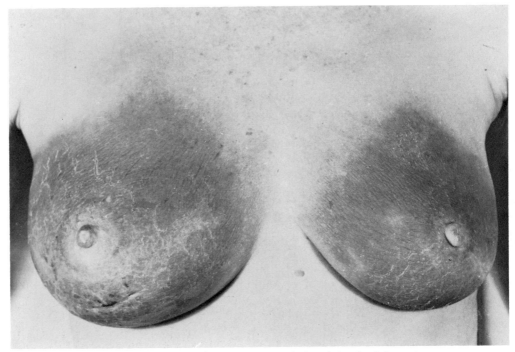

Figure 15–35.   Myelogenous leukemia involving both breasts.

leukemic infiltration developed in many body areas, and she died two months after the onset of her disease.

Leukemic involvement of the breast, as exemplified by these case histories, is often bilateral, and usually suggests an inflammatory process.

PLASMACYTOMA

There are occasional soft part tumors composed of plasma cells that are not associated with plasma cell myeloma. None has been reported in the breast. There are, however, two case reports by Cutler and by Rosenberg and his associates, of tumor composed of plasma cells developing in the breast as the first manifestation of plasma cell myeloma.

REFERENCES

Abrikossoff, A. I.: Ueber Myome, ausgehend von der quergestreiften willkürlichen Muskulatur. Virchows Arch. f. path. Anat., 260:215, 1926.

Abrikossoff, A. I.: Weitere Untersuchungen über Myoblastenmyome. Virchows Arch. f. path. Anat., 280:723, 1931.

Adair, F. E., Craver, L. F., and Herrmann, J. B.: Hodgkin's disease of the breast. Surg., Gynec. & Obst., 80:205, 1945.

Aronson, W.: Malignant cystosarcoma phyllodes with liposarcoma. Wisconsin M. J., 65:184, 1966.

Aulisio, A.: Un caso di mioblastomioma granulo-cellulare della mammella. Rassegna internaz. clin. e terap., 36:479, 1956.

Bachulis, B. L., Old, J. W., and James, A. G.: Postmastectomy lymphangiosarcoma in a patient with carcinoma of the rectum. Am. J. Surg., 113:289, 1967.

Baes, H.: Angiosarcoma in a chronic lymphedematous leg. Dermatologica, 134:331, 1967.

Bangle, R., Jr.: A morphological and histochemical study of granular-cell myoblastoma. Cancer, 5:950, 1952.

Barber, K. W., Jr., Harrison, E. G., Clagett, O. T., and Pratt, J. H.: Angiosarcoma of the breast. Surgery, 48:869, 1960.

Batchelor, G. B.: Haemangioblastoma of the breast associated with pregnancy. Brit. J. Surg., 46:647, 1959.

Bellini, F.: Linfosarcoma e reticolosarcoma della mammella; contributo casistico. Tumori, 42:737, 1956.

Berg, J. W., De Crosse, J. J., Fracchia, A. A., and Farrow, J.: Stromal sarcomas of the breast. Cancer, 15:418, 1962.

Bertrand, I., and Lataix, P.: Localisation mammaire de la lympho-granulomatose maligne. Presse méd., 60:1383, 1952.

Bilynskii, B. T., and Shegedin, I. E.: Myoblastic myoma simulating recurrence of breast cancer. Vopr. onkol., 11:101, 1964.

Blackwell, B.: Acute leukemia presenting as a lump in the breast. Brit. J. Surg., 50:769, 1963.

Botham, R. J., McDonald, J. R., and Clagett, O. T.: Sarcoma of the mammary gland. Surg., Gynec. & Obst., 197:55, 1958.

Bowers, W. F., Schear, E. W., and Le Golvan, P. C.: Lymphangiosarcoma in postmastectomy lymphedematous arm. Am. J. Surg., 90:682, 1955.

Breckenridge, R. L.: Liposarcoma of the breast. Am. J. Clin. Path., 24:954, 1954.

Byrne, J. J., and Dean, M. A.: Granular cell myoblastoma of the breast. Am. J. Surg., 100:98, 1960.

Chu, F. C. H., and Treves, N.: The value of radiation therapy in postmastectomy lymphangiosarcoma, Am. J. Roentgenol., 89:64, 1963.

Colberg, J. E., and Hubay, C. A.: Granular cell myoblastoma—a problem in diagnosis. Surgery, 53:226, 1963.

Craig, J. M.: Leiomyoma of the female breast. Arch. Path., 44:314, 1947.

Crawford, E. S., and DeBakey, M. E.: Granular-cell myoblastoma. Cancer, 6:786, 1953.

Cruse, R., Fisher, W. C., and Usher, F. C.: Lymphangiosarcoma in postmastectomy lymphedema. Surgery, 30:565, 1951.

Cutler, C. W.: Plasma-cell tumor of the breast with metastases. Ann. Surg., 100:392, 1934.

Danese, C. A., Grishman, E., Oh, C., and Dreiling, D. A.: Malignant vascular tumors of the lymphedematous extremity. Ann. Surg., 166:245, 1967.

De Crosse, J. J., Berg., J. W., Fraccia, A. A., and Farrow, J.: Primary lymphosarcoma of the breast—review of 14 cases. Cancer, 15:1264, 1962.

Dembrow, V. D., and Adair, F. E.: Lymphangiosarcoma in the postmastectomy lymphedematous arm. Cancer, 14:210, 1961.

De Navasquez, S., and Horton, R. E.: Liposarcoma of the breast. Guy's Hosp. Rep., 96:57, 1947.

Door, H. D.: Secundair lymfangiosarcoom. Nederlands Tijdschrift voor Geneeskunde, 107:1344, 1963.

Doremus, W. P., and Salvia, G. A.: Lymphangiosarcoma in the postmastectomy lymphedematous arm. Am. J. Surg., 96:576, 1958.

du Roy, R. M., and Sawyer, K. C.: Lymphosarcoma of the breast; discussion and presentation of a case. Am. Surgeon, 25:489, 1959.

Eby, C. S., Brennan, M. J., and Fine, G.: Lymphangiosarcoma: a lethal complication of chronic lymphedema. Arch. Surg., 94:223, 1967.

Eisler, P.: Die Muskeln des Stammes. In Bardeleben, Handbuch der Anatomie des Menschen, Jena, Gustav Fischer, 1912, vol. 2, part 2, first section, p. 109 (platysma) and p. 471 (sternal muscle).

Ende, M.: Lymphangiosarcoma—report of a case. Pacific Medicine and Surgery, 74:80, 1966.

Enticknap, J. B.: Angioblastoma of the breast complicating pregnancy. Brit. M. J., 2:51, 1946.

Enzinger, F. M., and Winslow, D. J.: Liposarcoma, a study of 103 cases. Virchows Arch. f. path. Anat., 335:367, 1962.

Evans, R. W.: Rhabdomyosarcoma of breast. J. Clin. Path., London, 6:140, 1953.

Ferraro, L. R.: Lymphangiosarcoma in postmastectomy lymphedema. Cancer, 3:511, 1950.

Fisher, J. H.: Postmastectomy lymphangiosarcoma in the lymphedematous arm. Canad. J. Surg., 8:350, 1965.

Friedman, R. M., and Hurwitt, E. S.: Granular cell myoblastoma of the breast. Am. J. Surg., 112:76, 1966.

Froio, G. F., and Kirkland, W. G.: Lymphangiosarcoma in post-mastectomy lymphedema. Ann. Surg., 135:421, 1952.

Fry, W. J., Campbell, D. A., and Coller, F. A.: Lymphangiosarcoma in postmastectomy lymphedematous arm. Arch. Surg., 79:440, 1959.

Garbay, M., et al.: Angiomes et angio-sarcomes du sein. J. de chir., 77:226, 1959.

Gelin, G., Gomez, F., and Gross, G.: Leucose tumorale simulant un abcès du sein. Bull. Soc. méd. hôp. Paris, 68:376, 1952.

Giacomelli, V., and Re, A.: Studio statistico sulle affezioni displastiche della mammella in rapporto all'età. Tumori, 25:213, 1951.

Gray, G. F., Jr., Gonzales-Licea, A., Hartmann, W. H., and Woods, A. C.: Angiosarcoma in lymphedema—an unusual case of Stewart-Treves syndrome. Bull. Johns Hopkins Hosp., 119:117, 1966.

Gray, S. H., and Gruenfeld, G. E.: Myoblastoma. Am. J. Cancer, 30:699, 1937.

Gulesserian, H. P., and Lawton, R. L.: Angiosarcoma of the Breast. Cancer, 24:1021, 1969.

Haagensen, C. D., and Stout, A. P.: Granular cell myoblastoma of mammary gland. Ann. Surg., 124:218, 1946.

Hall-Smith, S. P., and Haber, H.: Lymphangiosarcoma in postmastectomy lymphoedema. Proc. Roy. Soc. Med., 47:174, 1954.

Halpert, B., and Young, M. O.: Lipoma of the mammary gland. Arch. Path., 42:641, 1947.

Harrington, S. W., and Miller, J. M.: Lymphosarcoma of the mammary gland. Am. J. Surg., 48:346, 1940.

Herrmann, J. B.: Lymphangiosarcoma of the chronically edematous extremity. Surg., Gynec. & Obst., 121:1107, 1965.

Herrmann, J. B., and Ariel, I. M.: Therapy of lymphangiosarcoma of the chronically edematous limb. Am. J. Roentgenol., 99:393, 1967.

Horn, R. C., and Stout, A. P.: Granular cell myoblastoma. Surg., Gynec. & Obst., 76:315, 1943.

Howard, W. R., and Helwig, E. B.: Angiolipoma. Arch. Dermat., 82:924, 1960.

Hume, H. A., Erb, W. H., and Stevens, L. W.: Lymphangiosarcoma following radical mastectomy. Surg., Gynec. & Obst., 116:117, 1963.

Hummer, C. D., Jr., and Burkart, T. J.: Liposarcoma of the breast. Am. J. Surg., 113:558, 1967.

Jackson, A. V.: Metastasising liposarcoma of the breast arising in a fibroadenoma. J. Path. Bact., 83:582, 1962.

Jernstrom, P., and Fry, K.: Granular cell myoblastoma of the mammary gland. Am. J. Clin. Path., 26:1055, 1956.

Jernstrom, P., and Sether, J. M.: Primary lymphosarcoma of the mammary gland. J. A. M. A., 201:503, 1967.

Jessner, M., Zak, F. G., and Rein, C. R.: Angiosarcoma in postmastectomy lymphedema. Arch. Dermat. & Syph., 65:123, 1952.

Kappey, F.: Das angioplastische Sarkom bei chronischen Lymphöden nach Ablatio mammae. Chirurg, 38:59, 1967.

Kay, S.: Lymphosarcoma of the female mammary gland. Arch. Path., 60:575, 1955.

Keefer, G. P., and Vastine, J. H.: Lymphangiosarcoma in lymphedematous arm after mastectomy. Radiology, 77:722, 1961.

Khanna, S. D., Manchanda, R. L., Saigal, R. K., and Rathee, A. S.: Hemangioendothelioma (angiosarcoma) of the breast. Arch. Surg., 88:807, 1964.

Khodadadeh, M., and Johnson, R.: Lymphangiosarcoma arising from postmastectomy lymphedema. J. A. M. A., 186:1087, 1963.

Kirschner, H.: Ueber einen Fall von maligne entartetem Myoblastenmyom der Mamma. Bruns Beitr. z. klin. Chir., 204:87, 1962.

Kreitner, H., and Ulm, R.: Einfaches lokales Lymphom der Mamma (Lymphozytom der Mamma). Krebsarzt, 5:212, 1950.

Krückmeyer, Von K., and Scholz, H.: Ueber ein angioblastisches Sarkom bei chronischem Lymphödem nach Mamma-Radikaloperation (Stewart-Treves Syndrom). Zentralbl. f. Gynäkologie, 89:229, 1967.

Kückens, H.: Ein lokales Lymphogranulom der Brust in Form eines Mammatumors. Beitr. z. path. Anat. u. z. allg. Path., 80:135, 1928.

Lattes, R.: Sarcomas of the breast. J. A. M. A., 201:531, 1967.

Libcke, J. H.: Leiomyoma of the breast. J. Path., 98:89, 1969.

Lowbeer, L.: "Granular cell myoblastomas" of unusual locations (Bronchus, breast, chest wall). Am. J. Path., 29:611, 1953.

McClanahan, B. J., and Hogg, L., Jr.: Angiosarcoma of the breast. Cancer, 7:586, 1954.

McConnell, E. M., and Haslam, P.: Angiosarcoma in postmastectomy lymphoedema; a report of 5 cases and a review of the literature. Brit. J. Surg., 46:322, 1959.

McDivitt, R. W., Stewart, F. W., and Berg, J. W.: Tumors of the breast. In Atlas of Tumor Pathology, Washington, D. C., Armed Forces Institute of Pathology, 1967, Series 2, Fascicle 2.

McFarlane, A.: Liposarcoma of the breast. Brit. J. Surg., 45:106, 1957.

McGregor, J. K.: Hodgkin's disease of the breast. Am. J. Surg., 99:348, 1960.

Mackenzie, D. H.: Angiosarcoma (haemangioblastoma) of the breast. Brit. J. Surg., 49:140, 1961.

Mackh, G.: Das Stewart-Treves Syndrom. Bruns Beitr. z. klin. Chir., 214:235, 1967.

McClanahan, B. J., and Hogg, L., Jr.: Angiosarcoma of the breast. Cancer, 7:586, 1954.

McSwain, B., and Stephenson, S.: Lymphangiosarcoma of the edematous extremity. Ann. Surg., 151:640, 1960.

McWilliams, C. A., and Hanes, F. M.: Leukemic tumors of the breast mistaken for lymphosarcoma. Am. J. M. Sc., 163:518, 1912.

Malik, M. I., and Samter, T. G.: Postmastectomy lymphangiosarcoma. Wisconsin M. J., 66:510, 1967.

Mallory, F. B.: The results of the application of special histological methods to the study of tumors. J. Exper. Med., 10:575, 1908.

Mallory, T. B.: Case 35321 (Hemangio-sarcoma of the breast). New England J. Med., 241:241, 1949.

Melnick, P. J.: Fibromyoma of the breast. Arch. Path., 14:794, 1932.

Meyer, R.: Myoblastentumoren ("Myoblastenmyome" Abrikossoff). Vichows Arch. f. path. Anat., 287:55, 1932.

Middleton, W. S.: Some clinical caprices of Hodgkin's disease. Ann. Int. Med., 11:448, 1937.

Millo, L.: Liposarcoma della mammella. Arch. ital. di patholog. e clin. dei tumori, 2:610, 1958.

Moscovic, E. A., and Azar, H. A.: Multiple granular cell tumors ("Myoblastomas"). Cancer, 20:2032, 1967.

Mulcare, R.: Granular cell myoblastoma of the breast. Ann. Surg., 168:262, 1968.

Nelson, W. R., and Morfit, H. M.: Lymphangiosarcoma in the lymphedematous arm after radical mastectomy. Cancer, 9:1189, 1956.

Nemoto, T., Stubbe, N., Gaeta, J., and Dao, T.:

Pathogenesis of lymphangiosarcoma following mastectomy and irradiation. Surg., Gynec. & Obst., 128:489, 1969.

Norris, H. J., and Taylor, H. B.: Sarcomas and related mesenchymal tumors of the breast. Cancer, 22:22, 1968.

Oberman, H. A.: Primary lympho-reticular neoplasms of the breast. Surg., Gynec. & Obst., 123:1047, 1966.

Oberman, H. A.: Sarcomas of the breast. Cancer, 18:1233, 1965.

O'Brien, J. E., and Stout, A. P.: Malignant fibrous xanthomas. Cancer, 17:1445, 1964.

Oettle, A. G., and Blerk, P. J.: Postmastectomy lymphostatic endothelioma of Stewart and Treves in a male. Brit. J. Surg., 50:736, 1963.

Ogilvy, W. L., Franklin, R. H., and Aird, I.: Angioblastic sarcoma in postmastectomy lymphoedema. Canad. J. Surg., 2:195, 1959.

Ottow, B.: Ueber solitäre gestielte Fibroma der Brustwarzen. Zentralbl. f. Gynäk., 63:503, 1939.

Ozzello, L., Stout, A. P., and Murray, M. R.: Cultural characteristics of malignant histiocytomas and fibrous xanthomas. Cancer, 16:331, 1963.

Pack, G. T., and Tabah, E. J.: Dermatofibrosarcoma protuberans, Arch. Surg., 62:391, 1951.

Patrick, R. S., Jarvie, J., and Miln, D. C.: Haemangioblastoma of breast — a report of 3 cases. Brit. J. Surg., 45:188, 1957.

Pohl, W.: Ueber eine histologisch zunächst gutartige Geschwulst der Mamma mit sehr malignem Verlauf (Lymphozytoma mammae). Klinische Medizin, 3:863, 1948.

Powell, E. B.: Granular cell myoblastoma. Arch. Path., 42:517, 1946.

Rajchev, R., Krustev, B., and Andreev, V.: Lymphangiosarcoma in lymphedema after mastectomy (in Russian). Khirurgia, 16:231, 1963.

Randall, K. J., and Spalding, J. E.: Primary Hodgkin's disease of breast. Guy's Hosp. Rep., 94:137, 1945.

Ravich, A., Stout, A. P., and Ravich, R. A.: Malignant granular cell myoblastoma involving the urinary bladder. Ann. Surg., 121:361, 1945.

Rawson, A. J., and Frank, J. L.: Treatment by irradiation of lymphangiosarcoma in postmastectomy lymphedema. Cancer, 6:269, 1953.

Re, A., Zingo, L., and Veronesi, U.: Un caso di linfangiosarcoma postmastectomia. Tumori, 51:261, 1965.

René, L., et al.: Un cas de syndrome de Stewart-Treves. Bull. Soc. franç. de dermat., 70:9, 1963.

Riddell, R. J.: Lymphangio-endothelioma of the arm following radical mastectomy for carcinoma of the breast. Australian and New Zealand J. Surg., 30:228, 1961.

Robinson, J. M., and Castleman, B.: Benign metastasizing hemangioma. Ann. Surg., 104:453, 1936.

Roccamonte, G.: Rara localizzazione mammaria de un mioblastomioma granulo-cellulare. Rassegna internaz. Clin. e terap., 45:544, 1965.

Rosenberg, B. M., Attie, J. N., and Mandelbaum, H. L.: Breast tumor as the presenting sign of multiple myeloma. New England J. Med., 269:359, 1963.

Sailer, S.: Sarcoma of the breast. Am. J. Cancer, 31:183, 1937.

Salm R.: The nature of the so-called postmastectomy lymphangiosarcoma. J. Path. Bact., 85:445, 1963.

Sasano, N., et al.: Granular cell myoblastoma of the breast. Jap. J. Cancer Clin., 10:593, 1964.

Schilling, J.: Ein Fall von ungewöhnlich grossem Hautpapillom der Mamma. Deutsch Ztschr. f. Chir., 254:64, 1940.

Schmidt, E. C., Ambler, J. T., and Wroth, R. L.: Multiple granular cell myoblastomas. Maryland M. J., 8:287, 1959.

Seitz, A.: In Halban-Seitz, Biologie und Pathologie des Weibes, Berlin und Wien, Urban und Schwarzenberg, 1924–29, vol. 5, part 2, p. 1290.

Shore, J. H.: Haemangiosarcoma of the breast. J. Path. Bact., 74:289, 1957.

Simon, M. A.: Granular cell myoblastoma. A. J. Clin. Path., 17:302, 1947.

Sirsat, M. V., and Vakil, V. V.: Granular cell myoblastoma of the breast. Indian J. Path. Bact., 7:174, 1964.

Southwick, H. W., and Slaughter, D. P.: Lymphangiosarcoma in postmastectomy lymphedema. Cancer, 8:158, 1955.

Spalding, J. E.: Adeno-lipoma and lipoma of the breast. Guy's Hosp. Rep., 94:80, 1945.

Stein, L.: Granular cell myoblastoma of the breast. Arch. Surg., 87:703, 1963.

Stein, R. J.: Fibroleiomyoma of the breast. Arch. Path., 33:72, 1942.

Steingaszner, L. C., Enzinger, F. M., and Taylor, H. B.: Hemangiosarcoma of the breast. Cancer, 18:352, 1965.

Sternby, N. H.: Gynning, I., and Hogeman, K. E.: Postmastectomy angiosarcoma. Acta. chir. Scandinav., 121:420, 1961.

Stewart, F. W., and Treves, N.: Lymphangiosarcoma in postmastectomy lymphedema. Cancer, 1:64, 1948.

Stout, A. P.: Granular cell myoblastoma of the breast. J. Missouri M. A., 44:342, 1947.

Stout, A. P.: Hemangio-endothelioma. Ann. Surg., 118:445, 1943.

Stout, A. P.: Mesenchymoma, the mixed tumor of mesenchymal derivatives. Ann. Surg., 127:278, 1948.

Stout, A. P., and Bernanke, M.: Liposarcoma of the female mammary gland. Surg., Gynec. & Obst., 83:216, 1946.

Stout, A. P., and Lattes, R.: Tumors of the soft tissues. In Atlas of Tumor Pathology, Washington, D.C., Armed Forces Institute of Pathology, 1966, Series 2, Fascicle 1.

Stringer, P.: Reticulosarcoma of both breasts. Brit. J. Surg., 47:51, 1959.

Strong, L. W.: Leiomyoma of the breast. Am. J. Obst. & Gynec., 68:53, 1913.

Taylor, H. B., and Helwig, E. G.: Dermatofibrosarcoma protuberans. A study of 115 cases. Cancer, 15:717, 1962.

Thür, W.: Zur Kenntnis seltener Geschwulstformen der weiblichen Brustdrüse (Lymphosarkom, Spindel-zellensarkom). Virchows Arch. f. path. Anat., 265:96, 1927.

Tibbs, D.: Metastasizing haemangiomata; a case of malignant haemangio-endothelioma. Brit. J. Surg., 40:465, 1953.

Toni, G.: Su un raro caso di rabdomiosarcoma mammario. Arch. ital. pat. clin. dei tumori, 1:174, 1957.

Tuta, J. A., and Schmidt, F. R.: So-called myoblastoma. Arch Dermat. & Syph., 46:225, 1942.

Vandaele, R., and Van Craeynes, T. W.: Lymphangiosarcome sur lymphoedème primitif du bras. Bull. Soc. franç. de dermat., 70:122, 1963.

Vos, P. A.: Lymphangiosarcoma in postmastectomy lymphoedema. Arch. chir. neerl., 4:197, 1952.

Wilson, R.: Lymphangiosarcoma in the postmastectomy lymphedematous arm. Canad. J. Surg., 5:208, 1962.

Chapter Sixteen

Tumors of the Skin and the Accessory Glands of the Skin Over the Breast

Any of the lesions that develop in the skin and from its accessory glands may of course appear in the skin over the breast. Their only special interest in this situation is their simulation of lesions of the mammary gland. For this reason it seems worthwhile to present examples of several of these lesions of the skin of the breast that I have seen.

EPITHELIOMA

Epitheliomas are unusual in skin over the breast, perhaps because this area gets so little ultraviolet light. We have only two examples in our Presbyterian Hospital data. Both were basal cell epitheliomas. One of these is summarized as follows.

Mrs. H. W. developed a lesion of the skin of the right mammary region when she was 62, fifteen years after bilateral radical mastectomy had been performed for bilateral primary mammary carcinoma.

There was no evidence of recurrent or metastatic mammary carcinoma. The skin of the thorax, both in front and in back, showed scattered senile keratoses.

In the skin of the right mammary region, just lateral to the vertical mastectomy scar, there was a scaly, reddish, slightly raised, 2 cm. lesion. Biopsy showed it to be a basal cell epithelioma. It was

treated with irradiation and had not recurred 11 years later when she was last seen.

MOLES AND NEVI

Moles, either pigmented or nonpigmented, may develop in the skin over the breast. There is of course no more reason for excising them from the skin over the breast than elsewhere. However, when moles enlarge and become darker in color the suspicion of melanoma arises. The most deceptive lesion in this class is the so-called epidermoid type of nevus. It may simulate a melanoma and lead the surgeon to unnecessarily radical surgery, as in the following case.

A. B., a housewife aged 64, came to the Presbyterian Hospital complaining of a tumor of the skin of her right breast. She had had a "black spot" in the skin over the breast for many years. Four weeks previously it had begun to enlarge and had ulcerated.

Examination showed a slightly raised tumor of the skin just medial to the areola of the right breast (Fig. 16–1). The medial half of the surface of the lesion was covered by intact epithelium and was bluish-black. The lateral half of its surface was ulcerated. There were no enlarged axillary nodes. I assumed that the lesion was a melanoma, and not wishing to do a biopsy for fear of producing metastases, I performed a simple mastectomy and an

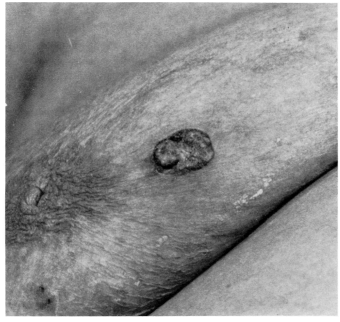

Figure 16–1. Seborrheic keratosis of the skin over the breast.

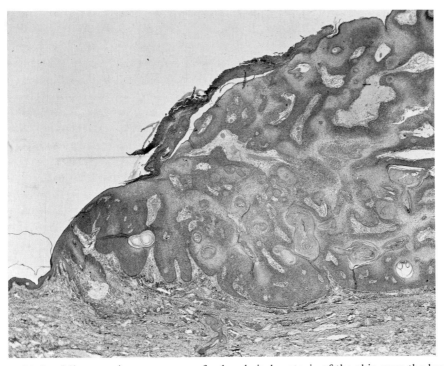

Figure 16–2. Microscopic appearance of seborrheic keratosis of the skin over the breast.

axillary dissection. To my surprise the lesion was only a papillary epidermoid nevus, or so-called seborrheic keratosis (Fig. 16-2).

MIXED TUMORS OF SWEAT GLAND ORIGIN

The so-called "mixed tumor" that develops in salivary glands is well known to pathologists. The identical tumor develops from sweat glands in the dermis of the skin over the breast, but it is rare. We have had only two of these lesions among our own patients, and we have studied eight others sent to us in consultation.

These tumors are very superficial, lying at the junction of the dermis and the subcutaneous tissue. They are very sharply delimited and encapsulated. They are made up of small cuboidal cells forming tubules and irregular clefts. These same cuboidal cells trail out in strands and sheets to form a stroma which

has extensive areas of cartilaginous metaplasia.

The lesion as it occurred in one of our patients, a housewife aged 34, is typical. It was situated beneath the skin of the upper inner sector of the breast, and was movable and very well delimited. It measured 2.5 cm. in diameter. It was excised locally and did not recur. Its general configuration is seen in Figure 16-3. The transition between its cartilaginous and epithelial elements, which give it a "mixed" character, is shown in Figure 16-4.

In one of these mixed tumors of sweat gland origin in the breast which we studied, the epithelial elements, arranged in tubules, predominated, and there was very little cartilaginous metaplasia (Fig. 16-5).

Smith and Taylor have reported eight of these tumors, and agree that they are entirely benign. They suggest that they are intraductal papillomas with chondroid and osseous metaplasia. We, however, are convinced that

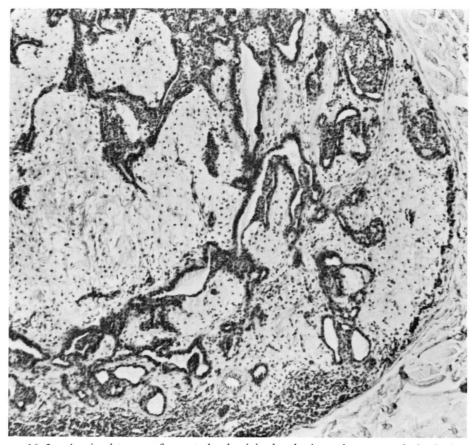

Figure 16-3.   A mixed tumor of sweat gland origin developing subcutaneously in the breast.

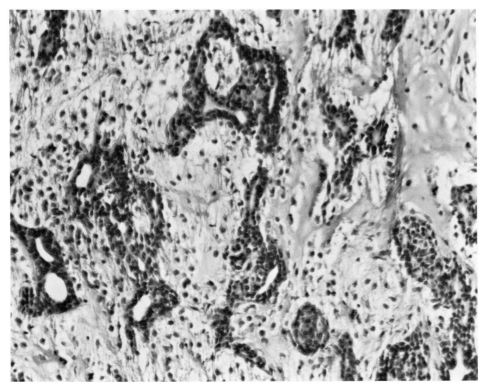

Figure 16–4. Transition between epithelial and cartilaginous elements in a mixed tumor of sweat gland origin.

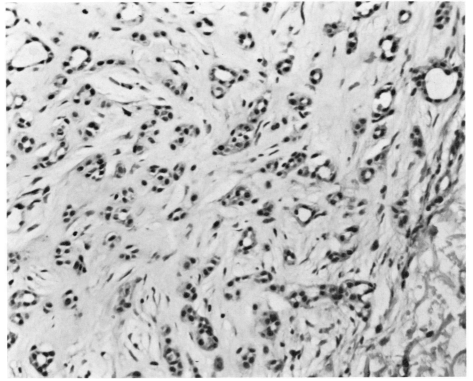

Figure 16–5. A mixed tumor in which epithelial elements in tubular formation predominate.

they are identical with the mixed tumors of salivary gland origin and that they develop from sweat glands when they occur in the subcutaneous region of the breast.

These lesions should not be confused with the malignant epithelial tumors containing cartilage and bone that develop in the breasts of dogs, mice, and human beings. They are carcinomas exhibiting metaplasia. I will discuss this special type of human breast cancer in Chapter 32.

MELANOMA

Malignant melanoma of the skin over the breast is a rare lesion. Cases have been reported by Stephenson and Byrd, and by Nyst. In our clinic we have had four patients with this lesion. Two of them were my own patients, and they illustrate the natural history of the disease so well that it is worthwhile summarizing their stories.

CASE 1

E. H., a housewife aged 63, came to the Presbyterian Hospital for a tumor of her right nipple. She had had a "reddish-brown wart," 5 mm. in diameter, close to her right nipple for 18 years, without any change in its size or color. One month previously it had begun to enlarge, and changed from its original reddish-brown to black. One week previously its surface had "cracked" and since then it had bled intermittently.

From the surface of the right nipple and the adjacent areola a black elevated lesion projected (Fig. 16-6). It measured 2.3 cm. in diameter. Its surface was irregular and crusted. There was a moderately enlarged movable lymph node in the right axilla. A chest film was negative and no melanin was found in the urine.

A diagnosis of malignant melanoma was made, and a radical mastectomy was performed. No preliminary biopsy was done because of the fear of producing metastases. Study of the operative specimen confirmed the diagnosis of malignant melanoma (Fig. 16-7). There were metastases in two of 15 axillary lymph nodes.

Three years later the patient developed anorexia, weakness, and left epigastric fullness. There was free fluid in the abdominal cavity and a mass in the left lower quadrant. At exploratory laparotomy the peritoneal cavity was found to be studded with black nodules of metastatic melanoma. The patient died 46 months after her first symptom of melanoma.

It is of interest to point out that this melanoma developed from the areolar epithelium, and not from the nipple. I have found no reliable report of a melanoma originating on the nipple.

CASE 2

Mrs. K. B., a housewife aged 38, had had a slightly elevated dark brown mole about 1 cm. in diameter in the skin of the upper inner sector of her right breast for as long as she could remember. It began to itch, and although there was no change in its appearance, her surgeon removed it with a narrow margin of the surrounding skin, using local anesthesia. To his surprise it proved to be a typical

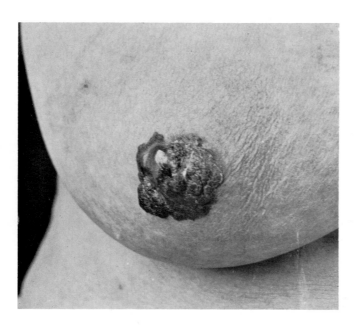

Figure 16-6. Malignant melanoma of the areola.

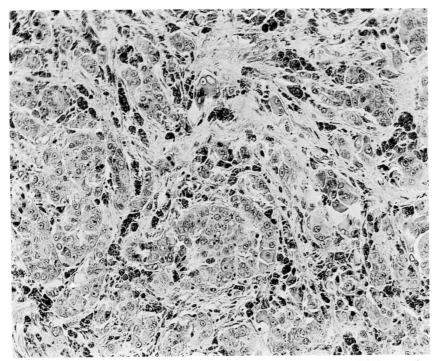

Figure 16–7.   Microscopic appearance of malignant melanoma of the areola.

malignant melanoma. The tumor extended down into the dermis. There was a separate focus of tumor cells deep in the dermis that suggested lymphatic permeation.

She was admitted to the Presbyterian Hospital, and one month after the local excision, under general anesthesia, her right axilla was dissected using a transverse incision. A wide area of skin and underlying breast tissue was then excised from the region of the previous local excision of the melanoma in the upper inner sector of the breast. The line of excision of skin skirted the area of local excision by 5 cm., and the skin flaps were dissected back an additional 5 cm. on all sides. A skin graft was used to cover the defect.

Microscopic studies showed no evidence of melanoma in the excised skin and the underlying breast, and no metastases were found in the 24 axillary lymph nodes.

The patient had had no recurrence when last seen seven and one-half years later.

The two other patients in our clinic records with melanoma of the skin over the breast were treated in a manner similar to my second patient. In both the melanoma was small and was very widely excised, and in both axillary dissection did not reveal metastases. These two patients have had no recurrence three years and four years, respectively, after operation.

SWEAT GLAND ADENOMA

Since sweat glands are found in the areola and in the skin over the breast, neoplasms might be expected to develop from them. Such neoplasms are rare, however, and apparently always benign. Moulonguet and Erjavec have described a sweat gland adenoma of the areola. We have studied two of these lesions of the skin of the breast. A summary of the features of one of these cases follows.

M. H., an adolescent Negress aged 16, came to the Presbyterian Hospital complaining of a tumor of the left breast. Eighteen months previously she had first noted a "pimple" in the skin over the lower inner sector of the breast. It had steadily increased in size and finally become ulcerated.

The appearance of this lesion is shown in Figure 16–8. It was a firm papillary tumor 2.5 cm. in diameter, projecting 1 cm. above the surrounding skin. Its surface was ulcerated.

It was excised with an ellipse of surrounding skin and proved to be a sweat gland adenoma (Fig. 16–9). There had been no recurrence 13 years later.

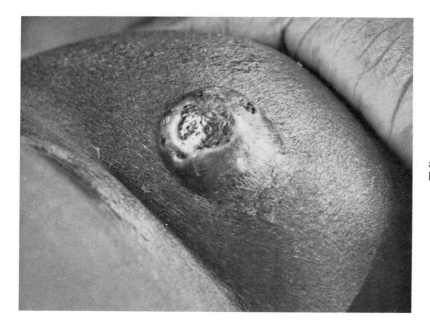

Figure 16–8. Sweat gland adenoma projecting from the lower portion of the breast.

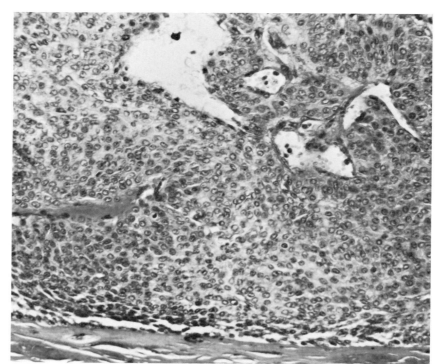

Figure 16–9. Microscopic appearance of a sweat gland adenoma of the skin of the breast.

REFERENCES

Allen, C. A.: So-called mixed tumors of the mammary gland of dog and man. Arch. Path., 29:589, 1940.

Moulonguet, P., and Erjavec.: Les tumeurs bénignes des glands mammaires accessoires rétroaréolaires. J. Chir., 67:689, 1951.

Nyst, M. E.: Malignant mammary melanoma. Nederl. T. Geneesk., 108:495, 1964.

Sicard, A., BenSahel, H., and Batisse, F.: Les tumeurs à stroma remanié du sein. J. de chir., 81:5, 1961.

Smith, B. H., and Taylor, H. B.: The occurrence of bone and cartilage in mammary tumors. Am. J. Clin. Path., 51:610, 1969.

Stephenson, S. E., Jr., and Byrd, B. F.: Malignant melanoma of the breast. Amer. J. Surg., 97:232, 1959.

Chapter Seventeen

Infections in the Breast

Most of the infections that occur in human tissues may localize in the breast, where the chronic types of infection may be distinguished only by the fact that since the blood supply of the breast is comparatively poor, their course may be unusually indolent. I do not propose to deal with their diagnosis in detail, but only to point out some of the main features of the more frequent types of infection.

LACTATIONAL MASTITIS

A common complication of nursing is the development within a breast of a localized area of inflammation, which becomes painful, and is indurated and tender to palpation. There is often a slight elevation of temperature. The usual treatment is to stop the nursing and give an antibiotic, preferably erythromycin (250 mg., four times a day) for five to seven days. The great majority of these limited areas of inflammation in a lactating breast will subside with this regimen.

I have observed that most of them subside even when nursing is continued, and since I believe that nursing is advantageous to the mother I favor at least trying to continue. Of course, if any purulent discharge from the nipple is seen, nursing should be abandoned.

Many cases of mastitis follow a cracked nipple that presumably provided entry for the infection. It is not uncommon to be able to trace an infection to skin pustules or to a paronychia in the baby.

LACTATIONAL BREAST ABSCESS

Occasionally mastitis in the lactating breast evolves into an obvious inflammation. The skin usually becomes reddened and edematous. Fluctuation can sometimes be observed. There is often a considerable elevation of temperature. If mastitis persists for more than five days after adequate antibiotic treatment, a deeply situated abscess should be suspected, even if not clinically evident.

When an abscess forms it should be drained by incision; antibiotic therapy alone is not sufficient. Occasionally repeated aspiration of the pus with a large-bore needle will suffice.

An obvious abscess such as that shown in Figure 17–1 should be adequately drained under general anesthesia in the operating room. A curved incision in the skin lines—not a radial incision—should be used. A Penrose drain should be left in place for at least 72 hours. The pus from the abscess should be cultured and the appropriate antibiotic selected on the basis of sensitivity tests. Almost all breast abscesses developing in our present-day hospital environment are caused by coagulase-positive *Staph. aureus*. Sensitivity tests show a large proportion of these organisms to be resistant to penicillin. In a 1959

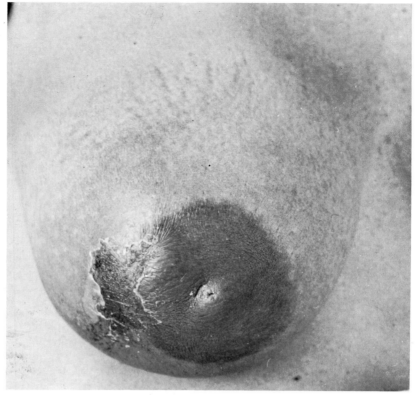

Figure 17–1. Typical lactation abscess.

study by Knight and Nolan at the Royal In-firmary in Edinburgh, 93 per cent were re-sistant to penicillin, 55 per cent resistant to streptomycin, and 1 per cent resistant to chloromycetin. Today, in the Columbia-Pres-byterian Medical Center, approximately 60 per cent of coagulase-positive *Staph. aureus* are resistant to penicillin, but only a very few are resistant to the synthetic penicillins—lin-comycin and oxacillin.

The antibiotic to which an organism in a given breast abscess is sensitive should be given in full dose for at least seven to ten days, to hasten the resolution of the asso-ciated cellulitis. Almost always this therapy proves to be sufficient, provided that the ab-scess has been diagnosed before it has ex-tended widely or produced massive necrosis in the breast, and provided that it has been drained adequately.

Knight and Nolan make the point in their study that breast abscess is a more protracted disease today than formerly. The average du-ration of the disease in their series of 100

cases was 50 days. They suggest that when the disease is caused by organisms resistant to antibiotics the natural course of the disease is changed unfavorably. Necrosis and pus formation are retarded and fibrosis is in-creased, with the result that a thick fibrous wall forming around the abscess prevents its collapse and resolution.

Soltau and Hatcher emphasize the role of cracked nipples in the etiology of breast ab-scess.

The use of stilbestrol to stop lactation when an abscess develops is favored by some (Knight and Nolan) but deprecated by others (Sawyer and Walker). We usually do not use it. If nursing is stopped and adequate support provided for the breasts, lactation soon ceases. It is debatable whether giving stilbes-trol actually favors the resolution of a breast abscess.

Lesions resembling abscess which develop in a non-lactating breast should be regarded with suspicion. They are probably not simple abscesses but may be duct ectasia, chronic recurring subareolar infection associated with metaplasia of the duct epithelium, or carcinoma.

SEBACEOUS CYST

Sebaceous cysts are not uncommon in the skin over the breast. Here, as elsewhere, they are recognized by their superficial situation, their circumscribed character, and by the dilated sebaceous duct orifice in the overlying skin.

There are two special points to be noted regarding the diagnosis of sebaceous cyst of the skin over the breast. At the periphery of the mammary gland, particularly along its medial border, where it extends as a very thin sheet almost to the midline of the sternum, a small carcinoma lies so close to the skin surface that it simulates a sebaceous cyst and has often been mistakenly excised locally without the surgeon having any suspicion that he was dealing with carcinoma.

Sebaceous cysts in the skin over the breast, when they become infected, may be accompanied by a considerable amount of induration and by such well-developed signs of inflammation that abscess or even the inflammatory type of carcinoma is suggested. Figure 17–2 shows such an infected sebaceous cyst of the skin over the breast, occurring in a woman aged 44, who came to the Presbyterian Hospital complaining of a tender tumor of the breast of one week's duration. The tumor measured 2 cm. in diameter and was firm but not hard. The skin over it was red. It was locally excised, and the wound closed with a small drain left in place for 48 hours.

TUBERCULOSIS OF THE BREAST

Tuberculosis of the breast is perhaps less frequent than it was a generation ago when tuberculosis was more ubiquitous. The diagnosis may be made less often because modern pathologists have come to realize that a great variety of granulomatous processes, including sarcoid and fungus disease, produce microscopic pictures indistinguishable from tuberculosis. In our laboratory, at least, the diagnosis is not now made without clinical findings which make the diagnosis presumptive, such as proven tuberculosis of the cervical or axillary nodes or subjacent chest wall, or when tubercle bacilli are demonstrated in the breast lesion, or in culture, or when guinea pig inoculation is positive. With these restrictions the diagnosis of tuberculosis of the breast has been made only five times in our laboratory between 1938 and 1967, during which a total of approximately 8000 breast specimens were studied. Schaefer reported finding only two examples of the disease among a total of 2141 breast specimens studied between 1949 and 1954 at the New York Hospital. Wilson and MacGregor have recently described five cases of tuberculosis occurring in a population of half a mil-

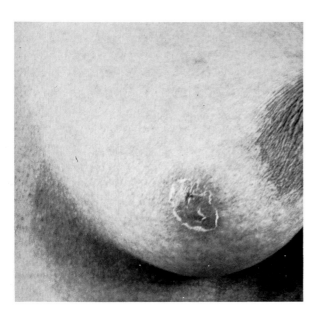

Figure 17–2. Infected sebaceous cyst of the breast.

lion over a 15 year period. The rarity of the disease today can be contrasted with reports of a generation ago, such as those of Cheever, and Shipley and Spencer, who found that about 1.5 per cent of the breast lesions seen in their clinics were tuberculosis.

The best modern discussions of tuberculosis of the breast, such as those of McKeown and Wilkinson, and Wilson and MacGregor, divide the cases into primary and secondary types. The primary cases are those in which the breast lesion is the only manifestation of tuberculosis. The secondary cases are those in which there is demonstrable tuberculosis elsewhere. In some the disease extends into the breast by continuity from involved axillary nodes or through the chest wall. Two of McKeown and Wilkinson's five cases, and three of Wilson and MacGregor's five cases, were of the primary type.

Younger pregnant women are predisposed to the disease. Two of McKeown and Wilkinson's patients, and three of Wilson and MacGregor's patients, were young and pregnant.

The breast lesion caused by tuberculosis may present as a fluctuant abscess, usually central in location, or as a firm poorly delimited tumor with associated skin retraction, which clinically resembles carcinoma. Discharge of pus from the nipple is not uncommon. Some lesions form fistulas. Leborgne described what he regards as the radiographic features of the disease. Despite these facts, tuberculosis of the breast has been mistaken for carcinoma and radical mastectomy done.

The following are examples of the primary and secondary types of tuberculosis of the breast from the files of our department.

Primary Tuberculosis of the Breast

Mrs. A. D., a Negro woman of 20, developed a painful tumor of her right breast. There was an associated sticky yellowish discharge from the nipple. The tumor grew larger as she waited four months before coming to the hospital.

On admission, she had a firm round movable tumor in the central sector of her right breast. A simple mastectomy was done.

Eighteen years later a large firm node was removed from her right axilla.

Both the breast lesion and the axillary node showed the microscopic picture of tuberculosis; and acid-fast bacilli were demonstrated in both lesions.

The patient at no time had any other manifestation of tuberculosis.

Secondary Tuberculosis of the Breast

Mrs. L. F., a Negro housewife aged 21, came to the Presbyterian Hospital with a tumor of the right breast. Her disease had begun with a sharp inspiratory pain under the breast two months previously. This called her attention to the tumor. It had doubled in size since she had discovered it. She had lost 10 pounds in the previous three months.

Examination showed a thickening over the fifth right costochondral junction. From this thickening a sessile tumor extended upwards into the lower middle sector of the breast. It measured 5 cm. in diameter and was round and seemingly encapsulated. I thought it fluctuant. There were no palpable axillary nodes. X-ray films showed a bulbous expansion of the anterior end of the fifth rib, with a central area of radiolucency. There was no evidence of pulmonary tuberculosis.

At operation the tumor was exposed, and a small incision made into it showed that it contained caseous and purulent material. The process was firmly attached to and seemed to originate from the chest wall in the region of the fourth interspace and the fifth costochondral junction. This area of the chest wall and the costal cartilage and rib were excised in continuity with the tumor. Microscopically the tumor proved to be a tuberculous abscess originating from tuberculosis of the rib.

The patient recovered without incident. Five years later she went through a pregnancy normally. It is interesting to note, however, that 11 years after her chest wall tuberculosis had been excised, she developed pulmonary tuberculosis.

Wilson and MacGregor emphasize that the conservative treatment of breast tuberculosis is long and expensive, even with the help of modern chemotherapy, because the lesion tends to persist and reappear with subsequent pregnancies. They therefore advise simple mastectomy.

COINCIDENT CARCINOMA AND TUBERCULOSIS OF THE BREAST

Carcinomas and tuberculosis of the breast are occasionally found coincidentally in the same patient. In 1926 Smith and Mason collected reports of 18 such cases and described one that they observed. Grausman and Goldman have described two indubitable cases. More recently, Schultze-Jena has reported four such cases.

The rare finding of carcinoma in one breast and tuberculosis in the other has been described by Scherer. Villard and Martin reported one case in which the two diseases coexisted not only in the breast but in the axillary lymph nodes. The latter finding is not rare. In our laboratory we have found microscopic tuberculosis in axillary lymph nodes as well as axillary metastases of carcinoma in a number of cases. The old concept that the two diseases are antipathetic to each other is certainly unsound.

RECURRING SUBAREOLAR ABSCESS

This is a special type of recurring low-grade infection of the subareolar region. It usually develops in younger women but has no relationship to lactation. Atkins emphasized its relationship to inverted nipples, but I have often seen the disease in women whose nipples were apparently normal.

The disease begins as a comparatively localized area of inflammation of the subareolar area which goes on to form a small abscess. It is usually treated ineffectively with antibiotics, and is finally incised and drained, if it does not rupture spontaneously. The small drainage sinus finally heals.

This cycle is repeated over and over again at intervals of a few months, sometimes over a period of years. A sinus often develops close to the base of the nipple, and closes intermittently, only to open again when the infection flares up.

Surgeons who do not understand the pathology of this lesion are sometimes driven to the desperate and entirely unnecessary extreme of excising a substantial sector of the central area of the breast together with the nipple, or even of amputating the breast.

In 1951 Zuska and his associates wrote a good clinical description of the disease, and recognized a basic fact of its pathology, namely, that the lining epithelium of the nipple duct or ducts leading down to the abscess undergoes squamous metaplasia. Unfortunately they confused this phenomenon with an entirely different breast lesion — so-called comedo-mastitis.

Atkins, a few years later, reported 28 cases. He emphasized the characteristic clinical features of the lesion and described his method of treatment, which consisted of laying open the diseased duct from the nipple surface to the abscess site, and allowing the wound to heal by granulation.

Patey and Thackray in 1958 wrote an excellent description of the squamous metaplasia of the nipple ducts which is regularly found in this disease, and described their method of local excision of the affected duct or ducts together with the abscess.

A paper by Toker describes the squamous metaplasia in more detail.

Kleinfeld has recently written an excellent description of the clinical features of the disease, its pathology, and its treatment.

To understand the pathology of the disease, the reader might refresh his knowledge of the anatomy of the nipple as shown in Figures 1–16, 1–17, and 1–18. The so-called milk sinuses, which are the terminal dilated portions of the main collecting ducts, have characteristic longitudinal accordion-like pleats which make it possible for them to dilate greatly and fill up with milk in nursing. They are normally lined with two layers of cuboidal epithelium. The milk sinuses extend the entire length of the nipple and terminate in funnel-shaped ampullae which open on the surface of the nipple. The ampullae are lined with squamous epithelium and in the resting breast are plugged with keratin debris.

In recurring subareolar abscess the milk sinus leading down to the abscess at the base of the nipple is greatly dilated. Its epithelium lining has undergone squamous metaplasia, and it is plugged with keratin. Figure 17–3 shows such a dilated milk sinus near the base of the nipple in a patient with recurrent subareolar abscess.

These abscesses often break through to the skin at the base of the nipple, and a sinus forms. This process is shown diagrammatically in Figure 17–4.

Our method of dealing with this disease is as follows. If the patient comes for consultation with an acute flare-up of the infection we drain the abscess as simply as possible. When the inflammation has subsided we do an elective excision under general anesthesia in the operating room. We use a circumareolar incision to turn up an areolar flap and expose the base of the nipple. We excise the diseased dilated milk sinus or sinuses within the nipple, together with the site of the previous abscesses and the surrounding fibrosis at the base of the nipple. We do not hesitate to excise the majority of the milk sinuses if it is not clear which are diseased.

This small operation, if carefully done, is almost invariably successful, and does minimal damage to the breast.

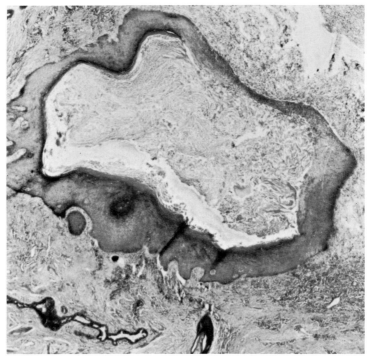

Figure 17-3. Dilated milk sinus lined with metaplastic squamous epithelium and filled with keratotic debris, in recurrent subareolar abscess.

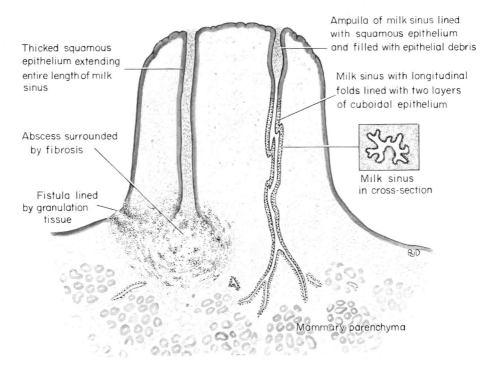

Thicked squamous epithelium extending entire length of milk sinus

Ampulla of milk sinus lined with squamous epithelium and filled with epithelial debris

Milk sinus with longitudinal folds lined with two layers of cuboidal epithelium

Abscess surrounded by fibrosis

Fistula lined by granulation tissue

Milk sinus in cross-section

Mammary parenchyma

Figure 17-4. Recurring subareolar abscess shown diagrammatically.

SARCOID OF THE BREAST

The localization of sarcoid in the breast is very unusual, even in the northern European countries where sarcoid is more frequent. Scott, as well as Stallard and Tait, have reported single cases from England, and Dalmark has described a third case from Denmark.

At the Francis Delafield Hospital we have had a patient with sarcoid in the breast, and generalized sarcoidosis.

S. C., a 53 year old Negro woman, was admitted to the hospital because of a lump in the left breast of two years' duration. Inquiry revealed no symptoms other than a progressive exertional dyspnea and a paroxysmal cough.

On physical examination her blood pressure was 200/120. A hard mass was palpable in the upper outer quadrant of the left breast with retraction of the overlying skin. An enlarged node was felt in the left axilla, and palpation of the neck and groins revealed a diffuse lymphadenopathy. The heart was enlarged but no abnormal physical findings were demonstrated in the lungs.

Serologic tests were positive for syphilis. A chest roentgenogram revealed cardiac enlargement, widening and calcification of the aorta, and an extensive infiltrative process in the right lung, with atelectasis of the right upper lobe.

The tuberculin skin test was negative, and several sputa were negative for acid-fast bacilli and tumor cells. Biopsy of the breast tumor and the internal mammary nodes in the upper three interspaces was performed. The breast tumor was a carcinoma. The internal mammary nodes contained no carcinoma, but a node from the first interspace showed sarcoid. A left radical mastectomy was done. The microscopic examination of the operative specimen revealed sarcoid in both the mammary gland and the axillary lymph nodes. Figure 17–5 shows the sarcoid in the mammary fat. The carcinoma was of limited extent in the breast, and had not metastasized to the axillary nodes.

After discharge from the hospital the patient's pulmonary symptoms increased. She was given a course of cortisone as antisarcoid therapy.

Three months after operation the patient developed an acute episode of abdominal pain for which she was readmitted as an emergency. She was thought to have a dissecting aortic aneurysm.

Treatment consisted of prophylactic digitalization, antibiotics, and cortisone, and within the next two months she showed a definite improvement. A chest roentgenogram showed considerable decrease of the pulmonary shadows.

She was readmitted for the third time seven months after operation, with another acute episode of pain involving the precordium and neck, and she expired soon after admission.

Postmortem examination revealed the cause of

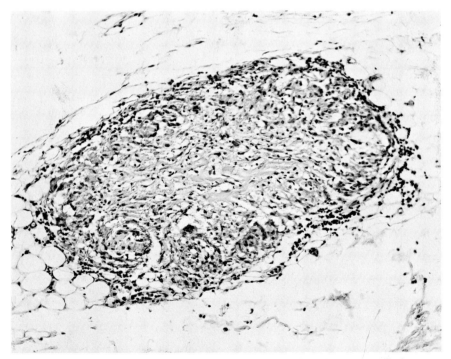

Figure 17–5.   Microscopic appearance of sarcoid in the mammary fat.

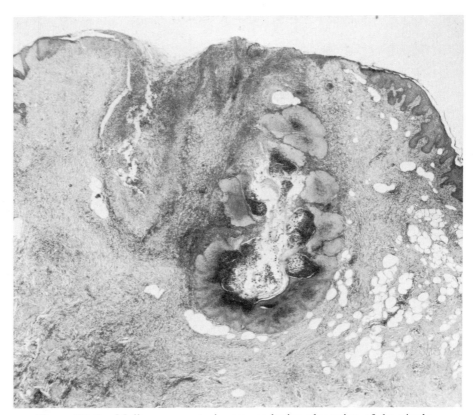

Figure 17–6.   Molluscum contagiosum producing ulceration of the nipple.

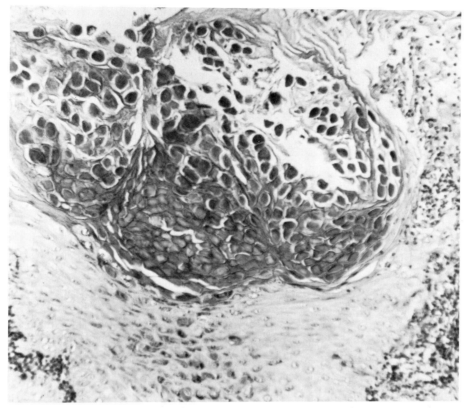

Figure 17–7. Characteristic molluscum bodies in the squamous epithelium of a dilated milk sinus in the nipple.

the death to be a dissecting aneurysm of the aorta. In addition sarcoidosis, involving the lungs, spleen, liver, lymph nodes, and tongue, was found.

MOLLUSCUM CONTAGIOSUM OF THE BREAST

Lattes has studied a unique example of molluscum contagiosum that occurred in the nipple of a middle aged woman. There was a small ulcer of the nipple surface, and beneath it the characteristic molluscum bodies were seen in the squamous lining of the dilated terminal portion of a milk sinus (Figures 17–6 and 17–7).

SYPHILIS OF THE BREAST

Both primary chancre and secondary gumma are so rarely seen in the breast, even in large clinics for syphilis, that their clinical characteristics are not well defined. The one feature of gumma that is common to most of the credible case reports is ulceration. The best descriptions, with good illustrations, of both lesions have been published by Kampmeier.

Reviews of previously reported cases of gumma of the breast, and descriptions of new cases, have been published by Adair, by Komori, by Braunstein and Woolsey, and by Whitaker and Moore. A good many of the reported cases must be regarded as of a doubtful nature. It is certainly impossible to differentiate gumma from other granulomatous processes on either clinical or microscopical grounds. In our laboratory Lattes takes the sound position that the only proof of gumma is the regression of the lesion with antisyphilitic treatment. We have no such acceptable case in our records.

HYDATID DISEASE OF THE BREAST

Hydatid cysts of the breasts have been described in countries in which the disease is endemic. Uriburu in Argentina, who is familiar with hydatid disease, observed only one hydatid cyst in a series of 1000 patients with breast disease. He pointed out that although Herrera-Vegas collected reports of 970 cases of hydatid disease in his 1901 book on the subject, only two patients had the disease in the breast.

Reddy and Rao have reported cases of hydatid disease of the breast from India.

RARE TYPES OF INFECTION IN THE BREAST

Some of the very rare types of infection in the breast, and the authors who have described them, follow: filariasis (McFee); blastomycosis (Köhlmeier and Kreitner); sporotrichosis (Jung); leprosy (Furniss); scleroderma (Coleman); and actinomycosis (Georgiades and Anezyres; Trempe).

REFERENCES

Adair, F. E.: Gumma of the breast; its differential diagnosis from carcinoma. Ann. Surg., 79:44, 1924.

Atkins, H. J. B.: Mammillary fistula. Brit. M. J., 2:1473, 1955.

Bernard, E., Delavierre, P., and Israël, L.: La tuberculose mammaire. Rev. de la tuberc., 25:366, 1961.

Braunstein, A. L., and Woolsey, R. D.: Gummatous mastitis. Am. J. Syph., Gonor. & Ven. Dis., 24:43, 1940.

Cheever, D.: Tuberculosis of the mammary gland. Surg. Clin. North America, 1:919, 1921.

Coleman, M.: Scleroderma simulating carcinoma of the breast. Brit. J. Surg., 25:61, 1937.

Dalmark, G.: Lymphogranulomatose bénigne. Acta Chir. Scandinav., 86:169, 1942.

Deaver, J. B., and McFarland, J.: The Breast: Its Anomalies, its Diseases, and their Treatment. Philadelphia, Blakiston, 1917.

Furniss, A. L.: Leproma in female breast presenting as carcinoma. Indian M. Gaz., 87:304, 1952.

Georgiadis, D., and Anezyres, N.: Primary actinomycosis of the breast. Hellen. Cheir., 8:803, 1961.

Grausman, R. I., and Goldman, M. L.: Tuberculosis of the breast. Am. J. Surg., 67:48, 1945.

Herrera-Vegas, M., and Cranwell, D. J.: Los Quistes Hidatídicos en la Republica Argentina. Buenos Aires, Ed. Coni Hermanos, 1901.

Jung: Disseminierte Gilchristsche Blastomykose und Sporotrichom der Mamma mit Bild- und Kulturdemonstration. Arch. f. Dermat. u. Syph., 191:482, 1950.

Kampmeier, R. H.: Syphilis of the breast; chancre and gumma. Am. Pract., 1:395, 1947.

Kleinfeld, G.: Chronic subareolar breast abscess. J. Florida M. A., 53:21, 1966.

Knight, I. C. S., and Nolan, B.: Breast abscess. Brit. M. J., 1:1224, 1959.

Köhlmeier, W., and Kreitner, H.: Blastomykose der Mamma. Wien. klin. Wchnschr., 65:13, 1953.

Komori, M.: Ueber einen Fall von Gumma der Brustdrüse. Zentralbl. f. Chir., 66:1441, 1939.

Leborgne, R.: Estudio radiológico de la mastitis tuberculosa. Tórax, 3:61, 1954.

McFee, W. F.: Filarial lymphatic varix of the breast. Ann. Surg., 94:135, 1931.

McKeown, K. C., and Wilkinson, K. W.: Tuberculous disease of the breast. Brit. J. Surg., 39:420, 1952.

Monro, J. A., and Markham, N. P.: Staphylococcal infection in mothers and infants. Maternal breast abscesses and antecedent neonatal sepsis. Lancet, 2:186, 1958.

Noack, H.: Die Mastitis puerperalis in der Penicillinära. Geburtsh. & Frauenh., 15:224, 1955.

Patey, D. H., and Thackray, A. C.: Pathology and treatment of mammary-duct fistula. Lancet, 2:871, 1958.

Reddy, D. J., and Rao, V. K.: Hydatid disease of the breast. Indian J. Surg., 21:253, 1959.

Sandison, A. T., and Walker, J. C.: Inflammatory mastitis, mammary duct ectasia, and mammillary fistula. Brit. J. Surg., 50:57, 1962.

Sawyer, C. D., and Walker, P. H.: A bacteriologic and clinical study of breast abscess. Surg., Gynec. & Obst., 99:368, 1954.

Schaefer, G.: Tuberculosis of the breast. A review with the additional presentation of ten cases. Am. Rev. Tuberc., 72:810, 1955.

Scherer, F.: Ueber die Tuberkulose der Brustdrüse. Deutsche Ztschr. f. Chir., 258:40, 1943.

Schultze-Jena, B. S.: Ueber die Tuberkulose der Brustdrüse in der Nachkriegszeit. Zentralbl. f. allg. Path. u. path. Anat., 88:52, 1951.

Scott, R. B.: The sarcoidosis of Bœck. Brit. M. J., 2:777, 1938.

Shipley, A. M., and Spencer, H. R.: Tuberculosis of the mammary gland. Ann. Surg., 83:175, 1926.

Smith, L. W., and Mason, R. L.: The concurrence of tuberculosis and cancer of the breast. Surg., Gynec. & Obst., 43:70, 1926.

Soltau, D. H. K., and Hatcher, G. W.: Some observations on the aetiology of breast abscess in the puerperium. Brit. M. J., 2:1603, 1960.

Stallard, H. B., and Tait, C. B. V.: Bœck's sarcoidosis. Lancet, 1:440, 1939.

Toker, C.: Lactiferous duct fistula. J. Path. Bact., 84:143, 1962.

Trempe, F.: Actinomycose mammaire primitive. Canad. J. Surg., 1:210, 1958.

Uriburu, J. V.: La Mama. Buenos Aires, Edit. Cientifica Argentina, 1957.

Verhaeghe, M., et al.: Quatre observations de tuberculose du sein. Lillechir., 15:187, 1960.

Villard, E., and Martin, J. F.: Coexistence de cancer et de tuberculose du sein et des ganglions axillaires. Bull. Assoc. Franç. p. l'étude du cancer, 22:128, 1933.

Whitaker, H. T., and Moore, R. M.: Gumma of the breast. Surg., Gynec. & Obst., 98:473, 1954.

Wilson, T. S., and MacGregor, J. W.: Tuberculosis of the breast. Canad. M. A. J., 89:1118, 1963.

Zuska, J. J., Crile, G., Jr. and Ayres, W. W.: Fistulas of lactiferous ducts. Am. J. Surg., 81:312, 1951.

Chapter Eighteen

Thrombophlebitis of the Superficial Veins of the Breast

One of the interesting aspects of clinical diagnosis is that comparatively infrequent lesions pass unnoticed until someone describes them well. Then at once many clinicians identify the lesion, and a rash of reports appear in the medical literature. So it has been with superficial phlebitis of the veins over the breast. Although good case reports of this disease were published in 1922 by Fiessinger and Mathieu in France, and by Williams and by Daniels in our country a decade later, this lesion is today called Mondor's disease because he described the clinical picture of the disease so well before his fellow Parisian surgeons in 1939. In 1947 Leger collected reports of 22 cases. More recently, good descriptions of cases have been published by Hughes, by Lunn and Potter, by Feldman et al., by Karlan and Traphagen, by Musgrove, by Johnson, Wallrich, and Helwig, by Oldfield, by Grow and Lewison, and by Honig and Rado.

Frequency

This lesion is apt to be regarded as disease of the breast and it thus comes to the attention of surgeons in breast clinics. In our own breast clinics where we see approximately 750 new patients with breast complaints yearly, only a half-dozen will have Mondor's disease. It is not a common lesion.

Etiology

Musgrove believes that trauma is responsible, because all three of his patients gave a definite history of local trauma. One carried a heavy typewriter under her arm, another swept vigorously in a curling game, while the third did strenuous exercises. Most case reports, however, do not mention any definite trauma, and in my own patients with the disease I have not been able to elicit a history of trauma.

An exception must be made for operative trauma; in a number of case reports the thrombophlebitis has developed about three weeks subsequent to excision of a benign breast lesion, and has affected a vein caudad to the operative site.

Almost one quarter of the patients with thrombophlebitis of the anterolateral chest wall have been males. In several of them there has been a history of local trauma.

In one of Lunn and Potter's five cases there was a coexisting, but presumably unrelated, carcinoma of the breast.

343

Diagnosis

The patient develops acute pain in the general region of the thrombosed vein, and, palpating the area, discovers a tender cord-like tumor. In the great majority of cases the vein that, together with its branches, is affected, is a superficial one which drains the lateral aspect of the breast and the hypochondrium. The anatomists have appropriately called it the thoracoepigastric vein. It extends diagonally upwards and laterally from the hypochondrium over the lateral aspect of the breast up to the lower end of the anterior axillary fold.

When the thrombophlebitis is well developed, one can see, in a good light and with the arm raised, a shallow groove extending upwards across the outer breast towards the axilla (Fig. 18–1). This groove is accentuated with slight caudad traction upon the anterolateral chest wall below the breast, as in Figure 18–2.

Palpation reveals a cord-like thickening beneath the groove or grooves. This is the thrombosed vein. The groove is produced by the fibrosis surrounding the vein, which pulls surrounding tissue in toward it, as well as actually shortening the vein so that it bowstrings.

The thrombosed vein is painful and very tender at the onset of the process. The tenderness gradually diminishes over a period of three or four weeks.

After six or eight weeks all trace of the lesion has usually disappeared.

In a small proportion of cases the vein affected is not one along the lateral aspect of the breast, but a vein or its branches extending from the lower inner sector of the breast toward the epigastrium.

The veins involved by the process are very

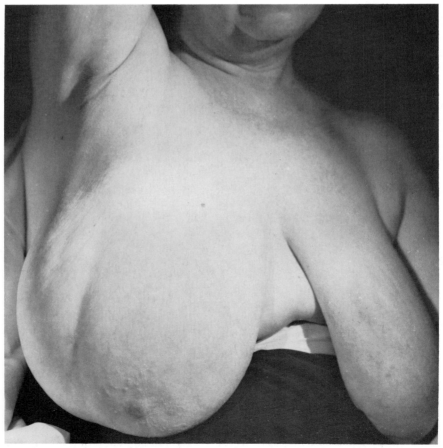

Figure 18–1. Thrombophlebitis of the thoracoepigastric vein producing a groove across the lateral aspect of the breast.

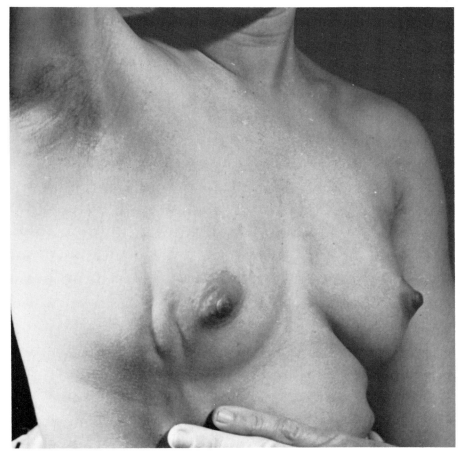

Figure 18–2.   Grooves across the lateral aspect of the breast, due to thrombophlebitis of branches of the thoracoepigastric vein, accentuated by caudad traction.

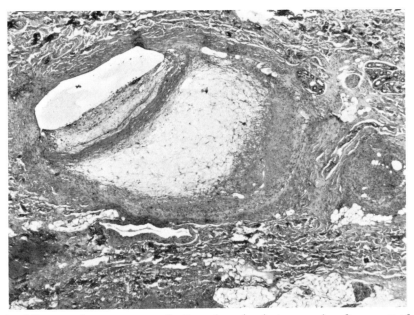

Figure 18–3.   Microscopic appearance of a thrombosed vein two weeks after onset of symptoms.

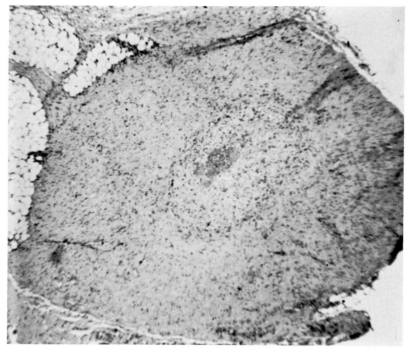

Figure 18–4. A later stage in the process of thrombophlebitis. The wall of the vein is greatly thickened and its lumen is replaced by a fibrous plug.

superficial. They lie only 3 or 4 mm. below the skin surface, just below the superficial layer of the superficial fascia.

Microscopic studies show that the involved vein is thrombosed. Figure 18–3 shows one of these veins excised two weeks after the onset of the disease. When the process is older, as in another excised vein, shown in Figure 18–4, the wall of the vein is greatly thickened, and its lumen replaced by a fibrous plug.

Treatment

Mondor's disease is self-limited, and requires no treatment. Since the diagnosis is usually obvious I have not done a biopsy of the lesion in the patients I have seen.

The importance of the lesion is only that it may be confused with carcinoma or some other lesion of the breast, and a biopsy done unnecessarily.

REFERENCES

Daniels, W. B.: Superficial thrombophlebitis; a new cause of chest pain. Am. J. M. Sc., *183*:398, 1932.

Feldman, S., Mahl, M., Friedman, D., and Dunewitz, A. L.: Mondor's disease. New York State J. Med., *54*:387, 1954.

Fiessinger, N. and Mathieu, P.: Thrombo-phlébites des veines de la paroi thoraco-abdominale. Bull. et mém. Soc. méd. d. Hôp. de Paris. *46*:352, 1922.

Grow, J. L. and Lewison, E. F.: Superficial thrombophlebitis of the breast. Surg., Gynec. & Obst., *116*:180, 1963.

Honig, C. and Rado, R.: Mondor's Disease — superficial phlebitis of the chest wall. Ann. Surg., *153*:589, 1961.

Hughes, E. S. R.: Sclerosing peri-angiitis of the lateral thoracic wall. Australian and New Zealand J. Surg., *22*:17, 1952.

Johnson, W. C., Wallrich, R., and Helwig, E. B.: Superficial thrombophlebitis of the chest wall. J.A.M.A., *180*:103, 1962.

Karlan, M., and Traphagen, D. W.: Superficial phlebitis of the breast. Am. J. Surg., *94*:981, 1957.

Leger, L.: Phlébite en cordon de la paroi antéro-latérale du thorax. Presse méd., *55*:859, 1947.

Lunn, G. M., and Potter, J. M.: Mondor's disease (subcutaneous phlebitis of the breast region). Brit. M. J., *1*:1074, 1954.

Mondor, H.: Tronculite sous-cutanée subaiguë de la paroi thoracique antéro-latérale. Mém. Acad. de chir., *65*:1271, 1939.

Musgrove, J. E.: Subcutaneous phlebitis of the breast (Mondor's Disease). Canad. M.A.J., *85*:36, 1961.

Oldfield, M. C.: Mondor's disease. A superficial phlebitis of the breast. Lancet, *1*:994, 1962.

Williams, G. A.: Thoraco-epigastric phlebitis producing dyspnea. J.A.M.A., *96*:2196, 1931.

Chapter Nineteen

Spontaneous Necrosis of the Breast

Spontaneous necrosis of the breast is a lesion so rare that it hardly deserves a separate chapter, yet it cannot properly be included with any other breast lesion.

It consists of massive necrosis of the most dependent portion of the breast—or usually both breasts—presumably on the basis of thrombosis. It has come to light only since anticoagulant therapy with dicumerol has been employed. Verhagen, in 1954, reported 13 examples of superficial necroses of soft tissues following the use of this drug. In one of his patients the breast was affected. In 1961 Kipen reported three cases of breast necrosis. In two patients the necrosis was unilateral. In the third patient there was almost total gangrene of both breasts.

Sustersic, in 1962, described a case in which a patient with chronic heart disease was given both sulphonamide and penicillin. She developed necrosis of the most dependent portions of both breasts. The exact cause remained unknown.

We have no examples of spontaneous breast necrosis in our clinic.

REFERENCES

Kipen, C. S.: Gangrene of the breast—a complication of anti-coagulant therapy. New England J. Med., *265*:638, 1961.
Sustersic, Z.: Ueber eine spontane beiderseitige Nekrose der Mamma. Chirug, *33*:485, 1962.
Verhagen, H.: Local haemorrhage and necrosis of the skin and underlying tissues during anti-coagulant therapy with Dicumarol or Dicumacyl. Acta med. Scandinav., *148*:453, 1954.

Chapter Twenty

The Frequency and Age Distribution of Mammary Carcinoma

An appreciation of the true frequency of a disease is basic in the attack upon it. Clemmesen is the foremost modern student of the epidemiology of cancer, and his observations on this subject are worth the reader's attention. The two basic types of data needed are of course mortality data and incidence data. Although the registration of deaths and certification as to the causes of death became obligatory in most western countries toward the end of the last century, reasonably accurate mortality data have been available for less than 50 years. Data as to the actual incidence of the various forms of cancer are much more recent. The first effective national registry for cancer was established in Denmark under Clemmesen's leadership in 1942. Similar cancer registries were established in England in 1945, in Norway in 1952, in Finland in 1953, in Iceland in 1954, and in Sweden in 1958. In the United States a comprehensive cancer registry for the state of Connecticut was organized in 1935; another for the State of New York (exclusive of its largest cities) was organized in 1940; and a limited one for the State of California was set up in 1942. The incidence data from the Connecticut registry are the most complete in the United States, and I will rely chiefly upon them in the present discussion.

348

Mortality from Breast Cancer

The World Health Organization began, in 1956, to publish death rates for mammary carcinoma for a number of countries, and Pascua reviewed them and made some interesting observations. In 1966 Segi published the mortality data for the years 1950-1963 for cancer of the breast from 24 selected countries, and computed death rates by age adjusted to a Japanese standard population. His study emphasizes the striking variations in the toll of breast cancer in different countries. I reproduce Segi's chart comparing the age-adjusted death rates for breast cancer in 24 countries for the years 1964-65 (Chart 20-1), as well as his chart showing the trend of mortality rates between 1950 and 1965 in 18 selected countries (Chart 20-2).

There are, of course, several secondary factors that may have a considerable influence in determining the death rate from breast cancer. The educational status of women, reflecting the stage of advancement at which breast cancer is diagnosed, as well as the expertness of treatment, may play a considerable role. Nevertheless, there is no escape from the fact, so well shown in Segi's data, that breast cancer is very much less frequent in Japan than in most countries. It is

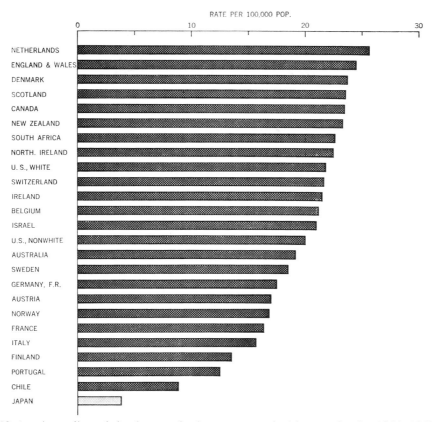

RATE PER 100,000 POP.

Chart 20-1.   Age-adjusted death rates for breast cancer in 24 countries for 1964–1965 (Segi).

equally evident from Segi's data that breast cancer has recently been increasing in some western countries such as Iceland, Germany, Austria, and Italy.

During the past decade there have also been a number of reports of the frequency of breast cancer in ethnic groups not included in Segi's study (Smith and his associates—Navajo; Strode—Hawaii; Prates—Mozambique; Annamunthodo—Jamaica; Piyaratn—Thailand; Higginson and Oettlé—South Africa; Muir—Singapore; Shani and his associates—Israel; Habibi—Iran; Chaklin—Russia; Sobin—Afghanistan).

Mammary carcinoma in our own country is one of the great diseases. In 1966 there were 27,304 deaths from it. In order of frequency as a cause of death in women it stands fifth, as shown in Table 20-1. Among forms of cancer in women it is exceeded as a cause of death only by cancer of the digestive system.

Those who rely entirely on death rates have stated that we are not making any prog-

ress with the control of breast cancer in the United States. That this is not true is shown by a study of the incidence rates for the disease.

Table 20-1.   SOME LEADING CAUSES OF DEATH AMONG WOMEN IN THE UNITED STATES, 1966

Cause	Rate per 100,000	Number
Atherosclerotic heart disease	226.5	226,336
Cancer of digestive organs	44.6	44,527
Hypertensive heart disease	30.7	30,697
Influenza and pneumonia	28.1	28,050
Cancer of breast	27.3	27,304
Diseases of the arteries	26.6	26,575
Diabetes	20.4	20,434
Motor vehicle accidents	14.5	14,475
Cancer of cervix and corpus	13.5	13,396
Cancer of respiratory system	9.5	9,448
Cirrhosis	9.3	9,314
Tuberculosis	2.0	2,023

Source: Vital Statistics of the United States (1966) Vol. II, Mortality, Part A. Table 1–22, U.S. Department of Health, Education and Welfare, Public Health Service, National Center for Health Statistics.

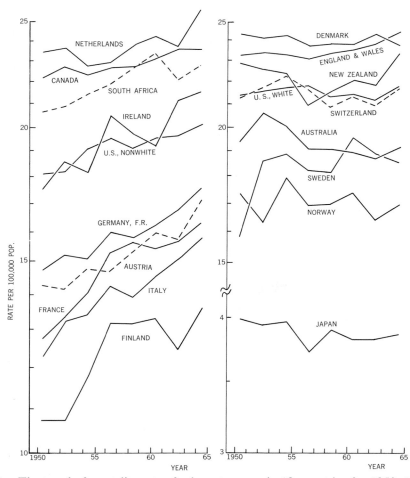

Chart 20–2. The trend of mortality rates for breast cancer in 18 countries for 1950–1965 (Segi).

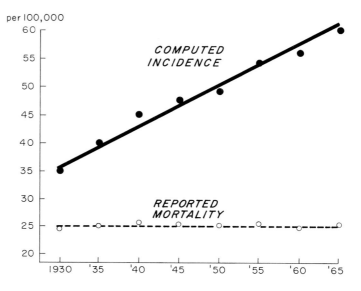

Chart 20–3. Computed age adjusted incidence rates for breast cancer in females in Connecticut compared with age-adjusted mortality rates for breast cancer in the United States (Schneiderman-Biometry Branch, National Institutes of Health).

The Incidence of Breast Cancer

Incidence rates have several advantages over death rates in studying breast cancer. Mortality rates take no account of the cured patients. Mortality and incidence rates for specific age groups can be computed, but in a slowly progressing disease like breast cancer the age of onset is necessarily somewhat earlier than the age of death.

The best indication that we are making progress in the control of breast cancer in our country comes from a comparison of age-adjusted mortality rates and incidence rates for this disease. In Chart 20–3 the computed age-adjusted incidence rates for Connecticut are plotted against the United States age-adjusted mortality rates. It is true that the death rates for the last 35 years have changed very little. But the incidence rates over the same period of time have risen strikingly. There is no escape from the conclusion that we are curing a higher proportion of women with the disease, either because it is recognized at an earlier and more curable stage, or because our methods of treatment have improved. This is an encouraging fact.

Age Distribution Studies

Below the age of 25 breast cancer is so infrequent — only about 0.2 per cent of the patients with the disease are in this group — that it has no practical importance. It begins

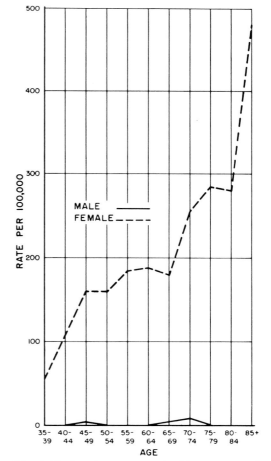

Chart 20–4. Age-specific incidence rates for breast cancer in Connecticut, 1964.

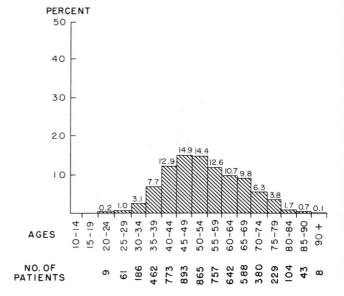

Chart 20–5. The age distribution of 6000 patients with breast cancer. Columbia-Presbyterian Medical Center, 1916–1966.

to have a considerable frequency after the age of 30, and steadily increases throughout the remainder of the life span. Chart 20-4 shows the age specific incidence rates for breast cancer in Connecticut in 1964.

Since the number of patients that we see in the more advanced age groups is smaller, the actual number of old patients who come to us with breast cancer is smaller. Chart 20-5 shows the distribution by age of 6000 patients with mammary carcinoma coming to our clinics between 1916 and 1966.

One of the interesting and unsolved phenomena regarding the age at which women get breast cancer is the occurrence of a break or pause in the steadily rising incidence of the disease with advancing age, which occurs about the time of the menopause. Clemmesen discovered this phenomenon in his 1948 analysis of the Danish registry data. There was a slight but definite depression between 47 and 52 years, in the steeply ascending incidence curve. This "hook" in the incidence rate has been found in data from many other sources.

De Waard and his associates, studying this bimodal age distribution of breast cancer in the data of the Netherlands Cancer Registry, have concluded that the bimodal age distribution can be explained by the fact that breast cancer patients can be divided into two groups as regards hormonal equilibrium. One group consists of patients with adrenocortical estrogen disturbance as evidenced by obesity, hypertension, and decreased glucose toler-

ance. The second group of patients do not have these symptoms.

In Clemmesen's latest Danish data for the years 1935-1957, the "hook" persists (Chart 20–6). It is most pronounced in ever married

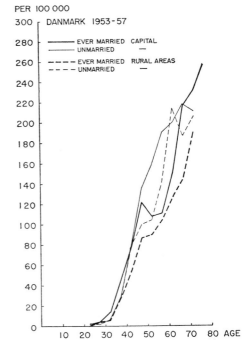

Chart 20–6. Incidence rates for breast cancer in Danish women at various ages (Clemmesen).

women, and was absent in unmarried women, living in Copenhagen. It is less pronounced in women from the rural areas. Clemmesen suggests that this "hook" phenomenon is, in some as yet unknown manner, associated with the menopause.

REFERENCES

Annamunthodo, H.: Observations on cancer of the breast in Jamaica. West. Ind. M.J., 7:93, 1958.

Average annual incidence rates per 100,000 population by age and site, 1945-47, 1949-51. Bureau of Cancer Control, 2 mimeographed reports, Albany, State of N.Y., Dept. of Health.

Cancer in Connecticut, 1935-1962. Hartford, Connecticut, State Department of Health, 1968.

Cancer Registration and Survival in California. State of California, Department of Public Health, 1963.

Chaklin, A. V.: Geographical differences in the distribution of malignant tumours. Bull. W.H.O., 27:237, 1962.

Clemmesen, J.: Carcinoma of the breast. Symposium. I. Results from statistical research. Brit. J. Radiol., 21:583, 1948.

Clemmesen, J., and Nielsen, A.: The social distribution of cancer in Copenhagen, 1943-1947. Brit. J. Cancer, 5:159, 1951.

Clemmesen, J.: Statistical Studies in the Aetiology of Malignant Neoplasms. Copenhagen, Munksgaard, 1965, Vol. 1.

Cutler, S. J.: The role of a population-based registry in the epidemiology of cancer of the breast. In Segaloff, A., Meyer, K. K., and DeBakey, S.: Current Concepts in Breast Cancer, Baltimore, Williams and Wilkins, 1967, page 10.

Denoix, P. F., et al.: Documents statistiques sur la morbidité par cancer dans le monde. Monographie de l'institut national d'hygiène, no. 1, Paris, Ministère de la santé publique, 1952.

de Waard, F., Baanders-van Halewijn, E. A., and Huizinga, J.: The bimodal age distribution of patients with mammary carcinoma. Cancer, 17:141, 1964.

Dorn, H. F., and Culter, S. J.: Morbidity from cancer in the United States; I. Variation in incidence by age, sex, race, marital status, and geographic region. Public Health Monograph, no. 29, Washington, U.S. Dept. of Health, Educ., and Welfare, 1955.

Epidemiological and Vital Statistics Report, Vol. V, nos. 1 & 2, Jan., Feb., 1952. World Health Organization, Geneva, 1952.

Gerhardt, P. R., Goldberg, I. D., and Levin, M. L.: Incidence, mortality, and treatment of breast cancer in New York State. New York State J. Med., 55:2945, 1955.

Habibi, A.: Cancer in Iran. J. Nat. Cancer Inst., 34:553, 1965.

Haenszel, W.: Cancer mortality among the foreign-born in the United States. J. Nat. Cancer Inst., 26:37, 1961.

Higginson, J., and Oettlé, A. G.: Cancer incidence in the Bantu and "Cape Colored" races of South Africa: report of a cancer survey in the Transvaal (1953-55). J. Nat. Cancer Inst., 24:589, 1960.

Lilienfeld, A. M., and Johnson, E. A.: The age distribution in female breast and genital cancers. Cancer, 8:875, 1955.

Muir, C. S.: Male and female genital tract cancer in Singapore. Cancer, 15:354, 1962.

Pascua, M.: Trends of female mortality from cancer of the breast and cancer of genital organs. Bull. W.H.O., 15:5, 1956.

Pirquet, C.: Allergie des Lebensalters, Leipzig, Georg Thieme, 1930.

Piyaratn, P.: Relative incidence of malignant neoplasms in Thailand. Cancer, 12:693, 1959.

Prates, M.: Malignant neoplasms in Mozambique. Brit. J. Cancer, 12:177, 1958.

Segi, M., Fujisaku, S., and Kurihara, M.: Geographical observation on cancer mortality by selected sites on the basis of standardised death rate. Gann, 48:219, 1957.

Segi, M., and Kurihara, M.: Cancer Mortality for Selected Sites in 24 Countries. Sendai, Japan, Tohoku Univ. School of Medicine, 1966.

Segi, M., and Kurihara, M.: Cancer in Japan from the viewpoint of geographical pathology. Tohoku J. Exp. Med., 72:169, 1960.

Shani, M., Modan, B., Steinitz, R. and Modan, M.: The incidence of breast cancer in Jewish females in Israel. J. of Israel Med. Assn. (Hebrew), 71:337, 1966.

Smith, R. L., Salsbury, C. G., and Gilliam, A. G.: Recorded and expected mortality among the Navajo, with special reference to cancer. J. Nat. Cancer Inst., 17:77, 1956.

Sobin, L. H.: Cancer in Afghanistan. Cancer, 23:678, 1969.

Strode, J. E.: Tumors of the breast occurring in Hawaii. Ann. Surg., 144:872, 1956.

Steiner, P. E.: Cancer, Race and Geography. Baltimore, Williams and Wilkins, 1954.

Stiner, O.: Die Sterbefälle an Brustkrebs in der Schweiz von 1091 bis 1934. Bull. schweiz. Vereinig. f. Krebsbekämpf., 2:102, 1935.

Stocks, P.: Studies of cancer death rates at different ages in England and Wales in 1921 to 1950: Uterus, breast, and lung. Brit. J. Cancer, 7:283, 1953.

Chapter Twenty-One

The Etiology of Breast Cancer

Carcinoma of the breast is one of the types of cancer concerning which a considerable amount of knowledge bearing on its causation has been accumulated. We do not yet know its ultimate cause but we have identified a number of factors which influence its occurrence.

The Comparative Biology of Breast Carcinoma

Mammary carcinoma occurs in only a few species of wild or domesticated mammals. It is seen rarely in rats and rabbits. It is frequent only in mice and dogs, species which, it must be pointed out, live in association with man, the only other mammal afflicted with the disease.

The general characteristics of mammary carcinoma are so similar in the mouse, the dog, and in man, that it is very likely that the etiology of the disease is the same in all three species. To begin with, the natural history of the disease, its localized origin from the mammary epithelium, its regional spread, and its metastases, are similar in all three species, although the disease evolves more slowly, and is less likely to metastasize and can therefore be said to be less malignant, in the dog and the mouse than in man. Histologically, the disease has similar basic histologic features in all three species. It is true that special forms of epithelial metaplasia—squamous metaplasia, cartilaginous metaplasia and sarcomatoid metaplasia—occasionally seen in mouse carcinomas, and frequently seen in dog carcinomas, are a rare phenomenon in human carcinoma of the breast.

As the century turned, Jensen of Copenhagen learned how to transplant mammary carcinoma occurring spontaneously in the mouse. In 1903 he reported transplantation through 19 generations of mice over a period of two and a half years. His experiments opened the modern epoch of experimental cancer research, and particularly, research concerning breast carcinoma.

Mammary carcinoma in the mouse was at once seized upon as a means of studying cancer in general. The research was carried on mainly in three laboratories: at the Pasteur Institute in Paris by Borrel, at Paul Ehrlich's new Institute for Experimental Therapy at Frankfurt am Main, and in the London laboratories of the Imperial Cancer Research Fund. Ehrlich was soon diverted from cancer research to the chemotherapeutic attack upon trypanosome disease. Bashford and Murray, who organized the English laboratory in 1904, persevered and made it the first modern laboratory devoted exclusively to cancer research. As such it was the forerunner of the many cancer research laboratories of today. Bashford and Murray began with a study of animal tumors in general and went on to an intensive and prolonged investigation of the mouse tumors, including mouse mammary carcinoma. The most important finding from this period of cancer research was that the disease is transplanted by living carcinoma cells. They will live only in animals of the same species, and best in animals of the same strain. Their growth characteristics do not change during countless transplantations and vicissitudes. The mouse mammary carcinoma has become the standard experimental tool of the modern cancer research worker, upon which he tests the effects of all types of therapeutic agents. Provided that he transplants a mammary carcinoma of known character, using a careful standard technique, into a "pure" strain of mice, it is a remarkably reliable experimental tool.

The value of mouse mammary carcinoma as an experimental tool has been greatly enhanced by careful selective brother to sister inbreeding. Strains of mice have been developed in which the incidence of spontaneous mammary carcinoma is very high—as high as 95 per cent of the females developing the disease. Similarly, strains of mice have been bred in which only a fraction of 1 per cent develop the disease. Maude Slye deserves the credit for this basic discovery, the result of long years of patient work in her Chicago laboratory. Many of these high and low mammary carcinoma strains of mice are now bred in laboratories all over the world. Even after hundreds of generations of selective breeding they cannot be said to be genetically pure, and will revert toward a common type unless the selective breeding is continued.

The rat has recently become an interesting experimental means of studying mammary carcinoma. Although adenofibromas occur spontaneously in selected strains of aged rats (Curtis, Bullock, and Dunning) breast carcinoma is exceedingly rare. Shay and his associates discovered in 1949 that mammary carcinoma could be induced in rats by the gastric instillation of methylcholanthrene. Huggins and his associates have used this method to study the influence of various hormonal factors upon the disease.

Although mammary carcinoma is very common in dogs the disease has not been much studied experimentally, probably because the life cycle of the dog is so long, and the expense of maintaining a dog colony so considerable.

I shall attempt to review our present knowledge of the several etiologic factors in carcinoma of the breast in animals as well as in man, including those of proven significance as well as those of only theoretical importance.

The Mammary Tumor Virus

In 1936 Bittner made the remarkable discovery that in mice the development of mammary carcinoma is dependent upon a factor transmitted by the mother in her milk to her offspring. Mice from a low mammary carcinoma strain, foster-nursed by a mother of a high mammary carcinoma strain, developed the disease with a high frequency. The converse was equally true: foster nursing of high mammary carcinoma strain mice by mothers belonging to a low mammary carcinoma strain markedly diminished the frequency of the disease in them. Bittner concluded from his discovery, which was soon confirmed in other laboratories, that an extrachromosomal factor present in the milk played an important part in the transmission of mammary carcinoma.

The next and obvious step was to identify, isolate, and characterize this factor, which was probably a virus. At Columbia University a team of chemists, physicists, and biologists began work on the problem soon after Bittner's discovery.

We had the advantage of a large and carefully controlled mouse colony, including two selectively inbred strains, ideally suited for studying the mammary tumor virus. One was our RIII strain of white mice which I had originally obtained from Lacassagne's Paris laboratory in 1933. About 90 per cent of the females of this high mammary carcinoma strain develop the disease. Our contrasting strain was the C57 black strain which I had obtained in 1935 from H. J. Bagg. In this strain mammary carcinoma very rarely occurs.

It soon became apparent from our own studies as well as from those of a number of other laboratories that the milk factor was a virus. It is present in the mammary carcinoma tissue itself, as well as in the mouse tissues in general, and in blood, although only in a very limited amount. By far the best source of the factor, however, is mouse milk. Andervont proved that the factor is present in semen and that it can be transmitted in this medium from male to female.

In experimental work the virus, whether obtained from milk or from tumor tissue, is ordinarily injected intraperitoneally into test animals of a known low mammary carcinoma strain. A remarkable feature of the milk factor is its long latent period, for if the experimental induction of the disease is to be successful, mice no more than two, or at the most three, weeks of age must be used. Mammary carcinoma then develops at a mature age for the mouse, at a mean of approximately twelve months.

Dan H. Moore, who directed the physical studies carried out by our group, eventually found better facilities to continue them at Rockefeller University. He has recently moved to new and enlarged laboratories at the Institute for Medical Research, Camden, New Jersey, where our Columbia RIII and C57 strains of mice are re-established.

In Moore's view it has now been firmly established that mouse mammary carcinoma is transmitted by a virus, which is easily recognized in the electron microscope. It usually proliferates in the mammary epithelial cells but can, occasionally, be found also in the male genitalia. By cross-breeding of strains, it can be shown that some males of strains having a very high incidence can transmit the disease to the offspring. Foster nursing of high mammary tumor strains on mothers who do not have the virus usually causes a large drop in the tumor incidence but does not completely eradicate it. The data indicate that a weak form of the virus can be in some way carried by the ovum, possibly by genome integration. The amount of ovum transmission varies greatly in different strains of mice.

Moore and his associates, Charney and Sarkar, have recently described the chemical and morphologic characteristics of the virus, and their methods of isolating, purifying, and transmitting it. During the last year they have greatly improved their procedures for quantitating the biological activity of the virus. The assay time has been reduced from over a year to under two months. This has resulted from development of methods for obtaining large quantities of highly purified virus from mouse milk, and from the production of strong antiviral rabbit serum.

The confirmation of the role of a virus in the transmission of mammary carcinoma in mice at once raises the question of a virus being the cause of human breast cancer. Is there enough evidence of the possibility that a mother may transmit the disease to her child by breast feeding to discourage the practice?

In his early efforts Moore failed to find the mammary tumor virus in human milk, but during the past two years he has identified it in 6 per cent of the samples of milk from 100 American women who did not have a family history of breast cancer. In milk from 10 other American women with a family history of breast cancer the virus particles were seen in 60 per cent. They were present in 39 per cent of the samples of milk from 46 Parsee women, members of the closely interbred Bombay sect who have a great deal of breast cancer.

There is very little direct evidence that breast feeding transmits mammary cancer in women. Wood and Darling described a remarkable family in which the occurrence of numerous breast carcinomas in four generations had a suggestive relationship to nursing history. I have taken careful nursing histories on my patients with breast carcinoma ever since Bittner's discovery, and I am convinced that most women do not know whether or not they were breast-fed. The milk virus, if it does exist in human beings, is certainly such a small particle that putting an infant to breast even once would be enough to transmit it. We have induced mammary carcinoma in mice by feeding 1 drop of milk to a young mouse. In studying the question in human beings we need to know that the individual was never put to breast even once. Patients do not know such details of their infancy. They often are ignorant of whether or not they were ever nursed in the conventional sense of the word. A long-range inquiry on the influence of nursing in the subsequent lives of present-day infants is being carried out at the University of Minnesota but it will be at least 50 years before their data can begin to have any meaning. Until there is more solid evidence on this point I believe that we must continue to encourage breast feeding because of its known advantages for both mother and child.

The Induction of Breast Cancer by Chemicals

The polycyclic hydrocarbons were first shown to induce mammary cancer in virus-free female mice by Bonser and Orr in 1939. They injected methylcholanthrene subcutaneously and obtained breast cancer. Later they also induced breast cancer with the same chemical instilled intranasally and painted on the skin. As I have already mentioned, Shay and his associates in 1949 induced breast cancer in rats by gastric instillation of methylcholanthrene.

Breast cancer has also been induced in mice with dimethylbenzanthracene (Howell, Marchant, and Orr), and with dibenzanthracene and benzpyrene (Jull).

Some of the aromatic amines produce cancer of the breast in mice (Armstrong and Bonser), and rats (Cantarow, Stasney, and Paschkis).

A great deal of experimental work has been done in mice and rats in which the polycyclic hydrocarbons have been administered in conjunction with various procedures modifying the hormonal physiology. The results of these studies are best described in the monograph *Human and Experimental Breast Cancer* by Bonser, Dossett, and Jull, who did much of the original work.

These polycyclic hydrocarbons which induce breast cancer in small laboratory animals have a structural similarity to the steroid hormones. Some of the hydrocarbons have physiologic effects in animals similar to those produced by estrogens. For example, benzanthracene and benzpyrene produce vaginal keratinization in mice.

Much more chemical and physiologic work must be done before any conclusions regarding breast cancer in humans can be drawn from these experimental studies in animals.

The Inheritance of Breast Carcinoma

The discovery of the mouse mammary carcinoma virus, and proof that it is the principal factor in transmitting the disease in mice have not obscured the fact that hormonal influences and genetic factors are also concerned. The importance of genetic factors has been shown by Heston and his associates, who freed C3H high mammary cancer strain mice of the virus by caesarian delivery and foster nursing by mothers of a strain that did not carry the virus. Nevertheless, 38 per cent of these mice developed breast carcinoma, and transmitted it to successive generations.

In further studies of the gene control over the transmission of mouse mammary carcinoma, Heston and his associates presented evidence that several genes are concerned.

In human beings a genetic factor in breast cancer, if it exists, is not concentrated and defined by long-continued inbreeding, and we should expect it to be less apparent. Never-

theless, careful studies of the occurrence of the disease in special families have revealed some very convincing data. For example, in 1866, the distinguished French surgeon, Paul Broca, who had a deep interest in anthropology and heredity, reported the incidence of cancer in his own family. He traced the cause of death of all 38 members of five generations of his family who died between 1768 and 1856. Ten of the 24 women died of cancer of the breast. Since then many family histories have been reported in which breast cancer is abnormally frequent. One of the most extensive of these studies of the history of breast cancer in a family is that carried out by Stephens and his associates for Kindred 107. Thirteen cases of breast cancer have been found in this family, all concentrated in four of its eight branches. The disease was inherited by the females as a simple Mendelian dominant trait.

Among the case histories of my own patients I have encountered several instances of striking familial prevalence of breast cancer. Three such family pedigrees are shown in Chart 21-1.

Statistical studies of the incidence of mammary carcinoma in relatives of women with the disease have been made during the last half century. This type of investigation presents great difficulties. In most studies, the incidence of breast cancer in the relatives of patients with cancer of the breast is obtained by questioning the patient or her relatives. The data in unit case histories of patients recorded by house staff and medical students are neither accurate nor complete enough to be useful. Only data obtained by a special interrogation of patients who know their family history are reliable. But even within these limitations the information is incomplete because many patients' relatives, particularly mothers, aunts, sisters, and daughters, are still alive at the time of investigation and may develop mammary cancer later on in life. The ultimate incidence of the disease in the patient's relatives must therefore be higher than this type of contemporary study reveals.

If, on the other hand, statistical study of the familial aspect of mammary cancer is based upon data obtained only from death certificates, it is likely that the occurrence of the disease in a number of women who were operated upon and cured will remain undiscovered because death certificates do not reveal such facts. Proportional mortality rates for mammary cancer in the general population

PEDIGREES OF BREAST CARCINOMA FAMILIES

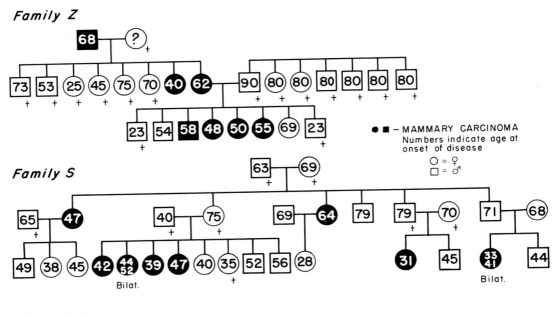

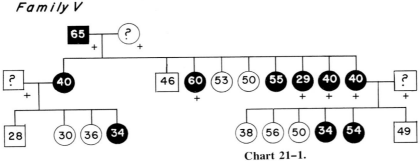

Chart 21–1.

are unreliable as a guide to the actual frequency of the disease for the same reason. Some statisticians are inclined to ignore the fact that a considerable proportion of mammary cancers are cured. Retrospective death certificate studies therefore also fail to reveal the whole truth regarding the familial character of the disease.

The problem of finding entirely suitable series in which to study the incidence of the disease in controls from the same ethnic, social, and economic groups as the probands is so great that it has defeated most investigations.

In view of these difficulties in obtaining adequate data regarding the familial inheritance of mammary carcinoma it is not surprising that statistical studies have led to different conclusions. It is, however, worthwhile to review briefly the most important of these studies. Waaler's Norwegian study (1932) consisted of an investigation of the causes of death in relatives of some 6000 patients with cancer, and a comparison of these data with the mortality for cancer in the Norwegian population as a whole. He found the incidence of cancer of the breast was much greater among sisters of patients with this disease than it was among sisters of patients with cancer, but not of the breast.

Wainwright, in 1931, reported a study of the frequency of cancer in parents, brothers and sisters of 784 women treated for mammary carcinoma. He used 576 well females between the ages of 45 and 70 as controls. Carcinoma of the breast was four times as frequent in mothers of patients with carcinoma of the breast as in the mothers of controls. Wainwright's study, although representing great personal effort, was not adequately controlled.

Wassink, in 1935, reported results of an extensive investigation of the frequency of cancer in the parents, brothers, sisters, grandparents, and first cousins of 660 Dutch women with mammary carcinoma. These 660 had a total of 301 relatives with cancer of all sites, of whom 192 were women and only 109 men. One hundred and twelve (59 per cent) of the 192 female relatives had mammary carcinoma. This finding represents a marked increase in cancer of the breast in female relatives of women with cancer of the breast. In the Dutch female population as a whole mammary cancer forms only 10 to 12 per cent of cancers of all sites in females.

Jacobsen, in his 1946 monograph *Heredity in Breast Cancer* described a detailed genealogical study of the families of 200 women with mammary cancer treated in Copenhagen hospitals. His investigations included grandparents, parents, uncles, aunts, brothers, and sisters. Among female relatives there were 71 cases of cancer of the breast, representing 35 per cent of cancers developing in all sites. In Jacobsen's control series of families of 200 women not having cancer, only eight cases of mammary cancer were found, representing only 18.6 per cent of all the cancers developing in all sites. Jacobsen's calculations showed the difference in the incidence of cancer of the breast in the two groups to be three times the standard error of the difference, and he concluded that it is "overwhelmingly probable that the development of cancer of the breast is due to hereditary predisposition." Jacobsen's data were subsequently studied and re-computed by Busk, Clemmesen, and Nielsen, and his main thesis confirmed. Busk also demonstrated that when a woman has a cancer of the right breast, her mother and sisters are predisposed not only to develop the disease but to develop it in the right rather than the left breast.

In 1948, Penrose, Mackenzie, and Karn reported their findings in a study of the occurrence of mammary cancer in the families of 510 patients with mammary cancer from University College Hospital and the London Hospital. They compared the observed and expected deaths from breast cancer among mothers (whose age at death was known) of 406 of their patients with this disease. The expected deaths were based upon the proportionate mortality for the disease in England and Wales according to age. Twenty-five patients' mothers died of cancer of the breast, although only 11.2 deaths would have been expected from this disease. Penrose and his associates therefore concluded that a familial predisposition does exist.

Smithers and associates followed the same method that Penrose used to study the familial pattern of cancer of the breast in data of the Royal Cancer Hospital. Among a total of 556 patients there were 29 whose mothers had died of the disease, although only 13.9 such deaths would have been expected. Smithers and his associates also concluded that there is a familial predisposition to breast cancer.

Buccalossi, Veronesi, and Pandolfi, in 1954, interviewed 230 of their patients with cancer of the breast in the National Cancer Institute of Milan to determine the frequency of the disease in relatives. They then compared their findings with the incidence of breast cancer as recorded in the family pedigrees of an equal number of controls who did not have mammary cancer. They did not state that their controls were strictly comparable, on social and economic levels, with their patients. However, they reported three times as many cases of cancer of the breast among relatives of their cancer patients, as among the relatives of their controls.

Woolf, in 1955, studied the frequency of cancer of the breast as recorded in death certificates, in mothers and sisters of Utah women who had died of cancer of the breast. Among 200 mothers four died of mammary cancer, although only 2.09 such deaths would have been expected on the basis of proportionate mortality rates in the United States. Among 561 sisters eight died of this disease although 3.19 such deaths would have been expected.

Anderson and associates reported, in 1958, a study of the frequency of cancer of the breast in relatives of 544 women with the disease from the University of Minnesota Hospitals, and in a control group consisting of relatives of the husbands of their patients. They obtained information by interviews and letters, as well as from death certificates. They compared the observed numbers of cases in relatives of patients who had cancer of the breast with the expected number of cases as determined by morbidity and mortality rates, and by a combination of the two, as well as with the observed number of cases in relatives of their controls. They could not prove that there was a higher rate of mammary cancer among mothers of their patients, but sisters showed a significantly higher incidence of the disease.

Macklin, in 1959, relied upon death certificates to determine the incidence of mammary cancer in relatives of 295 Columbus, Ohio, women who had cancer of the breast, and in relatives of a control series of women who had cancer elsewhere than in the breast, and in the relatives of another control series of women who did not have cancer. She chose controls as best she could from similar social, economic, and cultural levels. Macklin also made elaborate studies of expected mammary cancer rates based upon U.S. mortality data. Among the mothers of her patients with breast cancer Macklin found 11 with the disease as compared with 5.6 expected. In her cancer-free control series only three mothers developed mammary cancer as compared with 4.58 expected. Eleven sisters of her mammary cancer patients developed the disease when only 4.47 were expected. In her cancer-free control series 3 sisters developed mammary cancer as compared with 2.79 expected cases. Macklin concluded that cancer of the breast is significantly more frequent in relatives of women who have the disease.

Murphy and Abbey, in 1959, reported a study of the frequency of mammary cancer in two generations of women. One series of 200 women had mammary cancer. A control series did not have the disease. The patients with cancer of the breast were from Philadelphia hospitals, and the controls were dental school patients. The data were obtained from interviews, hospital records, and death certificates. Murphy and Abbey concluded that their study revealed no statistically significant differences in frequency of breast cancer in mothers and sisters of the patients in their two series.

Commenting on the lack of unanimity among these students of the heredity of mammary cancer, Clemmesen, who is the leading modern authority on the statistical aspects of cancer, states: "It is difficult to avoid the impression that the scale of such studies . . . has not yet reached a size matching their task. . . . Nevertheless, as a general conclu-

sion it would seem that heredity of breast cancer has in man been found too often to be explained as due to coincidental occurrence, and is probably as real as in the mouse."

In the hope of adding helpful data regarding the familial character of mammary carcinoma I began many years ago questioning patients regarding their family history. Not all patients know their family histories well enough to supply reliable information, so that some selection of data has been necessary. Nevertheless I have reasonably dependable information from a total of 1802 patients with mammary cancer regarding the occurrence of the disease in their families. The majority of patients were private, but they came from a wide variety of ethnic, social, and economic groups.

The diagnoses in relatives who had a breast removed for what was stated to have been cancer have not been checked by records from other hospitals, and no search of the cause of death in death certificates has been made. The magnitude of such a task has been beyond me.

Although the unit case histories in our hospital go back to 1916 and provide an exceptionally complete body of data regarding breast cancer, they do not provide information that helps much in questions related to heredity. The diversity of ethnic groups and the shifting unstable nature of some elements of the new York City population also present great handicaps in studying heredity.

We also lack a satisfactorily matched control series of family histories of women who did not have mammary cancer. Ethnic origin, social and economic status, age, marital status, parity, breast feeding history, and history of endocrine therapy, are some factors which should be matched in selecting a control series. No student of the problem has yet provided a control series in which all these fundamentally important factors are satisfactorily matched.

The simplest of the many different aspects of familial inheritance is the frequency of the disease in mothers, daughters, and sisters of the women who develop it. My data concerning this relationship are summarized in Table 21–1.

The fact that 9 per cent of the mothers of my patients with mammary carcinoma had the same disease is a striking indication of its familial character. We know that between 4 and 5 per cent of parous women in this coun-

Table 21–1. Breast cancer in the mothers, daughters, and sisters of female patients with breast cancer*

Patients with breast cancer who gave a reliable family history	1,802
Patients with breast cancer who did not have a history of breast cancer in the family	1,337
Patients with breast cancer whose mothers had had breast cancer	162, or 9 per cent
Patients with breast cancer who had daughters who had developed breast cancer	14 (15 daughters)
Patients with breast cancer who had sisters who had developed breast cancer	138 (159 sisters)

*Modified from Papandrianos, E., Haagensen, C. D., and Cooley, E.: Ann. Surg., *165*:10, 1967.

try today develop carcinoma of the breast. Nine per cent is therefore twice the normal frequency of the disease.

There is good reason for believing that this is a minimal, not a maximal, figure. Cancer of the breast is the most easily recognized of all cancers and is so rarely confused with other breast lesions that the possible error in diagnosis is of no statistical importance. Many of the mothers of my patients were still alive at the time I obtained the family history by interviewing the patient, and it is likely that some of them will have developed cancer of the breast subsequently. A much higher pro-

portion of the sisters of my patients were still alive and exposed to the risk of developing the disease subsequently. Anderson and his associates reported that a third of the sisters of their probands were still living at the time their study was carried out. Any estimate of the expected incidence of breast carcinoma in sisters of patients with this disease therefore becomes much more problematical.

It is possible to compare my findings regarding the frequency of breast carcinoma in mothers and daughters, as well as sisters, with the findings of others who have studied the question in comparatively large series of patients. Table 21–2 shows the data of Penrose and Smithers who used death certificates as a basis for their studies, as well as Anderson's data, and my own data, both of which were based upon interviews with patients and relatives.

It is difficult to explain the divergence between Anderson's findings and my own. Both data were obtained by interviewing patients and their relatives. There was, however, one difference in the method employed. My data were obtained from the patient at the time of her initial medical consultation. Anderson's data were obtained at a separate interview of the patient by a nonmedical questioner, subsequent to her initial medical consultation and usually after she had been operated upon.

Age of Onset

One aspect of the familial pattern as revealed in my data which I wish to present in more detail, is the age at which the disease appears.

Table 21–2. Mammary carcinoma in mothers and sisters of probands with mammary carcinoma*

Author	Type of Data	No. Probands	Observed No. Mothers	Expected No. Mothers	Observed No. Sisters	Expected No. Sisters
Penrose, McKenzie and Karn	Death cert.	406	25 (6.1%) of (406)	11.12	23 (7.5%) of (307)	6.97
Smithers *et al.*	Death cert.	556	29 (5.2%) of (556)	13.9	16 (3.5%) of (460)	not est.
Anderson, Goodman, and Reed	Interviews and death cert.	440	9 (2%) of (440)	13.9	48 (4.3%) of (1,108)	30.2
Papadrianos, Haagensen, and Cooley	Interviews	1,802	162 (9.0%) of (1,802)	not est.	159	not est.

*From Papadranos, E., Haagensen, C. D., and Cooley, E.: Ann. Surg., *165*:10, 1967.

In 1948, two years after Jacobsen had published his monograph on *Heredity in Breast Cancer*, his colleague Busk reviewed the original data and gave special attention to age of onset of the disease in probands with cancer of the breast and their female relatives. In Jacobsen's data there were 22 pairs of mothers and daughters with cancer of the breast, and the daughters developed the disease at a mean age of 10.3 years earlier than their mothers. Morse, in 1951, noted almost exactly the same difference of age of onset in a series of 13 mothers and daughters in our data.

Bucalossi and Veronesi, in 1957, reported the age of onset in 58 pairs of mothers and daughters. It averaged 4.17 years earlier in the daughters.

Busk calculated the correlation coefficients for the ages of onset of breast cancer in the probands and their female relations in his data. He found statistically significant differences in the ages of onset for groups of mothers and daughters, paternal aunts and nieces, and grandmothers and grand-daughters. But he was "doubtful whether they indicate a tendency of anticipation in the material."

Anderson and his associates also discussed this question of the age of onset in the relatives of their probands with the disease and concluded that they had no evidence that the disease develops earlier in daughters of mothers who have it.

Thus there remains some doubt as to whether or not the transmission of a predisposition to mammary cancer carries with it a tendency to develop the disease at an earlier age. The statistical demonstration of this difference in age of onset is complex. It must be kept in mind that carcinoma of the breast increases in frequency with advancing age,

and that the daughters in this mother-daughter relationship tend to be younger than their mothers at the time the study is carried out. Other daughters of the same mothers may still be alive and well, but some may develop cancer of the breast when they are older. This would change somewhat both the ultimate incidence and the mean age of onset of the disease in the daughters as a group. Some surviving mothers, even though the number still alive at the time of the study is much smaller, may also subsequently develop mammary cancer, and this would change, but to a lesser degree, the ultimate incidence and the mean age of onset of the disease in the mothers as a group. The ideal way of getting at the true incidence of breast cancer and its true age of onset in both mothers and daughters would be to use data from families in which the mother and all her daughters are dead, and to supplement information from death certificates with information gathered by interviews with surviving members of the family. But death certificates do not give the age of onset of breast cancer when it is the cause of death, and I have already pointed out above that death certificates alone are not an adequate guide because they do not reveal the occurrence of mammary carcinoma in those who were cured of it. And surviving members of present-day American families can usually supply information as to the occurrence of disease only in their own immediate relatives. This is particularly true of those who have migrated from abroad.

Table 21-3 presents my own data concerning age of onset of mammary carcinoma. It will be seen that 25.8 per cent gave a history of mammary carcinoma occurring in female relatives. Unfortunately, I lack the exact age of onset of the disease in a good many of the

Table 21–3.   AGE OF ONSET OF MAMMARY CARCINOMA IN PATIENTS WITH FEMALE RELATIVES OF DIFFERENT GENERATIONS WHO ALSO DEVELOPED THE DISEASE*

	Number	Per cent	Average Age
1. Female patients with mammary carcinoma interviewed	1,802	100.0	52.3
2. Those reporting no known mammary carcinoma in female relatives	1,337	74.2	52.8
3. Those reporting mammary carcinoma in one or more female relative	465	25.8	50.9
4. Those reporting mammary carcinoma in female relatives of an earlier generation (grandmothers, mothers or aunts)	306	17.0	48.7
5. Those reporting mammary carcinoma only in members of a succeeding generation (daughters, nieces, granddaughters)	17	0.9	68.4
6. Those reporting mammary carcinoma in members of their own generation (sisters or cousins) but not in those earlier generations	142	7.9	53.8

*From Papadrianos, E., Haagensen, C. D., and Cooley, E.: Ann. Surg., *165*:10, 1967.

relatives of my patients, but I nevertheless have enough data on the question of age of onset to be of interest.

The mean age of onset in my entire series of patients with mammary carcinoma was 52.3 years. It was 52.8 years in those who did not have a history of mammary carcinoma in their female relatives. It was 50.9 years in those who reported the occurrence of mammary carcinoma among female relatives. This difference of less than two years is barely significant statistically. But the mean age of onset in those reporting mammary carcinoma in female relatives of an earlier generation—that is, grandmothers, mothers, and aunts—was only 48.7 years. The difference between 52.8 and 48.7 years is highly significant statistically.

In my data there were a total of 182 pairs of mothers and daughters with mammary carcinoma developing at a known age. This total number of pairs results from adding to the

Table 21–4. AGE (IN YEARS) OF ONSET OF MAMMARY CARCINOMA IN MOTHERS AND DAUGHTERS.*

Mother	Daughter	Mother	Daughter	Mother	Daughter	Mother	Daughter
37	23	55	41	73	40	65	44
55	28	53	41	78	43	60	44
50	30	55	42	78	47	65	44
51	30	60	42	49	46	50	65
60	32	49	42	62	39	75	44
57	32	43	42	63	38	32	45
49	32	76	42	65	30	69	45
37	33	68	42	65	47	74	47
62	34	53	43	75	44	74	50
65	34	59	43	84	57	78	47
45	35	58	43	85	54	78	43
63	35	65	43	91	36	65	49
50	36	69	43	53	30	65	32
41	36	54	44	45	53	65	40
62	36	50	44	50	29	36	49
62	36	56	44	50	29	75	52
60	37	52	44	38	32	69	53
58	37	73	44	50	33	51	54
54	37	85	44	53	33	51	50
50	37	50	44	60	34	35	58
37	37	34	45	60	28	35	45
50	37	54	45	52	34	35	61
58	38	55	45	52	42	68	58
65	47	55	55	68	82	40	37
54	47	69	56	68	55	50	37
50	47	73	56	68	60	37	39
64	47	61	56	62	48	70	40
61	47	60	56	62	50	60	42
48	47	54	57	62	55	68	67
74	47	75	58	72	76	57	68
76	47	80	58	50	76	70	59
55	48	62	58	60	79	70	61
44	48	51	58	88	88	57	64
69	48	64	59	52	38	85	66
26	49	65	59	52	35	85	56
54	49	42	59	50	39	40	45
62	49	52	60	37	39	65	45
73	49	80	60	42	39	51	46
89	49	69	60	54	40	61	46
60	50	54	62	60	40	77	46
60	50	70	62	59	51	66	68
60	50	70	62	44	52	38	69
49	50	73	63	45	53	35	70
63	50	53	64	50	54	92	72
52	50	71	66	75	55	50	75
50	50	80	67				

Total number pairs of mother and daughter—182; mean age of mothers 59.7 years, mean age of daughters 47.5 years.
*From Papadrianos, E., Haagensen, C. D., and Cooley, E.: Ann. Surg., *165*:10, 1967.

pairs of patients and their mothers, additional pairs of sisters of patients and mothers of patients, as well as pairs consisting of patients and their daughters. Table 21–4 lists these data. The mean age of the mothers was 59.7 years; that of the daughters 47.5 years. This difference of 12.2 years is convincing evidence that mothers with mammary carcinoma pass on to their daughters a likelihood of developing the disease at an earlier age than they themselves get it. No matter how statisticians may interpret these data they are all too real to be ignored.

To my data regarding the age of mammary carcinoma for pairs of mothers and daughters, we should add the evidence regarding the age of onset of the disease for the aunts of my patients who developed it. This is presented in Table 21–5.

A comparison of the age of onset in mammary cancer developing in mothers, with the age of onset in maternal aunts, of my patients with the disease, is of special interest in terms of the etiology of mammary cancer. A mother and a maternal aunt may be assumed to have the same genetic constitution, and if the ages of onset of mammary cancer in both show a similar difference as compared with the age of onset in the patient (daughter and niece, respectively) this fact might be used as an argument for a genetic mechanism of transmission. If, however, mammary carcinoma is transmitted from mother to daughter by a virus present in mother's milk, then a difference in the age of onset observed between the patient and her mother would not be expected between the patient and her maternal aunt.

My data concerning the age of onset of mammary carcinoma in both paternal and maternal aunts of my patients with the disease are shown in Table 21–5. There were 66 pairs of maternal aunts and nieces who developed the disease at a known age. These maternal aunts were an average of 10.6 years older than their nieces when they got the disease. The age of onset in paternal aunts was 10.7 years higher on the average than that of their nieces, but there were only 32 such pairs with known ages in my data.

The fact that the age of onset of mammary cancer in mothers and aunts of my patients is similar, being approximately 11 to 12 years older than the age of onset in our patients, suggests that the disease is transmitted by a genetic mechanism rather than by a virus in the mother's milk.

Table 21–5.   AGE OF ONSET OF MAMMARY CARCINOMA IN AUNTS AND THEIR NIECES[*]

Aunt	Niece	Aunt	Niece
Maternal Aunts			
60	33	b55	46
75	33	81	48
48	37	70	48
42	38	b70	48
50	35	72	52
b50	42	42	53
56	37	70	54
65	39	79	50
65	40	b59	50
33	41	60	52
70	42	b60	52
45	43	75	52
36	44	50	55
68	40	55	57
60	42	60	59
65	43	50	56
50	44	b50	45
56	45	50	60
55	45	62	60
52	45	70	61
76	46	62	60
50	46	75	67
65	47	78	68
63	43	47	44
55	39	59	50
47	39	73	40
47	40	58	54
50	48	55	68
65	48	55	71
60	49	65	79
83	49	b65	79
60	45	50	83
61	46	60	45
Paternal Aunts			
50	34	57	52
30	33	50	53
50	35	92	54
35	40	47	57
45	40	59	57
45	42	b59	41
70	46	80	54
49	46	50	65
70	47	55	70
60	49	50	32
58	49	44	36
57	45	b45	36
63	46	65	44
b63	40	42	40
c63	49	47	31
70	48	47	33

Total number of pairs of maternal aunts and their nieces—66; mean age of maternal aunts 60.6 years, mean age of nieces 50.0 years.

Total number of pairs of paternal aunts and nieces—32; mean age of paternal aunts 56.0 years, mean age of nieces 45.3 years.

[*]From Papadrianos, E., Haagensen, C. D., and Cooley, E.: Ann. Surg., 165:10, 1967.

It is also of interest to compare the age of onset of mammary carcinoma in my patients with the age at which it developed in their sisters. Ninety of my patients reported the ages at which a total of 106 of their sisters had developed the disease. The age of onset in my patients was 51.5 years; it was 49 years in their sisters. This is not a statistically significant difference, and it is what might be expected in sisters, for they should have the same genetic constitution and environmental background.

My conclusion is that mammary carcinoma is a familial disease. When it appears in a family the succeeding generation of women are not only predisposed to develop it, but they develop it approximately 10 to 12 years earlier. Clinicians should be alert to these possibilities.

The fact that the difference in age of onset between mothers and daughters, and aunts and nieces, is similar, is an argument in favor of a genetic rather than a viral mechanism for the transmission of mammary cancer.

From my data I venture to suggest two other conclusions which I cannot substantiate statistically because of the infrequency of the phenomena. I suggest that when there is a strong family history of breast carcinoma the males as well as the females develop the disease with an abnormally high frequency. It will be noted that in Chart 21–1 which presents the pedigrees of three such families there were a total of 25 individuals with breast carcinoma, of which three were males. This is a ratio of 12 males to 100 females with the disease rather than the ratio of 1 male to 100 females which occurs in the general population.

My second conclusion is that the women in these breast cancer families have an abnormally high frequency of bilateral breast cancer. This is more difficult to prove but I have the impression that it is true.

Twin Studies

Theoretically the study of the occurrence of breast cancer in twins should provide an important test of the role of a genetic factor in the disease. In monozygotic twins the proportion of cancers of the breast in both of the twins should be higher than in dizygotic twins if the genetic factor is responsible.

Macklin was one of the first, in 1940, to review reports of the occurrence of neoplasms in twins. She found two reports of breast cancer in both twins in a total of 53 pairs of monozygotic twins who developed tumors. Among 35 pairs of dizygotic twins who developed tumors, there were likewise two female pairs in whom both twins had breast cancer. Macklin herself collected 17 examples of tumors developing in twins. Both twins in one of her 10 pairs of monozygotic twins had breast cancer. None of the seven pairs of dizygotic twins had the disease.

Nielsen and Clemmesen in 1958 reported their studies of a total of 336 pairs of Danish twins. They found only one pair of monozygotic female twins, both of whom had cancer of the breast. There were no pairs of dizygotic twins with breast cancer.

Harvald and Hauge in 1963 reported another study of an even larger number of Danish twins. Among 164 pairs of monozygotic twins in whom cancer developed, there were 4 pairs in whom both twins had cancer of the breast. Among 340 pairs of dizygotic twins of the same sex with cancer, there were six pairs in whom both twins had breast cancer.

Clemmesen has concluded that neither of the Danish studies of large numbers of twins has revealed statistically significant support for the concept that genetic factors play an important role in the transmission of cancer.

Parity and Breast Carcinoma

The effect of parity upon the development of mammary carcinoma varies in different strains of mice. In the well-known A strain, for example, the incidence of the disease is high in mice that are bred, but very low in unbred mice. In the C3H mice and in our own RIII strain the incidence of the disease is very high in the breeders, but in unbred mice it is diminished by about one-third.

Bagg showed that the interference with the normal mammary gland function in mice which occurs when the newly born litters are removed from the mother and she is at once again bred increases the incidence of mammary carcinoma in mice of low–mammary carcinoma strains.

Parity protects women against mammary carcinoma. It has been known since 1842, when Rigoni-Stern studied the occurrence of breast cancer in Verona, that the disease is more frequent in unmarried women and in nuns. In a modern counterpart of Rigoni-Stern's study, Taylor, Carroll and Lloyd surveyed the records of three orders of nuns in Massachusetts and New York, and in 1959 reported that the lifetime risk of breast cancer in nuns is between 1.4 and 1.5 greater than it is for women in the total population.

In 1926 Lane-Claypon reported a study of a variety of features in a series of 508 women with breast cancer from London and Glasgow hospitals, and in 509 controls. She found a higher proportion of single women in her series of cancer patients than in her series of controls. In the cancer series those who had married were married later, and they had fewer children, full allowance being made for their age at marriage and the duration of marriage.

Gilliam in 1951 studied the marriage and pregnancy records of 849 patients with breast cancer in New York, Missouri, and New Orleans hospitals. He found that as a group they had fewer pregnancies and fewer live births than women in the general population.

In two English studies of large series of hospital patients with breast cancer (Harnett's 2529 cases and Smithers' 1762 cases) approximately 22 per cent of the patients were unmarried. This is significantly higher than the expected figure of 17 per cent of unmarried women in the general English population.

Logan in 1953, studying English mortality data for breast cancer, found that the mean annual death rate for that disease for married women with children was 52.6 per 100,000, whereas the rates for single, and married childless women with the disease were 74.6 and 69.7, respectively. An important aspect of his findings was the fact that in women under the age of 35 the breast cancer–fertility relationship is reversed; the rate for married women with children was 3.5 per 100,000, as opposed to 2.1 for single women, and 2.5 for married, childless women.

In 1955 Dorn and Cutler reported similar findings in a study of United States mortality data for breast cancer. They found that married women under the age of 30 are as likely to succumb to the disease as single women, but that married women between the ages of 30 and 65 consistently have a lower death rate from breast cancer than do single women.

Lilienfeld in 1956 reviewed the relationship of the frequency of breast cancer to marital status as reported in the New York State Cancer Registry. He found that the age-specific incidence rates were almost identical for single and married women up to the age of 40. Thereafter, breast cancer was more frequent in single women.

Versluys reviewed the Dutch data on this question in 1955. He found that after the age of 45, Dutch single women more often die of breast cancer than those who are married, and that a low mortality rate for the disease is correlated with a high fertility.

Van der Werff, studying Belgian data in 1956, reported that single women and married women without children have more breast cancer than women with children.

Segi and his associates in 1957 found that in their series of 577 Japanese patients with breast cancer the proportion of single women was greater than it was in the general population, in all age groups. Their patients with breast cancer also married later and had fewer children than women in the general population.

Norwegian data concerning 1548 women with breast cancer published by Rennaes and Holan confirm the greater frequency of the disease in unmarried as compared with married women (Chart 21–2), and also the great diminution of the frequency of the disease as the number of children increases (Chart 21–3).

Schwartz, Denoix, and Rouquette studied 284 French patients with breast cancer and 568 controls paired for social status, and reported that the cancer patients had fewer children and a shorter total lactation period than the controls.

Stocks, in 1957, reviewing the official mortality data for England and Wales, reported that when the mortality for breast cancer was taken as 100, the comparative mortality for single women was 136, that for infertile married women 139, and that for fertile married women 93.

Maurer and Minder in 1958, studying 2001 patients with breast cancer treated in Erlangen and Bern, found that single women were more predisposed to the disease than married women.

Clemmesen's Danish Cancer Registry data regarding the incidence of breast cancer are the most extensive available. They show that below the age of 35 unmarried women have somewhat less breast cancer than married women, but that after 35 the disease is considerably more frequent in unmarried women.

The fact that the incidence of breast cancer decreases with the number of children is so well-established that MacMahon in 1958 was

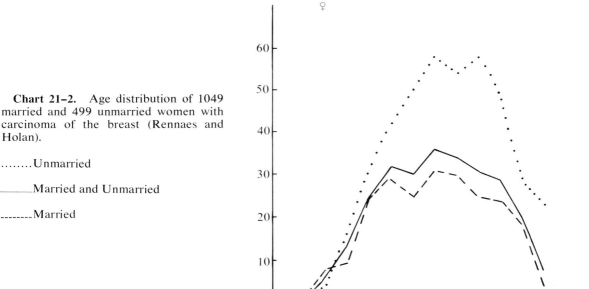

Chart 21–2. Age distribution of 1049 married and 499 unmarried women with carcinoma of the breast (Rennaes and Holan).

........Unmarried

_____Married and Unmarried

-------Married

led to study the relationship of the rising incidence of breast cancer during recent decades to contemporary changes in fertility rates in England, Wales, and Connecticut. He found that in all these areas the number of live births per 100,000 women has been rising since about 1906. He concluded that the increasing incidence of breast cancer cannot be explained by changes in fertility.

Among the most interesting contributions regarding carcinoma of the breast are the studies of Indian women by Khanolkar and Paymaster. Indians are sharply divided by the caste system into groups with different

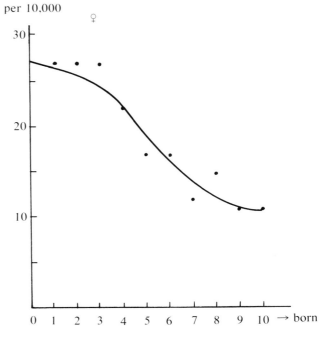

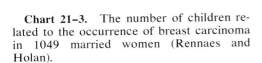

Chart 21–3. The number of children related to the occurrence of breast carcinoma in 1049 married women (Rennaes and Holan).

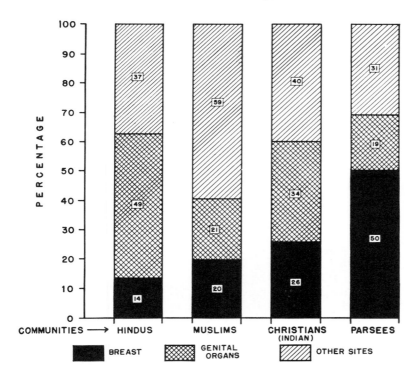

Chart 21–4. The frequency of different forms of cancer in Indian social groups, according to Paymaster.

economic and social traditions and customs. The Parsees are a small group with close interbreeding. They are well-to-do, marry late, at an average age of 25, and have few children, whom they often do not nurse. Hindu women are poor, marry early, at an average age of 16, and have numerous children, whom they usually nurse. Breast cancer is much more frequent in Parsee women, as Paymaster's chart shows (Chart 21–4).

Menstruation and Breast Cancer

There is no evidence that the origin of carcinoma of the breast is associated with any functional hormonal derangement in the women who develop it. We do not have any proof that they have increased production of estrogen or progesterone. There are, however, convincing data showing that women who develop mammary carcinoma have had an abnormally long menstrual life, with more menstrual cycles. If we accept the hypothesis that with each menstrual cycle there is a phase of hormonal growth stimulus to the mammary epithelium, and that abnormal repetition of this cyclic growth stimulus might be an etiologic factor in mammary carcinoma, the fact that women who develop the disease

have had more cycles than those who do not develop it merits our attention. The number of menstrual cycles that a woman in a primitive society has is comparatively small because she becomes pregnant as soon as she is fertile, and thereafter does not often menstruate because she is usually pregnant or nursing a baby. We know that breast carcinoma is more frequent in women who have no children and in those who have their first child late in life, that the likelihood of the disease diminishes as the number of children increases, and that breast feeding protects the mother to some degree against breast cancer. All of these factors, excepting the age of the mother at the time the first child is born, obviously limit the total number of menstrual cycles.

We do have a good deal of data as to the duration of menstrual life in women with breast carcinoma. In 1926, Lane-Claypon studied this question and found that the total duration of menstrual life in her series of 233 patients with breast cancer was longer than in women in her control series. Wainwright, in his duplication of Lane-Claypon's inquiry, found that the menopause was on the average 1.3 years later in his 401 patients with cancer than in his 402 controls who did not have the disease. Heiberg and Heiberg reviewed the menstrual histories in a series of 517 Danish women with breast carcinoma and concluded that the menopause occurred later in this group than in normal women. Olch reached a similar conclusion from a review of the case histories of 342 women with breast cancer. Smithers reported the mean total duration of menstrual life in a series of 290 women with breast cancer to be 34.6 years, which is significantly longer than that of Lane-Claypon's breast cancer series as well as Lane-Claypon's control series.

Bucalossi and his associates compared the total duration of menstrual life in 4000 patients with breast cancer in their Milan Cancer Institute with the duration of menstrual life in 2788 patients who did not have breast cancer, and found it to be slightly longer for the former. MacMahon and Feinleib, in 1960, published a study of the age at which menopause occurred in 340 New York City patients with mammary carcinoma, and in a carefully matched group of clinic patients who did not have the disease. They found that the menopause occurred significantly later in the breast cancer patients.

In the same year, Wynder, Bross, and Hirayama published another epidemiologic study of breast cancer, including data regarding menstruation. Their main data were based upon interviews with 632 New York Memorial Hospital Caucasian patients with breast cancer, and an equal number of controls who did not have the disease. There was no significant difference as regards the age of puberty in the two groups, but the menopause occurred on an average ten months later in the breast cancer patients.

This study included a small subgroup of 116 Japanese women with breast cancer, and an equal number of matched controls. A remarkable feature of the histories of those Japanese women of both groups was the short total length of their menstrual life. It was only about two-thirds that of American women, who have much more breast cancer.

Breast Feeding

One of the most interesting questions we face today is the role of breast feeding in the etiology of breast cancer.

It was during the Jurassic period, about 160,000,000 years ago, that mammals evolved on our planet. Their mammary glands provided a superior source of food for their progeny, and gave mammalian offspring an important advantage in the struggle for existence. Today we are abruptly abandoning this practice of breast feeding which goes so far back in our biologic heritage. My daughter, Mrs. Alice Gerard, in her recent book on breast feeding, has emphasized the fact that as recently as 50 years ago the overwhelming majority of women nursed their children. From her study of breast feeding in our Columbia-Presbyterian Medical Center, she estimates that only about 3 per cent of American women in metropolitan areas today nurse their babies for as long as six months. It would be strange if this abrupt and drastic change in breast function did not have some repercussion in terms of breast disease.

Until recently there has not been much dependable data correlating the risk of developing breast cancer with the number of children nursed and the length of time they were breast-fed. Lane-Claypon, in 1926, carefully studied these questions in a series of 213 patients with breast cancer in London and Glasgow hospitals and in 245 control mothers who did not have the disease. She found that 14.6 per cent of the children in the cancer series had not been breast-fed, whereas only 7.4 per cent of the children in the control series had not been nursed.

Smithers recalculated her results, including stillbirths and correcting the cancer series to the same family size distribution as the controls, and the difference between the two series was still about 7 per cent. Her own study of the lactation histories of 321 mothers with breast cancer in the Royal Cancer Hospital gave a figure of 18.63 as the percentage of children not breast-fed.

Wainwright in 1931 duplicated Lane-Claypon's study in hospital patients in New York and Pennsylvania, interviewing 665 women with breast cancer and 539 controls who did not have the disease. Wainwright found that 28.2 per cent of the married women in his cancer series had not nursed while only 15.7 per cent of the women in his control series had not nursed.

In the early 1960's several more detailed studies of breast feeding were published. MacMahon and Feinleib studied 258 patients with breast cancer and an equal number of controls matched for eight variables, and found no significant differences in the two groups of women as regards the total duration of nursing and the proportion of women in each group who nursed.

Table 21–6. Results of matched study of breast cancer cases and controls

	Breast Cancer	Controls
Mean months nursed	17.8 ± 1.43	22.2 ± 1.18
Mean years menstruated	29.1 ± 0.40	27.6 ± 0.48
Mean age at natural menopause	49.7 ± 0.28	47.2 ± 0.39
Mean age at artificial menopause	41.6 ± 1.04	40.4 ± 0.92

Levin, M. L., et al.:Amer. J. Public Health, *54*:580, 1964.

Wynder and his associates studied the significance of nursing in 632 New York Memorial Hospital patients with breast cancer and 1235 control patients. He reported no significant difference in the proportion who had not breast-fed children — 22 per cent of the cancer patients had not done so as compared with 23 per cent of the controls.

This same study included the results of Hirayama's interviews with 116 Japanese women with breast cancer and an equal number of controls matched for age. The controls had nursed considerably longer than the cancer patients. In both groups of women the proportion of women who nursed their babies was very high, 96 per cent in the cancer group and 97 per cent in the control group.

During the same year, Kamoi published a special study of the relation of breast cancer to lactation in 816 Japanese women with the disease and 1239 controls. In patients over the age of 40 Kamoi found that the total lactation period was significantly longer in the controls than in the cancer patients.

There have been other studies from the Far East and Middle East that suggest that breast feeding has a role in the development of breast cancer. Marsden reported that in Malaya the disease is more frequent in Chinese and Malayan women. It is appreciably less frequent in Indian women, who more often breast-feed their children. In Israel, Shani and his associates have recently analyzed 1610 cases of breast cancer diagnosed between 1961 and 1963. They report that the disease was much more frequent among European-born women than among those coming from Africa and Asia. The European women had a lower birth rate and nursed their children less.

The most penetrating study of the relationship of breast cancer to lactation was that published by Levin and his associates in 1964. They studied the nursing histories of their patients at the Roswell Park Memorial Institute between 1957 and 1962, and of an equal number of controls matched for the same variables that MacMahon and Feinleib had used. The results of Levin's matched study of breast cancer cases and controls are shown in Table 21–6.

Levin also compared the data regarding total number of menstrual years, number of lactation years, and number of pregnancy years for his New York controls with the same factors for the Japanese controls as compiled by Segi, Kamoi, and Hirayama (Table 21–7).

Study of this table shows that the New York women had an average of two children and spent an average total of 1.2 years nursing them. The Japanese women had an average of 3.2 children and spent an average total of 6.4 years nursing them. In view of the fact that cancer is at least 5.5 times more frequent among New York women than among Japanese women, these differences in

Table 21–7. Data regarding menstrual years, lactation years, and pregnancy years in control series of patients without breast cancer

Country of Origin	Number Menstrual Years	Number Lactation Years	Number Pregnancy Years	Number Postmenopause Years
United States				
Levin, 1964	30.2	1.2	1.8	3.8
Japan				
Segi, 1957	19.9	7.0	3.3	6.8
Wynder and Hirayama, 1960	23.5	5.8	2.4	5.3
Average Segi & Wynder	21.7	6.4	2.9	6.0

Table 21–8. PARITY AND BREAST FEEDING—PERSONAL SERIES OF CASES, 1956–1957

Age Group	Without Breast Cancer					With Breast Cancer				
	Number	Per cent with Children	Average Number Children	Per cent Nursed Children	Months Average Total Lactation	Number	Per cent with Children	Average Number Children	Per cent Nursed Children	Months Average Total Lactation
41–50	738	73.0	1.5	19.0	1.5	391	77.3	1.5	21.0	1.7
51–60	440	65.8	1	26.0	2.7	315	65.0	1.3	32.0	3.1
61–70	157	72.0	1.6	55.0	8.8	169	68.0	1.4	43.0	7.8
71–80	35	65.8	1.4	43.0	7.3	92	68.5	1.6	49.0	11.1
80+	1	0	0	0	0	14	85.7	2.7	64.2	23.9
Over 40	1271	71.0	1.4	28.0	3.1	981	70.9	1.4	31.8	4.4

menstrual history, parity, and lactation are striking.

Levin was impressed by these data and devised an elaborate statistical method of analyzing them for the "dynamic risk" of developing breast cancer. He reached the conclusion that both nursing and menstrual activity are related to the development of the disease.

I have been collecting data regarding parity and lactation history for many years from my own patients. My data for the last 10 years, based on my own interviews with a total of 2252 patients over the age of 40, are presented in Table 21–8. They included 981 patients with mammary carcinoma, and 1271 women who did not have the disease but consulted me for other breast conditions. I have used these women who did not have breast cancer as controls, and have matched them for age with the breast cancer patients. They also match in a general way as to social class because all were private patients.

It is apparent that in my own data there are no statistically significant differences as regards number of children and total lactation time between my patients with cancer and the controls.

McMahon has just reported an international study of the lactation history of seven different ethnic groups of women, in Boston, Glamorgan, Athens, Slovenia, São Paulo, Taipei, and Tokyo. Hospital patients with and without breast cancer were interviewed. These data, like my own, reveal no significant differences in the lactation histories of those who had breast cancer and those who did not. McMahon concludes that his data "fail to confirm the hypothesis of the protective effect of lactation." He suggests that socioeconomic status and other factors may be responsible.

Although it is apparent that individual lacta-

tion histories do not reveal a correlation with breast carcinoma, the basic fact remains that in populations in which women almost always nurse their babies, and do so for a long time, the incidence of breast cancer is strikingly low. McMahon's own data demonstrate this fact for Athens, Slovenia, Taipei, and Tokyo.

Until the dilemma of these conflicting data is resolved, I cannot ignore the basic truth that in ethnic groups breast feeding appears to protect against breast cancer, and I believe that it is my duty as a physician to advise breast feeding and to do all I can to help women succeed with it.

Hormonal Treatment and the Etiology of Breast Carcinoma

It is well known that the physiology of the mammary gland is controlled by the ovarian, adrenal, and pituitary hormones. This fact led investigators to study the relationships of these hormones to the development of mammary carcinoma. Here again the mouse has been the main experimental subject. Cori was the first, in 1927, to show that the removal of the ovaries in very young female mice of high carcinoma strains entirely prevents the development of mammary carcinoma.

Another method of studying the etiologic role of hormones in mammary carcinoma is, of course, to administer them to mice. Lacassagne, in 1933, was the first to treat mice with estrogen. He produced carcinoma of the breast in three male mice of the RIII strain. Subsequent studies by Bonser showed that this phenomenon occurs only in male mice of the high mammary carcinoma strains. The hormone produces what corresponds to a female breast in males, and in such a breast carcinoma develops as it does in females of the strain. Estrogen does not induce breast carcinoma in males of low mammary carcinoma strains. In our Columbia laboratory Randall and I also showed that the administration of estrogen to female mice in excessive and prolonged dosage does not modify the inherent strain tendency to develop mammary carcinoma, except to induce the disease at an earlier age in high mammary carcinoma strain mice. The mean age at which our RIII bred female control mice developed the disease was 12.1 months. Estrogen-treated RIII females developed it at a mean age of 8.1 months. Female mice of our C57 strain, in which mammary carcinoma does not normally occur, did not develop the disease when treated with estrogen.

Hall and Moore have recently studied the effects of administering estrogen to genetically identical hybrid male mice which they had castrated. The mice were the offspring of two high mammary carcinoma strains — C3H and A. One group of mice had been freed of the mammary carcinoma virus by foster-nursing and selective breeding. The other group carried the virus. When the mice carrying the virus were given estrogen, mammary carcinoma developed. This treatment did not produce the disease in the mice that did not carry the virus.

These experiments make it clear that the mammary carcinoma virus has a dominant role in the development of mammary carcinoma in mice, and that estrogen is a secondary factor in the production of the disease.

Another type of hormonal effect in mice is that caused by the administration of androgen. If given in large doses over a prolonged period of time to young female mice of high mammary carcinoma strains, androgen will prevent the development of mammary carcinoma. This effect is the result, we may assume, of the suppression of ovarian function by the overwhelming dosage of androgen.

The role of the pituitary gland in the etiology of mammary carcinoma in mice has recently been much studied. The basic importance of the pituitary in all matters concerning the breast has been known since Gomez and Turner, in 1937, showed that neither estrogen nor progesterone would induce breast growth in hypophysectomized small laboratory animals. Gardner and White were able to produce breast growth in hypophysectomized mice by administering the mammotrophin fraction of the pituitary hormone in combination with estrogen. Nandi found that the somatotrophin pituitary fraction in combination with estrogen had a similar effect. He and his associates extended their studies to the relationship of the pituitary to mammary carcinoma in mice, and have shown that in some strains of hypophysectomized mice, combinations of the pituitary and ovarian hormones induce the disease. Mühlbock has reported that pituitary implants alone induced mammary carcinoma in several strains of mice that presumably did not carry the mammary tumor virus. In our own laboratory we were unable to induce the disease with pituitary implants in our C57 mice, which we know do not carry the virus.

We can conclude from these experiments that the pituitary hormones play a role as yet not fully understood in the genesis of mammary carcinoma in mice.

In women, oophorectomy appears to lower the incidence of subsequent mammary carcinoma. Herrell found, in the Mayo Clinic data, that only 1.5 per cent of a total of 1906 women with breast carcinoma had had their ovaries removed earlier in life, whereas 15.4 per cent of a control series of 1,011 consecutive female patients over the age of 40, who did not have breast carcinoma, had had bilateral oophorectomy. Feinleib has recently published a study of the occurrence of breast carcinoma among 6908 women subsequent to oophorectomy or sterilization by irradiation at the Peter Bent Brigham Hospital and the Free Hospital for Women between 1920 and 1940. Among 1278 women who had bilateral oophorectomy before the age of 40, only six developed mammary carcinoma, although 24 would have been expected to develop the disease. This is a highly significant statistical difference.

The question of whether or not the administration of estrogen may induce carcinoma of the human breast is complex and difficult — but very pertinent today. Millions of women are taking estrogen in various hormonal combinations as a contraceptive, and many older women are being given estrogen to alleviate menopausal symptoms.

There have been striking isolated cases, such as the one described by Auchincloss and myself, in which the long continued administration of estrogen preceded carcinoma of the breast, and in which pathologic study showed, in addition to the carcinoma, a great variety of types of epithelial proliferation in both breasts. The epithelial proliferation in such a case is almost certainly the result of the intense estrogen stimulation, but we are not justified in assuming that the carcinoma also was induced by the estrogen.

There are unfortunately no adequate long-term follow-up studies of women who have taken estrogen for a long period of time. Retrospective studies of this question are difficult because, with rare exceptions, women do not know precisely which estrogen they have been taking, in what dosage, and for how long. Prospective case studies with complete medical data and a follow-up of at least 50 years for the young women and 25 years for the menopausal women are needed to settle this question. It will be a long time before they are available.

Hertz has recently warned against the carcinogenic potential of steroid contraceptives now so widely used. He points out that the estrogen-progesterone combination used in these preparations gives a characteristic clinical estrogen response, including a tendency to fluid retention, a degree of nausea and malaise, and fullness of the breasts. The clinical phenomena produced by the contraceptive preparations are more marked than normal cyclic manifestations, and justify the assumption that the estrogen administered in this way exceeds normal endogenous estrogen.

One of these estrogen-progesterone preparations (Ethynerone) has produced neoplastic changes in the breasts of dogs. No one can predict what the distant effects upon the human breast of long continued estrogen stimulation, such as the contraceptive preparations provide, will be.

Since we know that administering estrogen to female mice of the inbred high mammary carcinoma strains results in the appearance of the disease at an earlier age, one way of searching for an earlier indication of the danger of giving estrogen to women might be to study the data regarding breast cancer in women to see if there is a shift of the incidence of the disease toward a younger age.

In the meantime we must try to assess the risk of taking estrogen as best we can. We certainly should not give estrogen to women of the five different groups who are known to be predisposed to develop mammary carcinoma. They are:

1. Those with a familial history of the disease.

2. Those who have had gross cystic disease.

3. Those who have had carcinoma in one breast.

4. Those with lobular neoplasia (lobular carcinoma *in situ*).

5. Those with multiple papilloma.

Men are very often given estrogen in large doses for carcinoma of the prostate. These patients provide an ideal experimental group to test the ability of estrogen to induce breast cancer in the male. Their breasts enlarge strikingly, chiefly because of increase of the fibrous stroma of the breast, multiplication of ducts, and proliferation of their lining epithelium. Fully developed gland fields are not seen.

It might be expected that these changes would in some instances give rise to mammary carcinoma, and cases have in fact been reported in which this sequence is assumed to have occurred (Keller; Gibba; Jakobsen; Graves and Harris; Claisse and Daymas; McClure and Higgins; Corbett and Abrams; Howard and Grosjean; Reimann-Hunziker; Gardini; Abramson and Warshawsky).

It is unfortunately a fact that carcinoma of the prostate is similar histologically to some forms of carcinoma of the breast, and that it is difficult at times to distinguish the metastases of prostatic carcinoma to the breast from primary breast carcinoma. Campbell and Cummins, as well as Benson, have described breast lesions which they interpreted as metastases from prostatic carcinoma, and they suggest that the cases that have been reported as primary breast carcinoma developing as a result of stilbestrol are also examples of metastasis of prostatic carcinoma. Campbell and Cummins found histochemical acid phosphatase studies helpful in identifying metastases from prostatic carcinoma. Reiner and his associates emphasized, however, that this test has not entirely solved the problem. The technique is complex, and interpretation difficult.

It must be kept in mind that primary carcinoma of the breast has a small but appreciable frequency in males, and that very rarely it might develop independently of the existence of another disease in a patient being given estrogen. This might be the explanation in a case reported by Baierl. The patient did not have prostatic cancer. He was treated with stilbestrol for a gastric ulcer and developed a breast carcinoma for which radical mastectomy was done.

A recent case report by O'Grady and McDivitt may settle this controversial question. Their patient was a 77 year old man with a carcinoma of the prostate who had been given diethylstilbestrol for six years in doses that varied from 10 to 20 mg. daily for most of the time. This soon produced marked bilateral gynecomastia. After four years of estrogen therapy an erosion of the right nipple developed, and biopsy was done two years later. Characteristic Paget's carcinoma of the nipple epidermis was found. Radical mastectomy was done. Extensive intraductal carcinoma, typical of Paget's carcinoma of the female breast, with axillary metastases, was found. In view of the great rarity of Paget's carcinoma of the male breast there can scarcely be any reasonable doubt that in this patient it was caused by the estrogen treatment.

The Relationship of Inflammation and Trauma of the Breast to the Development of Mammary Carcinoma

Lane-Claypon made a careful study of the relationship of puerperal mastitis, nonsuppurative as well as suppurative, to the development of cancer of the breast, and found no evidence that these lesions predisposed to cancer.

In any series of cases of breast cancer many instances will be found of the patient attributing her carcinoma to antecedent trauma to the breast. In her 1926 series of cases Lane-Claypon had a strikingly high percentage (26.8 per cent) of patients who claimed antecedent breast injury. Since cancer is somewhat more common in the left than in the right breast, Lane-Claypon, who believed that trauma does predipose to breast cancer, suggested that its left-sided predominance is a result of the fact that right-handed persons protect the right breast from being traumatized.

Spratt and Donegan reported that 11.7 per cent of their patients with breast cancer gave a history of antecedent trauma to the breast. In the series of breast cancer patients studied by Wynder, Bross, and Hirayama 9 per cent stated that the affected breast had been traumatized.

From my own experience with mammary carcinoma I doubt that trauma is a factor in its causation. It is the most natural thing in the world for a scientifically uncritical patient to attribute any and all disease to trauma. Most patients with breast cancer whose case histories have provided the data for reports

such as Lane-Claypon's are uneducated ward patients, prone to prejudice and suggestion. The leading question regarding antecedent trauma put to them by the intern taking the history no doubt often suggests this easy explanation for their disease to them. In the case histories of breast carcinoma that I have myself taken it has been a rare thing for the patient to give a definite and precise story of antecedent breast trauma.

The Relationship of Benign Tumors of the Breast to Mammary Carcinoma

The most debated of all questions regarding the etiology of mammary carcinoma is its relationship to the various benign tumors of the breast, adenofibroma, cystic disease, intraductal papilloma, etc. The problem has been discussed by Charteris, Dawson, Ducuing et al., and Lewison and Lyons. I have dealt with this question in relation to each of the various benign lesions separately, in the chapters devoted to them.

The Relationship of Noncancerous Disease in Organs Other than the Breast to Mammary Carcinoma

Studies of the possible relationship of carcinoma of the breast to a wide variety of noncancerous lesions of organs other than the breast have been made, without finding any statistically significant correlation. Some of the lesions that have been investigated follow: pituitary adenoma (Steiner and Dunham); adrenal adenoma (Flynn and Halliday); granulosa cell tumor of ovary (Finkler); diabetes (Repert); acanthosis nigricans (Curth).

It has recently been suggested that women with thyroid disease are predisposed to breast cancer (Repert; Bogardus and Finley; Humphrey and Swerdlow). Adequate demographic studies of this question are not yet available.

On the other hand, Levy and Levy, as well as Repert, report that patients who have had thyroidectomy for thyroid disease develop breast cancer less often than women in the general population.

Modern laboratory studies of thyroid function measured by radioactive iodine uptake and total plasma iodine levels have not, however, revealed any abnormality in patients with localized breast cancer (Edelstyn, Lyons, and Welbourn; Sicher and Waterhouse; Cappelli and Margottini). In advanced metastatic disease, with metabolic disturbances, thyroid function is depressed as might be expected.

The Relationship of Cancer of Organs Other than the Breast to Mammary Carcinoma

The question of the association of malignant disease in the breast with that in other organs has been intensively studied. (Schreiner and Wehr; Bugher; Burke; Holmqvist and Nelson; Wassink; Slaughter; Curran and Kilroy; Englebreth-Holm; Larson and Kunz; Leidinger; Mider et al.; Watson; Moertel, Dockerty, and Baggenstoss; Einhorn and Jakobsson; Cook).

In studying this question it should first of all be pointed out that certain types of cancer are characterized by multiple and usually consecutive foci of the disease in the organ or epithelial area in which they develop. Cancers of the skin and intraoral mucosa are notorious for their multiplicity. Carcinoma of the colon and breast are multiple to a lesser degree. Because of this multiple nature, statistical studies should count these special types of cancer as single foci even when they are multiple.

Watson carried out an admirable follow-up study of the occurence of multiple cancer in a total of 16,626 patients in Saskatchewan. On the basis of the man-years' exposure to risk, his computations did not reveal a constitutional tendency to develop a second cancer.

One type of study of this frequency of multiple primary cancer is exemplified by that of Einhorn and Jakobsson in which the occurrence of diverse types of primary malignant tumors is studied in a series of patients treated for a single form of cancer. They studied 1675 patients with carcinoma of the lip, and reported that during an exceptionally long follow-up the incidence of new primary cancers of other types in the younger age groups was considerably higher than can be ascribed to chance. In the older age groups the incidence approached that attributable to chance.

All these studies of the multiplicity of cancer have failed to establish any general predisposition to the disease. It is probable that the reasons for differences in its frequency will be found in environmental and social circumstances, rather than in racial or genetic influences.

It has frequently been suggested that there is a tendency for the incidence rates for different types of cancer to counterbalance each other, and that there is a reciprocal relationship between the frequency of breast cancer and cancer of the cervix of the uterus. It is well established, for example, that in Puerto Rico where breast cancer is relatively uncommon, cancer of the cervix is common, while in Ireland breast cancer is frequent and cancer of the cervix infrequent. Clemmesen has refuted this concept of a total cancer mortality for women by showing that in the Danish data for the years 1951 to 1957, the rates for both breast and uterine cancer were very high.

There is, however, one form of cancer that seems to be more frequent in women with breast cancer — carcinoma of the endometrium. Taylor was the first, in 1931, to report an association between endometrial carcinoma and carcinoma of the breast. Since there is a good deal of evidence that carcinoma in both these organs may be to a degree hormone-dependent, an increase in one type might well be accompanied by a higher rate for the other. Cook, in his study of 4271 multiple cancers collected from the literature and the case material of the Ellis Fischel State Cancer Hospital, found 786 patients with cancer of the breast and endometrium. He calculated that this frequency was 1.6 times greater than that expected. Bailar reported the experience with endometrial cancer in 2358 residents of Connecticut diagnosed between 1935 and 1951. These patients had a 60 per cent greater incidence of breast cancer than would have been expected.

MacMahon and Austin have studied the question in the long-term follow-up data of the Boston Hospital for Women. A total of 869 women with endometrial carcinoma seen between 1920 and 1959 were included in their study. A 30 per cent increase in carcinoma of the breast over the expected number of cases was found. This excess of breast cancer was limited to the women who were 60 or more years of age at the time of diagnosis of endometrial carcinoma.

All these data suggest that women who develop carcinoma of the breast should be followed with special emphasis upon detection of carcinoma of the endometrium, and vice versa.

REFERENCES

Abramson, W., and Warshawsky, H.: Cancer of the breast in the male, secondary to estrogenic administration; report of a case. J. Urol., 59:76, 1948.

Allaben, G. R., and Owen, S. E.: Adenocarcinoma of the breast coincidental with strenuous endocrine therapy. J.A.M.A., *112*:1933, 1939.

Anderson, V. E., Goodman, H. O., and Reed, S. C.: Variables Related to Human Breast Cancer. Minneapolis, Univ. of Minnesota Press, 1958.

Andervont, H. B., and Dunn, T. B.: Influences of heredity and the mammary tumor agent on the occurrence of mammary tumors in hybrid mice. J. Nat. Cancer Inst., *14*:317, 1953.

Archer, B. H.: Incidence of peripheral malignancy in Simmonds' disease, with special reference to cancer of the breast. New York State J. Med., *53*:328, 1953.

Armstrong, E. C., and Bonser, G. M.: The carcinogenic action of 2-acetyl-amino-fluorene on various strains of mice. J. Path. Bact., *59*:19, 1947.

Bagg, H. J.: The functional activity of the breast in relation to mammary carcinoma in mice. Proc. Soc. Exper. Biol. & Med. *22*:419, 1925.

Baierl, W.: Zur Frage der Mammacarcinom-Manifestierung nach Cyren-B-Behandlung beim Mann. Med. Klin., *48*:1284, 1953.

Bailar, J. C., 3rd.: The incidence of independent tumors among uterine cancer patients. Cancer, *16*:842, 1963.

Benson, W. R.: Carcinoma of the prostate with metastases to breasts and testes. Cancer, *10*:1235, 1957.

Bittner, J. J.: Some possible effects of nursing on the mammary gland tumor incidence in mice Science, *84*:162, 1936.

Bogardus, G. M., and Finley, J. W.: Breast cancer and thyroid disease. Surgery, *49*:461, 1961.

Bonser, G. M.: The effect of oestrone administration on the mammary glands of male mice of two strains differing greatly in their susceptibility to spontaneous mammary carcinoma. J. Path. Bact., *42*:169, 1936.

Bonser, G. M., Dossett, J. A., and Jull, J. W.: Human and Experimental Breast Cancer. London, Pitman Med. Pub. Co., 1961.

Bonser, G. M., and Orr, J. W.: The morphology of 160 tumors induced by carcinogenic hydrocarbons in the subcutaneous tissues of mice. J. Path. Bact., *49*:171, 1939.

Boselli, P. L., and Maconi, F.: Influenza della condizione di nulliparità o di fertilità delle pazienti sull' insorgenza del carcinoma della mammella. Minerva chir., *15*:878, 1960.

Broca, P.: Traité des Tumeurs. Paris, Asselin, 1866.

Bucalossi, P., Catania, V. C., Pellegris, G., and Veronesi, U.: Il significato della lunghezza della vita mestruale nell' insorgenza del cancro della mammella muliebre. Tumori, Milano, *43*:538, 1957.

Bucalossi, P., and Veronesi, U.: Some observations on cancer of the breast in mothers and daughters. Brit. J. Cancer, *11*:337, 1957.

Bucalossi, P., Veronesi, U., and Pandolfi, A.: Il problema dell'ereditarieta neoplastica nell'uomo. 2. Il cancro della mammella. Tumori, Milano, *40*:365, 1954.

Bugher, J. C.: Probability of chance recurrence of multiple malignant neoplasms. Am. J. Cancer, *21*:809, 1934.

Burkard, H.: Gleichzeitige und gleichartige Geschwulsbildung in der linken Brustdrüse bei Zwillingsschwestern. Deutsche Ztschr. f. Chir., *169*:166, 1922.

Burke, M.: Multiple primary cancers. Am. J. Cancer, *27*:316, 1936.

Busk, T.: Some observations on heredity in breast cancer and leukemia. Ann. Eugenics, *14*:213, 1947–1951.

Busk, T., Clemmesen, J., and Nielsen, A.: Twin studies and other genetical investigations in the Danish cancer registry. Brit. J. Cancer, *2*:156, 1948.

Campbell, J. H., and Cummins, S. D.: Metastases, simulating mammary cancer, in prostatic carcinoma under estrogenic therapy. Cancer, *4*:303, 1951.

Campbell, J. H., Cummins, S. D., Kirk, D. L., and Mathews, W. R.: Secondary breast cancer of prostatic origin. J.A.M.A., *179*:458, 1962.

Cantarow, A., Stasney, J., and Paschkis, K. E.: The influence of sex hormones on mammary tumors induced by 2-acetaminofluorene. Cancer Research, *8*:412, 1948.

Cappelli, L., and Margotttini, M.: Thyroid function in cancer patients. Internat. Union against Cancer, *20*:1493, 1964.

Charney, J., Pullinger, B. D., and Moore, D. H.: A rapid assay for Bittner virus by the immunologic detection of virus antigen in the milk of inoculated mice. Proc. Am. A. for Cancer Research, *9*:13, Abstract no. 47, 1968.

Charteris, A. A.: On the changes in the mammary gland preceding carcinoma. J. Path. & Bact., *33*:101, 1930.

Claisse, R., and Daymas: Tumeur mammaire d'évolution rapide, au cours du traitement d'un cancer de la prostate par les oestrogènes de synthèse. Bull. et mém. Soc. méd. d. hôp. de Paris *67*:1137, 1951.

Clayson, D. B.: A working hypothesis for the mode of carcinogenesis of aromatic amines. Brit. J. Cancer, *7*:460, 1953.

Clemmesen, J.: On cancer incidence in Denmark and other countries. *In* Report on Oxford Symposium, 1950, Internat. Union against Cancer, 7(Spec. vol.):24, 1951.

Clemmesen, J.: Statistical Studies in Malignant Neoplasms. Copenhagen, Munksgaard, 1964.

Clemmesen, J.: The status of genetical studies in human cancer. Brit. J. Cancer, *3*:474, 1949.

Clemmesen, J., and Nielsen, A.: Incidence of malignant diseases in Denmark, 1943–47. Internat. Union against Cancer, *8*:140, 1952.

Cook, G. B.: A comparison of single and multiple primary cancers. Cancer, *19*:959, 1966.

Corbett, D. G., and Abrams, E. W.: Bilateral carcinoma of male breasts associated with prolonged stilbestrol therapy for carcinoma of the prostate. J. Urol., *64*:377, 1950.

Cori, C. F.: Influence of ovariectomy on spontaneous occurrence of mammary carcinomas in mice. J. Exper. Med., *45*:983, 1927.

Curran, J. F., and Kilroy, E. A.: Co-existent primary carcinoma of the fallopian tube and of the breast. New England J. Med., *236*:64, 1947.

Curth, H. O.: Cancer associated with acanthosis nigricans; review of the literature and report of a case of acanthosis nigricans with cancer of the breast. Arch. Surg., *47*:517, 1943.

Curtis, M. R., Bullock, F. D., and Dunning, W. F.: A statistical study of the occurrence of spontaneous tumors in a large colony of rats. Am. J. Cancer, *15*:67, 1931.

Dargent, M.: Carcinoma of the breast in castrated women. Brit. M. J., *2*:54, 1949.

Dawson, E. K.: "Precancerous conditions" of the breast. Brit. J. Radiol., *21*:590, 1948.

Denoix, P. F.: Rapports entre l'âge au premier symptome et certains aspects de la vie biologique de la femme dans une série de cancers de l'utérus et du sein. Bull. Inst. nat. d'Hygiène, 6:573, 1951.

Denoix, P. F., Schützenberger, M. P., and Denoix, G.: Contribution à l'étude du rôle des facteurs héréditaires dans le cancer. Bull. Inst. nat. d'Hygiène, 8:247, 1953.

Dobrovolskaïa-Zavadskaïa, N.: Heredity of cancer. Am. J. Cancer, 18:357, 1933.

Dorn, H. F.: The Statistical Approach to the Epidemiology of Cancer. Proceedings of the Second National Cancer Conference, 2:1103, 1952.

Dorn, H. F., and Cutler, S.: Morbidity from Cancer in the United States. Public Health Monograph, No. 29, 1955.

Ducuing, J., Bimes, C., and Estrade, J.: La question du potentiel dégénératif des lésions bénignes du sein. Bull. Assoc. franç. p. l'étude du cancer, 39:424, 1952.

Edelstyn, G. A., Lyons, A. R., and Welbourn, R. B.: Thyroid function in patients with mammary cancer. Lancet, 1:670, 1958.

Einhorn, J., and Jakobsson, P.: Multiple primary malignant tumors. Cancer, 17:1437, 1964.

Engelbreth-Holm, J.: Om Hyppigheden af dobbeltsidig Brystkraeft og om Brystkraeftens Samentraef med andre Kraeftformer. Ugesk. f. laeger, 104:456, 1942.

Feinleib, M.: Breast cancer and artificial menopause: a cohort study. J. Nat. Cancer Inst., 41:315, 1968.

Finkler, R. S.: Granulosa cell tumor of the ovary with a carcinoma of the breast. Am. J. Obst. & Gynec., 36:1064, 1938.

Flynn, R., and Halliday, J. H.: Adenoma of the adrenal gland and carcinoma of the breast. M. J. Australia, 2:497, 1953.

Ganz, E.: Ist der Brustkrebs bei ledigen oder verheirateten Frauen häufiger? Strahlentherapie, 61:190, 1938.

Gardini, G. F.: Ginecomastia con degenerazione cancerigna in prostatico dopo trattamento estrogeno. Oncologia, 1:129, 1948.

Gardner, W. U., and White, A.: Mammary growth in hypophysectomized male mice receiving estrogen and prolactin. Proc. Soc. Exper. Biol. & Med., 48:590, 1951.

Garfinkel, L., Craig, L., and Seidman, H.: An appraisal of left and right breast cancer. J. Nat. Cancer Inst., 23:617, 1959.

Gerard, A. H.: Please Breast-Feed Your Baby. New York, Hawthorn Books, 1970.

Gibba, A.: Carcinoma mammario bilaterale comparso in corso di terapia estrogena per cancro prostatico. Urologia, 19:180, 1952.

Gilliam, G.: Fertility and cancer of the breast and of the uterine cervix. Comparisons between rates of pregnancy in women with cancer at these and other sites. J. Nat. Cancer Inst., 12:593, 1951.

Gomez, E. T., and Turner, C. W.: Hypophysectomy and replacement therapy in relation to the growth and secretory activity of the mammary gland. Res. Bull., Missouri Agric. Exper. Station, No. 259, 1937.

Graves, G. Y., and Harris, H. S.: Carcinoma of the male breast with axillary metastasis following stilbestrol therapy; report of a case treated by radical mastectomy. Ann. Surg., 13:411, 1952.

Haagensen, C. D., and Randall, H. T.: Milk induced mammary carcinoma in mice. Cancer Research, 5:352, 1945.

Haagensen, C. D., et al.: Treatment of early mammary

carcinoma. A cooperative international study. Ann. Surg., 157:157, 1963.

Habs, H.: Krebs und Vererbung. Ztschr. f. klin Med., 135:676, 1939.

Hairstone, M. A., Sheffield, J. B., and Moore, D. H.: A study of B particles in the mammary tumors of strain A mice. J. Nat. Cancer Inst., 33:825, 1964.

Hall, W. T., and Moore, D. H.: Effects of estrogenic hormones on the mammary tissue of agent-free and agent-bearing male mice. J. Nat. Cancer Inst., 36:181, 1966.

Harnett, W. L.: A statistical report on 2529 cases of cancer of the breast. Brit. J. Cancer, 2:212, 1948.

Harvald, B., and Hauge, M.: Heredity of cancer elucidated by a study of unselected twins. J.A.M.A., 186:749, 1963.

Heiberg, B., and Heiberg, P.: Some investigations into the occurrence of carcinoma of the breast with special reference to the ovarian function. Acta chir. Scandinav., 83:479, 1940.

Herrell, W. E.: The relative incidence of oophorectomy in women with and without carcinoma of the breast. Am. J. Cancer, 29:659, 1937.

Hertz, R.: Experimental and clinical aspects of the carcinogenic potential of steroid contraceptives. Internat. J. Fertility, 13:273, 1968.

Heston, W. E.: Mammary tumors in agent-free mice. Ann. New York Acad. Sc., 71:931, 1958.

Heston, W. E., Vlahakis, G., and Deringer, M. K.: Delayed effect of genetic segregation on the transmission of the mammary tumor agent in mice. J. Nat. Cancer Inst., 24:721, 1960.

Hirayama, T., and Wynder, E. L.: A study of the epidemiology of cancer of the breast. II The influence of hysterectomy. Cancer, 15:28, 1962.

Holmqvist, I., and Nelson, A.: Ueber multiples Auftreten von Geschwülsten und Gewebsmissbildungen; eine statistische Untersuchung. Ztschr. f. Krebsforsch., 47:257, 1938.

Howard, R. R., and Grosjean, W. A.: Bilateral mammary carcinoma in male coincident with prolonged stilbestrol therapy. Surgery, 25:300, 1949.

Howell, J. S., Marchant, J., and Orr, J. W.: The induction of ovarian tumors in mice with 9–10 dimethyl 1-2 benzanthracene. Brit. J. Cancer, 8:635, 1954.

Huber, H.: Genitalkarzinom und Mammakarzinom als Multiplizitätstumoren. Strahlentherapie, 92:130, 1953.

Huggins, C., Briziarelli, G., and Sutton, H. Jr.: Rapid induction of mammary carcinoma in the rat and the influence of hormones on the tumors. J. Exper. Med., 109:25, 1959.

Humphrey, L. J., and Swerdlow, M.: The relationship of breast disease to thyroid disease. Cancer, 17:1170, 1964.

Jacobsen, O.: Heredity in Breast Cancer. A Genetic and Clinical Study of Two Hundred Probands. Copenhagen, Nyt Nordisk Forlag, 1946.

Jakobsen, A. H. I.: Bilateral mammary carcinoma in the male following stilboestrol therapy. Acta. path. et microbiol. Scandinav., 31:61, 1952.

Jensen, C. O.: Experimentelle Untersuchungen über Krebs bei Mäusen. Centralbl. f. Bakt., 34:28 & 22, 1903.

Jull, J. W.: The action of chemical carcinogens on the mouse breast. In International Symposium on Mammary Cancer, Perugia, Div. of Cancer Research, 1958, p. 423.

Kamoi, M.: Statistical study on the relation between breast cancer and lactation period. Tohoku J. Exper. Med., 72:59, 1960.

Keller, J.: Mammakarzinom nach Stilbenbehandlung eines Prostatakarzinoms. Zeitschr. f. ärztl. Fortbildg., 47:584, 1953.

Khanolkar, V. R.: Breast cancer in Bombay. Internat. Union against Cancer, 17:903, 1961.

Khanolkar, V. R.: Cancer in India. Internat. Union against Cancer, 6:881, 1950.

Kilgore, A. R.: Can injury cause breast cancer? Am. Surgeon, 20:1015, 1954.

Kistner, R. W.: The use of oestrogens and progestins during the perimenopause. South African J. of Obst. & Gyn., 6:1, 1968.

Korteweg, R.: Is there evidence that in the human an extra-chromosomal factor exists, which co-determines the susceptibility to breast cancers? Internat. Union against Cancer, 8:169, 1952.

Kranz, H.: Tumoren bei Zwillingen. Ztschr. f. indukt. Abstammungs und Vererbungsl., 62:173, 1932.

Lacassagne, A.: Influence d'un facteur familial dans la production par la folliculine de cancers mammaires chez la souris mâle. Compt. rend. Soc. de biol., 114:427, 1933.

Lane-Clayton, J. E.: A Further Report on Cancer of the Breast with Special Reference to Its Associated Antecedent Conditions. Reports on Public Health and Medical Subjects, no. 32, London, Ministry of Health, 1926.

Larson, C. P., and Kunz, G. G. R.: Multiple primary malignancies. Primary papillary carcinoma of the renal pelvis, ureter, and bladder, associated with primary adeno-carcinoma of the breast. Urol. & Cutan. Rev., 44:749, 1940.

Lasfargues, E. Y., Murray, M. R., and Moore, D. H.: Induced epithelial hyperplasia in organ cultures of mouse mammary tissues. Effects of the milk agent. J. Nat. Cancer Inst., 34:141, 1965.

Leidinger, H.: Ueber synchrone Primärkarzinome des Mastdarms und der weiblichen Brust. Krebsarzt, 3:285, 1948.

Levin, M. L., Sheehe, P. R., Graham, S., and Glidewell, O.: Lactation and menstrual function as related to cancer of the breast. Am. J. Public Health, 54:580, 1964.

Levy, J., and Levy, J. A.: Role of hypometabolic state in cancer. Am. Pract. & Digest Treatment, 2:522, 1951.

Lewison, E. F., and Allen, L. W.: Antecedent factors in cancer of the breast. Ann. Surg., 138:39, 1953.

Lewison, E. F., and Lyons, J. G.: The relationship between benign breast disease and cancer. Arch. Surg., 66:94, 1953.

Lilienfeld, A. M.: The epidemiology of breast cancer. Cancer Research, 23:1503, 1963.

Lilienfeld, A. M.: The relationship of cancer of the female breast to artificial menopause and marital status. Cancer, 9:927, 1956.

Logan, W. P. D.: Marriage and childbearing in relation to cancer of the breast and uterus. Lancet, 265:1199, 1953.

Lynch, C.: Studies on the relation between tumor susceptibility and heredity. J. Exper. Med., 39:481, 1924.

Lyons, M. J., and Moore, D. H.: Isolation of the mouse mammary tumor virus; chemical and morphological studies. J. Nat. Cancer Inst., 35:549, 1965.

Macklin, M. T.: An analysis of tumors in monozygous and dizygous twins. J. Hered., 31:277, 1940.

Macklin, M. T.: Comparison of the number of breast cancer deaths observed in relatives of breast-cancer patients and the number expected on the basis of mortality rates. J. Nat. Cancer Inst., 22:927, 1959.

Macklin, M. T.: Relative status of parity and genetic background in producing human breast cancer. J. Nat. Cancer Inst., 23:1179, 1959.

McClure, J. A., and Higgins, C. C.: Bilateral carcinoma of male breast after estrogen therapy. J.A.M.A., 146:7, 1951.

McFarland, J., and Meade, T. S.: Genetic origin of tumors supported by their simultaneous and symmetrical occurrence in homologous twins. Am. J. M. Sc., 184:66, 1932.

MacMahon, B.: Cohort fertility and increasing breast cancer incidence. Cancer, 11:250, 1958.

MacMahon, B., and Austin, J. H.: Association of carcinomas of the breast and corpus uteri. Cancer, 23:275, 1969.

MacMahon, B., and Feinleib, M.: Breast cancer in relation to nursing and menopausal history. J. Nat. Cancer Inst., 24:733, 1960.

McMahon, B., et al.: Lactation and breast cancer. Bull. Wld Hlth Org., 42:185, 1970.

Marsden, A. T. H.: The geographical pathology of cancer in Malaya. Brit. J. Cancer, 12:161, 1958.

Martynova, R. P.: The study of the role of the milk factor in the production of human breast cancer. Internat. Union against Cancer, 20:656, 1964.

Maurer, H. J., and Minder, R.: Statistischer Beitrag zur Frage des Follikelhormoneinflusses auf die Aetiologie des Mammakarzinoms. Ztschr. f. Geburtsh. u. Gynäk., 151:247, 1958.

Mider, G. B., Schilling, J. A., Donovan, J. C. and Rendall, E. S.: Multiple cancer: a study of other cancers arising in patients with primary malignant neoplasms of the stomach, uterus, breast, large intestine, or hematopoietic system. Cancer, 5:1104, 1953.

Moertel, C. G., Dockerty, M. B., and Baggenstoss, A. H.: Multiple primary malignant neoplasms. Cancer, 14:221, 1961.

Moore, D. H., Pillsbury, N., and Pullinger, B. D.: Titration of mammary tumor virus in fresh and treated RIII milk and milk fractions. J. Nat. Cancer Inst., 43:1263, 1969.

Moore, D. H., Charney, J., and Pullinger, B. D.: Mouse mammary tumor virus infectivity as a function of age of inoculation, breeding, and total lapsed time. J. Nat. Cancer Inst., 45:561, 1970.

Moore, D. H., et al.: Search for a human breast cancer virus. Nature, 1970 (in press).

Mühlbock, O., and Boot, L. M.: Induction of mammary cancer in mice without the mammary tumor agent by isografts of hypophyses. Cancer Res., 19:402, 1959.

Munford, S. A., and Linder, H.: Carcinoma of the breast in homologous twins. Am. J. Cancer, 28:393, 1936.

Murphy, D. P., and Abbey, H.: Cancer in Families. Cambridge, Harvard University Press, 1959.

Nandi, S., and Bern, H. A.: Relation between mammary-gland responses to lactogenic hormone combinations and tumor susceptibility in various strains of mice. J. Nat. Cancer Inst., 24:907, 1960.

Nielsen, A., and Clemmesen, J.: Twin studies in the Danish cancer registry, 1942–1955. Brit. J. Cancer, 11:327, 1957.

O'Grady, W. P., and McDivitt, R. W.: Breast cancer in a man treated with diethylstilbestrol. Arch. Path., 88:162, 1969.

Olch, I. Y.: Menopausal age in women with cancer of the breast. Amer. J. Cancer, 30:563, 1937.

Oliver, C. P., et al.: Relationship between pregnancies and age of occurrence of breast cancer in the human. Minnesota Med., 29:1230, 1946.

Oliver, C. P.: Studies on human cancer families. Ann. New York Acad. Sc., 71:1198, 1958.

Orr, J. W.: Mammary carcinoma in mice following the intranasal administration of methylcholanthrene. J. Path. & Bact., 55:483, 1943.

Papadrianos, E., Haagensen, C. D., Cooley, E.: Cancer of the breast as a familial disease. Ann. Surg., 165:10, 1967.

Parsons, W. H., and McCall, E. F.: The rôle of estrogenic substances in the production of malignant mammary lesions, with report of case of carcinoma of breast, possibly induced by strenuous estrogen therapy. Surgery, 9:780, 1941.

Pascua, M.: Trends of female mortality from cancer of the breast and cancer of the genital organs. Bull. World Health Org., 15:5, 1956.

Paymaster, J. C.: Cancer and its distribution in India. Cancer, 17:1026, 1964.

Paymaster, J. C.: Cancer of the breast in Indian women. Surgery, 40:372, 1956.

Paymaster, J. C., and Gangadharan, T.: Cancer in the Parsi community in Bombay. Internat. J. Cancer, 5:426, 1970.

Penrose, L. S., Mackenzie, H. J., and Karn, M. N.: A genetical study of human mammary cancer. Brit. J. Cancer, 2:168, 1948.

Phillips, R. B.: Identical cancers in identical twins. Proc. Staff Meet., Mayo Clin., 13:209, 1938.

Reimann-Hunziker, G.: Brustdrüsenkarzinom nach Ovocyclinbehandlung eines Prostatakarzinoms. Helvet. chir. acta, 15:242, 1948.

Reiner, L., Rutenburg, A. M., and Seligman, A. M.: Acid-phosphatase activity in human neoplasms. Cancer, 10:563, 1957.

Rennaes, S., and Holan, L.: Opptreden av brystkreft hos kvinner i forhold til alder ekteskap og barnetall. Nord. Med., 50:967, 1953.

Repert, R. W.: Breast carcinoma study: relation to thyroid disease and diabetes. J. Michigan M. Soc., 51:1315, 1952.

Rigoni-Stern, D.: Fatti statistici relativi alle malattie cancerose che servirono di base alle poche cose dette dal dott. Rigoni-Stern. Gior. servire progr. Pat. e terap., 2:507, 1842.

Rigoni-Stern, D.: Nota sulle ricerche del dottor Tanchou intorna la frequenza del cancro. Ann. Univ. Med., Milano, 110:484, 1844.

Santa Cruz, J. Z.: Cancer of the breast among Filipinos, Philippine J. Surg., 3:234, 1948.

Sarkar, N. H., and Moore, D. H.: The internal structure of mouse mammary tumor virus as revealed after tween-ether treatment. J. de Microscopie, 7:539, 1968.

Schreiner, B. F., and Wehr, W.: Multiple primary cancer as observed at the state institute for the study of malignant disease. Am. J. Cancer, 20:418, 1936.

Schwartz, D., Denoix, P. F., and Rouquette, C.: Enquête sur l'étiologie des cancers génitaux de la femme. Bull. Assoc. franç. p. l'étude du cancer, 45:476, 1958.

Segi, M., et al.: An epidemiological study on cancer in Japan. Gann, 48:supp., 1957.

Shani, M., Modan, B., Steinitz, R., and Modan, M.: The incidence of breast cancer in Jewish females in Israel. J. Israel Med. Assn., 71:337, 1966.

Shay, H., Aegerter, E. A., Gruenstein, M., and Komarov, S. A.: Development of adenocarcinoma of the breast in the Wistar rat following the gastric instillation of methylcholanthrene. J. Nat. Cancer Inst., 10:255, 1949.

Sicker, K., and Waterhouse, J. A. H.: Thyroid function in relation to mammary cancer. Brit. J. Cancer, 15:45, 1961.

Slaughter, D. P.: Multiplicity of origin of malignant tumors: collective review. Internat. Abstr. Surg., 79:89, 1944.

Slaughter, D. P.: Multicentric origin of intraoral carcinoma. Surgery, 20:133, 1946.

Smithers, D. W.: Cancer of the breast and the menopause, J. Fac. Radiologists, 4:89, 1952.

Smithers, D. W.: Family histories of 459 patients with cancer of the breast. Brit. J. Cancer, 2:163, 1948.

Smithers, D. W., Rigby-Jones, P., Galton, D. A. G., and Payne, P. M.: Cancer of the breast. Brit. J. Radiol., Supp. No. 4. 1952.

Spratt, J. S., and Donegan, W. L.: Cancer of the Breast. Philadelphia, W. B. Saunders, 1967, p. 26.

Steiner, P. E.: Cancer: Race and Geography. Baltimore, Williams and Wilkins, 1954, p. 161.

Steiner, P. E., and Dunham, L. J.: The anterior pituitary gland in women with carcinoma of the mammary gland, with report of a case of chromophobe adenoma. Am. J. Path., 19:1031, 1943.

Stephens, F. E., Gardner, E. J., and Woolf, C. M.: A recheck of kindred 107, which has shown a high frequency of breast cancer. Cancer, 11:967, 1958.

Stocks, P.: The epidemiology of cancer of the breast. Practitioner, 179:233, 1957.

Taylor, H. C., Jr.: The coincidence of primary breast and uterine cancer. Am. J. Cancer, 15:277, 1931.

Taylor, R. S., Carroll, B. E., and Lloyd, J. W.: Mortality among women in 3 Catholic religious orders with special reference to cancer. Cancer, 12:1207, 1959.

van der Werff, J.: The influence of age and marital state on the occurrence of mammary cancer. J. belge. Radiol. 39:706, 1956.

Versluys, J. J.: Marriage fertility and cancer mortality of the specifically female organs: mammary carcinoma. Brit. J. Cancer, 9:239, 1955.

Waaler, G. H. M.: Ueber die Erblichkeit des Krebses. Nord. med. tidskr., 4:761, 1932.

Wainwright, J. H.: A comparison of conditions associated with breast cancer in Great Britain and America. Am. J. Cancer, 15:2610, 1931.

Warthin, A.: The further study of a cancer family. J. Cancer Research, 9:279, 1925.

Wassink, W. F.: Cancer et hérédité. Genetica, 17:103, 1935.

Watson, T. A.: Incidence of multiple cancer. Cancer, 6:365, 1953.

Weitz, W.: Ueber die Erblichkeit des Krebses. Monatschr. f. Krebsbekämpf., 1:385, 1933.

Wood, D. A., and Darling, H. H.: A cancer family manifesting multiple occurrences of bilateral carcinoma of the breast. Cancer Research, 3:509, 1943.

Woolf, C. M.: Investigations on genetic aspects of carcinoma of the stomach and breast. Univ. of California Pub. in Public Health, 2:265, 1955.

Woolf, C. M., and Gardner, E. J.: The familial distribution of breast cancer in a Utah kindred. Cancer, 4:515, 1951.

Wynder, E. L., Bross, I. J., and Hirayama, T.: A study of the epidemiology of cancer of the breast. Cancer, 13:559, 1960.

Chapter Twenty-Two

The Natural History of Breast Carcinoma

THE PRIMARY FOCUS

Carcinoma usually appears clinically as a single focus in one breast. It is, however, true that we occasionally find two or more apparently separate foci of carcinoma when we section the operative specimens in the laboratory.

The Breast Affected

It is a puzzling fact that the left breast is more prone to development of cancer than the right breast. In all substantial data concerning the disease, this fact emerges. For example, Harnett, in a study of 2529 cases from London hospitals, found the ratio of left-sided to right-sided breast cancers to be 110. Smithers and his associates, in studying the question of laterality in a total of 1762

patients at the Royal Cancer Hospital, found the ratio of left-sided to right-sided breast cancers to be 114. In a total of 15,931 cases collected by Garfinkel and his associates in 1959 from many smaller series the ratio of left to right was 104.

Clemmesen found that in his Danish data, which included 16,217 women and 149 men with breast cancer, the ratio of left-sided disease to right-sided disease was 107 in the women and 113 in the men. Clemmesen found that this predominance of left over right-sided lesions did not vary with age or marital status.

The findings in our data from the Presbyterian Hospital during the years 1915 to 1955 are shown in Table 22–1. Our findings are identical with Clemmesen's.

Site Within the Breast

There are a number of large case series of breast cancer which include data as to the site of the tumor in the classical four sectors as well as the central region of the breast (Table 22–2). These data, however, are based upon written descriptions of the site of the tumor. They are not as precise as data based upon actual sketches of the breast or upon diagrams of the breast in which the various

Table 22–1. THE BREAST AFFECTED IN CARCINOMA. PRESBYTERIAN HOSPITAL, 1915–1955

Both Breasts Simultaneously	Right Breast	Left Breast	Ratio of Left Over Right
11	1430	1532	1.07

Table 22–2. SITE OF CARCINOMA WITHIN THE BREAST

Case Series	No. of Cases	Upper Outer	Lower Outer	Upper Inner	Lower Inner	Central	Diffuse	Axillary Tail
Lane-Claypon (1928)	1354	30.6%	8.9%	12.3%	4.3%	14.3%	4.7%	
Truscott (1947)	836	46.0%	12.0%	20.0%	5.0%	13.0%		4.0%
Harnett (1948)	2529	43.0%	9.6%	13.3%	4.4%	11 %	15.2%	
Nohrman (1949)	591	47.0%		18.0%		35.0%		
Smithers (1952)	662	47.7%	8.8%	14.8%	6.0%	22.8%		
Donegan (1967)	764	48.0%	11 %	16.0%	6.0%	17.0%		

breast sectors are specified. They are not precise enough for our modern studies of the significance of the exact site of the tumor in relation to the likelihood of metastasis to the different regional lymph node filters.

In our breast clinics we use a diagram for recording the clinical findings in mammary carcinoma in which the mammary region is divided into seven carefully delimited areas. Figure 22–1 shows the site of the primary tumor in terms of this diagram in my personal series of 1007 patients treated by radical mastectomy. It should be pointed out that we have chosen to record tumors that *impinge* upon the three critical areas G, E, and D, as being situated within these specific areas, even though the bulk of the tumor may be situated in an adjacent area. This rule is necessary if we are to assess the significance of tumor site accurately.

The upper outer sector of the breast is, in my own data as in those from other sources, the most frequent site of carcinoma. It may be argued that this sector contains a greater bulk of breast tissue than any of the other three quadrants; that is, it contains the greatest number of cubic centimeters of mammary gland exposed to the risk of carcinomatous change. This is a purely anatomic explanation, but I know of no other.

In our laboratory we are well aware that multiple foci of carcinoma are often found within the breast. Any pathologist who routinely takes multiple blocks of tissue for sectioning from different sectors of the breasts that he studies will be impressed with the fact that the disease often appears to originate simultaneously in a number of apparently independent foci. In our laboratory we have not made a special study of the frequency with which multiple foci are found.

Muir was one of the first to emphasize the multicentric nature of breast carcinoma. He noted that the multiple foci often had a regional distribution in the breast. Qualheim and Gall made a special study of 157 breasts utiliz-

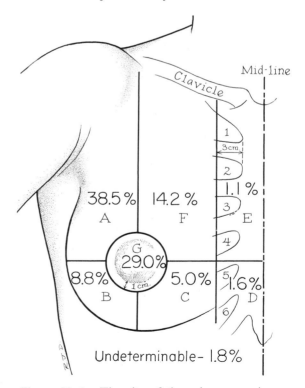

Figure 22–1. The site of the primary carcinoma within the breast in a personal series of 1007 patients.

ing large 8 x 12 cm. tissue blocks to determine the frequency of multiple sites of origin. They found multiple independent carcinomas, usually of microscopic size, in 54 per cent of these breasts.

This multiplicity of breast carcinoma is one of the reasons for removing *all* the breast when radical mastectomy is performed. When thick flaps are cut, as is the usual practice, a good deal of breast tissue is left on them, and I have no doubt but that some local recurrences in the flaps are explained by occult independent foci of carcinoma left behind in the mammary tissue on the flaps.

Size of the Primary Tumor

It was formerly the custom to record the size of tumors in the breast in terms of nuts or fruits. Fortunately, this practice is disappearing, but it has not been entirely replaced by careful measurement in terms of centimeters. There are, of course, two kinds of measurements, those made by the clinician before treatment, and those made by the pathologist

in his study of the surgical specimen. Both are important. The pathologist's measurement of the diameter of the tumor will in general be found to be about 1 cm. less than the clinician's.

The primary focus is sometimes discovered while it is very small. I have pointed out in discussing diagnosis that it is possible to detect a breast carcinoma by palpation when it is as small as 5 mm. in diameter, provided that it is not hidden in the depths of a large breast. Carcinomas smaller than this are found not by the clinician but by the pathologist in the course of his studies of tissue removed from the breast, usually for cystic disease or some other benign lesion. The following case is an example.

Mrs. E. M., a 44 year old widowed school teacher, was admitted to the Presbyterian Hospital for a tumor of the right breast of six weeks' duration. I had operated upon her mother at the age of 70 for a carcinoma of the breast.

Her tumor was a firm but movable 4 x 3 cm. mass in the right breast just beyond the areolar edge in the radius of 8 o'clock. There was questionable slight skin dimpling over the mass. At operation the tumor was found to be a group of blue-domed

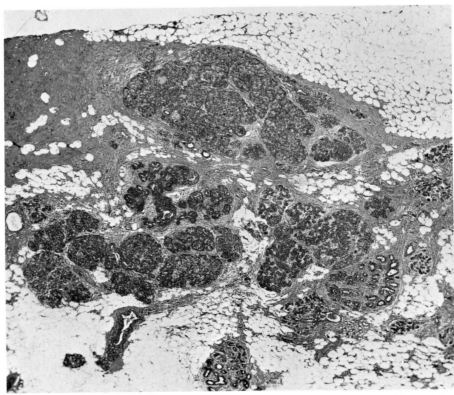

Figure 22–2.   A minute breast carcinoma discovered at microscopic examination of breast tissue removed for cystic disease.

cysts, the largest 1 cm. in diameter, lying in rather dense mammary tissue. The cysts and the adjacent breast tissue were excised. A frozen section revealed nothing suspicious. The wound was therefore closed.

Nothing suggestive of carcinoma was noted in the gross study of the specimen, but a number of blocks of tissue were cut for paraffin sections. The sections showed cystic disease and fibrosis. One section alone revealed a minute area of undoubted carcinoma. It is shown in low power magnification in Figure 22-2. Its total diameter was approximately 5 mm.

With this diagnosis a radical mastectomy was carried out. No residual carcinoma was found in the amputated breast, and there were no axillary metastases.

This case illustrates the value of meticulous pathologic study of surgical specimens from the breast. Several blocks of tissue are studied from small specimens received in our laboratory of surgical pathology, and when the entire breast is removed blocks are cut not only from the primary tumor and the adjacent breast tissue, the four sectors of the breast, the subareolar region, and the nipple, but also from any area that appears to be grossly abnormal. In this way one or two minute breast carcinomas are discovered in our laboratory every year.

The Rate of Growth of Breast Carcinoma

We have very little knowledge of the rate of growth of breast carcinoma as indicated by actual measurements of the increase in size of the untreated primary tumor. It might be supposed that each breast carcinoma has a growth rate that is more or less constant from the date of its origin as a mutation from a single cell. We know that some breast carcinomas grow slowly and others rapidly, but just what these growth rates are we do not know. Richards estimated that the *average* mammary carcinoma increases 1 cm. in size every three months. He correlated actual measurements of tumor size with patients' statements as to tumor duration in a series of 324 breast carcinomas, and drew up Table 22-3, which suggests that slowly growing tumors are much more curable than rapidly growing ones.

Collins has made some very shrewd and interesting speculations regarding the rate of tumor growth. He has observed that the time it takes for a pulmonary metastasis to double in size varies with different types of tumors.

Table 22-3. RATE OF GROWTH VS. SURVIVAL IN MAMMARY CARCINOMA*

Rate of Growth	Total No. of Cases	Alive After Five Years
SLOW Less than 1 cm. per 6 months	55	84 %
MODERATE 1 cm. per 6 months	104	63.5%
FAST More than 1 cm. per 3 months	139	18 %
RAPID (Inflammatory)	26	4 %
Total	324	43 %

*From Richards, G. E.: Mammary Cancer. Part 1. Brit. J. Radiol., *21*:109, 1948.

For breast carcinoma the doubling time was 28 days. Based on calculations of cell size, 30 doublings are required for a tumor originating from a single cell to reach a diameter of 1 cm. From these facts Collins assumes that most cancers have been present for a very long time before they become evident clinically.

Schwartz has used this biomathematical approach to study the growth rates of a series of primary pulmonary neoplasms. He reached the same conclusion as Collins, namely, that carcinomas have constant exponential growth rates which are reflected in fixed doubling times. These doubling times vary considerably with the individual neoplasm.

Ingleby studied the growth rates of a series of six mammary carcinomas roentgenographically. She estimated that the doubling time varied from 2.7 months to 15 months.

If breast carcinomas, like other neoplasms, have constant doubling times, we must face the fact that they are present for a very long time before they reach the minimal clinical size of about 1 cm. when they first become palpable. On the basis of Collins' estimate of a doubling time of 28 days, and Ingleby's minimal doubling time of 2.7 months, an average of approximately five years would be required for the tumor to reach a palpable size. Lesions with a slower doubling time would have a much longer latent period. These facts present an added challenge to us in terms of early diagnosis. They also provide an explanation for the long latent period in the development of recurrence in some cases.

THE SPREAD OF THE DISEASE IN
THE BREAST

The primary focus of carcinoma within the breast grows by division of its constituent cells which infiltrate the tissues of the breast. The infiltration tends to be along ducts, along fascial strands, and into the less resistant mammary fat. The carcinoma thus tends to have an irregular, or stellate, rather than a round outline, as in Figure 22–3, which shows an entire carcinoma in low magnification. There are, of course, certain types of carcinomas, which I will describe separately, that are exceptions to the rule. As the carcinoma cells multiply, they appear to stimulate proliferation of fibroblasts from the breast stroma, so that in the majority of breast carcinomas the carcinoma cells lie in a dense fibrous matrix. This fibrous matrix is what gives breast carcinomas their dense consistence. MacCarty believed that he could correlate the degree of fibrosis in and about breast carcinomas with their degree of malignancy, but we have not been able to confirm his theory. I will discuss this question of microscopic grading in Chapter 32.

Extension of the disease within the mammary ducts is often seen. I am not now referring to the special type of intraductal carcinoma in the milk sinuses of the nipple that characterizes the Paget's type of carcinoma; I refer to the extension of breast carcinoma within ducts in the region of the primary tumor and sometimes far into the other parts of the breast. Figure 22–4 shows carcinoma growing along a duct that has been cut longitudinally.

One of the striking microscopic features of breast carcinoma is malignant transformation of the epithelium of an entire lobule, the lobular architecture still being preserved. Figure 22–5 shows this kind of cancerization of a lobule. If carcinoma reaches the epithelium of the terminal acini by growing along the duct lumens, the process of intraductal spread must be a very extensive one, indeed. There is, of course, another possible explanation for the phenomenon, namely, that carcinomatous transformation develops as a generalized phenomenon throughout ducts and acini in a wide segment of the breast. This must be the way in which carcinomas that are primarily intraductal originate. In these neoplasms such

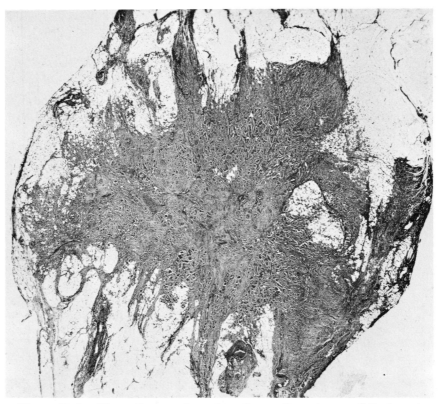

Figure 22–3.   The stellate configuration of a small carcinoma of the breast.

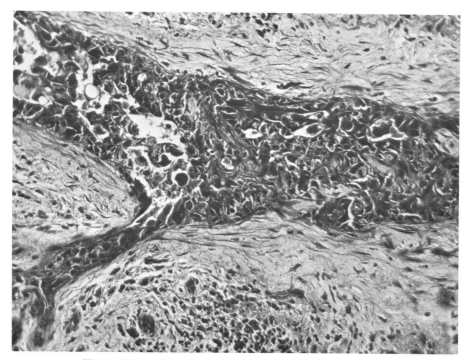

Figure 22–4. Mammary carcinoma growing along a duct.

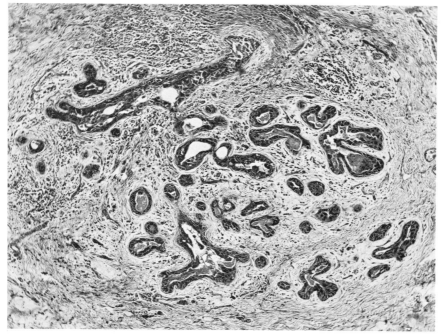

Figure 22–5. Mammary carcinoma involving an entire lobule.

a wide area of duct epithelium is involved that it is unreasonable to assume that the disease originated from a mutation in a single cell at one point in the epithelium of any one duct.

Carcinoma, extending locally in the breast, regularly infiltrates the mammary fat. Figure 22-6 shows this phenomenon. It would appear that fat offers very little resistance to the disease.

Extension of carcinoma within the breast also occurs through the lymphatics. Thorough microscopic study of breasts removed for carcinoma will occasionally reveal the disease in indubitable lymphatics, as seen in Figure 22-7, but it is sometimes difficult to be certain whether the focus of carcinoma cells is lying in a tissue space or in a lymphatic. One of the easiest types of lymphatic invasion to recognize is that which occurs in perineural lymphatics, as illustrated in Figure 22-8. In this regard, pathologists must take care not to confuse perineural carcinomatous invasion with benign epithelial invasion of nerves in the breast as described by Taylor and Norris, who found 20 examples of entirely benign epithelium situated beneath the

epineurium of breast nerves in studying a series of 1000 consecutive breast biopsies showing benign adenosis.

The periductal lymphatics of the breast also provide a route for the lymphatic spread of carcinoma. Figure 22-9 shows an embolus of carcinoma cells in a dilated periductal lymphatic.

Sampson Handley, whose studies of the lymphatic spread of breast carcinoma were among the most extensive that have been made, came to believe that the main direction of lymphatic spread in the breast is not centripetally to the subareolar plexus but vertically downward to the lymphatic plexus in the deep pectoral fascia underlying the breast.

Fraser, who carried out interesting studies of the spread of the disease in the breast by means of whole sections and key block sections, emphasized the frequency of infiltration along fascial planes. He pointed out that one side of a fascial line is often infiltrated while the other side is free, indicating that the cancer cells follow the lines of least resistance, and he emphasized the comparative immunity of muscle against invasion by carci-

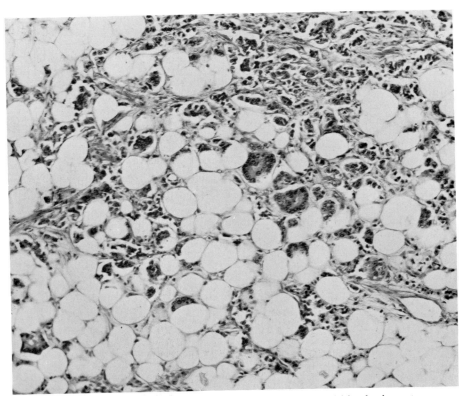

Figure 22-6. Mammary carcinoma infiltrating fat within the breast.

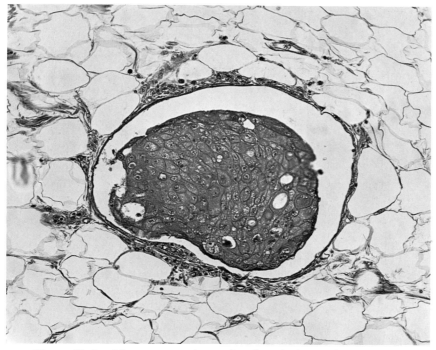

Figure 22–7.   Mammary carcinoma in a lymphatic within the breast.

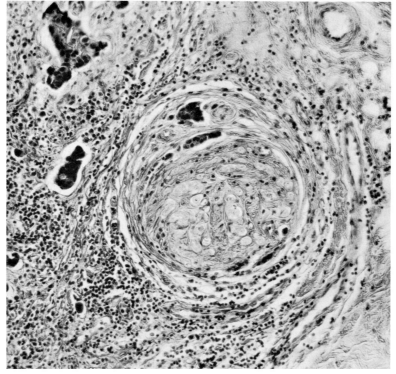

Figure 22–8.   Mammary carcinoma growing in perineural lymphatics.

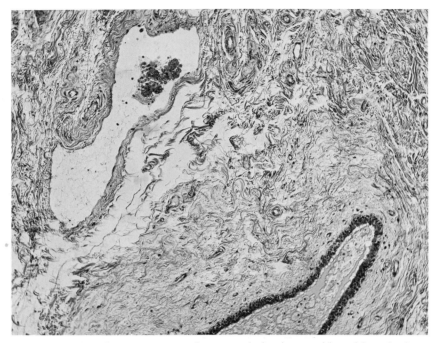

Figure 22–9.   A mammary carcinoma embolus in a periductal lymphatic.

noma cells. In advanced cases in which the cancer rests upon the pectoral muscle and infiltrates the pectoral fascia extensively, the muscle tissue itself is usually not involved.

Fraser found that lymphatic invasion occurs first in a vertical direction down through the whole thickness of the breast to the retromammary fascial plane, from whence the distribution is in a centrifugal direction. He stated "In whatever portion of the breast the primary tumor may originate, this scheme of primary vertical distribution is apparent." Figure 22–10, which is a drawing made from Fraser's photograph, shows this vertical lymphatic dissemination of a breast carcinoma downward to the pectoral fascia, as seen in a whole breast section.

Carcinoma also grows through the walls of blood vessels as it extends in the breast, and we sometimes see carcinoma emboli within the lumens of arteries as well as veins. Figure 22–11 shows a large carcinoma embolus in the lumen of a good-sized sclerotic artery. Figure 22–12 shows two small veins filled with carcinoma. Delbet and Herrenschmidt wrote a good description of a breast carcinoma that showed a special tendency to grow within blood vessels.

Vogt-Hoerner has recently studied the question of the direction of spread of carcinoma within the breast, in a series of 544

surgical specimens. Vertical as well as horizontal blocks of tissue from the nipple and subareolar area were studied microscopically to determine whether or not the carcinoma extended to this central area of the breast. Central spread was found in 250 of the cases. Among this group, 80 per cent had axillary metastases. In the 294 cases in which no central spread was found only 61 per cent had axillary metastases.

She classified the central spread as (1) lymphatic, (2) along connective tissue planes, and (3) intraductal. In the group with lymphatic spread, 53 per cent were found to have axillary metastases. When the disease extended along connective tissue planes there were axillary metastases in 35 per cent. When the spread was intraductal only 25 per cent had axillary metastases.

Vogt-Hoerner concludes that a considerable proportion of breast carcinomas tend to spread centrally to the subareolar region, and that this form of the disease is more apt to be associated with axillary metastases, particularly when the route of spread is through the lymphatics.

The truth probably is that mammary carcinoma spreads from the primary site within the breast both toward the central subareolar region and vertically downward to the retromammary plane. Our own observations of

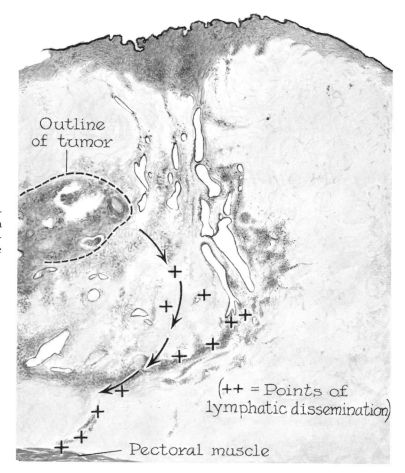

Figure 22–10. Lymphatic dissemination of breast carcinoma vertically downward to the pectoral fascia, as seen in a whole breast section.

Outline of tumor

(++ = Points of lymphatic dissemination)

Pectoral muscle

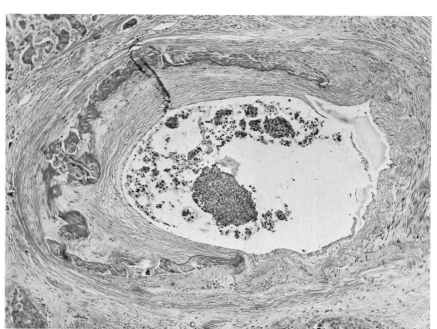

Figure 22–11. Mammary carcinoma in the lumen of a sclerotic artery within the breast.

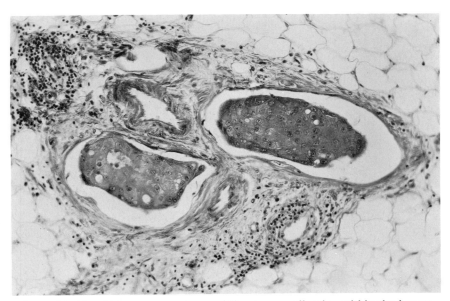

Figure 22–12.   Mammary carcinoma filling two small veins within the breast.

breast lymphatics during radical mastectomy, following subcutaneous injection of Direct Sky Blue dye, have convinced us that the lymphatics within the breast are more numerous than we had imagined, and that they are found extending from all sides of the operative field. We agree with Turner-Warwick that the grossly visible lymphatics run toward the axilla and not toward the subareolar region, but this fact does not invalidate Vogt-Hoerner's finding that there is microscopic spread toward the subareolar region in a considerable proportion of cases.

From a practical point of view these facts mean that the surgeon can never be certain of the extent of carcinoma within the breast, or of the direction of its spread. When he embarks upon the surgical removal of the disease he must carry the limits of his dissection as wide as the anatomic and functional limits permit and the results of his procedure justify.

Edema of the Skin

Edema of the skin over the breast is an important clinical phenomenon that develops in the course of breast carcinoma. It has been called pigskin by the English and peau d'orange by the French, but *edema* is a more accurate name because it identifies the nature of the phenomenon.

Edema is evident clinically by inspection of the skin in a good light. The openings of the skin glands, which are not normally visible, are clearly defined as small deep pits, as seen in Figure 22–13. The texture of the skin, as appreciated by very gentle palpation, is thickened and somewhat roughened.

Roentgenologists have recently become aware of the fact that thickened edematous skin is evident in their films. This is an expensive way of discovering a phenomenon that is easily appreciated clinically.

There has been surprisingly little attention given to the pathology of edema of the skin and its significance in mammary carcinoma. Leitch published a brief description of the microscopic findings many years ago, but no one has written adequately about it. In our laboratory we have long been interested in the pathologic mechanism by which edema of the skin is produced, and we have made a special effort over a period of years to study microscopic sections of the edematous skin in these cases. We have found that the skin is of course greatly thickened by edema in the corium. At an early stage of the process the lymphatics of the deep network in the corium are dilated and contain occasional emboli of carcinoma cells, as seen in Figure 22–14. At this early stage the edema involves only a limited area of the skin over the breast, usually the lower half of the areola or the skin just caudad to it. Gravity is no doubt a factor

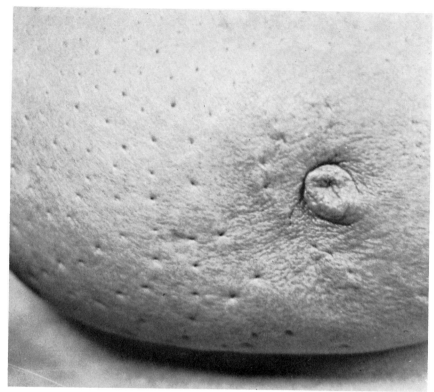

Figure 22–13. Edema of the skin of a breast containing carcinoma.

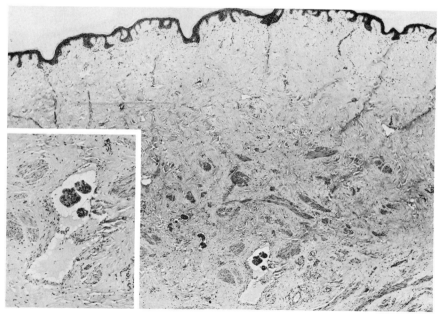

Figure 22–14. Carcinoma emboli in a dilated lymphatic deep in the corium of edematous skin. The insert at the left shows in higher magnification the dilated lymphatic with its emboli, from the lower central part of the section.

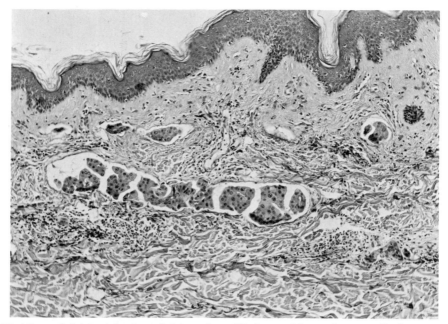

Figure 22–15. Superficial lymphatics of the corium filled up with carcinoma cells in a more advanced stage of edema of the skin.

in the predisposition of this area of skin over the breast to edema.

At a later stage, when skin edema is very extensive, the smaller, more superficial lymphatics, as well as the deeper ones in the corium, are filled by carcinoma cells, as seen in Figure 22–15. We infer that the deep lymphatics of the corium are at first partially blocked by embolism, and are finally solidly occluded by permeation with carcinoma cells. In edematous skin we have not seen carcinoma diffusely invading either the epidermis or corium. The disease is confined within the lymphatics, and it produces edema of the skin by blocking the lymphatics.

Infiltration and Ulceration of the Overlying Skin

In the course of its local infiltrative growth within the breast the carcinoma finally — in many patients who come for treatment late — reaches the overlying skin. Immobility of the skin over the tumor and localized redness are signs that infiltration of the skin has begun. Ulceration follows after a varying period of time. The typical ulcer has raised, reddish edges and a crusted, or necrotic, depressed base (Fig. 22–16). In the majority of patients

the ulcerated area enlarges very slowly and is not much of a surgical dressing problem. In occasional patients, however, the ulcerative process progresses more rapidly, and a large, foul-smelling, fungating tumor results, constituting an exceedingly difficult therapeutic problem. Hemorrhage, sometimes severe, is an occasional added complication. Figure 22–17 shows a long neglected, far advanced, massive breast carcinoma, solidly fixed to the chest wall, that bled profusely.

Satellite Nodules in the Skin over the Breast. One of the indications of comparatively extensive carcinomatous involvement of the breast itself is the appearance of satellite nodules of carcinoma in the skin of the breast. Figure 22–18 shows such nodules around a carcinoma of the lower portion of the breast. They are not a part of the phenomenon of widespread and distant metastasis to the skin seen in the terminal stage of breast carcinoma. They are a local manifestation of the disease in the breast, and result from extension of the disease along lymphatics, or ducts or fascial strands, which lead the carcinoma into contact with the skin at some little distance from the primary focus. They indicate, therefore, that the disease is widespread within the breast.

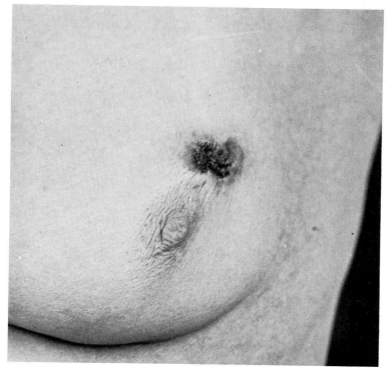

Figure 22–16. Small ulcer over a carcinoma of the breast.

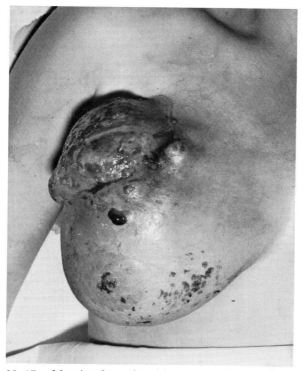

Figure 22–17. Massive fungating, bleeding carcinoma of the breast.

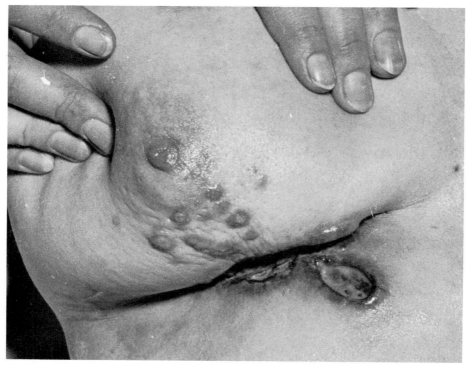

Figure 22–18.   Satellite skin nodules around an ulcerated carcinoma of the lower portion of the breast.

Carcinoma "Telangiectaticum" or "Erysipelatodes"

An unusual form of involvement of the skin in far-advanced breast carcinoma has been called carcinoma "telangiectaticum" or "erysipelatodes." Purplish-red, raised nodules appear in the skin over the breast, adjacent chest wall, or neck, and fuse to form broad reddish indurated areas. On microscopic study these nodules are seen to be dilated, thin-walled vessels situated very superficially in the epidermis and filled with carcinoma cells. The first good descriptions of this disease picture were written by Küttner, Rasch, Weber, Savatard, and Leavell and Tillotson. More recent case reports, by Pfahler and Case, Dawson and Shaw, Camiel and Bolker, and Ingram, include microscopic studies that attempt to determine whether the dilated tumor-containing vessels in the epidermis are capillaries or lymphatics. Dawson identified them as both blood and lymph vessels. Camiel and Bolker concluded that they are lymphatics. Ingram regarded them as small blood vessels.

This *telangiectatic* or *erysipelatoid* lesion should not be confused with the inflammatory type of breast carcinoma, as Chris has recently done. The former is a skin manifestation in far-advanced late mammary carcinoma, usually recurrent after mastectomy or irradiation. The latter is a primary clinical form of breast carcinoma in which the breast, from an early stage in the evolution of the disease, is enlarged and indurated, and the skin over it is generally reddened and edematous. I will deal with the inflammatory type of carcinoma in Chapter 31.

Carcinoma en Cuirasse

Velpeau's attention was first attracted in 1838 (he states) to a special form of carcinomatous involvement of the skin to which he gave the striking name *en cuirasse*. I cannot improve upon Velpeau's description.

It involves a single area, or sometimes several isolated small areas of subcutaneous tissue and skin. The involved area feels hard, rough, stiff, and thickened. It has an abnormal reddish color and stippled appearance. The skin looks as if it had been tanned, or as if a portion of stiff leather had replaced the natural skin. The small disseminated plaques have the same characteristics, and look like violet-red spots. . . .

Usually the larger plaques are surrounded by a multitude of these small ones. I have seen patients whose breasts were completely covered with the plaques and in whom the wooden-like change extended up to the hollow of the axilla on one side, towards the clavicle, and across the sternum to the other side. . . .

At its onset this primary scirrhus of the skin does not attract the attention of patients because it causes no pain and there is no exudate. Since the skin alone is affected, it is not noticed until it is fairly well advanced. The physician, however, should never be deceived, and I cannot too strongly urge him to be on guard when he notices in the skin over the chest of women patients, a yellowish-red marbling, or stippled gray patches scattered here and there, especially if they are permanent, and instead of being supple and disappearing with pressure, they are hard, thick, inelastic, or wooden-like. . . . Despite their benign appearance these spots are cancer of the worst kind. Although at first separate, they eventually fuse together, forming plaques of larger and larger size and finally a true cuirasse.*

When modern students of breast cancer such as Sampson Handley began to investigate carcinoma *en cuirasse* microscopically they found that the epidermis is atrophied, and the corium is greatly thickened by edema and fibrosis and by lymphocytic infiltration

---
*From Velpeau, A.: Traité des Maladies du Sein. Paris, Masson, 1858, 2nd. ed., p. 404.

around blood vessels and lymphatics. These changes, and the pigmentation which is such a striking feature of the lesion, are similar to those that develop in the lower legs of patients with lymphatic obstruction due to circulatory difficulties. At a later stage of carcinoma *en cuirasse,* when nodules and ulcers have developed in the involved skin, actual carcinomatous infiltration of the thickened skin is of course found.

The clinical characteristics of carcinoma *en cuirasse* are illustrated by the following case:

L. F., a 57 year old housewife, came to the Presbyterian Hospital in May, 1919, with a large carcinoma of the left breast with massive axillary metastases. A radical mastectomy was nevertheless done. Local recurrence appeared on the chest wall 20 months later, and evolved in the *cuirasse* shown in Figures 22–19 and 22–20. The *cuirasse,* outlined with a skin pencil, has involved the entire operative field and extended medially across the sternum to most of the skin over the opposite breast, upward over the clavicle to the supraclavicular skin, and laterally around to the skin of the back. The patient died four years and eight months after operation.

Fortunately, the *en cuirasse* form of carcinoma is not often seen today. The primary carcinoma can usually be controlled by either surgery or irradiation, and does not get out of hand as it did in Velpeau's time.

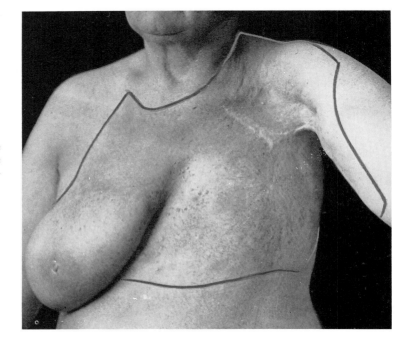

Figure 22–19. Carcinoma of the breast spreading through the lymphatics of the anterior surface of the thorax *en cuirasse.*

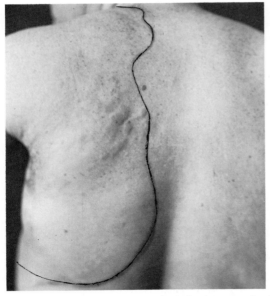

Figure 22-20. *En cuirasse* lymphatic spread of carcinoma around to the back.

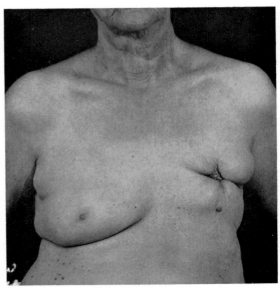

Figure 22-21. Breast contracted by carcinomatous fibrosis.

Carcinomatous Fibrosis of the Breast. The primary carcinoma in the breast does not always grow expansively and form a bulky, and sometimes ulcerated tumor. In occasional cases the fibrotic reaction in the breast to the presence of the carcinoma is so marked that the breast shrinks rather than enlarges. What was once a comparatively large, dependent, soft and movable breast becomes a hard, flattened, shrivelled organ, solidly fixed to the chest wall. Figure 22-21 shows this kind of carcinomatous fibrosis of the breast occurring in Mrs. R. P., an 82 year old widow.

She had first noted retraction of the left nipple 12 years previously. During the following years, the breast had slowly contracted. She had not consulted any physician and had no treatment. As the photograph shows, her left breast was greatly shrunken. It had not been destroyed by ulceration, because there was none, but by the slow process of replacement of the mammary fat and parenchyma. The areola could no longer be identified. The nipple was reduced to a papillary nubbin in the depths of a stellate depression. Beneath this central depression there was a firm 5 cm. tumor. The shrunken breast and the tumor within it were movable over the chest wall. A single, firm, movable, 1 cm. node was palpable in the axilla. Since this patient's slowly growing breast carcinoma gave her no symp-

toms it was not treated. She died two years after I first saw her, and 14 years after the onset of her breast carcinoma, of general debility.

THE SPREAD OF BREAST CANCER THROUGH LYMPHATICS

Embolism or Permeation

A description of the local extension and the regional lymph node metastasis of breast carcinoma must include a discussion of the method by which the disease extends along lymphatics. Until Sampson Handley carried out his studies of this question at the Middlesex Hospital in the early years of the twentieth century, it was generally assumed that carcinoma cells disseminate through lymphatics by embolism. All pathologists have occasionally seen these emboli in lymphatics in or adjacent to the primary tumor as well as in the peripheral sinuses of lymph nodes. The lymphatic trunks between the breast and the regional lymph nodes are usually found, however, to be free of carcinoma. It seems reasonable to conclude that the carcinoma emboli escape through them leaving no trace of their passage.

Handley concluded, however, that permeation rather than embolism is the usual method of dissemination. In his words, "Cancer spreads by permeating the lymphatic system like an invisible annular ringworm. The growing edge extends like a ripple, in a wider and wider circle, within whose circumference healing processes take place, so that the area of permeation at any one time is not a disc but a rim. . . . The advancing microscopic growing edge of the cancer, owing to the failure at isolated points of the defensive process of perilymphatic fibrosis, may leave in its track, here and there, isolated secondary foci, which give rise to secondary macroscopic metastases."

Handley documented his thesis with excellent descriptions and photomicrographs, and there can be no doubt but that in some patients, particularly those with advanced and terminal breast carcinoma, permeation of lymphatics is seen. It was such cases, in general, that Handley studied.

But the permeation theory has not withstood critical evaluation. Sampson Handley's contemporaries, such as Fitzwilliams and Fraser, equally devoted students of breast carcinoma, did not accept it, and continued to believe that embolism is the usual method by which breast carcinoma disseminates, at least in its earlier and operable stage. Present day pathologists in general take this view. It is certainly my own belief.

A special type of local extension of breast carcinoma to the liver through the epigastric angle was described by Sampson Handley. He pointed out that the lower inner border of the breast overlies the sixth costal cartilage, and that this point is only about an inch from the ensiform cartilage, where subperitoneal fat lies immediately beneath the fascia of the linea alba. In several cases which he illustrated with excellent drawings and photomicrographs. Handley traced breast carcinoma permeating lymphatics in the rectus sheath and muscle to reach the region of the tip of the ensiform cartilage. From the epigastric angle the disease penetrated the fascia of the linea alba and extended along the falciform ligament to reach the liver. I have shown these relationships in Figure 1–42. Although Handley's cases in which he demonstrated permeation of lymphatics along this route were advanced ones with extensive disease of the chest wall, there is no doubt that metastasis by embolism of mammary carcinoma cells occasionally occurs in earlier cases through this pathway to the liver.

Regional Lymph Node Metastases

At some point in its evolution breast carcinoma metastasizes through the lymphatic

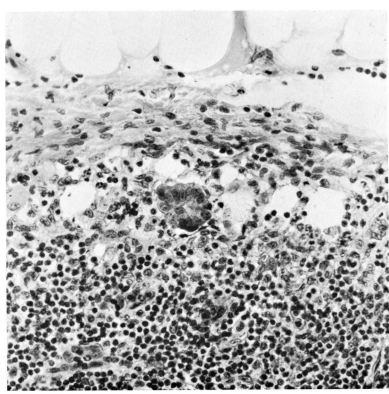

Figure 22–22. A small carcinoma embolus in the peripheral sinus of a lymph node.

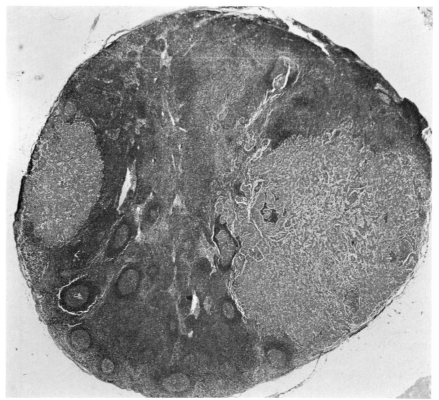

Figure 22–23. A lymph node invaded by two separate foci of metastatic carcinoma in the marginal sinuses on opposite sides of the node.

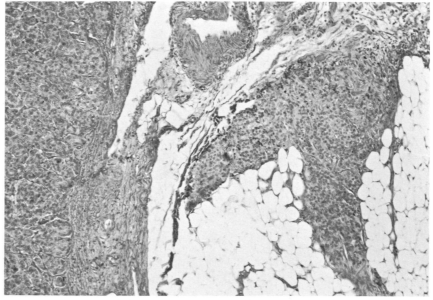

Figure 22–24. Metastatic carcinoma penetrating the capsule of a lymph node and infiltrating the surrounding fat.

Table 22–4. Results of multiple-level sections through lymph nodes in which single-level sections were negative

Author and Clinic	No. of Cases Studied	No. of Nodes per Case	Cases with Positive Nodes	
			Single-level	Multiple-levels
Saphir, O. (Chicago, Illinois)	30	5	0%	33%
Pickren (Presbyterian Hospital, N.Y.)	51	36	0%	22%

trunks which lead from the breast to the regional lymph nodes. Figure 22–22 shows a small embolus in the peripheral sinus of a lymph node, where these carcinoma cells proliferate and grow into the substance of the node. Figure 22–23 shows a lymph node in which carcinoma has penetrated deeply from two separate metastatic foci in the marginal sinuses on opposite sides of the node. Eventually the disease penetrates the capsule of the node and infiltrates the surrounding fat, as shown in Figure 22–24. The extent of the regional lymph node involvement is the most important single factor in determining the choice of treatment as well as the prognosis. It is a question that we have attempted to study with special care in our laboratory and I will present our findings in detail.

Although many lymph nodes containing metastases are enlarged, and the disease in them is grossly obvious, metastases are not infrequently found microscopically in very small lymph nodes measuring only a few millimeters in diameter.

The customary method of determining the presence of metastases in a lymph node has been to study microscopically one section through its greatest diameter. Because the volume of section cutting is so great that the technicians in laboratories are always pressed, usually only one section is cut through each node, even though it is obvious that we may well miss a small focus of carcinoma in an uncut part of a node. Saphir proved the inadequacy of one-level sectioning by an experiment in which he recut in serial sections the lymph nodes in a series of 30 cases of breast carcinoma in which previous single-level sections had not shown metastases. An average of 332 sections were cut through each node. By serial sections Saphir found metastases in 10, or 33 per cent, of the cases.

Pickren repeated and expanded this experiment in our laboratory by recutting the nodes in 51 cases in which previous one-level sectioning had not shown metastases. Pickren recut the nodes in serial sections, each 15 microns thick. An important point of difference between Saphir's and Pickren's studies is that Saphir had only an average of five nodes per case, while Pickren, who used the clearing technique for finding nodes, had an average of 36 per case. Pickren found metastases in 11, or 22 per cent, of his cases. These data are summarized in Table 22–4. They prove beyond doubt that our routine method of studying lymph nodes has missed metastases in a considerable proportion of cases. This is one explanation for the occasional appearance of distant metastases in patients in whom no axillary metastases were found. It is also a strong argument for meticulous and complete axillary dissection in breast carcinoma.

As the result of his study Pickren concluded that, since serial sectioning is impossible in the routine study of lymph nodes, a reasonable compromise would be to section all lymph nodes in three different levels, namely through their upper, middle, and lower thirds. He had found that the smallest number of sections that showed cancer cells was four if the serially sectioned node contained metastases. He assumed that if three levels were studied routinely, metastases would rarely be missed. Lattes has adapted Pickren's suggestion in our laboratories of surgical pathology.

Axillary Lymph Node Metastasis

The main route for lymphatic metastasis from breast carcinoma is through the axilla, the axillary nodes being the first to be involved in the regional lymphatic filter. I described the axillary lymphatic route in Chapter 1.

For a variable period of time the axillary

Table 22–5. Carcinoma of the breast, age of patient, and involvement of axillary nodes at operation. Personal series, 1935–1968.

Age	No. of Patients	Patients With No Axillary Node Involvement
Under 40	117	51%
40–49	312	57%
50–59	272	58%
60–69	203	54%
70+	103	55%
Total	1007	56%

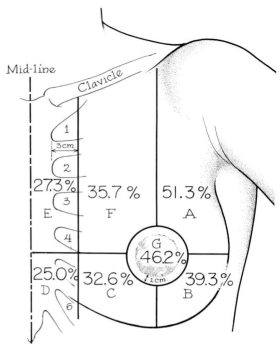

Figure 22–25. The frequency of axillary lymph node metastases from carcinomas of the different sectors of the breast in a personal series of 1007 patients.

nodes are usually the only regional nodes involved. The best proof of this is the fact that a considerable proportion of patients with not too extensive axillary node involvement are cured by radical mastectomy in which the axillary nodes, but none of the other regional lymph node groups, are removed.

Influence of the Age of the Patient on the Incidence of Axillary Metastasis. In keeping with the widely held belief that breast carcinoma is less malignant in old age we might expect the frequency of axillary metastasis to decrease with advancing age. Taylor and Nathanson found this to be true in their data. They reported that in a group of their patients under the age of 46, axillary node involvement was found in 77 per cent, whereas in a group of patients over the age of 60 only 57 per cent had axillary node involvement.

I have chosen to study this question in my own personal series of 1007 radical mastectomies because both the axillary dissection and the microscopic study of the surgical specimen were carried out with special care. Table 22–5 shows these data. They do not indicate that the age of the patient has any significant relationship to axillary metastasis.

The Relationship of the Site of the Primary Carcinoma in the Breast to Axillary Metastasis. It is of some practical importance to know how the site of the primary carcinoma in the breast influences the likelihood of metastasis to the axilla. To study this question I have again used my personal series of 1007 radical mastectomies in which the site of the primary tumor has been recorded precisely. These data, presented in Figure 22–25, show that axillary metastasis is more frequent from primary tumors of the upper outer sector. The primary tumors originating in the central sector of the breast metastasize

in approximately the same pattern as those in the upper outer sector. Lesions situated in the other sectors of the breast apparently have a somewhat lesser likelihood of metastasizing to the axilla.

The Influence of the Size of the Primary Carcinoma on Axillary Metastasis. In any series of patients with breast carcinoma there are some whose lesions are highly malignant and grow rapidly and metastasize to the axilla early. Other patients have carcinomas of lesser malignancy that grow more slowly and metastasize late to the axilla. Nevertheless, studies correlating the size of the primary carcinoma in the breast with the microscopic findings in the axillary nodes show that tumor size is an important factor in axillary metastasis.

Some skeptical students of breast carcinoma—usually those who have not had a great deal of personal experience with the actual treatment of the disease—suggest that most patients with even small primary tumors already have axillary metastases when they come for treatment.

For example, Park and Lees estimated that 60 per cent of the patients have metastasis

Table 22–6. Carcinoma of the breast, Columbia Clinical Classification stages *A* and *B*. Size of primary tumor correlated with axillary metastasis. Personal series of radical mastectomies, 1935–1968

Size of Primary Tumor (Clinical Measurement)	No. of Patients	Patients with Involved Axillary Nodes	
		No.	Per cent
No palpable tumor	26	5	19.2%
Less than 10 mm.	22	5	22.7%
10–19 mm.	119	29	24.4%
20–29 mm.	223	68	30.5%
30–39 mm.	180	84	46.7%
40–49 mm.	147	68	46.3%
50–59 mm.	101	61	60.4%
60–79 mm.	77	40	51.9%
80 mm. and over	27	14	51.9%
Total	922	374	40.6%

when their tumor first becomes palpable. McKinnon stated that axillary metastasis "is found in practically all cases of typical breast cancer no matter how small the lesion. . . ."

In reviewing these studies Gilliam has shown that a more sophisticated statistical approach might well produce different conclusions concerning the presence of metastasis in early stages of the disease. He concluded that 30 per cent is a more reasonable figure than Park and Lees' 60 per cent of axillary metastasis at onset of symptoms. Kraus also reviewed Park and Lees' studies and found their analyses unconvincing.

The data regarding the relationship of the size of the primary carcinoma to the frequency of axillary metastasis in my own series of 922 radical mastectomies performed on patients whose disease was classified as Clinical Stage A or B are shown in Table 22–6. I have included only the patients whose

disease was classified as Clinical Stage A and B, because in these patients clinical factors such as ulceration and edema of the skin, indicative of far advanced disease, are not present to influence judgment as to the extent of axillary involvement, and the significance of the size of the primary tumor can be studied by itself.

It is seen from these data that less than one-third of the patients whose primary tumor measured less than 3 cm. in diameter had axillary metastases. But about one-half of the patients whose tumors measured more than 3 cm. in diameter had involved axillary nodes.

Another way of studying the relationship of the size of the primary carcinoma to the extent of axillary metastasis is to correlate the size of the tumor with the number of involved nodes in cases in which axillary metastases were found. Table 22–7 shows these data in my personal series of radical mastectomies. It is evident that in patients who have axillary metastases the likelihood of having more involved nodes increases as the size of the tumor increases.

It is also interesting to study the relationship of tumor size and axillary metastasis in the early cases—the Stage A cases in our Columbia Clinical Classification. In these Stage A cases there are, of course, none with clinically involved axillary nodes. Table 22–8 presents these data. It shows that even in these early cases in which axillary metastases are considerably less frequent, their incidence is closely related to the size of the primary tumor.

The Route of Metastases Through the Axillary Lymph Node Filter. It is of considerable practical importance to know precisely how breast carcinoma extends through the axillary filter. This is a question which we have studied with special care.

Table 22–7. Carcinoma of the breast. Size of primary tumor in patients with axillary metastasis correlated with number of involved axillary nodes. Personal series of radical mastectomies, 1935–1968

Size of Primary Tumor (Clinical Measurement)	Total No. of Patients	No. of Patients With Involved Nodes	1 to 3 Nodes Involved		4 to 7 Nodes Involved		8 or more Nodes Involved	
			No. of Patients	Per cent	No. of Patients	Per cent	No. of Patients	Per cent
No palpable tumor	27	6	5	83.3%	—	—	1	16.7%
Less than 30 mm.	373	110	73	66.4%	16	14.5%	21	19.1%
30 mm. to less than 60 mm.	462	242	129	53.3%	54	22.3%	59	24.4%
60 mm. or larger	145	87	37	42.5%	16	18.4%	34	39.1%
Total	1007	445	274	54.8%	86	19.3%	115	25.8%

Table 22–8. Carcinoma of the breast, Columbia Clinical Classification Stage *A*. Size of primary tumor correlated with axillary metastasis. Personal series of radical mastectomies, 1935–1968

| Size of Primary Tumor (Clinical Measurement) | All Cases in the Series | | | Stage A, Columbia Clinical Classification | | |
| | No. of Patients | Patients With Involved Axillary Nodes | | No. of Patients | Patients With Involved Axillary Nodes | |
		No.	Per cent		No.	Per cent
No palpable tumor	27	6	22.2%	26	5	19.2%
Less than 30 mm.	373	110	29.5%	330	78	23.6%
30 mm. to less than 60 mm.	462	242	52.4%	306	120	39.2%
60 mm. and over	145	87	60.0%	63	24	38.1%
Total	1007	445	44.2%	724	226	31.2%

The cancerous emboli usually reach the central part of the axillary node filter first. Our data show that the nodes of the central group are not only the group most often involved, but also the group most often exclusively involved. The highest nodes in the filter, the subclavicular nodes, are the last to be involved, and have not, in our data, been alone involved.

Although we have been clearing the axillary dissection specimens in our laboratory of surgical pathology since 1951, our most accurate data are represented by our findings in a series of specimens studied between 1951 and 1954, to which I have referred in Chapter 1. The series includes 182 cases. Most of the work was done personally by Pickren. I have, therefore, used the findings in this special series to illustrate metastasis through the axillary lymphatic filter.

Metastases were found in 80 of these 182 specimens. The relative frequency of involvement and the proportion of nodes involved in each of the six different groups of axillary nodes are shown in Tables 22–9 and 22–10.

The Prognostic Significance of Metastasis in Different Axillary Lymph Node Groups. Table 22–11 presents the 10 year survival rates after radical mastectomy for patients with metastasis to the different groups of axillary nodes. Although this series of cases, in which Pickren studied the distribution of metastases in the different lymph node groups with special care, was small, the survival rates, as given, are probably representative. I have already emphasized the grave prognostic significance of metastases to the subclavicular nodes. The number of patients with metastasis to the external mammary group of nodes in this series of cases is too small to have any statistical significance. It is interesting, however, that metastasis to the other four axillary node groups have almost the same prognostic significance. The

Table 22–9. Axillary lymph node metastases in 182 cleared radical mastectomy specimens, 1951–1954. Relative frequency of Involvement of different axillary lymph node groups

| Axillary Lymph Node Group | All 182 Cases Studied | | | 80 Cases with Involved Nodes | | |
	No. of Cases with Nodes	No. of Cases with Involved Nodes	Per cent with Involved Nodes	No. of Cases with Nodes	No. of Cases with Involved Nodes	Per cent with Involved Nodes
External mammary	96	6	6.2%	41	6	14.6%
Scapular	152	15	9.9%	70	15	21.4%
Central	182	72	39.6%	80	72	90.0%
Interpectoral	97	17	17.5%	49	17	34.7%
Axillary vein	179	27	15.1%	80	27	33.8%
Subclavicular	169	15	8.9%	75	15	20.0%
Total	182	80	44.5%	80	80	100 %

Table 22–10. Axillary lymph node metastases in 182 cleared radical mastectomy specimens, 1951–1954. Proportion of nodes involved in different axillary lymph node groups

Axillary Lymph Node Group	All 182 Cases			80 Cases With Involved Nodes		
	No. of Nodes Found	No. of Nodes Involved	Per cent of Nodes Involved	No. of Nodes Found	No. of Nodes Involved	Per cent of Nodes Involved
External mammary	311	11	3.5%	139	11	7.9%
Scapular	1061	37	3.5%	534	37	6.9%
Central	2199	216	9.8%	1037	216	20.8%
Interpectoral	262	33	12.6%	158	33	20.9%
Axillary vein	1948	128	6.6%	987	128	13.0%
Subclavicular	641	45	7.0%	301	45	14.9%
Total	6422	470	7.3%	3156	470	11.7%

10 year survival rate for patients with metastases in all four node groups is approximately 30 per cent.

Metastasis to the Central Node Group. The central group regularly contained the largest number of nodes. The proportion of nodes involved was also much higher in this group (39.6 per cent) than in any other node group. Of the 80 cases in which metastases were found, the central group was involved in 90 per cent.

Göksel carefully studied a series of 46 radical mastectomy specimens with the clearing technique and reported a similar predominance of metastases to the central axillary node group.

It is interesting to note the site of metastasis when only a single node group was found to be involved (Table 22–12). There were 44 such cases in our data. In 38 of them it was the central group of nodes that was involved.

Vogt-Hoerner and Contesso have reported a similar experience in studying the site of solitary metastases to the axilla. They did not clear their specimens, and found an average of 18 nodes per specimen. In 35 cases in which there was a single node involved, and its site was known in terms of the same grouping of axillary nodes which I have used, the node was in the central group in 28 cases.

A frequent type of axillary lymph node involvement, in which only a few central nodes contain metastases, is illustrated in Figure 22–26.

Metastasis to the Interpectoral Node Group. It is also worthwhile to analyze the sequence of involvement of the groups of nodes in our data, particularly for two of the groups, the interpectoral and the subclavicular. It will be recalled from our discussion of the routes of lymphatic metastasis from the breast in Chapter 1 that the interpectoral nodes may provide a separate pathway to the subclavicular nodes at the apex of the axilla, by-passing the main axillary lymph node groups. Table 22–13 shows the node groups involved in 17 cases in which there were metastases in the interpectoral nodes. In none of these cases were metastases found only in the interpectoral and the subclavicular nodes.

Table 22–11. Results of radical mastectomy in 80 patients in whom axillary metastases were found by the clearing method, 1951–1954. Relationship of 10 year survival to group of axillary nodes involved.

Axillary Lymph Node Group	No. of Cases With Involved Nodes in Specified Group	Average No. of Involved Nodes in All Groups for these Cases	10 Year Survival	
			No.	Per cent
External mammary	6	9.0	1	16.7%
Scapular	15	13.1	4	26.7%
Central	72	6.3	21	29.2%
Interpectoral	17	8.6	5	29.4%
Axillary vein	27	12.8	7	25.9%
Subclavicular	15	16.2	1	6.7%
Total	80	5.9	25	31.2%

Table 22–12. Axillary lymph node metastases in 182 cleared radical mastectomy specimens, 1951–1954. Single node groups containing metastases

Axillary Lymph Node Group	No. of Cases With Metastases Only In Single Node Group	Per cent of All 80 Cases With Metastases
External mammary	2	2.5%
Scapular	1	1.2%
Central	38	47.5%
Interpectoral	3	3.7%
Axillary vein	0	0
Subclavicular	0	0

Our data indicate, therefore, that when breast carcinoma metastasizes through the interpectoral route, this pathway does not lead exclusively to the subclavicular group of nodes, but leads also to other node groups such as the central group and the axillary vein group. The close association of the lymphatics of the interpectoral route with branches of the thoracoacromial blood vessels, which originate in the area where the most medial of the axillary vein group of lymph nodes lie, makes it likely that the interpectoral lymphatics usually empty into these nodes.

The importance of removing these interpectoral nodes in radical mastectomy—and this can, of course, be achieved only by the removal of the pectoral muscles—is illustrated by the case for which the diagram of the axillary findings is shown in Figure 22-27. This patient is well 15 years after her radical mastectomy. In our series of 182 cases in which the distribution of axillary nodes was studied with special care, there were two others with solitary metastases in interpectoral nodes who have also survived more than 10 years.

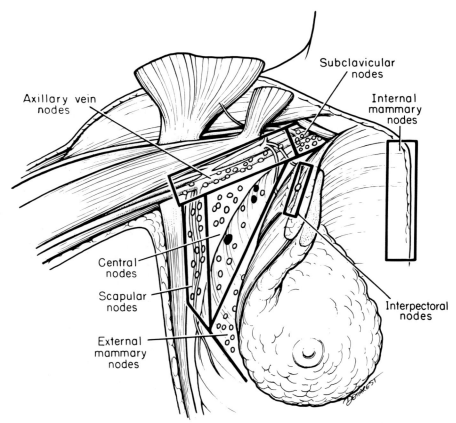

Figure 22–26. Diagram of the axillary lymph nodes found in a radical mastectomy specimen studied by the clearing method. A woman physician, aged 60, had a 2 cm. carcinoma of the central zone of her right breast. There were no palpable axillary nodes. Columbia Clinical Classification Stage A. A total of 70 axillary nodes were found. Three of the 20 nodes in the central group contained metastases. No postoperative irradiation or hormonal treatment was given. The patient was well 16 years later.

Table 22–13. AXILLARY LYMPH NODE METASTASES IN 182 CLEARED RADICAL MASTECTOMY SPECIMENS, 1951–1954. SEVENTEEN CASES WITH INTERPECTORAL NODE INVOLVEMENT

Case	No. of Nodes Involved in Different Node Groups						Total No. Involved Nodes	Total No. Nodes Found	Results of Treatment
	Sub-clavicular	Axillary vein	Central	Scapular	External mammary	Inter-pectoral			
1						1	1	61	10 year cure
2						1	1	58	11 year cure
3						1	1	58	12 year cure
4		1	4			2	7	44	10 year cure, then local recurrence
5			1			1	2	34	10 year survival with metastases
6			2			1	3	29	Died in 58 mos.
7			3			1	4	76	Died in 91 mos.
8			3			2	5	59	Died in 45 mos.
9			1			1	2	35	Died in 54 mos.
10		3	3			1	7	32	Died in 17 mos.
11		9	6			2	17	43	Died in 18 mos.
12		2	1	1		4	8	46	Died in 9 mos.
13	12	13	7	3		2	37	69	Died in 48 mos.
14	1	11	7			1	20	39	Died in 112 mos.
15	4		1		5	1	11	82	Died in 59 mos.
16	1		4	3		7	15	19	Died in 15 mos.
17	1			1		4	6	48	Died in 17 mos.

Average number of involved nodes per case — 8.6.
10 year survival rate — 29.4%.

Kay made a special study of metastasis to the interpectoral nodes and reported four similar patients in whom only the interpectoral nodes were involved and who were cured by radical mastectomy. Kay's specimens were not studied with the clearing method. He found interpectoral nodes in only 23 per cent of them as compared with the 53 per cent found in our series of cleared specimens.

Metastasis to the Subclavicular Group of Nodes. The subclavicular group of nodes, situated at the highest point, or apex, of the axillary lymph node filter, consists of three or four small nodes lying in the angle that the axillary vein forms with the chest wall before the vein passes beneath the tendon of the subclavius muscle. These subclavicular nodes constitute the last barrier in the axillary lymph node filter.

In our series of 182 radical mastectomy specimens studied with special care with regard to the distribution of axillary metastases, the subclavicular nodes were found to be involved in only 15 (Table 22–14).

Only the external mammary group of nodes was less frequently involved. But when the subclavicular nodes were involved, several other node groups always contained metastases. Also, when the subclavicular nodes were involved, the number of involved nodes in the axillary filter as a whole was large, averaging 16.2 involved nodes. The average number of involved nodes in all our 80 cases with axillary metastases was 5.9.

There was also a striking contrast between the numbers of involved nodes in cases in which the central group contained metastases as compared with the cases in which the subclavicular group contained metastases. In Table 22–15, which presents these facts, it will be seen that 80 per cent of the cases with subclavicular node metastases had eight or more involved nodes, whereas only 26.4 per cent of the cases with central node metastases had eight or more involved nodes.

The grave significance of metastasis to the subclavicular nodes is well illustrated by the diagram of the axillary findings in such a case, shown in Figure 22–28.

These facts regarding metastases in the subclavicular node group led us long ago to the conclusion that when these nodes are involved all hope of cure by surgery is gone. Under rare circumstances, one of these patients will survive as long as 10 years, but all eventually succumb.

It is not easy, in studying radical mastectomy specimens in the laboratory, to identify

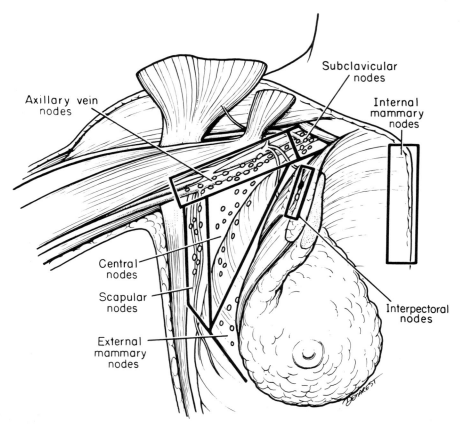

Axillary vein
nodes

Subclavicular
nodes

Internal
mammary
nodes

Central
nodes

Scapular
nodes

External
mammary
nodes

Interpectoral
nodes

Figure 22–27. Diagram of the axillary lymph nodes found in a radical mastectomy specimen studied by the clearing method. A woman aged 46 had a 3 cm. carcinoma of the central zone of the right breast. There was a 1 cm. firm movable axillary node, clinically involved. Columbia Clinical Classification Stage B. A total of 58 nodes were found. The only metastasis was in one of the two interpectoral nodes. No postoperative irradiation or hormonal therapy was given. The patient was well 15 years later.

the subclavicular nodes accurately. Even though the surgeon has marked the specimen carefully with a silk tie at the highest point, mistakes are apt to be made. In order to make certain that these subclavicular nodes are identified, I have for several years followed the practice of severing the small packet of areolar tissue containing these subclavicular nodes from the remainder of the specimen as soon as I have completed this part of the axillary dissection. This small mass of tissue is then studied separately.

PRELIMINARY BIOPSY OF THE SUBCLAVICULAR LYMPH NODES. It was this awareness of the grave prognostic significance of metastases in the subclavicular nodes that led us, in 1955, to begin to perform preliminary biopsy of these nodes in an effort to determine the extent of metastasis in the regional lymph node filter. The biopsy of apex of the axilla in

which these subclavicular nodes were removed, was combined with biopsy of the internal mammary nodes. With these biopsies we have acquired, during the last 13 years, a large amount of data regarding the frequency of metastasis in the subclavicular nodes and the correlation of involvement of these nodes with the various clinical features of breast carcinoma.

Our biopsies of the apex of the axilla have been fewer in number than our internal mammary biopsies, because we have not as often been in doubt regarding the extent of axillary involvement in operable cases as we have been regarding the presence of internal mammary metastases. In the axilla we have the help of axillary palpation to guide us; internal mammary metastases are always occult in patients in whom there is any question of surgical treatment. Although it has been difficult

Table 22–14. Axillary lymph node metastases in 182 cleared radical mastectomy specimens, 1951–1954. 15 cases with subclavicular node involvement

| Case | No. of Nodes Involved in Different Node Groups | | | | | | Total No. Involved Nodes | Total No. Nodes Found | Survival Time in Months to Death |
	Sub-clavicular	Axillary vein	Central	Scapular	External mammary	Inter-pectoral			
1	2	10	6				18	33	33
2	1	4	3				8	36	30
3	1	9	1				11	34	49
4	3	1	2				6	51	37
5	1	3	4	1			9	45	138*
6	6	5	3	5			19	42	20
7	1	3	10	2			16	41	67
8	5	6	8	9			28	38	93
9	4	19	13	5	1		35	42	8
10	12	13	7	3		2	37	69	48
11	1	11	7			1	20	39	112
12	4		1		5	1	11	82	59
13	1		4	3		7	15	19	15
14	1			1		4	6	48	17
15	2				2		4	46	15

Average number of involved nodes per case — 16.2.

*Intra-abdominal metastases developed after five years. Patient is living with disease after 12 years.

to follow a definite rule in the selection of patients for biopsy of the apex of the axilla, these biopsies have in general been performed in the three following groups of patients: (1) Clinical Stage A patients whose primary tumor is in the central sector or the lateral sectors of the breast (Zones G, A, and B) and measures more than 5 cm. in diameter; (2) patients with clinically involved axillary nodes (Columbia Clinical Stage B); (3) patients with more advanced disease.

When we were in doubt as to whether the clinical features of the patient's disease indicated that it was operable (Stages A and B) or inoperable (Stages C and D), we also often performed biopsy of the apex of the axilla.

We performed a total of 346 of these preliminary biopsies of the apex of the axilla from 1955 to 1966, inclusive. The patients constituted about 15 per cent of our patients with breast carcinoma coming to the Presbyterian and Delafield Hospitals during this period. The subclavicular nodes were found to be involved in 25.1 per cent of the patients in whom this type of biopsy was done.

In our experience with these 346 biopsies we learned a good deal regarding the pathology of metastasis to the subclavicular nodes. We usually found that from two to six small nodes were included in the packet of fat and areolar tissue that we excised from the apex of the axilla. In most instances it was impossible to guess whether or not the nodes contained metastases, because they were very small. Figure 22–29 shows six small nodes (twice their actual size) removed in one of

Table 22–15. Axillary lymph node metastases in 182 cleared radical mastectomy specimens, 1951–1954. 80 cases with involved nodes

| Axillary Lymph Node Group | No. of Cases with Involved Nodes | Cases with Given Total of Involved Nodes | | |
		1 or 2	3 to 7	8 or more
External mammary	6	50.0%	16.7%	33.3%
Scapular	15	6.7%	40.0%	53.3%
Central	72	45.8%	27.8%	26.4%
Interpectoral	17	29.4%	35.3%	35.3%
Axillary vein	27	0	37.0%	63.0%
Subclavicular	15	0	20.0%	80.0%
All groups	80	48.8%	27.5%	23.7%

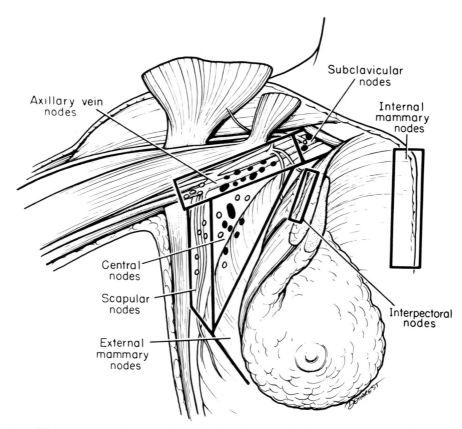

Figure 22–28.   Diagram of axillary lymph nodes found in a radical mastectomy specimen studied by the clearing method. A woman aged 71 had a 3 cm. carcinoma of the extreme upper outer sector of her right breast. There was marked retraction of the overlying skin. Two clinically involved, firm but movable 1 cm. nodes were present in the axilla. Columbia Clinical Classification Stage B. A total of 33 nodes, 18 of which contained metastases, were found.

Because of her extensive axillary node metastases the patient was given postoperative prophylactic irradiation. Despite this therapy she developed local recurrence and generalized metastases and died two years and eight months after operation.

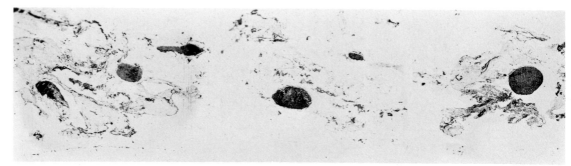

Figure 22–29.   Six small subclavicular lymph nodes removed from the apex of the axilla by preliminary biopsy.

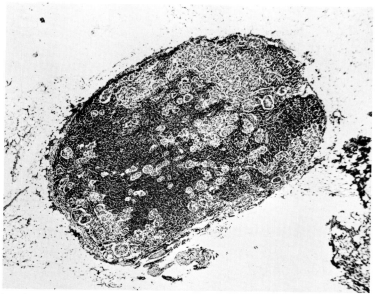

Figure 22–30.   A subclavicular lymph node partially replaced by metastatic breast carcinoma removed from the apex of the axilla by preliminary biopsy.

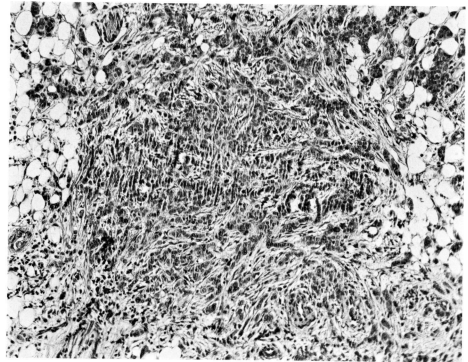

Figure 22–31.   Biopsy of the apex of the axilla showing metastatic breast carcinoma infiltrating areolar tissue.

Table 22–16. Biopsy of the apex of the axilla. Site of the primary breast tumor correlated with subclavicular node metastasis. Presbyterian and Delafield Hospitals, 1955–1966

Site of Primary Carcinoma	No. of Biopsies	Per cent Positive
Lateral sectors of breast (Zones *A* and *B*)	138	30.9%
Central zone of breast (Zone *G*)	158	24.0%
Medial sectors of breast (Zones *C, D, E,* and *F*)	50	12.0%
Total	346	25.1%

Table 22–17. Biopsy of apex of axilla. Size of the primary breast tumor correlated with subclavicular node metastasis. Presbyterian and Delafield Hospitals, 1955–1966

Site of Primary Carcinoma	No. of Biopsies	Per cent Positive
Under 3 cm.	56	32.1%
3 cm., but less than 5 cm.	107	16.8%
5 cm., but less than 8 cm.	133	25.6%
8 cm. or more	50	34.0%
Total	346	25.1%

Table 22–18. Biopsy of apex of axilla. Clinical findings in the axilla correlated with subclavicular node metastasis. Presbyterian and Delafield Hospitals, 1955–1966

Clinical Findings in Axilla	No. of Biopsies	Per cent Positive
No clinically involved nodes	88	4.5%
Clinically involved nodes less than 2.5 cm. in diameter and movable	112	19.6%
Clinically involved nodes 2.5 cm. or more in diameter, or fixed in axilla	146	58.2%
Total	346	25.1%

these biopsies. Three of them contain metastases. A metastasis in a small subclavicular node is shown in Figure 22–30.

In some patients in whom metastatic involvement of the apex of the axilla is more advanced, the planes of dissection are more difficult to define and the structures stick together. This often results from metastatic carcinoma infiltrating the areolar tissue of the region as shown in Figure 22–31.

Carcinomas of the medial sectors of the breast were less often associated with metastasis in the subclavicular nodes than carcinomas of the central and lateral zones of the breast (Table 22–16). This is, of course, what might be expected if we assume that the lymphatic route to the subclavicular nodes is shorter for carcinomas of the central and lateral sectors of the breast.

Our data relating the size of the primary carcinoma to the frequency of involvement of the subclavicular nodes (Table 22–17), shows no correlation.

The important correlation for biopsy of the apex of the axilla is, of course, with the clinical findings in the axilla. Our data are shown in Table 22–18. When there were no clinically involved axillary nodes, the subclavicular nodes were found to be involved in only 4.5 per cent of the patients in whom this type of biopsy was done. Among patients with clinically involved axillary nodes that were movable and less than 2.5 cm. in diameter, the subclavicular nodes were found to be involved in 19.6 per cent. But when there was more advanced axillary involvement, biopsy of the apex of the axilla was positive in 58.2 per cent.

Our Columbia Clinical Classification correlates very closely with the findings of this type of biopsy (Table 22–19), again confirming the validity of our classification.

Table 22–19. Biopsy of apex of axilla. Columbia Clinical Classification of breast carcinoma correlated with subclavicular node metastasis. Presbyterian and Delafield Hospitals, 1955–1966

Columbia Clinical Classification	No. of Biopsies	Per cent Positive
A	78	3.8%
B	98	20.4%
C	109	32.1%
D	61	47.5%
Total	346	25.1%

Extension to the Contralateral Axillary Nodes

Occasionally metastases appear in the nodes of the opposite axilla. This phenomenon is usually seen late in the course of carcinoma, when metastases have already developed elsewhere. Handley found it in 6 per cent of 422 autopsies. We have made a clinical diagnosis of contralateral metastases in about 4 per cent of our patients. Since the diagnosis was usually not proven by biopsy in these patients, this figure is only an approximate one.

It is of interest to speculate as to the lymphatic route by which the disease reaches the nodes in the opposite axilla. If we assume that the route is by way of the lymphatics of the skin, the disease should reach and involve the opposite breast before it reaches the lymph nodes of the opposite axilla.

In patients who have had radical mastectomy and have developed contralateral axillary node metastases we should, on the basis of this explanation, expect to find recurrence in the skin of the medial flap as well as disease in the opposite breast. But we have seen a number of patients with metastases in the nodes of the opposite axilla who did not have any evidence of regional skin recurrence, or of disease in the opposite breast. The following case in an example.

Mrs. A. W., aged 71, had discovered a tumor in her right breast six weeks before I first saw her. She had a 3 cm. carcinoma of the upper outer sector of her right breast. There were no palpable axillary nodes. Radical mastectomy was done. On microscopic study of the breast the carcinoma proved to be more extensive than clinical examination had suggested. There were multicentric foci throughout the entire upper half of the breast. Four of seventeen axillary nodes contained metastases.

She was well until five and a half years later when she was found to have a 3 cm. firm, movable, lower left axillary node. There was no evidence of local recurrence of her previous right-sided carcinoma and no detectable distant metastases. I could not make out anything abnormal in the left breast. I excised the left axillary node. On frozen section it was found to contain carcinoma. I assumed that there must be an occult second primary carcinoma in the left breast and performed a left radical mastectomy.

To our surprise, careful microscopic study of the left breast did not reveal carcinoma. Six of the 41 left axillary nodes contained carcinoma, however. The disease in these left axillary nodes closely resembled the carcinoma found in the right breast five and one-half years previously.

Within three months after the second operation widespread local recurrence developed in the skin of the anterior chest wall, in the operative fields of both radical mastectomies. She died while receiving irradiation 15 months after her second operation.

A case like this provides strong evidence that the carcinoma reaches the nodes of the opposite axilla by embolism or permeation through the deep lymphatic fascial plexus beneath the opposite breast. Emboli are swept through these deep lymphatics and reach the opposite axillary nodes before the disease has time to grow upward to invade the opposite breast.

Metastasis to the Supraclavicular Lymph Nodes

When metastases from carcinoma of the breast have reached the subclavicular nodes at the apex of the axilla, they are only 3 or 4 cm. from the lymph nodes of the "grand central" lymphatic terminus situated at the confluence of the subclavian and internal jugular veins. After these deeply situated grand central terminus nodes are involved, the disease extends in a retrograde direction to the supraclavicular lymph nodes above the clavicle, which are easily palpated. Thus, supraclavicular metastases become apparent to the clinician at an advanced stage of regional lymph node involvement.

Halsted was one of the first modern surgeons to understand the axillary-supraclavicular route for metastasis through the regional lymphatics, and to attempt to deal with these metastases surgically. Not long after he began to perform his epoch-making radical mastectomy, he added to it excision of the supraclavicular nodes. He tried a variety of techniques that would permit stripping the infraclavicular and supraclavicular portions of the subclavian vein clean of all lymph nodes and fat. At first he divided the clavicle, but later found this unnecessary. In 1898 he wrote "the supraclavicular region is almost invariably cleaned out." By 1907, when he reported his end results before the American Surgical Association, he had performed supraclavicular dissection as part of radical mastectomy in a total of 101 cases. He had also done the operation secondarily in 18 patients. In 44 of these 119 patients the supraclavicular nodes had been found to be involved. Yet only two of the 44 were cured for five years or more.

The poor results of supraclavicular dissection led Halsted's pupils to abandon it. It added a good deal of work to an operation that Halsted himself characterized as "a very great labor," and the number of cures attributed to it was very small. With the abandonment by most surgeons of the attack upon supraclavicular metastases, the importance of the supraclavicular route was lost sight of for a time.

In 1949 Dahl-Iversen of Copenhagen pointed out that supraclavicular lymph node recurrence was frequent in patients who developed recurrence following radical mastectomy. He tabulated the frequency of supraclavicular recurrence in several case series as shown in Table 22–20.

It was such data as these that led Dahl-Iversen and his associates in 1947 to begin to dissect out the supraclavicular nodes as part of radical mastectomy. Their first series consisted of 98 consecutive cases operated upon during 1947 and 1948. None of these patients had palpable supraclavicular nodes, but in 17 per cent metastases were found in the nodes removed by the dissection. These supraclavicular metastases were found exclusively among the 51 patients who had axillary metastases; the incidence of supraclavicular metastasis in this group was therefore 33 per cent.

Dahl-Iversen and his associates subsequently carried out supraclavicular dissection in two additional series of patients on whom they performed radical mastectomy (their third series and their fourth series). These two later series of cases included 176 additional patients. In these two series the incidence of supraclavicular metastases was much lower than in the first series of cases; supraclavicular metastases were found in only 8 per cent of the patients with axillary metastases. The explanation for the lower incidence of supraclavicular metastases in Dahl-Iversen's more recent case series is to be found in the comparatively favorable nature of his clinical material. The incidence of axillary metastases in his last two case series was only 42 per cent. In contrast the incidence of axillary metastases in my own contemporary personal series of radical mastectomies was 55.1 per cent. Dahl-Iversen's data regarding supraclavicular metastases in his several series of cases are combined in Table 22–21.

Just at this time my associates and I were acutely aware that our methods of determining the extent of metastasis to the regional

Table 22–20. FREQUENCY OF SUPRACLAVICULAR RECURRENCE AMONG PATIENTS WITH RECURRENCE FOLLOWING RADICAL MASTECTOMY

Author	Year	No. of Cases With Recurrent Carcinoma	Cases With Supraclavicular Recurrence
Dahl-Iversen	1927	48	27%
Todd & Dawson	1937	107	24%
Haagensen & Stout	1943	98	25%
Röden	1944	139	21%
Ducuing, Tailhefer, and Baclesse	1947	257	22%

lymph node filter were inadequate. Dahl-Iversen's emphasis upon metastasis in the supraclavicular lymph nodes, and Handley's demonstration of occult metastasis in the internal mammary lymph nodes, led us to do biopsies of these two lymph node groups as a separate preliminary step in determining the stage of advancement of the disease. In this manner we acquired data as to the frequency of supraclavicular metastases in a series of 110 patients (Table 22–22). Our cases did not form a consecutive series, and they represent the findings in comparatively advanced carcinoma of the breast because it was in such patients that we performed our supraclavicular biopsies.

By 1955 we had learned that biopsy of the supraclavicular nodes was not a critical enough measure of the extent of involvement of the regional lymph node filter to justify continuing it, and we abandoned it. In patients in whom the supraclavicular nodes as well as the internal mammary nodes were proved by biopsy to be free of metastases, and radical mastectomy was performed, the

Table 22–21. SUPRACLAVICULAR AND AXILLARY METASTASES. DAHL-IVERSEN'S 1ST, 3RD, AND 4TH SERIES

Extent of Metastases	No. of Cases	Per cent
Both axillary and supraclavicular nodes free	149	54.4%
Axillary nodes involved but not supraclavicular	102	37.2%
Supraclavicular nodes involved but not axillary	0	0.0%
Both axillary and supraclavicular nodes involved	23	8.4%
Total	274	100.0%

Table 22–22. RESULTS OF SUPRACLAVICULAR NODE BIOPSIES. PRESBYTERIAN AND DELAFIELD HOSPITALS, 1951–1955

Extent of Metastases	No. of Cases
Supraclavicular nodes involved, no internal mammary node biopsy	4
Supraclavicular nodes involved, internal mammary nodes free	2
Supraclavicular nodes involved, internal mammary nodes also involved	17
Supraclavicular nodes free, internal mammary nodes involved	15
Supraclavicular nodes free, internal mammary nodes also free	69
Supraclavicular nodes free, no internal mammary node biopsy	3
Total	110

subclavicular nodes at the apex of the axilla were sometimes found to be involved. The following case history illustrates this situation.

Mrs. M. R., a housewife aged 35, came to us complaining of a tumor of the left breast. She had a poorly delimited 6 cm. mass situated in the upper outer sector of her left breast. There were multiple lines of skin retraction below the lesion. In the axilla there were two firm, clinically involved lymph nodes, each about 1 cm. in diameter. The nodes were somewhat fixed to deeper structures in the axilla.

From these clinical findings I suspected that the disease might be inoperable. In an attempt to determine this question more accurately I did a biopsy of the primary tumor to prove that it was a carcinoma, and then excised the supraclavicular nodes, and the internal mammary nodes in the three upper interspaces. These nodes were not involved.

I went ahead with radical mastectomy. In dissecting the axilla I was distressed to find many small grossly involved nodes. Twenty-eight of the 30 axillary nodes, including four subclavicular nodes, contained metastases. The patient developed osseous and pulmonary metastases and died 10 months after operation. She should not have been operated upon.

The general conclusion from all these studies of the supraclavicular lymph nodes is that these nodes are involved in the last stage of the extension of breast carcinoma through the regional lymph node filter. If patients are properly selected for operation the number

who have involvement of the supraclavicular nodes is very small.

Metastasis to the Internal Mammary Nodes

The occurrence of metastases from carcinoma of the breast in the internal mammary lymph nodes has been known to pathologists for a long time. Handley found a description of such a metastasis in an autopsy report from the Middlesex Hospital cancer ward, dated October 22, 1806.

Pathologists must often have observed the picture seen in Figure 22–32. It shows the inner aspect of the sternum with enlarged internal mammary lymph nodes (indicated by arrows), replaced by metastases of mammary carcinoma, projecting inwardly beneath the

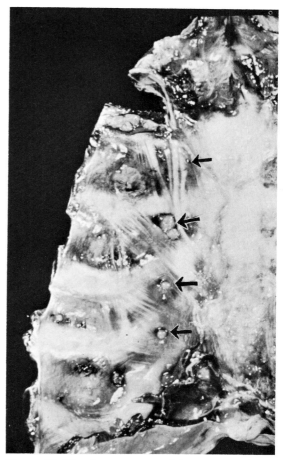

Figure 22–32. Inner aspect of the sternum showing internal mammary nodes enlarged and filled with carcinoma projecting inwardly at the sternal edge below the lower border of each of the upper four costal cartilages.

pleura at the sternal edge below the border of each of the upper four costal cartilages.

Since metastasis to the internal mammary nodes has only recently become well known, the pathologists in their older autopsy studies did not report their frequency. Smulders and Smets, however, in their 1960 study of the distribution of metastases of breast carcinoma in a series of 71 autopsies, reported finding involvement of the internal mammary nodes in 36.5 per cent of their cases.

The clinical manifestation of internal mammary metastasis is a firm, fixed mound-like tumor projecting from the inner end of one of the upper interspaces. Figures 22–33 and 22–34 show such a metastasis in the second interspace, in an anterior view and in profile.

Smithers and Rigby-Jones wrote an excellent description of this phenomenon and reported a series of 65 patients with breast cancer in whom parasternal metastases were observed at the Royal Marsden Hospital between 1937 and 1965. Göksel has also described this kind of recurrence very well.

In our breast clinics in the years before 1951 when we did not perform internal mammary biopsies for the purpose of detecting occult metastases to the internal mammary nodes, we saw parasternal recurrences all too often. We still see them occasionally because we have not performed biopsies of these nodes in all our patients. Sanger has reported our experience with parasternal recurrence.

In my personal series of 626 patients

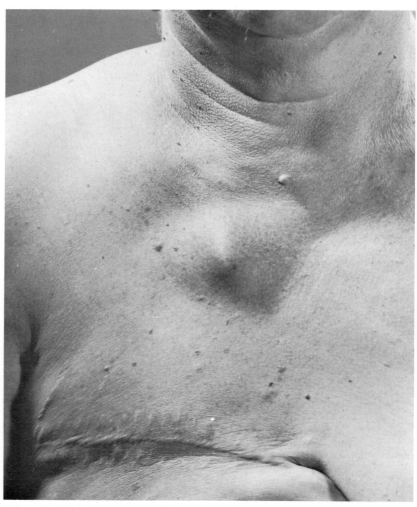

Figure 22–33. Parasternal tumor produced by metastasis to an internal mammary node in the second interspace.

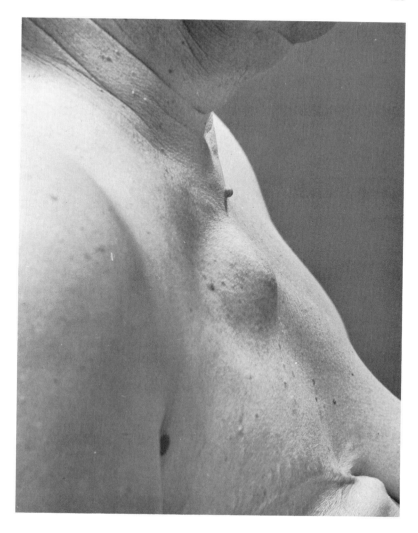

Figure 22–34. Profile of a parasternal tumor produced by metastasis to an internal mammary node in the second interspace.

treated by radical mastectomy and followed for a minimum of 10 years, 22 have developed these parasternal recurrences.

Parasternal recurrence may develop a very long time after radical mastectomy. In one of my patients 12.7 years, and in another 14.7 years, elapsed between operation and the appearance of the parasternal metastases.

In Smithers and Rigby-Jones' series of cases the average interval between mastectomy and the appearance of the parasternal recurrence was 3 years and 7 months.

Halsted was probably the first to attempt to excise the internal mammary nodes as part of the surgical attack on breast carcinoma.

In 1898 he wrote: "Dr. H. W. Cushing, my house surgeon, has in three instances cleaned out the anterior mediastinum on one side for recurrent cancer. It is likely, I think, that we shall in the near future remove the mediasti-

nal contents at some of our primary operations." Halsted never mentioned the matter again. What deterred him we can only guess.

Sampson Handley, whose studies of the routes of spread of breast carcinoma in the early years of this century were an important contribution to our knowledge of the disease, became sufficiently convinced from his clinical experience that metastasis takes place through the internal mammary route so that in 1922 he explored the mediastinum in six cases. He found involved internal mammary nodes in two of them. In 1927 Handley documented his belief in the importance of the internal mammary route of metastasis in a paper in which he described, among others, a remarkable case in which recurrences after radical mastectomy appeared at the inner ends of intercostal spaces, in one space after another from above downwards, until death

Table 22–23. Regional lymph node spread of breast cancer in relation to site of primary growth*

Node Involvement	Site of Primary Growth			
	Center and Inner Half of Breast	Outer Half of Breast	Total	Per cent
All nodes free	16	33	49	32.6
Axillary nodes only invaded	12	40	52	34.6
Internal mammary nodes only invaded	6	2	8	5.3
Both axillary and internal mammary nodes invaded	27	14	41	27.3
Total no. of cases	61	89	150	

*From Handley, R. S., and Thackray, A. C.: Brit. Med. J., *1*:61, 1954.

after twelve years. In this paper Handley stated his belief that *by the time the axillary nodes are enlarged the internal mammary nodes are frequently, and perhaps usually, invaded.*

The proof of this important rule has been provided by Sampson Handley's son, Richard Handley. Following his father as surgeon to the Middlesex Hospital he maintained an interest in the internal mammary route. In 1946 he began to dissect out the node in the second interspace at the completion of radical mastectomy. He shortly reported his findings in five cases. The axillary nodes and the second internal mammary node were both found to be involved in two, the internal mammary nodes alone in two, and neither axillary nor internal mammary nodes in the fifth case.

These results led Handley to adopt excision of the second or third internal mammary nodes as a routine at the completion of radical mastectomy. In 1949 he reported his findings in 50 cases. He found involvement of these nodes in 19. In three cases the internal mammary nodes alone were involved. Hand-

ley emphasized that he did not remove these nodes as a therapeutic measure, but to determine the extent of the disease.

Encouraged by his findings Handley extended his exploration to include all three upper interspaces. By 1954 he was able to report his findings in a total of 150 cases. This was the first large consecutive series of cases of breast carcinoma with information concerning the status of the internal mammary nodes. It is a landmark in our knowledge of the spread of the disease in the regional lymph node filters. I have reproduced the three most important tables in Handley's report (Tables 22–23 to 22–25).

With this series of cases Handley established three basic facts regarding the metastasis of breast cancer to the internal mammary nodes, which have not been modified by any of the studies since reported:

1. Internal mammary metastases are more frequent than has been suspected, being found in about 25 per cent of all patients with breast cancer whose disease is operable by general standards.

2. These metastases are more frequent

Table 22–24. Regional lymph node spread of breast cancer in relation to site of primary growth by quadrant*

Node Involvement	Site in Breast by Quadrants					
	Upper Inner	Lower Inner	Central	Upper Outer	Lower Outer	Total
All nodes free	11	4	1	28	5	49
Axillary nodes only invaded	6	2	4	34	6	52
Internal mammary nodes only invaded	4	0	2	2	0	8
Both axillary and internal mammary nodes invaded	10	7	10	13	1	41
Total	31	13	17	77	12	150

*From Handley, R. S., and Thackray, A. C.: Brit. Med. J., *1*:61, 1954.

Table 22–25. Relation of degree of axillary involvement to internal mammary invasion*

Extent of Axillary Invasion	No. of Cases	Cases with Internal Mammary Invasion
0 (free)	57	8(14%)
1 (light)	23	6(26%)
2 (moderate)	32	12(37%)
3 (heavy)	34	22(65%)

*From Handley, R. S., and Thackray, A. C.: Brit. Med. J., 1:61, 1954.

from tumors of the central zone and medial half of the breast, than from tumors of the lateral half of the breast.

3. Internal mammary metastases usually occur only after involvement of the axillary nodes, and the more numerous the axillary metastases, the greater the likelihood of internal mammary metastases.

Handley's striking findings concerning internal mammary metastases quickly stimulated American and European surgeons to remove these nodes therapeutically as part of their surgical attack on breast cancer. Within five years after Handley's first report, three different such case series, each totalling about 100 cases, were published. I will refer to them briefly to emphasize the point that the findings in all were very similar to Handley's.

Hutchinson, in Seattle, began to excise the internal mammary nodes in the upper three interspaces at the conclusion of radical mastectomy in his private cases. He followed Handley's technique of exposing the nodes in each interspace separately. His results are shown in Table 22–26.

In Italy in 1948, Margottini and Bucalossi began to exise the internal mammary nodes at the completion of radical mastectomy. They used a different technique, in which they removed the medial 2 cm. of the second and third costal cartilages, thus laying bare the internal mammary blood vessels and the accompanying lymphatic chain with its nodes, in the upper three interspaces. They then ligated the vessels as high as possible in the first interspace, and as low as possible in the third interspace, and excised all these tissues extrapleurally. Margottini and Bucalossi reported their findings in a series of 110 of these operations done in Rome and Milan as shown in Table 22–27.

In Copenhagen, Dahl-Iversen began to investigate the frequency of regional node metastasis in breast carcinoma. In his *first* series of 98 cases, studied during 1949, he performed a supraclavicular lymph node dissection in addition to radical mastectomy.

In 1951 he extended his studies to include the internal mammary nodes. He excised the internal mammary nodes in the upper three interspaces in a series of 57 patients in whom he also performed radical mastectomy. The nodes were excised from each interspace separately as Handley had done, without cutting the costal cartilages. This group of 57 patients constituted a *second* series for Dahl-Iversen.

In a *third* series of 76 patients, treated during 1951 and 1952, Dahl-Iversen and his associates excised the supraclavicular, as well as the internal mammary nodes, at radical mastectomy. A different method of excising the internal mammary nodes was used. The second, third, and fourth costal cartilages were cut across about 1 cm. from the sternal border, and the wall of the thorax was ele-

Table 22–26. Carcinoma of the breast; regional lymph node metastases. Hutchinson, 1949–1951.*

Extent of Metastasis	Site of Primary Carcinoma		Total Cases	
	Central and Inner Half	Outer Half	No.	Per cent
All nodes free	14	24	38	46.9
Axillary nodes only involved	2	20	22	27.2
Internal mammary nodes only involved	1	1	2	2.5
Both axillary and internal mammary nodes involved	3	16	19	23.4
Total	20	61	81	

*Data from Hutchinson, W. B., and Kiriluk, L. B.: Am. J. Surg., 92:151, 1956.

Table 22–27. Carcinoma of the breast; regional lymph node metastases.
Margottini and Bucalossi, 1948–1949*

Extent of Metastases	Site of Primary Carcinoma			Total Cases	
	Inner Half	Outer Half	Entire Breast	No.	Per cent
All nodes free	20	21	0	41	37.3
Axillary nodes only involved	18	25	1	44	40.0
Internal mammary nodes only involved	0	2	0	2	1.8
Both axillary and internal mammary nodes involved	9	11	3	23	20.9
Total	47	59	4	110	

*Data from Margottini, M., and Bucalossi, P.: Oncologia, *23*(2):70, 1949.

vated by means of gauze strips, to expose the internal mammary artery and veins and lymph nodes. These vessels, and the accompanying lymphatics and nodes, together with surrounding fatty tissue, were then excised extrapleurally from the lower edge of the first cartilage to the upper edge of the fifth. The series was made up of comparatively favorable cases: axillary nodes contained metastases in only 43 per cent of the patients. Unfortunately Dahl-Iversen did not include in his report of this series a detailed statement of the frequency of internal mammary metastases in relation to the site of the carcinoma in the breast.

In a *fourth* series of 100 patients reported in 1954, Dahl-Iversen combined excision of the supraclavicular and internal mammary nodes with radical mastectomy. This series was likewise composed of remarkably favorable cases, for only 41 per cent were found to have axillary metastases.

In order to learn as much as possible regarding the relationship of the frequency of internal mammary metastases to the site of the carcinoma in the breast in Dahl-Iversen's studies, I have combined his findings in his second and fourth series of cases into a single table (Table 22–28).

Like others whose data I have presented, I was myself stimulated by Richard Handley to investigate the internal mammary route of metastasis. Since I had been interested for many years in the problem of the proper selection of patients for operation, it was only reasonable that I should bring the new knowledge of the internal mammary route to bear on this question. We therefore began in 1951 to excise the internal mammary nodes not as a part of radical mastectomy but as a separate preliminary biopsy procedure. We intended to use our findings as an aid in classifying breast cancer as to its stage of advancement, and in the selection of treatment. Since our purpose was to determine the extent of metastatic spread to all the regional lymph nodes, we combined preliminary excision of the lymph nodes in the upper three interspaces with excision of the supraclavicular nodes. The first step in this biopsy procedure was, of course, excision of a small wedge of the primary breast tumor to make certain that it was a carcinoma. We called the procedure *triple biopsy.*

I have already explained, in discussing supraclavicular metastasis, why we abandoned preliminary supraclavicular biopsy in 1955, and substituted for it biopsy of the subclavic-

Table 22–28. Carcinoma of breast; regional lymph node metastases.
Andreassen, Dahl-Iversen, and Soerensen, 2nd and 4th series

Extent of Metastasis	Site of Primary Carcinoma		Total Cases	
	Medial	Lateral	No.	Per cent
All nodes free	31	48	79	51.6
Axillary nodes only involved	7	37	44	28.8
Int. mammary only involved	8	–	8	5.2
Axillary and int. mammary involved	11	8	19	12.4
Axillary and supraclavicular involved	–	3	3	2.0
Total number cases	57	96	153	
Percent of cases with internal mammary metastasis	31%	8.3%	17.6%	

ular nodes at the apex of the axilla. Thereafter we continued to perform preliminary biopsy, usually including biopsy of the internal mammary nodes, until 1968, when we reviewed our experience and decided to abandon internal mammary biopsy for reasons which I will explain in Chapter 33, when I discuss the treatment of breast cancer. In the 17 year period during which we performed these preliminary biopsies of the internal mammary nodes, we did them in more than a thousand patients. Metastases were found in 32.5 per cent.

There are several aspects of our experience with this phenomenon of internal mammary metastases that are worthwhile describing in some detail, even though our data have certain limitations. In the first place, our data are not derived from consecutive series of all our patients with breast cancer. Because of limitations on operating time, as well as economic restrictions, we have had to limit our preliminary biopsies to patients in whom we thought there was a greater likelihood of internal mammary metastasis. They constituted about one-third of all our patients with breast cancer. Although it has been difficult to follow a rule in a matter as complex as this, in general these patients have been the following: (1) clinical Stage A patients whose primary tumor is situated in the medial sectors, or the central sector, of the breast (Zones *C*, *D*, *E*, *F*, and *G*), and measures 3 cm. or more in diameter; (2) clinical Stage A patients whose primary tumor is situated in the lateral sectors of the breast (Zones *A* and *B*) and measures 5 cm. or more in diameter; (3) patients with more advanced disease.

We have also performed these preliminary biopsies of the internal mammary nodes in patients in whom our assessment of the clinical findings left us in doubt as to the stage of advancement of their disease in terms of our Columbia Clinical Classification. In this way we proved in a good many patients that their disease, which was apparently on the borderline between Columbia Clinical Stages B and C, was in fact unsuitable for radical mastectomy because of internal mammary metastases. Experience has taught us, however, that if the clinical features are clearly enough defined to permit accurate clinical staging, it should always take precedence over the findings of these internal mammary biopsies. When the clinical findings indicate that the disease has advanced to Stage C or D, radical mastectomy should not be performed even

though the internal mammary lymph node biopsies do not reveal metastasis.

Another disadvantage of our data concerning internal mammary metastasis is that we cannot correlate the occurrence of these metastases with axillary metastases in our cases. Because we have used the finding of internal mammary metastasis as a contraindication to radical mastectomy and have treated the patients in whom they were found with irradiation only, we do not know whether or not they had axillary metastases.

The experience of doing these 1007 internal mammary biopsies, and studying the tissue we have removed from the interspaces, has taught us much regarding the pathology of this type of metastasis. The close relationship of these metastases to the pleura is well shown in Figure 22–35. This makes extension of the disease beyond the limits of local chest wall resection a formidable hazard.

The process by which metastases reach these internal mammary nodes is illustrated by Figure 22–36. Here an internal mammary trunk lymphatic—shown in the lower portion of the microphotograph—is dilated and filled with emboli of carcinoma. It is feeding these emboli into the peripheral lymphatic sinus of the node.

At a more advanced stage, as shown in Figure 22–37, the node has been to a great extent replaced by carcinoma, which has broken out into the surrounding areolar tissue which it is infiltrating.

Small emboli of carcinoma cells also are carried, presumably by small lymphatics, into the areolar tissue of the interspace where they are surrounded by foci of lymphocytes (Fig. 22–38).

As it extends the disease may grow into and partially plug internal mammary blood vessels. Figure 22–39 shows a small artery with carcinoma in its lumen.

We have learned from carefully studying the tissue removed in these internal mammary biopsies, that the metastases may be exceedingly small. We do not do frozen sections on this tissue unless the interspace is grossly involved. We save every minute fragment of areolar tissue and the nodes which are removed, fix them in Bouin's fluid, and cut the blocks in at least three levels. Figure 22–40 shows tissue from the first interspace in which minute carcinoma emboli are seen in a very small lymphatic. This was all the carcinoma that was found, but its importance from the point of view of the patient's welfare has,

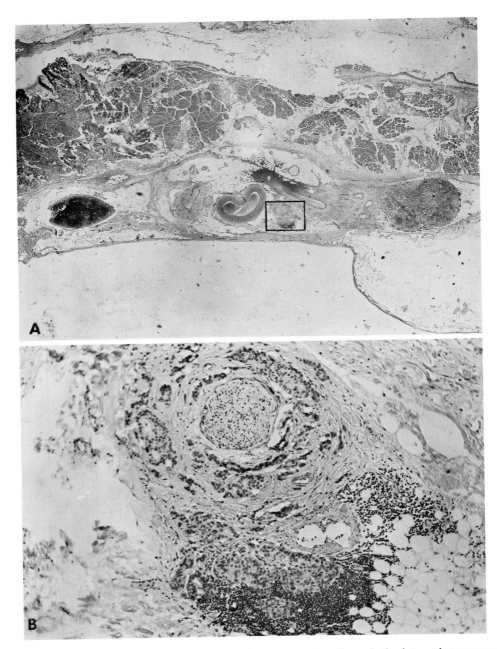

Figure 22–35. *A*, Low-power microscopic view of a cross section through the internal mammary region from a resection of the chest wall in this region for breast cancer. The internal mammary vessels are seen near the center of the photograph, with the intercostal musculature above and the pleura below. The darkly stained structure lying upon the pleura on the left is a grossly uninvolved lymph node. On the far right is another lymph node largely replaced by carcinoma.

B, High-power microscopic view of the small boxed area from *A*. In the upper central portion there is a nerve trunk surrounded by carcinoma cells, perhaps in lymphatics. In the lower portion there is a microscopic aggregate of lymphoid tissue containing foci of carcinoma.

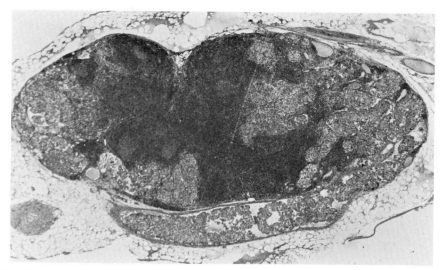

Figure 22–36. A dilated internal mammary lymphatic trunk filled with emboli of mammary carcinoma which it is carrying into an internal mammary lymph node.

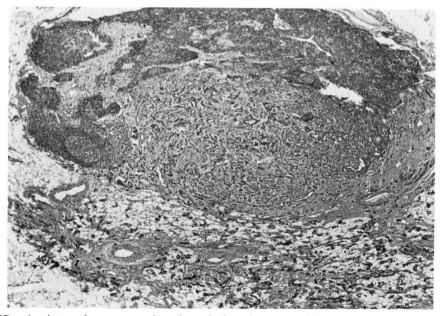

Figure 22–37. An internal mammary lymph node largely replaced by mammary carcinoma which is growing into the surrounding areolar tissue.

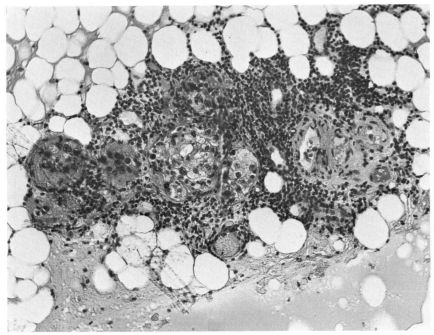

Figure 22–38. Emboli of breast carcinoma surrounded by a focus of lymphocytes in the areolar tissue of an interspace.

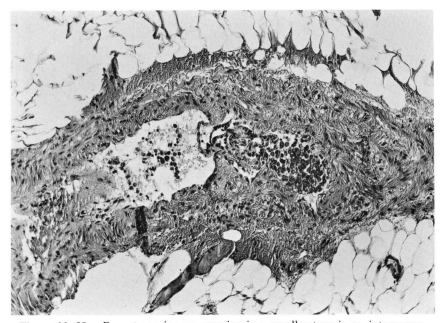

Figure 22–39. Breast carcinoma growing in a small artery in an interspace.

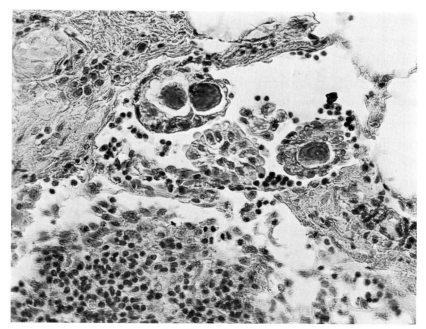

Figure 22–40. Emboli of breast carcinoma in a dilated lymphatic from the first interspace. This was all the carcinoma that was found at internal mammary biopsy.

of course, no relationship to its size. The patient had a 5 cm. carcinoma of the lower outer sector of her breast.

We have, of course, been particularly interested in correlating our findings in preliminary internal mammary biopsy, with the various clinical features of breast carcinoma, hoping to learn which ones are associated with metastasis to the internal mammary nodes.

One of the most important of these relationships is that concerned with the site of the primary tumor in the breast. Our data on this question are shown in Figures 22–41 and 22–42. It will be seen that although internal mammary metastases are less frequent in carcinoma of the upper outer sector of the breast, the frequency of metastases from tumors of the other sectors of the breast is rather similar, except that tumors of the center of the breast appear to be very likely to produce this kind of metastasis. Handley's most recent data based upon biopsies of the internal mammary nodes in 800 patients are almost identical (Fig. 22–43).

The size of the primary tumor also has a relationship to the likelihood of internal mammary metastases (Table 22–29). These nodes were involved three and one-half times more often when the primary tumor was 8 cm. or

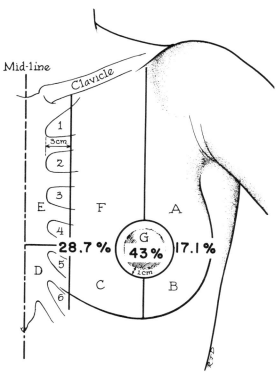

Figure 22–41. Internal mammary biopsy – the frequency of internal mammary metastasis from carcinomas of the inner and outer halves of the breast and its central sector in 1007 patients.

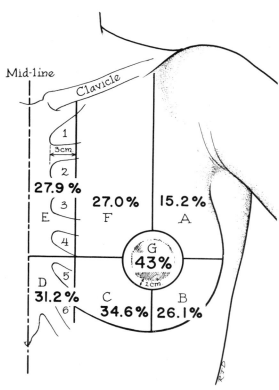

Figure 22–42. Internal mammary biopsy—the frequency of internal mammary metastasis from carcinomas of the different sectors of the breast in 1007 patients.

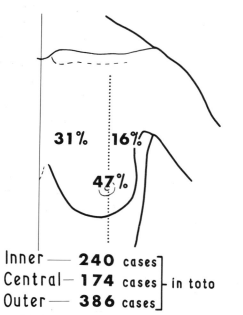

Inner — **240** cases ⎫
Central — **174** cases ⎬ in toto
Outer — **386** cases ⎭

Figure 22–43. Internal mammary biopsy—the frequency of internal mammary metastasis from carcinomas of the different sectors of the breast in 800 patients (Handley, 1969).

Table 22–29. INTERNAL MAMMARY BIOPSY. SIZE OF PRIMARY BREAST CARCINOMA CORRELATED WITH INTERNAL MAMMARY METASTASIS. PRESBYTERIAN AND DELAFIELD HOSPITALS, 1951–1966

Size of Primary Carcinoma	No. of Patients	Per cent with Internal Mammary Metastases
Under 3 cm.	153	16.3%
3 cm., but less than 5 cm.	333	20.1%
5 cm., but less than 8 cm.	355	39.4%
8 cm. or more	166	57.2%
Total	1007	32.5%

more in diameter, than when it was less than 3 cm. in diameter.

The most important factor determining the likelihood of internal mammary metastases is the status of the axillary lymph nodes.

Our data which, as we have pointed out, are based upon the findings in selected patients who are more likely to have internal mammary metastases, are shown in Table 22–30. It will be seen that when the axillary nodes were not clinically involved (we know that about one-third of these patients do in fact have axillary metastases) 19.6 per cent proved to have internal mammary metastases. When the axillary nodes were clinically involved but not large, internal mammary metastases were found in 33.5 per cent, and when there was advanced axillary involvement 50.2 per cent of the patients had internal mammary metastases.

Handley has more precise data regarding this relationship of internal mammary metastasis to axillary metastases, because he performed internal mammary biopsy on all his patients. We did so only in selected patients in whom we thought the internal mammary nodes might be involved. I reproduce his data (Fig. 22–44) which shows that 35 per cent of his 442 patients with axillary metastases had internal mammary metastases.

It is also interesting to correlate our findings regarding internal mammary metastases with the stage of advancement of the disease in our patients according to our Columbia Clinical Classification. Table 22–31 presents these data, and demonstrates the validity of our method of clinical classification. As the disease advances through Clinical Stages A

Table 22–30. INTERNAL MAMMARY BIOPSY. CLINICAL FINDINGS IN AXILLA CORRELATED WITH INTERNAL MAMMARY METASTASES. PRESBYTERIAN AND DELAFIELD HOSPITALS, 1951–1966

Clinical Findings In Axilla	No. of Patients	Per cent with Internal Mammary Metastases
Axillary nodes not clinically involved	438	19.6%
Clinically involved nodes less than 2.5 cm. in diameter, and movable	266	33.5%
Clinically involved nodes 2.5 cm. or more in diameter, or fixed in axilla	303	50.2%
Total	1007	32.5%

Table 22–31. INTERNAL MAMMARY BIOPSY. STAGE OF ADVANCEMENT MEASURED BY COLUMBIA CLINICAL CLASSIFICATION FOR BREAST CARCINOMA, CORRELATED WITH INTERNAL MAMMARY METASTASIS. PRESBYTERIAN AND DELAFIELD HOSPITALS, 1951–1966

Columbia Clinical Classification	No. of Patients	Per cent with Internal Mammary Metastases
Stage A	392	16.8%
Stage B	230	31.3%
Stage C	229	40.2%
Stage D	156	62.2%
Total	1007	32.5%

to D, the frequency of internal mammary metastasis steadily increases.

The true frequency of internal mammary metastases can only be determined from consecutive series of patients in whom the stage of advancement has been determined by careful clinical staging, and the internal mammary nodes in the upper three interspaces have been excised in all. Our own series of internal mammary biopsies does not meet this last requirement because it consists of selected patients with more advanced disease. But fortunately there are at least four large case series which approximately fulfill both requirements. They are shown in Table 22–32.

Handley's 800 patients are all carefully classified as Stage A and B, according to our Columbia Clinical Classification. Although Dahl-Iversen, Caceres, and Veronesi have not used our clinical classification, all follow our criteria of operability in selecting their patients for the extended radical mastectomy, which are very much the same as the criteria by which patients are classified as Clinical Stage A and B in our Columbia Clinical Classification. The findings as regards internal mammary metastases are strikingly similar in these four series, totaling 2667 cases.

These data confirm our own experience that the axillary nodes are first involved as breast cancer begins to metastasize through the lymphatics. As the extent of axillary involvement increases and the axillary filter is to some degree blocked, internal mammary metastasis occurs. The number of patients in whom only the internal mammary nodes are involved is small in unselected case series — varying between 3 and 5 per cent. When the cases with both internal mammary and axillary involvement are added to those who have only internal mammary metastases the total is between 20 and 25 per cent. At least one-fifth of all our patients with operable breast cancer therefore have these hidden metastases — a fatal complication of their disease unless treated effectively.

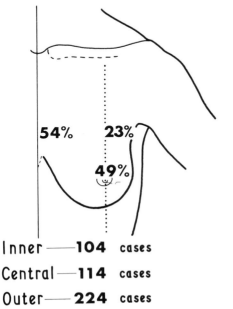

54% 23%

49%

Inner ——**104** cases

Central ——**114** cases

Outer ——**224** cases

Figure 22–44. Internal mammary biopsy — the frequency of internal mammary metastasis from carcinomas of the different sectors of the breast in 442 patients with axillary metastasis (Handley, 1969).

Table 22–32. RADICAL MASTECTOMY WITH INTERNAL MAMMARY BIOPSY OR DISSECTION. FREQUENCY OF INTERNAL MAMMARY METASTASES ALONE OR COMBINED WITH AXILLARY METASTASES

Author	No. of Cases	Internal Mammary Metastases Only	Internal Mammary and Axillary Metastases	Total Internal Mammary Metastases
Handley, 1969 (Columbia Clinical Stage A and B)	800	8%*	19%	27.2%
Dahl-Iversen, 1963	417	3.1%	13.7%	16.8%
Caceres, 1968	600	3.0%	16.0%	19.3%
Veronesi, 1968	850	5.1%	20.3%	25.4%

*In this series the proportion of patients wih metastases in the internal mammary nodes but not in the axillary nodes is exaggerated by the fact that when biopsy of the internal mammary nodes is done and they are immediately found to be involved, the axilla is not dissected and involvement of axillary nodes is, of course, not demonstrated.

DISTANT METASTASES THROUGH THE BLOOD STREAM

When breast carcinoma reaches the grand central lymphatic terminus at either side of the base of the neck, carcinoma emboli are emptied directly into the left or right innominate vein, from which they are carried through the right heart to the lungs.

Emboli that break loose from carcinoma that has grown into veins in the breast are swept in the venous stream either to the internal mammary veins or to the axillary veins. Both these sets of veins lead to the innominate veins, the superior vena cava, and the lungs. A third venous route to the lungs is through the intercostal veins which empty

Table 22–33. MOST FREQUENT SITES OF DISTANT METASTASES FROM CARCINOMA OF BREAST AT AUTOPSY

Organ	Kitain 1922 41 cases	Warren and Witham 1933 160 cases	Turner and Jaffe 1940 105 cases	Saphir and Parker 1941 43 cases	Walther 1948 186 cases	Abrams 1950 167 cases	Sproul Delafield Hospital 1955 100 cases	Smulders 1960 71 cases
Lungs	54%	59%	62%	65%	62%	77%	69%	72%
Liver	63%	58%		56%	35%	61%	65%	62%
Adrenals	27%	31%		41%	8%	54%	49%	51%
Kidneys	17%			14%	9%	13%	17%	15%
Spleen	7%	14%		23%	3%	17%	17%	8%
Pancreas	7%			11%	3%	14%	17%	8%
Ovaries	17%	9%		16%	4%	23%	20%	8%
Brain	9%			9%	6%	29%	22%	13%
Thyroid					8%	5%	24%	31%
Heart						8%	11%	3%
Diaphragm				14%		25%	11%	7%
Pericardium	5%			21%		35%	19%	31%
Pleura	63%	37%		23%		65%	51%	60%
Intestine							18%	
Peritoneum	19%	12%		9%		25%	13%	10%
Uterus							15%	4%
Mediastinal lymph nodes				32%		66%		
Peritoneal lymph nodes		72%		26%			76%	
Retroperitoneal lymph nodes				32%		44%		
Inguinal lymph nodes				7%		2%		
Bones	56%	44%	57%		47%	73%	71%	65%
Skin		39%		7%	1%	19%	30%	35%
No metastases	2%	5%		7%	12%		2%	

posteriorly into the azygos veins, which in turn terminate in the superior vena cava. These several routes by which carcinoma emboli reach the lungs are shown diagrammatically in Figure 1–28.

In view of the opportunity for carcinoma emboli to reach the lungs that these venous routes provide, it is not surprising that metastases to the lungs are very frequent in breast carcinoma. They are, in fact, the most frequent form of distant metastasis, being found in from 60 to 65 per cent of all autopsies in cases of mammary carcinoma. Table 22–33 shows the comparative frequency of distant metastases of breast carcinoma to various organs, as indicated in modern investigations. I have not included in this table the much quoted, antiquated nineteenth century data presented by Gross, Török, Paget, etc. These old data, largely based on gross pathology, cannot compare in accuracy with modern meticulous histologic studies. I have included our data from the Delafield Hospital, tabulated by Sproul, but not previously published.

Tumor Cells in the Blood Stream

Since 1955, when Engell reported that he frequently found tumor cells in the circulating blood of patients with malignant neoplasms (three with breast carcinoma) there has been a good deal of interest in the question of how often genuine tumor cells are found in the blood stream and what their significance actually is.

Some of those who have reported tumor cells in a very high proportion of cases have, without doubt, been mistaking immature or atypical cell forms of normal blood elements, particularly megalokaryocytes, for tumor cells. Alexander and Spriggs and Scheinin and Koinuniemi, as well as Fleming, have warned of this error.

As regards breast carcinoma cells in the blood stream, the most startling report was that of Candar and his associates who stated, in 1962, that if large enough samples of blood are studied, nearly all patients with breast cancer will be found to have tumor cells in their circulating blood. Among 20 patients from whom multiple samples of peripheral blood were taken during operation, they found tumor cells in 80 per cent. Long and his associates reported in 1960 that they found tumor cells in the peripheral blood of 24 per cent of 51 patients with breast carci-

noma. Watne and his associates reported finding tumor cells in the regional blood of 11.6 per cent of 60 patients with breast carcinoma, and in the peripheral blood of 4.9 per cent of 62 patients with the disease.

Alexander and Spriggs, on the other hand, did not find tumor cells in the circulating blood in a single patient with operable breast carcinoma. Fleming likewise failed to find indubitable tumor cells in blood drawn by catheter from the innominate vein before, during, and after operation, in nine patients with operable breast carcinoma and in one treated by irradiation. Fleming also carried out very interesting studies in three patients with metastatic breast carcinoma of the neck of the femur in whom nailing was done. A catheter was introduced into the saphenous vein and passed up into the common iliac vein. Samples of blood were taken through the catheter before the operation and at intervals during it. Showers of tumor cells were identified in the blood during the nailing. They disappeared soon after the nailing. Fletcher and Stewart carried out studies of tumor cells in prehepatic and posthepatic blood which suggest that the liver is an efficient filter for tumor cells reaching it via the portal vein.

These studies confirm what common sense has taught us, namely that breast carcinoma in its earlier and operable stages usually metastasizes through the lymphatics and only infrequently gets into the blood stream. They are a warning, however, that we must make every effort to avoid blood stream metastases by being as gentle as possible in palpation of the breast, and that our surgical attack should be carried out with gentle sharp dissection, avoiding traction and pressure upon the tissues being removed.

Lung Metastases

The carcinoma emboli that reach the lung through the right heart and the pulmonary arteries are caught and form tumor thrombi in the small arterial branches or in the capillaries. They are too large to filter through the pulmonary capillary network. Schmidt, who wrote a classical description of the process of pulmonary metastasis, thought that some of the carcinoma emboli that reach the lungs are choked and destroyed by the fibrosis that develops around them. Walther agrees with this opinion. He believes that latent lung metastases, appearing in some cases a number of years after successful mastectomy, evolve from emboli that have remained locked up in fibrosed tumor thrombi in the lungs. Certainly, many carcinoma emboli that reach the lungs survive and grow vigorously. They form the rounded tumor nodules that are so often seen grossly at autopsy. The roentgenologists call this the *nodular* form of pulmonary metastasis. Figure 22–45 shows a characteristic roentgenogram of this type of metastasis, with numerous round masses of varying size scattered throughout both lung fields.

In rare cases only a single metastatic nodule is seen. It presumably represents the only carcinoma embolus that has reached the lung, for the patient has no evidence of other distant metastasis and is cured by pneumonectomy.

The following is a summary of one of the two cases of this kind that I have observed.

Mrs. D. B., a widowed woman lawyer aged 54, consulted me July 25, 1945, for a tumor of her right breast that she had first discovered in February. Examination showed a hard, poorly delimited tumor measuring 3 cm. in diameter at the medial end of the inframammary fold of the right breast. Like most carcinomas of the inframammary

fold that I have studied, it was fixed to the underlying chest wall. Pectoral contraction brought out a definite notch in the contour of the breast in the vicinity of the tumor. A chain of 1 cm. movable nodes was palpated in the right axilla. Skeletal and chest roentgenograms showed no evidence of metastasis.

After biopsy to prove the carcinomatous nature of the tumor, radical mastectomy with the customary skin graft was done. Twenty-two axillary lymph nodes were found in the specimen. None contained metastasis.

The patient had no further evidence of disease until three and one-half years later, when, in January, 1949, a routine chest film showed a single well rounded density 2 cm. in diameter in the lower posterior portion of the upper lobe of her right lung. She had no symptoms whatever and we failed to persuade her to permit thoracotomy until eight months later, when new roentgenograms (Fig. 22–46) showed that the lung nodule had increased in size. When the chest was opened October 26, 1949, by Dr. Richmond Moore, the only tumor nodule that could be found was the one seen in the x-ray films. It was a rounded 3 cm. mass covered by normal visceral pleura and projecting slightly from the surface of the lower posterior portion of the upper lobe. Right upper lobectomy was done. The gross appearance of the resected lobe is shown in Figure 22–47. Microscopically

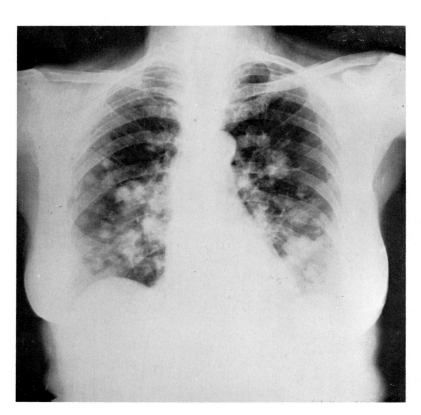

Figure 22–45. The roentgenographic appearance of the nodular type of bilateral pulmonary metastasis from mammary carcinoma.

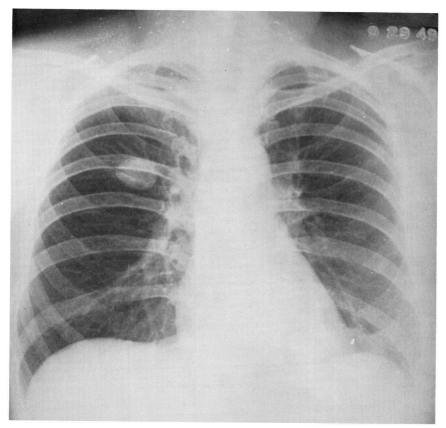

Figure 22–46. Solitary pulmonary metastasis from mammary carcinoma, as seen roentgenographically.

the tumor was carcinoma similar to the primary breast carcinoma removed four years and three months previously. The patient was well when last heard from in December 1965.

Seiler and his associates collected reports of solitary metastases to the lung treated by resection. This was successful in a number of patients, but none of them had had breast carcinoma.

The usual course of events when carcinoma emboli reach the lung is quite different. The emboli are numerous, and in the process of their expanding and infiltrating growth they break through the walls of the small pulmonary arteries or capillaries in which they have lodged. The disease then invades the structure of the lung diffusely, filling up the alveoli, blocking and permeating the lym-

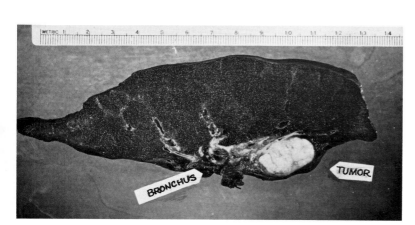

Figure 22–47. The gross appearance of the solitary pulmonary metastasis in the resected lung.

phatics, and growing into the pulmonary veins. Tumor fragments that break loose within the involved pulmonary veins are carried off back to the left heart and become carcinoma emboli in the systemic arterial circulation which carries them throughout the body. The viscera with a rich blood supply, such as the liver, spleen, and adrenals, and certain bones such as the vertebrae, are the most frequently involved. It was formerly thought that metastases to the spleen were significantly infrequent, but modern studies of this question show the spleen to be involved approximately as often as organs with a similar blood supply.

It follows from this concept of the process of blood stream metastasis that involvement of the lungs always precedes the development of blood-borne metastases in other parts of the body (an exception must be made for bone metastasis through the vertebral venous route which I shall discuss separately). Our clinical and autopsy evidence supports this premise. It must, of course, be understood that pulmonary metastases are not infrequently too small to be seen grossly or roentgenographically, and are found only by careful microscopic study of the lungs.

The nodular type of lung metastasis is remarkably silent clinically. If the parenchymal nodules are not associated with pleural involvement they produce no symptoms for months after they are first visible roentgenographically. Only when they have grown to a relatively large bulk do they begin to produce cough and some degree of dyspnea. With this type of pulmonary metastasis the respiratory symptoms are usually not the predominant ones in the terminal stage of the disease.

There is, however, another type of pulmonary metastasis of breast carcinoma that does produce important respiratory symptoms. It is the so-called lymphangitic type, characterized by permeation of the lymphatics and obliterative fibrosis around tumor thrombi in the small arteries of the lungs. This type of pulmonary metastasis is most often seen with carcinoma of the stomach, but we have seen it many times in patients with breast carcinoma at the Delafield Hospital. The most prominent symptom in these patients is dyspnea, which rapidly increases. It is accompanied by a productive cough, chest pain, and cyanosis. The patients fail rapidly and die with terminal edema of the lungs and pneumonitis. Roentgenograms of this lesion show streaks of increased density radiating out from the hilum diffusely into the lung fields. Both lungs are usually involved. Figure 22–48 illustrates the roentgenographic appearance of this type of metastasis.

At autopsy the findings do not show the massive involvement by carcinoma commonly seen with the nodular type of metastasis. The lungs are firm and edematous. Microscopic study shows the peribronchial and perivascular lymphatics to be filled with carcinoma cells. The small arteries and arterioles contain tumor thrombi and show a remarkable degree of fibrosis. It is these lymphatics distended with carcinoma and these fibrosed arteries that produce the linear x-ray shadows radiating from the hilum. Figure 22–49 shows the dilated lymphatics filled with carcinoma cells in the lungs of one of our patients with the lymphangitic type of metastasis. A summary of her case history follows.

R. B., was admitted to the Delafield Hospital in acute respiratory distress. She had had a left mastectomy in another hospital three years previously for carcinoma. Six weeks before admission she developed dyspnea. This rapidly increased until she could not walk or lie down, and she slept sitting up near a window. Edema of the legs had developed ten days before admission. Circulatory supportive treatment was given. Thoracentesis yielded 300 cc. of grossly bloody fluid from the left pleura. Nevertheless, her dyspnea and cyanosis increased and she died five days after admission to the hospital.

At autopsy the lungs showed marked congestion and edema but only small gross foci of metastatic carcinoma. There were metastases in many other organs. Microscopically there was extensive carcinomatous permeation of the lung lymphatics. The small pulmonary arteries contained tumor thrombi and showed marked fibrosis. There was also nonsuppurative lobular pneumonia.

Good descriptions of the lymphangitic type of pulmonary metastasis have been written by Wu, by Mueller and Sniffen, and by Hauser and Steer.

Some of the previous writers on the subject have assumed that the permeation of pulmonary lymphatics which is such a striking feature of this type of metastasis occurs in a centrifugal direction from the hilar nodes out into the lung fields, and that the metastases first reach the hilar nodes from the primary lesion via lymphatic routes. This assumption does not fit into our knowledge of the routes of spread of breast carcinoma. The posterior mediastinal, peritracheobronchial, and intrapulmonary lymph nodes that drain the lungs have no direct lymphatic connection with the

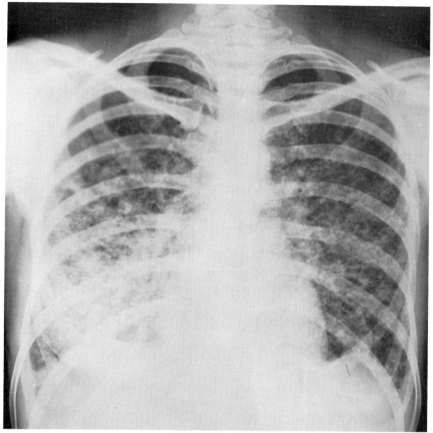

Figure 22–48. Roentgenographic appearance of the lymphangitic type of pulmonary metastasis from mammary carcinoma.

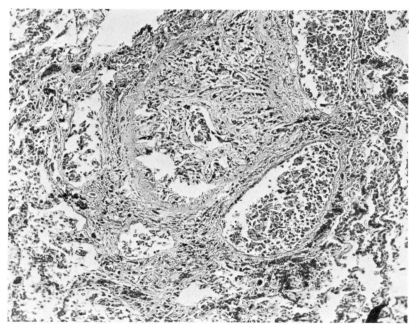

Figure 22–49. Dilated pulmonary lymphatics filled with carcinoma cells in the lymphangitic type of pulmonary metastasis from mammary carcinoma.

breast, and it is unlikely that lymphatic metastases from breast carcinoma go directly to them. It is more reasonable to think that the disease reaches the lungs via the usual venous route. The tumor thrombi in the pulmonary arteries are evidence of this fact. The peculiar feature of the lymphangitic type of metastasis is that an unusual fibrotic reaction to the presence of the carcinoma develops, and the fibrosis blocks lymph and blood vessels and permits the carcinoma to permeate the lymphatics in the normal centripetal direction of lymphatic drainage toward the hilar nodes, as well as peripherally toward the pleura.

Pleural Metastasis

Pleural involvement develops sooner or later in the great majority of patients with breast carcinoma metastases in the lungs. Abrams found pleural involvement at autopsy in 83.7 per cent of the cases with lung metastases. In some of these patients pleurisy, evidenced by pleuritic pain and pleural effusion, is the first sign that the disease has reached the lungs. There may be no roentgenographic evidence of the pulmonary parenchymal involvement at this stage. It may be assumed to exist, however, because the usual route of carcinoma to the pleura is from blood-borne emboli in the pulmonary arteries which grow and infiltrate the lung. From these parenchymal foci the disease permeates the superficial lymphatic network of the lung and reaches the pleura. Nodules of carcinoma beneath the

visceral pleura break through it, permitting carcinoma cells to escape into the pleural cavity and producing pleural effusion. In about 10 per cent of the cases the fluid is grossly bloody. Carcinoma cells can often be identified in this fluid when it is centrifuged and the cell block thus obtained studied microscopically. Luse and Reagan, in a special study of the cells of malignant tumors in effusions, were able to identify carcinoma cells in 66.6 per cent of their specimens of pleural fluid from patients with breast carcinoma.

The free floating carcinoma cells in the pleural effusion can presumably implant upon the surface of the pleura and grow, because nodules are much more frequently seen in the dorsal and basal portions of the pleural cavity where gravity would favor implantation.

Figure 22–50 shows a microscopic focus of breast carcinoma on the surface of the pleura, probably resulting from an implant.

It is of course possible for breast carcinoma that infiltrates the thoracic wall to penetrate through it and get into the pleural cavity by way of the parietal pleura. This is certainly an unlikely route in patients in whom effective treatment has eradicated the local primary disease, and no recurrence has developed on the chest wall.

In some patients the amount of pleural effusion is small, and the degree of fibrous thickening of the pleura great. In other patients the amount of serum that accumulates in the pleural cavities is very great. Two or three thousand ml. may be accumulated every day or so. Patients cannot tolerate this condition for long.

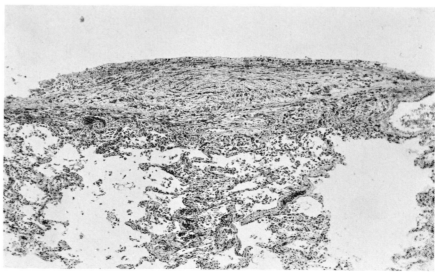

Figure 22–50. Microscopic appearance of a pleural focus of metastatic mammary carcinoma.

Esophageal Stenosis due to Mediastinal Lymph Node Metastasis

An infrequent but definite syndrome in advanced carcinoma of the breast is esophageal stenosis due to compression of the esophagus by mediastinal lymph node metastases. The main sympton is, of course, dysphagia.

Conklin reported three patients with this syndrome from our Delafield Hospital. All three had esophageal stenosis demonstrated by contrast roentgenograms and esophagoscopy. Two of the three also had supraclavicular recurrence associated with paralysis of the left recurrent laryngeal nerve. Two of the three patients were treated with irradiation to the area of esophageal compression, and the dysphagia improved.

Polk, Camp, and Walker have recently described this syndrome in six patients, and Atkins has described it in five patients.

Compression of the Superior Vena Cava by Metastases from Breast Carcinoma

Papillon and his associates have described a syndrome in which the superior vena cava was compressed by metastatic breast carcinoma, with the development of edema and cyanosis of the face and neck and dyspnea. They reported three such cases. Irradiation gave relief.

Metastasis to Bones

Metastasis of breast carcinoma to bone is probably as frequent as, if not more frequent than, metastases to lungs and liver. Since no pathologist has systematically investigated the frequency of metastasis in all the bones in which metastases are likely to be found, we do not really know what the true incidence of bone involvement is. At the most, pathologists have at autopsy taken sections at random from several of the vertebrae, and sometimes from ribs or pelvic bones. Kitain, and Turner and Jaffe reported bone involvement in some 56 per cent of cases. This figure is certainly too low. Abrams is nearer the truth with his figure of 77 per cent.

Unfortunately, roentgenograms do not give us as accurate information on this question as autopsy studies. Even when the entire skeleton is systematically studied a high percentage of bone metastases are not visualized. Forty years ago Chasin showed that in the vertebrae defects of from 1 to 1.5 cm. diameter, produced by experimentally removing portions of the spongiosa, could not be demonstrated by the usual anteroposterior roentgenograms. These findings were confirmed by Böhmig and Prévôt. Bachman and Sproul, at the Delafield Hospital, have carried out a similar but more precise study, correlating radiographic and autopsy findings. In a series of 59 autopsies Sproul found metastases in the vertebrae of 31. Bachman studied the vertebrae radiographically in these patients during the terminal stage of their disease, using the most elaborate techniques, including laminograms. At autopsy the vertebrae were dissected out and Bachman made roentgenograms of them. Nevertheless he was able to demonstrate metastases radiographically in only 15 of the 31 cases in which the microscope proved their presence. These findings are shown in Table 22–34.

As Bachman and Sproul's table shows, the

Table 22–34. Correlation of radiographic and autopsy findings*

No. of Cases	Pathological Findings	Radiographic Findings			
		Correct X-ray Diagnosis	Metastasis Not Visualized	False Positive	Total
28	No vertebral metastasis at autopsy	27	–	1	28
31	Vertebral metastasis at autopsy				
	osteoplastic	8	11	0	19
	osteolytic	4	1	0	5
	mixed	2	0	0	2
	intertrabecular	1	4	0	5
		15	16	1	31
59	Total cases	42	16	1	59

*From Bachman, A. L., and Sproul, E. E.: Bull. New York Acad. Med., *31*:146, 1955.

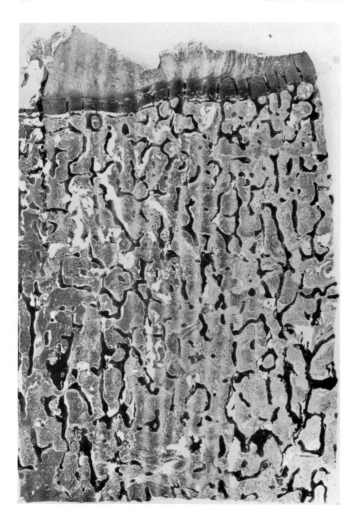

Figure 22–51. The intertrabecular type of mammary carcinoma metastasis to a vertebra.

degree of success with which roentgenograms reveal metastases in bone depends to a considerable extent upon the manner in which the disease grows in the bone. Roentgenologists have been accustomed to classify bone metastases from breast carcinoma as osteolytic or osteoplastic. This is too simple a classification. In terms of the actual pathology in the bones, we at the Delafield were taught by Sproul to distinguish four types of metastases. My illustrations for these four types are photographs of actual sections cut from vertebrae and decalcified and stained in the usual way.

1. The *intertrabecular type* (Fig. 22–51). Here the bone trabeculae, which are shown in black, are almost intact, but the marrow spaces between the trabeculae are filled with carcinoma. It is understandable why this type of metastasis cannot be detected roentgenologically. We subscribe fully to Schinz's state-

ment that, "The great majority of skeletal metastases merely cause a displacement of the bone marrow and do not produce any structural changes in the calcified bony tissue. They are not roentgenologically demonstrable."

2. The *osteolytic type* (Fig. 22–52). The bone trabeculae are to a large extent destroyed by the carcinoma. This change, in its early stage, may have the roentgenologic appearance of bone atrophy, but eventually its metastatic character is betrayed by the irregular defects that develop in the bone. In the vertebrae the pedicles, the spinous process, or the body, including part of the cortex, may be destroyed. The involved vertebrae are usually compressed and collapsed as the disease progresses. Figure 22–53 shows compression of the sixth and seventh dorsal vertebrae due to metastases. The roentgenologic appearance of osteolytic metastasis in

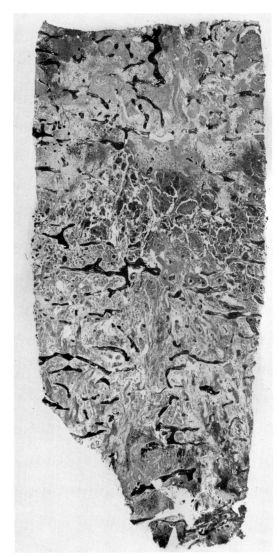

Figure 22–52. The osteolytic type of mammary carcinoma metastasis to a vertebra.

the pelvic bones and the upper end of the femur, and in the skull, is shown in Figures 22–54 and 22–55. The bones are seen to be riddled with irregular moth-eaten defects. The osteolytic type is overwhelmingly the most frequent type of bone metastasis of breast carcinoma that can be visualized roentgenologically.

In connection with the diagnosis of osteolytic metastases in the skull it should be kept in mind that venous lakes can closely simulate them. The bone defects produced by venous lakes may occur anywhere in the skull; they may be single or multiple, and they are occasionally surprisingly large. Figure 22–56

shows such a large venous lake, which at first view suggested a metastasis. The patient had an early breast carcinoma.

When a defect in the skull suggesting osteolytic metastasis is found in a patient whose breast carcinoma is not advanced, and in whom there are no demonstrable metastases in other bones, great caution should be exercised in making a diagnosis. Stereo views of the skull should be made. If the defect is a venous lake the views will often show the vascular channel leading into it. The fact that a presumed venous lake increases in size or that new ones develop over a period of years is not proof that they represent metastases. Taveras and Wood describe a case in which venous lakes increased in size and number over a 12 year interval.

3. The *osteoplastic type* (Fig. 22–57). The trabeculae are thickened. They coalesce to form irregular oseous masses. The bones assume an abnormally dense mottled or marbled appearance. Periosteal thickening may lead to an actual increase in the volume

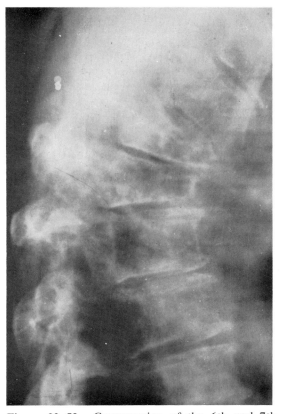

Figure 22–53. Compression of the 6th and 7th dorsal vertebrae due to osteolytic metastasis from mammary carcinoma, as seen roentgenographically.

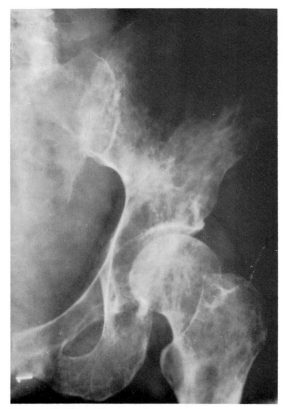

Figure 22–54. The roentgenographic appearance of osteolytic metastasis from mammary carcinoma to the pelvic bones and femur.

of the bone. Figures 22–58 and 22–59 show the roentgenographic appearance of the osteoplastic type of metastasis from breast carcinoma in the skull, and in the pelvic bones and the upper end of the femur. Not more than 5 to 10 per cent of bone metastases from breast carcinoma are of the osteoplastic type.

4. The *mixed type.* A fourth type of bone metastases might be called the mixed type (Fig. 22–60) in which the features of the other types are intermingled.

Metastases reach the bones through the blood stream. There are two routes. One is from metastases in the lungs that break through the pulmonary capillary network and are carried back to the left heart which pumps them through the arterial circulation to reach the bones. A second route to the bones, one that has not been recognized until recently, is through the vertebral system of veins. As I described in Chapter 1, the vertebral veins provide a route via the intercostal veins of the chest wall, directly to the spine, the pelvic bones, and the skull, a route

that is entirely separate from the route through the lungs and the systemic arterial circulation.

The venous circulation of the vertebrae, and its connections with both the intercostal veins and the lumbar veins of the systemic circulation, have been recently described and illustrated with superb anatomic preparations by Henriques. He has pointed out the importance of the vertebral veins as routes by which emboli from breast carcinoma reach the vertebrae directly via the intercostal veins.

The lower vertebrae contain particularly large quiet lakes of blood which provide a favorable environment for metastases which reach them, and it is understandable why they are the most frequent site of metastases from breast carcinoma.

Proof that carcinoma reaches the bones through the vertebral vein system is provided by cases in which bone metastasis occurs without lung involvement. The following is such a case.

Mrs. E. P., a housewife aged 39, consulted me on July 6, 1941, for a tumor of her right breast that she had discovered five days previously.

Examination revealed a 3 x 2 cm., firm tumor in the inner lower sector of the right breast, just beyond the areolar edge. There was retraction of the skin over the lesion. In the right axilla there was a single 1 cm., firm, movable node.

At operation frozen section showed the lesion to be a carcinoma. Radical mastectomy with Thiersch graft was carried out. Pathologic study of the specimen showed a moderately undifferentiated carcinoma. Twenty-three lymph nodes were dissected from the specimen. Three of these, two from the lower axilla and one from the apex of the axilla, contained metastasis.

She was well until September, 1944, when she began to have pain in the cervical region, suggesting metastasis. X-ray films at this time showed nothing more than "osteoarthritis" of the cervical spine, in the opinion of the roentgenologists. The pain in the cervical region persisted, although it was not severe. In March, 1945, she complained of pain in the left lateral chest region. Films at this time showed metastases in the seventh and ninth left ribs, as well as in the cervical spine. Radiotherapy to the cervical region and the left costal area gave her good palliative relief.

In May, 1945, she developed pain in the left elbow region, and films showed destruction of the medial condyle of the left humerus. This area was irradiated with relief of pain, and reduction in the size of the lesion in the bone.

She was comparatively well until February, 1947, when she began to have pain in the lower back. X-rays showed metastasis in T6. She was

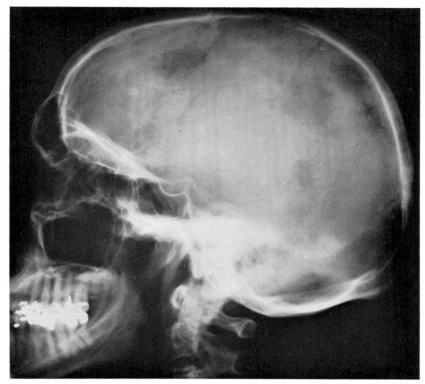

Figure 22–55. The roentgenographic appearance of osteolytic metastasis from mammary carcinoma to the skull.

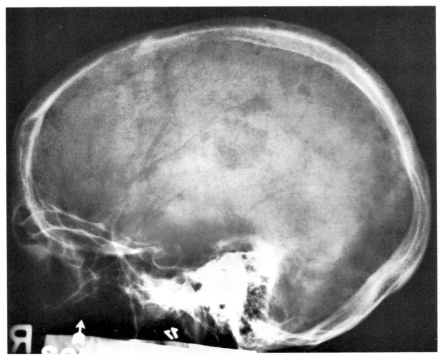

Figure 22–56. Large venous lakes suggesting metastasis in the skull of a woman with mammary carcinoma.

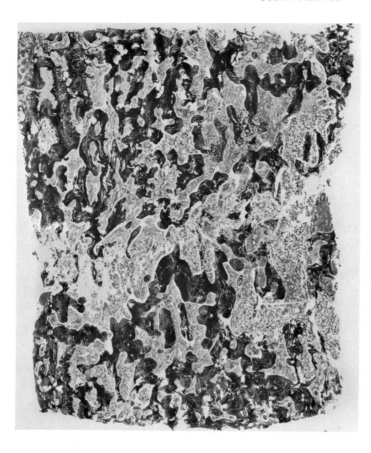

Figure 22–57. The osteoplastic type of mammary carcinoma metastasis to a vertebra.

admitted to the hospital again and the thoracic spine irradiated. This course of radiation relieved her somewhat, but not completely. She was therefore put for the first time upon testosterone, intramuscularly.

She had a relatively good summer during 1947 but was annoyed by the hoarseness and hirsutism which developed from the androgen. By October, 1947, however, the pain in her back and pelvis had increased. Films at this time showed progression of the metastases in the thoracic spine, T3, T6, T7, and T12 being involved. The fifth lumbar vertebra and the right ilium now showed involvement. She was admitted to the hospital again on October 30, 1947, and the lower spine and pelvis were irradiated with fairly good symptomatic relief. She continued to take testosterone.

During 1948, she continued to get along fairly well, although her x-rays showed progressive destruction of the pelvic bones and lumbar vertebrae. These bones were treated by irradiation with considerable relief. Films showed some filling in of a particularly large area of destruction in the right iliac bone. She continued to take androgen, although not regularly, and by mouth rather than intramuscularly. She objected strongly to the secondary changes which the androgen produced, although the fact that she looked and felt amazing-

ly well most of the time was without doubt to a considerable extent due to the hormone treatment. After July, 1948, she refused to take more hormone because of its unpleasant side effects.

In the early months of 1949, her back and legs were giving her almost no trouble. She was able to drive her car and be up and about most of the time. Her cervical spine and ribs now began to trouble her increasingly. The cervical vertebrae, particularly C4 and C5, showed a great degree of destruction, and she began to have forward dislocation of these vertebrae. She was given further radiation to the cervical spine, again with a fair degree or relief.

During the latter part of 1949, however, her neck pain became more and more troublesome. In October she was again admitted to the hospital and the cervical spine was again irradiated. An area of extensive destruction in the upper right femur was also treated at this time. She had fair relief from her leg and neck pain.

In the fall of 1950, she began to require morphine for the first time, but even with this, she was not comfortable. It was therefore decided in January, 1951, to do a unilateral lobotomy. This was performed by Dr. T. Scarff and gave her good relief of pain until February 6, when she had a spontaneous fracture of her right femur. From this

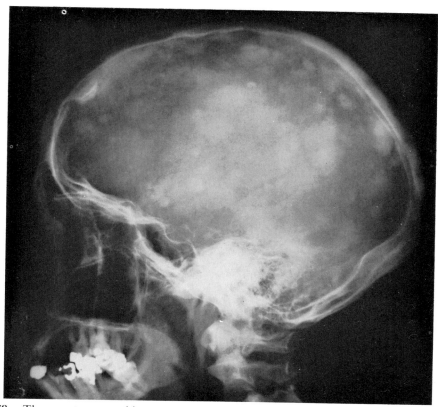

Figure 22–58. The roentgenographic appearance of osteoplastic metastasis from mammary carcinoma to the skull.

point on she required increasingly heavy sedation until her death on February 22, 1951, nine years and four months after radical mastectomy.

At autopsy widespread bone metastases, as well as nodular metastases in the liver, were found. The lungs, however, were entirely free of carcinoma, both grossly and microscopically. It is difficult to escape the conclusion that this patient's carcinoma reached her vertebrae, which were the first bones involved, through the vertebral system of veins. If the disease had reached the vertebrae through the caval route and the lungs, it should have been found in the lungs at death more than nine years later.

A generation ago Sampson Handley, in advancing his theory of the spread of carcinoma by lymphatic permeation, explained bone metastasis as the result of a process of continuous permeation of the lymphatics in fascial planes. Some students of the question, like Carnett and Howell, were convinced of the correctness of Handley's explanation, but most pathologists have opposed it. Piney, in an important study presented in 1922, was unable to demonstrate any lymphatics in

bone marrow, and he concluded that metastases to the bone marrow must be blood-borne. He explained the relative freedom of the distal bones of the limbs from carcinoma metastases as being a result of the absence of red marrow in these bones. The red marrow, according to Piney, is the place in which the bed of the blood stream widens, the course of the vessels becomes more complicated, and the conditions for the lodgment of emboli become correspondingly more favorable. The blood stream slows in the red marrow, and its solid elements, such as tumor emboli, settle at the periphery of the vascular bed and proliferate there.

According to Hanley's theory, the lymph nodes and fasciae in the region of distant bone metastases are assumed to have been involved by the permeation process before the disease reaches the bones. To test the validity of this theory, Willis made special studies of the lymph nodes and fascia regional to skeletal metastases. In 11 cases with metastases to the femur, he found the ingui-

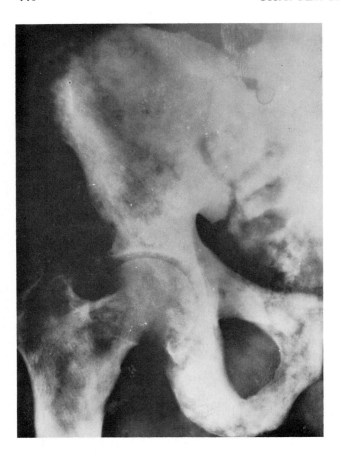

Figure 22–59. The roentgenographic appearance of osteoplastic metastasis from mammary carcinoma to the pelvic bones and femur.

nal lymph nodes to be involved in only one case. Moreover, thorough microscopic examination of the deep fascia from several parts of the thigh and buttock, and of the periosteum stripped from the bone near the metastases showed no evidence of cancer cells.

Handley wrote that: "The liability of a bone to cancer metastases increases with its proximity to the site of the primary growth." Modern x-ray and autopsy evidence have shown that this is not true in cancer of the breast. The sternum and ribs are not affected earlier and more frequently than other bones as Handley's theory would imply. The most extensive roentgenologic data on this point come from the Mayo Clinic where Sutherland and his associates studied the distribution of the lesions as shown by x-ray in a series of 628 breast cases of skeletal metastasis from breast carcinoma, and from the Ellis Fischel State Cancer Hospital where Staley studied skeletal metastases in 166 patients. The distribution of bone metastases in these two series of cases follows:

Bones involved	Sutherland	Staley
Pelvis	33.9%	59.6%
Lumbar spine	20.7%	53 %
Ribs	13.5%	61.4%
Femur	11.8%	46.4%
Shoulder girdle	5.3%	—
Skull	4.9%	34.9%
Thoracic spine	4.6%	39.1%
Humerus	2.8%	10.9%
Cervical spine	1.3%	7.2%
Lower extremity	0.1%	—
Upper extremity	0.8%	—

More accurate information as to which bones are most often involved by metastases in breast carcinoma has been derived from studies that utilize both roentgenologic and autopsy evidence, such as that by Lenz and Freid. Their data (Table 22–35) included 81 cases of breast carcinoma in which the existence of bone metastases had been proved roentgenologically or by autopsy. The predilection of the lower vertebrae and the pelvic bones to develop metastases is apparent from these data.

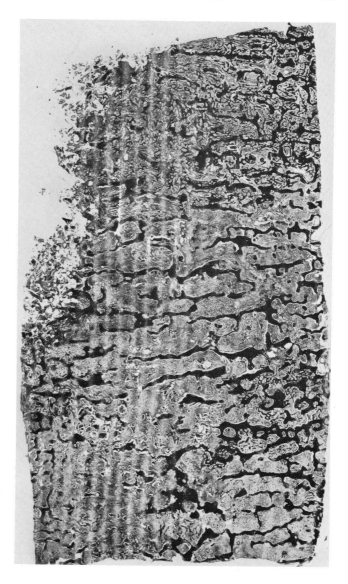

Figure 22–60. The mixed type of mammary carcinoma metastasis to a vertebra.

The smaller and the more peripheral the bones of the extremities, the less likely they are to be involved by metastases. Only in rare cases in which the entire skeleton is riddled with metastases, as in that described by Bendick and Jacobs, is involvement of the metacarpal bones and phalanges seen.

The diagnosis of bone metastases is often difficult because, as I have pointed out above, x-ray films fail to reveal them in the majority of cases until the metastases are far advanced. Pain, and less frequently tenderness in pressure or percussion over the diseased bone, are clinical signs of bone involvement. Tenderness is often present over metastases in ribs. Pain and tenderness are presumably due either to pressure of the metastases on the periosteum or to actual infiltration of the periosteum, since bone itself does not contain sensory nerves.

When the vertebrae are involved the patient at first complains of stiffness and pain in her back when she gets up or lies down. She may be perfectly comfortable when she lies quietly in bed. A jar, such as when she misses a step, or coughs or sneezes, may give her a sharp twinge of back pain. These symptoms intensify slowly but relentlessly. After a few weeks the patient is so uncomfortable that she consults an orthopedist. He obtains x-rays of her spine that are reported as negative, whereupon he assumes that she does not

Table 22–35. CARCINOMA OF THE BREAST; ANATOMIC DISTRIBUTION IN 81 CASES OF SKELETAL METASTASES*

General Localization	Per cent	Specific Localization	Per cent	Homolateral Heterolateral Bilateral	
Pelvis	62	Ischium	37		
		Ilium	58		
		Pubis	56		
Spine	59	Cervical	13		
		Dorsal	40		
		Lumbar	57		
		Sacral	38		
Femur	54			Bilateral	31
				Heterolateral	8
				Homolateral	5
Ribs	39			Bilateral	20
				Heterolateral	5
				Homolateral	7
Skull	35				
Humerus	27			Bilateral	11
				Heterolateral	5
				Homolateral	6
Scapula	16			Bilateral	8
				Heterolateral	4
				Homolateral	1
Clavicle	14			Homolateral	1
				Bilateral	5
				Heterolateral	6
Tibia	3			Homolateral	2
				Heterolateral	1
Sternum	1				
Radius	1				
Ulna	1				
Hands	1				
Fibula	1				
Bonds of feet	1				

*Data from Lenz, M., and Freid, J. K.: Metastases to the skeleton, brain, and spinal cord from cancer of the breast and the effect of radiotherapy, Ann. Surg., 93:278, 1931.

have metastases and advises back exercises or a back brace. In the patient who has had breast carcinoma he is very apt to be wrong.

It is important to realize that pain due to bone metastases often precedes roentgenologic evidence of the lesion by some months. Lenz and Freid described seven cases in which the pain preceded the roentgenologic visualization of the bone lesion by from six to twelve months. I have seen many patients with this sequence and I have learned that it is wisest to assume that bone metastases have developed, even though x-ray studies reveal nothing abnormal, in patients with breast carcinoma who develop back or leg pain, or pain over other bones, for which no other good explanation is apparent.

There are, of course, some patients whose bone metastases produce no pain at all. I have seen several whose skeletons were riddled with metastases, yet they did not complain of pain. I know of no adequate explanation for this paradox.

Pain due to vertebral metastases is often referred along the course of the cutaneous nerves. Thus the patient with metastases in

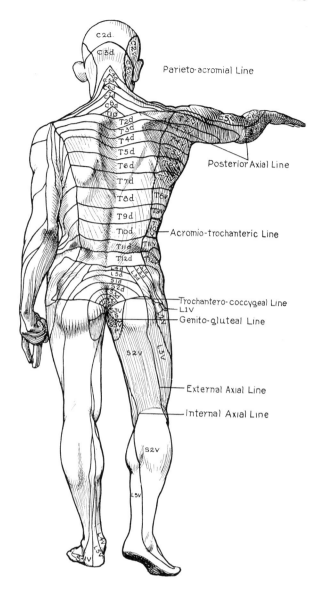

Figure 22–61. The cutaneous distribution of the spinal nerves—lateral view (Tilney and Riley).

the second and third lumbar vertebrae complains of pain radiating down the anterior and lateral aspects of the thigh.

The cutaneous distribution of the spinal nerves, and the areas to which pain from vertebral metastases is referred, are shown in Figures 22–61 and 22–62, reproduced from Tilney and Riley.

When breast carcinoma metastasizes to bone and destroys it extensively, important changes in calcium metabolism may occur, resulting in a dangerous clinical syndrome—hypercalcemia. In the early 1950's this syndrome was studied in several clinics (Lazlo et al.; Kennedy et al.; Myers et al.); its basic features were defined and its treatment worked out.

Calcium absorbed from the alimentary tract is deposited in the skeleton. Only a minute fraction exists in the body fluids—the normal serum calcium level ranging between 9 and 11 mg. per 100 ml. When bone is destroyed by metastatic breast carcinoma, the normal balance between deposition of calcium in and mobilization of calcium from bone is upset. Calcium accumulates in the blood serum faster than it can be excreted through the kidneys. If not corrected, this calcium imbalance results in renal insufficiency and death.

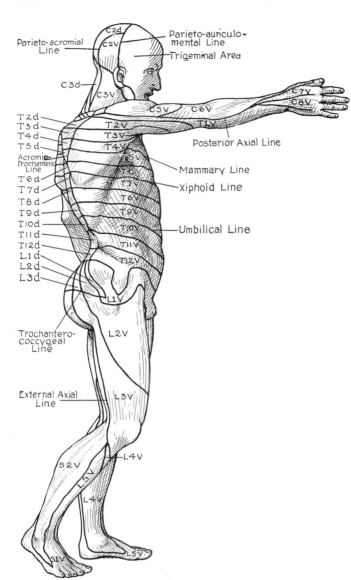

Parieto-acromial Line
C2d
C2V
Parieto-auriculo-mental Line
Trigeminal Area
C3d
C3V
C5V   C6V
C7V
C8V
T2d
T3d
T4d
T5d
T2V
T3V
T4V
T1V
Posterior Axial Line
Acromio-Trochanteric Line
T5V
T6V
Mammary Line
T6d
T7d
T7V
Xiphoid Line
T8d
T9d
T8V
T9V
T10d
T11d
T10V
Umbilical Line
T12d
L1d
L2d
L3d
T11V
T12V
L1V
Trochantero-coccygeal Line
L2V
External Axial Line
L3V
L4V
S2V
L5V
L4V
L5V
S1V

Figure 22–62. The cutaneous distribution of the spinal nerves—dorsal view (Tilney and Riley).

The symptoms of hypercalcemia are gastrointestinal (anorexia, nausea and vomiting), central nervous system disturbances (sleepiness, lethargy, stupor, disorientation, and coma), and a reduced urinary output. The patient, in a semi-comatose state, takes less and less fluid and becomes dehydrated. Deposition of calcium salts in the kidney increases, and renal function is further impaired. Uremia and death quickly follow.

The factors that precipitate hypercalcemia in patients with bone metastases from breast carcinoma are not yet fully understood. In some patients it is a spontaneous phenomenon resulting from very rapid bone destruc-

tion. Herrmann and his associates, and Kennedy and his associates, were among the first to point out that hypercalcemia may be precipitated by treatment with either androgen or estrogen. Kleinfeld reported three cases from our Delafield Hospital in which hypercalcemia developed probably as the result of stilbestrol treatment. Even small test doses of estrogen have been known to throw the patient into hypercalcemia. Jessiman and his associates report hypercalcemia developing after oophorectomy, after adrenalectomy, and after hypophysectomy.

The treatment of hypercalcemia consists of increasing the daily fluid intake to 5 or 6 liters, reducing the intake of calcium by eliminating milk and milk-products from the diet, and the administration of corticosteroids in the form of 20 to 40 mg. of prednisone daily. The response to treatment is usually dramatic; but in some patients this complication is immediately fatal despite vigorous treatment.

There have been a number of recent papers discussing hypercalcemia and reporting impressive case series. Jessiman and his associates reported 59 episodes of hypercalcemia which occurred in 33 patients in a series of 145 patients with metastatic breast carcinoma. Graham and his associates reported that 16.9 per cent of a series of 290 women with desseminated breast carcinoma whom they studied had hypercalcemia. Mannheimer described 59 episodes of hypercalcemia occurring in 40 patients. They represented about 10 per cent of the total number of patients with metastatic breast carcinoma treated in her clinic.

The mechanism of hypercalcemia is still imperfectly understood. Lemon has recently demonstrated increased parathormone activity in the serum of patients with hypercalcemia, and it has been suggested that some carcinomas may produce a parathormone-like substance that induces hypercalcemia.

Hypocalcemia also develops in rare instances, in patients with bone metastases from breast carcinoma. Hall and his associates have described this syndrome in three patients. All three had diffuse osteoblastic metastases. Their symptoms included anorexia, nausea, drowsiness, and muscular twitching, and coma. The administration of calcium by mouth and calcium infusions relieved the symptoms dramatically for a time.

Pathologic Fractures in Breast Carcinoma. Fracture of femurs, humeri, or ribs weakened by metastases of breast carcinoma is not infrequent. Compression fracture of vertebrae is less dramatic but is often seen in x-ray films of these patients. In Lenz and Fried's series of patients with bone metastases there were fractures of one or more bones in 26 per cent. In Copeland's series of such cases, 15 per cent developed fractures. Welch reported that 17 per cent of his series of these patients had fractures. Staley reported a much higher frequency of fracture in a series of 166 patients with bone metastases from breast carcinoma at the Ellis Fischel Hospital—48 per cent. Snell and Beals reported that in a series of 60 patients with breast carcinoma metastatic to the femur, 15

eventually had fractures. My own experience has been that pathologic fracture is less frequent. This may be because we use irradiation extensively for bone metastases, and if there is a large metastatic lesion in the humerus or femur we irradiate it prophylactically even though it is not causing pain.

Even though most of the substance of a long bone has been replaced by metastatic carcinoma at the site of one of these pathologic fractures, the normal healing process as expressed by callus formation is usually sufficient to achieve bony union if the fragments are adequately fixed. Figure 22–63A shows a pathologic fracture through a large metastasis in the humerus from a breast carcinoma. The site of the fracture was immobilized and irradiated, and good union resulted. Figure 22–63B shows its appearance a year later. Hummel described the pathologic aspects of this healing process in several cases.

It is therefore important to try to obtain healing of pathologic fractures. Today our orthopedists usually treat them by internal fix-

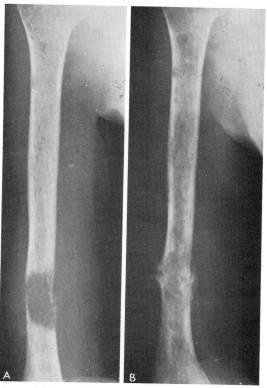

Figure 22–63. The roentgenographic appearance of metastasis from mammary carcinoma to the humerus. *A,* Pathological fracture through the metastasis. *B,* Immobilization and irradiation with good union one year later.

ation. They use an intramedullary nail for fractures of the shaft of the humerus or femur. Fractures of the neck or subtrochanteric region of the femur are fixed with a pin or screw and a long side plate. These patients are gotten out of bed very quickly. Pain is relieved and nursing care simplified. Phelan has described these methods of internal fixation of pathologic fractures.

It has been our practice to give irradiation to the lesion after fixation has been achieved. Irradiation relieves pain and we believe that it increases the patient's chances of regaining function of the limb.

Metastases to the Eye

In our Institute of Ophthalmology, Merriam has made a special study of metastatic tumors of the eye. He has had 40 patients with this condition. He has reviewed the more than 300 case reports of metastases to the eye. About 70 per cent originated from breast carcinoma. These metastases have a predilection for the posterior portion of the choroid. They produce failing vision, with eventual retinal detachment. Both eyes are often involved. Good illustrative case reports of choroidal metastases are found in papers by Bedell, Jensen, Dickson, and Stewart.

Bedford and Daniel reported metastasis of breast carcinoma to the extrinsic ocular muscles. Nicholls described two cases of metastasis to the optic nerve.

Merriam advises treatment by irradiation. About 50 per cent of the patients have good results, with preservation of vision.

Metastases to the Stomach and Duodenum

During recent years there have been reports from several clinics of metastasis of breast carcinoma to the stomach and duodenum. Although the phenomenon is not frequent, it has attracted attention because of the difficulty of distinguishing primary from secondary carcinoma in these organs. Hartman and Sherlock reported that in their series of 204 autopsies of patients with carcinoma of the breast, 18.1 per cent were found to have metastases to the stomach or duodenum.

Choi and his associates found metastases to the stomach in 8.1 per cent of their series

Table 22–36. Gastrointestinal metastases from breast carcinoma demonstrated in 337 autopsies*

Site of Metastasis	No. of Patients	No. Patients with Symptoms
Esophagus	20	6
Stomach	20	3
Small intestine	22	2
Colon	15	3
Rectum	3	2
Total	80	16

*Data from Asch, M. J., Wiedel, P. D., and Habif, D. V.: Arch. Surg., 96:840, 1968.

of 341 breast carcinomas. Fifteen of their 28 patients had gastrointestinal symptoms, including anorexia, nausea and vomiting, epigastric pain, gastrointestinal bleeding, and dysphagia. In nine of the patients these symptoms were severe enough to lead to roentgenologic studies, which showed abnormalities that were not diagnostic.

Graham and Goldman have described 21 cases in which there were metastases to the stomach or bowel revealed by exploratory laparotomy or autopsy in a series of 300 patients with advanced breast carcinoma; 11 patients had metastases to the stomach, nine had metastases to the small bowel, and 12 had metastases to the colon or rectum.

Asch, Wiedel, and Habif reviewed a series of 337 autopsies on patients who died of breast carcinoma in our Delafield Hospital and found 80 examples of gastrointestinal metastasis in a total of 57 patients. The sites of these metastases, and the frequency of symptoms which they produced, are shown in Table 22–36.

In their report Asch, Wiedel, and Habif also described 18 cases in which metastasis of breast carcinoma to the gastrointestinal tract produced symptoms requiring operation. The essential details of these 18 cases are shown in Table 22–37. Attention is called to the fact that three of the four patients with hematemesis had been receiving steroid therapy, and that it may play a role in this phenomenon.

Liver Metastases

The liver competes closely with the lungs as a frequent site of metastases from breast carcinoma. When metastases escaping from the lungs through the pulmonary veins get

Table 22–37. GASTROINTESTINAL METASTASES REQUIRING OPERATION

Age	Site	Symptoms	X-Ray Findings	Operation	Time Breast Lesion to GI° Symptoms	Time GI Symptoms or Operation to Death
37	Jejunum	Recurrent vomiting	Small intestinal series showed partial jejunal obstruction	Partial jejunectomy, gastrojejunostomy	6 yr	8 mo
33	Ileum	Abdominal pain, vomiting	Flat plate showed intestinal obstruction	Partial ileal resection, intussusception led by tumor mass	1 yr	?
42	Ileum	Abdominal pain, vomiting	Kinking of ileum on MA-tube study	Partial ileal resection	2 yr	10 mo
64	Colon	Narrow stool, rectal mass	Rectosigmoid narrowing on BA enema	Colostomy	5 yr	2 mo
35	Colon	Nausea, vomiting, obstipation	Flat plate showed obstruction, rectosigmoid obstruction on BA enema	Colostomy	12 yr	2 mo
85	Stomach	Hematemesis	...	50% gastrectomy after gastric hypothermia and 6-unit transfusion	2 yr	7 mo
42	Stomach	Abdominal pain	Pneumoperitoneum on abdominal x-ray film	Excision of perforated metastasis	2 yr	Living 9 mo postoperatively
37	Stomach	Disabling epigastric pain	Penetrating lesser curvature gastric ulcer	Biopsy of ulcer, vagotomy and pyloroplasty	6 yr	Living 13 mo postoperatively
57	Duodenum	Nausea, vomiting	Obstruction second portion duodenum by extrinsic mass on GI series	Gastrojejunostomy for retroperitoneal tumor invading stomach and duodenum	3 yr	Died postoperatively
63	Esophagus	Dysphagia, nausea, vomiting, left cord paralysis	BA swallow—extrinsic defect treated with radiotherapy	Gastrostomy one year after radiotherapy	5 yr	6 mo
53	Esophagus	Dysphagia	BA swallow showed narrowing	Gastrostomy	9 yr	2 mo
44	Stomach	Hematemesis melena	...	50% gastrectomy after 12-unit transfusion	4 yr	Died postoperatively
41	Stomach	Anorexia, nausea	Obstruction by infiltrating tumor on GI series	Total gastrectomy	1 yr	Died
50	Stomach	Vomiting	Antral constriction on GI series	50% gastrectomy	4 yr	7 mo
72	Stomach	Weakness, melena	Rigid antrum on GI series	50% gastrectomy	7 yr	24 mo
61	Colon	Frequent narrow stools	Multiple areas of constriction on BA enema	Laparotomy, biopsy, postoperative radiotherapy	1 yr	24 mo
58	Rectum	Constipation, rectal mass	...	Colostomy	6½ yr	2 mo
75	Rectum	Nausea, obstipation, rectal mass	Colonic dilatation on flat plate	Colostomy	1½ yr	Died postoperatively

*GI indicates gastrointestinal; MA, Miller Abbott; BA, barium.

Table 22–38. FREQUENCY OF METASTASES IN OVARIES REMOVED THERAPEUTICALLY FOR MAMMARY CARCINOMA

Author	No. of Patients Treated by Oophorectomy	Per cent of Ovarian Metastases
Sicard	38	28.9%
Kasilag and Rutledge	91	25.0%
Turksoy	26	30.7%
Lumb and Mackenzie	190	29.4%
Harris and Spratt	64	26.5%
Treves and Finkbeiner	191	30.0%

into the systemic arterial circulation they reach the liver through the hepatic artery. They grow to form spherical masses scattered throughout the liver substance. Figure 22–64 shows their usual appearance. Liver metastases usually produce few if any symptoms until an advanced stage is reached, when the liver may become so large as to cause abdominal distress. The obstructive jaundice that sometimes develops may be accompanied by pruritus.

Metastasis to the Brain

When the brain is examined and metastases carefully sought for they will be found to be fairly frequent in cases of carcinoma of the breast. Abrams found them in 29 per cent of his series of autopsies.

Metastases to the brain are important because of the therapeutic problem they present. They produce clinical signs of increased intracranial pressure such as headache and vomiting, disturbances of vision, and convulsive seizures, thus simulating primary brain tumors. Neurologic surgeons are well aware of this diagnostic problem. They also know that breast carcinoma is a frequent source of brain metastases, and they have learned to search for a primary breast lesion. Grant reported 15 of a series of 49 cases of metastasis to the brain as due to breast carcinoma, and Dunlap published a series of 95 secondary brain tumors, 28 of which were due to breast carcinoma.

These brain metastases may be situated in any part of the brain and they are usually multiple. This latter fact, and the presence of metastases elsewhere, usually makes craniotomy impractical. Rarely, brain metastases are solitary and cystic, as in the remarkable case described by Willis.

Metastasis to the Ovary

The ovaries have been found to contain metastases in approximately 20 per cent of autopsies of patients with breast carcinoma. In case series in which the ovaries have been removed therapeutically the frequency of metastases has surprisingly enough been higher. Even though the ovaries are grossly normal,

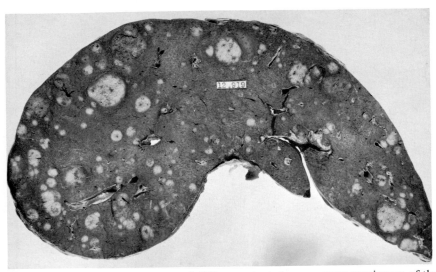

Figure 22–64. The gross appearance of diffuse metastatic mammary carcinoma of the liver.

careful microscopic study not infrequently reveals metastases.

Table 22–38 shows the per cent of ovarian metastases found in several series of patients treated by oophorectomy.

Metastasis to the Adrenals

From autopsy studies of the distribution of metastases in breast carcinoma it has been known that the adrenals are involved at death in as many as one-half of the patients. But the introduction of adrenalectomy as a therapeutic procedure which is done at an earlier stage in the natural history of breast carcinoma has made available much additional information concerning adrenal metastasis.

Table 22–39 shows the frequency with which adrenal metastases have been reported in several of the larger series of adrenalectomies.

It is of interest to add that in Lumb and Mackenzie's series of cases, which is much the largest yet reported, 15.7 per cent of the patients had unilateral adrenal metastases, and 23.8 per cent bilateral adrenal metastases.

In view of the fact that bilateral involvement of the ovaries is so frequent, it is to be expected that in some patients Addison's disease will develop. Galloway and Perloff have described such a case.

Metastasis to the Hypophysis

The likelihood of metastases of breast carcinoma to the hypophysis as reflected in the larger autopsy series was reviewed by Smulders. In his series of 71 autopsies the hypophysis was found to be involved in 28.1 per cent.

Table 22–39. FREQUENCY OF METASTASES IN ADRENALS REMOVED THERAPEUTICALLY FOR MAMMARY CARCINOMA

Author	No. of Patients Treated by Adrenalectomy	Per cent of Metastases
Huggins	56	25.0%
Pyrah	53	25.0%
Symington	82	23.0%
Tuaillon	155	30.4%
Aldrete	46	39.0%
Harris and Spratt	64	41.0%
Lumb and Mackenzie	235	39.1%

The development of therapeutic hypophysectomy has made much more data available on this question. Gurling, in 1957, reported that in his series of 44 hypophysectomies metastases were found in 25 per cent of the glands. The anterior lobe was the site of the metastases in 82 per cent of the involved glands, and the posterior lobe in 18 per cent. Pearson and Ray, in 1959, reported that in a series of 155 pituitaries studied microscopically, 15 per cent contained metastases. He has stated recently that in recent years, during which he has been more selective in choosing patients for hypophysectomy, the incidence of metastases has not been more than 7 per cent.

Less Frequent Forms of Metastasis

Carcinoma of the breast may metastasize to any part of the body, and there are many reports of unusual and bizarre metastases. Some of these follow: tongue (Fink and Garb); mandible (Sonntag; Lüdin; Burket; Pilheu and Fefer; Adair and Herrmann); parotid gland (Herrmann and Adair); gasserian ganglion (Fitzwilliams and Fell); maxilla (Blake and Blake;); placenta (Cross et al.); vagina (Held); umbilicus (Falkinburg and Savran); acoustic neuroma (Wong and Bennington); parathyroid adenoma (Woolner et al.); colon (Melnick and Rosenholtz); uterus (Krone and Englert; Benelli; von Szegvári et al.; Song; Birdsall et al.); vulva (Covington).

The Anemia of Cancer

At our Delafield Hospital, Hyman has carried out an interesting study of the anemia of cancer. The majority of the patients he studied had advanced breast carcinoma. He showed that the life span of erythrocytes is shortened in these patients, with the result that red cell destruction exceeds the capability of the marrow to replace red cells. Anemia develops and increases progressively as the carcinoma disseminates. Hyman suggests the existence of a specific hemolytic factor in patients with advanced cancer.

PRIMARY CARCINOMA IN THE SECOND BREAST

One of the important problems of breast cancer is involvement of the second breast. It

Table 22–40.   REPORTS OF PRIMARY CARCINOMA IN THE SECOND BREAST. CRUDE INCIDENCE RATES

Author	Year of Publication	Total No. Patients with Breast Carcinoma	Simultaneous Bilateral	Successive Bilateral
Kilgore	1921	1,100		1.1
Greenough	1921	639	0.7	1.6
McWilliams	1925	3,132	0.2	4.7
Berard	1939	645	1.5	1.6
Harrington	1946	6,559	1.0	3.4
Desaive	1949	1,259	0.7	3.6
Smithers	1952	1,777	0.6	2.4
Reese	1953	504		3.0
Hubbard	1953	275	1.1	3.4
Guiss	1954	1,521	0.1	1.0
Carroll and Shields	1955	173	0.6	4.6
Fitts and Patterson	1955	724	1.8	5.7
Kilgore et al.	1956	1,199		2.6
Moertel	1957	3,000	0.3	3.7
Kountz and Rogers	1961	355	2.0	2.5
Ruef and Ehlers	1962	1,200	0.3	1.5
Robbins and Berg	1964	1,458	0.3	6.5
Donnegan and Spratt	1967	704	1.0	2.0

may be involved by local extension from the disease in the first breast by permeation of lymphatics across the midline of the thorax, or by generalized metastases through the blood stream. Both of these phenomena are seen in advanced and terminal breast carcinoma.

When the disease is in an earlier stage and appears in the second breast, the distinction as to whether it is primary or secondary is more difficult. If the carcinomas in the two breasts are clearly of different microscopic types it may be presumed that they are of different origins. However, the majority of breast carcinomas are so much alike microscopically that it is often impossible to be certain that they are different. In practice the distinction has to be made on clinical grounds. Our rule is that a carcinoma in the second breast is classified as a new primary carcinoma when there is no evidence of local spread of the carcinoma in the first breast across the midline of the chest to the second breast and the carcinoma in the second breast is a solitary lesion. A second requisite is that there are no demonstrable distant metastases from the carcinoma in the first breast.

The threat of carcinoma in the second breast became real in a historical sense when the treatment of carcinoma in the first breast improved to the point where women survived long enough after the removal of the first breast to have time to develop a new primary carcinoma in the second breast. Kilgore, in 1921, was the first to study the magnitude of this threat. But he had only 5-year follow-up data, which we now know are clearly inadequate. As follow-up has improved, more significant data have become available. They are summarized in Table 22–40.

In addition to the difficulties in discovering the truth regarding carcinoma in the second breast due to inadequate follow-up, the statistical aspects of the problem are formidable. The more recent studies by Donegan and Spratt, and Robbins and Berg, are the only ones that bring modern statistical methods to bear on this problem.

The time relationship of carcinomas in the two breasts is also important in their classification. We do not classify a carcinoma detected in the second breast within six months after the treatment of a carcinoma in the first breast as successive to the first carcinoma. We classify it as synchronous with the first carcinoma. Considering the relatively slow rate of growth of most breast carcinomas it is most likely that the second cancer was present at the time the first one was noted, but escaped discovery.

A Personal Series of Cases of Carcinoma in the Second Breast

My personal series of 626 women with mammary carcinoma treated by radical mastectomy between the years 1935 and 1957 was particularly suitable for studying the complex question of carcinoma in the second breast because in all the patients the stage of advancement of the disease was carefully classified according to our Columbia Clinical Classification, the operation performed was always the same, and the follow-up, for a minimum of ten years, was virtually complete.

In my series of 626 women with breast carcinoma, 36 developed primary carcinoma in the second breast. In all but five the second primary was treated by radical mastectomy. In one of the patients not treated by mastectomy the carcinoma in the second breast was found only on postmortem examination. In a second patient the breast carcinoma was detected when she was admitted to the hospital for a cardiovascular accident; her breast carcinoma was not treated and she died of her cardiovascular disease after two years. Two patients were treated with radiotherapy alone because of distant metastases. The fifth patient was noted to have a carcinoma of the second breast at the age of 86. She had a simple mastectomy elsewhere.

The Concept of Breast Years of Follow-Up. In comparing the incidence of carcinoma of the second breast with the incidence of the disease in the general population, we must keep in mind that a women who has already had carcinoma in one breast has only one remaining breast in which the disease may develop. The women in the general population are exposed to the risk of developing it in two breasts. It seems therefore appropriate to introduce the concept of *breast-years* instead of *person-years*. A woman with one breast removed because of the first cancer contributes only one *breast-year* of follow-up.

Results of Treatment in Study Series. Of the total group of 626 women, four had bilaterally synchronous breast cancers and they have been excluded from the statistical evaluation.

The clinical classification, axillary lymph node status, and 10 year survival rates for the remaining 622 women in the series are given in Table 22–41. In 399, or 64 per cent, the disease was classified as clinical Stage A, and there was an overall 10 year survival rate of 70 per cent. In 153, or 25 per cent, the disease was classified as Stage B, and 41 per cent survived for 10 years or more. Three hundred and twenty-seven or 52 per cent of the women had no axillary lymph node metastases, and 74 per cent of these survived 10 or more years.

Table 22–41. RADICAL MASTECTOMY FOR BREAST CARCINOMA. PERSONAL SERIES OF CASES, 1935–1957. EXTENT OF AXILLARY METASTASIS AND 10 YEAR SURVIVAL*

Columbia Clinical Classification	No. Axillary Nodes with Metastases	No. of Cases	Per cent 10 Year Survivors
Stage A	No nodes involved	276	76%
	1–3 nodes involved	88	69%
	4–7 nodes involved	18	22%
	8 or more nodes involved	17	18%
		399	70%
Stage B	No nodes involved	37	70%
	1–3 nodes involved	50	43%
	4–7 nodes involved	33	36%
	8 or more nodes involved	33	9%
		153	41%
Stage C	No nodes involved	11	45%
	1–3 nodes involved	15	33%
	4–7 nodes involved	7	29%
	8 or more nodes involved	26	8%
		59	24%
Stage D	No nodes involved	–	–
	1–3 nodes involved	2	50%
	4–7 nodes involved	1	–
	8 or more nodes involved	8	13%
		11	18%
All Stages	No nodes involved	324	74%
	1–3 nodes involved	155	57%
	4–7 nodes involved	59	31%
	8 or more nodes involved	84	11%
		622	57%

*Four patients with bilateral simultaneous breast carcinoma were excluded, 3 in Stage A and 1 in Stage B.

Incidence of Primary Carcinoma in the Second Breast. Thirty-six primary carcinomas of the second breast developed in these 622 women. Table 22–42 shows the breast-years of follow-up in these 36 women classified by age group and the clinical stage of their disease. The average duration of the follow-up and clinical classification of the first breast cancer are correlated in Table 22–43. The incidence of cancers in the second breast is compared to the age-adjusted incidence of first breast cancers in women in the general population of New York State (New York City excluded) in Table 22–44. The expected number of breast cancers in the second breast is 9.8. The expected incidence rate per 100,000 breast-years is 79.25 (Table 22–45). The observed number of carcinomas of the second breast is 36 and the observed rate is thus seven times that

Table 22-42. BREAST-YEARS OF FOLLOW-UP IN 622 WOMEN WITH BREAST CARCINOMA TREATED BY RADICAL MASTECTOMY, BY AGE GROUP, CLINICAL STAGE, AND OCCURRENCE OF CARCINOMA OF SECOND BREAST

Age Group	Clinical Stage A			Clinical Stage B			Clinical Stage C			Clinical Stage D			Total		
	No. of Patients	Follow-up Breast Years	Second Carcinoma	No. of Patients	Follow-up Breast Years	Second Carcinoma	No. of Patients	Follow-up Breast Years	Second Carcinoma	No. of Patients	Follow-up Breast Years	Second Carcinoma	No. of Patients	Follow-up Breast Years	Second Carcinoma
25–29		0.00		3	1.50		1	0.50					4	2.00	
30–34	13	26.00		3	15.50		2	7.50					18	49.00	
35–39	38	106.50		12	40.00		6	20.00					56	166.50	
40–44	59	313.50		21	89.00	1	5	34.50	1	1	0.25		86	437.25	2
45–49	67	536.75	8	30	146.25		13	41.25					110	724.25	8
50–54	65	690.00	3	23	209.75	2	7	40.00		2	4.00		97	943.75	5
55–59	42	762.25	6	20	210.00	2	5	28.50		3	6.00		70	1006.75	8
60–64	40	674.00	3	10	192.50	1	8	35.50		2	5.00		60	907.00	4
65–69	37	498.25	3	15	149.00		8	37.00		1	4.50		61	688.75	3
70–74	24	389.75	1	11	141.25		3	39.00		1	7.00		39	577.00	1
75–79	9	276.50	1	3	90.00		1	26.50			9.00		14	402.00	1
80–84	5	158.50	3	1	35.00	1		13.50			4.50		6	211.50	4
85–89		59.50		1	8.50			2.00					1	69.50	
90–94		5.50			5.00									10.50	
95–99					4.50									4.50	
Totals		4496.50	28		1337.75	7		325.75	1		40.25	0		6200.25	36

Table 22–43. 622 PATIENTS TREATED BY RADICAL MASTECTOMY. IN BREAST CARCINOMA FOLLOWED FOR OCCURRENCE OF CANCER IN THE SECOND BREAST. STAGE OF CARCINOMA IN FIRST BREAST AND AVERAGE INTERVAL IN YEARS OF FOLLOW-UP

Columbia Clinical Classification	No. of Patients	Follow-up No. of Breast-years	Average Number of Years per Patient
Stage A	399	4496.50	13.3
Stage B	153	1337.75	8.7
Stage C	59	325.75	5.5
Stage D	11	40.25	3.6
Total	622	6200.25	10.0

Table 22–45. THE INCIDENCE OF BREAST CARCINOMA PER 100,000 BREAST YEARS

$$\text{Expected rate} = \frac{9.82778}{6200.25} \times 100,000 \times \frac{1}{2} = 79.25$$

Observed rate in carcinoma of the second breast =

$$\frac{36}{6200.25} \times 100,000 = 580.62$$

The observed rate of carcinoma in the second breast is thus $\frac{580.62}{79.25}$ or 7 times as large as in the general population of women in New York State. Standard Deviation = 14.03.

of the expected rate in women in the general populations of New York State. This difference in incidence rates is statistically highly significant; the standard deviation is 14.03.

No definite relationship was found between the patient's age at the time of her initial breast cancer and the chances of developing another primary cancer in the remaining breast (Table 22–46). Our data suggest that there is an incidence peak at the age of 45, but the overall incidence rates in the four age groups are not significantly different. If a cut-off point at 50 years is used, the incidence

rate for carcinoma of the second breast is 725 per 100,000 breast years for women under 50 years of age and 539 per 100,000 breast-years for those over 50. Respective incidence rates of 646 and 542 per 100,000 breast-years are found if age 55 is utilized as the cut-off point. These incidence rates are not significantly different. The incidence of carcinoma in the second breast when the carcinoma in the first breast occurred under the age of fifty is 17 times the normal incidence whereas the rate for women over fifty is 6 times the normal incidence (Table 22–47).

The incidence of carcinoma in the second breast is directly related to the clinical stage of the carcinoma in the first breast (Tables 22–48 and 22–49). The less advanced the clinical stage of the disease, the better the prognosis, and since the patient survives longer, the greater her chance of developing a carcinoma in her second breast. Women whose first breast carcinoma was classified as Stage D did not live long enough to develop a second primary breast cancer.

Table 22–44. EXPECTED NUMBER OF CARCINOMAS IN THE SECOND BREAST IF PATIENTS IN THIS STUDY WERE EXPOSED TO NEW YORK STATE RATES*

Age Group	New York State Rate per 200,000 Breasts per Year	Breast-years in Cohort	Expected No. Carcinomas
25–29	5.027	2.00	0.00010
30–34	16.716	49.00	0.00819
35–39	38.272	166.50	0.06372
40–44	71.290	437.25	0.31172
45–49	106.062	724.25	0.76815
50–54	117.358	943.75	1.10757
55–59	140.107	1006.75	1.41053
60–64	165.775	907.00	1.50358
65–69	200.541	688.75	1.38123
70–74	228.761	577.00	1.31995
75–79	265.922	402.00	1.06901
80–84	292.297	211.50	0.61821
85+	314.583	84.50	0.26582
Total		6200.25	9.82778

*Death Rates derived from *Life Tables for the Geographic Division of the U.S., 1949–51.* U.S. Dept. of Health, Education and Welfare. National Offices of Vital Statistics, vol. 41, no. 4, Table for white Females in the Middle Atlantic States, pp. 86–87.

Table 22–46. INCIDENCE OF CARCINOMA IN THE SECOND BREAST AND AGE OF PATIENT

Age	Breast-Years	Carcinoma in Second Breast	Incidence Rate per 100,000 Breast-Years
Less than 35	51.00	0	0
35–45	603–75	2	331
45–55	1668.00	13	779
55–65	1913.75	12	627
65+	1963.75	9	458
Total	6200.25	36	

These incidence rates are not significantly different.

Table 22–47. INCIDENCE OF CARCINOMA IN THE SECOND BREAST AND AGE OF PATIENT

Age	Breast-Years	No. Carcinomas Observed in Second Breast	Expected No. of Carcinomas per 100,000 Breast-Years	Ratio of Observed Expected
under 50	1379.00	11	$1.152 \times \frac{1}{2}$	$17\times$
over 50	4821.25	26	$8.676 \times \frac{1}{2}$	$6\times$

Carcinoma in the second breast occurred in 5.8 per cent of the 622 patients in our series of cases. The 399 patients whose disease in the first breast was classified as clinical Stage A had the highest frequency of carcinoma in the second breast, namely 7 per cent. Only 4.6 per cent of those whose disease was classified as clinical Stage B developed the disease in the second breast. For the patients with clinical Stage C carcinoma the frequency was still lower—only 1.7 per cent. Ninety-four, or 17 per cent, of the entire group of 622 women with breast carcinoma had a family history of breast cancer. Of the 36 patients who developed a carcinoma of the second breast, 12 or 33 per cent had a family history of breast carcinoma. These rates are significantly different.

The annual rate of new primary carcinomas in the second breast was an average of 2.1 carcinomas during the first ten years of follow-up. Thereafter the rate remained constant throughout 15 year follow-up (Table 22–50).

The average interval between the first and second primary breast carcinomas in our series of cases was 10 years—the range being from 2 to 20 years.

Characteristics of the 36 Women Who Developed Carcinoma of the Second Breast Compared With Those of the Entire Study Group. AGE. The average age of the entire group of 622 women was 51.9 years. The average age of the 36 patients who developed a carcinoma of the second breast was 58.7 years.

CLINICAL STAGE. Three hundred and sixty-seven, or 63 per cent, of 586 patients with carcinoma in one breast were classified in clinical Stage A. Thirty-two of 36, or 90 per cent, of the patients with carcinoma of the second breast were classified as clinical stage A. Thus there were significantly more clinical Stage A carcinomas in women with carcinoma of the second breast (Table 22–51).

AXILLARY NODE STATUS. Two hundred and ninety-eight, or 50 per cent, of 586 patients with one breast cancer had no axillary lymph node metastases. Twenty-one, or 68 per cent, of 31 patients with carcinoma of the second breast had no axillary lymph node metastases. Women with carcinoma of the second breast therefore had fewer axillary lymph node metastases than those with only one breast cancer (Table 22–52).

MICROSCOPIC CHARACTER. In the entire group of 626 patients with one breast cancer and followed for the occurrence of carcinoma of the second breast there was not a single patient with lobular carcinoma in situ. It has been our custom not to remove the breast for this lesion, which we prefer to call lobular neoplasia.

Characteristics of the First and Second Breast Carcinomas in the Same Patient. AGE. The mean age at the time of treatment of the carcinoma in the first breast was 47.1 years. The mean age at time of the second carcinoma was 58.7.

CLINICAL STAGE. Twenty-eight of the 36

Table 22–48. INCIDENCE OF CARCINOMA IN THE SECOND BREAST PER 100,000 BREAST-YEARS AND CLINICAL STAGE OF CARCINOMA IN THE FIRST BREAST

Columbia Clinical Classification	
Stage A	623 per 100,000 breast-years
Stage B	523 per 100,000 breast-years
Stage C	307 per 100,000 breast-years
Stage D	0 per 100,000 breast-years
Total group	580.6 per 100,000 breast-years

Table 22–49. RELATIONSHIP OF CLINICAL STAGE OF CARCINOMA IN THE FIRST BREAST TO FREQUENCY OF CARCINOMA IN THE SECOND BREAST

Stage	No. of Patients	No. Patients with Carcinoma in Second Breast
A	399	28 (7%)
B	152	7 (4.6%)
C	59	1 (1.7%)
D	11	0
Total	622	36 (5.8%)

Table 22–50. ANNUAL RATE OF CARCINOMAS IN THE SECOND BREAST BY YEARS OF FOLLOW-UP

Years After Carcinoma in First Breast	No. of Carcinomas in Second Breast
0–1	0
1–2	3
2–3	3
3–4	1
4–5	0
5–6	2
6–7	4
7–8	3
8–9	2
9–10	3
10–11	2
11–12	2
12–13	2
13–14	3
14–15	1

Table 22–52. AXILLARY NODE METASTASES IN PATIENTS WITH CARCINOMA OF FIRST BREAST AND PATIENTS WITH CARCINOMA OF SECOND BREAST

Axillary Findings	No. Patients with Carcinoma in First Breast	No. Patients with Carcinoma in Second Breast	Total No. Patients
No metastases	298	21	319
1 to 3 nodes involved	148	7	155
4 or more nodes involved	140	3	143
Total	586	31	622

carcinomas of the first breast were classified as clinical Stage A, whereas 32 of the 36 carcinomas of the second breast were classified as clinical Stage A.

AXILLARY LYMPH NODE STATUS. Twenty-six of the 36 patients had no axillary metastases from their first breast carcinoma, whereas 21 of 31 who had a radical mastectomy for their second breast carcinoma had no axillary involvement. The disparity in numbers is due to the fact that five patients who developed a carcinoma of their second breast did not have a second radical mastectomy.

SURVIVAL. In Table 22–53 cumulative probabilities of survival after radical mastectomy for a first breast carcinoma were computed for the entire group of 622 women and compared to age-adjusted survival rates of women in the general population of New York State.

Table 22–51. CLINICAL STAGE IN PATIENTS WITH CARCINOMA OF FIRST BREAST AND IN PATIENTS WITH CARCINOMA OF SECOND BREAST

Clinical Stage	No. Patients with Carcinoma in First Breast	No. Patients with Carcinoma in Second Breast	Total No. Patients
A	367	32	399
B	150	3	153
C	58	1	59
D	11	0	11
Totals	586	36	622

The same computation was done for the 36 women with carcinoma of the second breast, using the patients with only one carcinoma for controls (Table 22–54). The total number of breast-years for follow-up in this group is 246.

Curves for cumulative probabilities for survival of 622 women with one breast carcinoma and for the 36 women with carcinoma of the second breast are shown in Charts 22–1 and 22–2. Chart 22–1 shows the survival curves in 622 women who underwent radical mastectomy for carcinoma in one breast as well as for their age-adjusted controls from the general female population of New York State. The annual death rates for women with carcinoma of one breast are greater than that of the control population for the first eight years. After that there is no appreciable difference in the annual death rate and the two cumulative trends become essentially parallel. They remain so for an additional 12 years of follow-up. The annual death rate in these two groups is similar after eight years, and certainly after 10 years, following radical mastectomy, whatever the cause of death.

Chart 22–2 shows the cumulative survival curves of 36 women with carcinoma of the second breast. As controls we used women with carcinoma in one breast in our total group of 622, matched as closely as possible by age, extent of disease, and other characteristics.

The two survival curves are roughly comparable. The annual rate of dying from bilateral breast cancer is not appreciably different from the annual death rate due to one breast cancer. The small sample accounts for the unevenness of the curve. Of the 36 patients with carcinoma of the second breast, 16 were dead at the close of the study. The follow-up

Table 22–53. Cumulative probabilities of survival in 622 women treated by radical mastectomy for carcinoma of one breast compared to age-adjusted survival rates for women in the general population of New York State

Years after Operation	Women in General Population		Patients with One Breast Carcinoma	
	Death rate	Cum. Prob. of Survival	Death rate	Cum. Prob. of Survival
0–1	0.0153	0.985	0.0147	0.985
1–2	0.0173	0.968	0.0662	0.932
2–3	0.0190	0.950	0.0838	0.857
3–4	0.0214	0.930	0.0923	0.782
4–5	0.0226	0.909	0.0427	0.749
5–6	0.0234	0.888	0.0549	0.709
6–7	0.0250	0.867	0.0674	0.663
7–8	0.0268	0.844	0.0641	0.622
8–9	0.0291	0.820	0.0349	0.601
9–10	0.0293	0.796	0.0625	0.564
10–11	0.0315	0.771	0.0427	0.546
11–12	0.0311	0.747	0.0369	0.526
12–13	0.0326	0.723	0.0446	0.508
13–14	0.0358	0.698	0.0217	0.497
14–15	0.0375	0.672	0.0368	0.479
15–16	0.0411	0.645	0.0214	0.469
16–17	0.0430	0.618	0.0504	0.446
17–18	0.0437	0.591	0.0745	0.414
18–19	0.0428	0.566	0.0380	0.398
19–20	0.0431	0.542	0.1045	0.358

of patients with carcinoma of the second breast by necessity is variable. Of the 16 deaths, 8 were due to proven intercurrent disease at an average age of 74. Death due to breast cancer was responsible for the 8 other deaths at an average age of 56.6 years.

Discussion. Our overall crude rate of carcinoma of the second breast in patients who already had one breast carcinoma treated by radical mastectomy was 5.8 per cent. Among patients with clinical stage A carcinoma in one breast, 7 per cent developed carcinoma of the second breast, whereas none of our patients with clinical Stage D carcinoma in one breast developed the disease in the second breast. These data illustrate perfectly the effect of the composition of the case series upon the frequency with which carcinoma of the second breast is found. The more favorable the clinical stage of the first breast carcinoma the better the patient's chances for survival. Her longer follow-up period increases her chance of developing a carcinoma in her second breast. It is then not

Table 22–54. Cumulative probabilities of survival from carcinoma of the second breast in 36 women compared with survival from an initial breast carcinoma

Years after Operation	Patients with First Carcinoma		Patients with Carcinoma in Second Breast	
	Death rate	Cum. Prob. of Survival	Death rate	Cum. Prob. of Survival
0–1	0.0478	0.953	0.0284	0.972
1–2	0.0434	0.913	0.0303	0.943
2–3	0.0531	0.865	0.0689	0.880
3–4	0.0502	0.816	0.0000	0.880
4–5	0.0766	0.755	0.2351	0.783
5–6	0.0504	0.713	0.1176	0.696
6–7	0.0593	0.672	0.1428	0.604
7–8	0.0482	0.640	0.0833	0.556
8–9	0.0504	0.609	0.2000	0.455
9–10	0.0457	0.582	0.0000	0.455

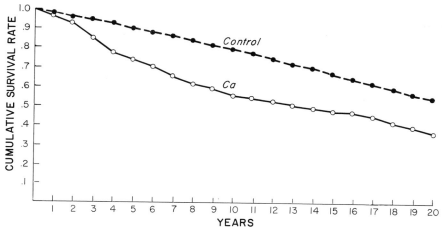

Chart 22–1. Cumulative probabilities of survival in 622 women treated by radical mastectomy for carcinoma of one breast, compared to age adjusted survival rates for women in the general population of New York State.

surprising to find a great deal of variation in the reported rates for carcinoma in the second breast. They range from 1.1 to 6.5 per cent (Table 22-40).

Incidence rates similarly fluctuate with variation as to the clinical stage of the disease. In our own study group the incidence of carcinoma of the second breast was 580.6 per 100,000 breast years. Patients with clinical Stage A carcinoma in the first breast had an incidence rate of 623 carcinomas of the second breast per 100,000 breast years whereas patients with clinical Stage D carcinomas of the first breast developed no carcinomas of the second breast. The incidence rate of carcinoma of the second breast reported by Robbins and Berg was 7.1 per 1000 patient years and that of Hubbard 5.8 per 1000 patient

years. The incidence rates of carcinoma of the second breast in our 622 patients is therefore almost exactly the same as that of Hubbard. It is lower than that reported by Robbins and Berg, despite the fact that in their patients the disease was more advanced as indicated by an incidence of axillary metastases of 60 per cent, compared with 48 per cent in our case series.

The adjustment for age is important in determining incidence rates. This adjustment for age is accomplished by comparing risks of developing carcinoma of the second breast in women who already have had one breast carcinoma, with the risk among the general population of developing the disease. In our 622 women the risk of developing a carcinoma of the second breast is seven times that in the

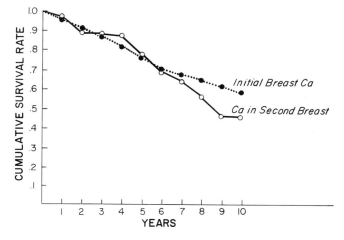

Chart 22–2. Cumulative probabilities of survival from carcinoma of the second breast in 36 women compared with survival from an initial breast carcinoma.

general population. Our figure of seven times normal risk compares roughly with that reported by Kilgore in 1921, as 4 times the normal risk. Since our computations are based upon "breast-years" rather than "person years" our figure should be twice as large. Robbins and Berg found that their patients had five times the risk of developing a carcinoma of the second breast compared to women in upper New York state.

The most important consideration regarding carcinoma in the second breast is whether or not it constitutes a separate and additional risk to the patient's life. Robbins and Berg, as well as Leis, have recently claimed that it does; Donegan and Spratt do not agree. In our own series we found no significant difference between the cumulative survival rates of patients with carcinoma of the second breast and those with only one breast carcinoma. Although our number of carcinomas of the second breast is small (36 with a total of 240 breast-years of follow-up) it is a group of patients who have been studied with great care. The original 626 patients make up a truly homogenous group. Their disease was carefully classified clinically, they all received the same surgical treatment, and the pathologic study of the surgical specimen was uniform and complete, including clearing of the axillary lymph nodes. All patients were followed by the same person and the follow-up was 99.3 per cent complete. There is no such series to be found in the literature.

The considerable incidence of carcinoma of the second breast led some surgeons to remove the second breast prophylactically. Bloodgood suggested it as long ago as 1921. More recently Pack, Leis, and Hubbard have advised simultaneous or subsequent removal of the second breast.

I disagree. Surgeons who know their patients well, and are humanists as well as scientists, know that her second breast is an important asset for a women who has lost one breast. The data from my personal case series, which I have presented here in detail do not indicate that a second breast carcinoma significantly lessens the patient's chances of survival. Our aim, I believe, should be to follow our patients who have had unilateral breast carcinoma with care, examining them, if possible, every three months. In this way we can expect to find carcinoma of the second breast at an early stage in those in whom it develops. If we perform a thorough radical mastectomy we can expect to cure them.

THE NATURAL DURATION OF CARCINOMA OF THE BREAST

An accurate concept of the natural duration of untreated carcinoma of the breast is essential to our understanding of variations in the course of the disease, as well as to our correct assessment of the value of different forms of treatment.

The distinguished English statistician, Major Greenwood, was the first to study the question adequately. In 1926 he analyzed data from hospitals in London, Glasgow, and Manchester regarding the length of life from the first symptom to death in 651 patients with breast carcinoma who received no treatment. The mean duration of life in these patients was 38.3 months.

Daland studied the course of breast carcinoma in 100 patients from two Boston hospitals to whom no surgical or radiation treatment had been given. The mean duration of life from the first symptom to death was 39.5 months.

Nathanson and Welch also reported the duration of life from onset to death in another series of 50 patients with breast cancer who had no treatment. Their findings agreed very closely with Daland's.

Forber studied a series of 64 patients with untreated breast cancer and found the mean duration of life from onset of symptoms was 39.3 months.

Wade tabulated the length of survival from onset of symptoms in a series of 26 patients who had no treatment. The mean survival time was 32.6 months.

Bloom has recently studied a remarkable series of 250 patients with untreated breast cancer in the records of the Middlesex Hospital Cancer Charity. These were patients with far advanced disease for the most part who came to the hospital to die, but detailed clinical records of their disease were kept. The series included patients admitted between 1805 and 1933.

Since irradiation, and more recently hormonal treatment, have come into general use it is very unusual to find patients who have had no treatment. It is therefore important that we draw that conclusions we can from these several case series.

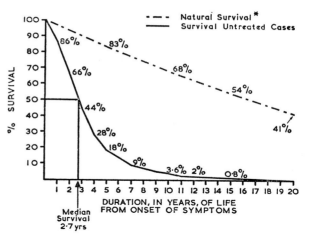

Chart 22–3. Survival of untreated breast cancer. Middlesex Hospital, 1805 to 1933 (250 cases).

The first conclusion is that spontaneous cure of breast carcinoma has not been observed. Spontaneous cure is a favorite armchair theory of those who lack practical experience with breast carcinoma. Those of us who work with the disease do not see spontaneous cures.

Bloom calculated the mean duration of life from onset of symptoms in the total of 1091 patients included in the studies I have referred to above and found it to be 38.7 months.

Bloom expressed the duration of life in his own series of untreated patients from the Middlesex Hospital in graphic form, comparing it with the natural survival term of the normal female population similarly distributed by age. I reproduce his chart (Chart 22–3).

There is great variation in the survival time of these patients who received no treatment. In a few the disease ran its course in as short a time as three months. In occasional patients the natural course of the disease was very

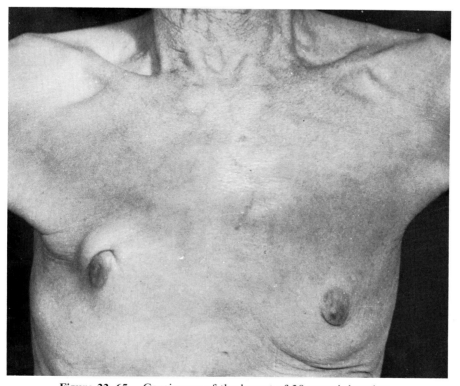

Figure 22–65. Carcinoma of the breast of 30 years' duration.

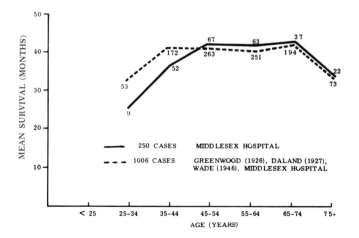

Chart 22–4. Untreated breast cancer. Mean duration of life from onset of symptoms related to age at onset.

long indeed. In Greenwood's data there were two women whose disease lasted 30 years. Daland referred to one patient who was still alive at the age of 80 after having had breast carcinoma for 35.5 years. Nathanson and Welch had one patient whose carcinoma lasted 15 years. One of Wade's patients lived for 22 years after her first symptom was noted and died at the age of 72. In Bloom's series the longest survival was 19 years.

A patient of my own illustrates the exceedingly slow course that carcinoma of the breast may take.

M. S., a widowed laundry worker in the Presbyterian Hospital, aged 64, complained on June 26, 1945, that she had a lump in her right breast. She stated that she had had it for about 17 years. Examination showed a 2 cm. hard tumor of the upper middle portion of her right breast. The tumor was relatively movable beneath the skin and over the chest wall. There were no retraction signs. There was a 5 mm. firm, movable node in the right axilla.

Biopsy showed the tumor to be a relatively undifferentiated carcinoma. The patient had advanced hypertensive cardiovascular disease, and since her breast disease was not giving her any symptoms it was decided not to treat it.

The patient's carcinoma progressed exceedingly slowly. By 1955, 10 years after her tumor had been biopsied, and 27 years after it had been discovered by the patient, it measured only 3 cm. in diameter. It had increased only 1 cm. in diameter in 10 years. Retraction signs, including distortion of the areola and nipple had, however, developed (Fig. 22-65). The axillary node measured about 8 mm. in diameter. She died in January, 1958, 30 years after she had first discovered her breast carcinoma.

In seeking for an explanation of the great variation in the course of breast carcinoma

two factors come to mind. The first of these is the effect of the degree of differentiation, that is, the biological character, of the tumor. We know very well how slowly well-differentiated carcinomas such as papillary carcinomas progress. On the other hand, highly malignant carcinomas, such as the inflammatory carcinomas, may run their entire course in a few months.

Bloom had graded a total of 86 of the tumors in the more recent patients in his series of untreated patients. His findings clearly show that the histologic character of the tumor bore a close relationship to the course of the disease. The total duration of life was more than twice as long for grade I tumors as it was for grade III tumors.

It is interesting to inquire as to the relationship of the age of the patient to her length of survival in these data. Bloom studied the question in his own series of cases, and in the cases reported by other authors. In all there was a somewhat lower mean survival time for patients under the age of 35 (Chart 22-4).

Bloom makes a final important point regarding the advantages of treatment for breast carcinoma, namely that these patients who had no treatment survived in discomfort and suffering. Seventy-three per cent had marked ulceration. Modern treatment may not cure, but it often relieves distressing symptoms, in addition to prolonging life.

REFERENCES

Abrams, H. L., Spiro, R., and Goldstein, N.: Metastases in carcinoma. Cancer, 3:74, 1950.
Adair, F. E., and Herrmann, J. B.: Unusual metastatic manifestations of breast carcinoma; metastasis to

the mandible with a report of five cases. Surg., Gynec. & Obst., *83*:289, 1946.

Aldrete, J. S., and Bohrod, M. G.: Adrenal metastases in cancer of the breast. Amer. Surg., *33*:174, 1967.

Alexander, R. F., and Spriggs, A. I.: The differential diagnosis of tumour cells in circulating blood. J. Clin. Path., *13*:414, 1960.

Andreassen, M., and Dahl-Iversen, E.: Recherches sur les métastases microscopiques des ganglions lymphatiques sus-claviculaires dans le cancer du sein. J. internat. chir., *9*:27, 1949.

Andreassen, M., Dahl-Iversen, E., and Sørensen, B.: Extended exeresis of the regional lymph nodes at operation for carcinoma of the breast and the results of a five-year follow-up of the first 98 cases with removal of the axillary as well as the supraclavicular glands. Acta chir. Scandinav., *107*:206, 1954a.

Andreassen, M., Dahl-Iversen, E., and Sørensen, B.: Glandular metastases in carcinoma of the breast; results of a more radical operation. Lancet, *1*:176, 1954b.

Anglesio, E., Calciati, A., and Pianarosa, M.: Changes of calcium, phosphorus, citrate, and alkaline phosphatases in metastatic breast cancer. Helvet. med. acta, *30*:116, 1963.

Asch, M. J., Wiedel, P. D., and Habif, D. V.: Gastrointestinal metastases from carcinoma of the breast. Arch. Surg., *96*:840, 1968.

Atkins, J. P.: Metastatic carcinoma to the esophagus. Ann. Otol. Rhin. & Laryng., *75*:356, 1966.

Bachman, A. L., and Sproul, E. E.: Correlation of radiographic and autopsy findings in suspected metastases in the spine. Bull. New York Acad. Med., *31*:146, 1955.

Baker, W. H., and Roth, S.: Hypercalcemia and mental confusion. New Eng. J. Med., *269*:801, 1963.

Bedell, A. J.: Bilateral metastatic carcinoma of the choroid Arch. Ophth., *30*:25, 1943.

Bedford, P. D., and Daniel, P. M.: Discrete carcinomatous metastases in the extrinsic ocular muscles. Amer. J. Ophthal., *49*:723, 1960.

Benelli, A.: Carcinoma mammario e metastasi uterina. Minerva ginec. (Torino), *14*:827, 1962.

Berg, J. W.: The significance of axillary node levels in the study of breast carcinoma. Cancer, *8*:776, 1955.

Birdsall, C. J., Dockerty, M. B., and Pratt, J. H.: Mammary carcinoma metastasis to uterine myoma. Obst. & Gynec., *23*:229, 1964.

Blake, H., and Blake, F. S.: Breast carcinoma metastatic to maxilla. Oral Surg., *13*:1099, 1960.

Blau, M., Spencer, H., Swernov, J., and Laszlo, D.: Utilization and intestinal excretion of calcium in man. Science, *120*:1029, 1954.

Bloom, H. J. G.: The natural history of untreated breast cancer. Ann. New York Acad. Sci., *114*:747, 1964.

Bloom, H. J. G., Richardson, W. W., and Harries, E. J.: Natural history of untreated breast cancer (1805–1933). Brit. Med. J., *2*:213, 1962.

Bodansky, O.: Serum phosphohexose isomerase in cancer. Cancer, *7*:1200, 1954.

Böhmig, R. and Prévôt, R.: Vergleichende Untersuchengen zur Pathologie und Röntgenologie der Wirbelsäule. Fortschr. Röntgenstr., *43*:541, 1931.

Bucalossi, P.: L'asportazione del linfonodi mammari interni nel trattamento del cancro mammario. Tumori, *47*:339, 1961.

Burket, L. W.: Jaw metastases in primary mammary carcinoma. Amer. J. Orthodontics, *27*:652, 1941.

Busk, T., and Clemmesen, J.: The frequencies of left- and right-sided breast cancer. Brit. J. Cancer, *1*:345, 1947.

Caceres, E.: Incidence of metastasis in the internal mammary chain in operable cancer of the breast. Surg., Gynec. & Obst., *108*:715, 1959.

Caceres, E.: Incidence of metastasis in the internal mammary chain in operable carcinoma of the breast and 5 year results. Internat. Union against Cancer, *19*:1566, 1963.

Caceres, E.: Personal communication, 1968.

Cain, H.: Hypophysenmetastasierung bei Mammacarcinomen mit Besonderheiten im Hypothalamus. Frankfurt. Ztschr. Path., *64*:142, 1953.

Camiel, M. R., and Bolker, H.: Carcinoma erysipelatodes, subepidermal lymphatic metastases confused with operative sequelae. Surg., Gynec. & Obst., *72*:635, 1941.

Campiche, P., and Lazarus-Barlow, W. S.: Malignant diseases of the breast: statistical study of the records of the Middlesex Hospital. Arch. Middlesex Hosp., *5*:83, 1905.

Candar, Z., Ritchie, A. C., Hopkirk, J. F., and Long, R. C.: The prognostic value of circulating tumor cells in patients with breast cancer. Surg., Gynec. & Obst., *115*:291, 1962.

Carnett, J. B., and Howell, J. S.: Bone metastases in cancer of the breast. Ann. Surg., *91*:811, 1930.

Carroll, W. W., and Shields, T. W.: Bilateral simultaneous breast cancer. A.M.A. Arch. Surg., *70*:672, 1955.

Caylor, H. D., and Hunt, V. C.: Bilateral adenocarcinoma of the breast. Ann. Surg., *89*:549, 1929.

Chasin, A.: Die Dimensionen der destruktiven Veränderungen in den Wirbelkörpern, die röntgenographisch bestimmt werden können. Fortschr. a. d. Geb. d. Röntgenstrahl., *37*:529, 1928.

Chris, S. M.: Inflammatory carcinoma of the breast. Brit. J. Surg., *38*:163, 1950.

Choi, S. H., Sheehan, F. R., and Pickren, J. W.: Metastatic involvement of the stomach by breast cancer. Cancer, *17*:791, 1964.

Ciambellotti, E.: Right and left localization of malignant neoplasms of the breast. Cancro, *14*:375, 1961.

Claus, H. G., and Matzker, J.: Oesophaguskompressionsstenosen als Spätfolge des Mammakarzinoms. Ztschr. Laryng., Rhin., Otol., *41*:559, 1962.

Cliffton, E. E., and Young, L. E.: Carcinoma of the breast. 5 to 20 year follow-up following radical mastectomy. Amer. J. Surg., *82*:185, 1951.

Collins, V. P., Loeffler, M. K., and Tivey, H.: Observations on growth rates of human tumors Amer. J. Roentgen., *76*:988, 1956.

Conklin, E. F.: Some unusual complications of metastatic carcinoma of the breast. Ann. Surg., *159*:489, 1964.

Copeland, M. M.: Bone metastases; study of 334 cases. Radiology, *16*:198, 1931.

Cordes, F. C.: Bilateral metastatic carcinoma of the choroid. Tr. Am. Ophth. Soc., *42*:181, 1944.

Covington, E. E., and Brendle, W. K.: Breast carcinoma with vulvar metastasis. Obst., Gynec., *23*:910, 1964.

Cross, R. G., O'Connor, M. H., and Holland, P. D. J.: Placental metastasis of a breast carcinoma. J. Obst. & Gynec. Brit. Emp., *58*:810, 1951.

Cullen, J. R., and Burns, J. E.: Bilateral breast cancer. Connecticut Med. J., *13*:1041, 1949.

Cussen, L. J.: Metastasis of malignant tumours to the adrenal gland. Med. J. Australia, *47*:39, 1960.

Dahl-Iversen, E.: Examen ultérieur de 109 malades ayant subi l'opération radicale du cancer du sein, concernant essentiellement le rapport entre la découverte microscopique et la fréquence de la récidive. Lyon chir., *24*:648, 1927.

Dahl-Iversen, E.: Recherches sur les métastases microscopiques des ganglions lymphatiques parasternaux dans le cancer du sein. J. Internat. chir., *11*:492, 1951.

Dahl-Iversen, E.: Recherches sur les métastases microscopiques des cancers du sein dans les ganglions lymphatiques para-sternaux et sus-claviculaires. Mém. Acad. de chir., *78*:651, 1952.

Dahl-Iversen, E.: An extended radical operation for carcinoma of the breast. J. Roy. Coll. Surg. (Edinburgh), *8*:81, 1963.

Daland, E. M.: Untreated cancer of the breast. Surg., Gynec. & Obst., *44*:264, 1927.

Davis, H. H., and Neis, D. D.: Distribution of axillary lymph node metastases in carcinoma of the breast. Ann. Surg., *136*:604, 1952.

Dawson, E. K., and Shaw. J. J. M.: Mammary cancer with generalized telangiectatic carcinoma ('carcinoma erysipelatodes'). Brit. J. Surg., *25*:100, 1937.

Delbet, P., and Herrenschmidt, A.: Note sur un cas de cancer hémophile. Bull. Assoc. franç, p. l'étude du cancer, *12*:664, 1923.

Desaive, P.: Le cancer mammaire bilatéral. J. de radiol. et d'électrol., *30*:335, 1949.

Dickson, R. J.: Choroidal metastases from carcinoma of the breast. Amer. J. Ophthal., *46*:14, 1958.

Donegan, W. L., and Spratt, J. S., Jr.: Cancer of the second breast. *In* Spratt, J. S., Jr., and Donegan, W. L.: Cancer of the Breast, Philadelphia, W. B. Saunders co., 1967, p. 179.

Dunlap, H. F.: Metastatic malignant tumors of the brain. Ann. Int. Med., *5*:1274, 1932.

Eggers, C., de Cholnoky, T., and Jessup, D. S. D.: Cancer of the breast. Ann. Surg., *113*:321, 1941.

Ehlers, P. N., and Ruef, J.: Uber pathologische Frakturen bei Mammacarcinom. Arch. f. klin. Chir., *300*:415, 1962.

Engell, H. C.: Cancer cells in the circulating blood. Acta chir. Scandinav., Supp. 201, 1955.

Falkinburg, L. W., and Savran, J.: Adenocarcinoma of the umbilicus secondary to carcinoma of the breast. Amer. J. Surg., *87*:795, 1954.

Fink, I., and Garb, J.: Carcinoma of the tip of the tongue; a case of metastasis from a malignant tumor of the breast. Amer. J. Surg., *62*:138, 1943.

Fitts, W. T., Jr., and Patterson, L. T.: Spread of mammary cancer. Surg. Clin. N. Amer., *35*:1539, 1955.

Fitzwilliams, D. C. L.: Carcinoma of the breast and its method of spread: embolism or permeation. Brit. J. Surg., *12*:650, 1925.

Fitzwilliams, D. C. L., and Fell, J. N.: Metastasis in gasserian ganglion following carcinoma of the breast. Brit. Med. J., *1*:387, 1939.

Fleming, J. A.: Tumour cells in the blood in carcinoma of the breast. Proc. Roy. Soc. Med., *56*:497, 1963.

Fletcher, W. S., and Steward, J. W.: Tumour cells in the blood with special reference to pre- and post-hepatic blood. Brit. J. Cancer, *13*:33, 1959.

Forber, J. E.: Incurable cancer; an investigation of hospital patients in eastern London. Gr. Britain Min. Health. Rep. Pub. Health & Min. Subj., No. 66, London, H. M. Stat. Off., 1931.

Fraser, J.: A study of the malignant breast by whole section and key block section methods. Surg., Gynec. & Obst., *45*:266, 1927.

Galloway, J. A., and Perloff, W. H.: Addison's disease secondary to adrenocortical destruction by metastatic carcinoma of the breast. Amer. J. Med., *28*:156, 1960.

Gandrille and Lauras: Cancer double à métastase inhabit-

uelle. Bull. et mém. Soc. d. chirurgiens de Paris, *41*:263, 1951.

Garfinkel, L., Craig, L., and Seidman, H.: An appraisal of left and right breast cancer. J. Nat. Cancer Inst., *23*:617, 1959.

Giacomelli, V., and Veronesi, U.: I linfatici mammari interni come sede e via di diffusione metastatica nel cancro della mammella. Tumori, *38*:375, 1952.

Gilliam, A. G.: A note on estimates of the rate of development of metastasis in patients with cancer of the breast. Surg., Gynec. & Obst., *94*:641, 1952.

Gjankovic, H.: Ueber den doppelseitigen Krebs der weiblichen Brustdrüse. Arch. f. klin. Chir., *194*:298, 1938.

Glomset, D. A.: The incidence of metastasis of malignant tumors to the adrenals. Amer. J. Cancer, *32*:57, 1938.

Göksel, H. A.: Postradical-mastectomy parasternal mass. Turkish J. Pediatrics, *6*:175, 1964.

Göksel, H. A.: Axillary lymph nodes in carcinoma of the breast. Turkish J. Pediatrics, *6*:250, 1964.

Graham, W. P., and Goldman, L.: Gastrointestinal metastases from carcinoma of the breast. Ann. Surg., *159*:477, 1964.

Graham, W. P., et al.: Hypercalcemia in carcinoma of the female breast. Surg., Gynec. & Obst., *117*:709, 1963.

Grant, F. C.: Intracranial malignant metastases. Ann. Surg., *84*:635, 1926.

Greenough, R. B.: Discussion: The incidence of cancer in the second breast. J.A.M.A., *77*:457, 1921.

Greenwood, M.: Report on the Natural Duration of Cancer. Reports on Public Health and Medical Subjects, no. 33, London, Ministry of Health, 1926.

Griboff, S. I.: Hypercalcemia secondary to bone metastases from carcinoma of the breast. I. Relationship between serum calcium and alkaline phosphatase values. J. Clin. Endocrinol., *14*:378, 1954.

Gross, S. W.: A clinical study of carcinoma of the breast and its treatment. Amer. J. Med. Sci., *95*:219, 1888.

Guiss, L. W.: The problem of bilateral independent mammary carcinoma. Amer. J. Surg., *88*:171, 1954.

Gurling, K. J., Scott, G. B. O., and Baron, D. N.: Metastases in pituitary tissue removed at hypophysectomy in women with mammary carcinoma. Brit. J. Cancer, *11*:519, 1957.

Haagensen, C. D., and Obeid, S. J.: Biopsy of the apex of the axilla in carcinoma of the breast. Ann. Surg., *149*:149, 1959.

Haagensen, C. D., et al.: Metastasis of carcinoma of the breast to the periphery of the regional lymph node filter. Ann. Surg., *169*:174, 1969.

Hall, T. C., Griffiths, C. T., and Petranek, J. R.: Hypocalcemia—an unusual metabolic complication of breast cancer. New Eng. J. Med., *275*:1474, 1966.

Halsted, W. S.: A clinical and histological study of certain adenocarcinomata of the breast. Ann. Surg., *28*:557, 1898.

Halsted, W. S.: The results of radical operations for the cure of cancer of the breast. Ann. Surg., *46*:1, 1907.

Handley, R. S.: The internal mammary lymph chain in carcinoma of the breast. Lancet, *2*:276, 1949.

Handley, R. S.: History and the parasternal lymphglands. Lancet, *1*:707, 1960.

Handley, R. S.: The early spread of breast carcinoma and its bearing on operative treatment. Brit. J. Surg., *51*:206, 1964.

Handley, R. S.: Indications and contraindications for mastectomy. J.A.M.A., *200*:610, 1967.

Handley, R. S.: Personal communication, 1968.

Handley, R. S., and Thackray, A. C.: Invasion of the internal mammary lymph glands in carcinoma of the breast. Brit. J. Cancer, *1*:15, 1947.

Handley, R. S., and Thackray, A. C.: The internal mammary lymph chain in carcinoma of the breast. Lancet, 2:276, 1949.

Handley, R. S., and Thackray, A. C.: Invasion of internal mammary lymph nodes in carcinoma of the breast. Brit. Med. J., *1*:61, 1954.

Handley, W. S.: Cancer of the Breast. London, John Murray, 1906.

Handley, W. S.: Parasternal invasion of thorax in breast cancer and its suppression by use of radium tubes as operative precaution. Surg., Gynec. & Obst., *45*:721, 1927.

Hanfling, S. M.: Metastatic cancer to the heart. Review of the literature and report of 127 cases. Circulation, *22*:474, 1960.

Harnett, W. L.: A statistical report on 2529 cases of cancer of the breast. Brit. J. Cancer, 2:212, 1948.

Harrington, S. W.: Survival rates of radical mastectomy for unilateral and bilateral carcinoma of the breast. Surgery, *19*:154, 1946.

Harris, H. S., and Spratt, J. S., Jr.: Bilateral adrenalectomy in metastatic mammary cancer. Cancer, *23*:145, 1969.

Hartmann, W. H., and Sherlock, P.: Gastroduodenal metastases from carcinoma of the breast. Cancer, *14*:426, 1961.

Hauser, T. E., and Steer, A.: Lymphangitic carcinomatosis of the lungs. Ann. Int. Med., *34*:881, 1951.

Held, E.: Métastases vaginales de cancers du sein et de l'estomac. Rev. franç. de gynéc. et d'obst., *34*:482, 1939.

Henriques, C. Q.: The veins of the vertebral column and their role in the spread of cancer. Ann. Roy. Coll. Surg. (Eng.), *31*:1, 1962.

Herrmann, J. B., and Adair, F. E.: Unusual metastatic manifestations of breast carcinoma. III. Metastatic involvement of preauricular lymph nodes and parotid gland. A report of five cases. Ann. Surg., *129*:137, 1949.

Herrmann, J. B., Kirsten, E., and Krakauer, J. S.: Hypercalcemic syndrome associated with androgenic and estrogenic therapy. J. Clin. Endocrinol., 9:1, 1949.

Hubbard, T. B.: Nonsimultaneous bilateral carcinoma of the breast. Surgery, *34*:706, 1953.

Huggins, C., and Dao, T. L.-Y.: Adrenalectomy and oophorectomy in treatment of advanced carcinoma of the breast. J.A.M.A., *151*:1388, 1953.

Hummel, R.: Zur Frage des Festigung von Spontanfrakturen bei Karzinometastasen im Knocken. Fortschr. Röntgenstr., *50*:529, 1934.

Hutchinson, W. B., and Kiriluk, L. B.: Internal mammary node investigation in carcinoma of the breast. Amer. J. Surg., *92*:151, 1956.

Hutchinson, W. B., Kiriluk, L. B., and Ansingh, H. R.: Surgical evaluation of carcinoma of the breast with axillary metastases. Amer. J. Surg., *107*:850, 1964.

Hyman, G. A.: Anemia in malignant neoplastic disease. J. Chronic Dis., *16*:645, 1963.

Hyman, G. A.: The anemia of cancer. Amer. J. Roentgenol., *79*:511, 1958.

Ingleby, H., Moore, L., and Gershon-Cohen, J.: Roentgenographic study of tumor growth rate of 6 early cancers of the breast. Cancer, *11*:726, 1958.

Ingram, J. T.: Carcinoma erysipelatodes and carcinoma telangiectaticum. A.M.A. Arch. Derm., *77*:227, 1958.

Jacox, R. F., and Tristan, T. A.: Carcinoma of the breast

metastatic to the bones of the foot. Arthritis, Rheum., *3*:170, 1960.

Jensen, A. F.: Bilateral metastasis to the eye following carcinoma of the breast. Amer. J. Ophthal., *24*:63, 1941.

Jessiman, A. G., Emerson, K., Jr., Shah, R. C., and Moore, F. D.: Hypercalcemia in carcinoma of the breast. Ann. Surg., *157*:377, 1963.

Kasilag, F. B., Jr., and Rutledge, F. N.: Metastatic breast carcinoma in the ovary. Amer. J. Obst. & Gynec., *74*:989, 1957.

Kastrup, H.: Das doppelseitige Mammacarcinom und seine Bedeutung zur Frage der Genese des Mammacarcinoms. Arch. f. klin. Chir., *206*:245, 1944.

Kay, S.: Evaluation of Rotter's lymph nodes in radical mastectomy specimens as a guide to prognosis. Cancer, *18*:1441, 1965.

Kennedy, B. J., Tibbetts, D. M., Nathanson, I. T., and Aub, J. C.: Hypercalcemia, a complication of hormone therapy of advanced breast cancer. Cancer Research, *13*:445, 1953.

Kennedy, C. S., Miller, E. B., and McLean, D. C.: Triple biopsy in carcinoma of the breast. J. Michigan Med. Soc., *62*:380, 1963.

Keyes, E. L., Jordan, E. J., and Wyatt, J. P.: Cancer of both breasts; 53 case reports. J. Missouri Med. A., *48*:385, 1951.

Kilgore, A. R.: The incidence of cancer in the second breast. J.A.M.A., *77*:454, 1921.

Kilgore, A. R., Bell, H. G., and Ahlquist, R. E., Jr.: Cancer in the second breast. Amer. J. Surg., *92*:156, 1956.

Kitain, H.: Zur Kenntnis der Häufigkeit und der Lokalisation von Krebsmetastasen mit besonderer Berücksichtigung ihres histologischen Baus. Virchows Arch. f. path. Anat., *238*:289, 1922.

Kleinfeld, G.: Acute fatal hypercalcemia. J.A.M.A., *181*:1137, 1962.

Kountz, S. L., Rogers, W. L., and Daniels, A. C.: Independent primary malignant neoplasms following mastectomy for breast carcinoma. Amer. J. Surg., *102*:312, 1961.

Kraus, A. S.: A review of the effectiveness of early treatment in breast cancer. Surg., Gynec. & Obst., *96*:545, 1953.

Kreyberg, L., and Christiansen, T.: Prognostic significance of small size in breast cancer. Brit. J. Cancer, *7*:37, 1953.

Krone, H. A., and Englert, R. G.: Metastasen eines Mammakarzinom im Endometrium uteri. Zentralbl. Gyn., *81*:969, 1959.

Küttner, H.: Beiträge zur Pathologie des Mammacarcinoms. Beitr. z. klin. Chir., *131*:1, 1924.

Lane-Claypon, J. E.: A Further Report on Cancer of the Breast with Special Reference to Its Associated Antecedent Conditions. Reports on Public Health and Medical Subjects, no. 32, London, Ministry of Health, 1926.

Laszlo, D., et al.: Mineral and protein metabolism in osteolytic metastases. J.A.M.A., *148*:1027, 1952.

Leavell, U. W., Jr., and Tillotson, F. W.: Metastatic cutaneous carcinoma from a breast; a clinical and pathologic study of a case showing three types of lesions. Arch. Dermat. & Syph., *64*:774, 1951.

Leis, H. P.: Bilateral mastectomy for carcinoma of the breast. J. Internat. Coll. Surg., *31*:329, 1959.

Lemon, H. M.: Abnormal circulating parathormone activity in advanced cancer. Proc. Amer. Assoc. Cancer Res., *3*:338, 1962.

Lenz, M., and Freid, J. R.: Metastases to the skeleton, brain, and spinal cord from cancer of the breast and the effect of radiotherapy. Ann. Surg., 93:278, 1931.

Long, L., et al.: Relationship of cancer cells in the circulating blood to operation. Arch. Surg., 80:639, 1960.

Lüdin, M.: Zahnfleischmetastase beim Brustkrebs; Röntgenbestrahlung. Strahlentherapie, 60:304, 1937.

Lumb, G., and Mackenzie, D. H.: The incidence of metastases in adrenal glands and ovaries removed for cancer of the breast. Cancer, 12:521, 1959.

Lund, R.: Et sjeldent tilfelle av dobbeltsidig cancer mammae. Nord. med. tidskr., 34:1058, 1947.

Luse, S. A., and Reagan, J. W.: A histological study of effusions. Cancer, 7:1167, 1954.

MacCarty, W. C.: Factors which influence longevity in cancer. Ann. Surg., 76:9, 1922.

McDonald, J. J., Haagensen, C. D., and Stout, A. P.: Metastasis from mammary carcinoma to the supraclavicular and internal mammary lymph nodes. Surgery, 34:521, 1953.

McKinnon, N. E.: Breast Cancer. Canad. J. Pub. Health, 42:88, 1951.

McWilliams, C. A.: Bilateral mammary cancer operations; ultimate results in 98 cases. Ann. Surg., 82:63, 1925.

Mannheimer, I. H.: Hypercalcemia of breast cancer. Cancer, 18:679, 1965.

Margottini, M.: Tecnica e indicazioni dello svuotamento linfoghiandolare sopraclaviculare nella cura del cancro della mammella. Oncologia, 22:281, 1948.

Margottini, M., and Bucalossi, P.: Le metastasi linfoghiandolari mammarie interne nel cancro della mammella. Oncologia, 23(2):70, 1949.

Massachusetts General Hospital: Cases from the medical grand rounds: case 273: breast carcinoma with hypercalcemia. Am. Pract., 5:83, 1954.

May, E., and Borm, D.: Hyperkalzämie und Mammakarzinom. Med. Klin., 57:2016, 1962.

Melnick, G. S., and Rosenholtz, M. J.: Metastatic breast carcinoma simulating ulcerative colitis. Amer. J. Roentgenol., 86:702, 1961.

Merriam, G. R.: Personal communication, 1969.

Meyer, P. C.: A statistical and histological survey of metastatic carcinoma in the skeleton. Brit. J. Cancer, 11:509, 1957.

Miller, E. B.: Five year review of carcinoma of the breast. Analysis according to the Columbia Classification. Ann. Surg., 163:629, 1960.

Moertel, C. G., and Soule, E. H.: The problem of the second breast: a study of 118 patients with bilateral carcinoma of the breast. Ann. Surg., 146:764, 1957.

Most, A.: Zur Metastasenbildung und Chirurgie des Brustkrebses. Arch. f. klin. Chir., 183:209, 1935.

Mueller, H. P., and Sniffen, R. C.: Roentgenologic appearance and pathology of intrapulmonary lymphatic spread of metastatic cancer. Amer. J. Roentgenol., 53:109, 1945.

Muir, R.: Evolution of carcinoma of mamma. J. Path. & Bact., 52:155, 1941.

Mustacchi, P., Pandolfi, A., and Bucalossi, P.: Bilateral mammary cancer in Italian women. J. Nat. Cancer Inst., 19:1035, 1957.

Myers, W. P. L.: Hypercalcemia in neoplastic disease. Cancer, 9:1135, 1956.

Myers, W. P. L., West, C. D., Pearson, O. H., and Karnofsky, D. A.: Androgen-induced exacerbation of breast cancer measured by calcium excretion. J.A.M.A., 161:127, 1956.

Nathanson, I. T., and Welch, C. E.: Life expectancy and incidence of malignant disease; carcinoma of the breast. Amer. J. Cancer, 28:40, 1936.

Nicholls, J. V.: Metastatic carcinoma of the optic nerve. Tr. Canad. Ophth. Soc., 24:18, 1961.

Nohrman, B. A.: Cancer of the breast. Acta Radiol., Supp. 77, 1949.

Paget, S.: The distribution of secondary growths in cancer of the breast. Lancet, 1:571, 1889.

Papillon, J., Pinet, F., and Bothier, F.: Le syndrome de la veine cave supérieure par métastase du cancer du sein. J. radiol. élect., 39:761, 1958.

Park, W. W., and Lees, J. C.: The absolute curability of cancer of the breast. Surg., Gynec. & Obst., 93:129, 1951.

Pearson, O. H., and Ray, B. S.: Results of hypophysectomy in the treatment of metastatic mammary carcinoma. Cancer, 12:85, 1959.

Pfahler, G. E., and Case, E. A.: Erysipelas carcinomatosum resembling radiodermatitis. Amer. J. Roentgenol., 35:804, 1936.

Phelan, J. T.: Treatment of pathologic fractures of the long bones from metastatic and primary ccancer. Cancer, 21:1233, 1968.

Pickren, J. W.: Significance of occult metastases. A study of breast cancer. Cancer, 14:1266, 1961.

Pilheu, F. R., and Fefer, S. A.: Mandibular metastasis secondary to a cancer of the breast. Semana med., 118:95, 1961.

Piney, A.: Carcinoma of the bone marrow. Brit. J. Surg., 10:235, 1922.

Polk, H. C., Jr., Camp, F. A., and Walker, A. W.: Dysphagia and esophageal stenosis. Cancer, 20:2002, 1967.

Pyrah, L. N.: Hormones in the treatment of cancer of the breast and prostate. Brit. J. Surg., 44:69, 1956.

Qualheim, R. E., and Gall, E. A.: Breast carcinoma with multiple sites of origin. Cancer, 40:460, 1957.

Rasch, C.: Carcinoma erysipelatodes. Brit. J. Dermat., 43:351, 1931.

Ray, B. S.: Personal communication, 1969.

Reese, A. J. M.: Bilateral carcinoma of the breast. Brit. J. Surg., 40:428, 1953.

Richards, G. E.: Mammary cancer, Part 1. Brit. J. Radiol., 21:109, 1948.

Robbins, G. F., and Berg, J. W.: Bilateral primary breast cancers. Cancer, 17:1501, 1964.

Ruef, J., and Ehlers, P. N.: Ueber 57 beobachtete doppelseitige Mamma-Carcinome. Arch. f. klin. Chir., 300:115, 1962.

Saghatoeslami, M., Khodarahmi, K., and Epstein, B. S.: Calcified intrahepatic metastases from carcinoma of the breast. J.A.M.A., 181:1139, 1962.

Sandberg, A. A., and Moore, G. E.: Examination of blood for tumor cells. J. Nat. Cancer Inst., 19:1, 1957.

Sanger, G.: An aspect of internal mammary metastases from carcinoma of the breast. Ann. Surg., 157:180, 1963.

Saphir, O., and Amromin, G. D.: Obscure axillary lymph node metastasis in carcinoma of the breast. Cancer, 1:238, 1948.

Saphir, O., and Parker, M. L.: Metastasis of primary carcinoma of the breast with special reference to spleen, adrenal glands, and ovaries. Arch. Surg., 42:1003, 1941.

Savatard, L.: Cancer en cuirasse. Brit. J. Dermat., 55:31, 1943.

Scheinin, T. M., and Koinuniemi, H. P.: The occurrence of cancer cells in blood. Surgery, 51:652, 1962.

Schilling, A., and Laszlo, D.: Rate of urinary calcium excretion following its intravenous administration as an indicator of bone metabolism. Proc. Soc. Exper. Biol. & Med., 78:286, 1951.

Schilling, A., and Laszlo, D.: Investigative tools in the study of calcium metabolism in man; balance studies, the calcium tolerance test, radioactive calcium, and complexing agents. Oral Surg., Oral Med., and Oral Path., 6:139, 1953.

Schinz, H. R., et al.: Roentgen-diagnostics. New York, Grune and Stratton, 1951–4, Vols. I & II.

Schmidt, M. B.: Die Verbreitungswege der Karzinome. Jena, Gustav Fischer, 1903.

Schmidt-Ueberreiter, E.: Carcinoma mammae utriusque. Arch. f. klin. Chir., 272:359, 1952.

Schmidt-Ueberreitre, E.: Histologische Feststellungen bei beidseitigen Mammacarcinomen. Arch. f. klin. Chir., 277:501, 1954.

Schwartz, M.: A biomathematical approach to clinical tumor growth. Cancer, 14:1272, 1961.

Seiler, H. H., Clagett, O. T., and McDonald, J. R.: Pulmonary resection for metastatic malignant lesions. J. Thoracic Surg., 19:655, 1950.

Sicard, A.: La fréquence des métastases ovariennes des cancers du sein. Presse Méd., 56:606, 1948.

Smithers, D. W., and Rigby-Jones, P.: Clinical evidence of parasternal lymph node involvement in neoplastic disease. Acta. radiol., Supp. 188:235, 1959.

Smithers, D. W., Rigby-Jones, P., Galton, D. A. G., and Payne, P. M.: Cancer of the breast. Brit. J. Radiol. Supp., No. 4, 1952.

Smulders, J., and Smets, W.: Les métastases des carcinomes mammaires. Fréquence des métastases hypophysaires. Bull. Assoc. franç. p. l'étude du cancer, 47:434, 1960.

Snell, W., and Beals, R. K.: Femoral metastases and fractures from breast cancer. Surg., Gynec & Obst., 119:22, 1964.

Song, J.: Metastatic carcinoma of the uterine cervix from primary breast cancer. J.A.M.A., 184:498, 1963.

Sonntag, E.: Beiträge zur Mund- und Kieferchirurgie. Deutsche Ztschr. f. chir., 223:236, 1930.

Staley, C. J.: Skeletal metastases in cancer of the breast. Surg., Gynec. & Obst., 102:683, 1956.

Stewart, D. S.: Progress of metastatic carcinoma of the choroid, secondary to mammary neoplasm. Brit. J. Ophthal., 44:53, 1960.

Stiles, H. J.: On the dissemination of cancer of the breast. Brit. Med. J., 1:1452, 1899.

Sutherland, C. G., Decker, F. H., and Cilley, E. I. L.: Metastatic malignant lesions in bone. Am. J. Cancer, 16:1457, 1932.

Swyer, A. J., Berger, J. S., Gordon, H. M., and Laszlo, D.: Hypercalcemia in osteolytic metastatic cancer of the breast. Amer. J. Med., 8:724, 1950.

Symington, T.: Endocrine Aspects of Breast Cancer. University of Glasgow, Edinburgh, Livingston, 1957.

Talbot-Déry, and Bonenfant, J. L.: Etude des cancers et de la distribution dans le matériel autopsique. Bull. Assoc. franç. p. l'étude du cancer, 48:666, 1961.

Taveras, J. M., and Wood, E. H.: Diagnostic Neuroradiology. Baltimore, Williams and Wilkins, 1964, p. 1221.

Taylor, H. B., and Norris, H. J.: Epithelial invasion of nerves in benign diseases of the breast. Cancer, 20:2245, 1967.

Taylor, G. W., and Nathanson, I. T.: Lymph Node Metastases. New York, Oxford University press, 1942, p. 24.

Tilney, F., and Riley, H. A.: The Form and Function of the Central Nervous System. New York, Hoeber, 1938.

Török, G. v., and Wittleshöfer, R.: Zur Statistik des Mamma-carcinoms. Arch. f. klin. Chir., 25:873, 1880.

Treves, N., and Finkeiner, J. A.: An evaluation of thera-peutic surgical castration in the treatment of metastatic recurrent and primary inoperable mammary carcinoma in women. Cancer, 11:421, 1858.

Trimble, F. H., Lewison, E. F., and Walewski, A. C.: First metastasis of breast cancer. Arch. Surg., 78:620, 1959.

Truscott, B. M.: Carcinoma of the breast. Brit. J. Cancer, 1:129, 1947.

Tuaillon, P., Bourgeois, M., Dargent, M., and Mayer, M.: Les métastases surrénaliennes dans le cancer du sein. Bull. Assoc. franç. p. l'étude du cancer, 50:139, 1963.

Turksoy, N.: Ovarian metastasis of breast carcinoma; a surgical surprise. Obst. Gyn., 15:573, 1960.

Turner, J. W., and Jaffe, H. L.: Metastatic neoplasms; clinical and roentgenological study of involvement of skeleton and lungs. Amer. J. Roentgenol., 43:479, 1940.

Urban, J. A.: Surgical excision of internal mammary nodes for breast cancer. Brit. J. Surg., 51:209, 1964.

Velpeau, A.: Traité des Maladies du Sein. Paris, Masson, 1858, 2nd. ed., p. 404.

Veronesi, U.: Removal of internal mammary nodes in cancer of the breast. Internat. Union against Cancer, 19:1560, 1963.

Vogt-Hoerner, G.: Propagations intramammaires dans les cancers du sein et rapports avec l'envahissement des ganglions lymphatiques axillaires. Bull. du cancer, 7:279, 1960.

Vogt-Hoerner, G., and Contesso, G.: Localisation anatomique du premier ganglion axillaire métastatique de cancer du sein. J. de chir., 86:37, 1963.

Von Szegvári, Von M., Szereday, Z., and Ormos, J.: In die Gebärmutter metastasierender Brustkrebs. Arch. Geschwulstforsch., 21:208, 1963.

Wade, P.: Untreated carcinoma of the breast. Brit. J. Radiol., 19:272, 1946.

Walther, H. E.: Krebsmetastasen. Basel, Schwabe, 1948.

Warren, S., and Witham, E. M.: Studies on tumor metastasis. 2. The distribution of metastases in cancer of the breast. Surg., Gynec. & Obst., 57:81, 1933.

Watne, A. L., Sandberg, A. A., and Moore, G. E.: The prognostic value of tumor cells in the blood. Arch. Surg., 83:190, 1961.

Weber, F. P.: Bilateral thoracic zosteroid spreading marginate telangiectasia. Brit. J. Dermat., 45:418, 1933.

Welch, C. E.: Pathological fractures due to malignant disease. Surg., Gynec. & Obst., 62:735, 1936.

Willis, R. A.: The Spread of Tumours in the Human Body. London, J. & A. Churchill, 1934.

Willis, R. A.: A solitary cystic metastasis in the brain from a carcinoma of the breast. J. Path. & Bact., 48:474, 1939.

Wong, T. W., and Bennington, J. L.: Metastasis of a mammary carcinoma to an acoustic neuroma. J. Neurosurg., 19:1088, 1962.

Woolner, L. B., Keating, F. R., Jr., and Black, B. M.: Primary hyperparathyroidism and metastatic breast carcinoma. Cancer, 11:975, 1958.

Wu, T. T.: Generalized lymphatic carcinosis ("lymphangitis carcinomatosa") of the lungs. J. Path. & Bact., 43:61, 1936.

Wuketich, S.: Das Erscheinungsbild der Lebermetastasen und seine differential-diagnostische Bedeutung. Beitr. z. path. Anat. u. z. allg. Path., 122:363, 1960.

Yeates, J. M.: Bilateral carcinoma of the breast. Med. J. Australia, 2:54, 1953.

Zeitlhofer, J.: Ueber die axilläre Lymphknotenmetastasierung des Brustdrüsenkrebses. Arch. f. klin. Chir., 272:429, 1952.

Chapter Twenty-Three

The Symptoms of Mammary Carcinoma

Women with breast carcinoma have almost always found their disease by themselves. With the modern practice of complete physical examination, however, physicians today discover breast carcinoma with increasing frequency, as I will document in the following chapter. An accurate knowledge of the symptomatology of this common disease is important for all physicians.

Table 23–1 presents a tabulation of the symptoms of breast carcinoma in four large European case series reported between 1926 and 1948.

For a closer inquiry into the frequency and sequence of symptoms in carcinoma of the breast I have utilized the records of my own 1669 private patients whom I saw between the years 1943 and 1967. I took these case histories personally. The symptoms of which these patients complained are shown in Table 23–2.

TUMOR

From these data it is seen that from 75 to 80 per cent of women with breast carcinoma become aware of their disease as a result of finding a breast lump. The discovery is almost always accidental. The patient's hand happens to encounter the tumor while she is bathing or dressing. The tumor that a carci-

Table 23–1. SYMPTOMS OF MAMMARY CARCINOMA

Symptom	Lane-Claypon 508 cases	Truscott 787 cases	Harnett 2529 cases	Kaae 500 cases
A lump first, no pain ever	39.0%	67.5%	} 77.4%	} 74.0%
A lump first, pain later	16.5%	16.0%		
Pain first	17.7%	10.0%	10.0%	12.0%
Nipple discharge	7.4%	7.5%	2.2%	2.7%
Nipple retraction	2.0%	3.0%	2.0%	4.2%
Nipple itching } Nipple erosion	1.0%			
Shrinkage of breast	2.0%			
Ulceration of skin of breast		0.5%		1.7%
Found by physician	1.0%	0.1%	1.6%	0.8%

Table 23-2. SYMPTOMS IN 1669 PERSONAL CASES OF CARCINOMA OF THE BREAST

	1943–1955			1956–1967		
	Primary	Secondary	Total	Primary	Secondary	Total
Lump	369	51	420	735	46	781
Pain in breast	40	54	94	48	6	54
Tenderness on pressure over breast	3	5	8	4	1	5
Abnormal sensation in breast	0	0	0	2	0	2
Skin dimpling	21	7	28	36	3	39
Skin ulceration	0	2	2	3	1	4
Nipple retraction	14	9	23	20	0	20
Nipple discharge	13	8	21	17	1	18
Nipple erosion	9	2	11	17	3	20
Nipple itching	4	5	9	3	2	5
Breast enlarged	3	2	5	14	1	15
Breast shrunken	2	2	4	0	0	0
Generalized hardness of breast	1	1	2	4	1	5
Redness of skin	1	6	7	9	6	15
Edema of skin	0	0	0	1	0	1
Skin nodules	0	1	1	0	0	0
Ecchymosis in skin	0	1	1	2	0	2
Axillary tumor	11	5	16	20	2	22
Pain in arm	1	0	1	0	0	0
Swelling of arm	1	0	1	2	0	2
Pain in back	2	0	2	1	0	1
Total	495	161	656	938	73	1011

No symptoms, disease discovered at physical examination

51 or 9.1 per cent   185 or 16.5 per cent

Total   546   1123

noma produces in the breast is more easily felt by the patient than most other types of breast tumor because of its hardness. The patient may not describe it as a lump but merely as an area of thickening. The important point is that she usually recognizes that she feels something abnormal. Patients occasionally find breast carcinomas as small as 5 mm. in diameter. This fact is striking evidence of the accuracy of their palpation.

It is impossible for me to assess with any accuracy the role of self-examination in the discovery of the breast tumor in my series of patients. I have for many years tried to encourage my patients to palpate their own breasts periodically, and to teach them how. But I have not made any systematic study of how many of them have actually done so. A considerable number have indeed found their tumor by self-examination, and I have the impression that most of these who did were women who had a special reason for trusting physicians—they were nurses, medical technicians, or doctors' relatives.

PAIN

Pain as a symptom of breast carcinoma has been studied by River and by Corry. Both of these authors have stressed the frequency of local pain in the primary breast lesion. River found it in 24 per cent of his patients, and Corry in 53 per cent. The latter presented an elaborate classification of the type of pain encountered. It was momentary and snatching (as if the breast had been suddenly pulled and then let go), or stabbing (single or multiple stabs), or continuous and aching (burning, gnawing, or dragging). The momentary and continuous types were about equally frequent.

My own experience with pain as a symptom of breast carcinoma has been rather different. I have found pain to be an uncommon primary symptom. In my personal series of 1433 patients who had symptoms, pain was the first symptom in only 88 patients, or 6.2 per cent. It has also been an infrequent secondary symptom, occurring in only 4.2 per cent of my patients. Pain, therefore, was a primary or secondary symptom in a total of only 10.4 per cent of my patients. There were, in addition, 13 patients who complained of tenderness on pressure as a primary or secondary symptom.

In taking histories from my patients I have been careful not to emphasize or suggest pain as a symptom. I ask the patient straight out what symptom called her attention to her breast. I suspect that leading questions may suggest pain to these frightened and receptive patients. The difference between Corry's data and my own can perhaps be explained by differences in the methods of questioning.

The one type of breast pain that is, in my experience, somewhat suggestive of carcinoma, is intermittent and sharp, and is felt in the region of the tumor. Patients have twinges of this kind of pain, usually occurring only infrequently, but of sufficient intensity to make them suspect breast disease. They describe it as sticking, stinging, shooting, stabbing, throbbing, or burning pain.

I am led to conclude that pain is not a very important symptom of breast carcinoma. Even in its most suggestive form it occurs too infrequently to be relied upon. If a woman past the menopause, at an age when the cyclical physiologic pain due to breast engorgement is not to be expected, experiences for the first time sharp pain localized in the breast, the fact should, of course, suggest the possibility of carcinoma to her physician. The physician's point of view regarding breast pain, however, is necessarily different from that of the layman. In our propaganda to the public I believe that we would do well to emphasize the fact that a lump is the all important warning sign of breast cancer, and that the lump is usually painless. Much of my own time is spent reassuring patients who come to me with nothing more than breast pain of physiologic origin.

RETRACTION

Retraction signs were noted only infrequently by our patients. In my personal series of 1669 patients, only 67 noted skin dimpling; four noted shrinkage of the breast. Only 43 noted retraction of the nipple. These retraction signs were usually discovered while bathing or dressing. A great many of my patients had perfectly obvious retraction signs and were entirely oblivious of them. It is unlikely that we will be able to teach patients to inspect their own breasts critically enough to enable them to detect breast carcinoma by means of the retraction signs that it so often produces.

REDNESS OF THE SKIN

There were 19 patients who noted redness of the skin over the breast in my personal series of carcinomas. In 11 of these in whom the whole breast was red, edematous, and indurated, the disease was classified as the inflammatory type and as inoperable. In two other patients, whose disease was also classified as Clinical Stage D and inoperable, there was redness involving about one-third of the skin over the breast, and in addition edema of lesser extent and a clinically involved axillary node 3 cm. in diameter. Both of these patients were treated by irradiation. One soon succumbed but the other is free of symptoms 12 years later.

In the other patients with redness of the skin, the disease was classified as operable, although comparatively advanced. In four of the six there was also edema of the skin involving less than one-third of the skin over the breast. The redness was more extensive than the edema, involving about one-half of the skin over the breast. In three of these patients the redness was transitory, disappearing with bed rest.

None of the six patients was cured, and I am inclined to regard redness of the skin of a sufficient degree to be noticed by a patient who has carcinoma as a sign of far advanced disease, even though the clinical picture is not that of the classical, inflammatory type of carcinoma.

NIPPLE DISCHARGE

The frequency of a spontaneous discharge from the nipple — watery, serous, or bloody — in carcinoma of the breast has been variously reported. One reason is, no doubt, that the patients with the nipple erosion of Paget's carcinoma, which of course oozes serum and blood, have been included by some authors with those having genuine discharge from the nipple ducts. Other authors have classified as having a nipple discharge those who squeeze the nipple and produce a few drops of serum or blood. In my view these phenomena should not be recorded as true nipple discharge.

Truscott reported that 7.5 per cent of his series of 787 patients with breast carcinoma had a nipple discharge, but I suspect that this comparatively high incidence can be explained by the inclusion of patients with phenomena such as I have mentioned above. Harnett comes nearer the truth with a 2.2 per cent incidence of nipple discharge in his series of 2529 cases. Hinchey reported that 3.2 per cent of his series of 742 patients with carcinoma had a nipple discharge. In Wolpers' series of 414 cases of carcinoma, 1.2 per cent had a bloody nipple discharge.

There are more reports of the reverse relationship, namely, the frequency of carcinoma in patients with nipple discharge. These reports can be divided into two groups, one with a high incidence of carcinoma and the other with a low incidence, depending upon the interpretation of the pathology of the papillary lesions. As an example of the former, Judd, as well as Gray and Wood from the Mayo Clinic, classified the lesions in 57 and 50 per cent, respectively, of their patients with a nipple discharge as malignant. I believe that most of these "malignant" lesions were benign papillomas. In another series of 219 patients with nipple discharge from the University of Iowa, Donnelly reported that 44 per cent had carcinoma; and Copeland and Higgins reported that 37 per cent of their series of 67 patients with a nipple discharge had carcinoma.

Examples of reports with a lower frequency of carcinoma among patients with nipple discharge, based upon more critical pathologic classification, are those from the Johns Hopkins Hospital by Hart in 1927, and by Lewison and Chambers in 1951. In Hart's series of 77 patients with a nipple discharge, 10.4 per cent had malignant lesions. In Lewison and Chambers' series of 114 patients with nipple discharge, 11.2 per cent had carcinoma. Kilgore and his associates reported 14 cases of carcinoma among a total of 103 patients with a bloody nipple discharge. Mercier and Redon found carcinoma in only 11.5 per cent of their 120 patients with a nipple discharge, while McPherson and MacKenzie reported that 12.5 per cent of their 72 patients with this symptom had carcinoma.

For studying this question of the frequency of breast carcinoma among patients who come for consultation because of a nipple discharge, I have used the data from my more recent patients — 1956 to 1967 — because I believe that I have continued to learn regarding the interpretation of nipple discharge and that this more recent experience has led me closer to the truth. Between 1956 and 1967 I saw 157 patients with nipple discharge. I analyzed my findings in detail in Chapter 5, but I can report here that only 18 or 11.5 per cent of these patients proved to have breast carcinoma. In seven it was serous, in 10 bloody, and in one it was watery.

These data lead me to the conclusion that discharge from the nipple occurs comparatively infrequently in breast carcinoma. When it does occur it is usually due either to benign intraductal papilloma which happens to be coincident with carcinoma, or to the papillary type of carcinoma. It is understandable that the papillary processes growing in the ducts in both of these lesions easily break off, and serum or blood escapes from the vessels in their stalks. In a few cases we did not find an explanation for the nipple discharge, but we can conjecture that our microscopic sections missed the papillary lesions in these cases.

NIPPLE EROSION

There were 31 patients in my personal series who noted erosion or crusting of the nipple due to the Paget's type of carcinoma. Fourteen of the 31 had itching of the eroded nipple, a symptom which I have found often present in Paget's disease. I will discuss this form of carcinoma separately in Chapter 29.

SYMPTOMS DUE TO METASTASES

In the present chapter I have been discussing the symptoms that patients with breast carcinoma develop that lead to the recognition of their disease. These symptoms for the most part, of course, originate from the primary lesion. In a small proportion of patients the initial symptoms are those produced by metastases.

In my personal series of patients there were 42 whose initial symptoms related to their axillary metastases. All had palpable primary breast tumors that they had not discovered. Thirty-eight complained of an axillary tumor, one of pain in the arm, and three of swelling of the arm.

Pain due to vertebral metastases is another type of initial symptom of breast carcinoma. The pain may be localized in the back or pelvis, or may radiate down the thigh. Cohn and Cohn called attention to this clinical syndrome in a paper describing four cases. Ducuing also emphasized the fact that bone pain, or even pathological fracture, may be the first sign of breast carcinoma.

In my personal series of patients there were three whose first symptom was back pain. All first consulted their internist for the back pain. He did a complete physical examination and found a breast tumor. The story of one of these patients is worth summarizing because it illustrates the difficulty of determining whether or not back pain is due to metastases.

Mrs. K. E., a housewife aged 51, consulted me for a breast tumor. It had been discovered by her internist to whom she had gone for help concerning low back pain. Her back pain had begun a year previously, but it had been increasingly troublesome during the last six months, and acute during the last month. It was centered over the central lower back, and occurred almost entirely with motion. Coughing and sneezing had recently produced it.

She had a 5 cm. tumor, with all the characteristics of a carcinoma, situated in the upper middle sector of the left breast. There was a 1 cm. movable left axillary node. Roentgenographic study of the lungs and skeleton showed no evidence of metastases. Being aware that the back pain might be due to metastases I asked an orthopedic consultant to study her. He concluded that she did not have vertebral metastases. I therefore performed a radical mastectomy. Three of 12 axillary lymph nodes contained metastases.

Her back pain got worse during the time she was in the hospital, and became so bad after she returned home that she never really got out of bed. She had to be readmitted two months after operation. New x-ray studies then showed extensive metastases in ribs, pelvic bones, and lumbar vertebrae. Irradiation was of little value and she died seven months after operation with widespread visceral and bone metastases.

DURATION OF SYMPTOMS

The length of time that elapses between the first symptom of breast carcinoma and diagnosis and treatment is an important fact. The accuracy of patients' statements as to the duration of their symptoms has been questioned. It is certainly true that some women are inaccurate in this regard. Either faulty memory or fear may cloud their statements. Individual women also vary greatly in their acuity of perception of any abnormality in their breasts. I have occasionally seen women who were entirely unaware of a carcinoma involving a large part of the breast. It is also true that the discovery of a tumor in the breast is usually accidental. The patient's hand encounters the tumor during bathing or dressing. This accidental discovery may occur soon after the tumor is large enough to detect or after it has been palpable for a considerable time. If duration of symptoms is to be treated statistically as a definite point in the evolution of breast carcinoma, all these

variables necessitate basing conclusions as to duration upon data from a large number of patients. If this is done, however, duration certainly has some significance.

The average delay in seeking medical advice by women with breast carcinoma has been astonishingly long. Table 23-3 lists the average duration of symptoms in a number of large case series. It is true that in general these data represent the course of events in women with breast cancer a generation ago. We hope that with modern educational efforts in our country this delay is decreasing.

In an effort to study this question I have put together in Table 23-4 data from the Presbyterian Hospital from 1915 to 1967, as well as Bloom's data from the Middlesex Hospital, and those from my personal series of patients from 1943 to 1967. These data are to me decidedly encouraging, and confirm my impression that women are today coming for consultation with the symptoms of breast disease a good deal more promptly than they did in the 1930's and 1940's. In those years, as the data from the Presbyterian and Middlesex hospitals indicate, only 16 to 18 per cent of patients came within a month, and only about 60 per cent came within six months. In my recent personal series of patients 46 per cent came within a month, and 80 per cent came within six months. This reduction in delay in consultation among patients with breast cancer in my own hospital cannot be explained by a change in the proportion of ward and private patients in the three series of cases. The 1915-1942 Presbyterian Hospital series contained both classes of patients. My personal series of patients

Table 23-3. DURATION OF SYMPTOMS OF MAMMARY CARCINOMA

Author	Year of Publication	Number of Cases	Average Duration of Symptoms in Months
Lane-Claypon	1926	508	20.5
Harrington	1933	4,038	17.4
Simmons, Daland, and Wallace	1933	?	9.2
Nathanson and Welch	1936	575	12.1
Truscott	1947	777	10.0
Nohrman	1949	1,042	8.8
Bloom	1950	423	8.3
Smithers et al.	1952	797	11.2
Haagensen	1956	1,420	10.7

Table 23-4. DURATION OF SYMPTOMS IN BREAST CARCINOMA

Duration of Symptoms	Presbyterian Hospital 1915-1942		Middlesex Hospital Bloom 1936-1949		Personal Series of Cases 1943-1955		Personal Series of Cases 1956-1967	
	Number Patients	Per cent Distribution Cumulated	Number Patients	Per cent Distribution Cumulated	Number Patients	Per cent Distribution Cumulated	Number Patients	Per cent Distribution Cumulated
Under 2 weeks	117	8.2	} 202	} 16	85	17.2	222	26.5
2 weeks to less than 1 month	136	17.8						
1–2 months	233	34.2			56	28.5	168	46.5
3–5 months	278	53.8	} 604	} 64	120	52.7	202	70.6
6–11 months	259	72	232	82	76	68.1	86	80.9
12–23 months	186	85.1	123	91	61	80.4	78	90.2
24–35 months	84	91	39	95	51	90.7	36	94.5
36–59 months	} 127		} 63		22	95.1	18	96.6
60 months or more		100		100	} 24	100	14	98.3
							14	100
Total number patients	1420		1263		495		938	
Mean duration of delay	10.7 months				7.5 months		4.9 months	

include about equal proportions of each group.

These facts lead me to believe that efforts to educate both women and physicians regarding breast cancer are having some success, and that they should be expanded.

THE IMPORTANCE OF DELAY

There is a group of skeptics who question the advantage of shortening the length of time women with breast cancer delay in seeking medical consultation. They suggest that delay is unimportant, and that the course of the disease is not influenced by treatment. Bloom has carried out the most thorough study of this question, using data from the Middlesex Hospital, correlating delay with a series of individual factors. Since I have similar data from the Presbyterian Hospital I have duplicated his studies of the relationship of delay to some of the different factors that he studied.

Delay and 10 Year Survival

In studying the relationship of different factors to survival, it has been, in our experience, more revealing to use 10 years as an end-point, than to use longer or shorter periods of time. When duration of symptoms as stated by the patient is correlated with 10 year survival as shown in Table 23-5, it is seen from both Bloom's and my own data

Table 23-5. DELAY AND 10 YEAR SURVIVAL

Delay in Months	Bloom (1936-1949)		Haagensen (1935-1957)	
	No. of Cases	10 Year Survival	No. of Cases	10 Year Survival
< 3 months	556	36%	328	60%
3–5 months	231	29%	107	54%
6–11 months	223	31%	78	54%
12–23 months	116	30%	59	58%
24–35 months	38	37%	28	54%
36 months +	61	38%	26	54%
	1225		626	

that patients who have delayed less than three months have a higher survival rate, but that their survival rate is less than 10 per cent higher than the survival rate for patients who delayed as long as 11 months. The surprising fact derived from these data is that longer delay has not been associated with a lower 10 year survival rate.

I agree with Bloom that a more penetrating study of the significance of delay than simple correlation with survival is necessary. The duration of disease as stated by the patient is not only inacurrate in many instances, but it of course represents only a small fraction of the total time that has elapsed following the original mutation from which the patient's carcinoma originated.

In the following pages I will present Bloom's data and my own data for a series of other individual factors related to delay. In comparing these data it should be kept in mind that my own series of cases consists only of patients who were carefully selected for treatment by radical mastectomy. Bloom has included in his tables all the Middlesex patients for whom pertinent data were available, including those not treated as well as those treated by a variety of methods. The differences in the data must be interpreted in view of this fundamental difference. Nevertheless, comparison is interesting and useful.

Delay and Tumor Size

The data correlating length of delay with tumor size in both Bloom's and my series of cases are shown in Table 23-6. It is clear from the data in both case series that patients delaying six months or more had larger tumors than those in whom the delay was less than three months. This difference is somewhat more marked in my data; 65 per cent of my patients who delayed from six to 11 months had tumors larger than 4 cm., whereas only 36 per cent of those who delayed less than three months had tumors larger than 4 cm.

Tumor Size and Survival. The data correlating tumor size with 10 year survival in both series of cases are shown in Table 23-7. The survival rates fall regularly and significantly as the size of the tumors increases. I have presented more detailed data correlating the size of the primary tumor with survival in my own series of cases in Chapter 33. The conclusion is inescapable that the size of the tumor significantly influences survival.

Delay, Tumor Size, and Survival. Both delay and tumor size are correlated with survival by Bloom for his data in Chart 23-1. I have constructed a similar table from my data (Chart 23-2). In Bloom's data the tumors with a duration of less than three months

Table 23–6. DELAY AND TUMOR SIZE

	Tumor Size									
	Bloom (1936–1949)					Haagensen (1935–1957)				
Delay in Months	< 1/2 in.	>1/2 < 1 in.	>1 < 2 in.	> 2 in.	No. of Cases	< 2 cm.	2–3 cm.	4–5 cm.	6 cm.+	No. of Cases
< 3 months	8%	38%	40%	14%	572	16%	48%	24%	12%	328
3–5 months	10%	36%	36%	18%	171	12%	35%	39%	14%	107
6–11 months	7%	24%	49%	20%	152	9%	26%	32%	33%	78
12 months +	7%	23%	46%	24%	149	11%	32%	32%	25%	113
					1044					626

Table 23–7. TUMOR SIZE AND 10 YEAR SURVIVAL

Bloom (1936–1949)			Haagensen (1935–1957)		
No. of Cases	Tumor Size	10 Year Survival	No. of Cases	Tumor Size	10 Year Survival
83	< 1/2 in.	46%	81	< 2 cm.	75%
346	> 1/2 < 1 in.	40%	252	2–3 cm.	67%
439	> 1 < 2 in.	33%	183	4–5 cm.	46%
176	> 2 in.	25%	110	6 cm. +	41%
1,044			626		

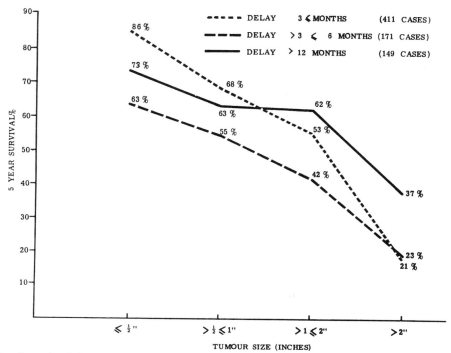

Chart 23–1. Length of delay, tumor size, and five year survival in patients with breast carcinoma treated by radical mastectomy (Bloom).

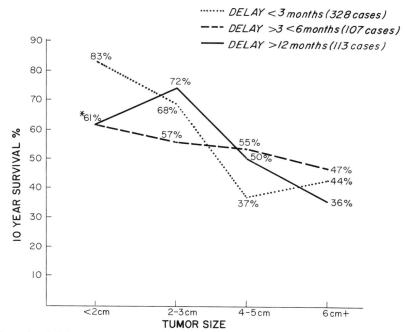

Chart 23–2. Length of delay, tumor size, and 10 year survival in patients with breast carcinoma treated by radical mastectomy (Haagensen).

show the greatest reduction in survival rate with increasing tumor size. In my data not only the tumors of short duration (less than three months) but also those of long duration (more than 12 months) have sharply reduced survival rates as they increase in size. The difference in Bloom's findings and my own may result from the fact that he reports five year survival and my survival time is 10 years. I cannot explain why the tumors with an intermediate duration (three to six months) in my data, show a comparatively less pronounced reduction in survival rates as they increase in size.

Delay and Axillary Involvement

The relationship of delay to microscopically proven axillary involvement in Bloom's data and in my own is shown in Table 23–8. Although Bloom's data show only a slightly higher incidence of axillary metastasis as the delay increases, my data show an increase of from 37 per cent to 59 per cent as delay is prolonged from one month to between 12 to 24 months. It is obvious from these data regarding axillary involvement that I have been more critical in selecting patients for operation than the surgeons at the Middlesex Hospital. The disease is earlier in my series of cases and my results are correspondingly better. This fact gives my series of cases added value in studying the significance of delay.

Delay and Extent of Axillary Involvement. I have shown in Chapter 22 that the degree to which the axillary lymph node filter is involved is in fact more important than whether or not there are axillary metastases. Bloom does not present data correlating delay with the extent of the axillary involvement. My own data on this relationship are presented in a simplified form in Table 23–9. It is apparent that the patients who delay less than a month have a definite advantage as to the extent of axillary involvement. Those who delay longer are twice as likely to have more than three axillary nodes involved.

Tumor Size and Axillary Involvement. Tumor size is correlated with axillary involvement in Table 23–10. In both Bloom's data and in my own the incidence of axillary metastases rises sharply as the size of the primary tumor increases.

Since tumor size increases with lengthening delay, it is to be expected that the patients who delay longer will more frequently have axillary metastases and that the extent of the axillary involvement will be greater.

Axillary Involvement and Survival. There is of course no single factor as important in determining 10 year survival after radical mastectomy for breast carcinomas as the simple fact of whether or not the axillary nodes were microscopically involved. This is well shown in Table 23–11, which presents these data for Bloom's series of cases and for my own.

Delay and Clinical Stage of Advancement

Study of the relationship of delay to the clinical stage of advancement of breast carcinoma is handicapped by the difficulties of clinical staging. Bloom's data are based on clinical staging with the old Manchester plan of staging, which I will discuss in Chapter 33. It has many defects. My own series of cases is staged with our Columbia plan of clinical staging, which is simpler and more precise. Nevertheless, I have presented Bloom's data and my own in Table 23–12.

Both case series show that the proportion of patients in the early stages decreases, while the proportion of cases in the later stages increases, as the delay lengthens. Bloom's patients who delayed more than three years constitute an exception to this rule. In this group there was a sharp increase in the proportion of Stage 2 lesions, suggesting a preponderance of carcinomas of relatively slow growth rate which, although long neglected, were still not far advanced. This was not apparent in my data.

There is, therefore, a good correlation between length of delay and clinical stage of advancement in both Bloom's data and my own.

Clinical Stage of Advancement and Survival. Bloom's data and my own correlating clinical stage of advancement and survival are presented in Table 23–13. In both case series it is obvious that as the disease advances through successive clinical stages the 10 year survival rate falls sharply.

Table 23–8. DELAY AND AXILLARY INVOLVEMENT

Bloom (1936–1949)			Haagensen (1935–1957)		
Delay	No. of Patients	Axillary Nodes Involved Microscopically	Delay	No. of Patients	Axillary Nodes Involved Microscopically
< 1 month	196	59%	< 1 month	195	37%
> 1 < 3 months	295	57%	1–2 months	133	51%
> 3 < 6 months	203	64%	3–5 months	107	47%
> 6 < 12 months	181	63%	6–11 months	78	58%
> 1 < 2 years	94	67%	12–23 months	59	59%
> 2 < 3 years	31	61%	24–35 months	28	57%
> 3 years	47	68%	36 months +	26	58%
Total	1,047	61%		626	48%

Table 23–9. DELAY AND EXTENT OF AXILLARY INVOLVEMENT
(Radical Mastectomy, Haagensen, 1935–1957)

Delay	No. of Patients	Patients with Microscopically Involved Nodes	Patients with More Than 3 Microscopically Involved Nodes
Less than 1 month	195	37%	14%
1–2 months	133	51%	26%
3–5 months	107	47%	23%
6–11 months	78	58%	29%
12–23 months	59	59%	25%
24–35 months	28	57%	32%
36 months or more	26	58%	23%
Total	626	48%	22%

Table 23–10. TUMOR SIZE AND AXILLARY INVOLVEMENT

Bloom (1936–1949)			Haagensen (1935–1968)		
Tumor Size	No. of Patients	Microscopic Axillary Involvement	Tumor Size	No. of Patients	Microscopic Axillary Involvement
< 1/2 in.	70	49%	< 2	167	23%
> 1/2 < 1 in.	280	49%	2–3 cm.	403	38%
> 1 < 2 in.	363	61%	4–5 cm.	248	52%
> 2 < 3 in.	104	76%	6–7 cm.	77	52%
> 3 in.	36	94%	8 cm. +	27	52%
Total	853	59%		922	40.6%

Table 23–11. AXILLARY INVOLVEMENT AND SURVIVAL

Microscopic Axillary Findings	Bloom (1936–1949)		Haagensen (1935–1957)	
	No. of Patients	10 Year Survival	No. of Patients	10 Year Survival
No metastases	497	55%	327	74%
Metastases	763	19%	299	39%
Total	1,260		626	

Table 23–12. DELAY AND CLINICAL STAGE OF ADVANCEMENT

	Bloom (1936–1949)					Haagensen (1935–1957)				
	Manchester Staging Distribution of Cases					Columbia Staging Distribution of Cases			
Delay in Months	Stage 1	Stage 2	Stage 3	Stage 4	Delay in Months	Stage A	Stage B	Stage C	Stage D
< 3 months	38%	44%	14%	4%	< 3 months	70%	22%	7%	2%
> 3 < 6 months	32%	41%	21%	6%	3–5 months	65%	23%	9%	2%
> 6 < 12 months	32%	34%	28%	6%	6–11 months	53%	27%	18%	3%
> 12 < 24 months	26%	36%	32%	6%	12–23 months	59%	31%	8%	2%
> 24 < 36 months	26%	13%	40%	21%	24–35 months	54%	32%	14%	0
> 36 months	18%	40%	29%	13%	36 months +	50%	35%	15%	0
Totals	419	495	267	74		402	154	59	11

Table 23–13. CLINICAL STAGE OF ADVANCEMENT AND SURVIVAL

Bloom (1936–1949)			Haagensen (1935–1957)		
Manchester Clinical Stage	No. of Patients	Per cent 10 Year Survival	Columbia Clinical Stage	No. of Patients	Per cent 10 Year Survival
1	419	55%	A	402	70%
2	495	25%	B	154	41%
3	267	20%	C	59	24%
4	74	3%	D	11	18%
Totals	1,255			626	

A Summary of the Relationship of Delay to the Course of Breast Carcinoma

Although an analysis of the simple relationship of the duration of symptoms of breast carcinoma to 10 year survival following radical mastectomy shows a significant advantage only for the patients who are treated within three months, careful correlation of the duration of symptoms with a series of other factors reveals that the disease undoubtedly becomes more unfavorable as delay lengthens. Smaller tumors are found less often, and larger tumors are more frequent. Patients with larger tumors have a lower survival rate. As the duration of symptoms lengthens, the frequency and extent of axillary metastasis increases. Increase in the size of the primary tumor is also associated with more axillary involvement. As delay increases the clinical stage advances, and in the more advanced clinical stages survival falls sharply.

Statistical studies thus support common sense when we urge careful attention to the symptoms of breast carcinoma, early medical consultation, and prompt diagnosis and treatment.

REFERENCES

Bloom, H. J. G.: Prognosis in carcinoma of the breast. Brit. J. Cancer, 4:259, 1950a.

Bloom, H. J. G.: Further studies in prognosis of breast carcinoma. Brit. J. Cancer, 4:347, 1950b.

Bloom, H. J. G.: The influence of delay on the natural history and prognosis of breast cancer. Brit. J. Cancer, 19:228, 1965.

Cohn, T. D., and Cohn, H.: Low-back pain as the presenting symptom of malignant breast tumors. New Eng. J. Med., 232:342, 1945.

Copeland, M. M., and Higgins, T. G.: Significance of discharge from the nipple in nonpuerperal mammary conditions. Ann. Surg., 151:638, 1960.

Corry, D. C.: Pain in carcinoma of the breast. Lancet, 1:274, 1952.

Donnelly, B. A.: Nipple discharge. Ann. Surg., 131:342, 1950.

Ducuing, J.: Les grands syndromes douloureux d'envahissement osseux dans le cancer du sein. Bull. Assoc. franç. p. l'étude du cancer, 29:36, 1940.

Gray, H. K., and Wood, G. A.: Significance of mammary discharge in cases of papilloma of the breast. Arch. Surg., 42:203, 1941.

Harnett, W. L.: A statistical report on 2529 cases of cancer of the breast. Brit. J. Cancer, 2:213, 1948.

Harrington, S. W.: Diagnosis and treatment of lesions of the breast. Amer. J. Cancer, 19:56, 1933.

Hart, D.: Intracystic papillomatous tumors of the breast, benign and malignant. Arch Surg., 14:793, 1927.

Higginson, J.: Patient delay with reference to stage of cancer. Cancer, 15:50, 1962.

Hinchey, P. R.: Nipple discharge. Ann. Surg., 113:341, 1941.

Judd, E. S.: Intracanalicular papilloma of the breast. Journal-Lancet, 37:141, 1917.

Kaae, S.: The prognostic significance of early diagnosis in breast cancer. Acta Radiol., 29:475, 1948.

Kilgore, A. R., Fleming, R., and Ramos, M. M.: The incidence of cancer with nipple discharge. Surg., Gynec. & Obst., 96:649, 1953.

Koeppler, D.: Ein örtliches, gewächsartiges Lymphogranulom der Mamma. Deutsche med. Wchnschr., 66:1220, 1940.

Lane-Claypon, J. E.: A Further Report on Cancer of the Breast with Special Reference to Its Associated Antecedent Conditions. Reports on Public Health and Medical Subjects, no. 32, London, Ministry of Health, 1926.

Lewison, E. F., and Chambers, R. G.: Clinical significance of nipple discharge. J.A.M.A., 147:295, 1951.

McKinnon, N. E.: Breast cancer. Canad. J. Pub. Health, 42:88, 1951.

McPherson, V. A., and MacKenzie, W. G.: Lesions of the breast associated with nipple discharge. Canad. J. Surg., 5:6, 1962.

Mercier, J., and Redon, H.: La valeur diagnostique des écoulements par le mamelon. Semaine d. hôp. Paris, Ann. Chir., 13:745, 1959.

Nathanson, I. T., and Welch, C. E.: Life expectancy and incidence of malignant disease; carcinoma of the breast. Amer. J. Cancer, 28:40, 1936.

Nohrman, B. A.: Cancer of the breast. Acta radiol., Supp. no. 77, 1949, p. 1.

River, L., et al.; Carcinoma of the breast; the diagnostic significance of pain. Amer. J. Surg., 82:733, 1951.

Robbins, G. F., and Bross, I.: The significance of delay in relation to the prognosis of patients with primary operable breast cancer. Cancer, 10:338, 1957.

Simmons, C. C., Daland, E. M., and Wallace, R. H.: Delay in the treatment of cancer. New Eng. J. Med., 208:1097, 1933.

Smithers, D. W., Rigby-Jones, P., Galton, D. A. G., and Payne, P. M.: Cancer of the breast. Brit. J. Radiol. Supp. 4, 1952.

Sutherland, R.: Cancer, the Significance of Delay. London, Butterworth, 1960.

Truscott, B. M.: Carcinoma of the breast. Brit. J. Cancer, 1-2:129, 1947.

Wolpers, C.: Die blutende Mamma. Arch. f. klin. Chir., 174:447, 1933.

Chapter Twenty-Four

The Diagnosis of Breast Carcinoma

In Chapter 5 I described methods of breast examination and the biopsy procedure I use to diagnose breast lesions in general. These methods are of course applied in diagnosing carcinoma. In the present chapter I wish to discuss our successes and failures in diagnosis, as well as certain special aspects of the problem in differential diagnosis that carcinoma presents.

It might be well to begin with an analysis of how cancer was detected in several different case series, including my own personal series of cases. Because in the latter cases I took the histories myself they are perhaps more complete than those for our Presbyterian Hospital ward patients taken by interns. Table 24–1 presents these data.

Table 24–1. Breast Carcinoma Discovered by Physicians During Routine Physical Examination

Year	Author	Number of Patients	Per cent of Carcinomas Discovered by Physicians
1926	Lane-Claypon	508	1.0%
1947	Truscott	787	0.1%
1949	Harnett	2529	1.6%
1948	Kaae	500	0.8%
1942	Haagensen Presbyterian Hospital	1033	5.9%
1943–1955	Haagensen Personal Series Presbyterian Hospital	546	9.1%
1956–1967	Haagensen Personal Series Presbyterian Hospital	1123	16.5%

The small proportion of patients in the European case series whose carcinomas were discovered by physicians at routine physical examination is perhaps explained by the fact that the patients in these series were largely ward patients, who usually did not have physical examinations unless they were ill. In our Presbyterian Hospital series, as well as in my personal series of cases, about half the patients were private patients, who presumably would have come for routine physical examination more often.

In this table I have divided my own data into two time periods—1943 to 1955 and 1956 to 1967—in an effort to see whether or not there has been any change in the proportion of carcinomas found by physicians performing routine physical examination. It would appear from my data that the proportion of carcinomas found by physicians has increased. In my 1943 to 1955 series of patients, 9.1 per cent of the carcinomas were found by physicians, whereas in my 1956 to 1967 series 16.5 per cent were detected in this way. I hope that this means that physicians are becoming more expert at detecting breast carcinoma. Mammography was not responsible for this change in my patients. The disease was detected by mammography in only five of the patients in my 1956 to 1967 series.

I must point out that the frequency with which physicians find carcinoma of the breast at physical examination of patients with no breast symptoms is directly proportional to their skill in examining the breast. Some physicians, who are not much interested in the problem of breast disease and who examine the breast inadequately, never seem to find breast carcinomas. On the other hand, I know two physicians, one an internist and the other an obstetrician, who have been especially interested in breast carcinoma and are unusually expert in breast examination, each of whom has found two or three unsuspected breast carcinomas every year. Almost all the carcinomas that they have found have been small and curable. Gynecologists and obstetricians have, of course, an exceptional opportunity to examine the breast; but not all of them take advantage of it.

DIAGNOSTIC ERRORS MADE BY PHYSICIANS

In any discussion of the diagnosis of breast carcinoma we should review our own failures in terms of missed diagnoses. I have studied the question in my personal series of cases.

Among the 1433 patients in my personal series of patients with breast carcinoma who came to me with signs or symptoms of the disease which they had themselves noted, there were 270 or 18.8 per cent in whom the diagnosis had previously been missed by a physician and wrong advice given. I have classified as wrong advice and treatment only such recommendations as all would agree to be obviously incorrect for carcinoma. In 19 per cent of these patients in whom the diagnosis had been missed, two or more physicians had erred. The added delay in diagnosis caused by the missed diagnoses in the 270 patients averaged 14 months.

I have attempted to analyze these errors by classifying them as follows:

1. Failure to examine a breast containing an obvious tumor while treating the patient for an unrelated disease.

The story of a recent patient illustrates this kind of error.

Mrs. A. L., a housewife aged 60, was admitted to the hospital for cardiac disease and a tumor of the breast. She had had heart trouble for 15 years, and had required digitalis and, during recent years, mercurial diuretics. She had been under the constant care of her local physician, who had examined her at least every two weeks and prescribed diuretics for her dyspnea and edema. Six months previous to her admission to our hospital, she had discovered a tumor of her right breast. She had not told her local physician about it, and since he had not examined her breasts on the many occasions when he had examined her heart, he had not found it.

She had an obvious 3 cm. carcinoma of the lower outer sector of her right breast. Because of her marginal cardiac reserve we chose to treat her with irradiation.

This error can be avoided to a degree by physicians examining the breasts as part of the general physical examination that they give every new patient. As Root has pointed out, however, when old patients, who are also old friends, drop in to a physician's office for a minor complaint, it is not easy to insist upon a general physical examination. The way to avoid missing something new in old patients is to follow the rule of doing a general physical examination, including examination of the breasts, at least every six months.

2. Failure of the physician, in his palpation of the breast, to feel the tumor that the patient had discovered and for which she came to consult him.

This mistake is illustrated by the experience of Mrs. C. D., aged 42, who happened to palpate her left breast as she lay in bed and discovered a small tumor in it. She went at once to her family doctor and pointed it out to him. He examined her breast but could not feel the tumor. He told her that there was "nothing wrong with her breast" and that she was "just nervous". He gave her "medicine to settle her nerves."

Six months later, the tumor persisting, she came to consult me. Her tumor, which was situated in the lower outer sector of the breast, was 2 cm. in diameter and entirely typical of a carcinoma.

This is the most difficult diagnostic error to avoid, because it depends upon palpatory skill, and not upon following rules. It is an all or none kind of error. If the patient has a tumor it must be investigated, but if no tumor can be felt, she is dismissed. When a patient states that she feels a tumor in her breast and her physician cannot feel it he should understand that he may be wrong and should insist that she return for re-examination in two or three months.

3. Mistaking a carcinomatous tumor of the breast for a breast infection.

This kind of mistake is more frequent since the discovery of antibiotics. It was made in the case of Mrs. L. H., aged 64.

Four months before she came to consult me, Mrs. L. H. had noted that her left nipple was becoming retracted. A month later she discovered a lump in the breast. Two months later the skin over the breast become red and hot and she consulted her family doctor. He diagnosed the lesion as an infection and prescribed sulfadiazine, and ice packs to the breast. With this treatment the inflammatory symptoms gradually disappeared, but the tumor persisted and she came to me for another opinion.

She had a large 10 cm. carcinoma with axillary metastases 2.5. cm. in transverse diameter. The redness had disappeared but limited edema of the skin remained.

This error can of course be avoided by biopsy. The existence of disease is obvious. Only its nature remains to be proved.

4. Wrongly diagnosing a carcinomatous tumor of the breast as a benign lesion, and failing to advise biopsy or excision.

A good example of this kind of error was found in the case history of Mrs. G. M., aged 44, a physician's mother-in-law, who consulted me for a tumor of her breast that she had discovered 24 months previously, while bathing. She had at once called it to the attention of her family doctor. He regarded it as benign and advised her to do nothing about it. He had been giving her weekly injections of estrogen for the previous two years because her menses had been irregular, and he continued this hormone therapy for a year after Mrs. M. had consulted him for her breast tumor. The tumor persisting, four other physicians—a surgeon, an internist, a gynecologist, and an otolaryngologist—were consulted regarding it. All diagnosed it as a cyst and advised no treatment.

The tumor nevertheless continued slowly to enlarge. When I saw Mrs. M., it measured 5 cm. in diameter, and although it was well delimited and comparatively movable in the breast like a cyst, it was hard, and there was slight dimpling of the skin evident in the forward bending position. At biopsy it proved to be a carcinoma.

This kind of error can be avoided by using aspiration or biopsy to prove the nature of every dominant tumor of the breast.

5. Disregarding a history of acute and sharp pain in the breast.

The following case illustrates the fact that even this infrequent symptom of breast carcinoma should not be ignored.

Mrs. R. K., aged 56, first developed a "sticking" pain in her right breast six months previously while in another hospital for a minor gynecological operation. She could not feel any tumor in her breast. She called the attention of her gynecologist to the breast pain and he told her that "it was nothing." After she returned home from the hospital the "sticking" pain recurred and she consulted two local physicians regarding it. The first told her that the pain was due to "a muscle strain" and gave her a salve. The second told her she had

"hardening of the arteries." She finally went to a public clinic from which she was sent to me.

I found that she had a small 2 cm. carcinoma in the upper outer sector of the breast—the region in which she had had the pain.

This error can be avoided by careful palpation of the breast in which the pain is centered.

6. Disregarding a definite retraction sign.

Three years before she came to consult me, Mrs. F. F., aged 52, had noticed a dimple in the lower portion of her left breast. She consulted her family physician about it. He said it was "old scar tissue—absolutely nothing to worry about." This reassured her until she noticed shrinkage of the breast as a whole two years later. But then her husband died and she had not got around to doing anything about her breast for another twelve months.

When I examined her, she had a 4 cm. carcinoma of the lower portion of the breast, fixed to the underlying tissues. The dimple had become a deep notch in the contour of the lower edge of the breast.

This error can be avoided by biopsy of the breast beneath an area of skin retraction. In almost all patients with retraction signs a tumor can be palpated. In two patients in whom there was definite skin retraction without a palpable tumor, however, I have biopsied the underlying breast. Although I did not find carcinoma in either of these patients, I believe that this practice is a sound one and that it will detect lesions that might otherwise be missed.

7. Failure to determine the cause of a nipple discharge.

The following case history is an example of the danger of disregarding a nipple discharge.

Mrs. H. H., a housewife aged 31, was referred to me by her physician. Ten months previously, while doing a routine physical examination, he had noted that watery fluid escaped from the right nipple during his palpation of that breast. This did not alarm him because he felt no tumor, and he took no action regarding it.

The nipple discharge—spontaneous, and always watery in character—continued for nine months. The patient then began to have pain in the breast and she returned to her physician who now found a tumor and sent her to me.

When I examined her, she had a 4 x 6 cm. tumor of the upper inner sector of the right breast with all the characteristics of a carcinoma. Cloudy fluid escaped from the nipple on palpation. There was a 1 cm. axillary node. The tumor proved on biopsy to be an intraductal papillary carcinoma and I performed a radical mastectomy. Five of 31 axillary nodes contained metastases.

8. Relying upon negative aspiration biopsy.

Those who use aspiration biopsy quite naturally come to depend upon it to exclude carcinoma. This leads them into missing carcinomas, as in the following case.

Mrs. L. M., aged 66, consulted me for a tumor in the upper part of her right breast that she had discovered two months previously. Her mother had had breast carcinoma and she was aware of the significance of a breast lump. She went to a surgeon who was a member of the staff of a breast service in a large special hospital for neoplastic disease—a man who had had extensive experience in the use of aspiration biopsy. He aspirated the tumor, and obtained tissue that his pathologist diagnosed as "negative." He assured the patient that her lesion was benign and advised her to go away for her summer vacation, as she had planned. The tumor continued to grow and two months later she consulted me.

When I saw her she had a clinically obvious breast carcinoma of the upper central portion of the right breast, measuring 6 cm. in diameter.

The way to avoid this error is to aspirate only clinically characteristic cysts. If my aspirating needle shows that the lesion is solid, and fluid is not obtained and the tumor remains, I proceed forthwith with incisional biopsy.

9. Relying on mammography rather than palpation.

Mrs. K. B., aged 39, secretary of a physician, discovered a "lump" in her left breast in May, 1965, and consulted her employer. He referred her for mammograms which were reported as showing a "cyst." Eight months later, when the lump was in her opinion larger, she was again sent for mammograms which were also negative.

In March, 1966, discouraged by her failure to get a diagnosis from her physician employer, she came to me. She had an obvious carcinoma of the upper outer sector of her left breast, 6 cm. in diameter, accompanied by skin retraction at several points.

Biopsy confirmed the diagnosis of carcinoma. Radical mastectomy was done. There were no metastases in 39 axillary lymph nodes.

Two years later, she had had no further evidence of breast carcinoma.

With the increasing use of mammography we see many patients in whom a definite dominant tumor had been palpated in the breast, which was not demonstrable by mammography. Physicians who do not palpate the breasts but instead send their patients for mammograms, as well as those who disre-gard the evidence of disease as revealed by palpation because it is not shown by mammograms, are very unwise. They will miss carcinomas.

Personal Diagnostic Errors

While pointing out the errors made by other physicians in the diagnosis of breast carcinoma I must not fail to point out my own. In the series of 1669 personal patients with breast carcinoma whom I studied between 1935 and 1967, I failed to diagnose the disease promptly in at least 17. I may, of course, have missed the diagnosis in other patients who consulted me, but I am thoroughly aware of my failure in these 17 patients.

I wish to present the histories of these 17 patients in some detail, and to analyze the reasons for my failures, in the hope that this kind of analysis will help others to avoid such errors. It is a heavy responsibility that we, as physicians, bear in the diagnosis of lesions of the breast. Each one of us must set for himself the highest standard of exactitude in the diagnosis of lesions of the breast, always seeking to improve our personal clinical skill and to discipline it by the pathologic diagnoses in our patients. We must also improve our medical education in regard to the diagnosis of breast lesions.

CASE 1

Mrs. M. O., a housewife aged 45, came to the Presbyterian Hospital in March, 1944, complaining of a tumor in the upper outer sector of her right breast that she had discovered while bathing. She had large, dense, dependent breasts. I examined her with care and failed to find the tumor. I dismissed her, and worst of all, I failed to ask her to return for another examination.

She returned of her own accord nine months later, in January 1945, again complaining of the breast tumor. This time I found the tumor. It was a small, 2 cm., firm, poorly delimited mass situated deeply in the upper outer sector of the right breast. Biopsy was done and the lesion proved to be a carcinoma. Radical mastectomy was performed. The carcinoma measured 1 cm. in diameter grossly. Metastases were found in one of nine axillary lymph nodes. The patient, fortunately, was well 22 years later.

CASE 2

Miss F. W., a 37 year old stenographer, consulted me in March, 1949, because she had begun, in January, to have pain in her right breast. The pain was centered in the outer portion of the breast, varied in type, and was accentuated during menstruation. In February she had become aware of a diffuse, barely palpable induration in the upper outer portion of the breast.

In my examination in March I found her right breast to be rather dense, but I did not make out any dominant tumor. I dismissed her.

She returned in July with a 6 cm., firm, poorly delimited tumor filling the outer middle sector of the breast. There was faint redness of the skin over the tumor, and a small area of edema of the skin caudad to it. There were several linear areas of retraction in the skin over the tumor. In the axilla there were several 0.5 cm. to 1 cm. hard nodes.

At biopsy the lesion proved to be a carcinoma. Radical mastectomy revealed metastases in 16 of 23 lymph nodes.

She developed right supraclavicular metastases in October, pulmonary metastases in December, and died in March, 1950.

Comment. My error in these two patients was to not give sufficient credence to their statements of having discovered a breast tumor by self-examination. I have since learned that patients can frequently palpate changes in the breast that I cannot detect. When a patient says that she has a tumor and I cannot palpate it, I do not stand on my dignity. I ask her to point it out to me and I search again for it.

CASE 3

Mrs. E. H., a widow aged 59, was sent to me in April, 1954, by her physician who had found, in the course of a routine physical examination, a small tumor of her left breast, of which the patient was entirely unaware.

In my examination I failed to find a tumor. The patient was vague as to how the supposed tumor had been found and as to its position in the breast. I further failed to insist upon learning her physician's name, and checking the discrepancy in our findings by talking with him.

She went back to her physician, who had the good sense to send her back to me asking me to re-examine her. When I did so in June I found the tumor, but only after she had pointed out its location to me. It was situated in the radius of 5 o'clock of the left breast, about 2 cm. beyond the areolar edge. It measured less than 1 cm. in diameter, but was firm and poorly delimited. There was a definite slight dimple in the skin over it when the arm was raised. I could feel the tumor easily when the patient sat up, but when she lay supine it disappeared into the soft subareolar breast tissue.

At biopsy it proved to be a carcinoma. Radical mastectomy showed metastasis in one of 18 axil-

lary lymph nodes. She was fortunately well 12 years later.

CASE 4

Miss J. O., a 72 year old retired teacher, was examined by Dr. Alice Baker who discovered a very small tumor beneath the caudad edge of the right areola and referred her to me in March, 1960. Her breasts were very atrophic and somewhat nodular. The tumor was only about 3 mm. in diameter and there was no associated retraction. I unwisely dismissed it as being only a nodule in the subareolar ridge. Five months later, Dr. Baker sent her back to me because the tumor was larger. It now measured 1 cm. in diameter and there was a suggestion of retraction over it. At biopsy it proved to be a carcinoma. There were no metastases in 19 axillary lymph nodes. She had had no recurrence of her carcinoma eight years later.

Comment. In both of these cases I failed to pay enough attention to the opinion of the referring physician. They were right and I was wrong. I have learned to respect the skill in breast examination of many physicians who refer patients to me.

CASE 5

Mrs. A. S., a housewife aged 53, consulted me in February, 1952, because during the previous two months she had occasionally noted a spot of blood on the left side of her brassiere.

I examined her left breast with care, giving special attention to the central subareolar area, but I could not make out any tumor. Neither could I find any pressure point that would produce a nipple discharge. I advised surgical exploration if and when the site of the presumed papilloma could be localized by repeated examination, and suggested that she return in three months for re-examination.

She did not come back to me but went to another physician after this period of time. He found that she had an undifferentiated carcinoma with axillary lymph node metastases.

CASE 6

Miss J. M., aged 34, was referred to me in November, 1957, because she had discovered a tumor in her left breast. It was a very well delimited, movable, soft 6 cm. adenofibroma situated in the upper outer sector of her left breast. I removed it through a circumareolar incision. She next consulted me in February, 1962, with the complaint that she had recently noted, on one occasion only, the discharge of a little bloody fluid from her left nipple. I examined her left breast with care but could feel nothing abnormal, nor could I find a pressure point producing a nipple discharge. I asked her to return for re-examination after a month but failed to convince her of the importance of doing so.

Although she continued to have occasional brownish nipple discharge, she did not consult me again until October, 1962, eight months later. Examination then showed a 1 cm. rounded tumor beneath the areola. At the edge of the breast in the radius of 5 o'clock there was a second 3 cm. rounded tumor with a similar well delimited contour. I did a biopsy of the subareolar tumor and found it to be a papillary carcinoma that invaded the duct system and the mammary parenchyma widely. There were no metastases in 37 axillary nodes.

In February, 1966, she developed metastases in her dorsal vertebrae, which were irradiated. In April, 1969, a parasternal internal mammary recurrence appeared, obviously originating from metastases in a node in the fourth or fifth interspace.

Comment. In the first of these patients with a nipple discharge but no localizing signs of disease, I made the mistake of failing to insist that she return for re-examination at monthly intervals. The three months interval that I suggested is too long. I failed to convince the second patient of the necessity for re-examination, and she waited too long.

The fact that only one out of every ten patients with a nipple discharge proves to have carcinoma should not diminish our alertness in making certain that the individual patient we are dealing with at the moment is not that one.

CASE 7

Mrs. L. S., an intelligent housewife, aged 43, consulted me under circumstances which led me in December, 1965, to examine her inadequately, and miss her breast carcinoma. I had excised an adenofibroma from the breast of her 18 year old daughter. In the daughter's hospital room, as I was sending the daughter home in her mother's care, the mother confessed to me that she had recently noticed that her own left nipple was retracted. She begged me to examine her then and there. I was at the end of a busy morning and short of time. I unwisely agreed to the mother's request, using the daughter's hospital bed as an examining table. I did not have good lighting and I probably missed the important fact that she had real nipple retraction. I did not palpate any tumor in the breast. I asked her to return for re-examination in three months.

She returned to consult me six months later. There was then no doubt about the presence of a tumor beneath her left areola. It was firm, poorly

delimited, and 3 cm. in diameter. The nipple was deeply retracted.

Biopsy revealed carcinoma. Radical mastectomy was done. There were no metastases in 49 axillary nodes. The patient is well three years later.

Comment. My mistake in this instance was being rushed and examining the patient under inadequate conditions. It is difficult enough to be accurate when one has adequate time and a quiet well equipped office.

CASE 8

Mrs. E. B., a housewife aged 33, consulted me in June, 1962, because of a small painful lump in her left breast which she had discovered three months previously. The tumor was a definite dominant tumor situated near the lateral edge of the left breast in the radius of 4 o'clock. It was only 5 mm. in diameter and was well delimited and movable in the surrounding breast tissue. Because of these characteristics and the comparative youth of the patient I thought it was an adenofibroma and advised her to return for re-examination in three months.

When she returned after four months the lesion was quite different. It now consisted of a chain of four small well delimited nodules. The one I had palpated four months previously was 1 cm. in diameter. The other three varied between 3 and 6 mm. in diameter.

I did a biopsy of the lesion, found it to be a well differentiated carcinoma, and performed radical mastectomy. There were no metastases in 40 axillary nodes.

Two years later she developed metastases in the cervical vertebrae, ribs, and pelvis, which were soon fatal.

CASE 9

Mrs. S. C., aged 41, consulted me in May, 1954, because another surgeon had found a small tumor in her left breast. I examined her and identified the tumor easily enough. It was situated in the outer sector of the breast in the radius of 3 o'clock about 6 cm. from the areola edge. It was rounded, well delimited, and firm, but it was not more than 3 mm. in diameter. It seemed movable within the surrounding breast tissue and there was no retraction over it. Chiefly because it was so small, movable, and well delimited, but also because the patient was reluctant to have it removed, I consented to observe it.

I examined her at six month intervals for five years until May, 1959. I then became convinced that the tumor was slightly larger, measuring about 8 mm. in diameter. I admitted her to the hospital, removed the small tumor, and found it to be a well-differentiated carcinoma, and did a radical mastectomy. There were no axillary metastases and she is well 17 years later.

Comment. In both of these patients I made the mistake of assuming that a very small well delimited and movable tumor occurring in a young woman was an adenofibroma. None of these features gives assurance that a tumor is not a carcinoma. Small well differentiated or circumscribed carcinomas may resemble adenofibroma very closely.

My studies of the age incidence of breast tumors have convinced me that carcinoma is so rare under the age of 25 that biopsy can be deferred until a convenient time. But in older patients carcinoma is more frequent and biopsy should be done promptly unless there are special contraindications.

The fact that the small carcinoma in the second patient did not show definite growth until five years had gone by is a warning against accepting the fact that a tumor does not grow as proof that it is benign.

CASE 10

Miss E. S. first consulted me in December, 1957, when she was 19. An adenofibroma had been excised from her right breast a year previously. She had a paternal aunt who had had breast carcinoma.

When I first examined her there was some irregular thickening along the line of the scar of her right breast operation but there was no dominant tumor in either breast. I next examined her in January, 1959, and found no breast disease.

She next consulted me again in July, 1967, because a new tumor had developed in her left breast. She was now 28 years old and had been married for four years. She had two children, aged 3 years and 1 year. She had nursed the first for 7 months and the second for 10 months. Examination now revealed a 1 cm. well delimited movable tumor situated just cephalad to the areola of her left breast. Because the new tumor had the characteristics of an adenofibroma, because she had already had one in her right breast, and because she was still in the age group when adenofibroma is common and carcinoma is rare, I assumed that this new tumor was another adenofibroma and I asked her to return for re-examination in two months.

When she returned in October, 1967, two additional small tumors measuring 3 and 10 mm. respectively were noted, situated just medial to the areola. They also had the character of adenofibromas. The fact that adenofibromas of the breast are frequently multiple and carcinomas are usually solitary strengthened my impression that all three tumors were adenofibromas.

When she was next examined in January, 1968, all three new tumors in the left breast were slightly larger and it was decided to excise them. The 1.5 cm. tumor situated medially to the areola was excised first and was found to be a circumscribed carcinoma. Radical mastectomy was done. All three of the tumors proved to be carcinomas of the same circumscribed type. There was a metastasis in one of 28 axillary nodes.

CASE 11

Mrs. D. F., a housewife aged 43, consulted me in March, 1955, because her breasts were large and nodular and her local physician thought he felt a dominant tumor in her left breast. Both her mother and a paternal aunt had had breast cancer.

At this time I found nodularity in the upper central portion of both breasts but no dominant tumor.

Six years later in April, 1961, she consulted me again. At this time there was a 1 cm. nodule in the upper central sector of her right breast that stood out among the other nodules. I admitted her to the hospital and did a biopsy but found only fibrosis.

I examined her at intervals of every three or four months. In November, 1962, I noted two prominent nodules in the upper central and middle outer sectors of her left breast. These did not seem as threatening as the similar nodule in the right breast on which I had done a biopsy the previous year.

When I next examined her five months later in April, 1963, the nodule in the upper central sector of the left breast had grown to be a definite dominant tumor, measuring 2 x 4 cm. Biopsy showed it to be a carcinoma. Radical mastectomy was done. There were no metastases in 23 axillary nodes.

Three years later she developed left supraclavicular metastases, and cerebral metastases to which she succumbed.

CASE 12

Mrs. M. W., a housewife aged 58, consulted me in June, 1960. She had been sent by her local physician who had found a tumor in her left breast. The patient insisted that she had had very "lumpy" breasts for many years.

Examination showed marked nodularity of the upper outer sector of both breasts. On the left side the upper outer edge of the area of nodularity was well delimited, and gave the impression of being a dominant tumor measuring 5 x 2 cm. There was no retraction. In a symmetrical area of the right breast there was a much smaller prominent nodule, measuring less than 2 cm. I admitted her to the hospital and did a biopsy of the left-sided tumor. It proved to be a characteristic area of fibrosis. Assuming that the similar smaller lesion on the right side was also fibrosis, I did not do a biopsy of it.

I examined her every few months and the right breast nodule did not change. She went abroad in November, 1962, and did not return to see me until November, 1963. I was then distressed to find that the right breast nodule had grown to become a 3 cm. dominant tumor. There was no retraction. In the right axilla there was a firm 1 cm. node. Biopsy confirmed the presence of carcinoma. Radical mastectomy was done. Sixteen of 24 axillary nodes contained metastases. She was given postoperative prophylactic irradiation to her chest wall, including the internal mammary area and her axilla. She had no recurrence of her carcinoma nine years later.

Comment. In all three of these patients I was prejudiced by the fact that a benign lesion had been excised — in one patient an adenofibroma, and in the other two patients areas of fibrosis. When new lesions developed which clinically resembled earlier benign lesions, I mistakenly assumed that they were similar in character.

I have learned from these experiences that in general every dominant tumor of the breast in women 25 years or older should be investigated by aspiration or biopsy, no matter what benign lesions the patient may have had.

CASE 13

Mrs. D. L., aged 65, was sent to me in December, 1961, by a physician who stated that a year previously he had found a small area of increased density in the outer middle sector of her right breast. In his opinion it had not changed during the year that he had followed it, but he was concerned and wished my opinion. The patient herself felt nothing abnormal in her breast.

I examined her carefully and could not make out anything more than a very small area of induration which I did not classify as a dominant tumor. It was agreed that a biopsy was not indicated but that her physician would examine her at regular intervals.

Thirteen months later I examined her again at his request and was still unable to identify a dominant tumor.

Eighteen months after my second examination she returned to me saying that she herself for the first time felt "something hard" at the site of the earlier area of induration. Examination now showed, at the site of this induration first noted three and one-half years previously, an easily recognizable 3 cm. carcinoma. She had a radical mastectomy at another hospital.

CASE 14

Mrs. H. W., a teacher aged 51, was sent to me in May, 1957, by her internist. She had called his attention to what she regarded as a questionable lump in her left breast which she had been aware of for five years. Her internist was not alarmed by it and neither was I. All that I could make out was increased nodularity in the upper outer sector of her left breast. I could not define a dominant tumor and there was no retraction or anything else

to suggest carcinoma. I did not believe a biopsy was indicated. It was agreed that her internist would examine her at regular intervals.

Two years and nine months later she came to see me again. She now had a definite 3 cm. carcinoma with some skin retraction at the site of the earlier "nodularity."

The diagnosis was confirmed at biopsy. Radical mastectomy was done and fortunately there were no metastases in 38 axillary nodes.

She is well 13 years later.

Comment. In both of these patients I palpated an abnormality in the breast, but it did not, in my opinion, constitute a dominant tumor requiring biopsy. In this decision I was of course wrong, but my error was perhaps excusable on the grounds that these patients' carcinomas were so small that it was not possible to recognize the need for biopsy. One cannot biopsy every abnormality in the breast. To do so would result in a great many unnecessary biopsies.

But I was entirely wrong in not insisting upon re-examining these patients myself at regular intervals. This kind of responsibility cannot be shared with the patient's physician, or indeed with anyone else.

CASE 15

Mrs. N. P., a teacher aged 49, consulted me in May, 1959, because ten weeks previously she had discovered a lump in her left breast. When I examined her I identified only a small area of what I regarded as increased nodularity in the outer middle sector of the breast. I did not classify it as a dominant tumor, and there was no retraction or any other sign suggesting carcinoma. I re-examined her after two months and found no change. I asked her to return again in six months. When she did the area of "nodularity" had become a definite dominant tumor, measuring 1.5 cm. in diameter.

Biopsy then revealed a well differentiated carcinoma. Radical mastectomy was done. There were no metastases in 22 axillary lymph nodes.

Comment. My error in this patient was in permitting a patient with a questionable area of nodularity to go without re-examination for six months. This is too long. Such a lesion should be re-examined every two months.

CASE 16

Mrs. J. M., aged 26, consulted me in September, 1961, complaining of a small tumor which she had discovered two months previously. She had a child, aged three years, whom she had not nursed.

Examination revealed a 1.5 cm. firm rounded tumor, fixed in the surrounding breast tissue in the upper central sector of her left breast. I advised excision and she was admitted to the hospital. When she was examined again the day before operation we could not palpate any breast tumor and she was discharged.

Three months later I examined her again and to my surprise I found the tumor to be exactly as I had originally palpated it in September. Puzzled by this sequence I asked her to return for another examination in three months, instead of recommending biopsy.

She did not return for three and one-half years. Then to my distress it was obvious that the tumor was a carcinoma, and had progressed to a comparatively advanced stage. The primary tumor measured 6 cm. in diameter. There was a 3 cm. movable axillary node. During the three and a half year interval during which I had not seen her she had had a second child, which she had not nursed.

Biopsy confirmed the diagnosis. Radical mastectomy was done. Two of a total of 32 axillary nodes contained metastases.

In December, 1966, she developed a left 1.5 cm. supraclavicular node which was assumed to be a metastasis and was irradiated.

In June, 1969, she had had no further evidence of disease.

CASE 17

Mrs. A. R., a housewife aged 51, consulted me in June, 1960, because her local physician had discovered a tumor of her left breast. She could not feel it herself. I found a poorly delimited area of increased nodularity in the upper outer sector of her left breast. She did not have, in my opinion, a dominant tumor. There was no retraction. I did not think biopsy was indicated.

I examined her again in two months and found no change. I asked her to return again in three months but she did not come back until a year later. At that time she had a well defined ovoid dominant tumor measuring 5 x 3 cm. at the site of what I had regarded as "nodularity." The tumor was nevertheless fairly movable within the breast and there was no retraction.

At biopsy the lesion proved to be a carcinoma. Radical mastectomy was done. There were no metastases in 54 axillary nodes. The patient had no recurrence of her disease nine years later.

Comment. I asked these two patients with lesions of questionable nature to return for early re-examination but they failed to do so. They both waited until their carcinomas were comparatively advanced.

When a patient has been asked to return for re-examination and she fails to do so, the consultant faces an insoluble dilemma. In our society where there is a free choice of physicians one can not very well telephone or write a patient and ask her to return. All that one can do to prevent this situation from develop-

ing is to take time to explain the diagnostic problem fully to every patient, to charge her only a reasonable fee, and to hope to inspire her confidence so that she will return for re-examination.

PROBLEMS IN DIFFERENTIAL DIAGNOSIS

Metastases of Mammary Carcinoma in Axillary Nodes Without a Palpable Breast Tumor

Occasionally mammary carcinoma metastasizes to axillary nodes, and forms a sizeable axillary tumor while the primary tumor in the breast is still too small to be palpable. In this sense these carcinomas are occult.

The great majority of isolated enlarged axillary nodes are, of course, inflammatory. Infrequently, such nodes are neoplasms, usually lymphoblastomas. Axillary metastasis from carcinoma of unknown primary site is very uncommon; yet, occult carcinoma of the breast must always be considered as the most likely diagnosis when a woman with an enlarged firm axillary node or group of nodes presents herself and no tumor can be found in the breast.

Another clinical form in which occult breast carcinoma manifests itself is as distant metastases in bone or viscera without an accompanying palpable tumor of the breast. The primary lesion is found only at autopsy. Horwitz, and Fitts and Horn, described cases of this type.

Halsted, a great expert in the diagnosis of breast carcinoma, as well as the originator of our modern operation, was the first to write of occult carcinoma of the breast. In his 1907 paper he described three cases. What he wrote is worth quoting:

I have twice seen extensive carcinomatous involvement of the axilla due to mammary cancer, which latter in neither instance became palpable or demonstrable for a considerable period after the axillary glands had attained conspicuous dimensions. In each case the "axillary tumors" had been removed, in one of them a year before, and in the other perhaps two years prior to my first examination which, though made in the most careful manner, failed to find the slightest evidence of cancer of either breast. In the course of a few months thereafter the mammary disease manifested itself in both patients.

A third patient was operated upon for enlarged glands of the axilla about two and a half years before she consulted me concerning the local axillary recurrence of the disease, and more especially to be relieved of severe neuralgic pains in the arms and legs. In this woman I found a large mass of axillary glands, which proved to be cancerous; but I found nothing in the breast except a quite definite parchment-like induration at the base of the nipple, which was retracted not at all, or merely to a barely appreciable degree.

During recent years there has been a flurry of papers regarding occult breast carcinoma. Good case reports have been presented by Rawls, Jackson, Cogswell, Rutkowski, Klopp, Fitts and Horn, Weinberger and Stetten, Rabinovitch, Huguet, Davidoff, Kaplan and Reinstine, Roux-Berger, Lamarina, and Larsen and his associates.

Pierce, Gray, and Dockerty reported that in a series of 41 women with isolated axillary adenopathy, biopsy had revealed metastatic adenocarcinoma of the axillary nodes in five. Three of the five were eventually shown to have occult breast carcinoma. In the other two women the primary carcinoma was not identified.

Atkins and Wolff reviewed their experience with nine patients with metastatic carcinoma in axillary nodes. In five a primary tumor was eventually found in the breast. In three of the five a considerable length of time (17, 10, and 9 months) elapsed between the biopsy which identified the axillary lesion as a probable breast carcinoma, and the appearance of the primary tumor in the breast. In four other patients mastectomy was not done and no primary source of the metastases was ever found.

Feuerman and his associates reported upon 14 patients with carcinoma in axillary lymph nodes. In 10, radical mastectomy was done; a primary lesion in the breast was found in seven. In four patients mastectomy was not performed, and the source of the metastasis was eventually found to be pancreatic carcinoma in one patient and gastric carcinoma in another; no primary carcinoma was ever found in the remaining two patients.

Until Owen, Dockerty, and Gray studied the question in the records of the Mayo Clinic, there had been no estimate of the frequency of the occult type of carcinoma of the breast. Among 5451 cases of breast carcinoma, they found 25, or 0.5 per cent, in which there was no breast tumor and no nipple discharge. The presenting symptom in these cases was an axillary tumor which proved on biopsy to be metastasis of adeno-carcinoma in lymph nodes. Radical mastectomy was then performed and an occult primary carcinoma found in the breast. None of the primary lesions was larger than 2 cm., and three were microscopic in size.

In the series of approximately 6000 breast carcinomas studied in the Presbyterian Hospital between 1916 and 1966 there were 18 cases in which the disease first manifested itself as an axillary metastasis with no palpable tumor in the breast. The essential features of these cases are shown in Table 24-2. There are several aspects of this group of cases that warrant discussion.

The duration of the axillary tumor was not so long as might be expected in view of its large size in most of the patients. Excepting one patient who admitted she had been aware of her axillary tumor for 18 months, the mean duration of the axillary tumor in the other 17 patients was only three months.

The axillary tumors were surprisingly large. In eight patients the axillary mass measured 5 cm. or more in diameter. The mean diameter was 4.7 cm. Three of four patients whose axillary metastases measured 5 cm. or more in diameter, and who were treated by radical mastectomy, were well more than 10 years later. Although the number of patients is small this experience suggests that our Columbia rule of classifying carcinoma of the breast as inoperable if the axillary metastasis is more than 2.5 cm. in diameter does not apply to the occult form of the disease.

The following case (Case No. 2 in Table 24-2), is a good example of the fact that occult breast carcinoma is operable even when the axillary metastasis is very large, provided that it is movable in the axilla.

Mrs. M. P., a widow aged 66, came to the Presbyterian Hospital because of a tumor of the left axilla that she had discovered two weeks previously.

In her left axilla there was a very large, firm, but movable tumor. It measured 8 x 5 cm. No tumor could be identified in the breast by Dr. Hugh Auchincloss, whose patient she was, or by several other examiners.

The axillary mass was first excised for diagnosis and was found to consist of two lymph nodes largely replaced by metastatic carcinoma. The larger measured 4.5 cm. and the smaller 1.2 cm. in diameter. Dr. Auchincloss then went ahead with radical mastectomy. On sectioning the mastectomy specimen a 1 cm. primary carcinoma was found in the upper outer sector of the breast. Sections of 15 axillary nodes dissected from the mastectomy specimen showed no metastases.

Table 24–2. Metastasis of mammary carcinoma in axillary lymph nodes without a palpable breast tumor. Presbyterian Hospital, 1916–1966

Case	Age of Patient	Axillary Tumor			Treatment	Pathology of Radical Mastectomy Specimen		End Results
		Duration	Clinical Features	Pathology		Breast	Axillary Contents	
1 (G.S.)	54	3 months	6 cm., movable	Carcinoma, 3 fixed nodes	Radical mastectomy	Grossly visible primary, 1 cm.	6 or 8 nodes involved	Generalized metastases, died in 4 months
2 (M.P.)	66	2 weeks	8 cm., movable	Carcinoma, 2 fixed nodes	Radical mastectomy	Grossly visible primary, 1 cm., upper outer sector	0 metastases, 15 nodes	Well, 25 years
3 (C.B.)	48	2 months	6 cm., movable	Carcinoma, 3 fixed nodes	1, Excision of axillary nodes; 2, radical mastectomy 64 months later	Grossly visible primary, 1 cm., upper outer sector	0 metastases, 19 nodes	Well, 15 years
4 (M.S.)	59	2 months	3 cm., movable	Carcinoma, 1 node	Radical mastectomy	No grossly visible primary; in 60 microscopic sections, two 5 mm. foci carcinoma, lower breast	1 of 17 nodes	Died other causes, 10 years, 4 months
5 (J.L.)	60	4 months	5 cm., movable	Carcinoma, 1 node	Radical mastectomy	No grossly visible primary; 6-mm. microscopic focus of carcinoma in subareolar area	0 mestastases, 40 nodes	Well, 11 years
6 (G.B.)	52	6 weeks	4 cm., movable	Carcinoma, 2 nodes	Radical mastectomy	Grossly visible primary, 1 cm., subareolar area	1 of 24 nodes involved	Well, 8 years
7 (J.R.)	50	4 months	5 cm., movable	Carcinoma, 1 node	Radical mastectomy	Grossly visible primary, 1.8 cm., beneath nipple	0 metastases, 20 nodes	Lung and bone metastases, died 7 years
8 (R.B.)	52	2 months	3 cm., movable	Carcinoma in 4 of 5 nodes	Radical mastectomy, postoperative irradiation	Grossly visible primary, 1 cm., upper inner sector	20 of 24 nodes involved	No local recurrence; pulmonary metastases, died 8 years
9 (B.F.)	47	4 months	3 cm., movable	Carcinoma, 1 node	Radical mastectomy	Grossly visible primary, 1 cm., upper central sector	3 of 38 nodes involved	Well, 5 years
10 (S.S.)	51	9 months	3 cm., movable	Carcinoma, 1 node	Radical mastectomy	No grossly visible tumor; 10 mm. microscopic focus of carcinoma in axillary prolongation	0 metastases, 30 nodes	Well, 2 years
11 (J.C.)	50	4 months	2 cm., movable	Carcinoma, 1 node	Radical mastectomy, postoperative irradiation	No grossly visible tumor; 10 mm. microscopic upper inner sector	26 of 46 nodes involved	Well, 18 months
12 (H.B.)	63	2 weeks	5 cm., fixed	Carcinoma in fused nodes	Radical mastectomy, postoperative irradiation	No grossly visible tumor; in 30 sections, one 5 mm. microscopic focus of carcinoma in upper outer sector	20 of 25 nodes involved	Local recurrence and metastases, died 12 months
13 (J.Q.)	40	6 months	4 cm., fixed	Carcinoma, 1 node	Radical mastectomy, postoperative irradiation	Grossly visible primary, 6 mm., lower inner sector	54 of 56 nodes involved	Local recurrence, pulmonary metastases, died 44 months

Table continued next page.

Table 24–2. Metastasis of mammary carcinoma in axillary lymph nodes without a palpable breast tumor. Presbyterian Hospital, 1916–1966 *(Continued)*

Case	Age of Patient	Axillary Tumor			Treatment	Pathology of Radical Mastectomy Specimen		End Results
		Duration	Clinical Features	Pathology		Breast	Axillary Contents	
14 (B.C.)	73	2 months	5 cm., fixed	Carcinoma in many fused nodes	Complete mastectomy	No gross or microscopic carcinoma	—	Local recurrence, skeletal and brain metastases, died 46 months
15 (H.N.)	35	4 months	8 cm., fixed	Carcinoma, 1 node	Irradiation	—	—	No primary demonstrated, died 47 months
16 (C.A.)	72	6 months	12 cm., fixed	Carcinoma, several fused nodes	Irradiation	—	—	No primary demonstrated, generalized metastases, died 6 months
17 (H.G.)	43	2 months	3 cm., several nodes movable	Carcinoma in several nodes	Irradiation because of bone metastases	—	—	Primary tumor of inframammary fold after 1 year, generalized metastases, died 45 months
18 (V.A.)	41	18 months	4 cm., movable	Carcinoma in 6 of 8 nodes	Irradiation	—	—	Primary subareolar tumor after 5 months, brain metastases, died 30 months

Although the carcinoma was undifferentiated in type, the patient is well 25 years after operation.

The most critical clinical prognostic factor in this series of 18 cases has been whether or not the axillary metastasis was fixed to the underlying tissue or to the overlying skin. In 13 of the patients the axillary metastasis was described as movable. Radical mastectomy was performed in 11. In nine of the 11 it was done more than five years ago. Eight of the nine survived more than five years. Three of the eight subsequently died with metastasis, seven, eight, and 10 years, respectively, after operation. But four of the eight patients are still well 8, 11, 15 and 25 years, respectively, after operation.

The axillary tumor was described as fixed in five of the patients. Three of the five were operated upon and all developed local recurrence and died within five years. I believe that irradiation would have been a better choice. Two other patients with fixed axillary metastases were treated by irradiation and succumbed after about the same length of time as those who had been operated. Our experience has, therefore, been that all the patients in this series whose axillary metastases were fixed succumbed, no matter how they were treated.

The following case (case no. 13 in Table 24–2) is a good example of the grave prognostic significance of fixed axillary metastasis.

Mrs. J. Q., a 40 year old housewife, had noted a small tumor in her left axilla six months before she came to the Presbyterian Hospital, and during the previous two months it had rapidly increased in size. On her admission to the hospital it measured 4 cm. in diameter. It was hard, and was solidly fixed to deeper axillary tissue. There was no palpable tumor in the breast.

Biopsy of the axillary mass was done and the mass was found to be metastatic from carcinoma in a node. The structure of the metastasis suggested origin from the breast. Radical mastectomy was done. On sectioning of the breast, a grossly visible primary tumor was found in its lower inner sector. A total of 56 nodes were found; 54 contained metastases. Postoperative irradiation was given. The patient developed local recurrence and pulmonary metastases and died after 44 months.

The question presented by an isolated axillary metastasis which microscopically resembles a metastasis from a breast carcinoma, although there is no palpable breast tumor, and no demonstrable primary anywhere else, is whether or not to perform radical mastectomy. In our breast clinics our surgeons facing this situation went ahead with mastectomy in 14 patients. Occult carcinoma was found in the breast in all but one of these patients. The details of the case (case no. 14, Table 24–2) in which the disease was not found in the amputated breast follow.

Mrs. B. C., a widow aged 73, had had an axillary tumor for two months. The tumor consisted of a group of firm, fixed nodes, measuring 5 cm. in diameter. The entire axillary mass was removed for biopsy. It was made up of many fused nodes filled with carcinoma resembling breast carcinoma.

A complete mastectomy was done. No grossly visible primary tumor was found in the breast. Although sections from 10 different blocks of tissue from different sectors of the breast were studied no focus of carcinoma was found.

The patient developed local recurrence, skeletal and brain metastases, and died 46 months after operation. Her course was so typical of breast carcinoma that it is likely that the primary focus in the breast was missed, and that more thorough microscopic study would have revealed it.

The occult impalpable primary focus of carcinoma in the breast in the 13 patients in whom it was found was grossly visible on sectioning the breast in eight. All the grossly visible primary lesions were small and measured approximately 1 cm. in diameter, with the exception of one which measured 1.8 cm.

In five other patients with no grossly visible primary tumor, very small microscopic primary foci of carcinoma were demonstrated. These foci would not have been found without the most painstaking pathologic study, in which many blocks of tissue were taken and many sections cut from them.

The following case (case no. 12, Table 24–2), illustrates the necessity for this kind of pathologic study.

Mrs. H. B., a housewife aged 63, came to the Presbyterian Hospital complaining of an axillary tumor which she said was of only two weeks' duration. The tumor was a hard mass, 5 cm. in diameter, solidly fixed in the axilla. There was no palpable tumor in either breast. A partial excision of the axillary mass was done. It consisted of fused nodes containing carcinoma that suggested mammary origin.

Radical mastectomy was performed. There was no grossly visible primary tumor in the breast. In one of 30 microscopic sections, from the lower inner sector of the breast, a single 5 mm. focus of carcinoma was found. It is shown in Figure 24–1. Twenty of a total of 25 axillary nodes contained metastases.

Although the patient was given postoperative irradiation she developed local recurrence and metastases, and died in 12 months.

It is of interest to note the site of the occult primary tumor in the breast. Its site was noted in 12 of the 13 patients in whom it was demonstrated. In three it was in the subareolar region, in four it was in the upper outer sector, in two it was in the upper inner sector, and in each of the remaining three the primary tumor was in a different sector of the breast. It is not surprising to me that the subareolar region was the most frequent site of these occult primary tumors. I have myself had more difficulty in palpating small tumors in this region than in any other sector of the breast.

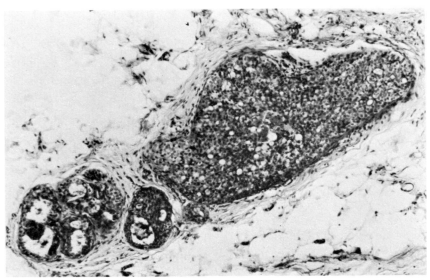

Figure 24–1. An occult 5 mm. microscopic primary focus of breast carcinoma which produced a 5 cm. axillary metastasis.

A final point of considerable interest concerning these occult breast carcinomas is the long latent period between the appearance of the axillary tumor and the development of a palpable tumor in the breast. Several clinicians, including Halsted and Roux-Berger, have emphasized this feature. Of our 18 cases there were three in which, the breast not having been removed, a primary tumor was detected in it 5 months, 12 months, and 64 months, respectively, after the axillary metastasis had been treated. The details of my own patient who had the longest latent period are worth presenting.

Mrs. C. B., a nurse aged 48, was admitted to the Presbyterian Hospital, for treatment of a tumor of the left axilla of two months' duration. Her past history was significant only in that 12 years previously a single cyst, 2 cm. in diameter, had been excised from just above the areola of her left breast.

In the lower left axilla there was a round, movable, 6 cm. tumor. The breast was examined by three of our surgeons specially skilled in the diagnosis of breast disease, none of whom could find a tumor. I also examined it and found nothing abnormal. The axillary tumor was excised locally and was found to consist of three encapsulated lymph nodes measuring 6 cm., 5 cm., and 3 cm., respectively. In all three the lymphoid tissue was almost entirely replaced by carcinoma, which resembled breast carcinoma. Although we recommended radical mastectomy on the grounds that there was probably an occult carcinoma in the breast, the patient demurred and we did not press the matter.

The patient's breasts were examined regularly by a skilled examiner, but it was not until five years and four months after the axillary metastases had been discovered that a tumor was found in the left breast. It was situated in the radius of 2 o'clock, about 6 cm. out from the areolar edge. It measured 2 cm. in diameter, and had the firm, poorly delimited character of a carcinoma.

I did a biopsy of the breast tumor, which lay deep in the substance of the breast, proved it to be a carcinoma, and performed a radical mastectomy. Study of the operative specimen showed the primary tumor to be only 1 cm. in diameter. It was a moderately undifferentiated carcinoma. There were no metastases in 19 lymph nodes. The patient was well 15 years later.

The inescapable fact in this case is that it took more than five years for the occult breast carcinoma to grow to a diameter of 1 cm. and become palpable, after it had given rise to large axillary metastases.

Our conclusion from this experience with 18 patients is that when careful microscopic study of the biopsy of the axillary tumor strongly suggests an origin from the breast, and no other source of the metastasis can be found, radical mastectomy should be done, provided that the axillary metastasis is not fixed in the axilla. The disease is incurable when there is axillary fixation, and irradiation is the reasonable method of treatment.

Heterotopic Apocrine Cysts in Axillary Lymph Nodes

A rare benign form of enlargement of axillary lymph nodes, which can simulate metastasis to axillary nodes from an occult carcinoma of the breast, is due to heterotopic apocrine cysts within the nodes. We have recently studied an example of this phenomenon which is unique in our case files. The patient was a woman aged 51 in whom my associate Kister found a firm 2.5 cm. axillary node. There was no palpable lesion in the breast. He removed the node fearing that it was a metastasis from an occult carcinoma in the breast.

The node contained cysts filled with debris. Microscopically the cysts were lined with flattened epithelium and filled with keratin (Fig. 24-2). Some of the keratin had escaped into the node and set up a granulomatous reaction with foreign body cells. The origin of the process was from small heterotopic apocrine cysts lined with the characteristic cylindrical acidophile epithelium. They were found not only in the large lymph node but in two of three small lymph nodes excised with it. Figure 24-3 shows one of these small heterotopic apocrine structures. As they enlarge, their epithelial lining becomes cuboid, but retains in places the characteristic apocrine snouts. Finally, the epithelium undergoes squamous metaplasia and fills the cyst with keratinized debris.

McDivitt, Stewart, and Berg mention having seen this phenomenon in an axillary lymph node in two cases, and assume that it represents "metastasis" of benign breast ducts.

Since the heterotopic elements in our case were so clearly apocrine it is likely that they originated either from the nearby subcutaneous apocrine glands of the axillary skin, or from the axillary extension of the breast. This is a theoretical point of no importance. What is important is that this lesion can simulate metastasis in an axillary lymph node.

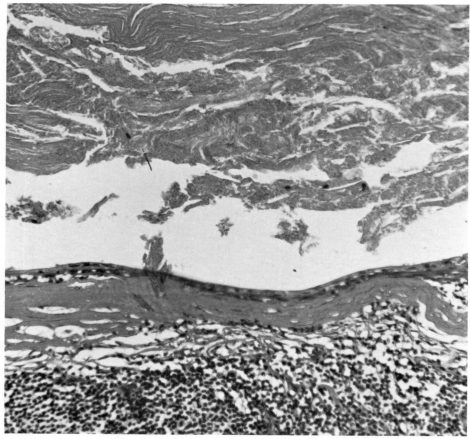

Figure 24–2.   Large heterotopic apocrine cyst filled with keratin debris in an axillary lymph node.

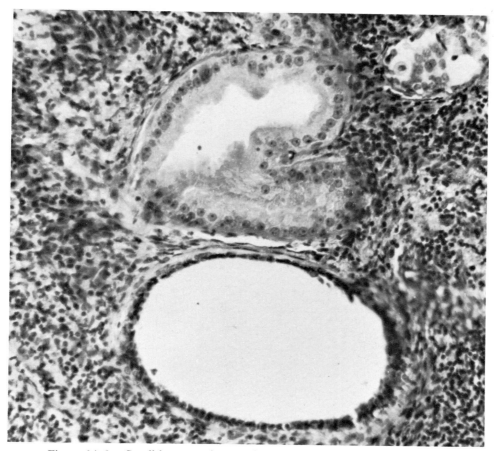

Figure 24–3. Small heterotopic apocrine cysts in an axillary lymph node.

Carcinoma in the Axillary Prolongation of the Breast

Another difficult type of breast carcinoma to diagnose is that arising in the axillary prolongation of the mammary gland. As I pointed out in Chapter 1, a good many women have such axillary mammary tissue. When carcinoma develops in it, the tumor is usually mistaken for lymph node disease. Mornard, Piccagli, Dickinson, Stringa, and Chiari have described cases of carcinoma arising in axillary mammary glands.

In the Presbyterian Hospital records we have several cases of this kind. Three of them are worth summarizing because they illustrate the special therapeutic problems which these cases pose.

CASE 1

Mrs. U. M., a Negro housewife aged 41, was admitted to the Presbyterian Hospital for a tumor of the left axilla. She was three months pregnant. She had first noted the axillary tumor 15 months previously, during a pregnancy that ended in a miscarriage. During the five months prior to her admission the axillary tumor had gradually increased in size.

Examination showed a stony hard, irregularly nodular tumor of the left axilla, measuring 4 x 6 cm. It was fixed to the deeper axillary structures and to the overlying skin. The skin attachment is shown in Figure 24-4. No tumor was palpable in either breast.

The axillary mass was excised and was found to be a carcinoma measuring 5 x 4 cm., arising in axillary mammary tissue. At the upper pole of the axillary specimen there were several large lymph nodes containing metastases. Radical mastectomy was performed. No carcinoma was found in the breast tissue removed by the mastectomy.

The patient received postoperative irradiation to the operative field and the supraclavicular area, and ovarian irradiation. She shortly miscarried. Twelve months after operation, however, local recurrence on the chest wall developed, and she died with widespread metastases to bones after another two years.

Comment. This patient's disease was inoperable in the sense that it formed a large fixed axillary mass. She should have been treated by irradiation rather than surgery.

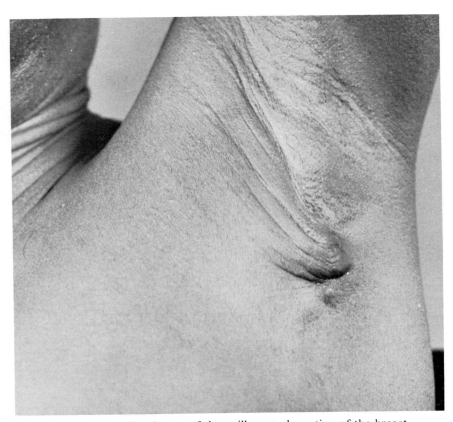

Figure 24-4. Carcinoma of the axillary prolongation of the breast.

CASE 2

Mrs. S. M. was a widow aged 50 when she developed a small axillary tumor. Her local physician incised it with the mistaken impression that it was a furuncle. The nodule persisted, and after ten months she was admitted to another hospital where it was excised locally through a transverse incision across the axilla. It was carcinoma arising in the axillary prolongation of the breast.

The patient then consulted me. I found a good deal of induration in the axilla at the site of the local excision. I assumed that this represented persisting carcinoma, and that there was no hope of getting the disease out of the axilla surgically. There was no palpable tumor in the breast, and no evidence of distant metastases.

She was treated by irradiation to the axillary and supraclavicular regions. She had no evidence of recurrence six years later.

Comment. If this patient's disease had been recognized when she first consulted a physician, and only a small biopsy done, it probably could have been treated successfully by radical surgery.

CASE 3

Mrs. H. F., came to the Francis Delafield Hospital at the age of 31 with three 1 cm. tumors in her right breast and two 3 cm. tumors in her left breast. The tumors had the clinical characteristics of adenofibroma. She had had two adenofibromas excised from her right breast when she was 24.

The two larger adenofibromas in the left breast were excised, and the small ones in the right breast were followed. They had not changed nine years later when she noted a small right axillary tumor. It was situated in the middle of the axilla. It was 1 cm. in diameter, firm, and although movable over the deeper structures of the axilla, it was fixed to the overlying skin. It was just beneath the skin. The resident surgeon was so convinced that it was a benign lesion of the skin that he excised it locally. It proved to be a small carcinoma arising in mammary tissue. It was a true primary carcinoma in the axillary prolongation of the breast.

The challenge in terms of surgical technique presented by a primary carcinoma in this axillary position was solved in this patient in a manner which I will describe in Chapter 34, where I discuss the technique of radical mastectomy.

No residual carcinoma was found in the breast removed in this patient. There were no metastases in 26 axillary lymph nodes.

The outstanding clinical feature of carcinomas developing in the axillary prolongation of the breast, exemplified in cases 2 and 3 that I have described above, as well as in several similar cases in our records, is that in its early stages while it is still small this lesion is usually mistaken for a lymph node or a benign subcutaneous axillary tumor. This is, of course, understandable in view of the fact that when mammary tissue extends up into the axilla it usually exists only as a thin subcutaneous layer. A carcinoma developing in it is necessarily subcutaneous.

Carcinoma Producing a Nipple Discharge but No Palpable Tumor

When a patient with a nipple discharge also has a breast tumor, or when a point in the breast can be found upon which pressure produces the nipple discharge, thus localizing the breast lesion and making it possible to place the exploratory incision in the appropriate sector of the breast, there is no doubt about what to do. The lesion should at once be investigated surgically.

But when there is no palpable tumor and no pressure point can be found, the surgeon's dilemma is a difficult one. If he explores the breast blindly and makes his circumareolar incision on the wrong side of the areola, opposite to that in which the diseased ducts are situated, he may not find the papilloma or the small carcinoma responsible for the nipple discharge. Surgeons of a generation ago could put off such patients and wait until the site of the lesion in the breast could be found by re-examination, because Hart, who had written one of the best papers on nipple discharge, had stated that in his Johns Hopkins data there was no case of breast carcinoma with a nipple discharge but no accompanying breast tumor.

Today, unfortunately, we know that such cases, although rare, do occur. Fitts and Horn have described four cases of breast carcinoma in which there was a nipple discharge but no breast tumor. Kilgore and his associates also referred to four such cases which they observed, although they describe only one of them.

In my personal series of 1669 patients with breast carcinoma (1943–1967) whose symptoms I have documented, there were 39 who had a nipple discharge. All but five also had a palpable tumor. These patients without a palpable tumor are so infrequent that I will present summaries of the case histories of all five.

The case histories of the first two patients are included in my series of personal diagnostic errors already described (Cases 5 and 6, p. 482). I missed the diagnosis initially in both.

The case histories of the other three patients follow.

Miss M. B., a spinster aged 69, consulted me because of a discharge from the right nipple. Ten months previously she had fallen and struck her breast slightly. Shortly thereafter she noted on two occasions a few drops of blood spotting her nightgown opposite her right nipple. This had recurred recently and led her to consult me.

Her breasts were symmetrical and no tumor was palpable in either one. On palpation of the right circumareolar region a pressure point, found at the radius of 8 o'clock, produced a drop of brown serous discharge from a duct in the center of the right nipple. Prompt surgical exploration was advised.

She was operated upon by my associate, David Habif. Through a circumareolar incision the collecting ducts leading to the base of the nipple from the outer sector of the breast were exposed. One of them was seen to be dilated and filled with dark blood. It was severed at the base of the nipple, and a cone of breast tissue surrounding it was excised. The gross study of the specimen revealed a friable, soft, yellowish tumor in the proximal portion of the dilated duct. The microscopic sections showed that there were multiple benign papillomas in several of the ducts, and in one, intraductal carcinoma.

Right radical mastectomy was done a week later. No residual papilloma or carcinoma was found in the specimen, and no metastases were found in 26 lymph nodes.

Eighteen months later Dr. Habif, in his examination of the patient, found a 5 mm. tumor in the left breast. It was situated 2 cm. from the areolar margin in the radius of 10 o'clock. There was dimpling of the skin over the tumor when the patient was in the forward-bending position. The tumor was excised and showed the same lesions as had been encountered in the right breast, benign intraductal papilloma and intraductal carcinoma. Since the patient was 71 and her breast disease was not regarded as much of a threat to her, only left complete mastectomy was done. In the amputated breast diffuse benign intraductal papilloma, but no more carcinoma, was found.

Mrs. J. B., a housewife aged 40, consulted me because of "congestion" of the lower half of the left breast. Her maternal grandmother had had breast carcinoma. Her fourth child had been born 15 months previously. She had not nursed any of her children.

On examining her, all that I found was that the lower half of her left breast was denser than the corresponding sector of her right breast. There was no true dominant tumor. I asked her to return in one month for re-examination. When she returned she reported that she had had a brownish discharge from her left nipple for several days following my examination. There was now a finely nodular area of increased density below and lateral to the areola, although I did not describe it as a true dominant tumor. There were no palpable axillary nodes.

Biopsy, however, revealed intraductal and papillary carcinoma. Radical mastectomy was performed. Thirty-four of 55 axillary nodes contained metastases.

Within 10 months she developed clinical evidence of carcinoma in the contralateral breast, and pulmonary and liver metastasis. She died three years after her mastectomy.

Miss E. G., aged 60, consulted me because she had developed a serous discharge from her right nipple. She had had a hysterectomy and removal of one ovary at the age of 34, and for many years had taken Premarin daily.

Examination revealed no tumor in the breast. Pressure on the medial side of the areola produced a serous discharge from a central duct. I explored the subareolar area through a medial circumareolar incision and found two dilated bluish ducts entering the base of the nipple. As I dissected them peripherally I found other ducts containing brownish soft papillary tumors and I realized I was probably dealing with papillary carcinoma. I terminated my dissection after removing tissue for pathologic study.

Permanent sections revealed multiple papillomatosis associated with papillary carcinoma of the apocrine papillary type. There were no metastases in 28 axillary nodes.

Two and one-half years later I found a 2 cm. firm tumor, fixed in surrounding breast tissue just lateral to the areola of her left breast. Biopsy revealed that she had the same disease in her left breast that she had had in her right breast. Radical mastectomy was done. Two of 27 axillary lymph nodes contained metastases.

She has had no recurrence six years after her left and three years after her right breast carcinoma.

My experience in these cases has forced me, reluctantly, to the conclusion that in patients with a spontaneous nipple discharge a surgical search for the lesion must be carried out with reasonable promptitude, even though there is no palpable tumor or pressure point to indicate the site of the disease. The great majority of these patients without localizing signs will have benign intraductal papilloma, and the surgical search for the papilloma will be greatly handicapped if it has to be attempted without any indication as to the radial position of the lesion in the circumareolar region. In order to minimize the number of cases in which exploration has to be done without such localizing information, I suggest the compromise of deferring operation for a month and examining the patients at weekly intervals during this period, searching for a pressure point that will betray the radial site of the lesion. In the rare lesion that proves to be a carcinoma, one month's delay will not add greatly to the hazard, while the task of finding the papillomas that produce the discharge in most of the patients will often be simplified by the localizing information found by repeated examination. Delay longer than one month is, however, unwise, for the possibility that the cause of the nipple discharge is carcinoma is remote but real.

In occasional cases the clinical circumstances in a patient with a history of spontaneous nipple discharge are such that surgical exploration is not reasonable. The following is such a case:

Mrs. G. L., a housewife, age 40, was sent to me in November, 1949. Her history was that since the age of 20 she had occasionally had slight bloody discharge from the nipples of both breasts. The discharge was sufficient to stain the sheets and her brassiere. From the age of 37 on, the discharge had almost completely disappeared. She came to consult me because within the month the discharge had begun again, this time from the right breast, from which there had been an occasional drop of dark blood.

On examination her breasts were normal. I could not make out any tumor in either breast. I could find no pressure point which would produce the discharge.

She has been followed at intervals and no tumor has developed in either breast. The discharge has disappeared. There was no evidence of disease in her breasts in January, 1955, more than five years after I first saw her.

A phenomenon that is not an indication for surgical exploration is the slight bloody nipple discharge that occurs from both breasts in some pregnant women. This is an expression of the intensity of the epithelial proliferation in the rapidly proliferating mammary epithelium. A milky secretion continuing long after lactation is apparently over is of course another physiologic phenomenon that does not require surgical investigation.

Hemorrhage Produced by Trauma Obscuring Carcinoma of the Breast

In our records we have several cases in which trauma to the breast produced ecchymosis. This led to the discovery of a tumor adjacent to the ecchymosis. Instead of assuming that the tumor was caused by hemorrhage and fat necrosis we fortunately did a biopsy and found the underlying carcinoma. The following case history illustrates this deceptive diagnostic problem.

Mrs. A. G., a housewife aged 54, with rather large dependent breasts, discovered a black and blue area in the skin of the inner portion of her left breast, and a lump beneath it. This was four weeks after she had been struck in the same breast by a ball. She could not recall any other trauma to the breast.

When I examined her a month after she had discovered the ecchymosis, a slight residuum of it was still visible in an area of skin about 6 cm. in diameter medial to the areola of the left breast. Just at the edge of the areola there was a 4 cm. firm, poorly delimited tumor, relatively fixed in the surrounding breast tissue. There was slight retraction of the skin just below and medial to the tumor.

I was afraid that the tumor was a carcinoma and that the hemorrhage had resulted from trauma to it. Biopsy and frozen section proved me correct. Radical mastectomy was, of course, performed. She never had recurrence of her breast carcinoma, but died six years later of other causes.

Duct Ectasia Simulating Carcinoma

The most difficult lesion to distinguish from carcinoma of the breast, because of the marked degree of fibrosis and the resulting retraction signs which it produces, is duct ectasia. I have described its characteristics in Chapter 10 but wish to emphasize again here that it is clinically indistinguishable from carcinoma. Among all the lesions that occur in the breast, it is the most likely to deceive the clinician into thinking that he must be dealing with a carcinoma and that it is safe to go ahead with radical mastectomy without a biopsy. The occurrence of this deceptive lesion in the breast is sufficient reason in itself to make it necessary always to perform a biopsy before carrying out mastectomy.

There are one or two features of duct ectasia which may suggest its presence. One is the fact that the tumor of duct ectasia usually lies in the central area of the breast beneath or close to the areola. A second point is that the signs of inflammation which evolve with this lesion are less acute than with an ordinary breast abscess, and more localized than with inflammatory carcinoma. Finally, the disease, unlike an ordinary abscess, occurs in women who have not recently lactated.

Lymph Nodes Within the Breast Area

In a number of patients I have performed a biopsy of a small tumor of the upper outer sector of the breast which I thought was a lesion of the breast itself, either a cyst or a carcinoma, and found that it was only an enlarged lymph node. The breast tissue normally extends laterally across the lower portion of the anterior axillary fold, and in women with good-sized breasts this upper outer margin of the breast may be rather thick. Occasionally an enlarged lower axillary lymph node will be found situated low along the edge of the pectoral fold, or near the edge of the pectoral fold upon the ventral surface of the pectoralis muscle, seemingly well within the limits of the upper outer sector of the breast. Such a lymph node, when covered by breast tissue, feels firm and only moderately well delimited. It cannot be distinguished clinically from a tense cyst or a small carcinoma.

Painful Costochondral Swelling (Tietze's Syndrome) Simulating Breast Carcinoma

Although Tietze's syndrome is not a disease of the breast at all, patients occasionally come with it, thinking that they have a breast lesion because they have a painful tumor in the breast area. Tietze, of Breslau, in 1921, first described the painful swelling of the costochondral cartilages which has become known by his name. Internists and thoracic surgeons were among the first to emphasize the importance of this lesion in a series of reports in the early 1950's (Gill, Jones, and Pollack; Beck and Berkheiser; Wehrmacher; Frey). Kayser, as well as Karon, Achor, and Janes, collected reports of a total of 159 cases by 1958. More recently, interesting discussions of this syndrome have been published by Barnes and Graham, by Landon and Malpas, by Skorneck, by Rawlings, and by Burch and De Pasquale.

Chest pain is the symptom that leads the patient to discover a tender mass which is in reality enlargement of one of the costochondral cartilages. The pain may be dull, or sharp enough to suggest angina pectoris if the lesion is on the left side. It often radiates laterally and is sometimes aggravated by coughing or deep breathing.

Many of the patients with Tietze's syndrome have had a recent respiratory infection, but beyond this fact the pathogenesis of the disease remains unknown. When one of these swollen cartilages has been removed no pathologic changes are seen.

The symptoms usually subside spontaneously after a few weeks or months. Nerve block for relief of the pain may be required.

The distinction between Tietze's syndrome and a tumor of the breast is easy enough if the diagnostician is familiar with the syndrome. It is exceedingly unusual for a breast neoplasm to produce as much pain as does Tietze's syndrome.

Metastatic Tumors of the Breast

Even though a breast tumor is malignant, and of epithelial origin, the possibility of its being a metastasis to the breast from a primary carcinoma in some other site must be kept in mind. This sequence, however, is infrequent. Dawson collected reports of 10 such cases and added one, an example of metastasis of carcinoma of the stomach to both breasts. Speert and Greeley, and Schumann described individual cases. Charache described six such cases, two originating in the ovary, one from a melanoma, and one each from kidney, adrenal, and uterine carcinomas. Wheelock and his associates reported two instances of metastasis of melanoma to the breast. Ibach found reports of 41 metastatic tumors of the breast, and described the fifth example of an ovarian carcinoma metastasizing to the breast. Sandison, reviewing a total of 1724 malignant and benign breast lesions in Glasgow, found eight that were metastatic—one from leukemia, two from lymphoblastomas, one from melanoma, and one each originating from bronchial carcinoma, leiomyosarcoma, gastric carcinoma, and renal carcinoma.

Sandison also studied at autopsy the breasts in 148 females who died of malignant disease other than that originating in the breast. Nine had metastases to the breast—two from bronchial carcinoma, one from pancreatic carcinoma, three from leukemia, and three from lymphoblastoma.

In their autopsy study of the breasts of 52 women who died of malignant disease other than that in the breasts in our hospital, Frantz and her associates found one metastasis to the breast from gastric carcinoma, one from cervix carcinoma, three from leukemia, and one from lymphosarcoma.

In our department of surgical pathology we have had two examples of metastasis of non-mammary malignant tumor to the breast, one a carcinoma of the thyroid and the other a carcinoid of the ileum. Brief summaries of these cases follow.

Mrs. H. M., a housewife aged 39, developed a nonproductive cough and weakness. When she came to the Presbyterian Hospital 10 weeks later, two lesions were found—a hard, 2 cm. fixed mass in the left lobe of the thyroid, and a 5 x 8 cm. oval shadow with well defined margins just below the middle of the left lung.

Biopsy of the thyroid tumor was done, and the tumor proved to be a poorly differentiated primary thyroid carcinoma. It was assumed that the lung lesion was a metastasis and irradiation to both the thyroid and the lung lesions was begun.

Two months after the diagnosis had been established, a tumor was found in the right breast. It was a hard, 3 cm. mass situated in the lower outer sector of the breast. There was retraction of the overlying skin. It was excised locally and proved to be metastatic thyroid carcinoma. The patient died with cerebral metastases four months after her cough had begun.

Mrs. K. B., a Negro housewife aged 55, came to the Presbyterian Hospital because of acute gastro-intestinal symptoms suggestive of cholecystitis. She proved not to have biliary disease, but physical examination revealed a 2 cm. firm but movable tumor of the upper outer sector of the right breast, with slight retraction of the overlying skin. The patient insisted that she had had the tumor for 17 years and that it had increased in size only very slightly during the past year.

Under general anesthesia a wedge of the tumor was excised for biopsy, and a frozen section diagnosis of carcinoma was made. Radical mastectomy was performed. When the primary tumor was studied with care in permanent section it was realized that its structure (Figs. 24–5 and 24–6) was that of a carcinoid tumor. Differential stains showed strongly positive argentaffin granules (Fig. 24–7) in many of the tumor cells, confirming this diagnosis. There were no metastases in 37 axillary lymph nodes.

The patient admitted that she had had an intestinal operation 10 years previously in the Wheeler Clinic in Lafayette, Alabama. The report from the clinic revealed that a portion of her ileum had been resected for a carcinoid tumor that had infiltrated all layers of the intestinal wall and metastasized to one mesenteric lymph node.

It was also learned that the patient had had an exploratory laparotomy at the Harlem Hospital two years previously for an abdominal mass. An enlarged nodular liver was found, containing tumor suggestive of carcinoid.

When last seen two years after her mastectomy the patient was surprisingly well.

This case is, therefore, an example of a very slowly evolving carcinoid of the ileum that metastasized to the breast and liver.

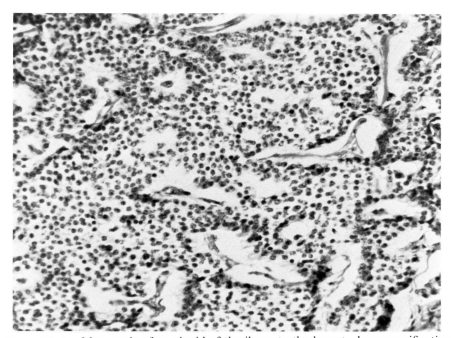

Figure 24–5.   Metastasis of carcinoid of the ileum to the breast—low magnification.

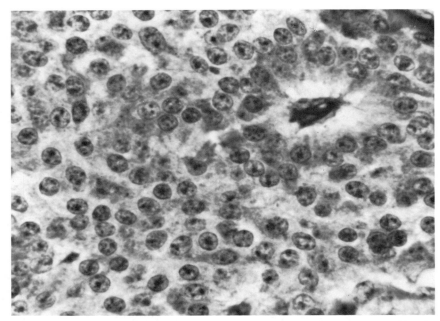

Figure 24–6.   Carcinoid of the ileum metastatic to the breast — high magnification.

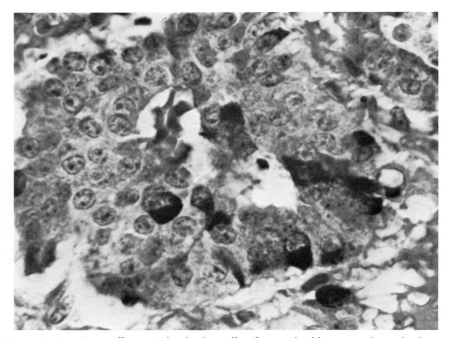

Figure 24–7.   Agentaffin granules in the cells of a carcinoid metastatic to the breast.

DIAGNOSTIC TESTS FOR BREAST CANCER

Unfortunately, there is no laboratory test, excepting, of course, microscopic study of tissue, that enables us to recognize carcinoma of the breast. Much clinical evidence suggesting that the steroid hormones play a part in the origin and growth of the disease has accumulated during recent years. Many efforts have been made to demonstrate abnormalities in the excretion of urinary steroids in patients with breast cancer. Although claims have been made, they have not won general confirmation.

In Chapter 5 I have discussed at some length mammography, infrared thermometry, and other techniques for diagnosing breast disease. All have only a very limited value.

GENERAL DIAGNOSTIC RULES

Although I invariably perform incisional biopsy to prove the nature of a breast lesion before carrying out any radical treatment, it is helpful for many reasons to develop as high a degree as possible of clinical skill in differentiating carcinoma from other breast lesions. The time and convenience saved in planning operative schedules by being able to guess the diagnosis fairly accurately is alone a sufficient reason for cultivating diagnostic skill.

I have discussed the clinical characteristics of most of the lesions of the breast in the preceding chapters, and all I can do at this point is to suggest some general rules that may help in differential diagnosis.

One of these rules is that the smaller the primary tumor, the more difficult is its clinical diagnosis. Carcinomas 1 cm. or less in diameter may not produce an appreciable degree of retraction, and they are very difficult to distinguish from cysts, adenosis, fibrous disease, etc. I have learned to be very cautious about predicting the nature of the very small breast lesions. Larger carcinomas are usually betrayed by their lack of delimitation, their relative fixation in the breast tissue, and the retraction that they produce.

Finally, the diagnostician is influenced to some degree by facts in the history of the individual patient. The fewer children a woman has had and the later in life she began to have them, the more likely she is to have breast carcinoma. The older she is, the more likely she is to have the disease. There are five special groups of women who are particularly predisposed to develop breast carcinoma:

1. Women with a family history of breast carcinoma
2. Women who have had breast carcinoma in one breast
3. Women who have had gross cystic disease of the breasts
4. Women with lobular neoplasia (lobular carcinoma in situ)
5. Women with multiple papilloma of the breast

SUMMARY

The price of skill in the diagnosis of breast carcinoma is a kind of eternal vigilance based upon an awareness that any indication of disease in the breast may be due to carcinoma. The physician's sympathy with a patient's distress, the seemingly benign physical character of a breast lesion, a natural desire to avoid all the hard work that goes into dealing with a carcinoma—all conspire to lull the physician into a state of mind in which he tends to think of the lesion as benign. When a biopsy is decided upon the surgeon must follow the strict rule of always explaining to the patient that the clinical evidence is not final, and that the definitive diagnosis is based upon the microscopic findings after biopsy. She must always be told of the possible necessity of radical mastectomy, and must give her approval. All these preparations, if they serve no other purpose, keep the surgeon alert to the threat of carcinoma.

REFERENCES

Atkins, H., and Wolff, B.: The malignant gland in the axilla. Guy's Hosp. Rep., 109:1, 1960.

Barnes, N., and Graham, J.: Parasternal chondrodynia (Tietze's syndrome). Ann. Int. Med., 51:57, 1959.

Beck, W. C., and Berkheiser, S.: Prominent costal cartilages (Tietze's syndrome). Surgery, 35:762, 1954.

Burch, G. E., and DePasquale, N. P.: Tietze's disease. Geriatrics, 19:61, 1964.

Charache, H.: Metastatic tumors in the breast. Surgery, 33:385, 1953.

Chiari, H. H.: Zur Frage des Karzinoms in aberrantem Brustdrüsengewebe. Brun's Beitr. z. klin. Chir., 197:307, 1958.

Cogswell, H. D.: Hidden carcinomas of the breast. Arch. Surg., 58:780, 1949.

Cogswell, H. D., and Czerny, E. W.: Carcinoma of aberrant breast of the axilla. Am. Surg., 27:388, 1961.

Davidoff, R. B.: Occult carcinoma of the breast. Geriatrics, 9:128, 1954.

Dawson, E. K.: Metastatic tumour of the breast, with report of a case. J. Path. Bact., 43:53, 1936.

Dickinson, A. M.: Carcinoma of the axillary tail of the breast. Amer. J. Surg., 49:515, 1940.

Dunn, J. E.: Epidemiology and possible identification of high-risk groups that could develop cancer of the breast. Cancer, 23:775, 1969.

Feuerman, L., Attie, J. N., and Rosenburg, B.: Carcinoma in axillary lymph-nodes as an indicator of breast cancer. Surg., Gynec. & Obst., 114:5, 1962.

Fitts, W. T., Jr., and Horn, R. C., Jr.: Occult carcinoma of the breast. J.A.M.A., 147:1429, 1951.

Frantz, V. K., Pickrin, J. W., Melcher, G. W., and Auchincloss, H.: Incidence of chronic cystic disease in so-called "normal breasts." Cancer, 4:762, 1951.

Frey, G. H.: Tietze's syndrome. Arch. Surg., 73:951, 1956.

Gill, A. M., Jones, R. A., and Pollak, L.: Tietze's disease. Brit. Med. J., 2:155, 1942.

Halsted, W. S.: The results of radical operations for the cure of cancer of the breast. Ann. Surg., 46:80, 1907.

Harnett, W. L.: A statistical report on 2529 cases of cancer of the breast. Brit. J. Cancer, 2:213, 1948.

Hart, D.: Intracystic papillomatous tumors of the breast, benign and malignant. Arch. Surg., 14:793, 1927.

Horwitz, T.: Widespread skeletal metastases from a primary carcinoma of the breast which was not demonstrable clinically. Bull. Hosp. Joint Dis., 9:65, 1948.

Huguet, J.: Les métastases précessive des cancers du sein, J. de radiol. et d'électrol., 34:192, 1953.

Ibach, J. R., Jr.: Carcinoma of the ovary metastatic to breast. Arch. Surg., 88:410, 1964.

Jackson, A. S.: Carcinoma of the breast in the absence of clinical breast findings. Ann. Surg., 127:177, 1948.

Kaae, S.: The prognostic significance of early diagnosis in breast cancer. Acta radiol., 29:475, 1948.

Kaplan, I. W., and Reinstine, H.: Occult carcinoma of the breast. Am. Surgeon, 20:575, 1954.

Karon, E. H., Achor, R. W. P., and Janes, J. M.: Painful nonsuppurative swelling of costochondral cartilages (Tietze's syndrome). Proc. Staff Meet., Mayo Clin., 33:45, 1958.

Kayser, H. L.: Tietze's syndrome. Amer. J. Med., 21:982, 1956.

Kilgore, A. R., Fleming, R., and Ramos, M. M.: The incidence of cancer with nipple discharge and the risk of cancer in the presence of papillary disease of the breast. Surg., Gynec. & Obst., 96:649, 1953.

Klopp, C. T.: Metastatic cancer of axillary lymph node without a demonstrable primary lesion. Ann. Surg., 131:437, 1950.

Lamarina, A.: Il carcinoma occulto della mammella. L'Osp. Magg. di Milano, 59:291, 1964.

Landon, J., and Malpas, J. S.: Tietze's syndrome. Ann. Rheumat. Dis., 18:249, 1959.

Lane-Claypon, J. E.: A Further Report on Cancer of the Breast with Special Reference to its Associated Antecedent Conditions. Reports on Public Health and Medical Subjects, No. 32, London, Ministry of Health, 1926.

Larsen, R. R., Sawyer, K. C., Sawyer, R. B., and Torres, R. C.: Occult carcinoma of the breast. Amer. J. Surg., 107:553, 1964.

McDivitt, R. W., Stewart, F. W., and Berg, J. W.: Tumors of the Breast. Atlas of Tumor Pathology. Washington, D. C., Armed Forces Institute of Pathology, Second Series, Fascicle 2, 1968, page 116.

Mornard, P.: Sur deux cas de tumeurs malignes des mamelles axillaires aberrantes. Bull. et mém. Soc. nat. de chir. de Paris, 21:487, 1929.

Motulsky, R. G., and Rohn, R. J.: Tietze's syndrome: cause of chest pain and chest wall swelling. J.A.M.A., 152:504, 1953.

Owen, H. W., Dockerty, M. B., and Gray, H. K.: Occult carcinoma of the breast. Surg., Gynec. & Obst., 98:302, 1954.

Piccagli, G.: Carcinoma mammario aberrante. Ann. ital. di chir., 17:241, 1938.

Pierce, E. H., Gray, H. K., and Dockerty, M. B.: Surgical significance of isolated axillary adenopathy. Ann. Surg., 145:104, 1957.

Rabinovitch, J., Rabinovitch, P., and Pines, B.: Silent carcinomas of the breast. Amer. J. Surg., 85:179, 1953.

Rawlings, M. S.: The "Rib syndrome." Dis. Chest, 41:432, 1962.

Rawls, J. L.: Extramammary breast carcinoma. Virginia Med. Monthly, 69:448, 1942.

Root, M. T.: Cancer from the family doctor's viewpoint. Connecticut Med. J., 13:619, 1949.

Roux-Berger, J. L.: Cancer du sein à debut clinique axillaire. Mém. acad. du chir., 77:436, 1951.

Rutkowski, J.: Cancer mammae latens. J. internat. chir., 10:415, 1950.

Sandisen, A. T.: Metastatic tumours in the breast. Brit. J. Surg., 47:54, 1959.

Schumann, H. D.: Retrograde Melanommetastasen der Mamma. Zentralbl. f. Chir., 77:1886, 1952.

Skorneck, A. B.: Roentgen aspects of Tietze's syndrome. Amer. J. Roentgen., 83:748, 1960.

Speert, H., and Greeley, A. V.: Cervical cancer with metastasis to breast. Amer. J. Obst. & Gynec., 55:894, 1948.

Stringa, U.: Sui tumori delle ghiandole mammarie aberranti. Minerva chir., 6:349, 1951.

Tietze, A.: Ueber eine eigenartige Haufung von Fallen mit Dystrophie der Rippenknorpel. Berl. klin. Wchnschr., 58:829, 1921.

Truscott, B. M.: Carcinoma of the breast. Brit. J. Cancer, 1:129, 1947.

Wehrmacher, W. H.: Significance of Tietze's syndrome in differential diagnosis of chest pain. J.A.M.A., 157:505, 1955.

Weinberger, H. A., and Stetten, DeW.: Extensive secondary axillary lymph node carcinoma without clinical evidence of primary breast lesion. Surgery, 29:217, 1951.

Wheelock, M. C., Frable, W. J., and Urnes, P. D.: Bizarre metastases from malignant neoplasms. Amer. J. Clin. Path., 37:475, 1962.

Lobular Neoplasia

In 1919 Ewing, in the first edition of his classic work, *Neoplastic Disease,* presented a photomicrograph of a lesion of the mammary lobule (his Fig. 184) which he described as "pre-cancerous change." He gave it no specific name, but it is obviously the lesion which I wish to discuss in the present chapter.

Foote and Stewart published the first adequate description of the lesion in 1941, and named it "lobular carcinoma in situ." In 1950, in Fascicle 34 of the Armed Forces Atlas of Tumor Pathology, *Tumors of the Breast,* Stewart amplified his description. He described two types of lobular carcinoma, the *noninfiltrating* and the *infiltrating* types.

Although the term "lobular carcinoma" has been generally accepted in the United States, a good deal of confusion exists among European pathologists as to what to name this lesion. Muir called it *epitheliosis.* Macgillivray, however, in a recent discussion of different types of epithelial proliferation in the breast uses epitheliosis to identify the common benign microscopic lesion which we call papillomatosis.

During the last 18 years a number of case reports of so-called lobular carcinoma have appeared (Godwin; Miller and Kay; Degrell; Haagensen; Benfield, Jacobson, and Warner). Two larger series of these cases have been repeatedly presented in recent years, one by Newman from the George Washington University Hospital, and another from the Memorial Hospital by Farrow, McDivitt, Hutter, Foote, and Stewart.

The correct choice of a name for a disease is important not only because it identifies it, but because the name connotes its characteristics and predicates its treatment. In our Department of Surgical Pathology we have come to believe that the name "lobular carcinoma in situ" is a most unfortunate choice for the disease entity which I discuss in this chapter. *Carcinoma* connotes an epithelial neoplasm which, once established in the breast, always grows progressively locally, and often metastasizes. "Lobular carcinoma in situ" is a lesion which evolves in premenopausal breasts but apparently regresses and disappears after the menopause. It does not metastasize. These characteristics, and others which I shall describe, make it imperative that surgeons and pathologists distinguish this lesion from true breast carcinoma; many are now performing mastectomy for it and including these cases in their reports of their results of treatment of breast cancer in general. A better name for this lesion would make surgeons consider the problem which the lesion presents more carefully. Lattes, the Director of our Department of Surgical Pathology, has suggested the name "lobular neoplasia," and we urge its adoption.

Pathology of Lobular Neoplasia

Since lobular neoplasia is a pathologic rather than a clinical entity, because it does not form a palpable tumor which can be identified clinically, I should begin my discussion of this lesion by describing its pathologic features.

The lesion cannot be identified grossly because the lobules and ductules involved by this type of epithelial proliferation are too small and too widely dispersed in the breast to form an aggregate visible with the naked eye.

The basic microscopic feature of lobular neoplasia is proliferation of the epithelium lining the acini of the mammary lobule and the small intralobular ductules. The acini in the resting mammary gland are lined by a single layer of small cuboidal cells. Outside of these epithelial cells there is a less well defined and less complete layer of myoepithelial cells. The acini have clearly defined lumens. The epithelial lining of the small ductules that emerge from the lobules is similar. In lobular neoplasia these cells lining the acini and ductules increase in size and number, although often maintaining a comparatively uniform size and shape. They crowd the acini, and the lumens are no longer seen.

A representative area of lobular neoplasia, involving several lobules, situated adjacent to a normal lobule, is shown in Figure 25–1. The contrast between the normal lobule and the solid pattern of the neoplastic lobules is obvious, making this an easy lesion for pathologists to recognize. When the lobules affected by this process are few and small and widely dispersed, as in the lesion shown in Figure 25–2, however, the pathologist may well miss it.

Although the uniformity of the proliferating cells in lobular neoplasia is a feature of this lesion, in some cases the cells vary more in size and shape and tend to be larger. On the basis of the extent to which the proliferating cells depart from the normal character of the acinar epithelium, lobular neoplasia can be classified into two types, which we are accustomed to call Types A and B. That shown in Figure 25–3 is Type A, and that in Figure 25–4, Type B. It is not always easy to draw a sharp line between the two. Both types are occasionally seen in the same lesion, and sometimes in the same microscopic field.

We do not have enough cases in which lobular neoplasia has been followed by carcinoma to correlate the microscopic type of

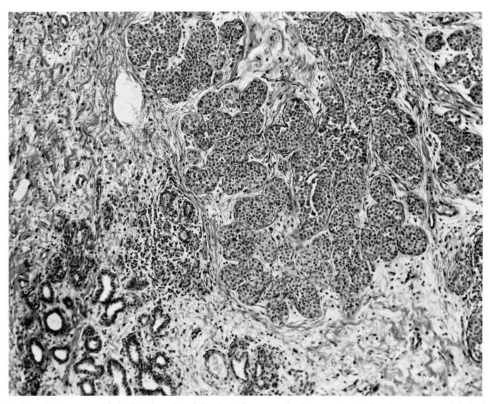

Figure 25–1. A group of lobules involved by lobular neoplasia, contrasted with a normal lobule in the lower left.

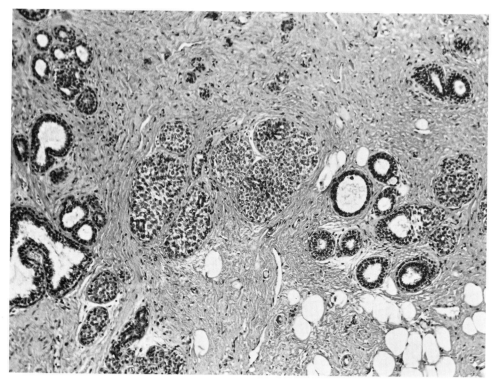

Figure 25–2. A smaller focus of lobular neoplasia.

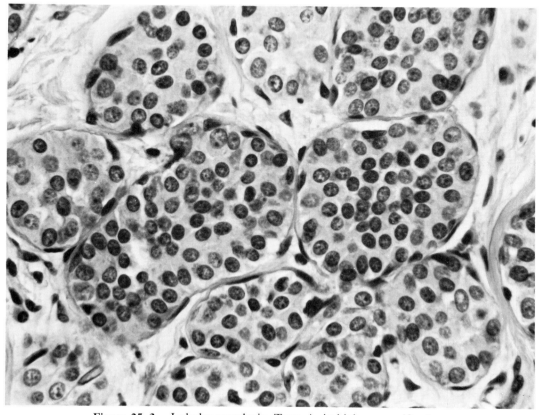

Figure 25–3. Lobular neoplasia, Type A, in higher magnification.

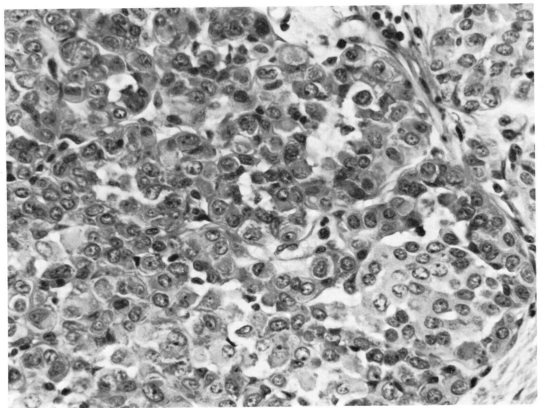

Figure 25–4. Lobular neoplasia, Type B, in which the cells are larger and vary more in size and shape. In the lower right portion there is a small round island of Type A in which the cells are smaller and more regular.

neoplasia with the frequency of carcinoma. We have regarded the Type A neoplasia as less threatening, and in such cases I have not removed the breast, whereas in some of the Type B lesions the proliferating cells have looked more malignant and I have done mastectomy. This distinction has not, however, been founded on proof, and is of questionable value.

The acini in these neoplastic lobules are enclosed by a delicate fibrillar reticulum which is well demonstrated in silver stains. There are no reticular fibrils between the individual proliferating epithelial cells in the acini. These features are seen in Figures 25–5 and 25–6 which show an average sized lobule and a large lobule affected by neoplasia.

The epithelium of the intralobular ductules is also involved in lobular neoplasia. Perhaps the earliest evidence of this lesion is the budding of small acini, solidly packed with the neoplastic epithelium, from intralobular ductules. This produces what we call the clover-leaf pattern. It is shown involving only part of

the periphery of a ductule in Figure 25–7, and involving the entire circumference of a ductule in Figure 25–8. A still more advanced stage of this process is seen in Figure 25–9. This clover-leaf pattern is a tell-tale sign of lobular neoplasia; whenever the pathologist sees it he should search for lobules of fully developed lobular neoplasia.

The neoplastic process extends from the lobules along the ductules emerging from them, filling up and blocking their lumens. Figure 25–10 shows this process.

Occasionally the epithelial lining of larger ducts is involved by this process. Figure 25–11 shows such a larger duct with the epithelial proliferation extending out from an involved lobule into the duct lining. In Figure 25–12 a large duct lined by neoplastic epithelium four or five layers deep is shown.

Lombird and Shelley have recently reported the distribution of lobular neoplasia within nine breasts studied in 2.5 cm. step blocks. They found the lesion to be concentrated in the upper quadrants, within 5 cm. of

(Text continued on page 512.)

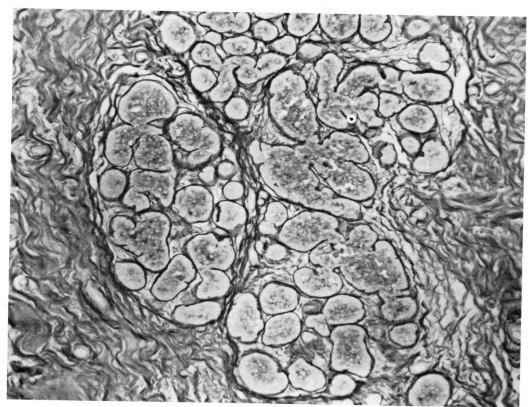

Figure 25–5. Silver stain showing the fibrillar reticulum of lobular neoplasia.

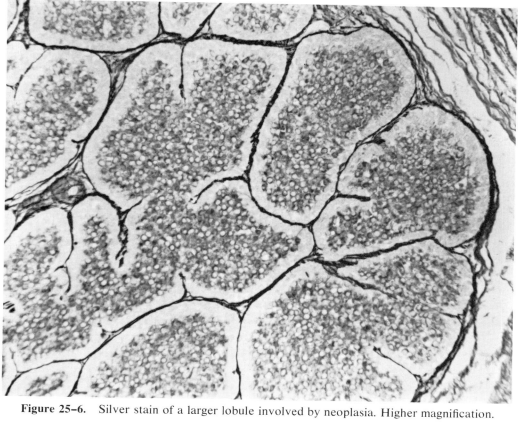

Figure 25–6. Silver stain of a larger lobule involved by neoplasia. Higher magnification.

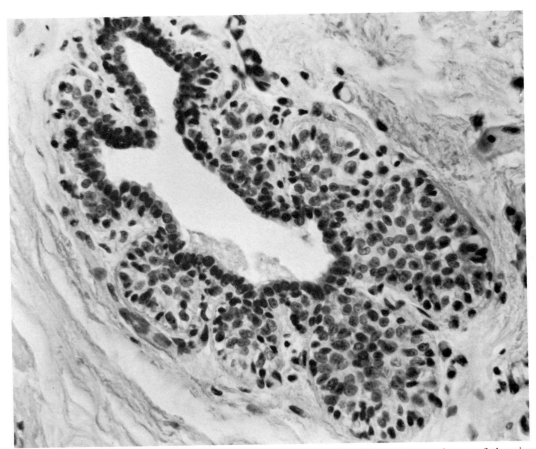

Figure 25–7. Lobular neoplasia beginning as a budding of small solid acini around part of the circumference of a ductule.

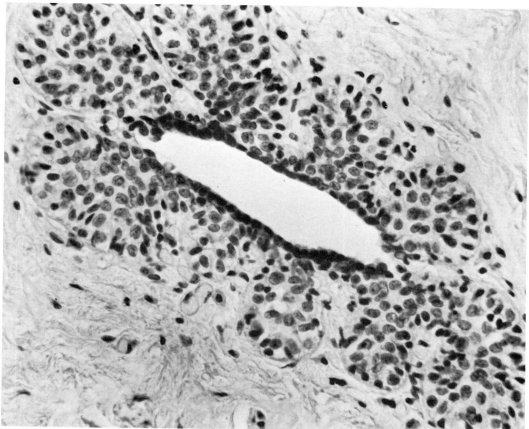

Figure 25–8. A further stage in the evolution of lobular neoplasia around a ductule, giving the clover-leaf pattern.

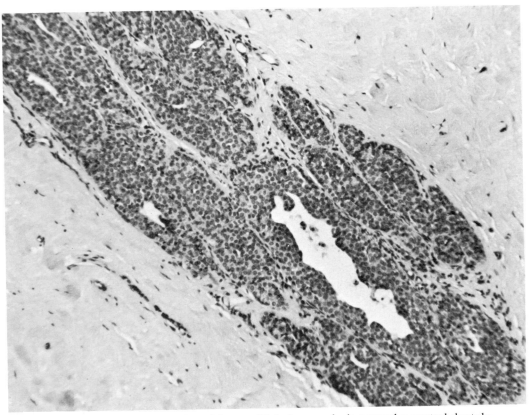

Figure 25-9. A fully developed focus of lobular neoplasia around a central ductule.

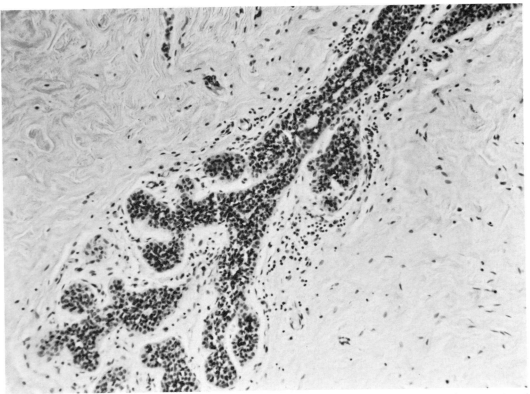

Figure 25-10. The neoplastic process has extended along a ductule leading away from an involved lobule.

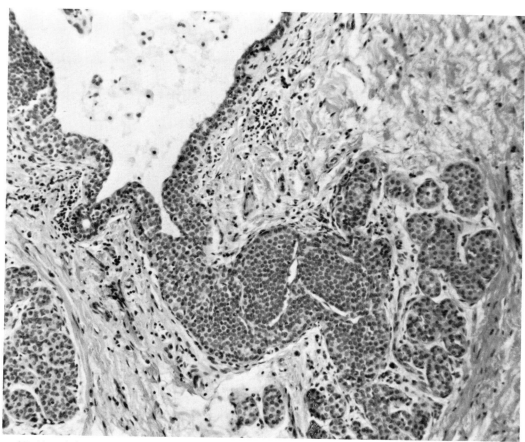

Figure 25–11.   A large duct in which the lining epithelium is involved by lobular neoplasia extending out from a lobule.

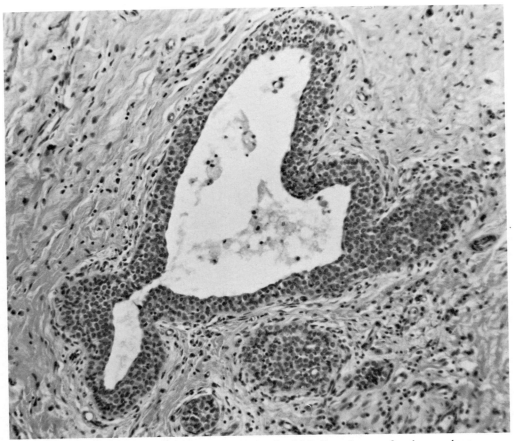

Figure 25–12.   A large duct with neoplastic epithelium four or five layers deep.

the nipple. Our experience has not been so simple. We have found lobular neoplasia in isolated foci in all sectors of the breast, and in other cases it has been seen involving the breast generally.

One of the interesting microscopic features of lobular neoplasia is that it is so often accompanied by adenosis, which is also a proliferative lesion of the mammary lobule. In approximately one-third of our cases of lobular neoplasia we have found some adenosis. Most pathologists are today fully familiar with adenosis and will not confuse it with lobular neoplasia unless the two lesions are intimately intermingled. This has been true of a number of our cases. In several the adenosis has predominated. Figure 25–13 presents, in low magnification, a microscopic field from one of these lesions. It shows four lobules grouped around a central area of fibrosis. The lobule in the lower left portion of the photograph is involved by neoplasia. The other three lobules show only adenosis. Figure

25–14 shows the neoplastic lobule in higher magnification.

Microscopic   Differential   Diagnosis. The accurate differentiation between lobular neoplasia and minor and insignificant epithelial proliferation within lobules and ductules depends upon technically perfect microscopic sections. Distortion due to poor fixation, cutting, or staining makes accurate diagnosis impossible.

There are two types of carcinoma that are apt to be mistaken for lobular neoplasia. One is well differentiated intraductal carcinoma growing in small rounded masses, as shown in Figure 25–15. The individual cells of this lesion are comparatively small and regular, like those of lobular neoplasia, but the carcinoma will, in some foci, have an obviously intraductal and sometimes cribriform pattern which betrays its nature.

Another lesion suggesting lobular neoplasia is well differentiated carcinoma growing peripherally along ducts down into the mam-

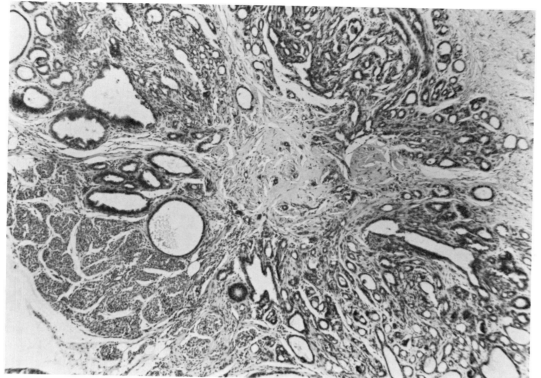

Figure 25–13. Four mammary lobules grouped around a central area of fibrosis. The lobule to the lower left is involved by neoplasia. The other three lobules show adenosis.

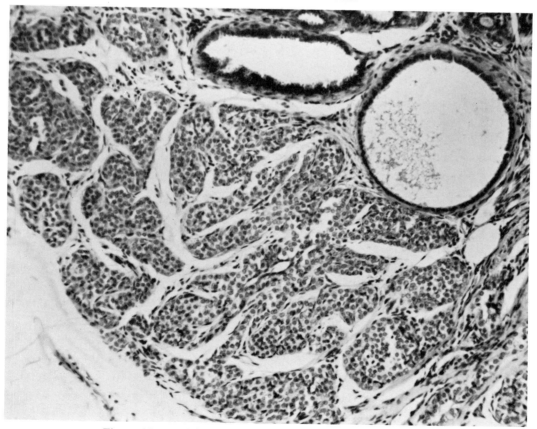

Figure 25–14. The neoplastic lobule in higher magnification.

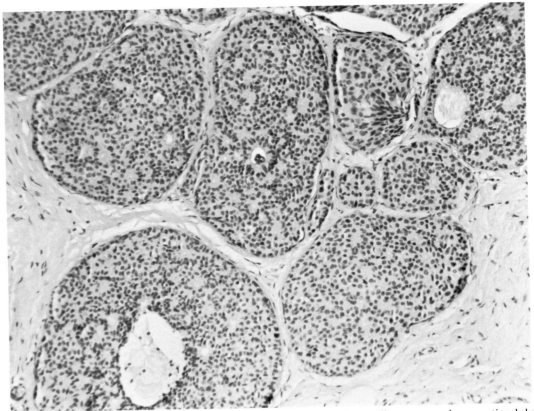

Figure 25–15. Well-differentiated intraductal carcinoma growing in small masses and suggesting lobular neoplasia.

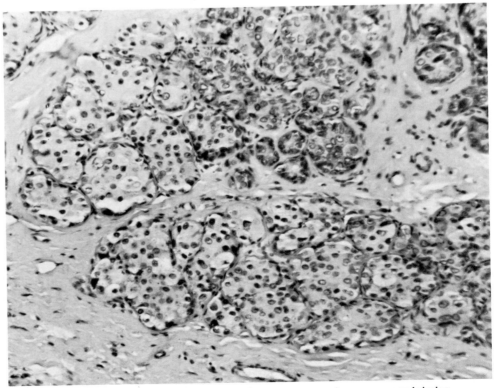

Figure 25–16. Well-differentiated carcinoma overgrowing mammary lobules.

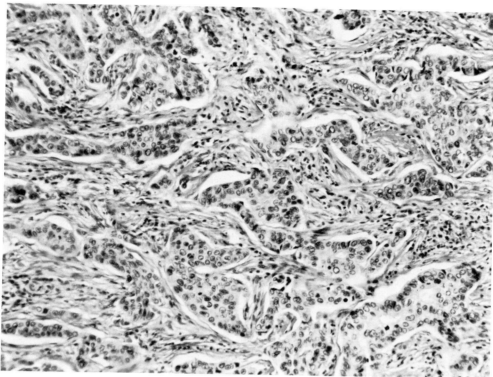

Figure 25–17. The obviously invasive portion of the carcinoma shown in Figure 25–16.

mary lobules. Figure 25–16 shows two lobules being overgrown by carcinoma of this type. The obviously invasive portion of this carcinoma, made up of similar cells, is shown in Figure 25–17.

The Classification of Lobular Neoplasia

It must be clearly understood that lobular neoplasia as I have described it above does not have the pathologic characteristics of carcinoma. There is no infiltration of the neoplastic epithelium outside of the lobules and ducts that are affected. Another un-carcinoma-like characteristic of lobular neoplasia is that we have never seen it metastasize. In our series of 55 patients with 61 breasts in which lobular neoplasia alone, unaccompanied by carcinoma, was found, there has been no regional lymph node or distant metastasis.

Breast carcinoma of various types does, of course, occur simultaneously with lobular neoplasia, but we then classify the lesion as carcinoma of whatever histologic type it may be. These lesions infiltrate and metastasize. Our series of a total of 118 patients in whom lobular neoplasia has been diagnosed includes

not only the 55 patients referred to above in whom lobular neoplasia unaccompanied by carcinoma was found, but also another 63 patients in whom both lobular neoplasia and some type of carcinoma were found co-existing simultaneously in the same breast. I will discuss this latter group of patients in the following chapter.

This distinction between simple lobular neoplasia and lobular neoplasia accompanied by carcinoma, is a fundamental one which all surgeons and pathologists must clearly understand if we are to clarify the problem of how to treat lobular neoplasia. Hutter and Foote have added to the confusion by failing to make this distinction in the text of their recent follow-up report of their series of cases. They state that 20 *cancers* (sic) developed subsequently in 46 patients in whom lobular carcinoma in situ had been demonstrated. In their accompanying table it appears that six of these *cancers* were merely simple persisting lobular neoplasia (lobular carcinoma in situ) and that only 14 were true infiltrating carcinomas.

Again, I point out that in the present chapter I am discussing the benign lesion which we prefer to call lobular neoplasia as it occurs alone. In the following chapter I will discuss several types of true infiltrating carcinoma that occur simultaneously with lobular neoplasia.

Frequency of Lobular Neoplasia

During the last 20 years—approximately the period during which we have recognized lobular neoplasia—we have identified it occurring unaccompanied by carcinoma in 61 breasts of 55 of our own patients (not counting cases sent to our department for consultation). This represents only a minute fraction of the breast specimens that we have studied during this period of time.

The truth is that these crude figures give us very little information as to true frequency of lobular neoplasia. All but two of our 61 breast specimens in which lobular neoplasia was found were only small biopsies or very limited local excisions, usually performed for cystic disease. The lobular neoplasia was an incidental microscopic finding. Although it has been a custom in our laboratory of surgical pathology to study serial blocks of tissue from these small specimens, the chances of finding lobular neoplasia in such a small portion of the total extent of a breast must be very small indeed.

Even when the entire breast is available for study, lobular neoplasia occurring alone without accompanying carcinoma is easily missed. In our mastectomy specimens we regularly study sections from all the quadrants of the breast and the nipple and subareolar area. A much more thorough microscopic search for lobular neoplasia was made in a number of the breasts in our series of cases. In four of these breasts, in each of which a total of from 70 to 367 microscopic sections were studied, only one single focus of lobular neoplasia in only one microscopic section was found in each breast!

Lombird and Shelley, in their recent discussion of this lesion, report that when an adequate (?) volume of breast tissue excised for biopsy is available, and a minimum of eight blocks of the tissue are studied, lobular neoplasia is found in 1.5 per cent of the patients with benign breast disease. This is a much higher frequency than we have found in our laboratory.

Certainly, the chances of finding lobular neoplasia by routine blind biopsy excision of a considerable portion of the breast are much too low to justify this procedure. The damage done to normal breasts by such injudicious surgery far outweighs the possible gain. Lombird and Shelley agree. They conclude that the incidence of lobular carcinoma in situ is far too low to warrant breast biopsy specifically in looking for this lesion.

Age Incidence

One of the most interesting features of lobular neoplasia, and one which is perhaps the key to the fundamental nature of this breast lesion, is its age incidence. All of the 55 patients in whom we found lobular neoplasia occurring alone were premenopausal; the youngest was 33, and the oldest 55, but the latter had menstruated within two months. The mean age of our patients was 44.4 years.

The fact that lobular neoplasia occurring alone is not found in postmenopausal women can only mean that, like gross cystic disease, it disappears when women enter this phase of life. Both lesions are in this sense hormone-dependent. Both also predispose to the subsequent development of carcinoma of the breast.

Bilaterality

Considering how incomplete our knowledge is as to the true frequency of lobular neoplasia not accompanied by carcinoma, we have found this lesion with a surprising frequency in both breasts.

In our series of patients we were able to study tissue from both breasts—usually only as local excision for cystic disease or some other benign lesion—in a total of 24 patients. Lobular neoplasia was found bilaterally in six, or 25 per cent. Its true bilateral incidence is probably considerably higher.

Clinical Features

Except for its special premenopausal age incidence, and its tendency to be bilateral, lobular neoplasia has no clinical features. When it occurs alone, not accompanied by carcinoma, it does not form a palpable tumor and therefore cannot be detected by clinical examination.

Snyder has claimed that mammography is helpful in the detection of lobular neoplasia chiefly because minute foci of microcalcification are seen in it. We have seen microcalcification occasionally in a variety of both benign and malignant lesions of the breast—cystic disease, adenosis, duct ectasia, and intraductal carcinoma. We have seen it only very rarely in lobular neoplasia occurring alone, unaccompanied by carcinoma, and we doubt that mammography is of practical value in identifying this infrequent lesion.

Carcinoma Subsequent to Lobular Neoplasia

That lobular neoplasia predisposes patients to the subsequent development of carcinoma there is no doubt. The question is to what degree it increases their chances of developing breast carcinoma. This question can be answered only by careful follow-up, for a long period of time, of patients in whom lobular neoplasia has been demonstrated by biopsy or excision of a portion of the breast, and mastectomy has not been done. When the breast is removed, carcinoma cannot, of course, develop in it. The opportunity of demonstrating the relationship of lobular neoplasia to the subsequent development of carcinoma in such a breast has, unfortunately, been lost. Since most surgeons and pathologists have been advocating mastectomy for lobular neoplasia the number of cases available to answer our question is small.

The longest series of pertinent cases published to date is that from Memorial Hospital, recently reported by Hutter and Foote. It includes 46 patients in whom lobular neoplasia alone, not accompanied by carcinoma, was originally demonstrated. They were followed for from four to 27 years. Six of them had had unilateral mastectomy. In the others—40 in all—neither breast was removed. In these 46 patients there were therefore a total of 86 breasts subject to the risk of subsequently developing carcinoma.

Ten, or 25 per cent, of the 40 patients in whom the breast containing the lobular neoplasia was not amputated, got carcinoma in it during the follow-up period. Four, or 8.7 per cent of 46 patients subsequently developed carcinoma in the contralateral breast. Carcinoma therefore occurred in a total of 14, or 16.3 per cent, of the 86 breasts subject to the risk of developing it.

From our Columbia-Presbyterian Medical Center we can report the follow-up, for from four to 24 years, of 49 patients in whom lobular neoplasia alone, not accompanied by carcinoma, was originally demonstrated. Both breasts were removed in two of the patients. The breast affected by the lobular neoplasia was removed in 25 others. Thus, in 49 patients, a total of 69 breasts were subject to the risk of subsequently developing carcinoma.

In eight, or 16 per cent, of our patients, it did develop. Five, or 23 per cent, of our 22 patients in whom the breast containing the lobular neoplasia was not amputated developed

Table 25–1. Follow-up of Lobular Neoplasia (Lobular Carcinoma in Situ) Occurring Alone, Not Accompanied by Simultaneous Carcinoma.

Data	Memorial Hospital, Hutter and Foote	Columbia-Presbyterian Medical Center, Haagensen and Lattes
No. of patients exposed to risk of developing breast carcinoma	46	47
Length of follow-up	4–27 years	4–24 years
Mean length of follow-up	?	9 years
Subsequent carcinoma in breast with lobular neoplasia not amputated	10 of 40 patients, 25%	5 of 22 patients, 23%
Subsequent carcinoma in contralateral breast	4 of 46 patients, 8.7%	4 of 47 patients, 8.5%
Total number breasts exposed to risk of developing carcinoma	86	69
Breasts in which carcinoma developed	14, or 16.3%	9 or 13%

carcinoma in it during the follow-up period. Four or 8.5 per cent, of our 47 patients have developed carcinoma in the contralateral breast. Thus the disease occurred in the contralateral breast in four, or 50 per cent, of the eight patients who developed it subsequent to the detection of lobular neoplasia. One of the patients in our series has developed bilateral breast carcinoma subsequent to the identification of lobular neoplasia. The intervals of time elapsing between the original demonstration of lobular neoplasia and the development of carcinoma in our patients were 3, 3, 3, 4, 4, 5, 7, 15, and 17 years. In terms of the total of 69 breasts exposed to the risk of developing carcinoma subsequent to the demonstration of lobular neoplasia, in our series of cases, the incidence of carcinoma has been 13 per cent.

One of the critical features of this kind of a follow-up study is the length of the follow-up period in the series of cases. Hutter and Foote followed their series of patients for from four to 27 years, but they do not state the average length of follow-up. In our series of cases, followed for from four to 24 years, the average length of follow-up for the 69 breasts exposed to the risk of developing carcinoma was nine years.

To recapitulate the follow-up findings from these two case series, it can be said that from about 25 per cent of the patients who had lobular neoplasia in one breast, and in whom the breast was not removed, subsequently developed carcinoma in this breast during a follow-up period of from four to 26 years. Carcinoma developed in the contralateral breast in about 8.5 per cent. These data are summarized in Table 25–1.

The Treatment of Lobular Neoplasia

Pathologists, impressed by the frequency with which true infiltrating carcinoma of the breast develops subsequent to the demonstration of lobular neoplasia of the breast, have generally advocated amputation of the breast in which the lobular neoplasia is found. Surgeons, most of whom are unaware of other basic facts concerning the natural history of this disease entity, have blindly followed the recommendations of their pathologists.

Both pathologists and surgeons should take a careful look at the following summary of the facts concerning this lesion and reconsider their therapy for it.

1. Lobular neoplasia alone, unaccompanied by simultaneous true carcinoma, occurs almost exclusively in the breasts of premenopausal women.

2. The chance of developing carcinoma during a subsequent 4 to 25 year period is approximately 25 per cent for the breast in which lobular neoplasia was found, and 8.5 per cent for the contralateral breast.

3. The interval between the demonstration of lobular neoplasia and the subsequent occurrence of carcinoma may be a long one—in some cases 15 or 20 years.

4. If a patient with lobular neoplasia is to be entirely safe she must have bilateral mastectomy.

5. Bilateral mastectomy is a bitter penalty for any woman—particularly for younger women. Pathologists are perhaps not as fully aware of this fact as the surgeons who have to care for these women.

6. The alternative of not removing either breast but carefully examining them at three month intervals offers a reasonable probability of detecting breast carcinoma at an early enough clinical stage to cure it in a high proportion of cases.

When I have presented these facts clearly and candidly to my patients in whom lobular neoplasia unaccompanied by carcinoma has been demonstrated they have, almost without exception, chosen not to have mastectomy. This has led me increasingly to be content to follow them with careful breast examination at three month intervals. Although the number of my patients in this category in whom carcinoma has subsequently developed is small—totaling only seven—I believe I have probably cured them all with radical mastectomy, performed when their carcinomas were detected. Six had no axillary metastases, and the seventh had only two axillary nodes involved.

Obviously we do not yet have enough long term follow-up data to know precisely how often and when true carcinoma of the breast follows lobular neoplasia. But as a humanitarian I prefer to consider the patient's point of view if I can do so without exposing her to unreasonable risk.

The following case history illustrates the advantage of this conservative point of view regarding the treatment of lobular neoplasia.

A 49 year old married woman consulted me in 1945 for a tumor of the right breast which she had discovered one month previously. Her mother and her maternal grandmother had had breast carcinoma.

Examination showed a well delimited, movable, soft tumor 3 cm. in diameter, situated just lateral to the right areola. There was also a 3 cm. tumor beneath the medial half of the left areola. This tumor was well delimited, but it was somewhat fixed in the surrounding breast tissue and was firm. Biopsies were done of both tumors on December 20, 1945. Both were found to be grossly typical cysts. The cysts, and a narrow margin of surrounding breast tissue on each side, were excised.

Three blocks of tissue from the *right*-sided lesion were studied, and showed nothing remarkable. Four blocks of the tissue of the *left*-sided lesion were studied. In one of these blocks, which included the cyst wall, there were several areas of proliferation of the acinar epithelium of an unusual type. It was classified merely as "hyperplasia."

Fifteen years later, in 1960, the patient discovered by self-examination, which she had practiced ever since her 1945 breast operation, a small tumor in her right breast. She did not consult me, however, until March 10, 1961. Her tumor was then 5 mm. in diameter and was situated at the caudad end of the circumareolar scar of the 1945 operation. The tumor was hard and poorly delimited, and there was definite retraction in the skin over it. There were no clinically involved axillary nodes. Skeletal and chest films were normal. The left breast was normal.

On March 17, 1961, biopsy of the new small tumor was done. Frozen section study showed it to be carcinoma, and radical mastectomy was performed. The gross extent of the carcinoma was only about 10 mm. A total of 53 blocks of tissue were studied. The primary carcinoma was a diffusely infiltrating type in which the tumor cells had some tendency to form acini. A second separate focus of infiltrating carcinoma was found. It was only 3 mm. in diameter and was situated in the upper outer sector of the breast, far from the primary tumor. In one block of tissue from the central portion of the breast a small focus of Type A lobular neoplasia was found. Twenty-six axillary nodes were found in the axilla. None contained metastases.

The original microscopic sections of the tissue removed in the 1945 operation were studied again. In the light of present knowledge the area of "hyperplasia" in one of the four blocks of tissue from the left breast was undoubtedly lobular neoplasia of Type A, which we had not recognized.

Twenty-five years after lobular neoplasia was found in her left breast this breast is normal. There has been no evidence of recurrence of the carcinoma in her right breast treated by radical mastectomy 14 years ago.

When I recently told this patient that I had not followed the current fashion of removing her left breast in 1945 she told me she was very pleased that I had not because she has had this left breast for the past 25 years, and she also had her right breast for 16 years after my initial operation.

REFERENCES

Benfield, J. R., Jacobson, M., and Warner, N. E.: In situ lobular carcinoma of the breast. Arch. Surg., 91:130, 1965.

Degrell, I.: Ueber das 'in situ' Karzinom der Mamma. Bruns' Beitr. f. klin. Chir., 202:334, 1961.

Ewing, J.: Neoplastic Disease, W. B. Saunders Co., Philadelphia, 1919, p. 473.

Farrow, J. H.: Clinical considerations and treatment of *in situ* lobular breast cancer. Amer. J. Roentgenol., 102:652, 1968.

Foote, F. W., and Stewart, F. W.: Lobular carcinoma in situ. Amer. J. Path., 17:491, 1941.

Godwin, J. T.: Chronology of lobular carcinoma of the breast. Cancer, 5:259, 1952.

Haagensen, C. D.: Lobular carcinoma of the breast. A precancerous lesion? Clin. Obstet. Gynec., 5:1093, 1962.

Hutter, R. V. P., and Foote, F. W.: Lobular carcinoma in situ. Long term follow-up. Cancer, 24:1081, 1969.

Lombird, P. A., and Shelley, W. M.: The spatial distribution of lobular in situ mammary carcinoma. J.A.M.A., 210:689, 1969.

McDivitt, R. W., Hutter, R. V. P., Foote, F. W., Jr., and Stewart, F. W.: In situ lobular carcinoma. J.A.M.A., 201:82, 1967.

McDivitt, R. W., Stewart, F. W., and Berg, J. W.: Tumors of the breast. Atlas of Tumor Pathology, Second Series, Fascicle 2. Armed Forces Institute of Pathology, Washington, D.C., 1968.

Macgillivray, J. B.: The problem of 'chronic mastitis' with epitheliosis, J. Clin. Path., 22:340, 1969.

Miller, H. W., Jr., and Kay, S.: Infiltrating lobular carcinoma of the female mammary gland. Surg., Gynec. & Obst., 102:661, 1956.

Muir, R.: The evolution of carcinoma of the mamma. J. Path. Bact., 52:155, 1941.

Newman, W.: In situ lobular carcinoma of the breast. Report of 26 women with 32 cancers. Ann. Surg., 157:591, 1963.

Newman, W.: Lobular carcinoma of the female breast. Report of 73 cases. Ann. Surg., 164:305, 1966.

Snyder, R. E.: Mammography and lobular carcinoma in situ. Surg., Gynec. & Obst., 122:255, 1966.

Stewart, F. W.: Tumors of the Breast. Atlas of Tumor Pathology, Section IX, Fascicle 34, Armed Forces Institute of Pathology, Washington, D.C., 1950.

Chapter Twenty-Six

Lobular Neoplasia and Simultaneous Carcinoma

Because it is a different pathologic and clinical entity, although probably of similar etiology, I will devote a separate chapter to lobular neoplasia and carcinoma occurring simultaneously in the breast. In our clinics of the Columbia-Presbyterian Hospital we have observed a total of 63 patients with this disease during the 20 year period between 1949 and 1969.

Frequency

This small group of carcinomas accompanied by lobular neoplasia constitutes less than one per cent of the breast carcinomas that we have studied during this period of time.

Age Incidence

All but three of these 63 patients were premenopausal. Their average age was 45.5 years. The youngest was 31. Three were postmenopausal; their ages were 60, 66, and 68 respectively. The two oldest patients, however, were both taking estrogen—one had been taking estrogen (Premarin) daily for 11 years, and the other, stilbestrol in substantial doses for a number of years. These two cannot therefore be regarded as physiologically post-

menopausal. Only the 60 year old patient was perhaps truly physiologically postmenopausal. Her case history was as follows:

Mrs. A. M. first came to our clinic when she was 50, because of multiple tumors of both breasts. Bilateral breast biopsies showed only gross cystic disease. When she was 53 her periods ceased. We do not know whether or not she subsequently took any estrogen. When she was 60 she was again admitted to our hospital for bilateral breast tumors. Biopsies revealed bilateral intraductal carcinoma. In the biopsy of the left breast lobular neoplasia, Type B, was also identified. X-ray studies revealed metastases in the spine and sacrum, and only irradiation treatment was given.

It is perhaps of some significance that this disease, in which lobular neoplasia occurs together with carcinoma, develops at an earlier average age than other forms of breast carcinoma. The average age at which carcinoma of all types has been diagnosed in my personal series of cases has been 51.9 years, that is about six and one-half years older than those patients in whom lobular neoplasia and carcinoma occurred simultaneously.

Pathological Classification

The lobular neoplasia accompanying the carcinoma in our cases of this disease did not differ from lobular neoplasia occurring alone as I have described it in the previous chapter, with one exception. When lobular neoplasia occurred alone, Type A lesions predominated in a ratio of three Type A to two Type B. When lobular neoplasia occurred together with carcinoma, the ratio of Types A and B was reversed: Type B predominated, in a ratio of three Type B to two Type A. It might be said therefore that the lobular neoplasia occurring simultaneously with carcinoma was more malignant-looking. But I have emphasized in the previous chapter that the classification of these lesions as to type is not exact.

The carcinomas accompanying the lobular neoplasia in this disease were a variety of types. I have classified the 74 carcinomas for which we had adequate microscopic sections, that occurred in our 63 patients, as follows: 35 small cell, 6 papillary, 18 intraductal, 2 tubular, 2 circumscribed, and 1 mucoid carcinoma, 3 well differentiated carcinomas, 2 moderately differentiated carcinomas, and 5 undifferentiated carcinomas. It will be seen that these carcinomas were a remarkable group—67 of the 74 were special types with comparatively favorable prognoses.

Carcinoma in the Contralateral Breast

Although only 24 of our 63 patients with simultaneous lobular neoplasia and carcinoma were treated more than 10 years ago, 15 of the 63 have already developed carcinoma in the contralateral breast. This is a remarkably high incidence of bilateral involvement. It is so high that we are justified in concluding that this combination of simultaneous lobular neoplasia and carcinoma, like lobular neoplasia when it occurs alone, has a special tendency to involve both breasts.

The carcinomas that developed in the contralateral breast were not always of the same pathologic type. In three, the original lesion was a small cell carcinoma but the contralateral lesion was intraductal.

Small Cell Carcinoma Accompanying Lobular Neoplasia

The 35 small cell carcinomas that occurred in association with lobular neoplasia in 33 patients constitute the largest and most inter-

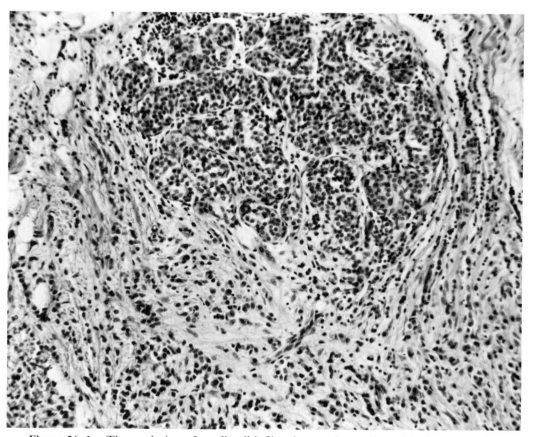

Figure 26–1. The evolution of small cell infiltrating carcinoma from lobular neoplasia.

esting group. Not only is this type of carcinoma a distinctive one pathologically, but it obviously evolves directly from the neoplastic process that affects the mammary lobules and ductules.

The proliferating epithelial cells which have packed the acini of the lobule break out and infiltrate the surrounding mammary stroma, giving the picture seen in Figure 26-1. On higher magnification, the identity of these invading cells with those which fill up the acini of the lobule is evident (Fig. 26-2). These cells infiltrate the breast diffusely, stringing out in single file as shown in Figure 26-3. The infiltration often produces a fibroblastic response in the breast stroma and the invading epithelial cells are compressed and distorted, as shown in higher magnification in Figure 26-4. They can easily be mistaken for fibroblasts and missed.

The growth pattern of these small cell carcinomas is not always uniform. The dominant pattern may be that of cells growing in irregular strands as shown in Figure 26-5, but in other areas the cells may grow in solid masses within ducts, as seen in Figure 26-6. The cell type in this lesion is more important than the pattern of cell arrangement.

All but one of these patients with small cell carcinoma accompanying lobular neoplasia had a palpable tumor with the usual characteristics of a carcinoma. The average diameter of the tumors was 2.8 cm., which is approximately the same as that of carcinomas of all types that have come to us during recent years.

Thirty of these carcinomas were treated by radical mastectomy. Axillary metastases were found in 11, or 37 per cent. This is a very low frequency of axillary metastases as compared with carcinomas in general.

Twelve of these patients were treated by radical mastectomy more than 10 years ago. Nine of the twelve, or 83 per cent, survived 10 years. Although this is a small number of patients, the data suggest that small cell carcinoma evolving from lobular neoplasia is a favorable type of carcinoma.

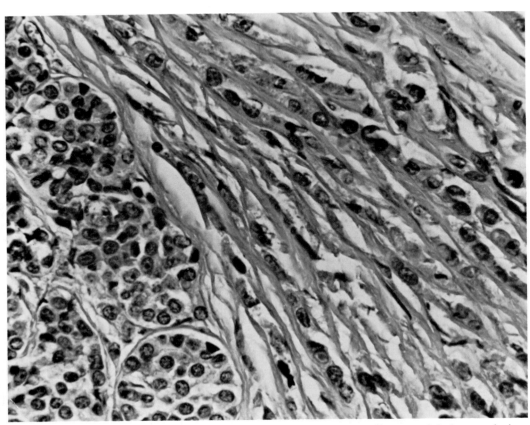

Figure 26-2. Small cell carcinoma infiltrating the breast stroma adjacent to lobular neoplasia.

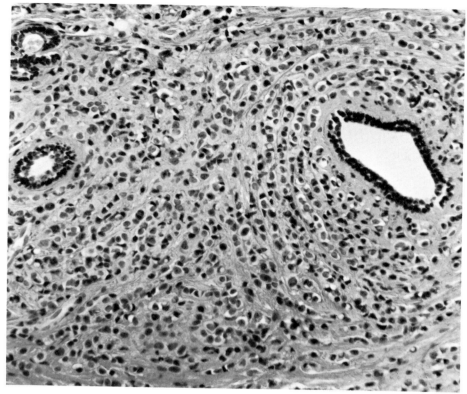

Figure 26–3. Small cell carcinoma diffusely invading the breast.

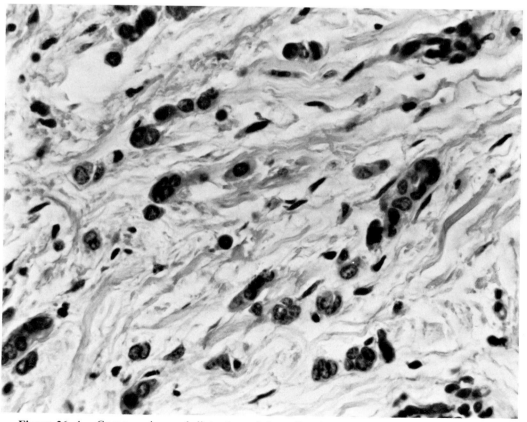

Figure 26–4. Compression and distortion of the cells of small cell carcinoma by fibrosis.

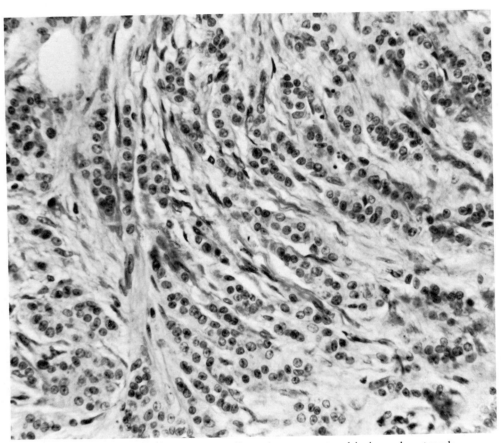

Figure 26–5.   The cells of small cell carcinoma arranged in irregular strands.

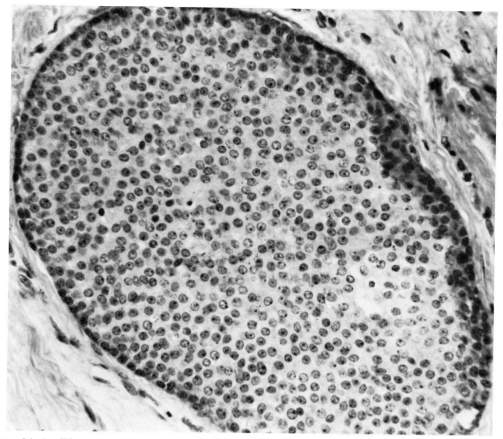

Figure 26-6. The cells of the same carcinoma shown in Figure 26–5 forming an intraductal pattern.

Other Types of Breast Carcinoma Accompanying Lobular Neoplasia

In 30 other patients a wide variety of types of breast carcinoma accompanied lobular neoplasia. There were a total of 39 carcinomas in these 30 patients, and all but 7 of them were favorable types. The intraductal carcinomas, 18 in all, were the most frequent.

In these 30 patients it was not possible to trace the origin of the carcinomas from the co-existing lobular neoplasia. Newman and others have made the assumption that when lobular neoplasia (lobular carcinoma in situ) and carcinoma occur together, it can be assumed that the carcinoma, whatever histologic type it may be, evolved from the lobular neoplasia. This assumption is, we believe, unjustified. Gross cystic disease and carcinoma are also often found in the same breast, but this fact does not warrant the conclusion that the latter evolves from the former. In fact, we

have no histologic evidence whatever that it does. Some basic factor in the mammary growth pattern predisposes to both diseases.

All these patients with carcinoma not of the small cell type accompanying lobular neoplasia had a palpable tumor produced by the carcinoma. These tumors averaged 2.2 cm. in diameter.

Thirty of these 39 carcinomas were treated by radical mastectomy. Axillary metastases were found in only 6, or 20 per cent. This low frequency of axillary metastases is in keeping with the favorable microscopic character of these carcinomas.

Eleven of these 30 patients with carcinoma of several different types and co-existing lobular neoplasia were treated by radical mastectomy more than 10 years ago. Eight, or 73 per cent, survived 10 years. While this number of cases is small, the facts suggest that these various types of carcinomas occurring together with lobular neoplasia have a favorable prognosis.

Chapter Twenty-Seven

Small Cell Carcinoma

Three different lesions of the breast form a triad and probably have in common some special etiology. The first is lobular neoplasia occurring alone in the breasts of premenopausal women, which I discussed in Chapter 25. The second, described in Chapter 26, is lobular neoplasia occurring simultaneously with true carcinoma of the breast, also in premenopausal women. The carcinomatous component of this lesion is often small cell carcinoma. The present chapter is devoted to the third lesion of the triad—small cell carcinoma occurring alone in the breasts of postmenopausal women.

Frequency, Age Incidence, and Bilaterality

Small cell carcinoma, occurring alone, without any other associated neoplastic process in the breast, is one of the most infrequent forms of breast carcinoma. Over the last 20 years, during which we have recognized this lesion as a special form of breast carcinoma, we have had only 17 examples, occurring in 16 patients.

Not only were all 16 patients postmenopausal, but as a group they were much older than our other patients with breast carcinoma. Their average age was 68 years. The youngest was 53, and the oldest 83.

Three of our 16 patients developed carci-

noma in both breasts. The interval between the appearance of the disease in the first and second breast was three years in two of the patients, and 11 years in the third patient.

Pathologic Features

These small cell carcinomas, which occur as a comparatively pure morphologic type in older patients, are identical with the small cell carcinoma component that occurs in association with lobular neoplasia in premenopausal women. Figures 26–3 and 26–4 in Chapter 26, which I have devoted to this form of carcinoma, illustrate small cell carcinoma adequately, but it is worthwhile emphasizing that this lesion, with its sparsely distributed small cells, often arranged in single file, is particularly easy to overlook in the fibrotic breasts of aged women. The carcinoma cells are passed over as fibroblasts. Figure 27–1 shows one of these lesions in which the small carcinoma cells are not at all prominent.

Etiology

The fact that these small cell carcinomas of aged women are morphologically identical with the small cell carcinoma component of the compound lesion of younger women in whom lobular neoplasia and small cell carci-

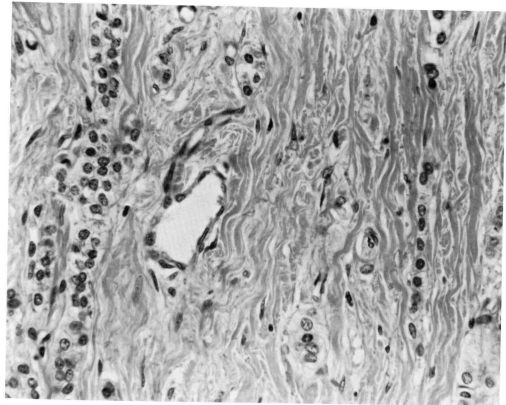

Figure 27–1. Small cell carcinoma. Sparse cells in single and double file are easily overlooked.

noma are combined, strongly suggests that both manifestations of small cell carcinoma are in some way associated with lobular neoplasia. We know that lobular neoplasia apparently disappears after the menopause, and it seems likely that it was present in the breasts of these aged women before they reached the menopause and then disappeared, leaving them with a predisposition to small cell carcinoma.

Clinical Features

These small cell carcinomas of aged women form a palpable tumor which is no different clinically from any other type of carcinoma. The average diameter of the 17 small cell carcinomas in our series was 3.5 cm., which is not significantly different from the diameter of other types of carcinoma coming to us during recent years.

Results of Treatment

Radical mastectomy was performed for 14 of our 17 small cell carcinomas. Axillary metastases were found in only 4 of the 14—that is, in 28 per cent. Moreover, the number of involved nodes was strikingly small—only one node contained metastases in three of the patients, while three of 39 nodes were involved in the fourth patient.

In seven of the 14 patients the radical mastectomy was done more than 10 years ago. Five of the seven, or 71 per cent, survived more than 10 years.

The number of cases in our group of small cell carcinomas is too small to have much significance, but when the comparatively low frequency of axillary metastases is considered in conjunction with the 10 year survival rate in these comparatively aged patients, the facts suggest that small cell carcinoma is perhaps a favorable form of carcinoma of the breast.

Chapter Twenty-Eight

The Papillary Type of Mammary Carcinoma

Mammary carcinoma that grows in a papillary form within dilated ducts and cysts deserves description as a separate type because it has both clinical and microscopic features which set it apart from other kinds of breast carcinoma. Very little has been written about the papillary type, and the character of the disease is, as a result, not well known. This anonymity is due to two facts. Papillary carcinoma is infrequent, and its microscopic differentiation from benign papilloma has given pathologists much difficulty.

Two useful papers dealing with this disease have recently appeared. Kraus and Neubecker at the Armed Forces Institute of Pathology collected reports of 21 cases. Veronesi reported 61 cases occurring among a total of 6300 carcinomas of the breast at the National Institute for the Study of Cancer in Milan.

Incidence

From our breast clinics at the Columbia-Presbyterian Medical Center we are able to report concerning a total of 130 of these lesions, representing about 2 per cent of the breast carcinomas that we have studied.

Age Distribution

The ages of our patients with papillary carcinoma averaged 54.4 years. This is older than the average age for all our patients with breast carcinoma, which was 50 years. It is definitely older than the average for my series of patients with benign intraductal papilloma, which was 48 years.

Clinical Features

Nipple Discharge. A nipple discharge occurred in only 44 of our 130 patients with papillary carcinoma. In 30 it was blood tinged, on some occasions at least. In the remaining 14 patients, the discharge was serous. Nipple discharge is, therefore, much less frequent in papillary carcinoma than in benign intraductal papilloma, in which about 80 per cent of my patients have had it.

Tumor. A tumor was present in all but three of our 130 patients with papillary carcinoma. There were several features of the tumors in these patients which distinguished them from the tumors of ordinary mammary carcinomas. In 87 of the 127 patients the tumor had a circumscribed or lobular contour, in contrast to the more diffuse, poorly delimited, contour of ordinary breast carcinoma.

Eighteen of the tumors were cystic. Several of these projected from the skin surface. In six the skin over the projecting tumor was reddened. Figure 28-1 shows one of these projecting cystic papillary carcinomas covered by intact but reddened epithelium.

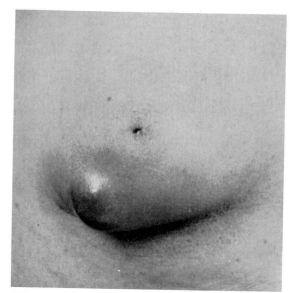

Figure 28–1. Redness of the skin over a papillary carcinoma of the breast.

two of our patients the skin over the projecting tumor broke down and ulcerated, as shown in Figure 28–2.

These papillary carcinomas were in general smaller than ordinary breast carcinomas, averaging only 2.9 cm. in diameter as compared with an average diameter of 3.7 cm. for operable breast carcinomas of all types in my 1943 to 1967 series of cases. Such a comparison is valid because almost all of these papillary carcinomas were operable.

Another type of tumor produced by papillary carcinoma consists of a zone of shotty nodules extending out from the subareolar area toward the periphery of the breast. The individual nodules are firm, discrete, movable within the breast, and about 5 mm. in diameter. Figure 28–3 reproduces my sketch of the clinical findings in such a papillary carcinoma.

In papillary carcinoma the tumor is more likely to be central than in ordinary breast carcinoma. In our series of 130 cases, the tumor was situated beneath, or adjacent to, the areola in 60, or 46 per cent. This central, as compared to a peripheral, origin indicates that papillary carcinoma has a predilection for the terminal portions of the mammary duct system. In my series of breast carcinomas as a whole only 29 per cent were situated in the central zone.

Retraction. Retraction signs, either skin dimpling or nipple deviation or retraction,

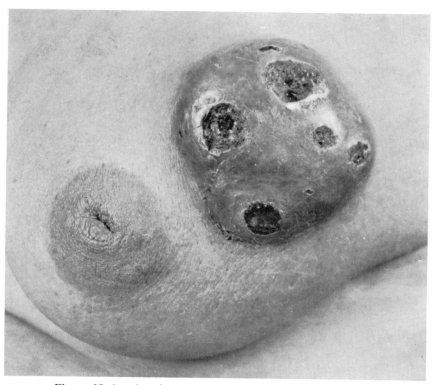

Figure 28–2. An ulcerated papillary carcinoma of the breast.

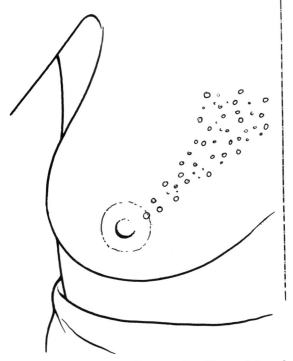

Figure 28–3. Hard, discrete, shot-like nodules of papillary carcinoma involving a pyramidal area of the upper inner sector of the breast.

were described in only 36 of our 130 patients with papillary carcinoma. In ordinary breast carcinoma retraction is much more frequent. The fact that papillary carcinoma grows largely within ducts and cysts no doubt accounts for the lesser degree of fibrosis and retraction that it produces.

Duration of Symptoms

The average duration of symptoms in our patients with papillary carcinoma was 12 months. Because these 130 patients with papillary carcinoma have come to us over such a long period of time — 1930 to 1968 — during which the duration of symptoms in our patients with breast carcinoma has decreased from 10.7 to 4.9 months, it is difficult to arrive at a figure with which to compare this duration of 12 months. It is obvious, however, that papillary carcinoma progresses more slowly than ordinary breast carcinoma, and that the duration of the disease is longer in those who have the papillary type.

Pathology

Surgeon and pathologist can gain important indications of papillary carcinoma from the gross appearance of the lesion. When papillary carcinoma grows in a cyst it is soft, friable, and hemorrhagic (Fig. 28–4). When the disease grows in dilated ducts involving a sector of the breast, the ducts stud the cut surface of the lighter colored breast tissue as circumscribed brownish or reddish nodules.

Another gross pathologic feature suggesting that a papillary lesion is carcinoma rather

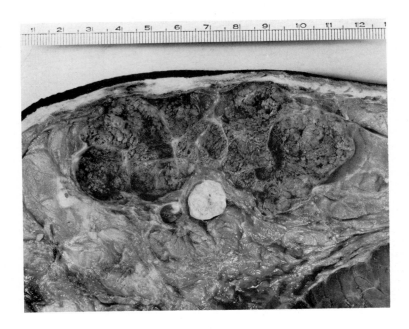

Figure 28–4. The gross appearance of a large papillary carcinoma growing within a cystic cavity, as seen in the mastectomy specimen.

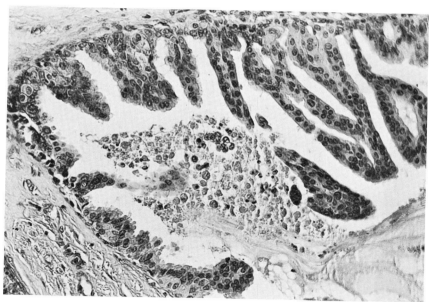

Figure 28–5. Papillary carcinoma in which the papillae do not have connective tissue cores.

than benign intraductal papilloma is involvement of a wide sector of the breast extending toward its periphery. In general, benign papillomas tend to be situated in the main ducts beneath the edge of the areola, or not very far out from it, and to be localized in extent.

The ultimate basis for classification of these papillary lesions as carcinomas rather than benign papillomas is, of course, their microscopic structure. Both the pattern in which they grow and the atypical character of their cells have a part in the distinction. The growth pattern is less important than the cytology. Among the papillary tumors that we have classified as carcinoma there were a number of very well differentiated lesions in which the growth pattern was virtually indistinguishable from that of benign intraductal papilloma. It has been stated that papillary lesions in which the papillae do not have connective tissue cores, such as that shown in Figure 28–5, are papillary carcinomas. But in many unquestioned papillary carcinomas the papillae have well developed cores, as in the lesion shown in Figure 28–6. In a few papillary carcinomas the supporting cores are very thick, as in Figure 28–7.

The length of the papillary processes has a bearing on the diagnosis only if they are very short. Long, branching, coreless papillae (Fig. 28–8) are a feature of many papillary carcinomas, and somewhat shorter papillae are commonly seen in these tumors (Fig. 28–9). But very short papillae, as shown in Figure 28–10, are characteristic of a special form of intraductal carcinoma which in our laboratory we have not classified as papillary. It is nevertheless true that this low papillary arrangement is also often seen in papillary apocrine carcinoma.

Another architectural feature of papillary carcinoma is the fusion of these short papillary processes as they line cystic cavities. In this way a cartwheel-like pattern is formed, which is an unmistakable sign of carcinoma. This pattern is seen in Figure 28–11.

In many papillary carcinomas there are areas in which the proliferating cells form solid masses, shown in low and higher magnification in Figures 28–12 and 28–13. The metaplastic process by which this solid form of carcinoma evolves from papillary carcinoma is shown in Figures 28–14 and 28–15.

The so-called cribriform pattern of growth is often seen in papillary carcinoma (Fig. 28–16). It appears to result from the fusion of the papillary processes. The cribriform pattern is an absolute indication of carcinoma, even if it is seen in only a minute portion of a breast lesion.

Some papillary carcinomas contain extensive areas of mucoid change, as seen in Figure 28–17. Although lakes of mucoid material are found in the connective tissue stroma of these lesions, it is probable that the mucoid material evolves from the carcinoma cells.

(*Text continued on page 538.*)

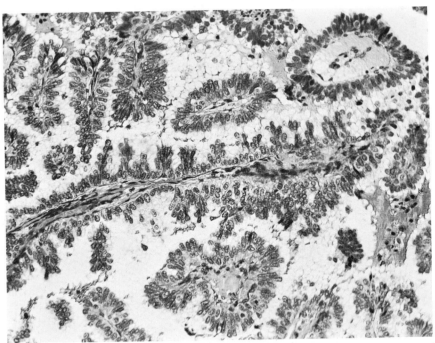

Figure 28–6.   Papillary carcinoma in which the papillae have well developed connective tissue cores.

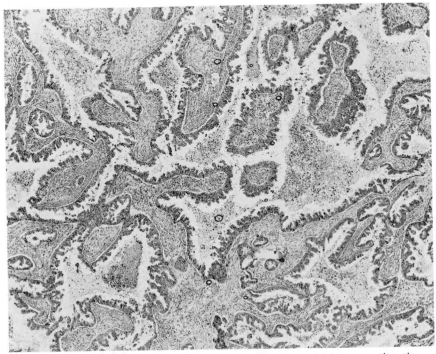

Figure 28–7.   Papillary carcinoma in which the papillae have thick connective tissue cores.

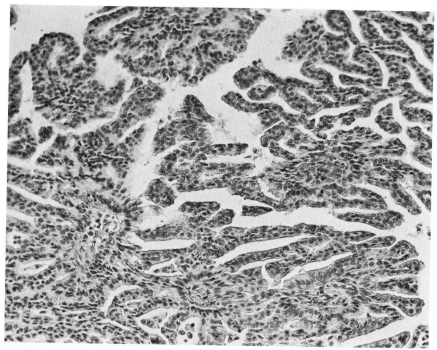

Figure 28–8.   Long, branching, coreless papillae in papillary carcinoma.

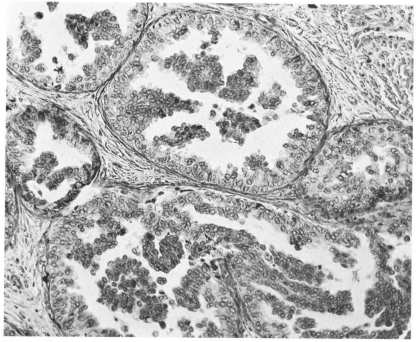

Figure 28–9.   Somewhat shorter papillary processes in papillary carcinoma.

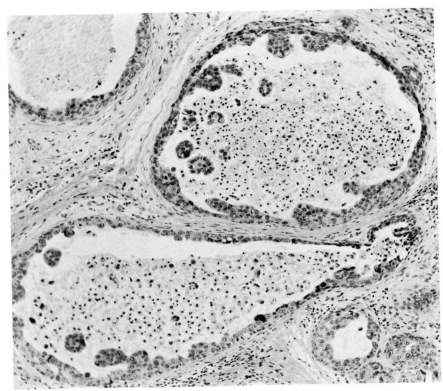

Figure 28–10. Very short papillae in intraductal carcinoma.

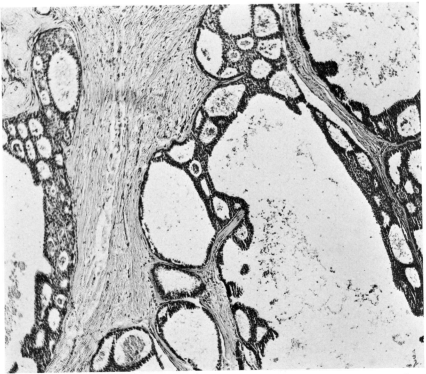

Figure 28–11. Papillary carcinoma in which low papillary processes have fused to form a cartwheel pattern lining dilated ducts.

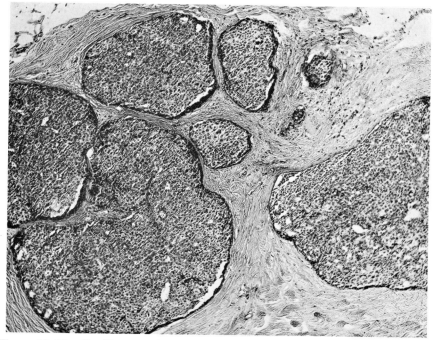

Figure 28–12. Papillary carcinoma growing in a solid pattern—low magnification.

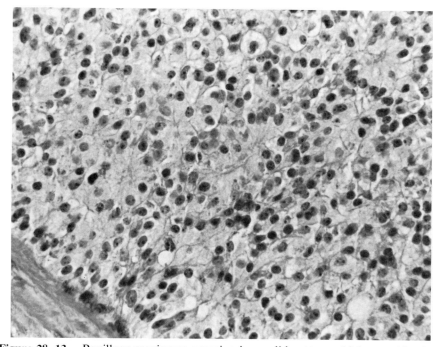

Figure 28–13. Papillary carcinoma growing in a solid pattern—high magnification.

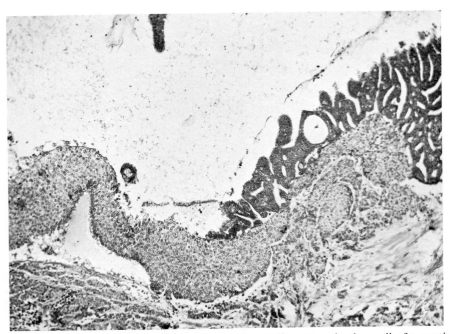

Figure 28–14. Transformation of a papillary to a solid growth pattern in the wall of a cystic space in a papillary carcinoma.

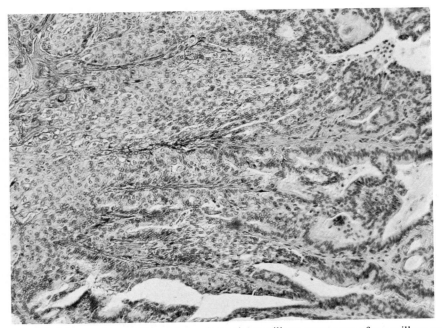

Figure 28–15. Solid masses of cells evolving from the papillary processes of a papillary carcinoma.

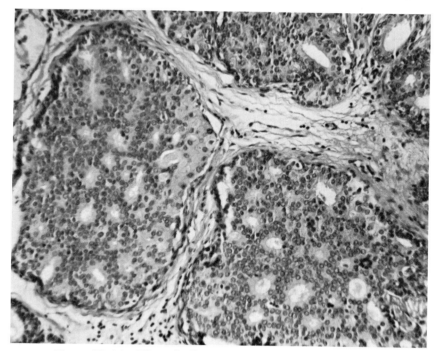

Figure 28–16. The cribriform pattern in papillary carcinoma.

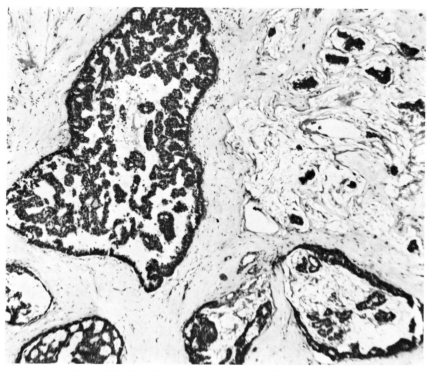

Figure 28–17. Mucoid change in papillary carcinoma.

Invasion of the stroma of the breast is, of course, an indication of malignancy when it is present, but it was not seen in a number of our well-differentiated, unquestionably malignant papillary lesions. If one could study serial microscopic sections from one of these tumors, evidence of invasion would probably be found. Invasion, as a histologic criterion by itself, is not a prerequisite for diagnosing a papillary lesion as a carcinoma.

The cytological criteria which constitute the most reliable basis for distinguishing between benign intraductal papilloma and papillary carcinoma include:

1. An abnormal degree of variation in the size and shape of the epithelial cells and their nuclei, and hyperchromatism of the nuclei. Frequent mitoses are an indication of malignancy when seen; but some of our indubitably malignant papillary tumors did not have them. Figure 28–18 shows an area in a papillary tumor where the large hyperchromatic cells and mitoses leave no doubt as to their carcinomatous nature.

2. A tendency for the proliferating cells to pile up several layers deep upon the papillary processes, with loss of the polarity of the nuclei. Figure 28–19 shows a papillary carcinoma in which the cells are arranged upon long branching papillary processes with well developed connective tissue cores. In a higher power view (Fig. 28–20) the cells are seen to be many layers deep. In Figure 28–21 a metastasis from this tumor to an axillary lymph node is seen to retain in part its papillary character.

This uniformly papillary type of carcinoma is usually the type found within a single cyst.

3. Although it is not an essential feature of papillary carcinoma, the great majority of these lesions are made up of cells of the so-called apocrine type, with cytoplasms which are larger and paler than the cells of most breast carcinomas. In Chapter 14 I described the origin of papillary carcinoma of the apocrine type from multiple papilloma. I must point out again that I could find no evidence in my data of papillary carcinoma originating from solitary papilloma. I do not mean to suggest that all papillary carcinomas are the apocrine type, but many are.

Kraus and Neubecker have discussed the special problems of distinguishing between benign papilloma and papillary carcinoma.

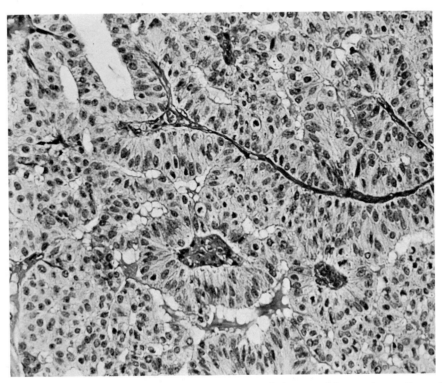

Figure 28–18. Papillary carcinoma with variation in size and shape and hyperchromatism of nuclei, and numerous mitoses.

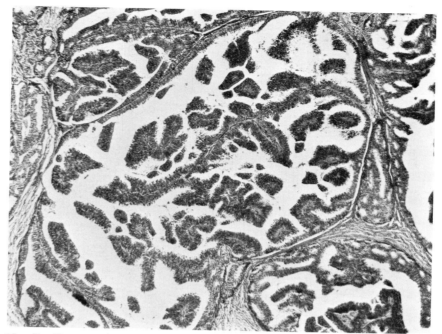

Figure 28–19. Papillary carcinoma in which the tumor cells are arranged on long, branching papillae.

They emphasize the microscopic differential features of the two lesions, as in Table 28-1.

While we agree with Kraus and Neubecker that hyperchromatic nuclei as well as the cribriform pattern of growth are important distinguishing features of papillary carci-noma, I must take issue with them regarding the other criteria in their list.

1. While two types of epithelial cells are often distinguishable in benign papillomas, there are a good many benign papillomas in which only one cell type is seen.

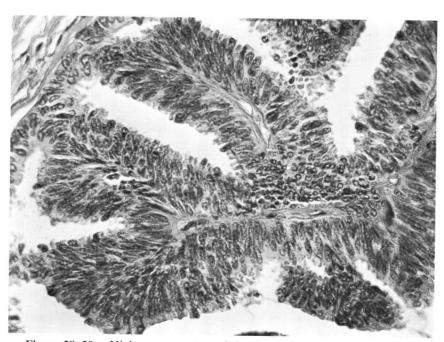

Figure 28–20. Higher power view of the tumor shown in Figure 28–19.

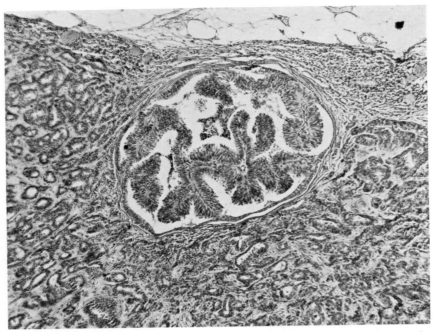

Figure 28–21. A metastasis in the marginal sinus of an axillary lymph node of the tumor shown in Figure 28–19.

2. Apocrine metaplasia is evident in many papillary carcinomas.

3. While it is true that the papillae in many papillary carcinomas do not have connective tissue stalks, we have studied a number of malignant papillary lesions in which the papillae had prominent stalks.

4. In some papillary lesions of proved malignant character, epithelial invasion is not demonstrable.

5. Particularly in the cystic form of papillary carcinoma, intraductal carcinoma in adjacent ducts is not found.

6. Sclerosing adenosis is a prominent feature of the breast tissue in the type of papillary carcinoma that originates from multiple papilloma.

The final proof that these papillary lesions that I have been describing are malignant is provided by the fact that they metastasize. In our 105 patients with papillary carcinoma treated by radical mastectomy 25 were found to have axillary lymph node metastases.

Although these tumors occasionally metastasize, they do not do so as often or as extensively as ordinary breast carcinomas. In my series of 1007 radical mastectomies axillary metastases were found in 44.3 per cent. Forty-five per cent of those who had axillary metastases had four or more axillary nodes involved. In the series of 25 patients with papillary carcinoma who had axillary metastases, only 32 per cent had four or more nodes involved.

Although only one-half of our 130 patients with papillary carcinoma have been followed for more than 10 years, eight of them have already developed carcinoma in the contralateral breast. I suspect that a longer follow up will reveal that this type of breast carcinoma involves both breasts with unusual frequency.

Table 28–1. DIFFERENTIAL DIAGNOSIS OF PAPILLARY BREAST TUMORS ACCORDING TO KRAUS AND NEUBECKER

Papilloma	Papillary Carcinoma
Two types of epithelial cells	Single type of epithelial cell
Nuclei normochromatic	Nuclei hyperchromatic
Apocrine metaplasia present	Apocrine metaplasia absent
Complex glandular pattern	Cribriform pattern
Prominent connective tissue stroma	Delicate or absent connective tissue stroma
Periductal fibrosis with epithelial entrapment	Epithelial invasion of stroma
Intraductal hyperplasia in adjacent ducts	Intraductal carcinoma in adjacent ducts
Sclerosing adenosis sometimes present in adjacent breast tissue	Sclerosing adenosis generally absent in adjacent breast tissue

We have learned not to try to distinguish between benign papilloma and papillary carcinoma by means of frozen sections: it is too difficult. We wait for permanent sections.

Treatment

Kraus and Neubecker fail to present 10 year follow-up data for their 21 patients with papillary carcinoma.

Veronesi reported 10 year follow-up data for 25 of his 60 patients with papillary carcinoma treated by radical mastectomy. Fifty-two per cent survived 10 years. This was a better survival rate than for ordinary breast carcinoma in his institute.

Review of the results of treatment in our series of cases leads us to the conclusion that papillary carcinoma is the least malignant and the most easily cured by surgery of all forms of mammary carcinoma. Sixty-four of our patients were treated more than 10 years ago. Forty-five, or 70 per cent, are known to have survived for more than 10 years. These end results are better than this simple 10 year survival rate indicates because there was one operative death, three patients were lost track of, and six are known to have died of intercurrent disease. All 10 patients are counted in the determination of this survival rate as succumbing to their carcinoma. These results are shown in detail in Table 28-2.

These results are the more remarkable because the good results in several of our patients were achieved with very limited surgery or delayed radical surgery, which, I believe, would have failed if the carcinoma had been an ordinary type. The results of the different methods of treatment are shown in Table 28-3.

Partial mastectomy as a primary method of treatment was successful in one patient. In a second patient treated in this way the disease

Table 28–2. TEN-YEAR RESULTS OF ALL METHODS OF TREATMENT OF PAPILLARY CARCINOMA OF THE BREAST, 1930–1958

Total number of patients treated more than 10 years ago	64
Operative death following radical mastectomy	1
Lost track of before 10 years	3
Died of intercurrent disease before 10 years	6
Died of unknown cause before 10 years	2
Died with metastases before 10 years	8
Survived 10 years	45

Table 28–3. METHODS OF TREATMENT IN PAPILLARY CARCINOMA AND 10-YEAR RESULTS, 1930–1958

Method of Treatment	No. of Patients	No. Surviving 10 Years
Primary radical mastectomy	46	30
Primary simple mastectomy	4	3
Primary partial mastectomy	1	1
Primary partial mastectomy, local recurrence, radical mastectomy	1	1
Primary local excision only	2	2
Primary local excision, local recurrence, simple mastectomy	1	1
Primary local excision, local recurrence, radical mastectomy	6	5
Irradiation only	1	0
Irradiation, later followed by simple mastectomy for persisting local disease	1	1
Irradiation, later followed by radical mastectomy for persisting local disease	1	1
Total	64	45

recurred locally after six years and radical mastectomy was done. This patient died of bone metastases seven years later.

Nine patients were treated primarily by local excision. Two of them, both feeble old women, aged 74 and 76, respectively, in whom more extensive surgery was regarded as hazardous, survived more than 10 years without recurrence. The other seven who were treated primarily by local excision developed local recurrence. One was then treated by simple mastectomy and died after 11 years, with cardiac disease. In the other six radical mastectomy was done. One of the six died of intercurrent disease seven years later. One died of bone metastases after 13 years. One died of pulmonary metastases after 16 years. The other three were well 14, 17, and 20 years later.

The slow course of papillary carcinoma is indicated by the fact that an average of 4.7 years elapsed before local recurrence developed in the 10 patients who were treated by local excision or partial mastectomy.

It is only fair, in defense of our surgeons, to point out why the initial treatment was only local excision or partial mastectomy in 11 of our patients with papillary carcinoma. In two aged patients it was thought that more extensive surgery would be hazardous. In the nine others the pathologist misdiagnosed the lesion as a benign papilloma. Some of these mistaken diagnoses were made as long as 30

Table 28–4. FREQUENCY OF AXILLARY METASTASES IN PAPILLARY CARCINOMA TREATED PRIMARILY BY RADICAL MASTECTOMY COMPARED WITH ALL BREAST CARCINOMAS IN MY PERSONAL SERIES OF RADICAL MASTECTOMIES, 1935–1968

Columbia Clinical Classification	Papillary Carcinoma		All Carcinomas in Personal Series	
	No. of Patients	Per cent with Axillary Metastases	No. of Patients	Per cent with Axillary Metastases
Stage A	36	16%	724	31%
Stage B	8	63%	198	75%
Stage C	1	100%	71	82%
Stage D	0	–	14	93%
Totals	45	23%	1,007	56%

years ago. We believe that we do better to-day.

Our findings as regards axillary metastases, and the 10-year survival rates, in our series of 45 patients with papillary carcinoma treated primarily by radical mastectomy, are presented in Tables 28–4 and 28–5. The frequency of axillary metastases in these papillary carcinomas was only about half that of carcinoma of no special type. The results in these papillary carcinomas are much better than a first glance at Table 28–5 indicates. If the operative death, the two deaths from intercurrent disease, and the three patients lost track of, had not been counted as deaths from carcinoma, the 10-year survival rate in our Clinical Stage A cases would have been 97 per cent.

These data indicate that radical mastectomy is a very successful method of primary treatment for papillary carcinoma. Less complete operations are apt to fail for two reasons. First, these lesions are often multicentric and may extend widely in the breast. All breast tissue should be removed, and this is best achieved with the sacrifice of a wide area of skin over the breast and a skin graft.

Second, papillary carcinomas do metastasize to the axilla, although less frequently than other types of carcinoma. No one can know which patient has axillary metastases for which an axillary dissection is imperative.

Unlike most types of breast carcinoma, the papillary form can sometimes be cured by a thoroughly radical surgical attack when it has recurred following inadequate surgery. The following case history illustrates this fact.

Mrs. D. P., a housewife aged 34, discovered a small movable tumor in the upper outer sector of the left breast in October, 1943. It was locally excised at a New York hospital and diagnosed microscopically as an intraductal papilloma. Eighteen months later local recurrence was noted. A second local excision was performed in another New York hospital. This time the surgeon removed a great part of the upper outer sector of the breast. Again the lesion was diagnosed microscopically as a papilloma.

One year after the second operation, and three and a half years after she had first found a tumor in her breast, a discharge from the nipple developed. It was usually serous, but occasionally blood-tinged.

In January, 1947, after another nine months had

Table 28–5. TEN-YEAR SURVIVAL FOLLOWING RADICAL MASTECTOMY FOR PAPILLARY CARCINOMA COMPARED WITH ALL BREAST CARCINOMAS IN MY PERSONAL SERIES OF CASES, 1935–1957

Columbia Clinical Classification	Papillary Carcinoma		All Carcinomas in Personal Series	
	No. of Patients	Per cent 10-Year Survival	No. of Patients	Per cent 10-Year Survival
Stage A	35	80%*	402	70%
Stage B	8	25%†	154	41%
Stage C	1	0%	59	24%
Stage D	0	–	11	18%
Totals	45	67%	626	57%

*One operative death, two deaths from intercurrent disease before 10 years, and three patients lost track of, are counted as deaths from carcinoma.

†Two deaths from intercurrent disease before 10 years counted as deaths from carcinoma.

elapsed, the patient first consulted me. I found a firm, poorly delimited tumor, measuring 5 × 6 cm., extending from the outer edge of the areola out into the upper outer sector of the left breast. In addition, the entire upper half of the breast was studded with small, movable, firm nodules, lying deep in the breast substance. I could not feel any enlarged axillary nodes.

My first step was to do a biopsy of the recurrent tumor in the upper outer sector of the breast. The tissue was studied by frozen sections, and unfortunately we relied upon them and decided that the lesion was indeed a benign papilloma. Because the lesion had recurred twice before, I chose to perform a simple mastectomy, including in my dissection the lowest group of axillary lymph glands.

We were distressed to find in study of paraffin sections that the tumor was a well-differentiated papillary carcinoma (Fig. 28–22). It had involved a great part of the breast. The widely disseminated shotty nodules that had been noted on palpation were all carcinoma, and the disease had extended down through the entire thickness of the breast to involve the pectoral fascia which had been excised with the breast. Metastases were found adjacent to two of the 13 axillary lymph nodes (Fig. 28–23). We were able to secure sections of the lesions removed at the two previous local excisions at other hospitals. It was apparent that the tumor had been a well-differentiated papillary carcinoma from the beginning.

With the diagnosis established, I at once performed a radical mastectomy, carrying out a specially wide removal of skin and subcutaneous tissues on the chest wall, which required very extensive skin grafting. No additional axillary metastases were found.

Twenty-two years later there had been no recurrence of her breast carcinoma.

A second case history of papillary carcinoma that I wish to summarize illustrates the slow course of the disease, which, in this instance, ended fatally.

Mrs. J. R., a nurse, aged 40, was admitted to the Presbyterian Hospital in February, 1938 for treatment of a tumor of her right breast of four months' duration. It was situated in the lower inner sector of the breast, measured 5 × 4 cm., and was well delimited and movable. It was excised locally and mistakenly diagnosed as a benign intraductal papilloma. We today recognize the lesion as well-differentiated papillary carcinoma.

Three and half years later, in September, 1941, she was again admitted to the hospital for a recurrence measuring 4 × 2 cm. at the site of the original tumor. Biopsy now led to the correct diagnosis of papillary carcinoma, and radical mastectomy was performed. The tumor was found to involve the breast very extensively, and there was a metastasis in one of the 20 lymph nodes removed in the axillary dissection.

In February, 1952, 10½ years after her radical mastectomy, enlargement of right supraclavicular and lower cervical nodes was noted, and a neck dissection revealed metastases from her breast carcinoma. She developed pulmonary metastases,

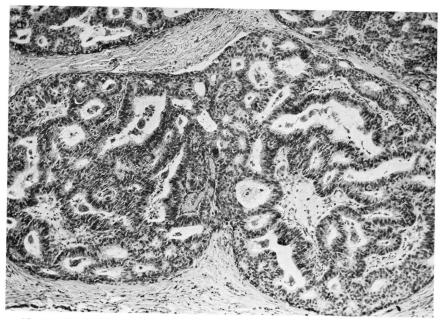

Figure 28–22. Well differentiated papillary carcinoma that recurred after local excision.

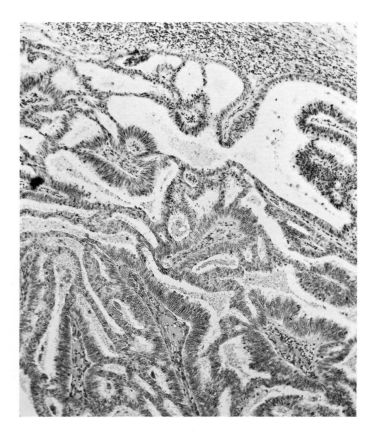

Figure 28–23. Metastasis to axillary node of papillary carcinoma shown in Figure 28–22.

and died in October, 1954, 16½ years after the onset of her papillary carcinoma.

Radiotherapy has not been a successful method of treatment in the three patients in our series of cases of papillary carcinoma in whom it was the primary treatment. It failed to control the local tumor, except temporarily, in all three. One patient died within a year with liver metastases, and the other two, whose tumors recurred locally one year and four years, respectively, after irradiation, were then treated by radical mastectomy and apparently cured.

REFERENCES

Gatchell, F. G., Dockerty, M. B., and Clagett, O. T.: Intracystic carcinoma of the breast. Surg., Gynec. & Obst., *106*:347, 1958.

Kraus, F. T., and Neubecker, R. D.: The differential diagnosis of papillary tumors of the breast. Cancer, *15*:444, 1962.

McDivitt, R. W., Stewart, F. W., and Berg, J. W.: Tumors of the Breast. Atlas of Tumor Pathology, Washington, D.C., Armed Forces Institute of Pathology, 1968, Second Series, Fascicle 2.

Veronesi, U., Giarrusso, A., and Guarino, M.: Il carcinoma papillifero della mammella. Tumori, *50*:421, 1964.

Chapter Twenty-Nine

Paget's Carcinoma of the Breast

More than a hundred years have gone by since Velpeau first described the lesion of the nipple that is today generally called Paget's disease, in the following words:

In two such cases, the crusts covering the nipple were thick, cracked, and adherent, and gave exit to a bloody discharge when an attempt was made to detach them. In one of the patients they were of a greenish, and in the other, of a yellowish-grey color.

In these, as in many other instances, the disease had lasted for several years, and was accompanied by itching, but without any marked inflammatory symptoms. Underneath the crusts there was neither fissure nor destruction of tissue, but simple excoriation. Everything indicated that the epidermis alone had undergone destruction, and that the free surfaces of the lobules and little glands of the organ were the seat of the disease. The nipple looked like a raspberry or strawberry, and rather suggested the idea of the granular neck of the uterus.

Velpeau could not have followed his patients, for he was unaware of any relationship of this nipple lesion to carcinoma. It was James Paget, in 1874, who first observed that the nipple erosion was associated with breast cancer. His terse clinical description of the disease, which follows, could scarcely be improved upon:

The patients were all women, various in age from 40 to 60 or more years, having in common nothing remarkable but their disease. In all of them the disease began as an eruption on the nipple and areola. In the majority it had the appearance of a florid, intensely red, raw surface, very finely granular, as if nearly the whole thickness of the epidermis were removed; like the surface of very acute diffuse eczema, or like that of an acute balanitis. From such a surface, on the whole or greater part of the nipple and areola, there was always copious, clear, yellowish, viscid exudation. The sensations were commonly tingling, itching, and burning, but the malady was never attended by disturbance of the general health. I have not seen this form of eruption extend beyond the areola, and only once have seen it pass into a deeper ulceration of the skin after the manner of a rodent ulcer.

In some of the cases the eruption has presented the characters of an ordinary chronic eczema, with minute vesications, succeeded by soft, moist, yellowish scabs or scales, and constant viscid exudation. In some it has been like psoriasis, dry, with a few white scales slowly desquamating; and in both these forms, especially in the psoriasis, I have seen the eruption spreading far beyond the areola in widening circles, or, with scattered blotches of redness, covering nearly the whole breast.

I am not aware that in any of the cases which I have seen the eruption was different from what may be described as long-persistent eczema, or psoriasis, or by some other name, in treatises on diseases of the skin; and I believe that such cases sometimes occur on the breast, and after many months' duration are cured, or pass by, and are not followed by any other disease. But it has happened that in every case which I have been able to watch, cancer of the mammary gland has followed within at the most two years, and usually within one year. The eruption has resisted all the treatment, both local and general, that has been used, and has continued even after the affected part of the skin has been involved in the cancerous disease.

The formation of cancer has not in any case taken place first in the diseased part of the skin. It has always been in the substance of the mammary gland, beneath or not far from the diseased skin, and always with a clear interval of apparently healthy tissue.

In the cancers themselves, I have seen in these cases nothing peculiar. They have been various in form; some acute, some chronic, the majority following an average course, and all tending to the same end; recurring if removed, affecting lymph-glands and distant parts, showing nothing which might not be written in the ordinary history of cancer of the breast.

The single noteworthy fact found in all these cases is that which I have stated in the first sentence, and I think it deserves careful study. For the sequence of cancer after the chronic skin-disease is so frequent that it may be suspected of being a consequence and must be always feared, and may be sometimes almost certainly foretold.

Incidence

Our Columbia-Presbyterian series includes 158 women and one man with Paget's carcinoma. This disease has constituted about 2.5 per cent of all our mammary carcinomas.

I discuss the special features of Paget's carcinoma in the male in Chapter 38.

Age Distribution

The mean age of our 158 women with Paget's carcinoma has been 53.9 years, which is slightly older than for our breast carcinomas of no special type, whose average age was 50. Studying the relationship of the age of our patients with Paget's carcinoma to the variety of the disease which they had, we found, however, that those who had only nipple changes (redness, roughness, or erosion) had an average age of 58, whereas those who had a breast tumor in addition to nipple changes or only a breast tumor had an average age of 49 (Chart 29-1). This age difference suggests that these two clinical types of Paget's carcinoma are somewhat different.

Pathology and Natural History

In discussing Paget's carcinoma it is desirable to deal first with the pathology of the disease, because its natural history and clinical classification can be understood only in the light of our knowledge of the pathologic process.

The first step in this direction was the microscopic recognition of the large cells with pale cytoplasms and prominent irregular nuclei, occasionally seen in mitoses, occurring singly or in clumps in the nipple epidermis, which we now call Paget's cells. Darier first

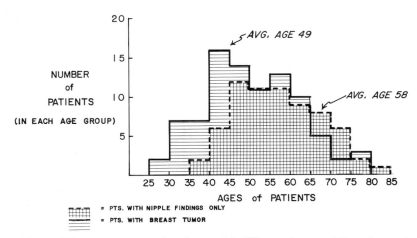

Chart 29-1. The average age of patients with different forms of Paget's carcinoma.

described these cells in 1889 but mistakenly regarded them merely as degenerated epidermal cells. There has since been much controversy regarding the nature of the cells but the fact is now established beyond any reasonable doubt that they are carcinoma cells that have invaded the epidermis of the nipple from carcinoma in the subjacent nipple ducts. It was Jacobaeus who, in 1904, first traced their origin from intraductal carcinoma in the nipple ducts. These Paget cells have a peculiar and special facility for invading epithelium—in the epidermis of the nipple as well as in the epithelial lining of nipple and mammary ducts. This invasive process has been well described during recent years by Simard, by Inglis, by Muir, by Toker, and by Sirtori.

If we adhere to the original descriptions of the disease by Velpeau and Paget it is one in which the epidermis contains the carcinoma cells we have come to call Paget's cells. I have therefore not included in our series several cases in which these cells are found in the ducts of the nipple but not in the nipple epidermis.

Paget's cells, in the earliest stage of their infiltration of the epidermis, are seen as isolated scattered units in the basal portion of the epidermis (Fig. 29-1). They are large cells with prominent, irregular, hyperchromatic nuclei, which are occasionally in mitosis. Their cytoplasms are very pale and finely granular. They are obviously malignant cells. Only a few isolated cells of this type need to be identified to establish the diagnosis. As invasion of the epidermis progresses, the Paget's cells form clumps and masses, as seen in Figure 29-2. Paget's cells may even form acini as shown in Figure 29-3.

Culberson and Horn pointed out an interesting feature of Paget's cells, namely, their tendency in occasional cases to have melanin granules in their cytoplasms. Usually the melanin is very limited in amount, and does not present a diagnostic problem. In infrequent cases—one of which was described by Culberson and Horn—the Paget's cells contain so much melanin that the lesion closely resembles a junctional type of melanoma. Pathologists who face this differential diagnosis

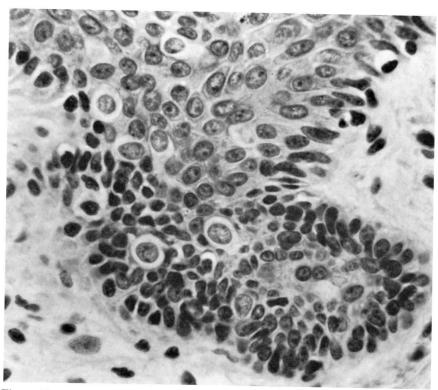

Figure 29-1. Isolated Paget's cells in the basal portion of the nipple epidermis.

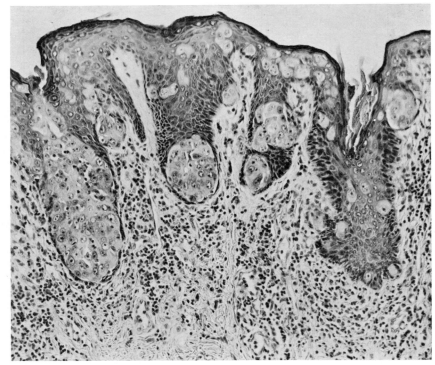

Figure 29–2.   Paget's cells invading the epidermis of the nipple more extensively.

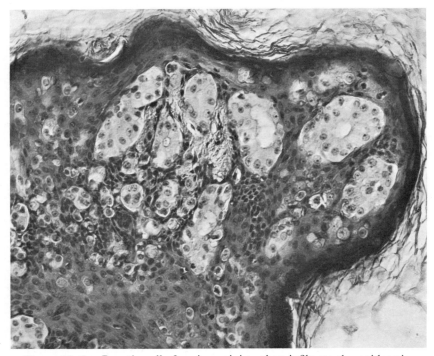

Figure 29–3.   Paget's cells forming acini as they infiltrate the epidermis.

can take comfort from the fact that, to my knowledge, malignant melanoma originating on the nipple itself has not been observed. Neubecker and Bradshaw have also discussed melanin in Paget's cells. Sagebiel has studied Paget's cells with the electron microscope. His findings support the epithelial origin of these cells and exclude their origin from the melanocytic system.

In their comparatively early stage of invasion of the nipple epidermis the Paget's cells produce no change in the naked-eye appearance of the nipple, although the patient may complain of itching or of a burning sensation in the nipple.

The next symptom in the sequence of clinical phenomena produced by invasion of the nipple by Paget's cells is often redness of the nipple surface. This may be so slight that the patient herself does not notice it, but it is occasionally obvious, as shown in Figure 29-4. The epithelium of this nipple is not eroded. It is merely reddened, and appears smoother than normal. Most clinicians are unaware of the significance of this phenomenon as an indication of Paget's carcinoma.

The microscopic features of this stage of the disease are shown in Figure 29-5. The cornified layer of the epidermis is intact, but Paget's cells have infiltrated the entire underlying thickness of the epidermis. In the dermis there are foci of lymphocytes.

Roughening and thickening of the epidermis are the next phases of the pre-erosive stage of Paget's disease in the nipple. This phase was exemplified in a patient of mine whose attention had been called to her nipple by itching. She noted that the surface of her nipple was somewhat roughened and thickened. This had not changed in two years when she consulted me. There was no erosion. I excised a small wedge of the nipple for biopsy. Figure 29-6 shows its microscopic character. The epidermis is replaced by Paget's cells except for a thin cornified layer which is intact. The Paget infiltration has extended down into the dermis and actually thickened the skin of the nipple.

In the next stage of Paget's disease, erosion of the nipple surface occurs. The most frequent story is that the patient next finds a brownish spot on her brassiere or nightgown, and on inspecting her nipple she discovers a small yellowish-gray, crusted area, or a tiny bright red erosion. Figure 29-7 shows such an erosion. The erosion often crusts over after being cleaned and treated with ointment of some kind. But after a few days or weeks it inevitably breaks open again. The enlargement of the erosion is so slow, however, that

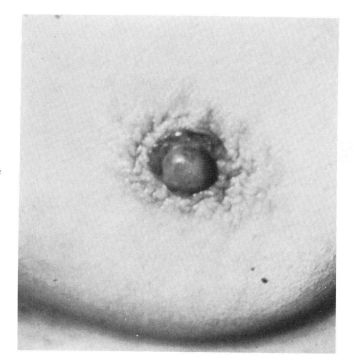

Figure 29-4. Redness of the nipple in the pre-erosive stage of Paget's carcinoma.

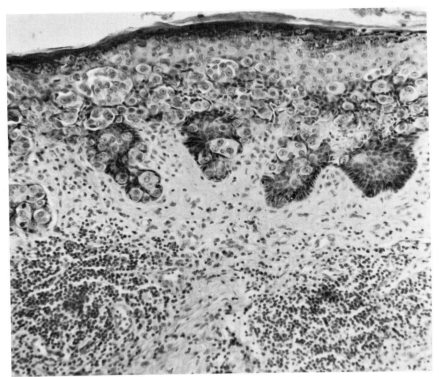

Figure 29–5.   Reddening of the nipple produced by infiltration of the epidermis by Paget's cells.

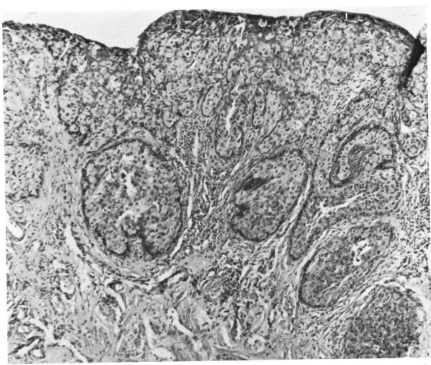

Figure 29–6.   Roughening and thickening of the nipple surface produced by infiltration of the epidermis by Paget's cells.

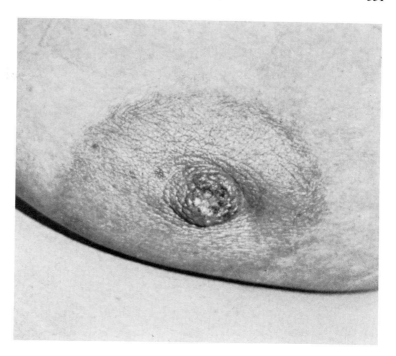

Figure 29–7. Erosion of the nipple surface in Paget's carcinoma.

many months may go by before much of the nipple surface is involved. It is difficult for the patient or her physician to believe that such a small and seemingly innocuous lesion can be cancer.

The nipple erosion is not always circular. It may take the form of a transverse crevice in the nipple. When the edges of the crevice are pulled apart its base has the characteristic bright red, granulomatous appearance.

The nipple discharge of which these patients with Paget's erosion of the nipple often complain is usually not a true discharge from nipple ducts, but only the serum or blood that oozes from the erosion. An occasional patient who has no erosion may have a true nipple discharge produced by the carcinoma growing in the ducts of the nipple.

Figure 29–8 shows the microscopic appearance of an eroded nipple in a patient in whom the erosion had been present for six years. The epidermis is completely replaced by Paget's cells, and is covered by a thin layer of fibrin. There is a heavy infiltration of lymphocytes in the dermis.

As time goes by the entire surface of the nipple is eroded, and it is flattened and distorted. The erosion extends out into the epidermis of the areola. The areola is contracted. The entire nipple and areolar area is covered with a crust, as seen in Figure 29–9.

The erosion may eventually involve a great part of the skin over the breast, as seen in Figure 29–10. In this patient the erosion had slowly extended during a seven year period. There was no palpable tumor in the breast. I performed radical mastectomy with a large skin graft. There were no involved axillary nodes. The patient survived for 19 years without any recurrence of her breast disease.

When nipple erosion has been present for a very long time and has involved the areola and the surrounding skin of the breast as in this patient, the outlines of both the nipple and areola are lost in scar tissue.

In occasional mammary carcinomas of no special type, the carcinoma extends upward through the breast until it reaches the nipple and areolar region and finally invades the overlying epidermis. This kind of contact invasion of the nipple epidermis should not be confused with the type described by Paget in which the carcinoma reaches the nipple epidermis via the duct system. The two types of invasion are also different clinically. In that due to contact invasion of the nipple by ordinary breast carcinoma the nipple is usually retracted and fixed to the underlying carcinoma. In the erosion of Paget's carcinoma the nipple continues to be erect and movable for a long time. It is destroyed only after the erosion involves the whole of the nipple epi-

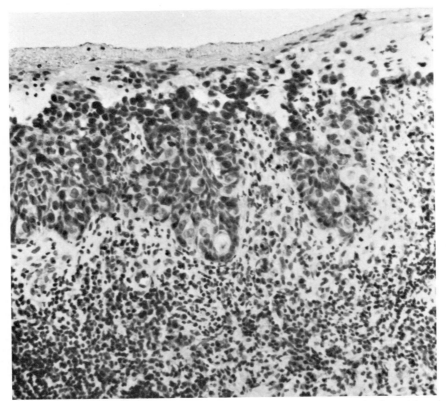

Figure 29–8. Erosion of the nipple surface produced by infiltration of the nipple epidermis by Paget's cells. The erosion is covered with a layer of fibrin.

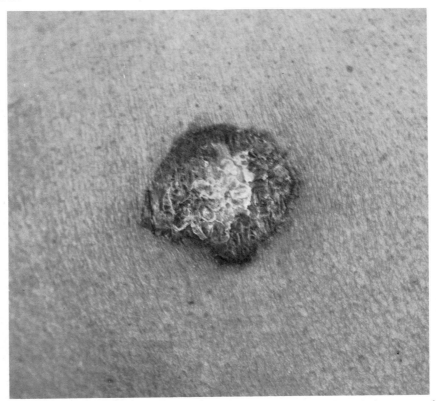

Figure 29–9. Paget's erosion that has destroyed most of the nipple and extended out over the contracted areola.

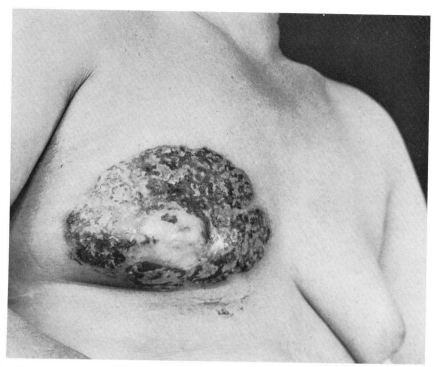

Figure 29–10. Extensive Paget's erosion of seven years' duration that has extended over a large portion of the skin of the breast.

dermis and extends out into the areola and the skin over the breast.

The question of the origin of the Paget's cells in the nipple epidermis has been much debated. Although a few cases have been reported in which Paget's cells were found only in the nipple epidermis, and it was therefore claimed that they had originated there, this finding can be explained as a consequence of incomplete study of the nipple ducts. In our laboratory we have no examples of Paget's carcinoma of the nipple epidermis in the female in which intraductal carcinoma was not found in the duct system of the nipple or breast.

We do, however, have a case of Paget's carcinoma in the male—our only one—in which Paget's cells were found only in the nipple epidermis. I describe this interesting case in detail in Chapter 38.

It can be said that there is today general agreement that in all cases of Paget's carcinoma the disease is found not only in the nipple epidermis but also in the nipple ducts, and that in the great majority of cases there is also intraductal carcinoma of the mammary gland itself.

Disagreement continues as to where in the duct system the intraductal carcinoma originates.

Cheatle devoted one-sixth of his book. *Tumours of the Breast,* to presenting the details of his study by the whole breast section method of his 17 cases of Paget's disease. This great effort did not solve the problem, because the cytology in whole breast sections is not the best, and because the sections were unfortunately cut vertically. It is obvious that the only method by which the relationship of lesions in the nipple and nipple ducts to lesions in the underlying breast ducts and in the breast as a whole can be accurately determined is by horizontal serial key block sections. The labor of studying a significant number of cases in this manner is so great that no one has attempted it.

Inglis has maintained that the disease is a special form of intraductal carcinoma that originates in the ducts of the nipple and spreads downward by continuity in the epithelium of the duct system, and thus produces the carcinoma so frequently found in the depths of the breast. There are two strong points that can be made against Inglis' concept. In our series of cases there are many in which there is extensive intraductal carcinoma in the breast itself, but only minimal involvement of the nipple ducts and epidermis. In such cases it would seem that the carcinoma must have developed first in the breast. Secondly, in our series of 148 cases of Paget's carcinoma in which we were able to carry out careful microscopic studies of the breast itself as well as the nipple and its ducts, there were only 17 in which we failed to find intraductal carcinoma in the breast itself. If Paget's carcinoma originates in the ducts of the nipple and grows downward into the breast, one would expect to find a much larger proportion of cases in which the underlying breast is not involved.

Muir, on the other hand, believes that the intraductal carcinoma of Paget's carcinoma is fundamentally no different from other breast duct carcinomas. It may originate in any part of the duct system and may arise in multiple independent foci. If it develops first in the ducts of the nipple it may spread to the nipple epidermis and produce Paget's erosion. If it develops in the ducts in the breast proper it may grow upward in the duct system to reach the nipple. To Muir, the Paget type of carcinoma is therefore merely "a rare complication of a quite common condition," i.e., intraductal carcinoma.

Sirtori has recently published an exhaustive review of the various theories concerning the site of origin of Paget's carcinoma, and has described his findings in 30 cases of his own, with excellent microphotographs.

Toker studied one example of Paget's carcinoma with serial sections. He traced the spread of an intraductal carcinoma situated deeply in the breast, upward in a single duct by continuous intraepithelial permeation to reach the nipple epidermis.

The relationship of carcinoma in the depths of the breast to involvement of the nipple is illustrated in Figure 29–11, which shows in low power magnification a vertical section of a breast in which Paget's cells are seen in the nipple epidermis (*A*), while in the depths of the breast there is a small infiltrating carcinoma (*C*). The two lesions are seen to be connected by a duct filled with carcinoma (*B*). The duct (*B*) which served as a pathway for the disease to reach the nipple epidermis is shown in higher magnification in Figure 29–12. These ducts in the nipple are generally referred to as *nipple ducts* or *lactiferous ducts*. They are in fact the specialized milk sinuses which I have described in Chapter 1, and, properly speaking, should be referred to by that name. Figure 29–13 shows a milk sinus filled with carcinoma leading up to its ampulla, lined with squamous epithelium, into which it empties. Parallel and to its right in

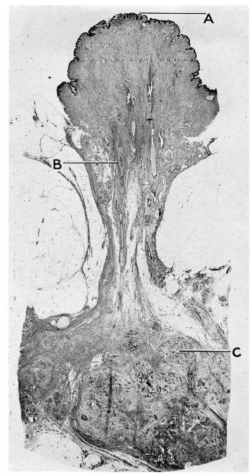

Figure 29–11. Low power vertical section through a breast containing Paget's carcinoma. *A*, Paget's cells in epidermis. *B*, Duct lined by intraductal carcinoma. *C*, Infiltrating carcinoma in the depths of the breast.

the photograph is a normal milk sinus with its pleated wall, cut vertically.

An early stage of involvement of a milk sinus by Paget's carcinoma (cut transversely), is shown in Figure 29–14. Beneath the normal two layers of cuboidal cells lining the milk sinus, around about three-quarters of its circumference, masses of paler and larger carcinoma cells have accumulated. They are growing upward in the wall of the milk sinus by permeation from the intraductal carcinoma in the underlying breast.

At a more advanced stage in the process, shown in Figure 29–15, the carcinoma cells have replaced the normal two-layered epithelial lining of the milk sinus and have piled up

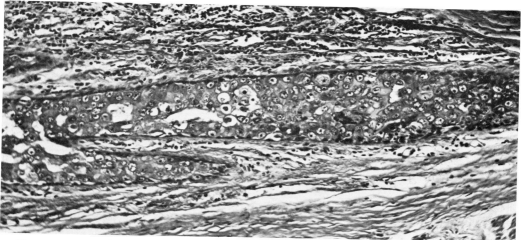

Figure 29–12. The duct at the base of the nipple (*B* in Figure 29–11) through which the carcinoma in the underlying breast reached the nipple epidermis.

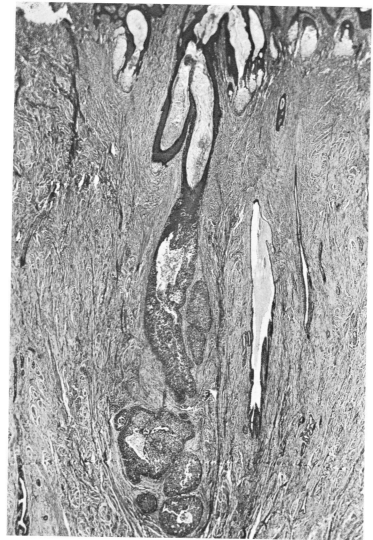

Figure 29–13. Intraductal carcinoma growing through a milk sinus up to the level of the epidermis in Paget's carcinoma.

many layers deep within it. At a still later stage (Fig. 29–16) the accordion-pleated configuration of the milk sinus is lost as it fills up with carcinoma cells. A collar of lymphocytes surrounds it.

A number of milk sinuses are usually involved by the disease. Figure 29–17 shows a transverse section through a nipple in which five of a total of 22 of the milk sinuses are involved. In one of my patients who had a nipple erosion for six years, and who had no gross or microscopic carcinoma in her breast, 18 of the 20 milk sinuses were involved by the disease. The fact that a number of milk sinuses are usually involved even when no carcinoma is found in the breast itself is a strong argument for the multicentric origin of Paget's carcinoma in the milk sinuses. In our 17 cases of Paget's disease in which no carcinoma was found in the breast itself, more than one milk sinus was involved in all but two cases. The case history of one of these two patients follows.

Miss C. T., an unmarried office worker aged 43, came complaining of "eczema" of the nipple which she had had for two years. When it first developed she consulted her physician, who gave her an ointment. The "eczema" healed temporarily but soon broke open again. Tar ointment had made it worse.

The nipple was erect, and normal in shape. The epithelium of the entire surface of the nipple was eroded, and appeared bright red and granular. The erosion also extended out onto the areola at one point. There was no tumor palpable in the breast. A 1 cm. firm axillary node was felt in the axilla.

Biopsy of the nipple erosion showed typical Paget's carcinoma. Radical mastectomy was then carried out.

The microscopic studies showed intraductal carcinoma in the terminal portion of a single milk sinus (Fig. 29–18) from which Paget's cells infiltrated the nipple epithelium extensively and produced a large erosion. More than 100 sections from the breast failed to show any carcinoma in it. There were no metastases in 49 lymph nodes.

This case, then, is an example of an early stage of the disease, the intraductal carcinoma being found only in a single milk sinus.

Carcinoma in the breast itself was found in 131 of our 148 cases of Paget's carcinoma in which we were able to study the breast. The lesion in the breast itself may be very small. When this is the case, very thorough microscopic study of the breast is required to find it. For many years it has been the tradition of our laboratory of surgical pathology to study

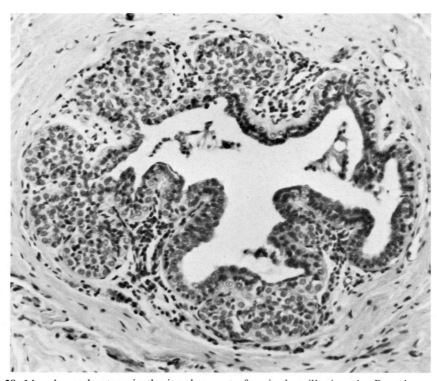

Figure 29–14. An early stage in the involvement of a nipple milk sinus by Paget's carcinoma.

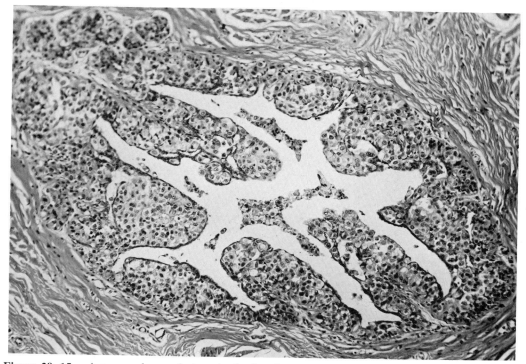

Figure 29–15. A more advanced stage in the involvement of a milk sinus by Paget's carcinoma.

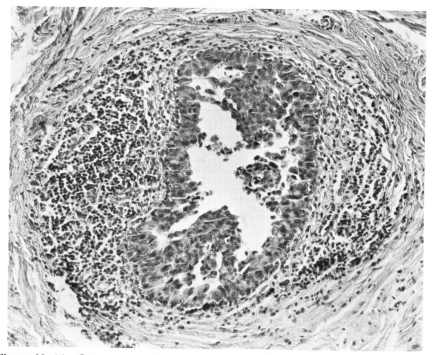

Figure 29–16. Later stage of involvement of a milk sinus by Paget's carcinoma.

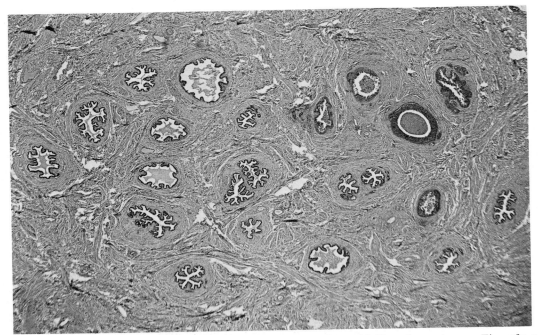

Figure 29–17. A transverse section through the nipple in a patient with Paget's carcinoma. Five of a total of 22 milk sinuses are involved by the disease.

breast specimens with great care. An average of about 20 microscopic sections from the nipple and breast are studied in each case, and occasionally many more. In one case of Paget's disease a total of 1092 sections were studied and no carcinoma was found in the breast itself.

The breast lesions in Paget's carcinoma are all of the intraductal type. Figure 29–19 shows a typical one. This does not mean to say that they are exclusively intraductal. Most of them invade the breast widely, as shown in Figure 29–20. There are many variations of the growth pattern of these intraductal carcinomas in Paget's disease. Figure 29–21 shows another common type.

The basic feature of the intraductal carcinomas of Paget's disease is their epidermotrophic character—their predilection to extend along ducts replacing the normal duct epithelium. They usually grow upward in the duct system to produce the lesion in the nipple epidermis that gives the disease its name. They also grow downward in the duct system of the breast to reach its ultimate with the lobule and replace the lobular epithelium. Figure 29–22 shows a mammary lobule in which the phenomenon has occurred.

The breast component of Paget's disease is not only intraductal, but it is often so widely dispersed in the breast that it must have originated in multiple foci. In a number of our cases several sectors of the breast were involved by the disease, although there was no dominant grossly visible tumor anywhere.

The ducts of the breast are occasionally much dilated, as seen in Figure 29–23. This is presumably the result of blocking of the main collecting ducts and the milk sinuses of the nipple by the carcinoma growing in them. Whatever the explanation, it is a phenomenon peculiar to Paget's carcinoma.

Classification of Paget's Carcinoma

On the basis of the natural history of Paget's carcinoma as I have described it, there are six different stages of the disease. I will define each stage and give an example of it.

1. Nipple Discharge

Mrs. R. L., aged 61, had noted a few spots of blood on her brassiere for six weeks. The nipple appeared to be normal, but compressing it produced a drop of serum from the orifice of a duct in

(Text continued on page 562.)

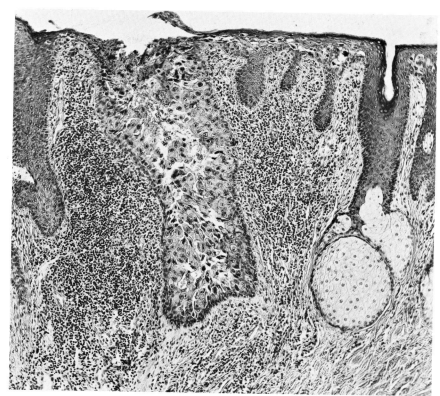

Figure 29–18. A single milk sinus involved by Paget's carcinoma as it terminates in the nipple epidermis.

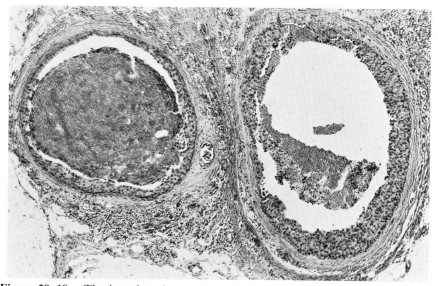

Figure 29–19. The intraductal type of carcinoma in the breast in Paget's disease.

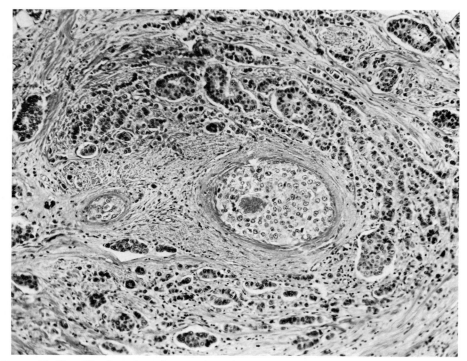

Figure 29–20. The intraductal type of carcinoma invading the breast in Paget's disease.

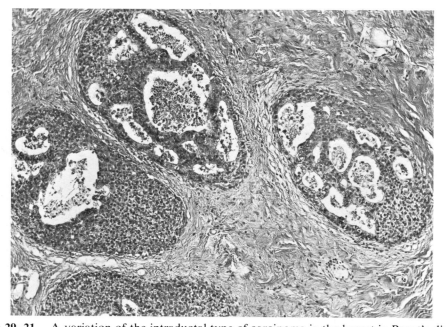

Figure 29–21. A variation of the intraductal type of carcinoma in the breast in Paget's disease.

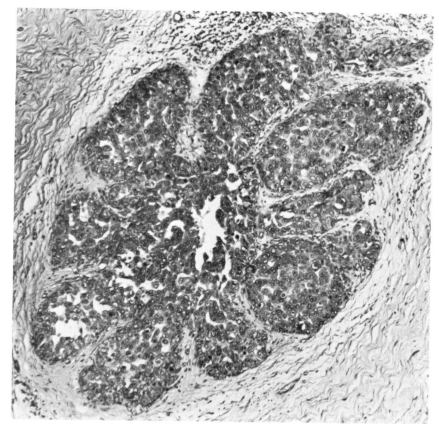

Figure 29–22. Paget's disease in which the intraductal carcinoma in the breast has extended peripherally in the duct system to finally involve a mammary lobule.

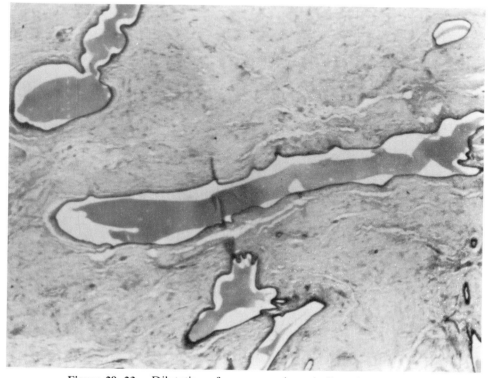

Figure 29–23. Dilatation of mammary ducts in Paget's carcinoma.

the center of the nipple surface. There was no palpable tumor in the breast, but a small area of skin retraction was evident just caudad to the areola. Biopsy of the breast tissue beneath this area of retraction revealed papillary intraductal carcinoma.

Radical mastectomy was done. There was a grossly visible tumor in the breast beneath the area of skin retraction. This lesion was an intraductal papillary carcinoma of the apocrine type. The lining of one of 22 milk sinuses was replaced by carcinoma cells. There were a few Paget's cells in the epidermis of the nipple at the point where this milk sinus terminated in it.

There were no metastases in 18 axillary lymph nodes.

This patient was treated in 1969 and no significant follow-up is yet available.

2. Reddening or Roughening of the Nipple Epithelium

Mrs. L. S., a 73 year old housewife, had noted redness of her left nipple for 4 months. The entire surface of the nipple was bright red, but the epithelium was smooth and intact. A biopsy of the nipple revealed that the epidermis was heavily infiltrated with Paget's cells, but its stratum corneum was intact. No tumor was palpated in the breast.

Radical mastectomy was done. Beneath the nipple in the center of the breast there was a firm area of grayish-white tumor which proved to be intraductal carcinoma. The lining of several of the milk sinuses in the nipple was replaced by carcinoma cells. There were no metastases in 12 axillary nodes.

The patient is well 12 years later.

3. Erosion of the Nipple Epidermis

Mrs. A. B., a 42 year old housewife, consulted me because her left nipple had been crusted and eroded for five months. She had previously consulted four physicians who had treated the nipple with a variety of ointments. The erosion involved the whole of the upper surface of the nipple and measured 1.5 cm. in diameter. There was no palpable tumor in the breast. Nipple biopsy confirmed the diagnosis of Paget's carcinoma.

Radical mastectomy was done. No grossly visible tumor was found in the breast. Paget's cells had infiltrated the entire thickness of the nipple epidermis and produced a shallow erosion. The linings of six out of a total of 22 milk sinuses in the nipple were replaced by carcinoma cells, and there was intraductal carcinoma in both the upper inner and outer sectors of the breast. No metastases were found in a total of 40 axillary nodes.

The patient is well 12 years later.

4. Redness or Roughness of the Nipple Epithelium and a Breast Tumor

Mrs. M. P., a housewife aged 57, came to me complaining of itching and roughness of her left nipple of two years' duration. She called the attention of her internist to these changes but he ignored them. Seven months before consulting me she had discovered a small tumor in the same breast, but again was reassured by her internist.

Examination showed that the epithelium of the nipple was roughened and slightly thickened, but not eroded. There was a 3 cm. tumor of the outer middle sector of the breast with the clinical characteristics of a carcinoma. There was a 5 mm. movable clinically involved axillary node.

Biopsy of the breast tumor was done, and its carcinomatous nature proved, and radical mastectomy was carried out. Paget's cells replaced and thickened the nipple epidermis but left it covered by a thin intact layer of the stratum corneum. Four of the nipple milk sinuses were filled with carcinoma cells. The breast tumor was an intraductal carcinoma. There were metastases in two of 29 axillary nodes.

The patient has no recurrence of her breast carcinoma 12 years later.

5. Nipple Erosion and a Breast Tumor

Mrs. S. N., aged 32, had noticed a very small "scab" on her left nipple five months previously. She consulted her family physician who prescribed an ointment, which did not help. Each time she bathed the scab came off and left a small erosion.

Examination in our clinic revealed a 5 mm. erosion of the nipple and also a 5 mm. firm tumor in the breast 3 cm. lateral to the areolar edge in the radius of 4 o'clock. There were no clinically involved axillary nodes.

At biopsy the breast tumor proved to be an intraductal carcinoma. Radical mastectomy was done. The nipple erosion was caused by Paget's involvement of the nipple. The lining of one of the nipple milk sinuses was replaced by carcinoma cells. There were also microscopic foci of intraductal carcinoma in the upper outer and lower outer sectors of the breast. Metastases were found in 5 of a total of 37 axillary lymph nodes. The patient was given prophylactic postoperative irradiation to the axillary, supraclavicular, and internal mammary areas. She has had no recurrence of her disease 10 years later.

6. Breast Tumor

Mrs. M. R., aged 73, discovered a tumor in her breast while dressing and came at once for consultation.

Examination revealed a 5 cm. tumor of the upper outer sector of the right breast. In the right axilla there were two movable but clinically involved 1 cm. nodes. The nipple was entirely normal.

Biopsy showed the breast tumor to be an intraductal carcinoma. On the same occasion biopsy of the internal mammary nodes in the upper three interspaces, and the nodes at the apex of the axilla showed them to be free of metastases.

Radical mastectomy was then done. Microscop-

Table 29–1. Clinical classification of Paget's carcinoma in 159 patients seen at Columbia-Presbyterian Medical Center, 1920–1969

Clinical Group	No. of Patients
1 – Discharge from nipple ducts	1
2 – Redness or roughness of nipple epidermis	5
3 – Erosion of nipple epidermis	62
4 – Redness or roughness of nipple epidermis plus a breast tumor	2
5 – Erosion of nipple epidermis plus a breast tumor	47
6 – Breast tumor	42
Total	159

ical study of the nipple showed Paget's cells in the epidermis. One of the milk sinuses of the nipple was lined by carcinoma cells. Three of a total of 31 axillary nodes contained metastases.

Two years after operation metastasis was demonstrated in a rib, and shortly thereafter involvement of the dorsal spine and brain became evident. She died two years and six months after operation.

Table 29–1 shows our 159 Columbia-Presbyterian cases of Paget's carcinoma classified into these six different clinical groups.

Diagnosis

Paget's carcinoma is the easiest form of breast carcinoma to detect because the nipple lesion frequently produces itching or burning which calls the patient's attention to it, and because it often takes the form of obvious crusting and erosion of the nipple. Unlike ordinary breast carcinoma, the Paget type is neither silent nor invisible. Nevertheless the diagnosis is missed more often, and treatment delayed longer, than in ordinary breast carcinoma. The data regarding delay and diagnostic failure in our series of cases of Paget's carcinomas are shown in Table 29–2. It will be seen that the average delay was 13 months. In the recent study of Paget's disease by Maier and his associates the average delay in diagnosis was 13.6 months. This is considerably longer than the average delay for breast carcinoma of no special type in our hospital over the same period of years, which was 8.4 months.

The frequency with which Paget's carcinoma had been missed by physicians in patients coming to us was much higher than for carcinoma of no special type. In 42 per cent of our patients with Paget's disease the diagnosis had been missed—often by several physicians whom the patient consulted one after another because the ointments and reassurance that they gave her did not help her nipple erosion. In my personal series of 1433 patients with breast carcinoma of all types who consulted me between 1943 and 1967, the diagnosis had been missed in 18.8 per cent. The medical profession's diagnostic record is therefore twice as bad in Paget's carcinoma as in ordinary breast carcinoma.

The fundamental reason for this bad diagnostic record is, I believe, the simple fact that it is difficult for both patients and physicians alike to realize that such a seemingly innocuous minute lesion on the surface of the nipple can be a manifestation of a vicious carcinoma. This is excusable on the part of

Table 29–2. Diagnostic record in 159 patients with Paget's carcinoma seen at Columbia-Presbyterian Medical Center, 1920–1969

Clinical Group	No. of Cases	Average Duration (Months)	Diagnosis Missed by Physicians	
			Number	Per cent
1 – Discharge from nipple ducts	1	1/4	0	—
2 – Redness or roughness of nipple	5	9	2	40%
3 – Erosion of nipple	62	14	32	52%
4 – Redness or roughness of nipple plus breast tumor	2	18	1	50%
5 – Erosion of nipple plus breast tumor	47	13.4	23	50%
6 – Breast tumor	42	11	7	17%
All Stages	159	13	65	42%
Personal series breast carcinoma, no special type, 1943–1967	1433	8.4*	270	18.8%

*1915–1967.

the patient, but on the part of the physician who fails to recognize the disease it is a sad reflection upon the inadequacy of our methods of medical education. These patients are often sent from one physician to another, frequently to dermatologists, and all sorts of misguided therapy—salves, cauterization, irradiation—are given without the true nature of the nipple erosion being discovered. In our own department of dermatology the diagnosis has often been missed. It is, of course, true that surgeons also sometimes fail to diagnose Paget's carcinoma, but in my experience dermatologists have been guilty more often than any other group of specialists.

Paget's carcinoma is most often mistaken for dermatitis of the nipple and areola. It is true that dermatitis, sometimes of the contact type due to irritation from clothes or cosmetics, sometimes due to bacterial infection, sometimes of unknown etiology, develops in the nipple and areola. But dermatitis is so much less frequent than Paget's carcinoma that every lesion of the nipple and areolar epithelium should be assumed to be carcinomatous until proven otherwise.

A rule that suggests itself to me is that all erosions and dermatitis-like lesions that involve *only* the nipple epithelium are carcinomatous. I have not seen one that was not. Lesions that involve the areola as well as the nipple epithelium and sometimes the skin of the breast are usually carcinomatous, but occasionally they are due to dermatitis. Erosions that involve the areola or the skin of the adjacent breast, leaving the nipple uninvolved, are not Paget's carcinoma. Figure 29-24 shows such an area of dermatitis involving only the areola.

Benign dermatitis of the nipple and areola has several features that suggest its benign nature. One of these is its rapid evolution. Within a few weeks it extends to involve a large portion of the areola. Figure 29-25 shows such a lesion.

The patient, Mrs. I. B., a Santo Dominican woman aged 22, came to me with this crusted, moist, granular, reddish lesion involving the nipple and almost the whole areola. She had had it for three months. The nipple was normal in shape. There was no tumor in the breast. A variety of ointments had not helped the lesion.

I did a biopsy of the lesion and proved that it was merely dermatitis. Cultures of the lesion grew out a pure hemolytic staphylococcus, coagulase positive. The application of a mild antiseptic ointment promptly cleared the lesion up.

Paget's carcinoma evolves very slowly in comparison to benign dermatitis. Many months would be required for Paget's erosion to extend over as wide an area.

A second feature of benign dermatitis is that it does not destroy the nipple. In cases of Paget's carcinoma that have extended out over the areola and to the skin of the breast the nipple is usually flattened and contracted by the fibrosis accompanying the carcinomatous infiltration.

Another condition that must be distinguished from Paget's carcinoma is benign intraductal papilloma of the nipple. This type of papilloma grows in the nipple ducts and some-

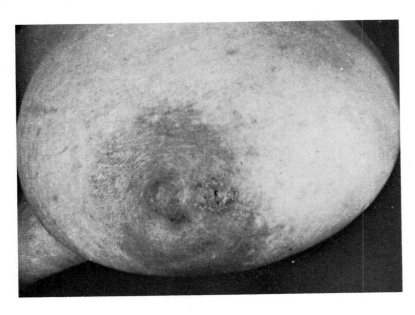

Figure 29-24. Dermatitis involving only the areola.

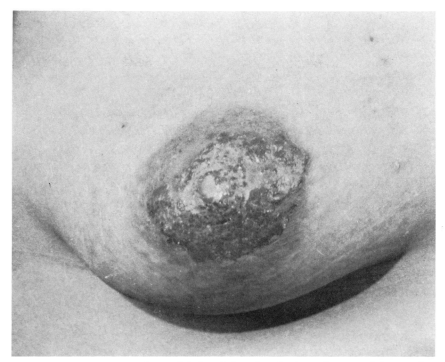

Figure 29–25. Acute dermatitis involving the nipple and most of the areola.

times projects out from them on the nipple surface as a reddish, granular, weeping lesion. Like Paget's carcinoma the lesion appears on the nipple surface. But unlike Paget's carcinoma, it forms a palpable mass that can be felt and often seen within the nipple.

Infrequently, women whose nipples have been long inverted will develop maceration and irritation of the nipple epidermis, and a discharge. This condition has no real similarity to Paget's carcinoma, and a routine of everting and cleaning the nipple will correct it.

The solution to the problem of prompt recognition of Paget's carcinoma is, of course, biopsy. Every area of redness, roughness, or thickening of the nipple epidermis, and every erosion no matter how minute and seemingly unimportant it may be, should at once be submitted to biopsy. If this simple rule were followed, Paget's carcinoma would often be diagnosed in its early stage and it would become the form of breast carcinoma with the most favorable prognosis.

The biopsy can properly be done in the office. The base of the nipple is infiltrated with Novocain and a small wedge, about 5 mm. in width, of the erosion is excised. A single silk suture across the incision controls the bleeding. This is the only form of breast carcinoma for which one may properly do a biopsy in the physician's office. For all other forms, biopsy should be done, as I have already emphasized, in the hospital operating room with all preparations made for radical mastectomy.

It is also essential to perform biopsies of erosions of the nipple to protect the patient against the surgeon's error of mistaking dermatitis for carcinoma and performing unnecessary mastectomy. Figure 29–26 shows an entirely benign dermatitis involving the nipple and the upper portion of the areola which had been present for one month. It was a crusted, exudative lesion. The attending surgeon mistakenly assumed that it was Paget's carcinoma and performed radical mastectomy without preliminary biopsy.

The following case histories are so typical of the difficulties women with Paget's carcinoma have in getting a correct diagnosis that it is worthwhile presenting them.

CASE 1

Mrs. K. S., a graduate nurse aged 54, felt a sudden momentary stinging pain in her left nipple.

After this episode the nipple began to itch, and two weeks later she first noted a small erosion on the surface of the nipple. She went to her family physician who told her that he was puzzled by the lesion. He gave her an ointment to apply. The erosion healed over partially but broke open again after a few weeks. Her physician then sent her to a radiotherapist who irradiated the nipple twice a week over a period of six months. When the erosion still persisted, her physician sent her to me.

I saw her for the first time seven months after her initial symptom. The surface of the nipple showed a moist, bright red, granular erosion, measuring 1 cm. in diameter. The breast was otherwise normal. No tumor was palpable. There were no enlarged axillary or supraclavicular lymph nodes.

A 5 mm. wedge of the erosion was excised under local anesthesia. It showed Paget's carcinoma in the epidermis. There was some squamous metaplasia of the carcinoma cells which was interpreted as the result of the irradiation.

Radical mastectomy was performed. Intraductal carcinoma was found in 20 of 21 milk sinuses, but nowhere else in the breast. There were no metastases in 31 axillary lymph nodes.

The patient is well 14 years later.

CASE 2

Mrs. B. K., a 57 year old housewife, developed itching of her left nipple and noticed a small erosion on it. She at once consulted her family physician who sent her to a dermatologist. During the next five and one-half years he treated it with various ointments and ultraviolet light. Neverthe-

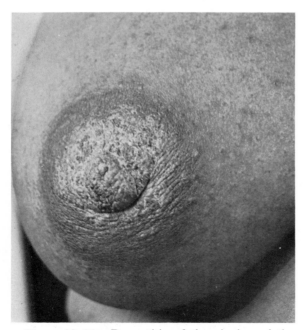

Figure 29–26. Dermatitis of the nipple and the areola mistaken for Paget's carcinoma.

less, the erosion gradually extended. Her son-in-law, a young physician, suggested that she might have Paget's carcinoma. The family physician disregarded this suggestion, but on the patient's insistence sent her to a second dermatologist, who treated the lesion with ointment for another six months. Finally, on the patient's insistence he did a biopsy of the lesion and found it to be Paget's disease, whereupon the patient came to me.

Her erosion now involved all of the nipple, and about one-third of the areola. There was no palpable tumor in the breast, and there were no clinically involved axillary nodes. Radical mastectomy was done. There was no grossly visible carcinoma in the breast and none was found microscopically. But 18 of a total of 20 of the nipple milk sinuses were lined by carcinoma cells, and the nipple was extensively infiltrated with Paget's cells. There were no metastases in 20 axillary nodes.

The patient is well six years later.

Treatment

If the concept of the pathology of Paget's carcinoma which I have presented is accepted—namely, that it is merely intraductal carcinoma involving the nipple epidermis, as well as the duct system of the nipple and the breast itself—its treatment must be the same as that for other breast carcinomas. There can be no logical defense for local excision or irradiation of the nipple lesion, or for simple mastectomy. These procedures have often been done for Paget's carcinoma, and even today continue to be advocated in some quarters. Local excision will fail to remove the carcinoma, found so often in multiple foci in the breast. Simple mastectomy will fail to remove axillary metastases of the carcinoma. Irradiation fails to destroy the carcinoma in the nipple and breast. I can present examples of the failure of these methods of treatment.

CASE 1

The Failure of Irradiation. Mrs. B. J., a housewife aged 50, came to me in May, 1954, for an erosion of the nipple. Seven years previously, in 1947, she had first developed a small erosion of the left nipple. She had consulted a surgeon who assured her the lesion was benign and sent her to a radiotherapeutist colleague. He treated the nipple with an unknown amount of irradiation. The lesion never entirely healed. It broke open at intervals and itched occasionally. Seven years later she finally came to me because her internist questioned the nature of the erosion.

The epithelium of her left nipple was thin and atrophic and in its center there was a 3 mm. erosion. There was no palpable tumor in the breast and no enlarged axillary lymph nodes. I did a biopsy of the nipple erosion and found characteristic Paget's cells in the epidermis. A radical mastectomy was done and showed intraductal carcinoma in the milk sinuses of the nipple as well as the breast. One axillary node contained metastases.

The patient is well 15 years later.

CASE 2

The Failure of Simple Mastectomy. Mrs. J. H., aged 64, developed an erosion of her left nipple but did not come for consultation until 18 months later. At this time the erosion involved the entire surface of the nipple and a sector of the areola. There was a firm, poorly delimited, 3 cm. tumor in the breast just beyond the areolar margin in the radius of 1 o'clock. In the axilla there were several clinically involved nodes between 10 and 15 mm. in diameter.

It was decided to treat her by simple mastectomy, with irradiation to the axilla. Pathologic studies of the breast showed the usual findings of Paget's carcinoma—involvement of the epidermis of the nipple, the milk sinuses of the nipple, and intraductal carcinoma of the breast.

The axillary nodes at first regressed with irradiation, but 21 months later they had grown to form a 5 cm. fixed mass. An axillary resection was then performed. Shortly thereafter she developed pleural and abdominal metastases and died 32 months after she first came for treatment. Autopsy showed local recurrence in the simple mastectomy site, and generalized metastases.

The surgeon is of course particularly tempted to perform only a simple mastectomy in patients with proven Paget's carcinoma manifested only by a nipple discharge, or by reddening, roughening, or erosion of the nipple epidermis, if there is no palpable tumor in the breast and there are no clinically involved axillary nodes. Review of our data now gives us a clear answer to this dilemma. Among a total of 56 patients with Paget's carcinoma evidenced only by these nipple changes, in whom there was no palpable breast tumor, and who were treated by radical mastectomy, three were found to have axillary metastases (Table 29–3). This is an incidence of axillary metastases of 5.4 per cent. Since failure to treat axillary metastases is fatal, and since we prefer surgical dissection to irradiation of the axilla for a number of reasons, we see no escape from the obligation of performing axillary dissection in all patients with the Paget's type of breast carcinoma. The disease is capable of metastasizing to the axilla even in its early stages. Figure 29–27 shows such an axillary metastasis.

Table 29–3. Paget's carcinoma. Frequency of axillary metastases in patients treated by radical mastectomy. Columbia-Presbyterian Medical Center, 1920–1969

Clinical Group	No. of Patients	Axillary Metastases	
		No. of Patients	Per cent
Nipple changes only (discharge, redness, roughness, or erosion)	56	3	5.4%
Nipple changes plus breast tumor	38	25	66.0%
Breast tumor only	39	21	54.0%
Totals	133	49	37.0%

In regard to the practice of performing a modified radical mastectomy in which the pectoral muscles are not removed, I can point out that in several of our patients the carcinoma in the breast was not only extensive but was situated deep in the breast very close to the pectoral fascia. Removing the pectoral muscles with the breast in cases of this kind surely diminishes the likelihood of local recurrence on the chest wall.

Even when radical mastectomy is done the results, as reported recently, in several comparatively small case series, have been poor (Colcock and Sommers; McGregor and McGregor; Helman and Kliman; Kay; Maier et al.; Rissanen and Holsti).

This generally unfavorable experience with Paget's carcinoma is surprising in view of the fact that this is one of the most slowly evolving forms of carcinoma, and, like other intraductal breast carcinomas, should give superior results. And indeed, in our experience as detailed in the data presented in Table 29–4, our results have been very good with radical mastectomy performed upon patients whose Paget's disease was operable, that is in Stage A or B according to our Columbia Clinical Classification. I am encouraged with our results with our type of thorough radical mastectomy in Paget's carcinoma and recommend it as the best treatment.

Paget's carcinoma is a fully malignant form of carcinoma of the breast and can produce occult internal mammary metastases. In keeping with our current plan of giving prophylactic irradiation to the internal mammary area in an effort to control such metastases I recommend that all patients with Paget's carcinoma who have a palpable breast tumor—

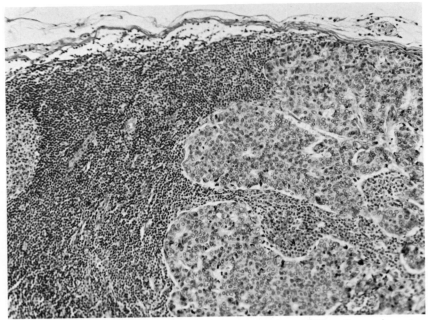

Figure 29–27. Axillary metastasis in an early stage of Paget's carcinoma.

Table 29–4. RADICAL MASTECTOMY FOR PAGET'S CARCINOMA.
COLUMBIA-PRESBYTERIAN MEDICAL CENTER, 1920–1959

Columbia Clinical Classification	Clinical Group	No. of Patients	Findings in Axilla	Per cent 10 Year Survival
Stages A and B	Nipple changes only (discharge, redness, roughness, or erosion)	26	No axillary metastases in 24 patients	83%
			Axillary metastases in 2 patients	50%*
	Nipple changes plus breast tumor	25	No axillary metastases in 12 patients	67%
			Axillary metastases in 13 patients	46%
	Breast tumor only	26	No axillary metastases in 14 patients	79%
			Axillary metastases in 12 patients	25%
Stages C and D	Nipple changes plus breast tumor	7	Axillary metastases in 7 patients	0%
	Breast tumor only	1	Axillary metastases in 1 patient	0%
Total		85		

*One patient died of cardiovascular disease 9 years postoperatively.

provided that the tumor is not less than 3 cm. in diameter and situated in the upper outer sector of the breast—be given this kind of irradiation. If axillary metastases are found at radical mastectomy, the patient should, of course, also be given such irradiation.

REFERENCES

von Braunbehrens, H.: Zur Strahlenbehandlung der Paget'schen Erkrankung der weiblichen Brust. Radiol. clin., Basel, 22:236, 1953.

Cheatle, Sir G. L., and Cutler, M.: Paget's disease of the nipple. Arch. Path., 12:435, 1931.

Cheatle, Sir G. L., and Cutler, M.: Tumours of the Breast. Philadelphia, J. B. Lippincott Co., 1931.

Ciprut, S., Roberts, T. W., and Volk, H.: Paget's carcinoma of the male breast. Ann. Surg., 154:1001, 1961.

Colcock, B. P., and Sommers, S. C.: Prognosis in Paget's disease of the breast. Surg. Clin. N. Amer., June, 1954, p. 773.

Culberson, J. D., and Horn, R. C., Jr.: Paget's disease of the nipple. Review of 25 cases with special reference to melanin pigmentation. Arch. Surg., 72:224, 1956.

Darier, J.: Sur une nouvelle forme de le psorospermose cutane; la maladie de Paget du mamelon. Compt. rend. Soc. de biol. Ser. 9, 1:294, 1889.

Dockerty, M. B., and Harrington, S. W.: Preclinical Paget's disease of the nipple. Surg., Gynec. & Obst., 93:317, 1951.

Handley, W. S.: On Paget's disease of the nipple. Brit. J. Surg., 7:183, 1919.

Helman, P., and Kliman, M.: Paget's disease of the nipple. Brit. J. Surg., 43:481, 1956.

Hutchin, P., and Houlihan, R. K.: Paget's disease of the male breast. Ann. Surg., 159:305, 1964.

Inglis, K.: Paget's Disease of the Nipple. London, Oxford Univ. Press, 1936.

Inglis, K.: Paget's disease of the nipple. Amer. J. Path., 22:1, 1946.

Jacobaeus, H. C.: Paget's Disease und sein Verhältniss zum Milchdrüsenkarzinom. Virchows Arch. f. path. Anat., 178:124, 1904.

Jopson, J. H., and Speese, J.: Paget's disease of the nipple and allied conditions. Ann. Surg., 62:212, 1915.

Kay, S.: Paget's disease of the nipple. Surg., Gynec. & Obst., 123:1010, 1966.

McGregor, J. K., and McGregor, D. D.: Paget's disease of the breast. Surgery, 45:562, 1959.

Maier, W. P., et al.: Paget's disease in the female breast. Surg., Gynec. & Obst., 128:1253, 1969.

Miller, M. W., and Pendergrass, E. P.: Some observations concerned with carcinoma of the breast. Amer. J. Roentgenol., 72:263, 1954.

Muir, R.: Further observations on Paget's disease of the nipple. J. Path. & Bact., 49:299, 1939.

Muir, R.: Paget's disease of the nipple and its relationships. J. Path. & Bact., 30:451, 1927.

Muir, R.: Pathogenesis of Paget's disease of the nipple and associated lesions. Brit. J. Surg., 22:728, 1935.

Neubecker, R. D., and Bradshaw, R. P.: Mucin, melanin, and glycogen in Paget's disease of the breast. Amer. J. Clin. Path., 36:49, 1961.

O'Grady, W. P., and McDivitt, R. W.: Breast cancer in a man treated with diethylstilbestrol. Arch. Path., 88:162, 1969.

Paget, Sir J.: On disease of the mammary areola preceding cancer of the mammary gland. St. Barth. Hosp. Reports, 10:86, 1874.

Pautrier, L. M.: Paget's disease of the nipple. Arch. Dermat. & Syph., 17:767, 1928.

Rissanen, P. M., and Holsti, O.: Paget's disease of the breast. Oncology, 23:209, 1969.

Rousset, J.: Maladie de Paget d'allure clinique et d'aspects histologiques inhabituelles. Bull. Soc. franç. de dermat. et syph., 58:585, 1951.

Sagebiel, R. W.: Ultrastructural observations on epidermal cells in Paget's disease. Amer. J. Path., 57:49, 1969.

Sarason, E. L., and Prior, J. T.: Paget's disease of the male breast. Ann. Surg., 135:253, 1952.

Simard, C.: La maladie de Paget du mamelon; cancer épidermotrope. Bull. Assoc. franç. p. l'étude du cancer, 19:50, 1930.

Sinckler, W. H., and Cooper, T. J.: Paget's disease of the male breast. Amer. J. Surg., 98:623, 1959.

Toker, C.: Some observations on Paget's disease of the nipple. Cancer, 14:653, 1961.

Treves, N.: Paget's disease of the male mamma. Cancer, 7:325, 1954.

Velpeau, A.: A Treatise on the Diseases of the Breast and Mammary Region; Translated from the French by Mitchell Henry. London, Sydenham Soc., 1856, p. 3.

Veronesi, U., Rabotti, G. C., and Sirtori, C.: Il carcinoma intraduttale epidermotropo della mammella, cosidetto morbo di Paget. Tumori, 41(supp.), 1955.

West, J. P., and Nickel, W. F., Jr.: Paget's disease of the nipple. Ann. Surg., 116:19, 1942.

Chapter Thirty

Circumscribed Carcinoma

A special type of breast carcinoma characterized clinically by its circumscribed form, and grossly by its soft and hemorrhagic appearance, is well enough known to students of breast disease; but very little has been written about it. Moore and Foote, as well as Richardson, called it "medullary" carcinoma and gave it a favorable prognosis. We prefer the name *circumscribed* carcinoma because of this striking clinical feature.

Frequency and Age Distribution

The circumscribed type of carcinoma is infrequent. In a series of 3000 breast carcinomas studied in our laboratory of surgical pathology between 1915 and 1950, 146 or approximately 2.5 per cent were of this type.

The youngest patient in our series of patients with this disease was 22, and the oldest 79. Their average age was 49 years, which is approximately two years younger than the average age of all our patients with breast carcinoma.

Clinical Features

The average duration of symptoms in our series of patients with circumscribed carcinoma was only 4.1 months, as compared with an average duration of 8.4 months for my personal series of breast carcinomas.

It has been my impression that circumscribed carcinomas are apt to be large, but a

review of the data concerning our 146 tumors did not confirm this impression. The average clinical diameter of our tumors was only 4.2 cm., which is approximately the same as the average diameter of ordinary breast carcinoma in our data. There were only nine very large tumors, measuring 10 cm. or more in diameter, in our series. Figure 30–1 shows one of these bulky circumscribed carcinomas.

Since circumscribed carcinoma attains the same size as other types of carcinoma in a shorter period of time, we are justified in concluding that the circumscribed type grows faster.

On palpation these tumors give the impression of being well delimited in the surrounding breast tissue, as might be expected from their grossly circumscribed character. They vary in consistence but are often softer than ordinary breast carcinoma. Even though they are relatively fixed in the breast tissue in which they lie, their remarkable delimitation has often betrayed the examiner into thinking them benign. I have made this mistake a number of times.

The skin over bulky circumscribed carcinoma is occasionally reddened, presumably as a reaction to the necrosis in these tumors. This redness has led some clinicians into classifying the lesion as inflammatory carcinoma. This is an unfortunate mistake because circumscribed carcinoma is a curable type of carcinoma and if it is operable should be treated surgically, whereas inflammatory carcinoma is incurable and should never be operated upon. Figure 30–2 shows a large cir-

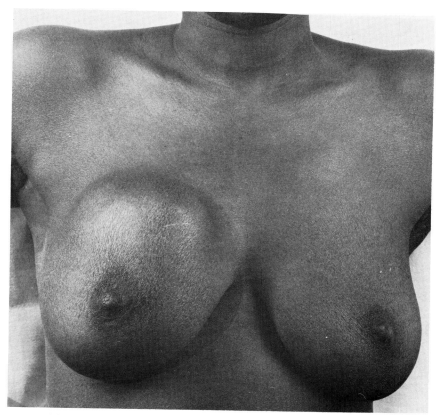

Figure 30–1. A bulky circumscribed carcinoma of the breast.

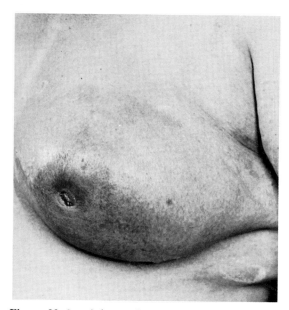

Figure 30–2. A large circumscribed carcinoma of the breast, with redness of the overlying skin.

cumscribed carcinoma with redness of the overlying skin simulating inflammatory carcinoma.

Fourteen of our 140 patients with circumscribed carcinoma developed primary carcinoma in both breasts. In six the lesion was of the circumscribed type in both breasts; in the other eight it was the circumscribed type in one breast and another type in the other breast. This is a higher frequency of bilateral involvement (10 per cent) than we have observed in most other types of breast carcinoma.

Pathological Features

These tumors are often so well delimited that they give the gross impression of having a capsule (Fig. 30–3). They do not, of course, have a true capsule; but a zone of encircling fibrosis and lymphocytic infiltration, as

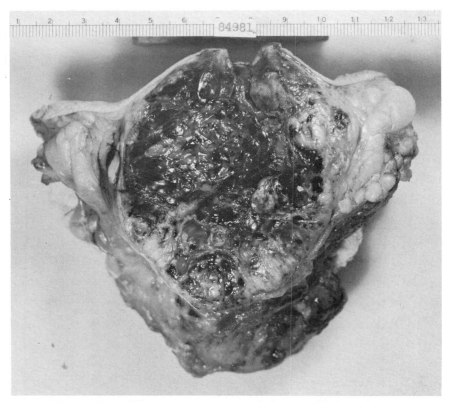

Figure 30–3. The gross appearance of circumscribed carcinoma.

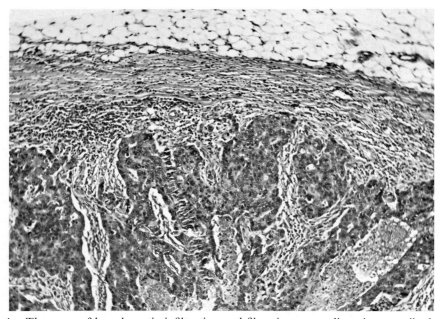

Figure 30–4. The zone of lymphocytic infiltration and fibrosis surrounding circumscribed carcinoma.

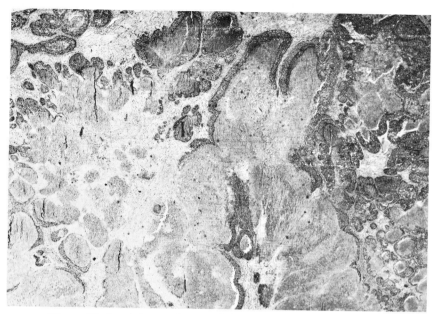

Figure 30–5. Advanced necrosis in circumscribed carcinoma.

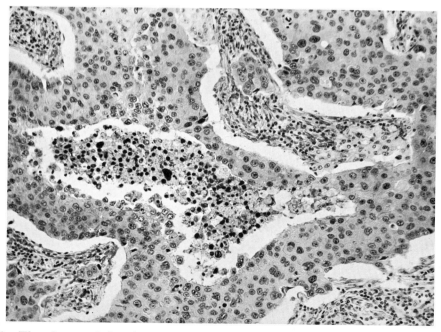

Figure 30–6. The characteristic microscopic appearance of circumscribed carcinoma. Broad bands of cells lie in a stroma containing many lymphocytes.

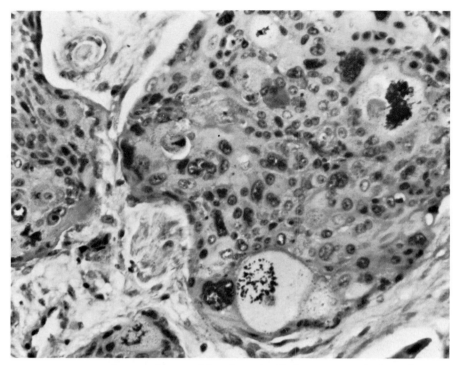

Figure 30–7.   Bizarre, giant, multinucleated cells in circumscribed carcinoma.

shown in Figure 30–4, gives this illusion. The cut surface of the tumor is often soft. When well nourished, the tumor is grayish-white. These carcinomas are, however, especially prone to necrosis. Their centers are often largely necrotic, and appear hemorrhagic and partly liquefied. When only a rim of visible carcinoma remains the lesion may be mistaken grossly for carcinoma within a cyst.

Circumscribed carcinomas have such a distinctive microscopic character that they are among the easiest of breast carcinomas to classify. They are made up of strands and masses of cells lying in a stroma that usually shows much degeneration. It is often heavily infiltrated with lymphatics, which become one of its striking features. In other examples of this type of carcinoma the degeneration has progressed so far that only acellular debris remains in some areas, as shown in Figure 30–5. In some of these tumors fibrosis has replaced the degenerated areas.

The tumor cells themselves lie solidly packed together without any intervening fibrillar matrix, and form broad anastomosing bands or masses of cells (Fig. 30–6). The individual cells are large, in general larger than in any other type of breast carcinoma. The nuclei are usually large and hyperchro-

matic, and vary greatly in size and shape. Bizarre giant and multinucleated cells are frequently seen (Fig. 30–7). Mitoses are numerous. Microscopically these tumors look highly anaplastic and malignant.

One of the interesting features of these circumscribed carcinomas is their tendency to develop squamous metaplasia. This metaplasia can be so marked that the pathologist is betrayed into thinking that he is dealing with squamous carcinoma. I have discussed and illustrated this phenomenon in Chapter 32. In our laboratory we have seen a total of 20 of these circumscribed carcinomas showing squamous metaplasia.

Treatment

In our series of 140 patients who had a total of 146 circumscribed carcinomas, 138 radical mastectomies were done. In an analysis of the regional lymph node findings and the results of treatment in a series of cases it is essential to classify the cases as to clinical stage of advancement. We rely upon our Columbia Clinical Classification for this purpose.

The frequency of axillary metastases in our

series of cases of circumscribed carcinoma treated by radical mastectomy is shown in Table 30–1. As compared with the frequency of axillary metastases in my personal series of breast carcinomas of all types treated by radical mastectomy, it was remarkably low— 31.9 per cent as compared with 56 per cent.

Although these circumscribed carcinomas metastasize less frequently to the axillary lymph nodes than breast carcinomas of no special type, the results of radical mastectomy in our series of circumscribed carcinomas have been approximately the same as my results in my personal series of radical mastectomies. They are compared in Table 30–2.

It should be pointed out that the number of patients succumbing to intercurrent disease before 10 years in this series of circumscribed carcinomas was unusually large—12 in all. Two additional patients died postoperatively. In comparing the results of treatment in different forms of carcinoma it is worthwhile comparing the adjusted survival rates obtained by excluding the patients who died postoperatively as well as those who died of intercurrent disease. When this is done the 10-year survival rates for circumscribed carcinoma in the present series of cases and for all types of carcinoma in my personal series of radical mastectomies are identical.

Although size is not a criterion in our Columbia Clinical Classification it is interesting to review the influence of tumor size in this series of circumscribed carcinomas. Seven of the nine tumors that were 10 cm. or more in diameter and were treated by radical mastectomy had no axillary metastases. However, only one of the eight who were operated upon more than 10 years ago survived 10 years.

Three of our patients with circumscribed

Table 30–2. 10-YEAR SURVIVAL FOLLOWING RADICAL MASTECTOMY FOR CIRCUMSCRIBED CARCINOMA COMPARED WITH ALL BREAST CARCINOMAS IN PERSONAL SERIES OF CASES, 1935–1957

Columbia Clinical Classification	Circumscribed Carcinoma		All Carcinomas in Personal Series	
	Number	Per cent 10-Year Survival	Number	Per cent 10-Year Survival
Stage A	57	67%	402	70%
Stage B	23	52%	154	41%
Stage C	11	27%	59	24%
Stage D	6	0	11	18%
Total	98	54%	626	57%
No. of postoperative deaths and deaths from intercurrent disease before 10 years	14		53	
Adjusted 10-year- survival rate		63%		63%

carcinoma were found to have internal mammary metastases by preliminary internal mammary biopsy more than 10 years ago. Two were treated by irradiation alone; one died of metastasis after five years, but the other is still alive without evidence of disease. The third patient had simple mastectomy and irradiation; she is well 10 years later.

Although the results of radical mastectomy in this disease have not proved to be superior to the results in other forms of breast carcinoma, I believe that radical mastectomy is much the best method of treatment that we have available for patients with circumscribed carcinoma classified as Clinical Stage A or B.

REFERENCES

McDivitt, R. W., Stewart, F. W., and Berg, J. W.: Tumors of the Breast. Atlas of Tumor Pathology, Washington, D.C., Armed Forces Institute of Pathology, 1968, Second Series, Fascicle 2.

Moore, O. S., Jr., and Foote, F. W., Jr.: The relatively favorable prognosis of medullary carcinoma of the breast. Cancer, 2:635, 1949.

Richardson, W. W.: Medullary carcinoma of the breast. Brit. J. Cancer, 10:415, 1956.

Schwartz, G. F.: Solid circumscribed carcinoma of the breast. Ann. Surg., 169:165, 1969.

Table 30–1. FREQUENCY OF AXILLARY METASTASIS IN CIRCUMSCRIBED CARCINOMA COMPARED WITH ALL BREAST CARCINOMAS IN PERSONAL SERIES OF CASES, 1935–1968

Columbia Clinical Classification	Circumscribed Carcinoma		All Carcinomas in Personal Series	
	Number	Per cent with Axillary Metastasis	Number	Per cent with Axillary Metastasis
Stage A	88	16.0%	724	31%
Stage B	31	61.3%	198	75%
Stage C	13	53.9%	71	82%
Stage D	6	66.6%	14	93%
Totals	138	31.9%	1,007	56%

Chapter Thirty-One

Inflammatory Carcinoma

Our systematized knowledge of this, the most terrible form of breast carcinoma, is relatively recent. Toward the end of the last century several surgeons of great experience, including Billroth and von Volkmann, had noted the exceptional malignancy of breast carcinomas evolving during pregnancy and had coined for them the term "mastitis carcinomatosa." Schumann, in 1911, described in detail a case of acute carcinoma mistaken for an abscess in a lactating breast, and collected the earlier case reports. Most of these cases were not examples of the disease that we today call inflammatory carcinoma, but the name "mastitis carcinomatosa," and the implied association with pregnancy and lactation, persisted and confused students of breast carcinoma until recently.

The clinical picture of inflammatory carcinoma as we know it today was defined in two excellent papers, the first by Lee and Tannenbaum in 1924, and the second by Taylor and Meltzer in 1938. Their papers so well established the disease as a special form of breast carcinoma that it is today known in all surgical clinics. If anything, the diagnostic criteria are interpreted too liberally and the diagnosis is made too frequently.

During the last decade several papers have been published dealing with the question of how best to treat inflammatory breast carcinoma. I will discuss them later on in this chapter.

Incidence

Between the years 1915 and 1968 a total of 89 patients with breast carcinoma which I have classified as the inflammatory type were seen in our medical center. They constituted about 1.5 per cent of all our patients with primary breast carcinoma. Inflammatory carcinoma, as we classify it, is therefore a comparatively rare disease. It constituted 1.3 per cent of Lee and Tannenbaum's series of breast carcinomas, 4 per cent of Taylor and Meltzer's series, and 1.7 per cent of Barber, Dockerty, and Clagett's series.

Predisposing Factors

There was no predilection of the disease in our series of cases for patients of a special race or age. The average age of our patients with inflammatory carcinoma was 49.5 years, as compared with 50 years for all our patients with breast carcinoma. Similarly, in Taylor and Meltzer's series of cases of inflammatory carcinoma the age distribution of the patients was the same as for breast carcinoma in general.

Pregnancy and lactation do not predispose to the inflammatory type of carcinoma, as early writers thought. In our series of 89 cases we have had only four patients in whom the disease developed during pregnancy or lactation. Occasional cases of this kind have been reported in other large case series.

Symptoms

Inflammatory carcinoma usually makes itself evident in a very different way from ordinary breast cancer. The patient's attention is called to her breast disease by tenderness or pain, and she discovers that her breast is abnormally firm and enlarged, and that the skin over it is reddened or dusky in color. Patients do not ordinarily recognize edema of the skin, so that even when it is extensive they usually ignore it. Only about half the patients are able to define a definite tumor in the breast.

The symptoms of which the patients in our series of 89 patients with inflammatory carcinoma complained, are shown in Table 31-1.

These symptoms increase rapidly in severity and the patient is soon forced to consult her local physician. In the patients with this disease whom we have seen during the last 10 years the average delay in seeking medical help has been only 2.5 months. Our patients with ordinary breast cancer who have consulted me during the same period have delayed, on an average, approximately twice as long.

Physical Features of Inflammatory Carcinoma

The essential clinical characteristics of the inflammatory type of carcinoma in its fully evolved state are enlargement and generalized induration of the breast, and redness and edema of the skin over it. In some patients the induration may be localized to one sector or one half of the breast. These lesions are never sharply delimited; they are so diffuse that it is very difficult to measure their size.

The redness of the skin, which is the most distinctive feature of inflammatory carcinoma, is not always a bright red. It is sometimes merely a flush of pink. The discoloration is not uniform over the breast. It tends to be more prominent over the most dependent part of the breast and it is often mottled in its distribution. We have not counted small zones of redness as justifying the diagnosis of inflammatory carcinoma. For example, the

Table 31-1. PRESENTING SYMPTOMS IN 89 PATIENTS WITH INFLAMMATORY CARCINOMA, 1915-1968

Presenting Symptom	No. of Patients
Localized tumor	51
Pain in breast or nipple	26
Enlargement of breast	43
Redness of skin	51
Tenderness	14
Generalized hardness	13
Increased warmth of skin	7
Edema of skin	12
Nipple discharge	7
Nipple retraction	12
Itching of nipple	3
Axillary tumor	8
Pain in axilla	4
Swelling of arm	3
Bone pain	1

skin over a limited area immediately over a rather superficial carcinoma is not infrequently red, and should not be regarded as a sign of inflammatory carcinoma. It is merely a local reaction to the underlying invading carcinoma. In a general way we have regarded as significant in terms of inflammatory carcinoma only redness that involves more than one-third of the skin over the breast. The redness usually extends steadily and after a few weeks affects the skin over most of the breast, and finally extends to the skin of the opposite breast. In its early stage the redness may diminish if the patient is put to bed for a few days, but it soon reappears.

The reddened skin in these patients often feels abnormally warm to the touch. This evidence in our series of cases cannot be evaluated very well since there were many different examiners. Unfortunately, no accurate skin temperature measurements were made in our cases.

Edema of the skin accompanies the redness, although it is usually less extensive.

Retraction of the nipple is seen in many of these patients. As the disease progresses the nipple epithelium becomes reddened and crusted.

Physiological signs of inflammation—elevated body temperature and leukocytosis—occur in very few of these patients with inflammatory carcinoma. In Taylor and Meltzer's series of 38 cases there were only five patients who had leukocytosis, and six who had a febrile course. The latter, however, all had some complication that might have been responsible. Similarly, in our series of patients there were only a few whose blood count or temperature was abnormal. Only one of our 65 patients in whom blood counts were done had leukocytosis. Three of them had elevation of body temperature. Axillary metastases are a regular feature of inflammatory carcinoma. Eighty-one of our 89 patients had clinical involvement of axillary nodes on admission, and in half of them the involvement was massive. By this we mean that the involved nodes measured more than 2.5 cm., in their greatest transverse diameter. In the 30 patients who were treated by radical mastectomy, making microscopic study of the nodes possible, all were found to have axillary metastases.

More distant metastases were found in 25 of our 89 patients when they came for consultation. Twelve had palpable subclavicular nodes, nine pulmonary metastases, five bone metastases, and one had brain metastases. The opposite breast was involved in two of our patients on admission, and became involved during the course of the disease in at least 25 other patients. In Taylor and Meltzer's series of 38 cases, 21 ultimately developed involvement of the opposite breast.

Figure 31–1 shows the characteristic appearance of inflammatory carcinoma.

The patient, Mrs. N. C., aged 46, noticed that her right breast was enlarging three months before she came to the Presbyterian Hospital. On admission the right breast was elevated in position on the chest wall, and formed a bulky, solid, firm mass fixed to the deeper structures. The skin over the lower portion of the breast was bright red, and there was reddish mottling of the skin over the remainder of the breast. The outline of the lower portion of the areola was lost in the red discoloration.

The nipple was flattened and broadened. There was edema of the skin over almost the entire breast. In the axilla there was a chain of large firm nodes extending high up, and fixed to the underlying chest wall.

The surgeon in charge of the patient, although realizing that her carcinoma was advanced, performed a so-called "palliative" radical mastectomy. He did not achieve palliation, however, for local recurrence developed within five months, and two months later a similar inflammatory carcinoma developed in the left breast. Left simple mastectomy was done but it did not check the progress of her disease. She died seven months after onset of her symptoms.

Differential Diagnosis

Abscess. The resemblance of inflammatory carcinoma to true inflammation is so close that it is often mistaken for, and treated as, an abscess. Many of our patients had been given antibiotics and the diagnosis delayed for several weeks. Finally, biopsy is done and the surgeon finds, instead of pus, dense hemorrhagic tissue which shows carcinoma on frozen section.

The chief clinical feature of infection or

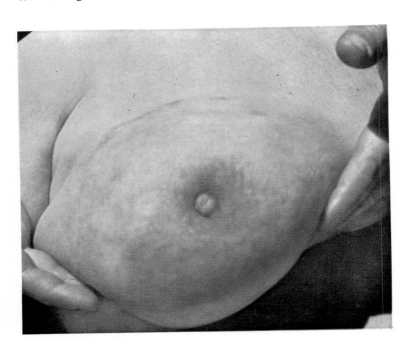

Figure 31–1. Inflammatory type of carcinoma.

abscess in the breast is that it occurs almost exclusively in the lactating breast. I have already indicated that inflammatory carcinoma is rare in the lactating breast. Infection and abscess are, moreover, more localized than inflammatory carcinoma, and are usually accompanied by leukocytosis and fever, which are infrequent in inflammatory carcinoma.

Duct Ectasia. In the advanced stage of the evolution of duct ectasia in which the irritative material has penetrated the duct walls and set up inflammation and even abscess in the breast, the process may suggest inflammatory carcinoma. These patients with duct ectasia are, like those with inflammatory carcinoma, older women, and their disease is not associated with lactation. An important difference between the two diseases is that the signs of inflammation produced by duct ectasia are apt to be more localized than those accompanying inflammatory carcinoma. Moreover, the inflammatory reaction of duct ectasia evolves very quickly, usually within a few days, and usually subsides spontaneously just as rapidly, thus solving the diagnostic problem.

Involvement of the Skin in Advanced Carcinoma. In the late stage of local extension of carcinoma of the breast, when the skin is invaded or ulcerated, secondary infection may produce redness and edema of the skin. Redness and edema of this type is at first of limited extent and evolves very slowly. Several authors have called this phenomenon "secondary inflammatory carcinoma." This only serves to confuse the recognition of true inflammatory carcinoma, which is, as I have emphasized, a separate disease *sui generis.*

Necrosis in the Circumscribed Type of Carcinoma. In Chapter 30 I have described the special form of breast carcinoma which we designate as the circumscribed type. It forms a large well delimited tumor which has a special tendency to break down and become necrotic centrally, perhaps because of the poor blood supply of this rapidly growing tumor. The necrosis is often followed by extensive redness and edema of the overlying skin. The clinical features suggest inflammatory carcinoma. It is of great importance to differentiate the two lesions because circumscribed carcinoma can often be cured by radical mastectomy and inflammatory carcinoma cannot. The key to this differential diagnosis is the pathology. The circumscribed

type of carcinoma is easy to identify in frozen section, and a biopsy will solve the problem.

The following case history illustrates the diagnostic dilemma that a necrotic circumscribed carcinoma presents.

Mrs. L. M., a 54 year old woman, was admitted to the Delafield Hospital for a tumor of the right breast that she had first noted only five weeks previously. It had grown rapidly and had become painful during the last three weeks.

Examination showed the right breast to be half again as large as the left, owing to the presence of a 10 cm. hard tumor which filled its center. The tumor was somewhat fixed to the underlying chest wall. The skin over the tumor was reddened, and over the lower half of the breast it was edematous. There were two 1 cm. enlarged, firm axillary nodes.

The lesion was classified as inflammatory carcinoma. Irradiation was decided upon, and to facilitate delivering the desired tumor dose the radiotherapeutists requested simple mastectomy. This was performed, the lower axillary lymph nodes being included in the dissection. Pathologic study of the specimen showed that the tumor occupied the center of the breast, was well delimited from the surrounding breast tissue, and was made up of soft, lobulated, yellowish-pink tissue. At its center there was a large cavity lined by necrotic tissue and filled with cloudy amber fluid. The tumor proved to be the circumscribed type of carcinoma, with extensive necrosis. It showed some squamous metaplasia. There were no metastases in 13 lymph nodes.

Irradiation treatment was completed without incident. The patient had no further evidence of breast carcinoma. She died two years later from carcinoma of the uterus.

Carcinoma en Cuirasse. Although carcinoma *en cuirasse* produces reddish discoloration of the skin, its resemblance to inflammatory carcinoma goes no further. *En cuirasse* is a very slow process in which the skin is thickened and fibrosed as the carcinoma advances in its deeper portion. There is no edema of the skin, and no acute signs suggesting inflammation.

Lymphoblastoma. Leukemic or lymphosarcomatous involvement of the breast can resemble inflammatory carcinoma very closely. The differentiation can be made only by biopsy.

Mammography in the Differential Diagnosis of Inflammatory Carcinoma. Berger has discussed the role of mammography in diagnosing the inflammatory type of carcinoma. The skin edema can, of course, be recognized as thickening of the skin which is easily visible in films of good quality. It seems to me, however, that edema is more readily recognized with the naked eye, and that beyond this, mammograms cannot reveal anything that is characteristic of this disease.

Pathology

Because most of the patients with inflammatory carcinoma are not operated upon, information concerning the pathologic characteristics of the lesion has been slow to accumulate. The studies of Hartmann and his associates, of Taylor and Meltzer, of Meyer, Dockerty, and Harrington, and of Chris are in agreement, however, that inflammatory carcinoma is not a special microscopic type. All the usual microscopic forms of carcinoma are found.

Our series of cases of inflammatory carcinoma, like these others, was made up of a wide variety of microscopic types. There were partly intraductal carcinomas, circumscribed carcinomas, scirrhous carcinomas, small cell carcinomas, and large cell carcinomas. A few formed mucin. Of the 59 tumors which we were able to study adequately mi-croscopically, one was well differentiated, 11 were moderately differentiated, and 47 were classified as undifferentiated. If it were possible to say that any single type of carcinoma predominated it would be the large cell type. The cells in this type have large pale cytoplasms, and prominent nuclei showing bizarre variation in size and shape. They form loosely arranged masses, without any intercellular fibrous stroma. In our series of cases there were 19 of the large-cell undifferentiated carcinomas among the 59 inflammatory carcinomas that we studied microscopically. Figure 31-2 shows a typical one.

One of the questions that arises concerning the histology of inflammatory carcinoma is how often these tumors show any microscopic evidence of the "inflammation" that characterizes them clinically. In our series of 59 cases there were only six in which there was an unusual degree of lymphocytic infiltration in and about the carcinoma.

The redness of the skin over the breast that characterizes this disease, like the edema that accompanies the redness, finds its explanation microscopically in the involvement of the subdermal lymphatics by the carcinoma. When the skin and subcutaneous tissue are

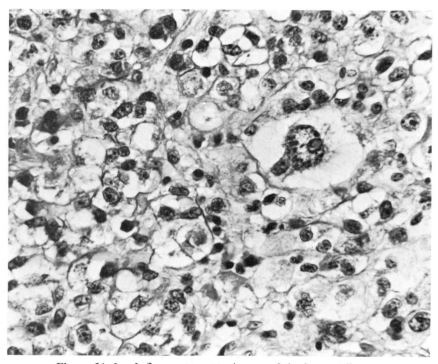

Figure 31-2.   Inflammatory carcinoma of the large cell type.

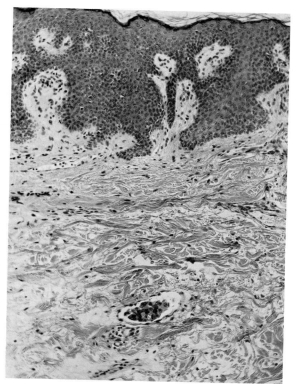

Figure 31–3. Carcinoma in a skin lymphatic in inflammatory carcinoma.

adequately studied microscopically, emboli of carcinoma cells will almost always be found in the superficial subdermal lymphatics. Figure 31–3 shows this phenomenon in one of our inflammatory carcinomas. Presumably, the redness of the skin is due to hyperemia in response to the presence of the carcinoma close beneath it. It may be asked why, then, is redness of the skin not always present when edema of the skin develops, as it does in a good many locally advanced carcinomas. I cannot answer this question except to suggest that the peculiarly malignant nature of these inflammatory carcinomas in some manner induces hyperemia of the skin.

The subdermal lymphatics are not the only ones involved in inflammatory carcinoma. The lymphatics of the breast itself are often dilated and filled with carcinoma cells. Figure 31–4 shows a group of dilated lymphatics deep in the breast parenchyma filled with carcinoma cells of the large cell type. We found dilated lymphatics containing carcinoma cells in two-thirds of our cases of inflammatory carcinoma. We also noted emboli of carcinoma cells in blood vessels in a number of our cases. These are further evidences of the extreme malignancy of this disease.

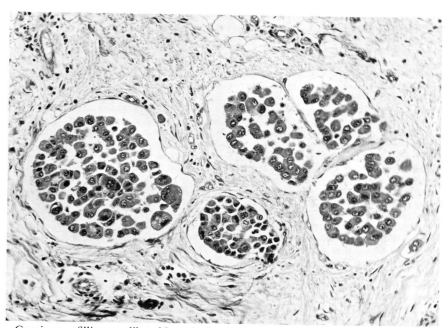

Figure 31–4. Carcinoma filling up dilated lymphatics in the breast in the inflammatory type of carcinoma.

Treatment

The papers by Lee and Tannenbaum, and Taylor and Meltzer, not only defined inflammatory carcinoma as a clinical entity, but they established the fact that the disease cannot be cured by surgery. Previously the surgical tradition of operating on all breast carcinoma had been applied with disastrous results to inflammatory carcinoma.

Lee and Tannenbaum reported that radical mastectomy in their four patients with inflammatory carcinoma was followed by prompt local recurrence and early death. The fate of Taylor and Meltzer's six patients treated by radical mastectomy was the same.

Our Presbyterian Hospital experience long ago provided data regarding the futility of surgical attack upon inflammatory carcinoma. By 1943, when Stout and I presented our *criteria of operability* for breast carcinoma we had enough data to be convinced that patients with the disease are categorically inoperable. Twenty patients who had it had been treated by radical mastectomy. Fifty per cent had developed local recurrence and all 20 had succumbed after an average survival of 15.5 months.

In 1952, Treves reviewed his own experience, and collected reports of a total of 262 cases of inflammatory carcinoma in which the treatment had been radical mastectomy. Only four patients had survived for as long as 5 years, and there were no long-term cures. Treves appealed to surgeons to stop doing radical mastectomy for this disease.

A series of papers dealing with the treatment of this disease published more recently show that radical mastectomy is nevertheless still recommended by some surgeons. Rogers and Fitts in 1956, and Barber, Dockerty, and Clagett in 1961, continued to advocate radical mastectomy, although the former were able to report only one eight-year survivor among 10 patients operated upon, and the latter had only five patients who survived five years among 50 treated by operation. Barber and his associates suggested that "bolder surgery" is needed for inflammatory carcinoma.

Other surgeons have been more realistic regarding the treatment of inflammatory carcinoma, and have recognized the futility of surgery in this disease. Byrd and Stephenson reported no five-year survivors among 12 patients in whom mastectomy was done. Richards and Lewison had no five-year survivors among 13 patients operated upon. Donegan had no five-year survivors among 12 patients treated by surgery.

In our own medical center, radical mastectomy has long since been abandoned as the treatment for inflammatory carcinoma, but a total of 29 of these operations were done in our hospital before this method of treatment was given up. We have cared for one other patient with inflammatory carcinoma who had had a radical mastectomy before consulting us. I am therefore able to present the end results of radical mastectomy in a total of 30 patients. Local recurrence developed in 7 per cent. All the patients succumbed to the disease and the average postoperative survival was 19 months. Only one patient survived longer than five years. She was a woman aged 49, who developed local recurrence and distant metastases following radical mastectomy, but whose disease was held in check for a considerable time by irradiation. She died 78 months after the onset of her disease, and 68 months after her operation. The course of the disease in this patient was certainly not typical of that of inflammatory carcinoma.

The following case history is representative of our experience with radical mastectomy in this disease.

Mrs. L. W. was a housewife aged 56. Three weeks before her admission to the Presbyterian Hospital she had developed throbbing and shooting pain in her right breast. It radiated to the axilla. With the onset of the pain she noted that her right nipple was retracted and that the skin around it was reddened, and the breast was enlarged.

Examination showed that the right breast was larger than the left and diffusely indurated. No definite localized tumor could be felt. The nipple was inverted and there was extensive redness and edema centered around the areola and involving at least one-half of the skin over the breast. A 1.5 cm. hard right axillary lymph node suggested metastasis. The disease was classified as inflammatory carcinoma.

Radical mastectomy was nevertheless done. Pathologic study showed the lesion to be a highly anaplastic carcinoma that had metastasized to eight of 21 lymph nodes. She was given postoperative irradiation but nevertheless local recurrence in the lateral skin flap was noted thirteen months after operation. Pulmonary metastasis became apparent two months later. She died 16 months after operation.

Most of us today are trying to see what can be accomplished in inflammatory carcinoma with irradiation, with hormonal treatment, or with a combination of the two methods. Wang and Griscom in 1964 reported their experience with supervoltage irradiation. They had treated 33 patients. Thirty had already died, and their average survival from the beginning of treatment was 18.5 months. This is almost the same survival time as in our 30 patients treated by radical mastectomy.

I must report that in our clinic we have been disappointed with the results of irradiation in this disease. During the last 15 years, 29 of our patients have been treated primarily with supervoltage irradiation. All these patients have also had some form of hormonal treatment. This is of course also true of the patients treated by radical mastectomy; all patients in whom surgery or irradiation fails are given hormonal treatment. Only one of our 29 patients treated primarily with irradiation remains alive. She came to us in February, 1968, with typical inflammatory carcinoma and was treated only with supervoltage irradiation. At this writing, in August, 1969, she has no evidence of active disease. All our other 28 patients with inflammatory carcinoma treated by irradiation have succumbed. They survived an average of 14.7 months after irradiation was begun.

It should be pointed out that most of these patients with inflammatory carcinoma have had large breasts. Carcinoma in large breasts has always been a difficult problem for the radiotherapeutists, and these patients with inflammatory carcinoma have done particularly badly. The primary lesion in the breast, and the axillary nodes, have diminished somewhat in size in a few of the patients, but the disease has progressed so rapidly in most of them that it has always been beyond the control of the radiotherapeutist. We have come to the pessimistic point of view of not attempting to give these patients as much irradiation as we usually administer, because it has regularly proved futile.

The various hormonal methods of treatment have also been disappointing. Oophorectomy in these patients does not give the palliation that it often provides for younger women with ordinary breast carcinoma. Dao and McCarthy recommend primary oophorectomy and adrenalectomy, but no one has treated enough of these patients with this method to have any statistically significant data regarding its comparative value.

The Inexorable Course of Inflammatory Carcinoma

We have seen that all methods of treatment fail to influence significantly the inexorable course of inflammatory carcinoma. The length of life from the first symptom to death is very much the same in most of the case series that have been reported, as shown in Table 31-2.

Our practice, for the present, is to avoid surgery in this terrible disease, to attempt to restrain it locally with the judicious use of irradiation, and to modify the patient's hormonal balance with combined oophorectomy and adrenalectomy. We have had one patient whom we have treated in this way who has survived longer than most of our other patients with inflammatory carcinoma. She was a 43 year old housewife who came to us in May, 1967, with a four weeks history of enlargement of her breast. It was obviously larger, and more firm, than her other breast. Just above and medial to the areola was a poorly defined 5 cm. tumor. Two-thirds of the skin over the breast was red and edematous. In the axilla there were two clinically involved axillary nodes, one 3 cm. and the other 1.5 cm. in diameter. Oophorectomy and adrenalectomy were done first, and followed by supervoltage irradiation. During a six week period 5475 R. were administered to the breast and chest wall through two tangential ports, and 5000 R. was given to the axilla and supraclavicular areas through a single port. Twenty-nine months later the patient has no

Table 31-2. INFLAMMATORY CARCINOMA. DURATION OF LIFE FROM FIRST SYMPTOM TO DEATH

Author	Number of Patients	Predominant Method of Treatment	Mean Total Duration of Disease
Taylor and Meltzer	25	Radical mastectomy	21.3 months
Lee and Tannenbaum	28	Radical mastectomy	2.4 months
Richards and Lewison	19	All methods	20.0 months
Byrd and Stephenson	19	All methods	16.0 months
Wang and Griscom	33	Irradiation	26.3 months
Barber, Dockerty and Clagett	53	Radical mastectomy	25.0 months
Donegan	38	All methods	18.5 months
Haagensen	87	All methods	19.0 months

evidence of active disease. We can only hope that this method of treatment will give better palliation in this terrible disease.

REFERENCES

Barber, K. W., Jr., Dockerty, M. B., and Clagett, O. T.: Inflammatory carcinoma of the breast. Surg., Gynec. & Obst., *112*:406, 1961.

Berger, S. M.: Inflammatory carcinoma of the breast. Am. J. Roentgenol., *88*:1109, 1962.

Byrd, B. F., Jr., and Stephenson, S. E., Jr.: Management of inflammatory breast cancer. South. M.J., *53*:945, 1960.

Chris, S. M.: Inflammatory carcinoma of the breast. Brit. J. Surg., *38*:163, 1950.

Dao. T. L., and McCarthy, J. D.: Treatment of inflammatory carcinoma of the breast. Surg., Gynec. & Obst., *105*:289, 1957.

Donegan, W. L., *In* Spratt, J. S., Jr., and Donegan, W. L.: Cancer of the Breast, Philadelphia, W. B. Saunders, 1967, p. 167.

Donnelly, B. A.: Primary "inflammatory" carcinoma of the breast. Ann. Surg., *128*:918, 1948.

Hartmann, H., Bertrand-Fontaine, T., and Guérin, P.: Les mastites carcinomateuses et leur traitement. Bull. Assoc. franç. p. l'étude du cancer, *24*:137, 1935.

Lee, B. J., and Tannenbaum, N. E.: Inflammatory carcinoma of the breast. Surg., Gynec. & Obst., *39*:580, 1924.

McDivitt, R. W., Stewart, F. W., and Berg, J. W.: Tumors of the Breast. Atlas of Tumor Pathology, Washington, D.C., Armed Forces Institute of Pathology, 1968, Second Series, Fascicle 2.

Meyer, A. C., Dockerty, M. B., and Harrington, S. W.: Inflammatory carcinoma of the breast, Surg., Gynec. & Obst., *87*:417, 1948.

Orbach, E.: Ueber Mastitis Carcinomatosa. Zentralbl. f. Chir., *58*:1258, 1931.

Richards, G. J., Jr., and Lewison, E. F.: Inflammatory carcinoma of the breast. Surg., Gynec. & Obst., *113*:729, 1961.

Rogers, C. S., and Fitts, W. T. Jr.: Inflammatory carcinoma of the breast. Surgery, *39*:367, 1956.

Schumann, E. A.: A study of carcinoma mastitoides. Ann. Surg., *54*:69, 1911.

Taylor, G. W., and Meltzer, A.: "Inflammatory carcinoma" of the breast. Am. J. Cancer, *33*:33, 1938.

Treves, N.: Castration as a therapeutic measure in cancer of the male breast. Cancer, *2*:191, 1949.

Treves, N.: Inflammatory carcinoma of the breast in the male patient. Surgery, *34*:810, 1953.

Treves, N.: The inoperability of inflammatory carcinoma of the breast. Surg., Gynec. & Obst., *109*:240, 1952.

Wang., C. C., and Griscom, N. T.: Inflammatory carcinoma of the breast. Clin. Radiol., *15*:167, 1964.

Chapter Thirty-Two

Special Pathological Forms of Breast Carcinoma

The special clinical features of small cell carcinoma, papillary carcinoma, Paget's carcinoma, circumscribed carcinoma, and inflammatory carcinoma to some degree set them apart from other breast carcinomas. The great majority of breast carcinomas possess no such characteristic clinical features. They do, indeed, show a great range in growth vigor, but we cannot classify them in this regard according to any generally accepted standards.

From the clinical point of view we can only group all other breast carcinomas together, and hope to sort out from among them, as our correlation of clinical characteristics with pathologic features improves, additional characteristic types of breast carcinoma.

This paucity of clinical types of breast carcinoma should not deter us from classifying breast carcinomas as to their pathologic types. In the present chapter I shall attempt this.

We believe that mammary carcinomas in general originate from the epithelium of the duct system. An exception must be made for small cell carcinomas, which I have described in Chapters 26 and 27. They can often be seen to originate from the epithelium of the lobules.

In our laboratory we classify carcinomas on a purely pathological basis—after sorting out the clinical types that I have described in the preceding chapters—into ten categories, as follows:

1. Intraductal carcinoma
2. Mucoid carcinoma
3. Apocrine carcinoma
4. Tubular carcinoma
5. Adenoid cystic carcinoma
6. Carcinoma with squamous metaplasia
7. Carcinoma with fibroblastic metaplasia
8. Carcinoma with cartilaginous and osseous metaplasia
9. Lipid-secreting carcinoma
10. Carcinoma of no special type

It will be noted that in our classification we do not include a division into noninfiltrating and infiltrating types of carcinoma. We believe that all these lesions are fully malignant carcinomas, capable of metastasizing and killing. The fact that we do not see, in the study of an individual tumor, any point at which the cells penetrate the duct wall or invade the breast stroma, does not, in our opinion, justify the conclusion that infiltration has not taken place. The exceedingly small portion of the total extent of the carcinomatous epithelium that we see in any individual carcinoma, even when a great many microscopic sections are studied, can only suggest in a general way whether or not infiltration has actually occurred. It cannot be regarded as decisive evidence. The statement by the pathologist that a carcinoma is "noninfiltrating" is apt to be taken literally by the surgeon as an indication that he may perform something less drastic than radical mastectomy. In this way the patient's chance of cure may be lost.

1. INTRADUCTAL CARCINOMA

By intraductal carcinoma we mean the carcinomas that appear to grow predominantly within the mammary ducts. The so-called comedo carcinoma is a prototype of intraductal carcinoma. But there are a number of other cell patterns of intraductal growth. We know that all are infiltrating and fully malignant even though we do not happen to see actual infiltration.

Papillary carcinoma and Paget's carcinoma are also types of intraductal carcinoma, but they have clinical features that characterize them and justify considering them separately (Chapters 28 and 29).

Intraductal carcinoma, in the sense that I here consider it, includes several forms of intraductal growth, often seen in the same tumor.

1. Comedo Intraductal Carcinoma. The ducts are dilated and filled with carcinoma cells. The centers of these cell masses have become necrotic. Grossly, the dilated ducts appear as small, yellowish-gray tubes from which the semisolid necrotic plugs can be expressed, as from a comedone (Fig. 32–1). Microscopically, the viable cells that rim the ducts in this form of carcinoma are so large, and show such a high degree of variation in size and shape and such hyperchromatism, that their malignant nature is obvious (Figs. 32–2 and 32–3).

2. Solid Intraductal Carcinoma. In this form the ducts are solidly filled with fully viable carcinoma cells (Fig. 32–4). The individual cells in this type are apt to be smaller and more uniform in size and shape.

3. Cribriform Intraductal Carcinoma. The cribriform pattern (Fig. 32–5) which identifies this form of intraductal carcinoma is one of the most easily identified of all types of breast carcinoma. Even when only one or two dilated ducts filled with cells growing in the characteristic cribriform pattern are seen, this is sufficient to justify the diagnosis of carcinoma.

Incidence

The frequency of intraductal carcinoma varies with the criteria which pathologists use to classify tumors in this category. A great many well differentiated carcinomas grow to some degree within ducts, but Dr. Stout pre-

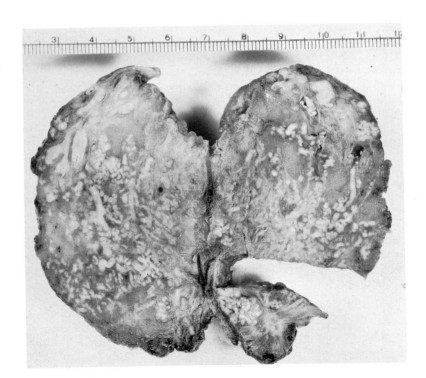

Figure 32–1. The gross appearance of the comedo form of intraductal carcinoma.

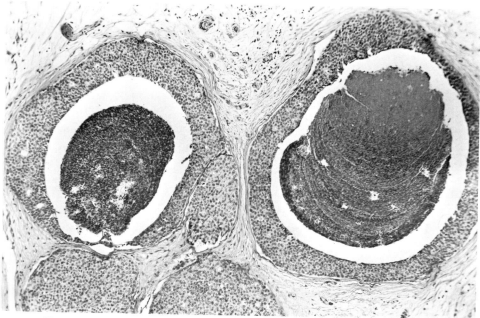

Figure 32–2. Comedones in the comedo form of intraductal carcinoma.

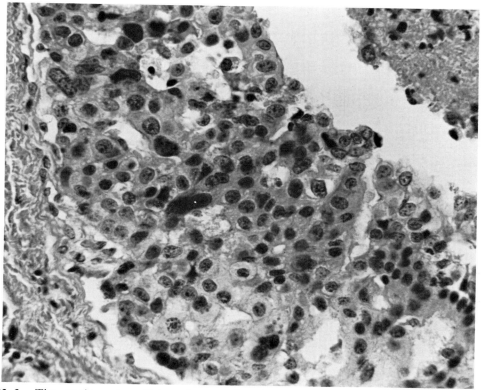

Figure 32–3. The carcinomatous lining of a comedone in the comedo form of intraductal carcinoma — higher power view.

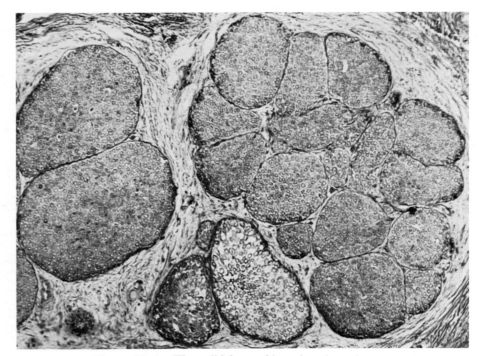

Figure 32–4.   The solid form of intraductal carcinoma.

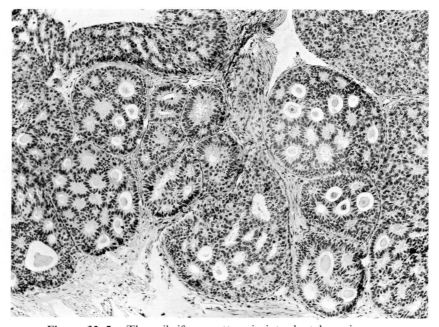

Figure 32–5.   The cribriform pattern in intraductal carcinoma.

ferred to classify as intraductal only those carcinomas in which at least 50 per cent of the carcinoma grew intraductally. I have followed this rule and have found a total of 195 intraductal carcinomas in 193 patients in our laboratory files, studied between 1931 and 1968. They constituted about 3 per cent of all our breast carcinomas during this period.

Age

The average age of our 193 patients with intraductal carcinoma was 49.6 years. This is very close to the average age for all breast carcinomas in our clinics—which was approximately 50 years.

Clinical Features

The average duration of symptoms in our 193 patients was 6.2 months, which is somewhat shorter than the average duration of 8.4 months for all types of carcinoma in my personal series of cases.

The average diameter of these intraductal carcinomas, measured clinically, was 3.5 cm., which is very similar to the 3.7 cm. average diameter of the carcinomas in my own personal series of cases.

These intraductal carcinomas have no special clinical characteristics which identify them. I have the impression that they are somewhat less apt to produce a marked degree of skin retraction, but I cannot document it.

Treatment

We have good evidence that these intraductal carcinomas are somewhat less malignant than breast carcinomas in general, derived from our data as to the frequency of axillary metastases, and the survival rate following radical mastectomy.

The frequency of axillary metastases in the total of 192 radical mastectomies performed for intraductal carcinomas in our series of cases is shown in Table 32–1. It will be seen that axillary metastasis was somewhat less frequent in the Clinical Stage A and B cases of intraductal carcinoma than it was in my personal series of radical mastectomies for all types of carcinoma.

The 10-year survival rates for our 146 pa-

Table 32–1. Frequency of Axillary Metastases in Intraductal Carcinoma Treated by Radical Mastectomy Compared with All Breast Carcinomas in My Personal Series of Radical Mastectomies (1935–1968)

Columbia Clinical Classification	Intraductal Carcinoma		All Carcinomas in Personal Series	
	Number	Per cent Axillary Metastases	Number	Per cent Axillary Metastases
Stage A	141	24%	724	31%
Stage B	36	70%	198	75%
Stage C	15	86%	71	82%
Stage D	0	–	14	93%
Total	192		1007	

tients with intraductal carcinoma treated by radical mastectomy more than 10 years ago are shown in Table 32–2. As compared with the survival rates in my personal series of radical mastectomies for all types of carcinoma, the patients with intraductal carcinoma did somewhat better. These results confirm our general impression that intraductal carcinoma is less malignant than breast carcinoma of no special type.

Radical mastectomy is clearly the preferred treatment. These are fully malignant tumors which often extend widely in the breast and metastasize to the axilla; and "modified" operations in which the entire breast is not removed and the dissected axilla is incompletely dissected risk failure.

The knowledge that the carcinoma which I have to deal with is an intraductal type and likely, therefore, to have a better prognosis,

Table 32–2. Ten-Year Survival Following Radical Mastectomy for Intraductal Carcinoma Compared with All Breast Carcinomas in My Personal Series of Radical Mastectomies (1935–1957)

Columbia Clinical Classification	Intraductal Carcinoma		All Carcinomas in Personal Series	
	No. of Patients	Per cent 10-Year Survival	No. of Patients	Per cent 10-Year Survival
Stage A	107	74%	402	70%
Stage B	29	62%	154	41%
Stage C	10	20%	59	24%
Stage D	0	–	11	18%
Total	146		626	

has sometimes influenced my decision as to treatment, as in the following case.

Mrs. N. O., aged 41, had first discovered a small tumor in her right breast four months previously. The tumor was situated just below and lateral to the nipple. Her family physician diagnosed "mastitis" and gave her estrogen. The tumor persisting, she was finally referred to a surgeon, who had operated upon her ten days previously. He had first excised the tumor locally for biopsy. It measured grossly 2 cm. in diameter and was a carcinoma. He had then performed a "mastectomy" through a transverse incision. When her family realized what had happened they brought her to consult me.

When I examined her the transverse incision was well healed. It was obvious that only the central part of the breast had been removed. Its peripheral portion remained undisturbed. I could not palpate any remaining tumor. The pectoral muscles had not been removed, and no axillary dissection at all had been attempted. I could not palpate any enlarged axillary or supraclavicular lymph nodes. Skeletal and chest x-ray films showed no evidence of metastasis.

Experience has taught me that in the usual breast carcinoma of no special clinical or microscopic type it is futile to try to save the patient after this kind of inadequate operative attack. The carcinoma has been implanted throughout the operative field, and any subsequent surgical attempt to get beyond it will not succeed. But in this particular patient I decided to attempt it, because her carcinoma was an intraductal type of the comedo variety.

In the radical mastectomy that I performed I carried out an unusually wide removal of skin and subcutaneous tissue. A large skin graft was required to close the defect on the chest wall. It took me 7½ hours to complete the operation.

A total of 57 lymph nodes were found in the operative specimen, and three of these contained metastases.

My hopes were fortunately justified. The patient is well 18 years after operation. She owes her cure, I believe, to the facts that her tumor was a comparatively favorable intraductal type and she had a meticulous and thorough radical mastectomy.

2. MUCOID CARCINOMA

Many carcinomas of the breast, when studied microscopically with the mucicarmine stain, will be found to contain mucin in varying amounts. Frantz studied the phenomenon and its prognostic significance. Barbieri and his associates have also carried out extensive histologic investigations of mucin formation in carcinoma. The mucin is usually present in the form of intracellular droplets, but occasionally it appears in small scattered pools. We do not classify such tumors as mucoid. We limit this designation to breast carcinomas in which the mucoid change is marked, forming large lakes of mucoid material, which are often visible grossly.

We prefer the term *mucoid* rather than colloid or gelatinous, which are more commonly used, for this form of breast carcinoma. Gelatinous is a purely descriptive term. Colloid is inaccurate. Mucoid is more appropriate, because it is today generally accepted that the material that characterizes this group of breast tumors is mucin that has accumulated by secretion from malignant epithelial cells. Fifty or more years ago, when there was a considerable interest in this group of tumors, and large series of cases were collected and studied and reported in two classical papers by Lange and by Gaabe, the question of whether the mucoid material originated from the stroma or the epithelium of the tumor was hotly debated.

Tellem and his associates have recently studied one of these mucoid carcinomas by histochemistry, electron microscopy, and tissue culture, and have clearly demonstrated that the mucin is produced by the carcinoma cells.

Incidence

True mucoid carcinoma as I have defined it is infrequent. In the largest case series (Lee et al.; Geschickter; Veronesi and Gennari; Melamed et al.; Norris and Taylor) mucoid carcinoma constituted only from 1 to 3 per cent of all breast carcinomas.

Our Columbia-Presbyterian series of 63 cases represents about 1 per cent of our entire series of breast carcinomas, during a 39 year period (1930 to 1969).

Age

The average age of our 63 patients was 55.5 years. This is definitely older than the average age for all breast carcinomas in our series (50 years). In Veronesi and Gennari's as well as Norris and Taylor's series, the patients were also older.

Clinical Features

Several of those who have written about mucoid carcinoma have emphasized the slow rate of growth and the large size of these tumors, but critical study of the data they have presented regarding these characteristics is not entirely convincing. Some of these tumors certainly grow slowly and attain a large size, but so do some ordinary breast carcinomas.

In our series of 56 patients with mucoid carcinoma treated by radical mastectomy the average duration of symptoms was 10.1 months, as compared with 8.4 months for my personal series of breast carcinomas. These facts suggest that mucoid carcinomas may grow somewhat more slowly than carcinomas of no special type.

Many mucoid carcinomas, on palpation, are remarkably well delimited, and some seem to be fluctuant. On these grounds I have several times mistaken them for cysts.

Halsted, in 1915, described a clinical sign that he had noted in four cases of mucoid carcinoma. He wrote, "there was conveyed to the finger on testing for elasticity a peculiar sensation which in the first instance made me apprehensive lest I had ruptured a possible capsule of the nodule . . . it might be defined as a delicate swish or crush of a jelly-like structure under tension, with the suggestion of a delicate bursting."

Halsted's gentleness and precision were well known and it is likely that most examiners would miss what he felt. I have never, myself, experienced this swishing or crushing sensation.

Pathology

Mucoid carcinoma can often be recognized grossly for its sharply delimited, seemingly encapsulated character, its soft and jelly-like consistence, and its mucoid, translucent appearance. Figure 32–6 shows the gross appearance of one of these tumors.

Microscopic study of these tumors indicates that the mucoid material is secreted by the tumor cells. These cells often have acidophilic cytoplasms and tend to form acini as in Figure 32–7. They are lost, to a varying degree, in the lakes of mucoid material that they secrete. In some tumors only scattered small groups of cells remain (Fig. 32–8).

It is important for pathologists to be on guard against mistaking adenofibromas showing extensive myxoid degeneration for mucoid carcinoma. It is very difficult to make good frozen sections from either of these tumors, and the pathologist is tempted to rely

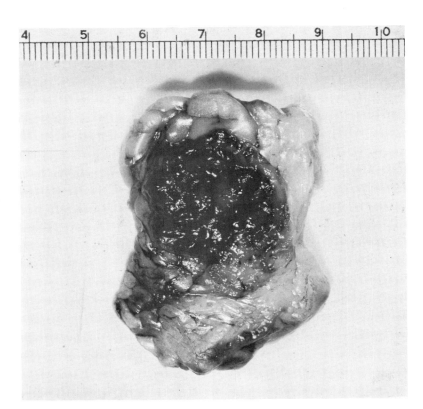

Figure 32–6. The encapsulated, soft, jelly-like gross appearance of mucoid carcinoma.

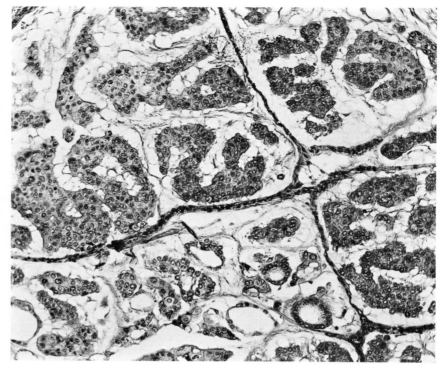

Figure 32–7. Characteristic microscopic appearance of mucoid carcinoma.

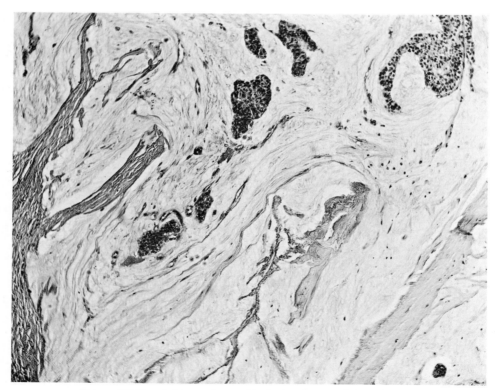

Figure 32–8. Advanced mucoid change in mucoid carcinoma.

on gross appearance. The adenofibromas are truly encapsulated, whereas the mucoid carcinomas do not have a real capsule. The cut surface of the adenofibroma bulges; the mucoid carcinoma does not. But the differential diagnosis should be made only on microscopic grounds.

Treatment

The three largest series of mucoid carcinomas yet reported provide evidence that suggests that this lesion is less malignant than breast carcinoma of no special type, but they do not give a clear indication of the comparative success of radical mastectomy in the disease. In Veronesi and Gennari's series of 73 cases of mucoid carcinoma treated by radical mastectomy, 35.6 per cent had axillary metastases, as compared with 58.4 per cent in their entire series of breast carcinomas. In the series of 97 patients who had an axillary dissection as part of this surgical attack, reported by Melamed and his associates, 41 per cent were found to have axillary metastases. Norris and Taylor's series of cases included 59 patients treated by radical mastectomy; 27 per cent had axillary metastases.

Although Veronesi reports that the 5-year survival rate for mucoid carcinoma was better than for other carcinomas in his series, he unfortunately includes no 10-year survival rates. Melamed and his associates reported that 35.6 per cent of their 90 patients treated by radical mastectomy survived 10 years, as compared with 29.4 per cent for all breast carcinomas. However, 26 per cent of Melamed's series of patients were lost to follow-up before 10 years. When the proportion of patients lost track of is as high as this, any conclusions regarding therapy are of doubtful value. Norris and Taylor present 10-year survival data for a total of 23 patients, after excluding patients who succumbed to operation and those lost track of. Radical mastectomy was apparently performed in only half the cases they report—the others being treated by simple mastectomy. On the basis of these meager and incomplete data, they suggest that the type of this disease which they classify as "pure mucinous carcinoma" should be treated by simple mastectomy. Their definition of "pure" was that no areas of "infiltrating" duct carcinoma were found in the gross or microscopic examination of the lesion.

The most important defect in these data concerning the treatment of mucoid carcinoma is that the patients were not classified as to the stage of clinical advancement of their disease. Without clinical staging it is impossible to assess the results of treatment.

The thoughtful surgeon who looks for solid facts upon which to base his choice of treatment will find small comfort from these data. Fortunately, I am able to present more complete data from our clinic as to the results of radical mastectomy in patients with mucoid carcinoma. A total of 62 patients with the disease were operated upon more than 10 years ago. The axillary findings, compared with those in my personal series of radical mastectomies for all types of breast carcinoma are shown in Table 32–3. The mucoid carcinomas metastasized to the axilla much less often than mammary carcinoma in general. In patients with Clinical Stage A and B carcinoma, the frequency of axillary metastases for mucoid carcinoma was only 16.4 per cent, as compared with 40.2 per cent for all types of carcinoma in my personal series of cases.

In Table 32–4 the 10-year survival rates for our 62 patients with mucoid carcinoma treated by radical mastectomy are compared with the survival rates for patients with carcinomas of all types in my personal series of cases. The survival rate for our patients with mucoid carcinoma whose disease was classified as Clinical Stage A was the same as the survival rate for all types of the disease in my personal series of cases. Some allowance should be made, however, for the fact that these patients with mucoid carcinoma were older, and four of the 48 patients in our clini-

Table 32–3. FREQUENCY OF AXILLARY METASTASES IN MUCOID CARCINOMA TREATED BY RADICAL MASTECTOMY, COMPARED WITH ALL BREAST CARCINOMAS IN MY PERSONAL SERIES OF RADICAL MASTECTOMIES (1935–1968)

Columbia Clinical Classification	Mucoid Carcinoma		All Carcinomas in Personal Series	
	Number	Per cent Axillary Metastases	Number	Per cent Axillary Metastases
Stage A	48	12.5%	724	31%
Stage B	7	43%	198	75%
Stage C	7	86%	71	82%
Stage D	0	–	14	93%
Total	62		1007	

Table 32–4. TEN-YEAR SURVIVAL FOLLOWING
RADICAL MASTECTOMY FOR MUCOID CARCINOMA
COMPARED WITH ALL BREAST CARCINOMAS IN
MY PERSONAL SERIES OF RADICAL MASTECTOMIES
(1935–1957)

Columbia Clinical Classification	Mucoid Carcinoma		All Carcinomas in Personal Series	
	No. of Patients	Per cent 10-Year Survival	No. of Patients	Per cent 10-Year Survival
Stage A	48	71%	402	70%
Stage B	7	43%	154	41%
Stage C	7	14%	59	24%
Stage D	0	–	11	18%
Total	62		626	

cal stage A group died of intercurrent disease before 10 years had elapsed. If these four patients are not counted as succumbing to their carcinomas, the 10-year survival rate for mucoid carcinoma becomes slightly better than the survival rate for all types of carcinoma in my personal series.

This slightly better survival rate for mucoid carcinoma is certainly not striking enough, however, to justify simple mastectomy or any "modified" type of mastectomy. These mucoid carcinomas are fully malignant, and any surgeon who performs less than a thorough and meticulous radical mastectomy for them is risking his patient's life unnecessarily.

3. APOCRINE CARCINOMA

The morphology of occasional breast carcinomas is so reminiscent of the "apocrine" or "pale" epithelium of the breast that we are tempted to infer that they originate from these cells. Lee and his associates; Higginson and McDonald; McDivitt, Stewart, and Berg; Wald and Kakulas; and Frable and Kay have all written about these tumors.

The cells of these carcinomas have the same large acidophilic cytoplasm as the apocrine cells of the normal breast (Fig. 32–9). They tend to grow within dilated ducts, which they line with low papillary projections (Fig. 32–10). On higher magnification the apocrine character of the tumor cells is obvious (Fig. 32–11). In other apocrine carcinomas the tumor cells form small regular acini (Fig. 32–12).

There are two special features of these "apocrine" carcinoma cells that may assist in identifying them. One is the tendency of the cells to extrude their cytoplasms into the gland lumen as snouts projecting from the medial poles of the cells. A second feature is

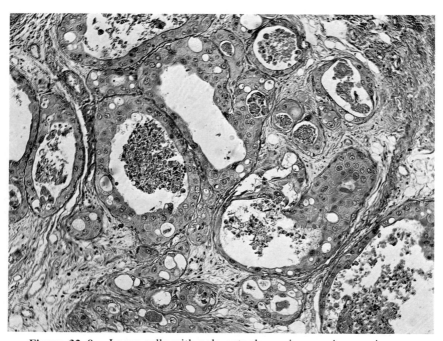

Figure 32–9. Large cells with pale cytoplasms in apocrine carcinoma.

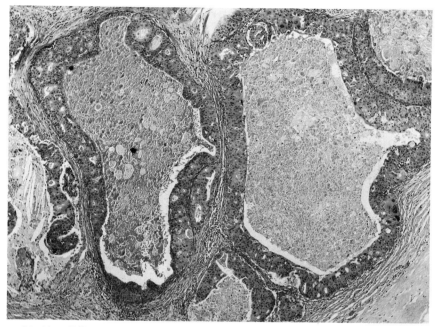

Figure 32–10.   Dilated ducts lined with apocrine carcinoma—low power magnification.

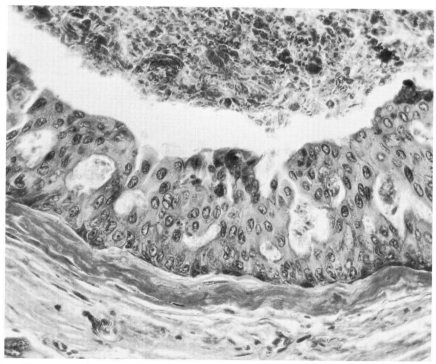

Figure 32–11.   The apocrine type cells lining dilated ducts in apocrine carcinoma—higher power magnification.

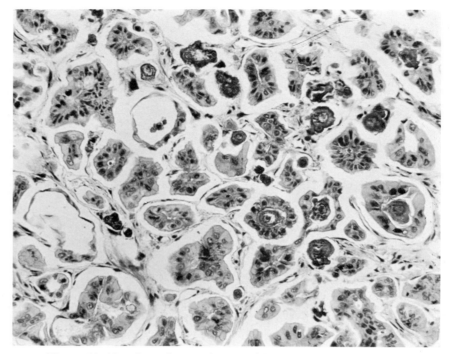

Figure 32–12. Apocrine carcinoma with a glandular arrangement.

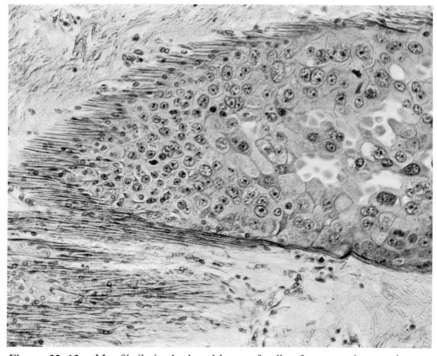

Figure 32–13. Myofibrils in the basal layer of cells of an apocrine carcinoma.

the presence of myofibrils in the bases of the peripheral layer of cells in ducts. These myofibrils are shown in Figure 32–13 in a phosphotungstic acid stain.

The carcinomas that we have been willing to classify as apocrine in our laboratory have been few. In reviewing 16 such tumors, we did not observe anything distinctive in their natural history. The number of our cases is too small to permit any conclusions regarding the results of treatment. In their series of 18 patients with this type of breast carcinoma, Frable and Kay were unable to demonstrate that the prognosis was better.

4. TUBULAR CARCINOMA

There is a rare type of carcinoma which has a tubular pattern and is probably best classified as a sub-variety of apocrine carcinoma. The cells are smaller than those of the apocrine carcinomas I have illustrated, but they have distinctly acidophilic cytoplasms and quite regular small nuclei. They form small tubules, often consisting of only a single layer of cells. Figures 32–14 and 32–15 show the structure of one of these tumors in low and high power magnification. The tumor cells often have apocrine snouts projecting into the lumens of the tubules, as shown in Figure 32–16.

McDivitt, Stewart, and Berg call this lesion "tubular carcinoma." Norris and Taylor have recently reported a series of 33 of these lesions, which they name "well differentiated carcinoma."

We have had too few examples of this type of tubular apocrine carcinoma to have an opinion as to its degree of malignancy. Norris and Taylor report that 10 of their 24 patients with this tumor treated by radical mastectomy had metastases, but they nevertheless suggest that it is a slowly growing lesion.

This lesion has such an orderly and seemingly innocuous character that its carcinomatous character is easily missed. The tubules lie in a rather dense fibrous stroma, which distorts them and may lead the pathologist to confuse the lesion with sclerosing adenosis. Another lesion for which tubular carcinoma may be mistaken is intraductal papilloma distorted by fibrosis.

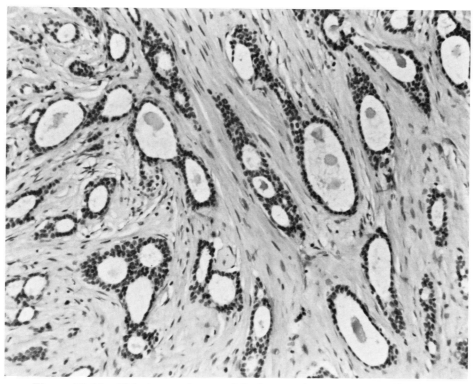

Figure 32–14. Tubular carcinoma of the breast—low power magnification.

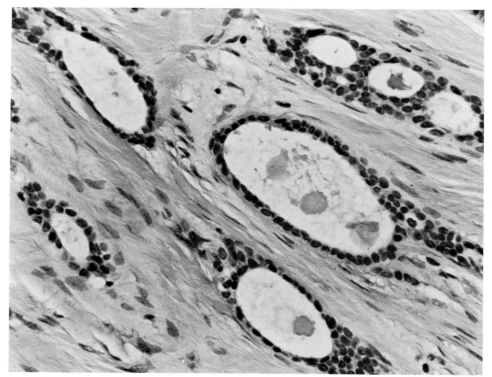

Figure 32–15. Tubular carcinoma of the breast—higher power magnification.

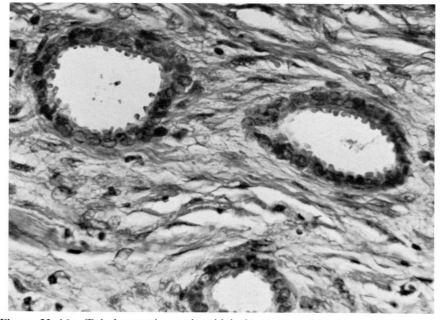

Figure 32–16. Tubular carcinoma in which the tumor cells have apocrine snouts.

I believe that tubular carcinoma should be treated by radical mastectomy. It certainly metastasizes to axillary lymph nodes, and less thorough operations risk incomplete removal of the lesion.

5. ADENOID CYSTIC CARCINOMA

One of the rarest forms of breast carcinoma is adenoid cystic carcinoma, which is identical in its histologic character with the tumors of the salivary glands called adenoid cystic carcinoma or cylindroma. Foote and Stewart described this form of breast carcinoma in 1946. Galloway and his associates collected reports of a total of 12 of these tumors and have described nine additional ones observed at the Mayo Clinic. Cavanzo and Taylor have recently reported 21 of these tumors from the Armed Forces Institute of Pathology.

Although there is no report of any of these tumors metastasizing to the regional lymph nodes, a patient who was treated by radical mastectomy by Nayer died with pulmonary metastases after 12 years.

Microscopically, these tumors certainly appear to infiltrate the breast, and Wilson and Spell describe local recurrence in one patient treated by simple mastectomy. Nine of the 21 patients reported by Cavanzo and Taylor had been treated more than five years previously; none had died of her breast tumor.

The pathologic feature of this lesion is unmistakable. The tubules of varying size lined by small comparatively regular cells are filled with mucoid material. The name "cylindroma" is appropriate. Figures 32–17 and 32–18 show a characteristic area in one of our tumors in low and higher power magnification.

We have recently studied three of these tumors in our laboratory of surgical pathology. Two were from patients sent to Lattes for consultation. The third was a patient of our own, a 39 year old nurse who found a tumor in her left breast. The tumor was only 15 mm, in diameter, and was well delimited. It was situated 6 cm. from the areolar edge in the radius of 2 o'clock. There was no skin retraction over it, and there were no clinically involved nodes.

The surgeon who biopsied it had thought it to be benign, but frozen section revealed that it was an adenoid cystic carcinoma. Radical mastectomy was done. There were no metastases in 39 axillary lymph nodes.

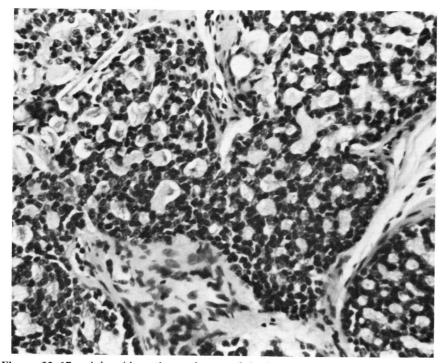

Figure 32–17. Adenoid cystic carcinoma of the breast—low power magnification.

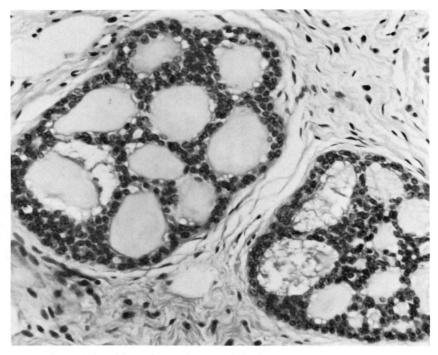

Figure 32–18.   Adenoid cystic carcinoma of the breast—higher power magnification.

6. CARCINOMA WITH SQUAMOUS METAPLASIA

Squamous metaplasia is occasionally seen in mammary carcinomas of mice. In human breast carcinoma it also occurs, as might be expected, but it is rare. During a 50 year period—1919 to 1969—only 20 mammary carcinomas with squamous metaplasia were recorded in the Presbyterian Hospital. All these tumors were of the circumscribed type. The squamous metaplasia occurred within the broad bands and masses of cells that characterize this form of breast carcinoma.

In these tumors the extent of the squamous metaplasia varied greatly. In some there were only scattered small areas of squamous transformation, such as that shown in Figure 32–19, found within masses of otherwise unremarkable carcinoma cells. It is apparent from the study of such tumors that the squamous areas in them develop by metaplasia. Even when the squamous change involves most of the tumor, and includes the development of intercellular bridges and epithelial pearls, the phenomenon is still only a metaplastic one. These tumors are not pure squamous cell epitheliomas developing as such within the breast.

Squamous cell epithelioma developing within sebaceous cysts in the skin over the breast may grow to a large size and simulate carcinoma of the breast, which, of course, it is not.

Good descriptions of breast carcinomas showing squamous metaplasia have been published by Loeb, by Brocq, Wolf, and Giet, by Foot and Moore, by Harrington and Miller, by Pasternack and Wirth, by James and Treip, by Willis, and by Arffmann and Hjgaard.

Review of our 20 cases of breast carcinoma showing squamous metaplasia does not reveal that these tumors have any distinctive clinical characteristics. The average age of the patients was 50. The average duration of symptoms was 6 months, which is rather shorter than the duration in ordinary breast carcinoma, if such a small series of cases permits any conclusion. The average size of these tumors by clinical measurement was 6.5 cm. Axillary metastases were found microscopically in only four of the 16 patients treated by radical mastectomy.

One of the patients was treated by irradiation and was well when last heard from 19

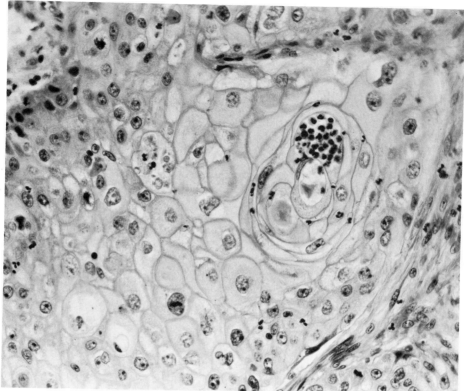

Figure 32–19. An area of squamous metaplasia in mammary carcinoma of the circumscribed type.

years later. Two other patients, both of whom had very large tumors and whose disease was regarded as inoperable, were treated by palliative simple mastectomy with excision of lower axillary nodes; they both succumbed within a year. The remaining 16 patients were treated by radical mastectomy; in 13 the operation was done more than 10 years ago. Eight, or 61 per cent, survived more than 10 years. These carcinomas characterized by squamous metaplasia are, to judge from our Presbyterian Hospital experience, by no means as hopeless as they have sometimes been reported to be.

7. CARCINOMA WITH FIBROBLASTIC METAPLASIA

In rare breast carcinomas of the solid circumscribed type, fibroblastic metaplasia may occur. We studied one such tumor sent to us by Wasdahl. The patient was a 70 year old woman whose breast tumor had metastasized extensively to the axilla. The primary lesion in the breast was the solid circumscribed type

of carcinoma with marked, spindle cell metaplasia. In the axillary metastasis this metaplasia was of such an extreme degree (Fig. 32–20), with gigantic, mostly spindle-shaped cells, that diagnosis of rhabdomyosarcoma had been suggested.

8. CARCINOMA WITH CARTILAGINOUS AND OSSEOUS METAPLASIA

Carcinomas showing cartilaginous metaplasia, and particularly those showing osseous metaplasia, are the rarest breast tumors. Such tumors have been well described by Biggs, by Kreibig, and by Robb and MacFarlane. Gonzalez-Licea and his associates have recently studied one of these rare tumors by both light and electron microscopy. Smith and Taylor have described 10 which they collected at the Armed Forces Institute of Pathology.

These tumors have been called carcino-sarcomas or "mixed tumors" by some writers, but we believe that they are primarily carcinomas, because no matter how predominant

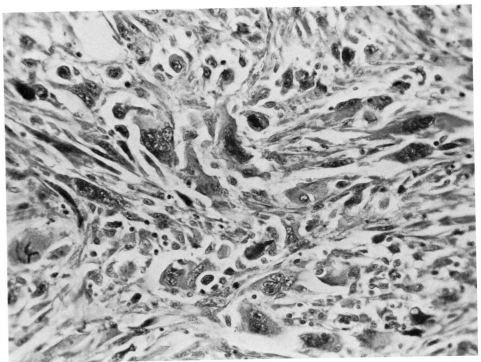

Figure 32–20.   Axillary metastasis showing an extreme degree of spindle cell metaplasia, originating from a circumscribed type of breast carcinoma.

the cartilage or bone may be in them, areas of indubitable carcinoma can be found. In mammary carcinomas of the dog, cartilaginous metaplasia is almost the rule. It is occasionally seen in mouse breast carcinoma. It is not unreasonable, therefore, to find it now and then in human carcinoma.

Cartilage was present in all eight of these tumors which we studied in our laboratory. It was scattered throughout the lesions, and transition from masses and cords of carcinoma cells to cartilage was obvious. Figure 32–21 shows this cartilaginous metaplasia in one of our cases. The patient was a 58 year old woman with a rapidly growing tumor which filled her breast and had metastasized to the axilla. Irradiation checked its growth somewhat, but the patient died within six months with pulmonary metastases.

Osseous metaplasia was present in association with cartilaginous metaplasia in three of our eight tumors.

The most recent example of a breast carcinoma with cartilaginous and osseous metaplasia that we have had is particularly striking as regards its microscopic features. The patient was a 50 year old Negro housewife who had discovered a tumor in the upper outer sector

of her right breast 8 months before she consulted us. It was a hard 6 cm. mass accompanied by marked retraction of the overlying skin. There was a 1.5 cm. firm axillary node. After biopsy, a radical mastectomy was performed. Only one of a total of 40 axillary nodes contained metastases.

There was no doubt about the basic carcinomatous nature of the lesion as indicated by its epithelial component shown in Figure 32–22. Some of the epithelial cells showed a very striking degree of variation (Fig. 32–23). There were scattered areas of cartilaginous and osseous metaplasia (Figs. 32–24 and 32–25). Altogether, the lesion gave the impression of great malignancy.

There is not enough information concerning the natural history of these rare tumors to draw any solid conclusions regarding their treatment. Certainly, they are more malignant than the carcinomas with squamous metaplasia. Six of Smith and Taylor's patients whose carcinomas showed cartilaginous or osseous metaplasia died. In one of our patients the lesion progressed with great rapidity and was fatal in eight months. Two of our other patients with this rare type of tumor are very recent ones.

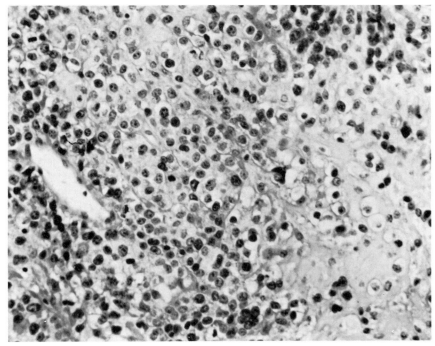

Figure 32–21. Mammary carcinoma with cartilaginous metaplasia.

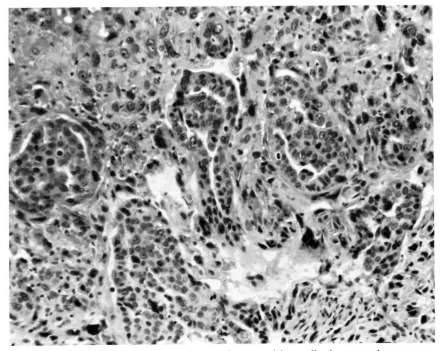

Figure 32–22. The epithelial component of a carcinoma with cartilaginous and osseous metaplasia.

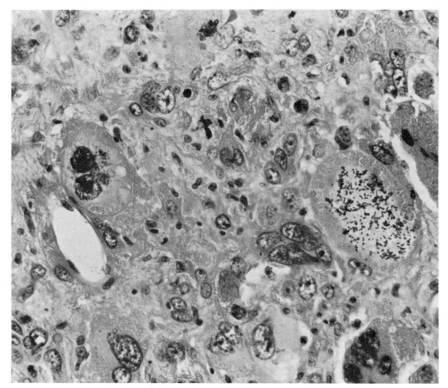

Figure 32–23. Striking variation in the cells of the epithelial component of a carcinoma with cartilaginous and osseous metaplasia.

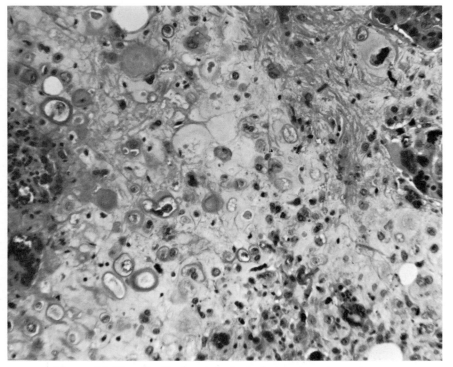

Figure 32–24. Cartilaginous metaplasia in a breast carcinoma.

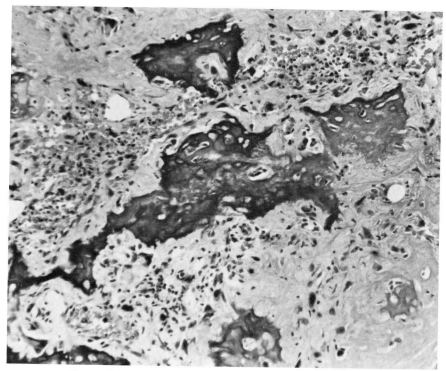

Figure 32–25. Osseous metaplasia in a breast carcinoma.

9. LIPID-SECRETING MAMMARY CARCINOMA

The fact that the epithelium of mammary ducts often contains lipid, and that this is a secretory and not a degenerative process, has been emphasized by Aboumrad, Horn, and Fine. They described clear cell carcinoma of the breast in which the flaming red stain revealed a large amount of lipid within the cytoplasm of the tumor cells, and suggest that clear cell lipid-secreting carcinomas of this kind may constitute 1 per cent of all breast carcinomas.

10. MAMMARY CARCINOMA OF NO SPECIAL TYPE

The great majority, in fact some 70 per cent, of our breast carcinomas have not been of any special microscopic type. Those showing a pronounced degree of desmoplasia might be called scirrhous, while the softer and more cellular ones might be called medullary, but these are broad descriptive terms that have, in our opinion, no definite significance as regards the natural history of the carcinoma to which they are applied. This brings us to the consideration of other methods of classifying breast carcinomas on the basis of their gross and microscopic characteristics.

Macroscopic Grading

A decade ago Nathan Lane, in our laboratory of surgical pathology, conceived a plan of classifying breast carcinomas into two groups on the basis of their macroscopic contour, as judged by naked eye or hand-lens examination of the histologic slides, as follows.

1. Well-Delimited Carcinomas. Those with a well-delimited rounded or lobulated contour, suggesting a "pushing" or apparently expansile type of growth. Figures 32–26 and 32–27 show two of these well-delimited carcinomas.

2. Irregular Carcinomas. Those with a serrated, grossly irregular, often stellate periphery, showing radial projections into the surrounding tissue. Figure 32–28 shows one of these irregular carcinomas in low magnification. Figure 32–29 shows a radial projec-

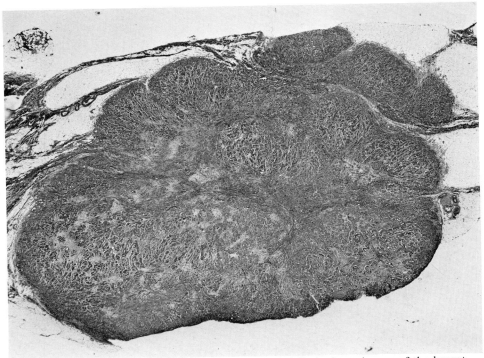

Figure 32–26. The rounded contour of a well delimited carcinoma of the breast.

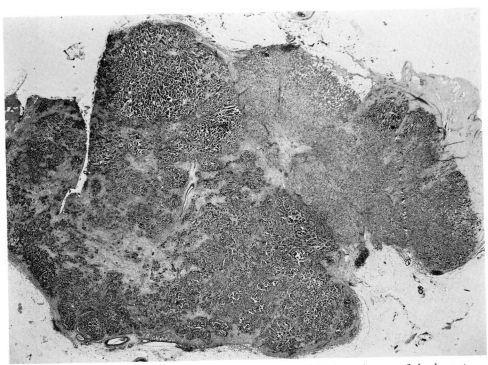

Figure 32–27. The lobulated contour of a well delimited carcinoma of the breast.

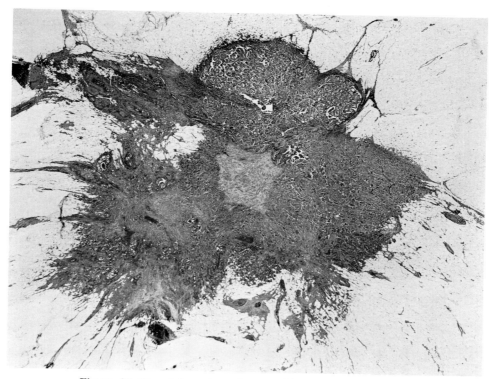

Figure 32–28. A breast carcinoma with an irregular contour.

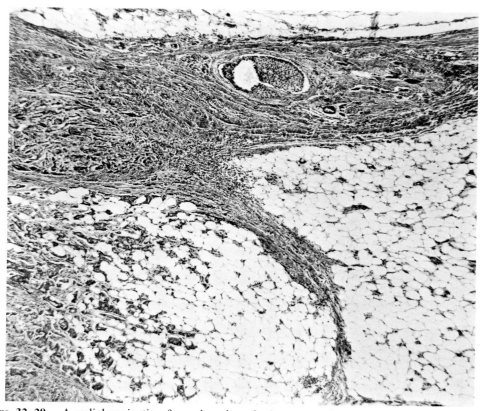

Figure 32–29. A radial projection from the edge of a breast carcinoma with an irregular contour.

Table 32–5. Relationship of macroscopic contour to the frequency of axillary metastases, and the end-results of treatment by radical mastectomy

	Carcinoma with Well-Delimited Contour (46 cases)	Carcinoma with Irregular Contour (158 cases)
Per cent with axillary metastases	41%	65%
Per cent 10 year clinical cures in patients with axillary metastases	74%	22%
Per cent 10 year clinical cures all cases	80%	38%

tion from the edge of such a lesion, in higher power magnification.

Lane and his associates tested the prognostic significance of this simple classification in a series of 241 of my personal cases of breast carcinoma. The uniform character of this series of cases, in terms of treatment and follow-up, make it particularly suitable for studying a question of this kind. In order to make their study as valid as possible Lane and his associates excluded the well known special types of carcinoma—papillary, intraductal, and mucoid—from the study.

In the remaining lesions of no special type, Lane and his associates found that the *well-delimited* carcinomas were one-third larger than the *irregular* carcinomas. Nevertheless, the frequency of axillary metastasis was significantly lower in the well-delimited carcinomas, and even when axillary metastases were present the end-results of radical mastectomy were strikingly better in the carcinomas with well-delimited contours, as shown in Table 32–5.

Lane's work has convinced us in our department of surgical pathology that his method of macroscopic grading is an important aid in determining the prognosis of breast carcinomas. We recommend it as a routine procedure in the study of all of these lesions.

Microscopic Grading

Microscopic grading has been the traditional method of estimating the degree of malignancy of breast carcinoma.

It was toward the end of the last century

that Hansemann, in his monograph "Studien über die Spezificität, den Altruismus und die Anaplasie der Zellen" first presented the idea that a scale might be drawn up to represent the degree of anaplasia, that is, the degree to which the morphology of a tumor departs from that of the mother cells from which it arises. He suggested the possibility that the degree of clinical malignancy of the tumor, as evidenced by its tendency to metastasize, might be correlated with its grade of anaplasia.

Hansemann's idea was tested extensively by American pathologists in the 1920's. Good evidence was accumulated that for a few special types of carcinoma, such as that in the cervix and in the rectum, the grade of anaplasia is a useful guide to the grade of malignancy.

Mammary carcinoma would seem to be an ideal form of cancer upon which to test the significance of histologic grading, since the disease is frequent, and abundant pathologic material is secured by radical mastectomy. Greenough's 1925 study of a series of cases from the Massachusetts General Hospital was the first attempt in this direction. He graded the tumors in 73 cases in which complete follow-up data were available, distinguishing three grades of anaplasia which he designated as low, medium and high malignancy. Hansemann himself, in estimating the grade of anaplasia of adenocarcinoma, had used loss of an adenoid arrangement of the cells, and the number of normal and atypical mitoses, as his criteria. Greenough, in his grading of breast carcinoma, followed Hansemann fairly closely. His criteria were the arrangement of the cells around an open gland lumen, the degree of secretory activity as indicated by the presence of vacuoles and droplets of mucoid material, the uniformity of size of cells and nuclei, the degree of hyperchromatism of the nuclei, and the number and irregularity of mitoses. When tumors were graded on this basis, Greenough found a striking relationship between the grade of anaplasia and curability. Sixty-eight per cent of his patients with Grade I tumors were alive five years after operation, and 33 per cent of those with Grade II tumors survived, whereas none of those with Grade III tumors lived for five years.

Similar studies, using Greenough's method of grading breast carcinoma, were shortly carried out by White, by Lee and Stubenbord, and by Smith and Bartlett. These studies in general confirmed Greenough's findings.

Table 32–6. MICROSCOPIC GRADE AND SURVIVAL: MATHEWS SERIES OF BREAST CARCINOMAS

Grade	No. of Cases	No. Surviving 5 Years	Per cent Surviving 5 Years	Average Length of Life of Those Dying Before 5 Years
1	40	32	80	3.4 years
2	66	25	38	2.3 years
3	48	6	13	1.5 years
Total	154	63	41	2.0 years

Meanwhile, at the Mayo Clinic, MacCarty had become interested in the grading of breast carcinomas. The histologic characteristics that MacCarty used as a basis for grading were, however, quite different from those suggested by Hansemann. MacCarty relied upon what he called "defensive factors." These included lymphocytic infiltration, and fibrosis and hyalinization, as well as cellular differentiation. MacCarty's pupils, Flothow and Heuper, applied and elaborated his method of grading breast carcinoma to case series. Their follow-up data were not complete and their conclusions were not convincing.

French pathologists became interested in relating the morphology of breast carcinoma to its prognosis through the studies carried on by Delbet. He was particularly interested in the prognostic significance of mucin secretion. He thought that the carcinomas that contained mucin were more benign. Leroux and Perrot, Moureau and Lambert, and Toro made similar studies of the significance of mucin secretion in breast carcinoma, and confirmed these findings. Frantz, in our laboratory, carried out a much more systematic study of the significance of mucin secretion in breast carcinoma. Although she was cautious in her conclusions, they tended to confirm the favorable prognostic significance of finding mucicarminophilic material in breast carcinomas.

In 1933 I myself attempted to determine the significance of histologic grading of breast carcinoma. I used for the study a remarkable series of 164 consecutive radical mastectomies performed by the late Dr. Frank Mathews. The follow-up was known in all but five of these patients. I studied in detail the prognostic significance of fifteen different histologic characteristics in the tumors of this case series. Six of these characteristics were found to have a probable relationship to the degree of malignancy as expressed by the end results of treatment. These significant characteristics were similar to those which Hanse-

mann originally proposed for the determination of grade of anaplasia. They were:

1. The tendency of the carcinoma to grow in a papillary pattern.
2. An intraductal type of growth, as illustrated by comedo carcinoma.
3. An adenoid arrangement of the cells.
4. Variation in size and shape of the nuclei.
5. The number of mitoses.
6. The presence of mucin.

The factors of fibrosis and lymphocytic infiltration emphasized by MacCarty and his pupils I found to be without prognostic significance. When Mathews' cases were graded on the basis of the six characteristics that I found to be significant, the correlation with five-year clinical survival was as shown in Table 32–6.

The pathologists of the Middlesex Hospital have made important contributions to the subject of microscopic grading of breast carcinoma. In 1928 Patey and Scarff, using as criteria the characteristics of the epithelial elements of the tumor, as formulated by Greenough, graded a series of 73 breast carcinomas. Encouraged by the results of this study, Scarff and Handley, in 1938, graded the tumors of a series of 172 patients for which they had a 10 year follow-up after radical mastectomy. Their study clearly showed that there is a close relationship between microscopic grade and end-results. Their findings are shown in Table 32–7.

Table 32–7. MICROSCOPIC TUMOR GRADE AND RESULTS OF RADICAL MASTECTOMY. SCARFF AND HANDLEY, 1938*

Microscopical Grade	No. of Cases	Per cent 10-Year Survival	Average Time Which Those Who Died Survived Operation
I	62	31%	37 months
II	66	11%	33 months
III	44	13%	29 months
Total	172		

*Data from Scarff, R. W., and Handley, R. S.: Lancet, 2:582, 1938.

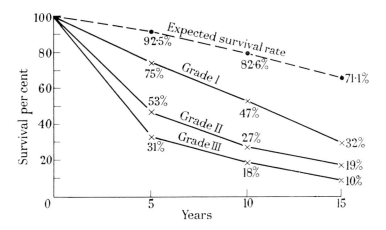

Chart 32–1. Microscopic grade of breast carcinoma and survival. (From Bloom, H. J., and Richardson, W. W.: Brit. J. Cancer, *11*:359, 1957. Reproduced with permission.)

Bloom has carried on microscopic grading at the Middlesex Hospital and has published two important papers on the subject in 1950 and 1957. The latter study, carried out with Richardson, and based upon 1544 cases, is the most comprehensive and helpful yet made.

Bloom and Richardson used the same general criteria for grading that had been followed in the earlier studies from their laboratory. They are the tendency of the tumor cells to form tubules, the pleomorphism of the tumor cells, and the frequency of hyperchromatic nuclei and mitoses. Points are awarded for each of these histologic factors, and three grades of malignancy are determined from the sum of these points. The relationship of microscopic grade to the results of treatment in these data is well shown in Chart 32–1.

Microscopic grading gives a more accurate prognosis when it is combined with information as to whether or not the axillary nodes were involved. Table 32–8 presents these

data from Bloom and Richardson's series of cases.

Stout himself graded the breast carcinomas treated by radical mastectomy in our clinic between 1915 and 1942. They totalled 1103. His findings, presented in Table 32–9, show a remarkable correlation between histologic grade and degree of malignancy as evidenced by the frequency of axillary metastases, as well as curability.

Schiødt has recently graded a series of 640 breast carcinomas from Copenhagen hospitals, using the Bloom-Richardson criteria. His findings are shown in Table 32–10. They are remarkably similar to those of Bloom and Richardson, and Stout.

As the years have gone by, microscopic grading has come to be generally accepted as an important method of estimating the degree of malignancy of breast carcinoma. It should be based upon the concept of anaplasia originally suggested by Hansemann—that is, the degree to which the carcinoma departs, both in its architecture and its cytology, from the normal breast epithelium. Grading should not be based upon the so-called defensive factors—lymphocytic infiltration and fibrosis. It should be simplified as much as possible. Elaborate systems of grading depending upon many microscopic features and employing four to five grades are not realistic. In order to avoid emphasizing the numerical aspect of grading, Stout preferred to use the terms *well-differentiated*, *moderately differentiated*, and *undifferentiated* to designate three grades, only, of malignancy. It is difficult to illustrate these three grades photographically because of the infinite variety of breast carcinomas. I have been content to show two extremes, a well-differentiated carcinoma in Figure 32–

Table 32–8. AXILLARY NODE INVOLVEMENT, MICROSCOPIC GRADE, AND 10-YEAR SURVIVAL. BLOOM AND RICHARDSON (1957)*

Status of Axillary Nodes	Microscopic Grade	No. of Cases	Per cent 10-Year Survival
Not involved	I	94	61%
	II	110	47%
	III	57	42%
Total		261	
Involved	I	81	51%
	II	178	14%
	III	138	9%
Total		397	

*Data from Bloom, H. J., and Richardson, W. W.: Brit. J. Cancer, *11*:359, 1957.

Table 32–9. RESULTS OF RADICAL MASTECTOMY BY MICROSCOPIC GRADE. STOUT, PRESBYTERIAN HOSPITAL, 1915–1942

Grade	No. of Cases	Per cent with Axillary Metastases	5-Year Clinical Cures	
			Number	Per cent
Grade I — well differentiated				
Limited to breast	52		45	86.5
With axillary metastases	32		21	65.6
Total	84	38.1	66	78.6
Grade II — moderately differentiated				
Limited to breast	165		114	69.1
With axillary metastases	257		89	34.6
Total	422	60.9	203	48.1
Grade III — undifferentiated				
Limited to breast	202		121	59.9
With axillary metastases	395		75	19.0
Total	597	66.2	196	32.8
All Grades				
Limited to breast	419		280	66.8
With axillary metastases	684		185	27.0
Total	1103	62.0	465	42.2
Unclassified	32		12	37.5
Grand total	1135		477	42.0

30, and an undifferentiated one in Figure 32–31.

Some pathologists, such as Stewart, prefer to base prognosis upon the "anatomical histological" type of mammary carcinoma rather than upon degree of anaplasia. To Stewart, the fact that a tumor is the papillary or the circumscribed type outweighs the significance of the degree of anaplasia that its cells exhibit.

"Appropriate anatomical histological classification," Stewart wrote, "obviates the need of grading."

It is of course true that classification of breast carcinomas into special clinical and anatomic types, as I have done in this and the preceding chapters, is of fundamental importance, but the great majority of breast carcinomas do not fall into any special type, and for them I believe that microscopic grading is a useful aid in estimating prognosis. In order to test this hypothesis I excluded a total of 337 tumors of the special types that I have described, from Stout's series of 1103 breast carcinomas that he graded microscopically. Table 32–11 shows his findings in grading the remaining 766 carcinomas of no special type. Both the frequency of axillary metastases and

Table 32–10. GRADE OF ANAPLASIA IN RELATION TO THE PATIENTS' FIVE-YEAR SURVIVAL. SCHIØDT, COPENHAGEN, 1950–1957*

Grade of Anaplasia	Number of Cases	Per cent of All	Alive 5 Years after Operation		Dead of M.C. within 5 Years of Operation		Dead from Other Cause than M.C.
			Number	Per cent	Number	Per cent	Number
I	129	20	113	87.5	6	4.5	10
II	358	56	236	66	106	29.5	16
III	153	24	57	37	92	59	4
Total	640	...	406	63	203	32	30

*From Schiødt, T.: Breast Carcinoma. A Histologic and Prognostic Study of 640 Followed-Up Cases. Copenhagen, Munksgaard, 1966.

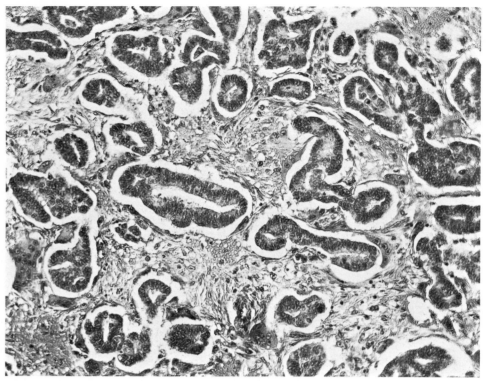

Figure 32–30. A well differentiated carcinoma of the breast. The comparatively regular cells are arranged in a glandular pattern.

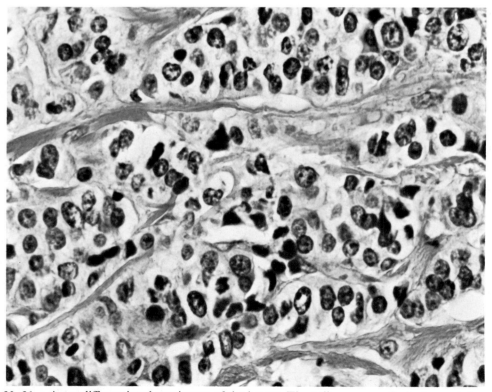

Figure 32–31. An undifferentiated carcinoma of the breast. The cells vary greatly in size and shape, often show mitoses, and are not arranged in any definite pattern.

Table 32–11. RESULTS OF RADICAL MASTECTOMY IN CARCINOMA OF NO SPECIAL TYPE BY MICROSCOPIC GRADE FOR PATIENTS TRACED FIVE YEARS FOLLOWING TREATMENT. STOUT, PRESBYTERIAN HOSPITAL, 1915–1942

Grade	No. of Cases	Average Clinical Size of Tumor (cm.)	Per cent with Axillary Metastases	Per cent Dying in less than 5 Years with no Evidence of Cancer	Five-Year Clinical Cures	
					Per cent	Standard Error of Percentage
Grade I – well differentiated						
Limited to breast	21	2.6			100.0	
With axillary metastases	20	4.4			65.0	±10.7
Total	41	3.4	48.8	2.4	82.9	± 5.9
Grade II – moderately differentiated						
Limited to breast	89	4.0			68.5	± 4.9
With axillary metastases	154	4.8			36.4	± 3.9
Total	243	4.5	63.4	5.3	48.1	± 3.2
Grade III – undifferentiated						
Limited to breast	147	4.1			62.6	± 4.0
With axillary metastases	335	5.8			19.1	± 2.1
Total	482	5.3	69.5	4.6	32.4	± 2.1
All Grades						
Limited to breast	257	4.0		6.2	67.7	± 2.9
With axillary metastases	509	5.5		3.9	26.1	± 1.9
Total	766	4.9	66.4	4.7	40.1	± 1.8

the per cent of clinical cures at 5 years are seen to be closely correlated with the microscopic grade.

Histologic grading has a practical value in the choice of treatment. When a patient has a very well differentiated carcinoma and her disease is on the borderline of inoperability, I have in several instances chosen to operate and I have cured her. With undifferentiated carcinomas I have learned that it is wiser not to operate on borderline cases.

Bloom has pointed out that it may eventually be possible to establish a correlation between the microscopic grade of breast carcinomas and their response to hormonal methods of treatment. He refers to the claim by Dao and Huggins that well-differentiated tumors respond better to adrenalectomy, although Cade did not confirm this relationship.

Another form of microscopic grading which has been studied recently is concerned with supposed "defense factors" of the host evidenced by lymphocytic infiltration in the primary tumor, and sinus histiocytosis in the axillary lymph nodes.

In 1953, Black, Kerpe, and Speer first proposed that sinus histiocytosis in regional lymph nodes is an indication of a defense mechanism by the host against breast cancer. In 1955 Black and his associates expanded this concept of "tumor retarding factors" to include lymphocytic infiltration in the primary tumor. Black and his associates have claimed that these microscopic phenomena are correlated with a more favorable prognosis.

Cutler has supported Black's thesis in several elaborate repetitions of Black's original study. Massé and Chassaigne, as well as Wartman, have also confirmed Black's findings. Hamlin has recently presented the most elaborate study of these microscopic factors suggesting host resistance to breast carcinoma. She combines her grading of "host defense factors" with grading as to malignancy in terms of degree of differentiation of the carcinoma, and claims that her elaborate method of point scoring correlates closely with survival.

On the other hand, Berg in 1956, and Moore, Chapnick, and Schoenberg in 1960, were unable to confirm Black's claim that sinus histiocytosis is an indication of a better prognosis. Di Re and Lane, in 1963, studied the relationship of sinus histiocytosis to 10-year survival in my personal series of 203 radical mastectomies performed between

Table 32–12. SINUS HISTIOCYTOSIS RELATED TO 10-YEAR SURVIVAL BASED ON 212 CASES WITHOUT AXILLARY LYMPH NODE METASTASES KISTER ET AL., 1969*

Degree of Sinus Histiocytosis	No. of Cases	Alive	Dead	Per cent 10-Year Survival
0–1	153	120	33	78
3	40	28	12	70
3–4	19	15	4	79
Total	212	163	49	77

$X^2 = 1.36$ (with 2 degrees of freedom) $p > 0.50$.
There is no significant difference among the three survival rates.
*From Kister, S. J., et al.: Cancer, 23:570, 1969.

Table 32–13. SINUS HISTIOCYTOSIS RELATED TO 10-YEAR SURVIVAL BASED ON 106 CASES WITH AXILLARY LYMPH NODE METASTASES. KISTER ET AL., 1969*

Degree of Sinus Histiocytosis	Cases	Alive	Dead	Per cent 10-Year Survival
0–1	76	44	32	58
2	17	8	9	47
3–4	13	6	7	46
Total	106	58	48	55

$X^2 = 1.08$ (with 2 degrees of freedom) $p > 0.58$.
There is no significant difference among the three survival rates.
*From Kister, S. J., et al.: Cancer, 23:570, 1969.

1935 and 1948. This series of cases is fortunately well-adapted to this kind of study because the patients were all classified by me as to the clinical stage of their disease, the operation was always my version of the radical mastectomy, and the follow-up was complete. Di Re and Lane found no correlation between the degree of sinus histiocytosis and 10-year survival, whether there were axillary metastases or not.

Kister and other members of our staff have recently carried out a more elaborate study of the significance of sinus histiocytosis, using a larger and still more selective group of my personal series of patients with breast carcinoma treated by radical mastectomy. Only Clinical Stage A cases were used in the study; there were 318 of these with adequate histologic sections. No correlation was found between the degree of sinus histiocytosis in the axillary lymph nodes and the 10-year survival rates in this very carefully controlled study. The data are presented in Tables 32–12 and 32–13.

Blood vessel invasion by breast carcinoma is still another microscopic phenomenon which has been studied in relation to prognosis. Teel and Sommers in 1964, and Friedell, Betts, and Sommers in 1966, reported a close correlation between blood vessel invasion and survival. In these studies, the clinical description of the patients, the methods of treatment, and length and completeness of follow-up were not clearly defined.

Kister and his associates studied the significance of vessel invasion in my series of personal radical mastectomies. The presence of blood vessel invasion was correlated with the 10-year survival in 328 patients whose

disease was classified as Stage A by our Columbia Clinical Classification. The data are presented in Table 23–14.

It is seen that no statistically significant difference was found in the 10-year survival rates of patients in whom blood vessel invasion was found, if axillary lymph node metastases were not present. Among the patients with axillary metastases in whom blood vessel invasion was found, the survival rate was strikingly reduced. This leads us to speculate that when there are metastases in axillary lymph nodes, blood vessel invasion in the lymph nodes may serve as a further source of dissemination of carcinoma cells via the blood stream. The arterial and venous circulation of lymph nodes is far greater than is commonly appreciated, and the lymphatic-venous relationship within lymph nodes is not fully understood.

Table 32–14. TEN-YEAR SURVIVAL FOLLOWING RADICAL MASTECTOMY RELATED TO BLOOD INVASION. KISTER ET AL., 1966*

Blood Vessel Invasion	Patients with Axillary Lymph Node Metastases†			Patients without Axillary Lymph Node Metastases‡		
	No. of Patients	10-Year Survival No.	Per cent	No. of Patients	10-Year Survival No.	Per cent
Present	30	10	33.3	40	28	70
Absent	78	48	62	180	140	77.8

*Data from Kister, S. J., et al.: Cancer, 19:1213, 1966.
†$\chi^2 = 5.83$, $0.01 < p < 0.02$
‡$\chi^2 = 0.67$, $0.3 < p < 0.5$

REFERENCES

Aboumrad, M. H., Horn, R. C., Jr., and Fine, G.: Lipid-secreting mammary carcinoma. Cancer, 16:521, 1963.

Arffmann, E., and Hjgaard, K.: Squamous carcinoma of the breast. J. Path. & Bact., 90:319, 1965.

Barbieri, G., Briziarelli, G., Olivi, M., and Squartini, F.: Carcinomi mucosi della mammella a genesi particolare. Lav. d. Ist. anat. e istol. pat., Perugia, 13:231, 1953.

Berg, J. W.: Sinus histiocytosis: a fallacious measure of host resistance to cancer. Cancer, 9:935, 1956.

Biggs, R.: The myoepithelium in certain tumours of the breast. J. Path. & Bact., 59:437, 1947.

Black, M. M., Kerpe, S., and Speer, F. D.: Lymph node structure in patients with cancer of the breast. Amer. J. Path., 29:505, 1953.

Black, M. M., Opler, S. R., and Speer, F. D.; Survival in breast cancer cases in relation to the structure of the primary tumor and regional lymph nodes. Surg., Gynec. & Obst., 100:543, 1955.

Black, M. M., Speer, F. D., and Opler, S. R.: Structural representations of tumor-host relationships in mammary carcinoma. Amer. J. Clin. Path., 26:250, 1956.

Bloom, H. J. G.: Prognosis in carcinoma of the breast. Brit. J. Cancer, 4:259, 1950.

Bloom, H. J. G.: Further studies on prognosis of breast carcinoma. Brit. J. Cancer, 4:347, 1950.

Bloom, H. J. G., and Richardson, W. W.: Histological grading and prognosis in breast cancer. Brit. J. Cancer, 11:359, 1957.

Brocq, P., Wolf, and Giet: Epithélioma du sein. Bull. et mém. Soc. anat. de Paris, 92:270, 1922.

Cade, S.: Adrenalectomy for hormone dependent cancers: breast and prostate. Ann. Roy. Coll. Surg., Eng., 15:71, 1954.

Cavanzo, F. J., and Taylor, H. B.: Adenoid cystic carcinoma of the breast. Cancer, 24:740, 1969.

Cheatle, Sir G. L., and Cutler, M.: Gelatinous carcinoma of the breast. Arch. Surg., 20:569, 1930.

Cutler, S. J., et al.: Prognostic factors in cancer of the female breast. II. Reproducibility of histopathologic classification. Cancer, 19:75, 1966.

Cutler, S. J., et al.: Further observations on prognostic factors in cancer of the female breast. Cancer, 24:653, 1969.

Dao, T. L.-Y., and Huggins, C.: Bilateral adrenalectomy in the treatment of cancer of the breast. Arch. Surg., 7:645, 1959.

Dawson, E. K.: Sweat gland carcinoma of the breast. Edinburgh Med. J., 39:409, 1932.

Dawson, E. K.: Carcinoma in the mammary lobule and its origin. Edinburgh Med. J., 40:57, 1933.

Dawson, E. K., and Tod, M. C.: Progress in mammary carcinoma in relation to grading and treatment. Edinburgh Med. J., 41:61, 1934.

Delascio, D., Assali, N. S., and Mastroianni, E.: Carcinoma gelatinoso da mama. Rev. de ginec. e d'obst., 39:131, 1945.

Delbet, P.: Sur un cas de cancer mammaire muci-sécrétant. Bull. Acad. de méd., Paris, 123:407, 1940.

Delbet, P., and Mendaro: Les Cancers du Sein. Paris, Masson et Cie., 1927.

Di Re, J. J., and Lane, N.: The relationship of sinus histiocytosis in axillary lymph nodes to surgical curability of carcinoma of the breast. Amer. J. Clin. Path., 40:508, 1963.

Eicke, W. J.: Ueber ein primär doppelseitiges Gallertcarcinom der Mamma mit sekundärer Verkalkung (Carcinoma psammosum). Ztschr. f. Krebsforsch., 47:498, 1938.

Ewing, J.: Classification of mammary cancer. Ann. Surg., 102:249, 1935.

Flothow, P. G.: Defensive factors in carcinoma of the breast. Surg., Gynec. & Obst., 46:789, 1928.

Foot, N. C., and Moore, S. W.: A fatal case of deep-seated epidermoid carcinoma of the breast with widespread metastasis. Amer. J. Cancer, 34:226, 1938.

Foote, F. W., Jr., and Stewart, F. W.: Lobular carcinoma in situ. Amer. J. Path., 17:491, 1941.

Foote, F. W., Jr., and Stewart, F. W.: Comparative studies of cancerous versus noncancerous breasts. Ann. Surg., 121:6, 197, 1945.

Foote, F. W., Jr., and Stewart, F. W.: A histologic classification of carcinoma of the breast. Surgery, 19:74, 1946.

Frable, W. J., and Kay, S.: Carcinoma of the breast. Histologic and clinical features of apocrine tumors. Cancer, 21:756, 1968.

Frantz, V. K.; The prognostic significance of intra-cellular mucicarminophilic material in carcinoma of the female breast. Amer. J. Cancer, 33:167, 1938.

Friedell, G. H., Betts, A., and Sommers, S. C.: The prognostic value of blood vessel invasion and lymphocytic infiltrates in breast cancer. Cancer, 18:164, 1966.

Gaabe, G.: Der Gallertkrebs der Brustdrüse. Beitr. z. klin. Chir., 60:760, 1908.

Galloway, J. R., Woolner, L. B., and Clagett, O. T.: Adenoid cystic carcinoma of the breast. Surg., Gynec. & Obst., 122:1289, 1966.

Geschickter, C. F.: Gelatinous mammary cancer. Ann. Surg., 108:321, 1938.

Gonzalez-Licea, A., Yardley, J. H., and Hartmann, W. H.: Malignant tumor of the breast with bone formation. Studies by light and electron microscopy. Cancer, 20:1234, 1967.

Greenough, R. B.: Varying degrees of malignancy in cancer of the breast. J. Cancer Research, 9:454, 1925.

Gricouroff, G.: Du pronostic histologique dans le cancer du sein. Bull. Assoc. franç. p. l'étude du cancer, 35:275, 1948.

Gricouroff, G., Zajdela, A., and Herrera Bendana, B.: Le cylindrome mammaire. Bull. Assoc. franç. p. l'étude du cancer, 51:277, 1964.

Guénin, P.: Le pronostic et le traitment des cancers du sein. J. de chir., 54:332, 1939.

Haagensen, C. D.: The bases for the histologic grading of carcinoma of the breast. Amer. J. Cancer, 19:285, 1933.

Halsted, W. S.: A diagnostic sign of gelatinous carcinoma of the breast. J.A.M.A., 64:1653, 1915.

Hamlin, I. M. E.: Possible host resistance in carcinoma of the breast: A histological study. Brit. J. Cancer, 22:383, 1968.

von Hansemann, D. P.: Studien über die Spezificität, den Altruismus und die Anaplasie der Zellen. Berlin, A. Hirschwald, 1893, p. 93.

Harrington, S. W., and Miller, J. M.: Intramammary squamous-cell carcinoma. Proc. Staff Meet. Mayo Clin., 14:484, 1939.

Heuper, W. C., and Schmitz, H.: Relations of histological structure and clinical grouping to the prognosis of carcinomata of the breast and uterine cervix. Ann. Surg., 81:993, 1925.

Higginson, J. F., and McDonald, J. R.: Apocrine tissue,

chronic cystic mastitis, and sweat gland carcinoma of the breast. Surg., Gynec. & Obst., 88:1, 1949.

James, T. G. I., and Treip, C.: Squamous-celled carcinoma of the breast. Brit. J. Surg., 42:650, 1955.

Kister, S. J., Sommers, S. C., Haagensen, C. D., and Cooley, E.: Re-evaluation of blood-vessel invasion as a prognostic factor in carcinoma of the breast. Cancer, 19:1213, 1966.

Kister, S. J., et al.: Nuclear grade and sinus histiocytosis in cancer of the breast. Cancer, 23:570, 1969.

Kreibig, W.: Zur Kenntnis seltener Geschwulstformen der weiblichen Brustdrüse. Virchows Arch. f. path. Anat., 256:649, 1925.

Lane, N., Göksel, H., Salerno, R. A., and Haagensen, C. D.: Clinico-pathologic analysis of the surgical curability of breast cancers. Ann. Surg., 153:483, 1961.

Lange, F.: Der Gallertkrebs der Brustdrüse. Beitr. z. klin. Chir., 16:1896.

Lee, B. J. Hauser, H., and Pack, G. T.: Gelatinous carcinoma of the breast. Surg., Gynec. & Obst., 59:841, 1934.

Lee, B. J. Pack, G. T., and Scharnagel, I.: Sweat gland cancer of the breast. Surg., Gynec. & Obst., 56:975, 1933.

Lee, B. J., and Stubenbord, J. G.: Clinical index of malignancy for carcinoma of the breast. Surg., Gynec., & Obst., 47:812, 1928.

Lepper, E. H., and Baker, A. H.: Diffuse intraductal carcinoma of the breast. Brit. J. Surg., 22:415, 1934.

Leroux, R., and Perrot, M.: Classification pronostique des cancers du sein. Bull. Assoc. Franç. p. l'étude du cancer, 21:37, 1932.

Leroux, R., and Perrot, M.: Pronostic histologique des cancers du sein. Bull. Assoc. franç. p. l'étude du cancer, 19:439, 1930.

Lewis, D. and Geschickter, C. F.: Comedo carcinoma of the breast: Arch. Surg., 36:225, 1938.

Loeb, P. W.: Ueber Adenocancroide. Frankfurt. Ztschr. f. Path., 25:154, 1921.

MacCarty, W. C.: Factors which influence longevity in cancer. Ann. Surg., 76:9, 1922.

McDivitt, R. W., Stewart, F. W., and Berg, J. W.: Tumors of the breast. Atlas of Tumor Pathology, Second Series, Fascicle 2, Washington, D.C., Armed Forces Institute of Pathology, 1968.

McLellan, P. G., Tennant, R., and Sarokhan, J.: Adenoid cystic carcinoma of the breast. Surgery, 33:905, 1953.

Massé, C., and Chassaigne, J. P.: Est-il possible de déterminer le pronostic du cancer du sein d'aprés l'examen histologique des ganglions axillaires? J. Méd. Bordeaux, 139:360, 1962.

Mathews, F. S.: Results of operative treatment of cancer of the breast. Ann. Surg., 96:871, 1932.

Melamed, M. R., Robbins, G. F., and Foote, F. W., Jr.: Prognostic significance of gelatinous mammary carcinoma. Cancer, 14:699, 1961.

Moore, R. D., Chapnick, R., and Schoenberg, M. D.: Lymph nodes associated with carcinoma of the breast. Cancer, 13:545, 1960.

Moureau, P., and Lambert, G.: Les facteurs de malignité dans les cancers du sein. Cancer, Bruxelles, 9:117, 1932.

Muir, R.: The evolution of carcinoma of the mamma. J. Path. & Bact., 52:155, 1941.

Nayer, H. R.: Cylindroma of the breast with pulmonary metastases. Dis. Chest, 31:324, 1957.

Norris, H. J., and Taylor, H. B.: Prognosis of mucinous gelatinous carcinoma of the breast. Cancer, 18:879, 1965.

Norris, H. J., and Taylor, H. B.: Well-differentiated carcinoma. Cancer, 25:687, 1970.

Pasternack, J. G., and Wirth, J. E.: Adeno-acanthoma sarcomatodes of the mammary gland. Amer. J. Path., 12:423, 1936.

Patey, D. H., and Scarff, R. W.: Position of histology in prognosis of carcinoma of breast. Lancet, 1:801, 1928.

Robb, P. M., and MacFarlane, A.: Two rare breast tumors. J. Path. & Bact., 75:293, 1958.

Saphir, O.: Mucinous carcinoma of the breast. Surg., Gynec. & Obst., 72:908, 1941.

Scarff, R. W., and Handley, R. S.: Prognosis in carcinoma of breast. Lancet, 2:582, 1938.

Schiødt, T.: Breast Carcinoma. A Histologic and Prognostic Study of 640 Followed-up Cases. Copenhagen, Munksgaard, 1966.

Smith, B. H., and Taylor, H. B.: The occurrence of bone and cartilage in mammary tumors. Amer. J. Clin. Path., 51:610, 1969.

Smith, G. V., and Bartlett, M. K.: Malignant tumors of the female breast. Surg., Gynec. & Obst., 48:314, 1929.

Teel, P., and Sommers, S. C.: Vascular invasion as a prognostic factor in breast carcinoma. Surg., Gynec. & Obst., 118:1006, 1964.

Tellem, M., Nedwich, A., Amenta, P. S., and Imbriglia, J. E.: Mucin-producing carcinoma of the breast. Cancer, 19:573, 1966.

Toro, N.: Classifica di malignità del carcinoma mammario; parte l. Arch. ostet. e ginec., 42:17, 1935.

Veronesi, U., and Gennari, L.: Il carcinoma gelatinoso della mammella. Tumori, 46:119, 1960.

Wald, M., and Kakulas, B. A.: Apocrine gland carcinoma (sweat gland carcinoma) of the breast. Australian and New Zealand J. Surg., 33:200, 1964.

Wartman, W. B.: Sinus cell hyperplasia of lymph nodes regional to adenocarcinoma of the breast and colon. Brit. J. Cancer, 13:389, 1959.

White, W. C.: Late results of operation for carcinoma of the breast. Ann. Surg., 86:695, 1927.

Wilson, W. B., and Spell, J. P.: Adenoid cystic carcinoma of the breast. Ann. Surg., 166:861, 1967.

Willis, R. A.: Squamous-cell carcinoma of predominantly fibrosarcoma-like structure. J. Path. & Bact., 76:511, 1958.

Wulsin, J. H., and Schreiber, J. T.: Improved prognosis in certain patterns of carcinoma of the breast. Colloid, medullary with lymphoid stroma, and intraductal. Arch. Surg., 85:791, 1962.

The Clinical Classification of Carcinoma of the Breast and the Choice of Treatment

There are only four methods of treatment for carcinoma of the breast that have any value. They are surgical removal, irradiation, alteration of the hormonal physiology, and chemotherapy. Each of these methods has definite limitations, both as to its inherent capacity to control carcinoma, and also as to the manifestations of the disease to which it can reasonably be applied. Surgical removal and irradiation are both local methods of treatment. It is not generally realized that modern intensive irradiation aiming at cure of primary breast carcinoma can only encompass a limited local area of tissue. The hormonal attack is, of course, a systemic one and has an effect upon carcinoma throughout the entire body. Chemotherapy is also a systemic method of treatment, but it has as yet only a small place in our armamentarium.

In discussing the choice of treatment for breast carcinoma I must at the outset state what I believe to be a basic premise. It is simply that surgery and radiotherapy are the only methods that cure. Hormonal and chemotherapeutic methods give only palliation and should not be considered when the disease is early enough to hope for cure. In the cases in which cure is possible, surgery is preferable for two basic reasons. First, when the surgeon succeeds in entirely removing the carcinoma the patient is better off than when her carcinoma has been irradiated, because the surgeon's success is permanent, whereas irradiation can usually hope only to lock up the carcinoma in a fibrous prison, from which there is a considerable chance of the disease escaping after a time and growing again in all its original vigor. Second, it is my experience that a skillfully performed radical mastectomy has less morbidity than skillfully applied intensive irradiation.

Each of these methods of attacking breast carcinoma penalizes the patient. They should never be used needlessly or futilely. The choice of the best method of treatment for the individual patient is therefore a matter of very great importance. It is based primarily upon the stage of advancement of the patient's disease as determined by precise clinical classification.

THE CLINICAL CLASSIFICATION OF BREAST CARCINOMA AS TO ITS STAGE OF ADVANCEMENT

It may seem unnecessary to define what is meant by the *clinical classification* of breast carcinoma, but I continue to encounter physicians who confuse *clinical classification* with *pathologic staging.* The two types of staging are of course entirely different. Pathologic staging is based upon the pathologist's microscopic findings. Stage 1 patients are those who have no axillary metastases, while Stage 2 patients are those in whom axillary metastases are found. Pathologic staging is done *after* treatment has been carried out, and it therefore has nothing to do with the initial decision as to whether or not to perform radical mastectomy.

The clinical classification of breast carcinoma as to its stage of advancement is based solely upon the clinical findings, and is necessarily carried out *before* treatment. Once the clinical stage of the disease in the individual patient is decided upon, it is, of course, never changed, no matter what the pathologic findings may be.

Clinical classification is difficult and complex. All classifications are necessarily pragmatic. They are based upon clinical experience, correlating the presence of specific clinical features of breast carcinoma with the pathologic findings and the results of different methods of treatment.

The need of some kind of practical clinical classification that would help select the patients with breast carcinoma who would benefit from operation was first appreciated by Steinthal. In 1905, in reviewing his results at Stuttgart with breast carcinoma, he found that there were certain clinical types of the disease in which operation was futile. He divided his cases into three groups or stages, as follows:

"*Stage 1.* Cases in which the tumor has apparently grown very slowly, is only a few centimeters in diameter, is situated entirely within the breast tissue and is not fixed to the skin, and in which there are only a few axillary nodes that are ordinarily not found until operation.

"*Stage 2.* Cases in which the tumor has definitely enlarged, has become adherent to the skin, and in which there are definitely palpable axillary nodes. Most patients who come to operation are in this stage.

"*Stage 3.* Cases in which the tumor involves a great part of the breast, has involved the skin as well as the underlying tissues, and in which the supraclavicular nodes are involved."

Steinthal found that none of his Stage 3 cases were cured by operation, and he therefore advised against it.

Staging originated in this way as a clinical guide to the selection of patients for surgery. Staging has since been elaborated, however, into complex classifications used to compare the results of different methods of treatment. This is a different problem from that of the selection of patients for operation.

Steinthal's staging was based, of course, upon clinical features. His concept was widely taken up in Germany and the Scandinavian countries in studying the results of methods of treatment. It was shortly emphasized by several of the Scandinavians that clinical findings are unreliable in distinguishing Stage 1 patients (those without axillary metastases) from Stage 2 patients (those with axillary metastases, but still operable). The Scandinavians substituted pathologic for clinical evidence as to the presence of axillary metastases and evolved a system of staging, combining both clinical and pathological criteria, which is still widely used. It is as follows:

Stage 1. Locally operable, no axillary metastases as determined by microscopic examination of all axillary nodes.

Stage 2. Locally operable, with axillary metastases proved microscopically.

Stage 3. Inoperable because of local extent of disease or because of distant metastases.

Portmann devised a more elaborate plan for staging breast carcinomas, again based on both clinical and pathological criteria. His plan follows:

"*Group or Stage I*
Skin—not involved
Tumor—localized in the breast and movable.
Metastases—none in axillary lymph nodes (microscopic examination) or elsewhere.

"*Group or Stage II*
Skin—not involved.
Tumor—localized in the breast and movable.
Metastases—few axillary lymph nodes involved (Microscopic examination); no other metastases.

"*Group or Stage III*
Skin—edematous; brawny red induration and inflammation not obviously due to infection; extensive ulceration; multiple secondary nodules.
Tumor—diffusely infiltrating breast; fixation of tumor or breast to chest wall; edema of breast; secondary tumors.

Metastases—many axillary lymph nodes involved or fixed; no clinical or roentgenologic evidences of distant metastases.

"Group or Stage IV

Skin—as in any other group or stage.

Tumor—as in any other group or stage.

Metastases—axillary and supraclavicular lymph nodes extensively involved, and clinical or roentgenologic evidences of more distant metastases."

This type of combined clinical and pathologic staging cannot, of course, be used to select the patients suitable for operation, because Stage I can only be distinguished from Stage II after the axilla has been dissected.

In response to the need of a purely clinical method of staging breast carcinoma a classification was evolved at the Christie Hospital and Holt Radium Institute in Manchester, and has been widely adopted in England. It has been called the Manchester System, and is as follows:

"Stage I. The growth is confined to the breast. Involvement of the skin directly over and in continuity with the tumour does not affect staging, provided that the area involved is small in relation to the size of the breast.

"Stage II. As in Stage I, but there are palpable mobile nodes in the axilla.

"Stage III. The growth is extending beyond the corpus mammae, as shown by:

    (a) the skin is invaded or fixed over an area large in relation to the size of the breast or is ulcerated:

    (b) the tumour is fixed to the underlying muscle or fascia.

Axillary nodes may or may not be palpable, but if nodes are present they must be mobile.

"Stage IV. The growth has extended beyond the breast area as shown by:

    (a) fixation or matting of the axillary nodes;

    (b) complete fixation of tumour to chest wall;

    (c) secondaries in supraclavicular nodes;

    (d) secondaries in opposite breast;

    (e) secondaries in skin wide of tumour;

    (f) distant metastases, e.g., bone, liver, lung, etc."

Smithers and his associates at the Royal Cancer Hospital devised a plan for staging which they believe to be an improvement over the Manchester plan. Their plan follows:

"Stage I. Tumour clinically confined to the breast.

No deep fixation.

Skin dimpling or nipple retraction, but no skin infiltration.

No significant* nodes palpable.

"Stage II. As in Stage I, except that mobile nodes of significance* are palpable in the axilla on the same side only.

"Stage III. As in Stages I and II, except that: the skin in infiltrated in direct continuity with the tumor and may be ulcerated, or—the tumor is attached to the underlying fascia or muscle:

    (a) without significant* palpable axillary nodes;

    (b) with mobile significant* palpable axillary nodes on the same side only.

"Stage IV. As in Stages I, II, and III, except that: mobile significant* supraclavicular nodes are palpable on the same side, or parasternal or intercostal nodes on the same side are detected; the tumour is firmly fixed to the chest wall; there are skin nodules confined to the skin over the breast, but not in direct continuity with the primary tumour; there is extensive peau d'orange; the axillary nodes are matted together, fixed deeply, or infiltrating the skin which may be ulcerated.

"Stage V. There is evidence of distant metastases beyond the area of the breast, or the regional lymphatic drainage included in Stage IV."

The International Classification

At the 1954 São Paulo meeting of the International Union against Cancer, a "Committee on Clinical Stage Classification and Statistics" was appointed which, under the leadership of Denoix, drafted a clinical classification for breast carcinoma which evolved into the well known T (tumor) N (nodes) M (metastases) classification and has been adopted by the International Union against Cancer. There have been several versions of this TNM clinical classification for breast carcinoma. The latest was published by the International Union against Cancer in 1969, with instructions to discard all previous versions of the classification. This recent version follows:

Primary Tumour (T)

In the breast the three main qualities which determine the T category are size, involvement of

---

*Clinically suggestive of metastasis.

T (Primary Tumour) Category

Determining Quality	T1	T2	T3	T4
Size	up to 2 cm.	2 – 5 cm.	5 – 10 cm.	10 cm.
Skin	not involved	dimpled	infiltrated or ulcerated	whole breast involved
Muscle and chest wall	not involved	not involved	muscle fixation	chest wall involved

skin and involvement of underlying tissues. There are four degrees of T and any quality can determine the degree of T, as indicated in the table above.

Regional Lymph Nodes (N)

The regional nodes for the breast are those in the axilla, though those in the parasternal region (internal mammary chain) may be of equal importance prognostically in many cases. The latter are however not as a rule accessible to clinical examination and therefore have at least initially to be disregarded in a general classification. Sometimes the localisation of the lymph nodes on the same side or contralateral side relative to the primary tumour has to be taken into account. The standard N classification is therefore as follows:

N0 No palpable lymph nodes
N1 Movable homolateral lymph nodes
N2 Movable contralateral or bilateral lymph nodes
N3 Fixed lymph nodes.

Distant Metastases (M)

The absence or presence of metastases is indicated by the letter M. M0 indicates that none can be detected clinically, M1 that metastasis other than to regional lymph nodes is present. If necessary M1 can be subdivided into further categories to indicate the type of metastasis, e.g., to bone, liver, lung, etc.

Stage-Grouping

Classification by T, N and M aims at a more precise recording of the apparent extent of the disease, and the combination of cases into several groups based on criteria which are statistically predictive can then be done. For breast tumours with four possible degrees of T, four degrees of N and two degrees of M, the number of groups, extending from T1 N0 M0 at one end of the scale to T4 N3 M1 at the other, is 32 (see table below).

The American Classification

An American Joint Committee in Cancer Staging, representing the American College of Surgeons and a number of other organizations, was organized in 1959, and by 1962 presented its plan for the clinical classification of breast carcinoma. The American plan follows the International plan fairly closely. The American plan is presented below.

T – Primary Tumor

T1   Tumor of 2 cm. or less in its greatest dimension
Skin not involved; or involved locally with Paget's disease
T2   Tumor over 2 cm. in size; or with skin attachment (dimpling of skin); or nipple retraction (in subareolar tumors).
No pectoral muscle or chest wall attachment.
T3   Tumor of any size with any of the following: skin infiltration, ulceration, peau d'orange, skin edema, pectoral muscle or chest wall attachment.

N – Regional Lymph Nodes

N0   No clinically palpable axillary lymph node(s) (metastasis not suspected)
N1   Clinically palpable axillary lymph nodes that are not fixed (metastasis suspected)
N2   Clinically palpable homolateral axillary or infraclavicular lymph node(s) that are fixed to one another or to other structures (metastasis suspected).

STAGE GROUPING

Clinical Stage	TNM Groups		No. of groups per Stage
I	T1 N0 M0	T2 N0 M0	2
II	T1 N1 M0	T2 N1 M0	2
III	T1 N23 M0	T2 N23 M0	
	T3 N0123 M0	T4 N0123 M0	12
IV	Any TN Symbols + M1		16

M — Distant Metastasis

M0   No distant metastasis
M1   Clinical and radiographic evidence of metastasis except those to homolateral axillary or infraclavicular lymph nodes.

Clinical Stages

STAGE I

No clinically palpable axillary lymph node(s) (metastasis not suspected) (N0).
(a) Tumor of 2 cm. or less in its greatest dimension (T1).
Skin not involved (T1); or involved locally with Paget's disease (T1).
No distant metastasis (M0).
T1, N0, M0; or

(b) Tumor over 2 cm. in size (T2); or
Skin attachment (dimpling of skin) (T2); or
Nipple retraction (in subareolar tumors) (T2).
No pectoral muscle or chest wall attachment (T2).
No distant metastasis (M0).
T2, N0, M0

STAGE II.

Clinically palpable axillary lymph node(s) that are not fixed (metastasis suspected) (N1)
(a) Tumor of 2 cm. or less in its greatest dimension, as in (Stage I T1).
Skin not involved, as in (Stage I T1); or Paget's disease, as in (Stage I T1).
No distant metastasis (M0).
T1, N1, M0; or

(b) Tumor over 2 cm. in size, as in (Stage I T2); or
Skin attached (dimpling of skin); or
Nipple retraction (in subareolar tumors) as in (Stage I T2); or
No pectoral muscle or chest wall attachment, as in (Stage I T2).
No distant metastasis (M0).
T2, N1, M0

STAGE III

(a) With no clinically palpable lymph node(s) (N0) (metastasis not suspected).
Tumor of any size with any of the following associated findings: skin infiltration, ulceration, peau d'orange, skin edema, pectoral muscle or chest wall attachment (T3).
No distant metastasis (M0).
T3, N0, M0; or

(b) With clinically palpable axillary lymph node(s) (N1), that are not fixed (metastasis suspected).
Tumor of any size with any of the follow-

ing associated findings: skin infiltration, ulceration, peau d'orange, skin edema, pectoral muscle or chest wall attachment (T3).
No distant metastasis (M0).
T3, N1, M0; or

(c) With clinically palpable homolateral axillary or infraclavicular lymph node(s) fixed to one another or to other structures (N2) (metastasis suspected).
No distant metastasis (M0).
T3, N2, M0

STAGE IV

Any stage of disease with distant metastasis (M1).

Summary

The following summary of clinical staging is presented.

STAGE   I T1, N0, M0; T2, N0, M0.
STAGE   II T1, N1, M0; T2, N1, M0 (includes all N1, M0 except for T3).
STAGE   III T3, N0, M0; T3, N1, M0; T3, N2, M0; T1, N2, M0; T2, N2, M0 and includes any combination of T1, T2, or T3, with N2 and M0.
STAGE   IV Any clinical stage of disease with distant metastasis (M1).

I could point out many individual faults in both the International and American classifications. One of the most important deficiencies of the International Classification is its failure to distinguish between axillary nodes that are not clinically involved and those which are. Any palpable node in the axilla is regarded as containing metastases and is classified as N1. Experienced clinicians know that many women who do not have breast carcinoma have small palpable but innocuous axillary nodes. When all patients with breast carcinoma who have such palpable but not clinically involved axillary nodes are classified as having Clinical Stage II carcinoma, the number of patients in Clinical Stage I is too small and the number in Clinical Stage II too large. Stages I and II approach each other.

Neither the International nor the American classification includes measurement of the size of clinically involved axillary nodes. There is a vital difference in the significance of a 1 cm. clinically involved axillary node and a 3 cm. clinically involved node. Such differences in size can be measured with reasonable accuracy. The extent of the disease in the axilla as judged by careful axillary palpation is the most important guide that we have in estimating the stage of advancement of breast carcinoma. It is essential to make use of all the information that can be gained from it.

In addition to these deficiencies of omission in the International and American classifications, both classifications are misleading as regards the significance of some clinical features of breast carcinoma. In both classifications a carcinoma is classified as T2 if there is skin dimpling. The fact is that skin dimpling can be demonstrated in most breast carcinomas if the examiner knows how to look for it and elicit it. It is related to the situation of the lesion in relation to the skin and not to prognosis.

The International Classification does not mention edema of the skin, which is without question the most important clinical sign of an advanced stage of the disease.

Both the International and the American classifications are confusing as regards fixation of the tumor to deeper structures. Both use pectoral muscle "attachment" or "fixation" as an indication of advanced disease, without specifying what these terms mean clinically. The truth is that it is exceedingly difficult to determine whether or not a carcinoma is fixed to the pectoral muscles *per se*, and in our own studies we have not been able to define this condition clinically. The International Classification uses "chest wall involvement," and the American Classification "chest wall attachment," as indication of advanced disease, again without specifying what these terms signify clinically. In our experience the only type of fixation of the tumor to deeper structures that is significant is firm fixation of the lesion to the underlying chest wall so that it cannot be moved over it; we call this *solid fixation* to the chest wall.

Both the International and the American plans have in common one outstanding disadvantage — their complexity. Both are so complex that they are entirely unworkable in the hands of the house staff physicians who have to do the day-to-day actual classification of the extent of the disease in patients as they enter the hospital. This has been our experience in our own breast clinics, and Richard Handley at the Middlesex Hospital tells me that his experience there has been similar. Even when he provided his house staff with a pocket version of the TNM classification they failed to use it correctly.

OUR COLUMBIA CRITERIA OF OPERABILITY

None of the plans that had been devised for the clinical staging of breast carcinoma and the choice of treatment seemed adequate to Dr. Stout and me when, some years ago, we began to search for a method of accurately selecting the patients who would benefit from classical radical mastectomy. The methods by which criteria for staging had been arrived at seemed, to us, wrong. They were based upon conjecture as to what "early" and "late," "operable" and "inoperable," breast carcinoma might be, rather than upon actual findings as to what types of cases had been cured by operation in carefully controlled case series.

We had been stimulated to search for criteria of operability by our experience in reviewing the results of treatment of breast carcinoma at the Presbyterian Hospital during the years 1915 to 1935. We were impressed by the frequency with which radical mastectomy had been performed upon patients with advanced disease, without any benefit. Several of the surgeons who had performed many of the mastectomies in the series held to the theory that patients should be operated upon and given their chance of cure no matter how small that chance might be. The practical application of this point of view led them to attempt to remove extensive breast carcinomas. These attempts and their results, carefully documented in our case histories, made the Presbyterian Hospital series of cases a particularly instructive one to study from the point of view of determining just which of the various clinical signs of advanced carcinoma of the breast are truly indicative of surgical incurability.

There are several features of the Presbyterian Hospital data concerning breast carcinoma that favored our inquiry. Our unit record system, established in 1915, made the case records easily available for study. The clinical descriptions of breast disease in our unit records have been exceptionally complete, and have usually been supplemented by drawings and photographs. Studies of the pathologic material, under Dr. Stout's direction, have been exceptionally thorough. Finally, our follow-up system has been so efficient that we known what has happened to virtually all our patients with breast carcinoma.

Dr. Stout and I had all these data concerning our series of breast carcinomas on punch cards when we undertook our study of the criteria of operability. With the punch card method it was easy to determine the statistical significance, as regards cure by operation, of various clinical signs of the extent of the disease. The significance of combinations of the various individual clinical signs was also studied. A large series of such correlations between clinical signs and the results of operation were worked out for the 1544 breast carcinomas coming to the Presbyterian Hospital between 1915 and 1942, inclusive.

There are four types of evidence which are concerned in the clinical classification of the extent of the disease in patients with breast carcinoma, and the choice of treatment. These are:

1. The local extent of carcinoma in the breast and in the tissues covering it and lying beneath it on the chest wall.

2. The presence and extent of metastases in the regional axillary, internal mammary, and supraclavicular lymph node filter.

3. The presence of distant metastases.

4. Constitutional factors in the patient.

In the search for more exact criteria of operability that Dr. Stout and I made in our 1915-1942 Presbyterian Hospital data—a search culminating in the list of criteria of operability that we published in 1943—our chief emphasis was upon the criteria related to the local extent of the carcinoma. The significance of each of the various clinical features of the local growth of breast carcinoma was considered separately in relation to the possibility of cure by radical mastectomy.

In our study we were at once struck by the fact that there were three local clinical features which, if present, always doomed the patient. These were (1) extensive edema of the skin over the breast, (2) satellite tumor nodules in the skin, and (3) the inflammatory type of carcinoma. There is no need to describe these three clinical features at this point. I have described edema of the skin over the breast and satellite skin nodules in Chapter 22 dealing with the natural history of breast carcinoma, and I have dealt with the inflammatory type of carcinoma separately in Chapter 31.

All our Presbyterian Hospital attempts at surgery for patients with any one of these three local clinical features have been disastrous. There were in our data a total of 59 patients (Table 33–1) in whom one or more of these three clinical features were present, and for whom radical mastectomy was done. Approximately 60 per cent of them had local recurrence in the operative field, and not a single one was well five years after operation. It is this experience which led up to classify patients with these three local features as *categorically inoperable.*

Our search in the Presbyterian Hospital data for *categorically inoperable clinical types of breast carcinoma* also led us, of course, to those groups of cases in which the disease had metastasized beyond the reach of the surgeon. There were three of these clinical groups: (1) those with distant metastases, (2) those with clinically evident parasternal or supraclavicular metastases, and (3) those with edema of the arm.

The futility of radical mastectomy when *distant metastases* are present needs no comment.

Table 33–1. RESULTS OF RADICAL MASTECTOMY IN CATEGORICALLY INOPERABLE GROUPS OF CASES. PRESBYTERIAN HOSPITAL, 1915–1942

Clinical Group		No. of Cases	5-yr. Local Recurrence		5-yr. Clinical Cure
			No.	Per cent	No. of Cases
I. Patients with local signs indicating categorical inoperability	Extensive edema of skin over breast	51	31	60.8	0
	Satellite nodules in skin over breast	7	4	57.1	0
	Inflammatory type of carcinoma	25	15	60.0	0
	Patients concerned	59	35	59.3	0
II. Patients with distant or regional node metastasis indicating categorical inoperability	Distant metastasis	10	2	20.0	0
	Regional parasternal or supraclavicular node metastasis	16	9	56.2	0
	Edema of arm	4	2	50.0	0
	Patients concerned	29	12	41.4	0
	Total no. of patients concerned	77	41	53.2	0

A parasternal mass in a patient with breast carcinoma means metastasis to an internal mammary node that has grown outward and involved the overlying tissues. This kind of advanced internal mammary metastasis is not curable by chest wall resection. We have done the operation for several patients with such clinically evident parasternal metastases—always unsuccessfully. Irradiation is a better method of treatment.

Patients with *supraclavicular metastases* that are clinically evident are likewise incurable by surgery in our experience. Approximately 4 per cent of our patients coming for treatment with primary breast carcinoma have had palpable supraclavicular metastases. Neither surgical nor irradiation attack upon clinically evident supraclavicular metastases has saved our patients. Twelve of them had supraclavicular dissection—all futilely. Eggers and his associates reported a similar experience.

From what we know today concerning the sequence of metastatic involvement of the regional lymph node barrier in carcinoma of the breast we must of course expect that conventional radical mastectomy will fail to cure patients with clinically evident supraclavicular metastases. The supraclavicular nodes are involved only after the nodes at the apex of the axilla or those of the internal mammary chain have become involved. The first supraclavicular node or nodes to be involved are the sentinel node or nodes lying deep in the base of the neck upon the confluence of the internal jugular and subclavian veins. These nodes are not palpable clinically until metastases in them have enlarged them greatly, and have extended in a retrograde manner to more superficially and more laterally situated supraclavicular nodes. By then the supraclavicular metastases are advanced and incurable by surgery.

The usefulness of prophylactic supraclavicular dissection as practiced long ago by Halsted, and more recently by Dahl-Iversen, is an entirely different question. I will discuss it separately in Chapter 34.

Edema of the arm develops in an untreated patient with carcinoma of the breast only when axillary metastases have progressed to the stage in which they partially block the lymphatic pathways through the axilla. A patient with such extensive axillary metastases cannot be cured by surgery. It was attempted in four such patients in our Presbyterian Hospital series of cases, and failed in all.

There were 29 patients in our Presbyterian Hospital series of cases with distant or regional lymph node metastases beyond the reach of the surgeon or with edema of the arm who were nevertheless treated by radical mastectomy (Table 33–1). Forty-one per cent had local recurrence and none was cured.

The total number of our patients falling into the clinical groups which Dr. Stout and I called *categorically inoperable* because not a single patient was cured by radical mastectomy, was 77. In studying the significance, in terms of cure by surgery, of various individual clinical signs of the local extent of carcinoma of the breast in our data, it seemed necessary to exclude these 77 categorically inoperable cases, lest their presence distort our interpretation of the significance of less critical clinical features. In the separate consideration of the significance of the several clinical signs of the local extent of the disease to which I now turn, the categorically inoperable cases have been excluded.

In studying the significance of individual local clinical features in our cases, we correlated the significance of each individual clinical feature, occurring *alone*, as well as *with any one of five grave signs* of advanced disease, with the results of radical mastectomy. These five grave signs of locally advanced breast carcinoma in the breast and in the axilla are ones which emerged in our studies as being the most important (excepting the signs of categorical inoperability which I have mentioned above). These five grave clinical signs of advanced breast carcinoma are:

(1) edema of the skin of limited extent, (2) skin ulceration, (3) solid fixation of the tumor to the chest wall, (4) axillary lymph nodes measuring 2.5 cm. or more in transverse diameter, and (5) axillary lymph nodes fixed to the overlying skin or the deeper structures of the axilla.

Our evidence concerning the prognostic significance of these five grave signs in patients treated by radical mastectomy is detailed below.

Edema of the Skin Related to Operability. I have already described, in Chapter 22, the blockage of the subdermal lymphatics by emboli of carcinoma cells which is the underlying cause of edema of the skin. The grave prognostic significance of this clinical sign is therefore understandable. In order to assess as accurately as possible the significance of edema we classified the cases with edema in two groups:

Table 33–2.   RESULTS OF RADICAL MASTECTOMY IN CASES WITH LIMITED EDEMA OF THE SKIN—CATEGORICALLY INOPERABLE CASES EXCLUDED. PRESBYTERIAN HOSPITAL, 1915–1942

Group of Cases	No. of Cases	Local Recurrence		5-yr. Clinical Cure	
		No.	Per cent	No.	Per cent
I. Total patients, radical mastectomy	1058	169	16	477	45.1
II. Limited edema *only*	75	24	32	17	22.7
III. Limited edema *with* any other grave sign of locally advanced disease	24	14	58.3	0	

1. Those in which the extent of the edema was limited to less than one-third of the skin over the breast.

2. Those in which the edema involved a larger area of skin.

I have already pointed out that none of our patients with the latter more extensive form of edema was cured by operation.

I am here concerned with the prognostic significance of edema of only limited extent. Table 33-2 shows our data regarding 99 cases in which this sign was present. In 75 patients in whom limited edema was the only evident sign of advanced disease, radical mastectomy achieved only approximately half the rate of cure that it achieved in our series of breast carcinomas as a whole. And in 24 patients in whom limited edema was associated with one or more of the other grave signs of locally advanced disease, operation did not cure a single one.

This experience indicated that even a limited amount of edema is an extremely grave prognostic sign, and that operation is contraindicated when skin edema of any extent is present.

Ulceration of the Skin Related to Operability. Ulceration of the skin over a carcinoma is merely a more advanced stage of the process of involvement of the skin by the disease. Ulceration becomes a grave sign of locally advanced disease because when this stage is reached in most cases, the disease has become obviously inoperable for other reasons. Our data, shown in Table 33-3, therefore include only 27 cases with ulceration of the skin in which radical mastectomy was done. Patients with erosion of the nipple are, of course, not included.

The results of radical mastectomy in our patients who have had ulceration of the skin, without any other sign of locally advanced disease, have not been as good as in our series of radical mastectomies as a whole. The number of cases in this group was, however, so small that these data were not very meaningful. My own more recent experience with ulceration of the skin has convinced me that it is indeed a grave local sign of advanced breast carcinoma, and I am opposed to radical mastectomy for these patients. Irradiation is a better form of treatment for them.

Fixation of the Carcinoma Related to Operability. In Chapter 5 I described the phenomenon of fixation of breast carcinoma to the underlying pectoral fascia and muscle and finally to the thoracic cage, and my classification of fixation in three degrees. First and second degree fixation are early evidences of fixation. Third degree fixation is the advanced stage in which the carcinoma is immovably fixed to the chest wall.

The surgeons who described the physical findings in the breast carcinomas in our Presbyterian Hospital data in years gone by did not in general distinguish the lesser degrees

Table 33–3.   RESULTS OF RADICAL MASTECTOMY IN CASES WITH ULCERATION OF SKIN—CATEGORICALLY INOPERABLE CASES EXCLUDED. PRESBYTERIAN HOSPITAL, 1915–1942

Group of Cases	No. of Cases	Local Recurrence		5-yr. Clinical Cure	
		No.	Per cent	No.	Per cent
I. Total patients, radical mastectomy	1058	169	16	477	45.1
II. Ulceration of skin *only*	14	2	14.3	5	35.7
III. Ulceration of skin *with* any other grave sign of locally advanced disease	13	4	30.8	0	

Table 33–4. RESULTS OF RADICAL MASTECTOMY IN CASES IN WHICH THERE WAS THIRD DEGREE FIXATION OF THE TUMOR TO THE CHEST WALL—CATEGORICALLY INOPERABLE CASES EXCLUDED. PRESBYTERIAN HOSPITAL, 1915–1942

Group of Cases	No. of Cases	Local Recurrence		5-yr. Clinical Cure	
		No.	Per cent	No.	Per cent
I. Total patients, radical mastectomy	1058	169	16	477	45.1
II. 3rd degree fixation, *only*	20	8	40	1	5
III. 3rd degree fixation *with* any other grave sign of locally advanced disease	27	10	37	1	3.7

of fixation which I have described. They recorded only solid fixation to the chest wall. I am therefore able to present data from our Presbyterian Hospital 1915–1942 series only in regard to third degree fixation. These data are shown in Table 33-4. There were a total of 47 patients with third degree fixation of their carcinomas. Whether or not the third degree fixation was associated with another grave sign of locally advanced disease made little difference; operation failed to cure in almost all.

There is one exception in regard to the grave prognostic significance of solid fixation. It is that carcinomas occurring in the inframammary fold are occasionally solidly fixed but are still not advanced and are perfectly curable by surgery. I will discuss the problem of these inframammary carcinomas separately, later on in the present chapter.

The Extent of Regional Lymph Node Metastases Related to Operability. Many years ago when Dr. Stout and I began analyzing our Presbyterian Hospital data in search of criteria of operability the only indications we had of the presence or extent of regional metastases in axillary, internal mammary, and supraclavicular lymph nodes were based upon palpation of these lymph node regions.

More recently we have biopsied the apex of the axilla and the internal mammary nodes in a large series of patients, and by correlating our findings in palpation of the axilla with the results of these biopsies we have improved our interpretation of our findings in axillary palpation. Nevertheless it is worthwhile to present these earlier data of ours relating our findings in palpation of the axilla to operability.

Massively Enlarged Axillary Lymph Nodes Related to Operability. Although axillary palpation is an inaccurate guide to the presence of metastases in axillary lymph nodes when the lymph nodes are small, palpation is highly accurate when they are large. We measure the transverse diameter, as carefully as we can, of nodes that we palpate in the axilla, and we classify them as *massively enlarged* when they measure 2.5 cm. or more in transverse diameter.

Our early data regarding the relationship of massively enlarged axillary nodes to operability are presented in Table 33-5. We had a total of 43 patients in this group, in whom radical mastectomy was done. Although the number of cases was small it was clear enough that the presence of massively enlarged axillary nodes was a grave sign. Par-

Table 33–5. RESULTS OF RADICAL MASTECTOMY IN CASES WITH MASSIVE ENLARGEMENT OF METASTATIC AXILLARY LYMPH NODES—CATEGORICALLY INOPERABLE CASES EXCLUDED. PRESBYTERIAN HOSPITAL, 1915–1942

Group of Cases	No. of Cases	Local Recurrence		5-yr. Clinical Cure	
		No.	Per cent	No.	Per cent
I. Total patients, radical mastectomy	1058	169	16	477	45.1
II. 2.5 cm. nodes *only*	24	3	12.5	9	37.5
III. 2.5 cm. nodes *with* any other grave sign of locally advanced disease	19	9	42.1	1	5.3

Table 33–6. RESULTS OF RADICAL MASTECTOMY IN CASES WITH FIXED METASTATIC AXILLARY NODES—CATEGORICALLY INOPERABLE CASES EXCLUDED. PRESBYTERIAN HOSPITAL, 1915–1942

Group of Cases	No. of Cases	Local Recurrence		5-yr. Clinical Cure	
		No.	Per cent	No.	Per cent
I. Total patients, radical mastectomy	1058	169	16	477	45.1
II. Fixed axillary nodes *only*	8	1	12.5	1	12.5
III. Fixed axillary nodes *with* any other grave sign of locally advanced disease	18	9	50	0	

ticularly when combined with another grave sign, these large axillary nodes were a contra-indication to operation.

Fixation of Axillary Lymph Nodes. As metastases grow in axillary lymph nodes the disease breaks through the capsule of the nodes and invades the axillary fat and connective tissue. The nodes finally become fused together and fixed to the chest wall deeply or to the skin of the axilla superficially. Fixation to the axillary skin may be apparent as a zone of skin dimpling.

Our data regarding the results of radical mastectomy in patients with fixed axillary lymph nodes containing metastases are shown in Table 33–6. The results of operation were so poor in all cases in which the axillary nodes were fixed, whether this feature was present alone or in association with one of the other grave signs of locally advanced disease, that we concluded that these patients should be treated with irradiation and not by surgery.

Dr. Stout and I also studied the prognostic significance of two other local clinical signs of advancing breast carcinoma—redness of the skin of the breast over the lesion, and involvement of the overlying skin by the carcinoma. Our data, which follow, did not indicate that these individual clinical phenomena have a grave prognostic significance.

Redness of the Skin Related to Operability. I have mentioned redness of the skin over breast carcinoma—when not of the inflammatory type—as being due to involvement of the skin by the disease or to necrosis in the tumor.

In Table 33–7 the results of operation in a total of 75 cases with redness of the skin are shown. Our cases of inflammatory carcinoma have been excluded, of course, from this table, together with other categorically inoperable cases. In our patients with redness of the skin unaccompanied by other clinical features of locally advanced disease, operation gave approximately as good results as it did in our series of cases of carcinoma as a whole. The local recurrence rate doubled and the cure rate was only half as good when redness was accompanied by any one of the five grave signs of locally advanced disease.

We concluded from this experience that *redness of the skin* over a carcinoma is, in itself, not a contraindication to operation. When it is accompanied by any one of the five grave signs of locally advanced disease, however, the results of surgery are so poor that irradiation is preferable.

Skin Involvement Related to Operabilty. Involvement of the skin over carcinoma, as we have used it in our classification, refers to those cases in which the skin over

Table 33–7. RESULTS OF RADICAL MASTECTOMY IN CARCINOMA WITH REDNESS OF THE SKIN—CATEGORICALLY INOPERABLE CASES EXCLUDED. PRESBYTERIAN HOSPITAL, 1915–1942

Group of Cases	No. of Cases	Local Recurrence		5-yr. Clinical Cure	
		No.	Per cent	No.	Per cent
I. Total patients, radical mastectomy	1058	169	16.0	477	45.1
II. Redness of the skin *only*	33	7	21.2	14	42.4
III. Redness of the skin *with* any one of 5 grave signs of locally advanced disease	42	17	40.5	8	19.0

the tumor has become fixed and immovable. It is tied down by fibrosis developing over the carcinoma or by actual infiltration of the derma by carcinoma cells. This is a clinical and not a pathologic criterion. Cases in which skin involvement has progressed to the point of ulceration are not included: they form a group which I have discussed separately.

Our results in a total of 116 cases with involvement of the skin are shown in Table 33–8. When such involvement was the only sign of locally advanced disease the results of operation were approximately the same as in our series of radical mastectomies as a whole. But when involvement of the skin was accompanied by any one of the five grave signs of locally advanced disease the cure rate was reduced by more than half.

Our data therefore indicated that involvement of the overlying skin by the carcinoma is in itself no contraindication to surgical treatment. When, in addition, any one of the five grave signs of locally advanced disease is present, surgery is usually unsuccessful and irradiation is preferable.

From the correlations of the clinical features of our Presbyterian Hospital breast carcinoma with the results of operation, which I have presented in Tables 33–1 to 33–8, Dr. Stout and I drew up a list of *clinical criteria of operability* which we tested and refined over a period of years, and presented in their final form in 1951. The only important change that we made in the final version of the criteria, as compared with the original version, was the omission of the interdiction of operation for carcinoma developing during pregnancy and lactation.

Clinical Criteria of Operability. Our *clinical criteria of operability* in their final form were as follows: Carcinoma of the breast in women of all age groups, who are in good enough general condition to withstand operation, should be treated by radical mastectomy, except when:

1. Extensive edema of the skin over the breast is present.
2. Satellite nodules are present in the skin over the breast.
3. The carcinoma is of the inflammatory type.
4. A parasternal tumor is present.
5. Proved supraclavicular metastases are present.
6. There is edema of the arm.
7. Distant metastases are demonstrated.
8. Any two, or more, of the following grave signs of locally advanced carcinoma are present:
   a. Ulceration of the skin.
   b. Edema of the skin of limited extent (less than one-third of the skin over the breast involved).
   c. Solid fixation of the tumor to the chest wall.
   d. Axillary lymph nodes measuring 2.5 cm., or more, in transverse diameter.
   e. Fixation of the axillary lymph nodes to the skin or the deep structures of the axilla.

It was fortunate indeed for the purposes of the inquiry as to operability that Dr. Stout and I were carrying out that several of our attending surgeons at the Presbyterian Hospital, spurred on by the most idealistic of motives, had performed radical mastectomy on types of cases which were clearly inoperable according to our criteria. In this manner our criteria have been well tested in our own hospital where our records are sufficiently complete to provide an adequate test. The application of our clinical criteria of operability to our Presbyterian Hospital 1915–1942 series of carcinomas treated by radical mastectomy is shown in Table 33–9.

Table 33–8. RESULTS OF RADICAL MASTECTOMY IN CASES WITH SKIN INVOLVEMENT — CATEGORICALLY INOPERABLE CASES EXCLUDED. PRESBYTERIAN HOSPITAL, 1915–1942

Group of Cases	No. of Cases	Local Recurrence		5-yr. Clinical Cure	
		No.	Per cent	No.	Per cent
I. Total patients, radical mastectomy	1058	169	16.0	477	45.1
II. Involvement of skin *only*	58	10	17.2	25	44.8
III. Involvement of skin *with* any one of the 5 grave signs of locally advanced disease	58	13	22.4	10	17.2

Table 33–9. Clinical criteria of operability applied to Presbyterian Hospital series of radical mastectomies, 1915–1942

Group of Cases	No. of Cases	5-yr. Local Recurrence		5-yr. Clinical Cure	
		No.	Per cent	No.	Per cent
I. Cases in which radical mastectomy was performed (1915–1942)	1135	225	19.8	477	42.0
II. Cases that would be classed as *inoperable*					
1. Categorically inoperable group	77	41	53.2	0	
2. Combinations of any two of five grave signs of locally advanced disease	43	18	42.0	1	2.3
III. Cases that would be classed as *operable*	1015	166	16.4	476	46.9

Study of this table shows that a total of 120 cases fall into the inoperable group, of which 77 were inoperable because they were in our so-called categorically inoperable class, while 43 were inoperable because two or more of the five grave signs of locally advanced carcinoma were present. Half of these 120 patients with inoperable disease who were nevertheless operated upon are known to have developed local recurrence. Only one was free of evidence of disease after five years, and she died of metastasis eight years after operation.

If the clinical criteria of operability which I have described had been followed in the selection of our Presbyterian Hospital cases for radical mastectomy, 120, or some 10 per cent, of the operations would have been avoided, without foregoing permanent cure in a single patient.

It may be asked what effect radical mastectomy had on the length of life in these patients whose carcinomas were inoperable. Table 33–10 attempts to answer the question from our data. It will be seen that the average duration of life from onset of symptoms to death was shorter in the patients with inoperable carcinoma who were treated by radical mastectomy than it was in those who were treated by simple mastectomy or by irradia-

tion. Those treated by irradiation lived slightly longer than the untreated patients in Wade's collected series. There are, of course, several possible interpretations of these facts, but they at least suggest that the more surgery performed upon patients with inoperable carcinoma the shorter will be their survival. This is in agreement with our understanding of the mechanism of metastasis. A surgeon dissecting in tissues infiltrated by carcinoma can be expected to produce showers of carcinoma emboli which should hasten death. I have observed this clinical phenomenon many times.

Our clinical criteria of operability have been tested and found useful not only in our own clinic but in various hospitals in this country and abroad (Tomlinson and Eckert; Wells; Dahl-Iversen and Soerensen; Kay and Poulos; Miller; Cheek; Göksel).

THE COLUMBIA CLINICAL CLASSIFICATION

From our early efforts to define the stage of advancement of breast carcinoma in which radical mastectomy is indicated, we came to appreciate the great need for a practical formal plan for clinical staging.

Table 33–10. Mean total duration of breast carcinoma — onset to death — in various groups of cases

I. 777 untreated cases collected by Wade from various published sources	38.55 months
II. 77 Presbyterian Hospital cases (1935–1942) classified as inoperable and treated by radiotherapy only	40.4 months
III. 38 Presbyterian Hospital cases (1915–1942) classified as inoperable but treated by simple mastectomy	37.4 months
IV. 120 Presbyterian Hospital cases (1915–1942) classified as inoperable but treated by radical mastectomy	33.0 months

Early carcinoma of the breast is very different from advanced breast carcinoma, and its treatment presents an entirely different problem. We do not have for mammary carcinoma any general method of treatment which is effective at all stages of the disease, as some antibiotics are curative for certain infectious diseases whatever their stage may be.

Without a workable method for clinical staging of breast carcinoma we cannot compare the results in case series treated by different methods. Unless the case series are staged accurately, differences in local recurrence and survival rates may be due to differences in the stage of advancement of the disease in the different case series. Comparisons then become as meaningless as a race without a starting line. We also needed an accurate plan for clinical staging to study the significance of a wide variety of clinical factors which influence the course of breast carcinoma, such as the age of the patient, the site of the primary tumor in the breast, the influence of pregnancy, etc. Unless series of patients whose breast carcinomas are at the same early clinical stage can be sorted out, the influence of such individual critical factors cannot be determined. In the majority of patients with breast cancer, the disease is advanced when they first consult a physician. The inevitable bad results in these patients with advanced disease obscure the effects of the special features which, in earlier clinical stages, influence the course of the disease.

Clinical staging also has great value as a guide to therapy. Our Columbia Clinical Classification is aimed particularly at distinguishing the early from the late stages of mammary carcinoma, because in these earlier stages the choice of treatment is much more critical. We believe that a thorough radical mastectomy is the best treatment for early breast carcinoma, and that irradiation, oophorectomy, and chemotherapy are unnecessary and harmful. In contrast, surgery does harm in advanced breast carcinoma. It is in these advanced stages that irradiation, hormonal methods, and chemotherapy should be used, one after another, in a carefully chosen sequence.

More than 20 years ago, Edith Cooley, who brought her training as a statistician to bear on the problem, and I, began to define a plan for the clinical classification of breast cancer as to its stage of advancement. We wanted a method of classification that was simple enough to be practical and so precisely worded that there could be no confusion about the meaning of the terms employed. After much testing, we evolved the Columbia Clinical Classification. It is shown in Table 33-11. It has been used in our own clinic and in several other clinics for a long enough time to convince us that it is comparatively simple to use and surprisingly accurate. It would be possible to devise a somewhat more accurate classification if other significant factors such as the age of the patient, the size, and the gross and histologic character of the tumor, were included, but the classification would then become to complex to be practical.

Much the most important part of any clinical classification of breast carcinoma as to its stage of advancement is the interpretation of the findings of axillary palpation. The palpation of the axilla is also the most difficult part of the clinical examination.

We have found our Columbia Classification much more accurate as regards the presence and extent of axillary metastases than we would have expected. I should mention

Table 33-11. THE COLUMBIA CLINICAL CLASSIFICATION

Stage A. No skin edema, ulceration, or solid fixation of tumor to chest wall. Axillary nodes not clinically involved.

Stage B. No skin edema, ulceration, or solid fixation of tumor to chest wall. Clinically involved nodes, but less than 2.5 cm. in transverse diameter and not fixed to overlying skin or deeper structures of axilla.

Stage C. Any one of five grave signs of advanced breast carcinoma:
1. Edema of skin of limited extent (involving less than one-third of the skin over the breast).
2. Skin ulceration.
3. Solid fixation of tumor to chest wall.
4. Massive involvement of axillary lymph nodes (measuring 2.5 cm. or more in transverse diameter).
5. Fixation of the axillary nodes to overlying skin or deeper structures of axilla.

Stage D. All other patients with more advanced breast carcinoma, including:
1. A combination of any two or more of the five grave signs listed under Stage C.
2. Extensive edema of skin (involving more than one-third of the skin over the breast).
3. Satellite skin nodules.
4. The inflammatory type of carcinoma.
5. Clinically involved supraclavicular lymph nodes.
6. Internal mammary metastases as evidenced by a parasternal tumor.
7. Edema of the arm.
8. Distant metastases.

Table 33–12. CLINICAL EXAMINATION OF AXILLA CORRELATED WITH INCIDENCE OF
MICROSCOPICALLY VERIFIED METASTASES. PERSONAL SERIES OF 1007
RADICAL MASTECTOMIES, 1935–1968

Columbia Clinical Classification	No. of Patients	Per cent with Metastases	Per cent with 1 to 3 Involved Nodes	Per cent with 4 to 7 Involved Nodes	Per cent with 8 or more Involved Nodes
Stage A. No clinically involved nodes	724	31.2%	21.7%	5.0%	4.6%
Stage B. Clinically involved nodes less than 2.5 cm. in diameter	198	74.7%	33.8%	19.2%	21.7%
Stages C and D. Clinically involved nodes 2.5 cm. or more in diameter, or fixed nodes	35	97.1%	34.3%	25.7%	37.1%
Stages C and D (all cases)	85	82.3%	24.7%	14.1%	43.5%

that when we palpate the axilla and find no clinically involved nodes (Clinical Stage A), we expect that microscopic study will reveal metastases in about one third of the cases, as shown in Table 33–12, which correlates the findings of axillary palpation with the incidence of microscopically verified axillary metastases in my personal series of 1007 radical mastectomies. This table also shows that extensive involvement of the axilla, as indicated by the involvement of eight or more nodes, has occurred very infrequently in Clinical Stage A cases. In contrast, axillary metastases were found in 74.7 per cent of Clinical Stage B cases, and eight or more nodes were involved in 22.7 per cent. These data indicate that our classification distinguishes fairly well between Clinical Stages A and B as regards the axillary findings.

Another indication of the reliability of our Columbia Clinical Classification regarding the axilla is seen in Table 33–13. Here the microscopic findings in the axilla are shown in four different series of patients classified by our clinical classification and treated by radical mastectomy. The percentages of cases with axillary metastases are remarkably similar. Considering the fact that in these data we are equating a classification based on palpation, with microscopic findings, our Columbia Clinical Classification performs astonishingly well.

We have been considering for some time the idea of refining our classification of our findings in axillary palpation by adding criteria concerning the presence of more than one clinically involved axillary node. When there are only two or three small clinically involved axillary nodes situated in the lower axilla we have not been greatly impressed by their un-

Table 33–13. RADICAL MASTECTOMY FOR MAMMARY CARCINOMA. FREQUENCY OF
MICROSCOPIC AXILLARY METASTASES

Columbia Clinical Classification	Butcher St. Louis 1950–1955		Miller Detroit 1951–1960		Dahl-Iversen and Tobiassen Copenhagen 1950–1955		Haagensen Columbia New York 1935–1955	
	No. of Cases	Per cent Ax. Met.	No. of Cases	Per cent Ax. Met.	No. of Cases	Per cent Ax. Met.	No. of Cases	Per cent Ax. Met.
Stage A	214	32.2%	315	29.5%	317	28.7%	344	32.2%
Stage B	135	75.5%	90	84.4%	69	76.8%	138	76.0%
Stage C	48	89.5%	60	76.7%	26*	46.2%	63	76.2%
All stages	397		465		412		545	

*This number of cases is too small to have any statistical significance.

toward prognostic significance. But when there is a chain of clinically involved axillary nodes extending high into the axilla, even though the individual nodes are not as large as 2.5 cm. in diameter, we have learned that the axilla will usually be found to be extensively involved. The number of patients in this group is, however, small. We do not yet have enough data to justify adding this criterion to our Columbia Clinical Classification. What we have done, as a practical solution to our dilemma in deciding about the operability of these patients with several nodes or a chain of nodes, is to perform preliminary biopsy of the nodes of the apex of the axilla. In a number of such patients we have found metastases in the subclavicular nodes. We have treated these patients with irradiation alone.

Our Columbia Clinical Classification has been used as the basis for a cooperative international study of the 5 and 10-year results of treatment of early breast cancer by seven different methods. Baclesse also presented his 5-year results for his remarkable series of patients treated by irradiation only and classified by our Columbia Classification; unfortunately, he did not live to present his 10-year results in our cooperative study.

The 10-year results are much more significant than 5-year results. This fact is evident in Chart 33–1 which presents a 20-year survival curve for all females derived from U. S. Life Tables, together with a survival curve for my completely documented series of cases

of mammary carcinoma treated by radical mastectomy. In determining the survival curve for all females, survival curves for females of specific age groups were worked out from U. S. Life Tables for 1949–1951. A weighted average of these survival curves was then taken. It is apparent from this chart that the gap between the survival curve for all women and the survival curve for women with breast carcinoma treated by radical mastectomy continues to widen between 1 and 10 years after operation. But between 10 and 20 years the survival rates for all women, and for those with breast carcinoma, are parallel.

Another survival curve (Chart 33–2), constructed in the same way from British mortality data, and another completely documented series of cases treated by a different method (Williams and Stone), shows that women with breast carcinoma continue to succumb at an abnormal rate until about 9 years after treatment.

These data indicate that 10 years is probably the best interval at which to assess the results of treatment of breast cancer. Five years is too early in the course of this relatively slowly progressive disease to evaluate treatment. Nothing is gained in the accuracy of the evaluation by waiting until 15 years because by this time the increasing toll of deaths from intercurrent disease tends to obscure the truth of what has been accomplished by treatment.

In a study of this kind, of the end-results of

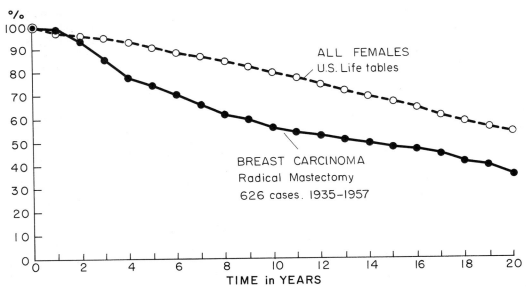

Chart 33–1. Survival curve for normal women and for those with carcinoma of the breast treated by radical mastectomy.

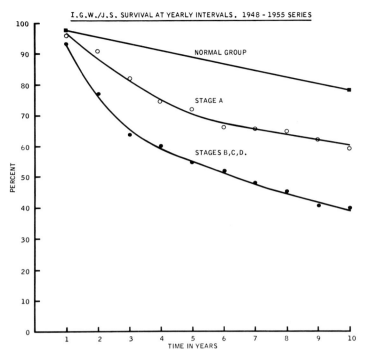

Chart 33–2. Survival curve for normal women and for those with carcinoma of the breast in different stages treated by total mastectomy with axillary dissection followed by irradiation (Williams and Stone).

different methods of treatment, all patients treated are of course included, and all are counted as dying of breast cancer even when it is known that they died of intercurrent disease. It is also essential that follow-up be virtually complete if a true picture of the results of treatment is to be presented.

In our cooperative international comparison of results we were able to include data as to the frequency of local recurrence in five of the seven case series. In a comparison of local recurrence rates it is essential to classify local recurrence as to type. Parasternal recurrence, usually in one of the upper three interspaces and solidly fixed to the chest wall, develops from internal mammary metastases which were missed and untreated. Recurrence in the skin flaps or the axilla following mastectomy represents carcinoma not removed by the surgeon, or not controlled by irradiation if it was the treatment.

I present the detailed findings of our "Cooperative International Study of the Treatment of Early Mammary Carcinoma" in Chapter 34 because that is where the various surgical methods of treatment are discussed. Our study is, to my knowledge, the first comparison of different methods of treatment that meets reasonable standards for this kind of an

investigation—including accurate and detailed case records, all case series classified clinically by a simple and precise method, adequate pathologic study of the surgical specimens, and a complete follow-up for at least 10 years.

In recent papers by Zippin, by Cutler and Myers, and by Cutler, Zippin, and Myers the International and the American classifications were compared in studying the extent and prognosis of breast carcinoma in 2039 patients treated in 12 different hospitals. These authors are apparently unaware of the inadequacy of their data. The descriptions of physical findings in unit case records of this type from general hospitals where special clinics for breast disease did not exist were no doubt made by comparatively inexperienced internes. In accordance with the TNM classification all palpable axillary nodes were interpreted as representing metastases, no effort being made to distinguish between clinically uninvolved and involved palpable nodes. No mention is made of the different surgical techniques used, the numbers of axillary nodes found in the surgical specimens, and other such fundamentally important details. The statistician-authors of these papers lose their way in a maze of statistics, none of which is valid be-

Table 33–14. Conservative radical mastectomy for mammary carcinoma. Crude survival rates in 250 cases. Comparison of Columbia and TNM clinical staging (R. S. Handley – Middlesex Hospital)

COLUMBIA

Stage	No. of Patients	5-yr. Survival		10-yr. Survival	
		Total	Per cent	Total	Per cent
A	127	93	73.2	69	54.3
B	98	57	58.0	41	41.8
C	21	5	23.8	4	18.0
D	4	nil	0	nil	0
Total	250	155	62.0	114	45.6

TNM

Stage	No. of Patients	5-yr. Survival		10-yr. Survival	
		Total	Per cent	Total	Per cent
1	93	64	68.8	48	51.6
2	103	66	64.0	52	50.5
3	52	25	48.0	14	26.9
4	2	nil	nil	nil	nil
Total	250	155	62.0	114	45.6

cause their basic data are inadequate. The *clinical* classification of the stage of advancement of breast carcinoma is necessarily based upon *clinical* expertise.

The best comparison of the practical value of the TNM and Columbia methods of clinical classification of breast carcinoma has been made recently by Handley, and I am indebted to him for permission to include his data (Table 33–14) and the graphs (Chart 33–3) which he has made from them. The spread according to prognosis is much better in the Columbia Classification. In the TNM Classification there is no statistically significant difference between the results in Clinical Stages I and II. This is to be expected, be-

cause in the TNM system no effort is made to distinguish critically between uninvolved and involved axillary nodes as we do in our Columbia Clinical Classification. Since this determination of axillary involvement is the most important aspect of clinical staging, the TNM system fails badly.

The best indication that both the International and American plans are impractical is the fact that no one has succeeded in drawing useful conclusions as to which is the best method of treating breast carcinoma from comparisons of the results in case series classified by the International and American plans and treated by different methods. This is the primary purpose of all efforts to classify breast carcinoma. Unless these clinical classifications make it possible to answer this question they are useless.

Regional Lymph Node Biopsy

Our efforts to classify breast carcinoma clinically, and to select the patients for whom radical mastectomy offers the best hope of cure, left us very much aware that clinical classification alone is not always an adequate guide to the extent of the disease. Our ideal should be to perform radical mastectomy only for those patients whom we can cure; and we have failed to cure approximately 40 per cent of the patients we have selected for operation.

We have been aware for a long time that there are two important weaknesses in the selection of patients for operation on the basis of clinical classification alone. One is a lack of a dependable method for determining

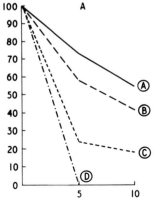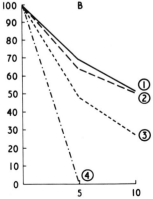

Chart 33–3. Conservative radical mastectomy for mammary carcinoma. Percentage crude survival in 250 patients. Handley, 1970. *A,* Columbia Clinical Classification; *B,* TNM Clinical Classification.

the existence of occult regional lymph node metastases at the periphery of the operative field—in the nodes at the apex of the axilla, and in the internal mammary nodes. The other weakness was our inability to detect distant metastases in bone. By employing biopsy we have attempted to remedy both of these defects in our method of selection of patients for operation. In substituting criteria based on pathologic evidence of the spread of the disease, for our clinical criteria based on clinical examination, we have improved our ability to select the patients who can be cured by operation.

In my account in Chapter 22 of the routes of metastases of mammary carcinoma, I described regional lymph node metastases occurring first in the mid-axillary nodes. After the axillary lymph node filter has been partially blocked, metastases are found in the internal mammary lymph nodes in the upper three interspaces with increasing frequency. The third stage in the process of lymphatic extension is involvement of the nodes at the apex of the axilla. Finally, carcinoma emboli reach the deep inferior cervical sentinel nodes at the confluence of the internal jugular and subclavian veins, either through the subclavian lymphatic trunks from the axilla, or through the internal mammary lymphatic trunks.

Internal Mammary Biopsy

I have told in Chapter 22 how Richard Handley's demonstration of the frequency of occult internal mammary metastases stimulated us in 1951 to begin to perform preliminary biopsy of the internal mammary nodes for the purpose of improving our selection of patients for radical mastectomy. When we found these nodes to be involved we treated our patients with irradiation alone, because our knowledge of the surgical pathology of internal mammary metastases and the technical limitations of surgical excision of these nodes had convinced us that extending the surgical attack to include removal of the internal mammary nodes would not improve the rate of cure. These internal mammary biopsies were always preceded, of course, by a small incisional biopsy of the primary tumor in the breast to prove that we were dealing with carcinoma.

The technique of internal mammary node biopsy is not familiar to most surgeons. It requires the ability to deal with minute structures in a very small operative field which must be kept bloodless.

Although we began by exploring only the second interspace, as Handley had done, we soon realized that all the upper three interspaces should be explored if an accurate estimate of the presence of internal mammary metastases is to be had.

The skin incision (Fig. 33–1) is made along the edge of the sternum from the lower edge of the first rib to the upper edge of the fourth rib. We investigate one interspace at a time, beginning with the second, because it is easiest to explore and because it is the interspace in which involved nodes are most often found. The pectoralis major muscle is detached from the sternum, and from the costal cartilages of the interspace being explored. In this step great care is necessary to identify and secure the perforating vessels and their branches. If hemostasis is not complete, bleeding will obscure the small operative field and make dissection of the internal mammary vessels impossible.

Then the intercostal muscle is excised from between the costal cartilages for a distance of about 4 cm. out from the sternal edge, creating a small rectangular window into the internal mammary area. A very thin layer of fascia roofs over the areolar tissue in which the internal mammary vessels and lymphatic trunks and small lymph nodes lie. This film of fascia is incised and the delicate process of removing the areolar tissue, and what lymph nodes can be found, is begun. This is achieved best, in my hands, with what I call the micro-peanut. This is made by rolling a bit of fine-meshed gauze into a ball about 3 mm. in diameter and clamping it in the tip of a fine-curved Halsted hemostat. Figure 33–2 shows one of these instruments. The areolar tissue surrounding the internal mammary vein or veins and artery is cleared from these vessels with these micro-peanuts, and removed with fine thumb-forceps. As the interspace is cleared one, or sometimes two, small nodes will usually be encountered. They are often not more than 2 to 4 mm. in diameter. They may be partially hidden beneath the edges of the costal cartilages or the sternum, from which they have to be fished out with a fine curved Halsted hemostat. This is an essential instrument in performing this dissection.

When the dissection is completed the internal mammary vessels lie bare upon the pleura, beneath which the lung can be seen moving.

In a few cases we have put a small hole through the pleura during the dissection but no harm has come from it. When this has occurred we take care to have a postoperative x-ray film of the chest to make sure no appreciable amount of air remains in the pleural cavity. If necessary, we aspirate it. One precaution which will minimize the chance of entering the pleura is not to carry the dissection of the interspace more than 3 cm. laterally from the sternal edge.

We close the subcutaneous fat and the skin in layers over the dissected interspaces, without drainage.

Every minute bit of areolar tissue removed from each interspace, as well as the lymph nodes, is put at once into a small bottle of Bouin's fixative kept at the operating table. These small pieces of tissue dry out very quickly if left lying about on gauze, and the cellular detail is ruined. We embed these tissues in paraffin and cut them in a number of levels.

We utilize frozen sections only if we find

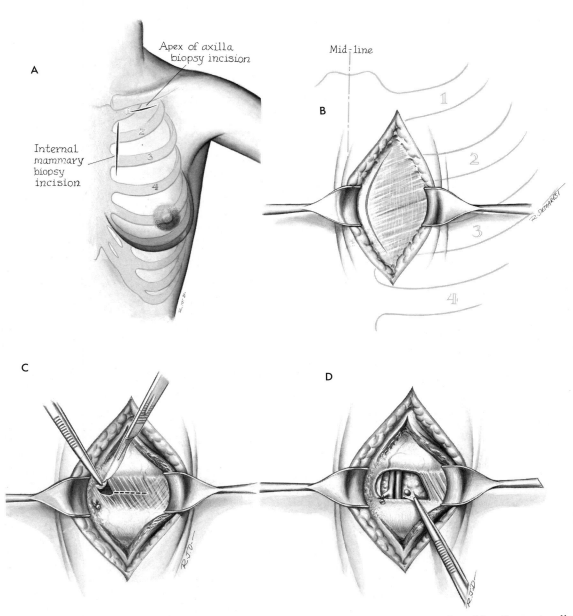

Figure 33–1. Technique of internal mammary biopsy. *A*, The skin incision; *B*, detaching the pectoralis major muscle to reveal the interspace; *C*, excising the intercostal muscle to expose the contents of the interspace; *D*, dissection of the areolar tissue and lymph nodes from the interspace.

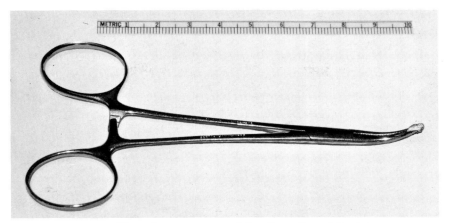

Figure 33–2.   The micro-peanut used for dissection of the interspace.

grossly evident disease in an interspace. If we find metastasis in the first interspace explored, we terminate our biopsy. Otherwise we usually explore all three upper interspaces. We leave the first interspace to the last because it is the most difficult. This difficulty is due partly to the fact that it is usually narrower than the others, and partly because this interspace is inclined toward the base of the neck instead of being in the horizontal plane of the chest wall as are the other interspaces. This inclination makes access to it more difficult.

In patients in whom internal mammary metastases were not found, radical mastectomy consequently was delayed for a few days. We have no evidence that this delay was harmful. When metastases were found in these internal mammary nodes, it was our practice to treat the patient with irradiation only. However, in occasional patients in whom the primary breast tumors were very large or persisted and grew after irradiation, simple mastectomy was performed.

Selection of Patients for Internal Mammary Lymph Node Biopsy.   We did our internal mammary lymph node biopsies only in a selected minority of our patients with breast carcinomas, usually those in whom the clinical findings led us to believe that these nodes were likely to be involved. Although it was difficult to follow a rule in a matter as complex as this, these patients generally were the following:

1. Clinical Stage A patients whose primary tumors were situated in the medial sectors or the central sector of the breast (zones C, D, E, F, and G) and measured 3 cm. or more in diameter.

2. Clinical Stage A patients whose primary tumors were situated in the lateral sectors of the breast (zones A and B) and measured 5 cm. or more in diameter.

3. Patients with more advanced disease.

We also performed these preliminary biopsies of the internal mammary nodes in patients in whom our assessment of the clinical findings left us in doubt regarding the stage of advancement of their disease in terms of our Columbia Clinical Classification. In this way, we proved in a good many patients that their disease, which was apparently on the borderline between Clinical Stages B and C, was in fact unsuitable for radical mastectomy because of internal mammary metastases. However, experience taught us that if the clinical features are defined clearly enough to permit accurate clinical staging, it always should take precedence over the negative findings of these internal mammary biopsies. We have learned that when the clinical findings indicated that the disease had advanced to Stage C or D, radical mastectomy should not be performed even though the internal mammary lymph node biopsies did not reveal metastasis.

In 1967, after we had performed preliminary internal mammary lymph node biopsy in selected cases for 17 years, and had done the procedure in a total of 1007 patients, we reviewed our findings. I have presented them in detail in Chapter 22, and they have been discussed in a recent paper dealing with the whole subject of "The Metastasis of Carcinoma of the Breast to the Periphery of the Regional Lymph Node Filter."

Internal Mammary Node Metastasis and Choice of Treatment.   There are several aspects of the phenomenon of metastasis to the internal mammary nodes which bear on the choice of treatment of breast carcinoma and which are worthwhile emphasizing again here.

The first point is the frequency of these occult internal mammary metastases. Reference to Table 22–32 (p. 426) shows that at least 20 per cent of all patients with carcinoma in Clinical Stages A and B—that is operable disease—have these metastases. They are entirely undetectable except by biopsy, and most surgeons have hitherto ignored them. They must ignore them no longer if they are to hope to improve their results with breast carcinoma.

The second point is that the most important factor determining the likelihood of internal mammary metastases is the status of the axillary nodes. In the early stage of breast carcinoma, before metastases reach the axillary nodes, internal mammary metastases are unusual—being found in only 3 to 5 per cent of patients. But when the axillary lymph node filter is involved and to some degree blocked by metastases, the direction of lymphatic flow turns more toward the internal mammary lymph node filter and these nodes are increasingly involved. Thus the patients with internal mammary metastases usually have comparatively advanced breast cancer, and on this basis, their prognosis is in general unfavorable. It is to be expected that the results of treatment of these patients will be poor, and indeed they are.

There have been, in general, three different therapeutic plans for dealing with internal mammary metastases. (1) The radical surgical attack is extended to include excision of the internal mammary nodes. When they are found to be involved, prophylactic irradiation is given. (2) Biopsy of the internal mammary nodes is the first step of the surgical attack. When they are found to be involved, mastectomy only is performed, and the axilla and internal mammary area are irradiated. (3) Preliminary internal mammary node biopsy is done. When involvement is found, no further surgical therapy is performed. Treatment is by irradiation alone. This is the plan we have used in our clinic.

The extended radical mastectomy, in which an attempt is made to excise internal mammary metastases, has several technical handicaps. Even in the small percentage of cases in which surgical excision conceivably might succeed, the attempt is often doomed to failure because the nodes in the first interspace are involved. The line of dissection for an excision of the internal mammary filter together with the chest wall must be carried through the first interspace; if there are metastases in this narrow interspace, there is no reasonable hope of succeeding because the dissection has to be carried through disease. When metastases exist in the internal mammary filter, the first interspace is involved in one half to two thirds of the cases.

A correlated disadvantage of the addition of internal mammary node dissection to radical mastectomy is the technical limitation to the thoroughness of radical mastectomy which is imposed by removal of the internal mammary sector of the chest wall. The skin flaps must be cut thick and no skin graft can be used because the closure of the defect in the chest wall must be secure. We believe that these features of radical mastectomy are important, and we are unwilling to abandon them.

Although the extended radical mastectomy can be done without prohibitive mortality, the operation undoubtedly penalizes the patient more than does the classical radical mastectomy.

These objections to the addition of chest wall excision of the internal mammary node area to radical mastectomy are confirmed by the poor results of the procedure. Table 33–15 shows results obtained by two surgeons who have had very extensive experience with the operation—Caceres and Veronesi. They have presented their 10-year results in series of operable patients with breast carcinomas in whom the internal mammary nodes were found to be involved. Their results with the extended operation cannot be attributed entirely to the surgical attack because patients who had internal mammary involvement also received postoperative prophylactic irradiation. In our opinion a 10-year survival rate of only 13 per cent for this drastic operation, which has a real morbidity even though its mortality is negligible, does not justify it. We predict that the extended radical mastectomy will not survive long in the surgeons' repertoire.

Handley (1969) has used a more moderate attack, combining both operation and irradiation. For patients whose disease is Stage A or B according to our Columbia Clinical Classification, he commences mastectomy by turning back skin flaps. He next begins removal of the breast at the midline, dissecting it off the inner portion of the pectoralis major muscle. At this point, biopsies of the medial

Table 33–15. TEN-YEAR SURVIVAL—OPERABLE CARCINOMA OF THE BREAST WITH INTERNAL MAMMARY METASTASES*

Author	Treatment	No. Cases with Internal Mammary Metastases	Per cent 10-yr. Survival
Handley, 1969 Columbia Clinical Classification Stages A and B	Biopsy of internal mammary nodes. Simple or radical mastectomy plus irradiation	98	15.0%
Caceres, 1968	Extended radical mastectomy, excision of chest wall, internal mammary region plus irradiation	54	13.0%
Veronesi, 1968	Extended radical mastectomy, excision of chest wall, internal mammary region plus irradiation	46	13.0%
Haagensen, 1969 Columbia Clinical Classification Stages A & B	Biopsy of internal mammary nodes plus irradiation	79	13.9%

*Urban's series of extended radical mastectomies unfortunately cannot be included because his data are presented in a different form.

ends of the upper three intercostal spaces are performed. If metastases are found, he terminates the procedure by removing only the breast. Postoperative irradiation is given to the axillary and internal mammary regions. In a series of 98 patients with proved internal mammary metastases treated by either a simple or modified radical mastectomy followed by irradiation, Handley's 10-year survival rate was 15 per cent. He himself emphasizes that these results are the same as those achieved by Caceres and Veronesi.

Our own results in patients proved to have internal mammary metastases by preliminary biopsy are also shown in Table 33–15. They have been achieved by irradiation alone. In our series of 79 patients, the 10-year survival rate was 13.9 per cent. This is essentially the same as the survival rate achieved by extended radical mastectomy plus irradiation and by Handley's conservative surgical attack.

We must face up to the fact that all methods of dealing with internal mammary metastases which have been tried to date have failed badly. If we are to improve our results with breast carcinoma, we must find a more effective method of controlling these occult internal mammary metastases. In our recent paper we proposed a new plan of treatment which we hope will improve our results. We abandon our preliminary internal mammary biopsy. Instead, we will follow our radical mastectomies with prophylactic irradiation to the internal mammary region. However, patients will not receive this prophylactic internal mammary irradiation if their disease is in Stage A in our Columbia Clinical Classification and if the primary tumor is less than 3 cm. in diameter and is situated in the outer half of the breast. Data from our series of internal mammary node biopsies in such patients (Table 33–16) suggest that the likelihood of having internal mammary node metastases in this special group of patients is very small. Handley has also studied the relationship of the site and size of the primary tumor to internal mammary metastasis. His

Table 33–16. BREAST CARCINOMA: COLUMBIA CLINICAL CLASSIFICATION STAGE A, INTERNAL MAMMARY NODE BIOPSY. SIZE AND POSITION IN BREAST OF PRIMARY TUMOR. PRESBYTERIAN AND DELAFIELD HOSPITALS, 1951–1966

Size of Primary	Inner Half of Breast, Zones C, D, E, and F			Center of Breast, Zone G			Outer Half of Breast, Zones A and B			Entire Breast		
	Cases	Positive	Per cent	Cases	Positive	Per cent	Cases	Positive	Per cent	Cases	Positive	Per cent
Less than 3 cm.	38	3	8%	22	2	9%	20	1	5%	80	6	8%
3 cm. or more	112	25	22%	135	28	21%	65	7	11%	312	60	19%
Totals	150	28	19%	157	30	19%	85	8	9%	392	66	17%

Table 33–17. Breast Carcinoma: Columbia Clinical Classification Stage A, internal mammary node invasion. Size and position in breast of primary tumor (R. S. Handley—Middlesex Hospital)

Size of Primary Carcinoma	Inner Half of Breast			Center of Breast			Outer Half of Breast			Entire Breast		
	Cases	Positive	Per cent	Cases	Positive	Per cent	Cases	Positive	Per cent	Cases	Positive	Per cent
1 inch and under	69	13	19%	17	2	12%	88	5	6%	174	35	20%
Over 1 inch	45	11	24%	23	8	35%	45	7	16%	113	26	23%
Totals	114	24	21%	40	10	25%	133	12	9%	287	61	21%

data (Table 33–17) also show that small tumors of the upper outer sector of the breast infrequently produce internal mammary metastases.

All patients in whom pathologic study of the surgical specimen reveals axillary metastases will, of course, be given this prophylactic internal mammary irradiation.

This new plan of treatment might give us better results for two reasons. The first is that we would largely avoid the error of missing and not treating occult internal mammary metastases. With our previous policy of preliminary internal mammary node biopsy, we have missed a good many of these metastases because we did not perform our biopsy in a large enough proportion of our patients. The second possible reason why our new policy may give us better results is that we may have been disseminating the disease with our internal mammary node biopsies.

The postoperative prophylactic irradiation to the internal mammary region that we propose for those treated with this new plan will be delivered to a comparatively small area limited above by the lower edge of the clavicle, below by the lower edge of the fourth costal cartilage, medially by the midline of the sternum, and laterally by a line parallel to and 4 cm. lateral to the sternal edge. To this area, we propose to deliver a tissue dose of 5000 to 6000 rads of high intensity irradiation at a depth of 3 cm. from the skin surface in a protracted dosage pattern over five to six weeks. This kind of irradiation penalizes the patient very little.

The small size of the internal mammary nodes, and their situation within a limited area only 3 or 4 cm. below the skin surface, probably explain why metastases in them are particularly vulnerable to this kind of irradiation. This has been our experience even in patients in whom internal mammary metastases have progressed to the stage where they form a parasternal tumor (Guttmann; Sanger). We have a number of these patients whose parasternal nodules have been treated only by irradiation, and they are well many years afterwards. Surgical procedures in the internal mammary region, with consequent fibrosis and perhaps surgical spread of the disease, probably diminish the effectiveness of irradiation to internal mammary metastases.

Apex of Axilla Biopsy

When the usefulness of preliminary internal mammary biopsy to determine the stage of breast carcinoma in selected cases became apparent to us we devised an additional type of biopsy of the periphery of the regional lymph node filter—biopsy of the apex of the axila. Our purpose was to make our determination of the extent of involvement of that regional lymph node filter more complete. Radical mastectomy invariably fails to cure when the lymph nodes at the apex of the axilla—the subclavicular nodes—are found to be involved. This is to be expected in view of the position of these subclavicular lymph nodes at the very apex of the axilla in the cleft between the axillary vein and the chest wall. There is literally no margin between these nodes and the adjacent structures which it is not reasonable to remove. It is a general rule of cancer surgery undertaken in any region of the body that if surgical excision is to succeed it must include a reasonable margin of uninvolved tissue beyond the cancer. This is lacking when the subclavicular nodes are involved.

There is another reason why there is no hope of cure when the subclavicular nodes are involved. The distance between involved subclavicular nodes and the grand central lymphatic terminus at the base of the neck where the subclavian lymphatic trunks empty into the confluence of the internal jugular and subclavian veins, is only about 3 cm. The likelihood that emboli from metastases in the subclavicular nodes have reached the venous stream at the time any treatment is contemplated is therefore very great. Whatever is done is only palliative, and we do not believe that any radical surgery is justified.

We realized that if we could determine by preliminary biopsy whether or not the subclavicular nodes are involved we would have an additonal method of determining the stage of advancement of breast carcinoma and we would be able to classify our cases more accurately. In 1955 we therefore added biopsy of the apex of the axilla to our preliminary biopsy procedure for selecting patients, which now could be called a triple biopsy, because the first step must of course be incisional biopsy of the primary tumor in the breast. Depending upon which group of nodes at the periphery of the regional lymphatic filter seemed most likely to be involved, we next performed biopsy of the internal mammary nodes or the nodes at the apex of the axilla. If grossly involved nodes were found in the first group to be explored, the third biopsy step was of course omitted.

Our apex of axilla biopsies have been fewer in number than our internal mammary biopsies, because we have not as often been in doubt regarding the extent of axillary involvement in operable cases as regarding the presence of internal mammary metastases. In the axilla we have the help of axillary palpation to guide us; internal mammary metastases are always occult in patients in whom there is any question of surgical treatment.

Although it has been difficult to follow a definite rule in the selection of patients for these biopsies, the apex of axilla biopsies have in general been performed in the three following groups of patients:

1. Clinical Stage A patients whose primary tumor is in the central sector or the lateral sectors of the breast (Zones G, A, and B) and measures more than 5 cm. in diameter.

2. Patients with clinically involved axillary nodes (Clinical Stage B).

3. Patients with more advanced disease.

When we were in doubt as to whether the clinical features of the patient's disease indicated that it was operable (Stages A and B) or inoperable (Stages C and D), we also often performed apex of axilla biopsy.

Biopsy of the nodes at the apex of the axilla is done through a short 6 to 8 cm. incision made just below and parallel to the middle of the clavicle. The pectoralis major muscle is retracted caudad and severed from its attachment to the clavicle. The deep axillary fascia is exposed, the highest part of the axillary vein identified, and the fascia incised caudad to it. This defines a small area between the axillary vein and the chest wall containing areolar tissue, in which are embedded a few small subclavicular nodes. This areolar tissue and the nodes in it are removed for biopsy. The operative field at the completion of this biopsy is shown in Figure 33–3. As with the tissue removed in internal mammary

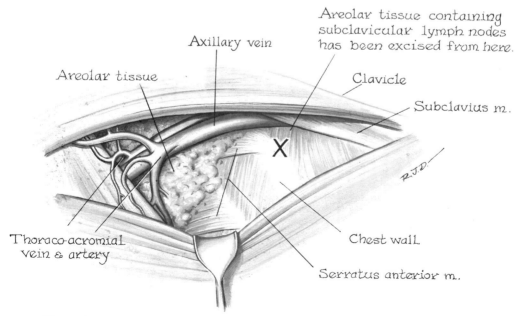

Figure 33–3. The operative field at completion of biopsy of the apex of the axilla.

biopsy, frozen sections should not be done on this tissue unless large grossly involved nodes are found.

We performed a total of 346 of these preliminary apex of axilla biopsies between 1955 and 1966, inclusive. The patients constituted about 15 per cent of our patients with breast carcinomas coming to the Presbyterian and Delafield Hospitals during this period. The subclavicular nodes were found to be involved in 25.1 per cent of the patients in whom this type of biopsy was done. They were, of course, patients whose disease was comparatively advanced.

In patients whose disease is classified as Clinical Stage A or B, the nodes at the apex of the axilla are less often involved. Between 1955 and 1959 we found metastases in only 10 of the 109 patients who had biopsy of the apex of the axilla. In these 10 no further operative procedure was done, and they were treated by irradiation alone. Nine succumbed to their disease after an average survival of 62 months. The tenth patient is still alive without obvious recurrence after 11 years. I believe that the apex of axilla biopsy was useful in these 10 patients in sparing them futile radical mastectomy. We will continue to perform preliminary biopsy of the apex of the axilla in patients in whom the extent of clinical involvement of the axilla suggests that the subclavicular nodes may be involved. This includes patients with more than one clinically involved axillary node and those who have a chain of such nodes extending high in the axilla, as well as those in whom it is questionable whether their involved axillary node is 2.5 cm, or more in diameter or fixed. When the subclavicular nodes are found to be involved, we will continue to treat these patients with irradiation alone because we know that they generally are incurable by surgical procedures.

Supraclavicular Lymph Node Biopsy

In Chapter 22 I reviewed the data concerning metastases to supraclavicular lymph nodes, emphasizing that these nodes are involved in the last stage of the extension of breast carcinoma through the regional lymph node filter. We have learned that if the extent of the disease is carefully assessed by our Columbia Clinical Classification, and biopsy of the apex of the axilla performed as a preliminary step in those patients in whom classification is doubtful, the number of patients whose disease is in Clinical Stage A or B and who develop supraclavicular metastases after radical mastectomy is very small. It is so small that preliminary biopsy of the supraclavicular nodes, as well as dissection of the supraclavicular region as part of radical mastectomy, is unjustified.

When a patient whose breast carcinoma is being classified as to stage of advancement has a palpable clinically involved supraclavicular node, we of course excise it, and if it is involved we treat the patient only with irradiation because we know that her disease is incurable by surgery.

The Site of Carcinoma in the Breast Related to Choice of Treatment

In our criteria of operability, and in our Columbia Clinical Classification, we have not given the site of the primary tumor in the breast any role.

Very few data as to the significance of the site of the carcinoma have been published. Smithers did not find any statistically significant differences in the survival rates for carcinoma of the different sectors of the breast in data from the Royal Cancer Hospital. Truscott reported that the five-year survival rate in the Middlesex Hospital data was slightly lower for lower inner sector carcinomas. Nohrman found in the Radiumhemmet data that Stage I carcinomas of the medial portion of the breast had a definitely poorer prognosis than Stage I carcinomas situated elsewhere in the breast. Urban and Baker, reviewing the Memorial Hospital data, found that carcinoma of the central and medial areas of the breast gave somewhat lower rates of cure than their breast carcinomas in general. They did not, however, present their actual rates of cure for tumors of the outer sectors of the breast, and they did not define their criteria for classification as to site in detail. Their data are therefore not very helpful.

Fisher and his associates have recently published data from 45 hospitals in which the site of the breast carcinoma is correlated with the five-year survival rate in 1005 patients. The method of recording the site of the tumor in the breast in this study is too complex to be practical and the data are not meaningful.

For the purpose of studying the relationship of the site of the primary tumor to the results of radical mastectomy I have turned again to my personal series of radical mastectomies. Since we are concerned with the significance of a single factor, namely the site of the tumor, we have excluded the patients who died of intercurrent disease before 10 years after operation. These data are shown diagrammatically in Figure 33-4, and in detail in Table 33-18.

These data show that the results of radical mastectomy are essentially the same wherever the primary tumor may be situated in the breast. The low survival rate for Zone D tumors and the high survival rate for Zone E tumors are not statistically significant because the numbers of patients are too small.

Carcinoma in the Inframammary Fold. As I emphasized in Chapter 5, the inframammary fold is a transverse ridge of denser tissue across the lower edge of the breast. Here the edge of the breast is bound down tightly to the deep fascia of the thoracic wall. A carcinoma developing in the inframammary fold is therefore often abnormally fixed to the underlying fascial planes of the chest wall, as compared with carcinoma elsewhere in the breast.

In order to study the operability of these carcinomas of the inframammary fold, and

Table 33-18. CARCINOMA OF BREAST. SITE OF PRIMARY TUMOR IN BREAST CORRELATED WITH 10-YEAR SURVIVAL. PERSONAL SERIES OF RADICAL MASTECTOMIES, 1935-1957, EXCLUDING 53 PATIENTS DYING OF INTERCURRENT DISEASE BEFORE 10 YEARS

Site of Tumor in Breast	No. of Patients	10-Year Survival No.	10-Year Survival Per cent
Upper Outer — Zone A	235	146	62.1%
Lower Outer — Zone B	45	28	62.2%
Lower Inner — Zone C	34	24	70.6%
Lower Parasternal — Zone D	9	5	55.6%
Upper Parasternal — Zone E	10	8	80.0%
Upper Inner — Zone F	74	47	63.5%
Central — Zone G	157	93	59.2%
Not Evident Clinically*	9	8	88.9%
Total	573	359	62.6%

*8 of the 9 in this group had Paget's carcinoma without a palpable tumor, and 7 of the 8 survived 10 years. The ninth patient had a microscopic focus of carcinoma found when her breast was removed for cystosarcoma.

particularly the significance of fixation of these tumors to the underlying chest wall, I selected a series of 26 of them from our records. I took care to choose cases in which the degree of attachment of the tumor to the underlying chest wall was clearly defined.

When an inframammary carcinoma is small, and lies within a prominent dense inframammary fold, it is not always easy to identify. Fortunately, almost all these carcinomas produce well defined retraction of the overlying skin, which either is obvious with simple inspection when the patient lies prone on the examining table, or can be elicited by molding the breast as shown in Figures 33-5 and 33-6.

When these carcinomas are larger, like that shown in Figure 33-7, their nature is obvious. It should be kept in mind, however, that a simple sebaceous cyst, like that shown in Figure 33-8, can resemble carcinoma in this location, and biopsy must always be done before radical surgical attack.

The main point of interest regarding these inframammary fold carcinomas is whether or not their fixation to the underlying chest wall renders them incurable by surgery. In this series of 26 which I studied, 24 had been treated by radical mastectomy more than 10 years previously. One of the 24 died of a cardiovascular accident eight years after operation, and is therefore properly excluded in a study of the significance of a single clinical factor like fixation.

I have defined two degrees of fixation of

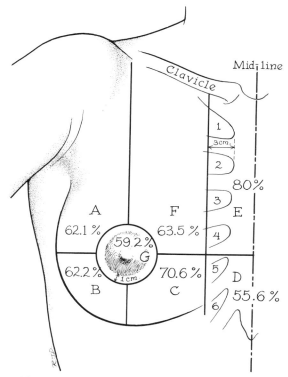

Figure 33-4. Ten-year survival rates for carcinoma in different sectors of the breast. Haagensen, personal series of radical mastectomies, 1935-1957.

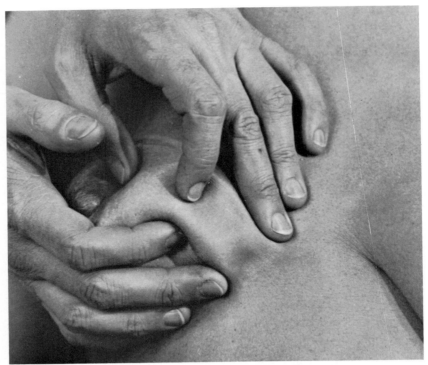

Figure 33–5. Skin retraction over a small carcinoma of the inner end of the inframammary fold.

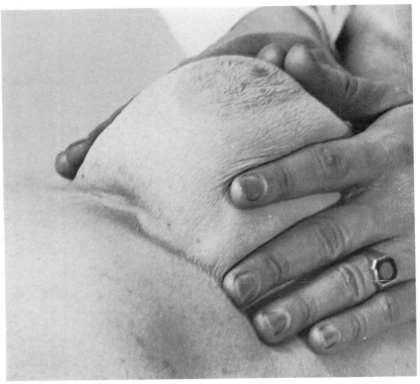

Figure 33–6. Skin retraction over a small carcinoma of the middle of the inframammary fold.

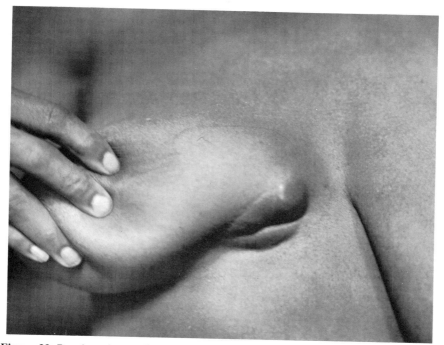

Figure 33–7.   An advanced carcinoma of the inner end of the inframammary fold.

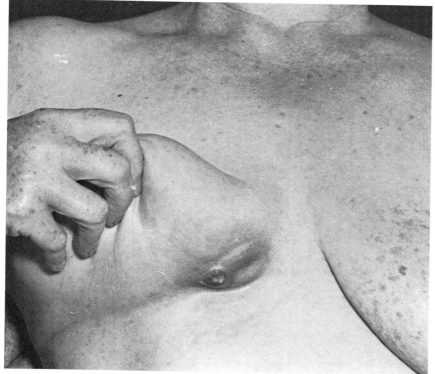

Figure 33–8.   An ulcerated sebaceous cyst of the inframammary fold of the breast simulating a carcinoma.

these carcinomas to the underlying structures of the chest wall. The first is *relative fixation*, in which movement of the breast over the chest wall is clearly diminished but not entirely abolished. The second is when the lesion is *solidly fixed* to the underlying structures.

The 10-year survival rates for radical mastectomy, and the frequency of axillary metastases, are correlated with the clinical stage in our series of inframammary carcinomas in Table 33-19. In the clinical classification of these cases the factor of the fixation of the tumor to the underlying chest wall has been disregarded. The presence of fixation to the underlying chest wall in these cases is correlated with 10-year survival in Table 33-20.

From these data it would appear that neither relative nor solid fixation to the chest wall is a contraindication to radical mastectomy for these inframammary fold carcinomas. Five of our 9 patients with relative fixation of their carcinomas, and four of the 9 patients whose carcinomas were solidly fixed to the chest wall survived 10 years after radical mastectomy. We have in the past regarded solid fixation of carcinoma to the chest wall as a contraindication to radical mastectomy. In the future we must make an exception for solidly fixed carcinomas of the inframammary fold. If there are no other contraindications these carcinomas should be classified as Clinical Stage A or B and treated by radical mastectomy.

There is, of course, one additional fact regarding carcinomas situated in the medial portion of the inframammary fold that may influence choice of treatment—they are very close to the internal mammary lymphatic route and metastases to the internal mammary nodes may be more frequent. There is some suggestion of this in our series of cases.

Table 33-19. TEN-YEAR SURVIVAL AFTER RADICAL MASTECTOMY AND FREQUENCY OF AXILLARY METASTASES IN CARCINOMA OF THE INFRAMAMMARY FOLD ACCORDING TO CLINICAL STAGE

Columbia Clinical Classification°	No. of Cases	Per cent with Axillary Metastases	Per cent 10-Year Survival
Stage A	15	20%	73%
Stage B	6	83%	17%
Stage C	2	100%	0%
Total	23		

*In classifying these cases the factor of fixation has been disregarded.

Table 33-20. FIXATION OF INFRAMAMMARY CARCINOMA CORRELATED WITH 10-YEAR SURVIVAL FOLLOWING RADICAL MASTECTOMY

Columbia Clinical Classification	Degree of Fixation to Chest Wall	Number Surviving 10 Years
Stage A	None – 3 patients	2
	Relative fixation – 6 patients	5
	Solid fixation – 6 patients	4
Stage B	None – 1 patient	1
	Relative fixation – 2 patients	0
	Solid fixation – 3 patients	0
Stage C	None – 1 patient	0
	Relative fixation – 1 patient	0

Two of our six patients with Clinical Stage B inframammary fold carcinoma developed clinically evident parasternal internal mammary metastases, three and four years, respectively, after radical mastectomy. Axillary metastases were present in both. In our new plan of treatment for mammary carcinoma these patients with carcinoma of the inframammary fold will all receive postoperative irradiation to the internal mammary area.

Our results with radical mastectomy in patients with carcinoma of the inframammary fold whose disease was classified as Clinical Stage A certainly justify the operation. Baclesse, however, reported the end-results in seven of these patients with inframammary fold carcinoma who were treated by irradiation alone, or by local excision of the primary tumor and irradiation. Six survived more than five years.

The Size of the Carcinoma Related to the Choice of Treatment

The size of the primary carcinoma in the breast is not a criterion in our Columbia Clinical Classification because we have learned that, like several other clinical features of breast carcinoma, it does not have a dominant influence upon prognosis. The International Clinical Classification uses four different categories of size for the primary tumor, and in so doing adds greatly to the complexity of the classification without adding much to its accuracy.

The size of the primary tumor does, of course, influence the results of treatment to some degree. To determine the extent of its influence we need data in which tumor size is correlated with 10-year survival rates. Bloom

Table 33–21. RADICAL MASTECTOMY FOR BREAST CARCINOMA. AVERAGE CLINICAL SIZE OF PRIMARY TUMOR. PERSONAL SERIES OF 626 PATIENTS, 1935–1957

Columbia Clinical Classification	Average Size of Primary Tumor
Stage A	3.0 cm.
Stage B	4.5 cm.
Stage C	5.8 cm.
Stage D	6.5 cm.
Average diameter	3.7 cm.

is one of the few who have provided such data. In Table 23–7 (p. 472) I have presented his data as well as that from my own personal series of cases.

Fisher has recently studied tumor size and prognosis in a series of 2000 cases of breast carcinoma collected from 45 different institutions. It is hardly to be expected that data from such a large number of different clinics, where the type of treatment must have varied

greatly, and the length of follow-up was only five years, can be as informative as data from a single clinic with a uniform treatment policy and a complete 10-year follow-up.

The data from my personal series of radical mastectomies shows very clearly that as breast carcinoma advances in terms of our Columbia Clinical Classification, the average size of the primary tumor increases (Table 33–21). But we now treat our patients with Clinical Stage C and D carcinoma by irradiation, not surgery. Thus the patients whose carcinomas are classified as Clinical Stage A and B are the only ones in whom the size of the primary tumor may be of practical value to us in relationship to the results of radical mastectomy.

In order to look more carefully into this relationship, I have studied it in my personal series of radical mastectomies by excluding the patients who died from intercurrent disease before 10 years after operation. In studying the significance of a single factor such as tumor size, the exclusion of these cases

Table 33–22. CARCINOMA OF BREAST BY CLINICAL STAGE. SIZE OF PRIMARY TUMOR CORRELATED WITH 10-YEAR SURVIVAL FOLLOWING RADICAL MASTECTOMY (PERSONAL SERIES OF CASES—1935–1957) EXCLUDING 53 PATIENTS WHO DIED OF INTERCURRENT DISEASE BEFORE 10 YEARS

Columbia Clinical Classification	Tumor Size	No. of Patients	Number 10-Year Survivors	Per cent 10-Year Survival
Stage A	Under 2 cm.	69	58	84.1%
	2–3 cm.	172	141	82.0%
	4–5 cm.	93	60	64.5%
	6 cm. or more	32	21	65.6%
	Total	366	280	76.5%
Stage B	Under 2 cm.	3	3	100.0%
	2–3 cm.	47	22	46.8%
	4–5 cm.	57	23	40.4%
	6 cm. or more	33	15	45.5%
	Total	140	63	45.0%
Stage C	Under 2 cm.	2	1	50.0%
	2–3 cm.	8	4	50.0%
	4–5 cm.	16	1	6.2%
	6 cm. or more	30	8	26.7%
	Total	56	14	25.0%
Stage D	Under 2 cm.	—	—	—
	2–3 cm.	2	—	0.0%
	4–5 cm.	3	1	33.3%
	6 cm. or more	6	1	16.7%
	Total	11	2	18.2%
All Stages	Under 2 cm.	74	62	83.8%
	2–3 cm.	229	167	72.9%
	4–5 cm.	169	85	50.3%
	6 cm. or more	101	45	44.6%
	Total	573	359	62.7%

sharpens the focus of the inquiry. Table 33-22 presents these data.

It is clear that for Clinical Stage A carcinomas the 10-year survival rate for tumors less than 4 cm. in diameter was significantly better—approximately 20 per cent better—than for carcinomas 4 cm. and larger. This is, however, the only definite conclusion that can be drawn from these data regarding the significance of tumor size. In Clinical Stage B the survival rates for tumors of different sizes were the same. We do not believe that these facts justify making tumor size a criterion in our Columbia Clinical Classification.

DISTANT METASTASES RELATED TO OPERABILITY

No one would deny that the demonstration of distant metastases in carcinoma of the breast is a contraindication to radical mastectomy. Yet many women are operated upon who have them. I cannot excuse a surgeon who performs radical mastectomy without having had roentgenograms of the chest. In addition, all patients whose disease has advanced beyond Clinical Stage A should have skeletal films. In our clinic they have revealed distant metastases in occasional patients, each time avoiding a futile radical mastectomy.

Unfortunately, as I have pointed out in Chapter 22, x-ray study is a crude and inaccurate method of demonstrating metastases. Over and over again, x-ray study fails to reveal metastases, yet they become evident within a year or two after radical mastectomy. Such metastases were undoubtedly present at the time of operation. We greatly need more efficient methods of demonstrating occult metastases in the bones and viscera.

At the Francis Delafield Hospital we have been attempting to develop new methods of demonstrating metastases in bones. We first studied the usefulness of bone marrow aspiration, utilizing the crest of the ilium. The smears made from the aspirated material were prepared as blood smears and studied by our hematologist and pathologist. Hyman summarized our results with this method. It did not yield as high a degree of accuracy as we had hoped. For example, in a series of 41 patients in whom skeletal metastases from breast carcinoma were demonstrated radiographically, aspiration of the iliac crest revealed carcinoma cells in only 10.

Trephine Biopsy in Determination of Distant Metastases

A method of trephine biopsy developed in the Francis Delafield Hospital by Dr. Wolfgang Ackermann has, however, proved much more successful. It has been used chiefly for biopsying the lower vertebrae, which are, of course, the commonest site of osseous metastases. Dr. Ackermann secures, with this method, a perfectly adequate cylinder of vertebral marrow. This is fixed and sectioned like any tissue specimen. Figure 33-9 shows such a biopsy specimen from a lumbar vertebra containing metastatic mammary carcinoma.

Dr. Ackermann's description of his method, summarized from his recent paper, follows.

Instruments. None of the available bone trephine instruments was satisfactory, and new ones had to be designed. The construction of the instruments was turned over to an instrument manufacturer in this particular field. Stainless steel was used for the construction of all parts, with the exception of the Luer attachments which are chrome-plated. After some initial improvements the final set was completed. It is composed of:

1. PERFORATOR (Fig. 33-10B and C). It has an over-all length of 4.5 cm. Its top is a 3 mm. thick, flat, solid, round, and knurled disc 18 mm. in diameter; its solid shaft, which is 2.5 mm. in diameter, ends with a 1 cm. long, three-edged, sharp-pointed cutting tip. The perforator serves for cutting skin and dense fasciae down to the muscles. It does it with ease, causing hardly any bleeding, unlike the knife customarily used.

2. LOCATOR (Fig. 33-10D). It has an over-all length of 15 cm. Its shaft is 2 mm. in diameter. Its top is like that of the perforator, but its 1 cm. long tip, which gradually narrows down to a dull point, has a smooth surface.

3. TREPHINE GUIDE (Fig. 33-10D). It is a tube with an over-all length of 14 cm. At its upper end is a 15 mm. long Luer needle-hub, to be used if additional Novocain to anesthetize the periosteum is needed. The outer surface of the tube, beginning at 4 cm. from the lower end, is graduated in 1 cm. intervals up to 10 cm. Its outside diameter is 2.5 mm., and its inner diameter readily admits both the locator and the trephine.

The purpose of the locator is to direct the trephine guide to the area to be biopsied.

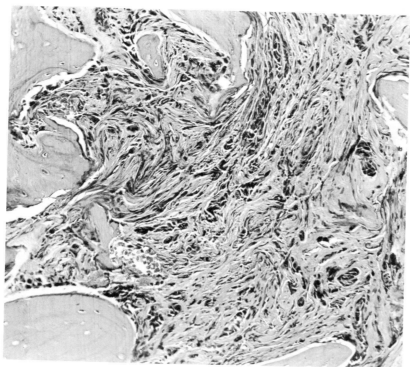

Figure 33–9. Tissue from a lumbar vertebra obtained by trephine biopsy, showing metastatic breast carcinoma.

When the locator is completely inserted into the trephine guide, both are combined as a unit, and as such the unit is inserted into the opening made in the skin by the perforator.

When in use as a unit the 1 cm. long tip of the locator protrudes beyond the trephine guide. Because of its dull point, it can easily advance the unit forward through muscles and thin fasciae, but not through nerves or blood vessels, which are not injured by the non-cutting instruments if limited force is applied.

4. TWO TREPHINES (Fig. 33–11*B*). One is short and the other long. The short trephine is a tube with an over-all length of 16.75 cm. At its upper end is a Luer needle-hub, for eventual bone marrow aspiration. Below the needle-hub is a knurled disk. This disk has the same dimensions as the disks of the perforator and the locator. While the disks of the perforator and locator serve to facilitate their insertion, the trephine disk is used to facilitate cutting into the bone by a rotating motion. The ouside diameter of the trephine is 2 mm. and its inner diameter is 1.5 mm. Its tip has a serrated edge, and it represents a circular saw with six very fine sharp teeth beveled on the leading edge for cutting. The inner bore is straight to permit easy advancement of the core-like specimen up the trephine.

The long trephine is exactly the same as the short one, except that it is 1.25 cm. longer. Thus it has an over-all length of 18 cm.

5. TWO EXTRUDERS (Fig. 33–11*D*). One is short and the other long. They actually are stylets for the corresponding trephines, with the sole purpose of extruding the specimens. They, too, are topped with knurled disks, which are 7 mm. in diameter, reinforced to facilitate expelling of the specimens.

Technique. On May 12, 1954, the first vertebral trephine biopsy was performed on a patient. It was carried out in the Department of Radiology, with the patient on an x-ray table and under a Novocain-block anesthesia. No difficulties of any kind were encountered. The procedure has since undergone a number of modifications. At present the technique is being performed as follows:

1. One-half hour before the operation takes place the patient receives an intermuscular injection of 100 mg. of Demerol for sedation.

2. Immediately upon arrival in the Roentgenologic Department the patient is placed on the x-ray table in the prone position, with

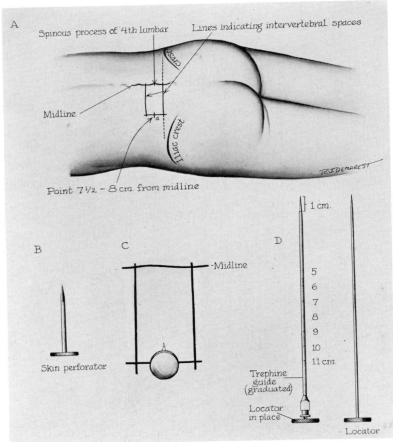

Figure 33–10. Trephine biopsy. *A*, Landmarks of L-4 to be biopsied; *B*, perforator with its three-edged tip; *C*, perforator in situ; *D*, locator without and with trephine guide combined as a unit, with graduations in centimeters, and a 1 cm. long smooth tip.

an extra pillow under the lower abdomen so that the spinous interspaces are widened and the landmarks more easily established (Fig. 33–10*A*).

3. With a dermatograph, a line is drawn across the lower back at the level of the margins of both iliac crests. This line passes either over the body of L-4 or, as it does most of the time, over the fourth interspace between L-4 and L-5.

4. A line is drawn along the midline over the lumbar spinous processes down to the sacrum.

The left side of the patient is routinely preferred for the biopsy because on the left the aorta is situated more anteriorly than the vena cava on the right. There is therefore less chance of injuring the aorta when the left side is used than of injuring the vena cava when the right side is used. There is also the fact that the right kidney, being topographically

lower than the left, can be more easily damaged.

5. Lines are drawn along the interspaces above and below the vertebra to be biopsied. These lines, which are parallel to each other, extend from the midline laterally for a distance of 8 cm., except in patients who weigh 100 pounds or less, in whom a distance of only 7 cm. is used. The lateral ends of these parallel lines are then connected by a perpendicular line, and at its center a cross is marked. This is the entrance point for the nerve block, as well as for the perforator.

6. The skin of the back is prepared, as for any other operation, and the area is draped.

7. At the cross mark a skin wheal is followed by a paravertebral nerve block with 10 to 15 ml. of 1 per cent Novocain, without adrenalin if only one vertebra is biopsied. The posterior root must be included in the nerve block because a branch of it supplies

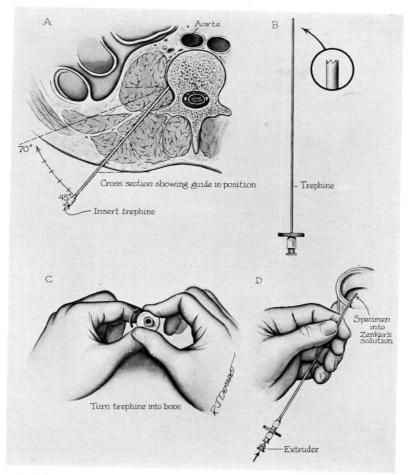

Figure 33–11. Trephine biopsy. *A*, Angulation range of the trephine guide on a cross section; *B*, trephine and its serrated tip (insert); *C*, trephining procedure; *D*, inspection of extruded specimen prior to placing in Zenker's solution.

the periosteum—the most sensitive structure involved in this operation—as well as the bone proper.

8. Immediately upon completion of the paravertebral block, the perforator is introduced at the cross mark through the skin and thick fasciae down to the muscles for a depth of 3 cm.

9. The locator, together with the trephine guide as a unit, is inserted through the track thus established, and advanced medially and downward, at an angle of about 45 degrees until the body of the vertebra is encountered, usually at a depth of 8 to 9 cm. In emaciated people the distance is 6 to 7 cm.

10. The point of the locator is bored into the cortex of the vertebra to make it stay in place for the radiographic check.

11. Roentgenographs in anteroposterior and lateral views are taken, and the position of the instrument is checked in the wet films.

If, unlike that in Figure 33–12, its position does not appear satisfactory, the necessary adjustment is made. The locator can easily be swung up or down, forward or backward, changing the angulation to a more or less acute bend. The topographical relations of the instrument to the nerve roots as well as to the large vessels must always be kept in mind.

12. The trephine guide, which in the unit is 1 cm. shorter than the locator, is advanced for that distance and brought into contact with the vertebral body. It is held fast in that position by the left index finger and thumb.

13. The locator is removed and replaced by the short trephine, which is brought into contact with the vertebral body. With gentle pressure, the trephine is slowly driven through the periosteum and cortex and into the marrow by rotation of its knurled disk.

14. Roentgenographs are taken in two

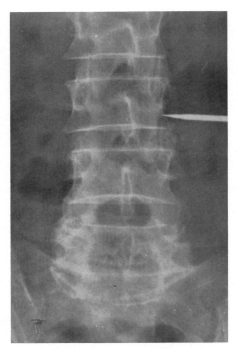

Figure 33–12. The tip of the locator bored in the cortex of L-3 in a satisfactory position for biopsy.

views for the second time. The wet films are again checked for the exact location, as well as for the angulation of the trephine. Figure 33–13 shows the trephine driven about half way in the body of L-3.

15. The trephine is now rotated several times clockwise, without dislodging it, in order to break off the core-like specimen. The trephine is then withdrawn with a continuous slow rotating motion.

16. The trephine guide, still being in contact with the vertebral body, is now adjusted as to the most desired angulation. The long trephine is then introduced both through the guide and through the track cut by the short trephine through the cortex, and bored into the vertebra to its full length.

Because the long trephine cuts more deeply into the vertebral marrow than the short trephine, it obtains a specimen not only from a different location but also at a different depth. This second specimen therefore has less cortical bone and more marrow.

17. The long trephine is now left in place, and by means of the extruder the specimen from the short trephine is expelled into the bottle of Zenker's solution.

18. The long trephine is removed, and the

specimen is expelled from it by the extruder, and its characteristics are observed.

This procedure of obtaining two specimens can, if necessary, be repeated once or twice on the same vertebra, either above or below the area just biopsied, thus giving the pathologist specimens not only from different depths but also from different levels.

Since metastases in bones are nearly always multiple, it may be desirable to do biopsies of more than one vertebra. If the second vertebra to be biopsied is adjacent to the first one, the procedure is carried out from the same entrance point by directing the instrument upward or downward at an acute angle in relation to the midline (Fig. 33–14). This maneuver must, of course, be preceded by a nerve block of the corresponding root.

Our experience with the trephine biopsy method convinces us that it should be used whenever pain suggests bone metastases and their presence can not be confirmed by roentgenographs. In this way the presence of metastases can be proven and the patient spared a futile radical mastectomy.

Trephine biopsy can also be of value in ruling out vertebral metastases, thereby saving the patient from unnecessary radiotherapy. There is an infrequent nonneoplastic lesion of the vertebrae characterized by the development of a dense area of sclerosis in the vertebral body. These lesions are usually single and fairly large. They are situated contiguous to the edge of the vertebrae. Their etiology is unknown, but in several instances they have been associated with disc disease. When they occur in a patient who has breast carcinoma, they naturally suggest the osteoblastic type of metastasis. If there is any clinical reason to doubt this diagnosis, trephine biopsy should be done. Ackermann and Schwarz have described several of these cases in which trephine biopsy was of decisive value. One of them is summarized.

The patient had had a breast carcinoma without axillary metastases operated upon 13 years previously. She returned complaining of lower back pain. In her x-ray films a single area of increased density was seen in the body of the second lumbar vertebra. This was diagnosed by the roentgenologist as metastasis. Fortunately for the patient, we were doubtful of the nature of the vertebral lesion, first because her carcinoma had been a favorable one operated upon long ago, and second, because of its x-ray appearance. A trephine biopsy revealed only sclerotic bone with no evidence of metastasis.

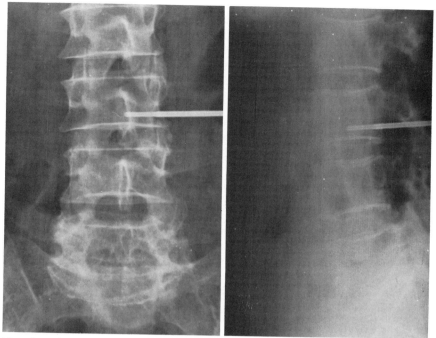

Figure 33–13.   Anterior-posterior and lateral views of the trephine driven halfway into the body of L-3.

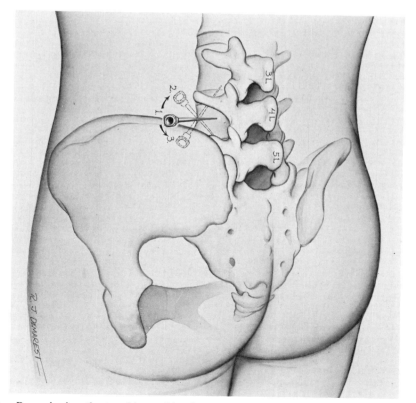

Figure 33–14.   By swinging the trephine guide alone or in combination with the locator tip up or down, from the same entrance point, biopsies of two or even three vertebrae can be performed at one operation.

The Detection of Bone Metastases with Radioisotope Techniques

During recent years efforts have been made in a number of clinics to utilize radioisotopes to identify bone metastases (Corey et al.; Gynning et al.; Pearson et al.; Ackerman; Sklaroff and Charkes; Charkes et al; Briggs; Rubin and Ciccio). Strontium-85, which is concentrated to some degree in metastases in bone, has been the isotope most used. But the method is complex and expensive, and the evidence gained from it is so difficult to interpret and so uncertain that it has not been widely adopted. My own experience with it, although limited to a few cases, has not convinced me of the practical value of the radioisotope technique.

In some clinics it is the custom to carry out serum calcium determinations in all patients with breast carcinoma, searching for evidence of bone metastases. Disturbances of calcium metabolism of course develop in patients with advanced breast carcinoma and extensive bone metastases. However, I have not seen abnormal calcium levels in patients whose disease had not advanced beyond Clinical Stage A or B, and who had no clinical evidence of bone metastases. Calcium studies are thus of no value as criteria of operability.

CONSTITUTIONAL FACTORS RELATING TO CHOICE OF TREATMENT

There are three factors in the constitution, so to speak, of patients with carcinoma of the breast, which play a role in the choice of treatment. They are (1) youth, (2) old age and debility, and (3) pregnancy and lactation.

Breast Carcinoma in Children

Below the age of 20, carcinoma of the breast is a medical curiosity. In Pirquet's monumental tabulation of English mortality data that included 70,257 deaths from breast carcinoma, there was one case of a child under the age of 5 years, one case of a child between the ages of 10 and 14, and five cases of children between the ages of 15 and 19.

During the last 60 years, there have been only six single case reports of breast carcinoma occurring in children between the ages

of 6 and 14 which were sufficiently detailed and justified the conclusion that the lesions were genuine mammary carcinomas. Four of these were in girls (Thompson; Levings; Sears and Schlesinger; Haagensen) and two were in boys (Simmons; Hartman and Magrish). Hartman and Magrish's report and mine were the only one that include follow-up. In 1966, McDivitt and Stewart reported seven additional cases sent to them in consultation. All were girls between the ages of 3 and 15. These lesions were unquestioned infiltrating carcinomas. McDivitt and Stewart pointed out that all the seven tumors they studied showed eosinophilic droplets of secretion within the cytoplasm, although the surrounding breast tissue showed no secretory activity. Care must be taken to distinguish these carcinomas occurring in adolescents from malignant hemangioendothelioma, which develops in this same age group. A highly malignant tumor occurring in a 15 year old girl, described by Chauvel and Renaud, was probably a hemangioendothelioma.

Although these lesions look like ordinary breast carcinomas they do not behave as such. Only one of the 13 lesions I have referred to metastasized. This was the one described by Hartman in a 6 year old boy. Radical mastectomy was performed and metastasis found in one of 21 axillary nodes. The child was well 11 years later.

Equally significant is the fact that local excision has cured these carcinomas in three of the four patients in which it was used in McDivitt and Stewart's series of cases, and also in the case I have reported. In McDivitt and Stewart's case in which local excision failed, the patient had a 1 cm. tumor excised at the age of three. Two years later a second local excision for recurrence was performed. A second local recurrence developed six years later. Mastectomy was then apparently successful.

The history of the patient whose lesion was studied in our laboratory illustrates very well the fact that these carcinomas in children are not malignant in the usual sense of the word, and suggests that local excision is the appropriate treatment.

A. J. S. first came under the observation of Dr. George H. Semken when she was 9 years and 7 months of age. She had had a tumor of the right breast since the age of 5 years. It was situated beneath the edge of the areola, and extended lateral to it, between the radii of 8:30 and 11 o'clock.

Dr. Semken observed the tumor for some six

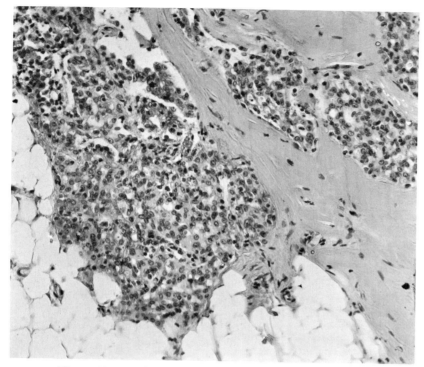

Figure 33–15. Carcinoma of the breast in a girl aged 15.

years, until the patient was 15 years and 10 months old, and the tumor had grown to about 3 cm. in diameter. The right breast, in which the tumor was situated, was retarded in development. On April 12, 1945, he excised the tumor locally. Dr. Stout described it as a firm, sharply circumscribed nodule enclosed in a little fat. It measured 25 × 18 × 13 mm. Microscopically, it was a carcinoma composed of strands and cords of epithelial tumor cells that showed very little tendency to form acini, but anastomosed, one with another, to infiltrate the surrounding fat (Fig. 33–15). Mitoses averaged one in every five or six high power fields.

Twenty-five years later the patient is well. There has been no recurrence of the breast tumor despite the fact that only a very limited local excision had been done. She has had two children, but has not nursed them.

The fact of the rare occurrence of these carcinoma-like, clinically comparatively benign lesions of the breasts in children does not justify the excision of a tumor developing beneath the areola in a child. As I have pointed out in Chapter 3, in occasional children the breast begins to develop precociously and unilaterally as a small nubbin of tissue beneath the areola. If the surgeon excises this supposed *tumor*, he removes the breast.

Breast Carcinoma Between Puberty and the Age of Thirty

The incidence of carcinoma of the breast is very low under the age of 30. In our own series of 6000 patients only 1.2 per cent were under 30. There were 72 of them. Their age distribution is shown in Table 33-23.

These carcinomas of the breast in women under 30 had no special clinical features except that they were larger than the carcinomas of older women. In my personal series of

Table 33–23. AGE DISTRIBUTION OF 72 PATIENTS WITH BREAST CARCINOMA BETWEEN PUBERTY AND THE AGE OF 30

Age	No. of Patients
20	1
21	1
22	1
23	4
24	4
25	9
26	5
27	10
28	10
29	27

patients of all ages the average diameter of their carcinomas by clinical measurement has been 3.7 cm; in this series of women under 30 the average diameter was 5.3 cm. I have not included in this computation four patients in whom the entire breast was involved by the lesion.

Our data regarding the duration of symptoms in these women under 30 are not accurate enough to be worth comparing with the duration in my personal series of cases. But since the tumors of the younger group of women were so much larger, I believe it is reasonable to assume that the carcinomas in these women under 30 grew faster than breast carcinomas in older women.

Nine of the 72 women under 30 are known to have developed another primary carcinoma in the contralateral breast. This is a very high incidence of bilateral carcinoma, considering the comparatively short time that most of these patients survived.

Another important aspect of carcinoma of the breast in young women is the frequency with which it is associated with pregnancy. Thirteen of our 72 patients under 30 were pregnant. Pregnancy certainly adds to the gravity of the disease, as I will demonstrate in a subsequent discussion of this problem.

These carcinomas of the breast developing in our series of 72 women under this age of 30 were of all the usual pathologic types. Only one feature merits mention, namely, that a total of 8, or 11 per cent, were the circumscribed type. This is several times the normal frequency of this type of carcinoma. It is in agreement with our finding, reported in Chapter 30, that patients with the solid circumscribed type of breast carcinoma are younger than patients with breast carcinomas of other microscopic types.

Studies of case series of breast carcinoma in young women published during the last 25 years reveal marked variation in the survival rates. Smithers reported a five-year survival rate of 25 per cent for his patients in the age group of 21 to 30, as compared with a 36.5 per cent five-year survival rate for patients of all age groups. Nohrmann's experience was similar: the five-year survival rate in the 21 to 30 age group in his series of patients was 22 per cent, as compared with 40 per cent for patients of all ages. In contrast, Harrington reported that the five-year survival rate in a series of 88 women from 20 to 29 years of age was 60 per cent, as compared with a survival rate of 47 per cent for 5314 women

aged 30 years or older. Richards, in his series of 906 cases, also found the prognosis to be better in the younger than the older group. Macdonald and Wilcox, reviewing a series of 55 cases of breast carcinoma in women 30 years of age or younger, found the five-year survival rate to be 43.4 per cent, which was somewhat better than "that reported in large series of patients of all ages." The largest series of breast carcinomas in young women reported is that of Treves and Holleb. They had a total of 124 patients under the age of 31 treated by radical mastectomy. The five-year survival rate for these young women was 41 per cent, as compared with a five-year survival rate of 39.6 per cent for 13,000 Memorial Hospital patients of all ages. Treves and Holleb concluded that "breast cancer in young women offers a prognosis equal to that of older women."

More recent papers by White, by Berndt et al., and by Moore and Lewis present results in small series of women 30 years of age and younger. The five-year survival rates range from 35.9 to 48 per cent.

There are three defects common to all these reports of case series of younger women with breast carcinoma. (1) The patients have not been carefully classified as to the clinical stage of advancement of their disease; (2) ten-year follow-up data are not provided; and (3) the results of treatment in these young women are not compared with the results in older patients whose carcinomas were classified in the same way.

From our clinic we have a series of 72 patients under the age of 30 with breast carcinoma. In all patients, the stage of advancement of the disease has been classified by our Columbia Clinical Classification. Fifty-nine of them had 66 breast carcinomas and applied for treatment more than 10 years ago. The end-results are known in all 59. They are shown in Table 33-24.

Reviewing our results with the treatment of breast carcinoma in our patients under the age of 30, as shown in this table, the first point to emphasize is that the only patients who survived 10 years were treated by radical mastectomy. The second point is that in all but one of the 17 patients who survived 10 years, their disease was classified as Clinical Stage A. The 10-year survival rate for radical mastectomy in these Clinical Stage A cases was 51 per cent.

I can best evaluate these results of radical mastectomy in our patients under the age of

Table 33–24. CARCINOMA OF THE BREAST BELOW THE AGE OF 30.
10-YEAR SURVIVAL BY CLINICAL STAGE AND TYPE OF TREATMENT.
COLUMBIA-PRESBYTERIAN HOSPITAL, 1912–1960

Columbia Clinical Classification	Treatment	No. of Patients	Axillary Findings	Number Surviving 10 Years	Per cent Surviving 10 Years
Stage A	Radical mastectomy	31	No axillary metastases, 22	14	51%
			Axillary metastases, 9	2	
	Irradiation	1		0	0
	No treatment	1		0	0
Stage B	Radical mastectomy	4	Axillary metastases, 4	1	25%
	Simple mastectomy and irradiation	1		0	0
	Irradiation	1		0	0
Stage C	Radical mastectomy	2	Axillary metastases, 2	0	0
	Irradiation	3		0	0
Stage D	Radical mastectomy	7	Axillary metastases, 7	0	0
	Irradiation	8		0	0
Total		59		17	30%

30 by comparing them with the results of this operation in my personal series of all patients classified by age and clinical stage as presented in Table 33-25.

In this compilation I have excluded the patients who succumbed to intercurrent disease—a method of sharpening the focus upon the significance of a single factor.

The number of our patients under 30 was large enough to have significance in a comparison of results only in Clinical Stage A. In this clinical stage 51 per cent of our 59 patients under 30 treated by radical mastectomy survived 10 years (Table 33-24), as compared with 76.4 per cent of the patients over 30 in my personal series of cases (Table 33-25). This fact confirms my own clinical impression that the prognosis for breast carcinoma in these young women is not as good as it is in our older patients. Radical mastectomy is, of course, the correct treatment for these young patients, but the prognosis should be guarded.

The following history of a patient of mine illustrates, however, that even in these young women radical mastectomy sometimes succeeds surprisingly well.

Mrs. H. S., a 29 year old housewife, whose elder sister had succumbed at this same age to carcinoma of the breast and whose mother had also died of the disease, came to me in March, 1940, with a history of a tumor of her right breast of six weeks' duration. It was situated in the lower outer sector of the breast, measured 2.5 cm. in diameter, and was hard and fixed in the surrounding breast tissue. There were no clinically involved axillary nodes. Radical mastectomy was performed after incisional biopsy had proved that the lesion was a carcinoma. Twenty-five axillary nodes did not contain metastases.

Eight months later I found a new tumor in her left breast. It was situated in the upper outer sector of the breast, measured 2.5 cm. in diameter, and had the characteristics of a carcinoma. There were no clinically involved axillary nodes. Incisional biopsy was done and the new lesion proved to be an independent carcinoma of the contralateral breast. At radical mastectomy 28 axillary nodes were found. None contained metastases.

Table 33–25.   CARCINOMA OF BREAST BY CLINICAL STAGE. AGE OF PATIENT CORRELATED WITH 10-YEAR SURVIVAL FOLLOWING RADICAL MASTECTOMY. PERSONAL SERIES OF CASES, 1935–1957, EXCLUDING 53 PATIENTS WHO DIED OF INTERCURRENT DISEASE BEFORE 10 YEARS

Columbia Clinical Classification	Age	No. of Patients	No. Surviving 10 Years	Per cent Surviving 10 Years	No. of Patients Excluded
Stage A	Under 30*	1	1	100.0%	
	30–64	310	242	78.1%	
	65 and over	55	37	67.3%	
	Total	366	280	76.5%	36
Stage B	Under 30*	3	1	33.3%	
	30–64	115	54	47.0%	
	65 and over	22	8	36.4%	
	Total	140	63	45.0%	14
Stage C	Under 30*	1	—	0.0%	
	30–64	46	10	21.7%	
	65 and over	9	4	44.4%	
	Total	56	14	25.0%	3
Stage D	Under 30*	—	—	—	
	30–64	8	—	0.0%	
	65 and over	3	2	66.7%	
	Total	11	2	18.2%	—
All Stages	Under 30*	5	2	40.0%	
	30–64	479	306	63.9%	
	65 and over	89	51	57.3%	
	Total	573	359	62.7%	53

*In this personal series of cases the numbers of patients under the age of 30 are too small to have any significance.

It is interesting to recount that the patient had had no children after eight years of marriage when she developed these bilateral breast carcinomas. Despairing of having children of their own, she and her husband adopted a child five years later. Two years later, in 1947, she became pregnant and was delivered of a normal child.

She is well 30 years after her bilateral breast carcinomas were treated by radical mastectomy.

Carcinoma of the Breast in Old Age

As the life expectancy of elderly women continues to lengthen, more of them develop breast carcinoma, and clinicians increasingly face the problem of how to treat their disease. They often decide to treat their elderly patients with breast carcinoma less vigorously than their middle-aged patients, assuming that the progress of the disease in aged patients is less rapid than in younger patients and the aged patients will succumb to intercurrent disease before their breast carcinomas trouble them. Surgeons also fear that their aged patients cannot withstand radical mastectomy. Both of these assumptions are probably false, and need to be critically tested.

There are surprisingly few published data correlating the age of patients with breast carcinoma with long-term survival rates. Spratt and Donegan, in studying their series of 704 patients, found no statistically significant differences in the age-specific five-year survival rates after radical mastectomy, corrected for natural mortality. Ratzkowski and Hochman correlated age with the length of survival in a series of 338 patients who had inoperable breast carcinoma. They found no statistically significant differences in the length of survival in the different age groups. Kraft and Block reviewed their experience in treating 75 women over the age of 75 who had breast carcinoma, and concluded that the disease is not less malignant in these aged patients. Axillary metastases were found in 66 per cent of their aged patients treated by radical mastectomy, while 55 per cent of their patients of all ages had them.

The results in my own personal series of patients with breast carcinoma treated by radical mastectomy, as presented in Table 33–25, which correlates them with age, provide useful information regarding the comparative malignancy of the disease in older patients. In both Clinical Stage A and Clinical Stage B, patients 65 years of age and older had a 10 per cent poorer 10-year survival rate than patients between the ages of 30 and 64 years. This difference cannot be explained by intercurrent disease because, as best we could, we excluded from the tabulation the patients dying from intercurrent disease. The facts suggest that breast carcinoma may be more malignant when it occurs in older patients.

The data from my personal series of 1007 patients treated by radical mastectomy (1935–1968) show no significant difference in the frequency of microscopically verified axillary metastases in the different age groups. These data were presented in Table 22–5 on page 400.

There is a widely held impression that elderly patients cannot withstand radical mastectomy. For example, Berg and Robbins found at the Memorial Hospital that operation carried a definitely increased operative mortality in the older age group, and advised the use of extended simple mastectomy. Hosbein and Mithoefer, on the other hand, have emphasized that modern supportive measures have made it possible to perform radical mastectomy on most elderly patients with breast carcinoma, and they recommend the radical operation.

I can best document my opinion that most aged patients can withstand radical mastectomy, provided the operation is gently and skillfully performed, by again referring to my experience in my personal series of patients. In this series of consecutive radical mastectomies performed between 1935 and 1957 there were a total of 109 patients 65 years of age or older. In 103 of them the operation was my usual radical mastectomy. One of the best indications of the thoroughness of radical mastectomy is the time the surgeon devotes to it. My average operating time in my personal series of patients of all ages is 330 minutes. In the 103 patients 65 years of age or older in whom I did my radical mastectomy it was 247 minutes, or 83 minutes less. This was achieved by making a special effort to hasten the dissection without omitting any of its principal features. I have no doubt but that saving this amount of operating time in these elderly patients makes good sense.

In three of my 109 patients who were 65 years of age or older the breast was large and there was sufficient skin to perform an adequate excision and close the wound primarily without a skin graft. This shortened the oper-

ating time somewhat: it was 190, 180, and 255 minutes, respectively. None of these patients developed local recurrence.

In three other aged patients in my series of 109, the operation was somewhat modified to reduce the risk involved. The details of these three cases follow:

CASE 1

Mrs. A. W., aged 78, had had degenerative joint disease and hypertension for some years, but was nevertheless fairly active. She had typical Paget's erosion of the left nipple, but no palpable breast tumor and no clinically involved axillary nodes.

Because of the presumed limited extent of her carcinoma, and her comparatively advanced age, the operation was modified by leaving the pectoralis major intact, and dividing the pectoralis minor. The operating time was 270 minutes. There were no metastases in 18 axillary nodes.

The patient did well postoperatively and had had no recurrence 10 years later.

CASE 2

A housewife aged 72 had had moderately severe hypertensive cardiovascular disease for seven years and had taken digitalis intermittently. Her carcinoma was situated in the upper outer sector of her left breast. It was 4 cm. in diameter and was accompanied by marked skin retraction. There was a 1-cm. clinically involved axillary node.

It was decided to limit the operative attack somewhat because of her cardiovascular disease. Accordingly, the pectoralis major was not removed. The pectoralis minor was cut across to give access to the upper axilla. Twenty-one axillary nodes were removed: three from the central group of nodes contained metastases. The skin flaps were brought together without a graft. Operating time was 190 minutes.

The patient stood the operation well. She had no recurrence of her breast carcinoma but died of a cerebral hemorrhage 6 years and 2 months after her mastectomy.

CASE 3

Mrs. A. P. was 89. She was, except for crippling arthritis, in comparatively good health. Her carcinoma was 5 cm. in diameter and was situated in the upper central portion of her left breast. There was a 1 cm. clinically involved axillary node.

Because of her advanced age a limited operation was done in which the pectoralis major was not removed. Only the lateral half of the axilla was dissected. Twenty-five nodes were removed. None contained metastases. The wound was closed without skin grafting. Operating time was 200 minutes.

She stood the operation well. There was never any recurrence of her carcinoma. She died of cardiovascular disease within one month of her 100th birthday, 11 years after her mastectomy.

Our experience has taught us that neither moderately advanced cardiovascular disease nor advanced age are today contraindications to radical mastectomy. With expert anesthesia and careful preoperative and postoperative care these patients tolerate operation well, provided that the dissection is performed gently and with exact hemostasis.

It may be wise to curtail the extent of the operation somewhat in exceptional cases, but even in these cases the operation must include careful removal of the entire breast and dissection of the axilla.

There is no place, in my opinion, for simple mastectomy. If this is done, it must be supplemented by irradiation. It is more difficult for these aged and decrepit patients to get through protracted daily irradiation for 6 or 8 weeks than it is to have a skillfully performed radical mastectomy.

Elderly patients should be gotten out of bed earlier than younger patients. We try to get them up by their fourth to sixth postoperative day.

Patients who have had previous thrombophlebitis must be watched with special care for recurrence of the thrombophlebitis and for embolism. They probably should be given anticoagulation therapy prophylactically beginning on the second postoperative day.

Diabetes is common in these elderly patients with cardiovascular disease. Its management presents no special problem.

There were no operative deaths and no serious postoperative complications in the 109 patients of age 65 and over in my personal series of radical mastectomies. While good fortune has no doubt played a part in the record, I have made a great effort to care for my patients personally.

Carcinoma of the Breast in Pregnancy

Carcinoma of the breast developing during pregnancy or lactation is a dread disease. All experienced clinicians are aware of its grave prognosis. Yet it can sometimes be cured. Our need today is to find criteria which will enable us to select the patients in whom cure by radical mastectomy is possible.

As I have emphasized above, the search for such criteria of operability for breast carcinoma has been one of our main objectives for many years at the Columbia-Presbyterian Medical Center. When Dr. Stout and I re-

viewed the results of the treatment of breast carcinoma in our clinic 28 years ago, we found that no patient in whom the disease had appeared during pregnancy or lactation had been cured. To be sure, the total number of such patients operated upon was small. There were only 20, and 19 had microscopically proved axillary metastases.

About the same time (1937), Harrington reported his results with radical mastectomy in a much larger series of cases of breast carcinoma developing during pregnancy or lactation. The outcome was almost as bad in his case series. He reported upon a total of 24 patients in whom the disease appeared during pregnancy and radical mastectomy revealed axillary metastases; none was cured. In 54 other patients, the disease was diagnosed during lactation, and radical mastectomy revealed axillary metastases; 10.4 per cent of those traced (number traced not stated) survived 10 years. It should be added that Harrington in his report also included 14 cases in which radical mastectomy had been done and no axillary metastases had been found: 40 per cent of those traced (number traced not stated) survived 10 years.

These facts led us to conclude in 1943 that radical mastectomy was not justified in patients with breast carcinoma developing during pregnancy or lactation.

We did not persist long with this point of view, however. Within a few years, several patients with breast carcinoma in pregnancy who had been operated upon in our clinic survived for a longer time, and we began to doubt the validity of our interdiction of operation. We were also influenced by the fact that surgeons from other clinics, stimulated by our emphasis upon this bad prognosis of breast carcinoma in pregnancy, convinced us that occasionally these patients could be cured by operation. In 1949, we withdrew our objection to radical mastectomy for breast carcinoma in pregnancy; and pregnancy has never since been included among our contraindications to operation. Looking backward from the vantage point of 28 years of further intensive experience with breast carcinoma, we can only emphasize that our error was the result of drawing conclusions from too small a series of cases.

It might still be argued, of course, that "error" is too strong a word. In his contemporary report, Harrington stated that, of the patients that he was able to trace, only 14.5 per cent survived for 5 years and only 8.7 per cent survived for 10 years (number traced not

Table 33–26. RESULTS OF TREATMENT OF BREAST CARCINOMA DURING PREGNANCY

Year	Author	Status of Patient	No. of Cases	5-Year Results
1929	Kilgore	Pregnancy and lactation	49	17% Well
1937	Harrington	Pregnancy and lactation	92	14.5% Survival*
1955	White	Pregnancy and lactation	27	33.3% Survival
1956	Haagensen	Pregnancy and lactation	31	32% Well
1962	Holleb and	Pregnancy	45	33% Well
	Farrow	Lactation	72	29% Well
1968	Peters	Pregnancy	187	33% Survival
1964	Rosemond	Pregnancy	37	38% Survival

*Based not upon the number of patients operated upon but upon the number traced. The actual number traced was not stated.

stated). With such a low 10-year survival rate, was radical mastectomy justified? Today we have more precise methods of selecting our patients for radical mastectomy and we can confidently expect a higher survival rate. But in 1942 the prognosis for breast carcinoma in pregnancy or lactation was grim indeed, and a surgeon might well search his conscience as to whether it was justifiable to inflict the hard penalty of radical mastectomy upon 100 women to achieve the prolonged survival of only eight of them. It must be kept in mind that irradiation alone — then as now — will probably give a 10-year survival rate at least as good as this.

Fortunately, carcinoma of the breast is very infrequent during pregnancy and lactation, and this paucity of case material makes it difficult to accumulate case series of significant size. Table 33–26 shows seven of the largest original case series reported during the last 30 years.

A review of these and other case series referred to in the references shows that during the last 15 years the usual experience has been that approximately one third of the patients who have mastectomy for carcinoma of the breast developing during pregnancy of lactation survive five years.

Study of these case series will reveal no statistically significant difference between end-results in patients whose disease was diagnosed during pregnancy and those in whom it was diagnosed during lactation. This is indeed what might be expected. We know that breast carcinoma usually grows comparatively slowly, and that at the time it is ordinarily discovered as a dominant tumor in the breast it has been present for a long time — probably several years. During pregnancy, moreover, the normal physiologic increase in the size and density of the breasts makes recognition of a tumor more difficult, and car-

cinoma is usually recognized at a more advanced stage than in nonpregnant women. Therefore, it can be assumed that when a carcinoma is diagnosed during lactation, it was present, although undiagnosed, during the preceding pregnancy. For statistical purposes, I have defined lactation, in the context of reporting the end results of our treatment of these patients, as the 12 month period following parturition, irrespective of whether the mother nursed her child or not.

Our Columbia-Presbyterian series of patients with breast carcinoma associated with pregnancy, who were admitted to our clinic during the period 1915 to 1965, totals 71.

There are several features of the group of patients worth noting (Table 33–27). The average age of our patients was 33.4 years. This agrees with the average age in other case series. Since these patients are in the childbearing age, they can be expected to be younger than other patients with breast carcinoma.

The average duration of symptoms in our series of patients when they came for admission was 12 months, which is about 3½ months longer than for our series of breast carcinomas as a whole. The reason why these women with carcinoma developing during pregnancy and lactation delay longer in coming for treatment is unquestionably that the

Table 33–27. CARCINOMA OF THE BREAST ASSOCIATED WITH PREGNANCY. COLUMBIA-PRESBYTERIAN MEDICAL CENTER, 1915–1965

Number of cases	71	
Average age	33.4	years
Average duration of symptoms before admission	12	months
Those with inoperable disease according to our clinical criteria	45	per cent

patients themselves, as well as the physicians they consult, usually assume that the breast tumor is an abscess or some other non-neoplastic lesion associated with the pregnancy.

The following is a typical story.

M. B., a housewife aged 40, who had had one previous pregnancy, became pregnant for the second time in November, 1942. Six months later she discovered a small hard tumor below the nipple of her left breast. She consulted her obstetrician about it and he advised her to ignore it. She was delivered in July, 1943, and nursed the baby until November, 1943. During all this time the breast tumor continued to enlarge slowly but gave her no pain. Her obstetrician continued to ignore it.

In March, 1944, the tumor began to pain her and her obstetrician decided to operate. In his description of his operation he wrote that he had "excised" the tumor under local anesthesia. He described it as being hard, not encapsulated, and adherent to the overlying skin. He was apparently content with his pathologist's diagnosis of "fibroadenoma." The tumor continued to grow, however, and the obstetrician's suspicions were finally aroused and he sent her to the Presbyterian Hospital in November, 1944.

Examination at that time, two years after the tumor had first been discovered, revealed the left breast to be contracted and deformed. The breast was solidly fixed to the chest wall. The whole central and lower portion of the breast was occupied by a hard tumor measuring 6 × 5 cm. At its lateral and caudad edge the tumor involved the skin and there was a small area of ulceration. The scar of the previous operation crossed the lower part of the breast. There were no clinically involved axillary nodes, and x-ray films of the chest and skeleton were negative.

The lesion was an obviously far advanced and inoperable carcinoma. A small biopsy of the ulcerated area confirmed this diagnosis. Curiously enough, study of the microscopic section of the tissue removed by the obstetrician at the original operation showed only normal breast tissue. The

conclusion seemed inescapable that in his "excision" under the difficulties of local anesthesia, he had somehow removed only breast tissue adjacent to the tumor. He was guilty of ignoring an obvious breast tumor for 15 months, and when he attempted to prove its nature by operation, he failed to get a piece of the carcinoma.

The patient was treated by irradiation, which held the local lesion in check, but did not control the bone metastases in her spine which shortly appeared. She died in November, 1947.

The stage of the disease in our 71 patients was comparatively advanced. This is evidenced by the fact that 45 per cent were inoperable by our clinical criteria. This was the most advanced group of cases in our series of breast carcinomas, excepting the inflammatory type.

Forty-eight of our 71 patients with breast carcinoma associated with pregnancy were treated with our version of the radical mastectomy, and followed for a minimal period of 10 years. I have studied the end-results in this group of cases relative to three different factors: (1) the clinical stage of advancement of the disease; (2) the age of the patients; and (3) the microscopic type of mammary carcinoma.

The significance of the clinical stage of the disease in terms of end-results of radical mastectomy in our series of 48 cases of carcinoma of the breast diagnosed during pregnancy or lactation is shown in Table 33-28, in which the 10 year survival rates for our patients with carcinoma during pregnacy are compared with those for the patients in my personal series of patients as a whole, by clinical stage.

It is seen that the 10-year survival rate for the patients in Clinical Stage A whose carcinomas were associated with pregnancy is only 10 per cent less than the survival rate in my series of patients as a whole. In the

Table 33–28. TEN-YEAR RESULTS OF RADICAL MASTECTOMY CORRELATED WITH CLINICAL STAGE. COLUMBIA-PRESBYTERIAN MEDICAL CENTER

	Breast Carcinoma During Pregnancy and Lactation (1915–1959)			Personal Series of Breast Carcinomas (1935–1957)	
Columbia Clinical Classification	No. of Patients	No. Surviving 10 Years	Per cent Surviving 10 Years	No. of Patients	Per cent Surviving 10 Years
Stage A	20	12	60%	402	70%
Stage B	11	3	27%	154	41%
Stage C	8	1	12.5%	59	24%
Stage D	9	0	0	11	18%
Total	48	16	33%	626	54%

Table 33–29. LONG-TERM RESULTS OF RADICAL MASTECTOMY FOR CARCINOMA OF THE BREAST IN PREGNANCY. COLUMBIA-PRESBYTERIAN MEDICAL CENTER, (1915–1959)

Columbia Clinical Classification	No. of Cases	Microscopic Axillary Findings	Results after 10 Years
Clinical Stage A	20	No axillary metastases, 13 patients	Six patients well without recurrence 23, 22, 18, 15, 13, 10 years, respectively. E.S., aged 31, developed new carcinoma in contralateral breast one year after original carcinoma. There were no axillary metastases. She is well 22 years later. E.S., aged 30, well until developed new carcinoma contralateral breast with axillary metastases after 11 years. Died 1 year later. R.Z., aged 30, well until abdominal metastasis developed after 11 years. Died 1 year later.
		Axillary metastases, 7 patients	A.W., aged 42, had 5 of 24 axillary nodes involved. She was given prophylactic postoperative irradiation. Well 14 years and then developed pulmonary metastases. Died 15 years later. A.S., aged 34, had 8 of 23 axillary nodes involved. She also had prophylactic postoperative irradiation. Well for 18 years, then developed new carcinoma in contralateral breast for which she refuses treatment. D.R., aged 40, had 6 of 20 axillary nodes involved. Pleural metastases after 6 years. Oophorectomy. Living with recurrence 11 years after mastectomy.
Clinical Stage B	11	No axillary metastases, 1 patient	A.C., aged 24, well without recurrence, 10 years.
		Axillary metastases, 10 patients	C.B., aged 39, had a single small embolus of carcinoma in 1 of 21 axillary nodes. Died of liver metastases after 16 years. A.H., aged 39, living with metastases, 11 years.
Clinical Stage C	8	No axillary metastases, 1 patient	
		Axillary metastases, 7 patients	G.G., aged 32, had 13 of 25 axillary nodes involved. No irradiation. Well 14 years.
Clinical Stage D	9	No axillary metastases, no patients	
		Axillary metastases, 9 patients	
All clinical stages	48	No axillary metastases, 15 patients	Eight well 23, 22, 22, 18, 15, 13, 10, 10 years, respectively.
		Axillary metastases, 33 patients	One well 14 years.

more advanced clinical stages, however, the survival rate for the pregnant patients is only about one-half the rate in my series of patients as a whole.

Closer study of our results, as detailed in Table 33–29, unfortunately reveals that although the 10-year survival rate for our patients whose disease was associated with pregnancy was 33 per cent, recurrence and contralateral breast carcinoma after 10 years have been unusually frequent in these pregnant patients. Only nine patients of the original 48 — that is, 19 per cent — are at present free of evidence of breast carcinoma. It is also interesting to note that eight of these nine did not have axillary metastases.

The ages of our patients who developed carcinoma of the breast during pregnancy and were treated by radical mastectomy are shown in Table 33–30. The numbers of patients in these different age groups in our data are clearly too small to permit any conclusions as to the bearing of age upon the results of treatment.

The third, and perhaps the most important factor which I wish to correlate with the end-results of radical mastectomy in pregnant or lactating patients is the microscopic type of the disease. There are, of course, a number of microscopic forms of the disease which experience has taught us to associate with an improved prognosis. These several favorable

Table 33–30. CARCINOMA OF THE BREAST IN PREGNANCY. COLUMBIA-PRESBYTERIAN MEDICAL CENTER (1915–1959). AGE OF PATIENTS CORRELATED WITH 10-YEAR SURVIVAL AFTER RADICAL MASTECTOMY, CLINICAL STAGE A

Columbia Clinical Classification	Age	No. of Patients	Per cent Surviving 10 Years
Clinical Stage A only	20–29	2	50%
	30–39	14	64%
	40–49	4	50%

microscopic types are grouped together in Table 33–31, and the end-results in these favorable types contrasted with the end results for the other microscopically less favorable types. It is a striking fact that all but one of our patients who have apparently been cured have had microscopically favorable types of carcinoma.

There was an additional feature of the natural history of breast carcinoma developing during pregnancy in our 48 patients, namely, a high incidence of a second new carcinoma in the contralateral breast. This occurred in four of our patients 6 months, and 1, 11, and 18 years, respectively, after the carcinoma in the breast originally involved had been cured by radical mastectomy. All four patients had well-differentiated carcinomas and in all the disease was classified as Clinical Stage A.

Of course our series of cases is too small for this incidence of 8.7 per cent of new carcinomas in the contralateral breast to have

Table 33–31. CARCINOMA OF BREAST IN PREGNANCY. COLUMBIA-PRESBYTERIAN MEDICAL CENTER. TEN-YEAR RESULTS OF RADICAL MASTECTOMY (1915–1959) CORRELATED WITH MICROSCOPIC TYPE OF CARCINOMA

	Microscopic Type	No. of Patients	No. Surviving 10 Years
Microscopically favorable cases	Intraductal	13	7
	Papillary	2	1
	Small cell	1	1
	Circumscribed	7	4
	Grade I, no special type	3	2
	Total	26	15
Microscopically unfavorable cases	Grade II, no special type	6	1
	Grade III, no special type	16	0
Total – all cases		48	16

any statistical significance, but the fact is worth noting.

The data I have reviewed leave no doubt that carcinoma of the breast developing during pregnancy is a more malignant disease. With rare exceptions it is curable by radical mastectomy only when it has not progressed beyond Clinical Stage A of our Columbia Clinical Classification, and when it is a microscopically favorable type. This last criterion is so important that I suggest that when the microscopic type cannot be determined accurately by frozen section, the decision as to whether or not radical mastectomy is to be performed be delayed until the lesion can be accurately classified from permanent microscopic sections.

Peters, whose series of patients with breast carcinoma associated with pregnancy is the largest yet reported, has pointed out an interesting relationship of the phase of pregnancy at which treatment of the carcinoma was begun, to the five-year results of treatment. In a series of 28 patients treated during the first half of pregnancy the survival rate was 48 per cent whereas it was only 11 per cent in 28 other patients treated during the last half of pregnancy. Peters emphasizes that the dramatic difference in results was not due to any difference in the delay from onset of disease to treatment in the two groups.

The effect of the termination of pregnancy in patients who develop breast carcinoma remains controversial. There is no statistical proof that the prognosis is improved by termination, yet most surgeons favor it. I have usually favored terminating the pregnancy when carcinoma is diagnosed during the first half of pregnancy, but the problem involves so many factors such as how much the child is desired, and the stage of advancement of the carcinoma, that no rules are applicable. In a recent patient of ours whose carcinoma was far advanced and inoperable, and whose child was just viable, it was delivered by cesarean section, and oophorectomy was performed, with a dramatic regression of her carcinoma.

Pregnancy Subsequent to Breast Carcinoma

The effect of subsequent pregnancy in women who have been treated for breast cancer is another much debated question. Although several students of this problem (White and White; Devitt et al.; Peters) have reported survival rates for patients with subsequent pregnancy which were apparently better than average, their data are not based upon large enough numbers of patients whose disease was accurately classified as to stage of advancement, and who were followed for a long enough time.

Lacking satisfactory statistical evidence, I fall back on my clinical impression that pregnancy soon after carcinoma of the breast adds an unreasonable hazard. If any carcinoma remains in the patients, the flood of estrogen of placental origin is likely to set it on fire. I have seen this happen in a number of patients.

The following case history illustrates the phenomenon.

Mrs. H. J., aged 26, a housewife with two children, 5 and 2 years of age, came to the Delafield Hospital in April, 1969 complaining of a tumor in her right breast which she had had for a year. It was a typical breast carcinoma 9.5 cm. in diameter. In the right axilla there was a group of clinically involved axillary nodes 3 cm. in diameter. Her disease was classified as Clinical Stage C.

She was treated by irradiation with comparatively satisfactory regression of both the primary tumor and the axillary metastases. At the end of 1969 the patient was feeling very well.

Early in January, 1970, she suddenly began to have severe pain in her lower back, and right hip and knee. She could not walk. X-ray studies showed widespread lytic metastases in many bones. Her last menstrual period had been December 13. Laparotomy was done on January 30th with the intention of performing adrenalectomy and oophorectomy. Pregnancy of 10 to 12 weeks duration was found. Oophorectomy was done and the pregnancy terminated.

The acute onset of pain due to bone metastases, which must have been present for a considerable time, was probably due to the stimulation of her carcinoma by the excess of estrogen associated with her pregnancy.

As a working rule I suggest that a patient who has had a Clinical Stage A breast carcinoma of a favorable microscopic type, in whom no axillary metastases were found at radical mastectomy, and in whom careful study reveals no evidence of recurrence, may undertake pregnancy after three years. All others had better delay for 10 years or avoid pregnancy altogether.

SUMMARY

This chapter, devoted to the clinical classification of breast carcinoma as to its stage of

advancement, and the various special factors which enter into the choice of treatment, has been a long one, because the subject is an exceedingly important one. The choice of treatment is just as critical as the actual details of the treatment itself.

With the exception of the special forms of carcinoma that I have discussed above, I am firmly convinced that the Halsted radical mastectomy is the best treatment for carcinoma of the breast when the disease is sufficiently limited in extent so that cure is possible.

From all our efforts to classify breast carcinoma as to its stage of advancement by clinical methods, I have learned that radical mastectomy is the treatment of choice only for patients whose disease is classified as Clinical Stage A or B. If there is doubt as to whether the patient's axillary findings by palpation place her disease in Clinical Stage C instead of Stage B, preliminary biopsy of the nodes of the apex of the axilla will help settle the dilemma, and I recommend it.

All patients whose disease is classified as Clinical Stage C or D, as well as those in whom the nodes at the apex of the axilla are found to be involved, should be treated primarily by irradiation.

I will discuss the use of irradiation as a primary and as an auxiliary method of treatment in Chapter 35.

I have often been criticized, and the results of my radical mastectomy explained away, by critics who accuse me of "selecting" my patients for operation. They do not understand that meticulous study of patients, and critical selection of treatment appropriate to the clinical stage of advancement of their disease, is basic. *My aim is to operate only upon patients whom I can cure, because experience has convinced me that in patients whom surgery will fail to cure, irradiation is to be preferred.* I have defined in great detail just how the patients in my personal series of radical mastectomies have been selected. I urge my critics to adopt these methods of selection, and to test the validity of the criteria for operability which I have defined. This is the way to better patient care, which is our mutual aim.

REFERENCES

Abrão, A., Silva Neto, J. B. Da, and Mirra, A. P.: Cancer de mama na gravidez e lactaçao; considerações em tôrno de 10 casos. Rev. paulista de med., 45:563, 1954.

Ackerman, N. B.: The diagnosis of cancer with radioisotopic techniques. Surg., Gynec. & Obst., *118*:1333, 1964.

Ackermann, W.: Vertebral trephine biopsy. Ann. Surg., *143*:373, 1956.

Ackermann, W.: Application of the trephine for bone biopsy. Results in 635 cases. J.A.M.A., *184*:11, 1963.

Ackermann, W., and Schwarz, G. S.: Non-neoplastic sclerosis in vertebral bodies. Cancer, *11*:703, 1938.

American Joint Committee for Cancer Staging and End Results Reporting: Clinical Staging System for Cancer of the Breast. Chicago, Illinois, 1962.

Andreassen, M., Dahl-Iversen, E., and Soerensen, B.: Glandular metastases in carcinoma of the breast. Lancet, *1*:176, 1954.

Baclesse, F.: Les localisations sus-mammaires du cancer du sein. Traitement et résultats. Radiol. Clin., *32*:349, 1963.

Berg, J. W., and Robbins, G. F.: Modified mastectomy for older, poor risk patients. Surg., Gynec. & Obst., *113*:631, 1961.

Berndt, H., et al.: Einfluss des Alters auf die Prognose des Mamma-Carcinoms. Chirurg, *32*:401, 1961.

Betson, J. R., Jr., and Golden, M. L.: Cancer and pregnancy. Amer. J. Obst. Gynec., *81*:718, 1961.

Briggs, R. C.: Detection of osseous metastases. Cancer, *20*:392, 1967.

Brooks, B., and Proffitt, J. N.: The influence of pregnancy on cancer of the breast. Surgery, *25*:1, 1949.

Brown, R. N.: Carcinoma of the breast followed by pregnancy. Surgery, *48*:862, 1960.

Bunker, M. L., and Peters, M. V.: Breast cancer associated with pregnancy or lactation. Amer. J. Obst. Gynec., *85*:312, 1963.

Byrd, B. F., Jr., Bayer, D. S., Robertson, J. C., and Stephenson, S. E., Jr.: Treatment of breast tumors associated with pregnancy and lactation. Ann. Surg., *155*:940, 1962.

Caceres, E.: Personal communication, 1968.

Charkes, N. D., Sklaroff, D. M., and Young, I.: A critical analysis of strontium bone scanning for detection of metastatic cancer. Amer. J. Roentgenol., *96*:647, 1966.

Chauvel and Renaud, M.: Cancer du sein à marche rapide, ayant la structure d'un épithéliome à végétations dendritiques observé chez une jeune fille. Bull. Soc. anat. de Paris., *91*:245, 1921.

Cheek, J. H.: Survey of current opinions concerning carcinoma of the breast occurring during pregnancy. Arch. Surg., *66*:664, 1953.

Cheek, J. H.: Management breast. Texas Med., *66*:44, 1970.

de Cholnoky, T.: Mammary cancer in youth. Surg., Gynec. & Obst., *77*:55, 1943.

Corey, K. R., et al.: Detection of bone metastases in scanning studies with calcium-47 and strontium-85. J. Nucl. Med., *3*:454, 1962.

Cutler, S. J., and Myers, M. H.: Clinical classification of extent of disease in cancer of the breast. J. Nat. Cancer Inst., *39*:193, 1967.

Cutler, S. J., Zippin, C., and Asire, A. J.: The prognostic significance of palpable lymph nodes in cancer of the breast. Cancer, *23*:243, 1969.

Dahl-Iversen, E.: Carcinoma of the Breast. Copenhagen, Official Tr. Northern Surg. A., 1951, p. 150.

Denoix, P. F., et al.: Clinical Stage Classification of Malignant Tumors of the Breast. Internat. Union against Cancer (1956 draft).

Devitt, J. E., Beattie, W. G., and Stoddart, T. G.: Carcinoma of the breast and pregnancy. Canad. J. Surg., *7*:124, 1964.

Eggers, C., de Cholnoky, T., and Jessup, D. S. D.: Cancer of the breast. Ann. Surg., *113*:321, 1941.

Fisher, B., et al.: Cancer of the breast: size of neoplasm and prognosis. Cancer, *24*:1071, 1969.

Fisher, B., Slack, N. H., and Ausman, R. K.: Location of breast cancer and prognosis. Surg., Gynec. & Obst., *129*:705, 1969.

Göksel, H. A.: Radical mastectomy for mammary carcinoma. Turkish J. Pediatrics, *6*:116, 1964.

von Gusnar, K.: Zur Frage einer neuen Schwangerschaft nach Radikaloperation eines Brustkrebses. Chirurg., *13*:82, 1941.

Guttmann, R. J.: Survival and results after 2-million volt irradiation in the treatment of primary operable carcinoma of the breast with proved positive internal mammary and/or highest axillary nodes. Cancer, *15*:383, 1962.

Gynning, I., Langeland, P., Lindberg, S., and Waldeskog, B.: Localization with Sr-85 of spinal metastases in mammary cancer and changes in uptake after hormone and roentgen therapy. Acta radiol., *55*:119, 1961.

Haagensen, C. D.: Cancer of the breast in pregnancy and during lactation. Amer. J. Obst. Gynec., *98*:141, 1967.

Haagensen, C. D.: The treatment and results in cancer of the breast at the Presbyterian Hospital, New York. Amer. J. Roentgenol., *62*:328, 1949.

Haagensen, C. D.: The treatment of carcinoma of the breast. New York State J. Med., *55*:2797, 1955.

Haagensen, C. D., et al.: Treatment of early mammary carcinoma—a cooperative international study. Ann. Surg., *157*:157, 1963.

Haagensen, C. D., et al.: Treatment of early mammary carcinoma—a cooperative international study. Ann. Surg., *170*:875, 1969.

Haagensen, C. D., et al.: Metastasis of carcinoma of the breast to the periphery of the regional lymph node filter. Ann. Surg., *169*:174, 1969.

Haagensen, C. D., and Cooley, E.: Radical mastectomy for mammary carcinoma. Ann. Surg., *157*:166, 1963.

Haagensen, C. D., and Stout, A. P.: Carcinoma of the breast; results of treatment. Ann. Surg., *116*:801, 1942.

Haagensen, C. D., and Stout, A. P.: Carcinoma of the breast; criteria of operability. Ann. Surg., *118*:859 and 1032, 1943.

Haagensen, C. D., and Stout, A. P.: Carcinoma of the breast; results of treatment, 1935–1942, Ann. Surg., *134*:151, 1951.

Handley, R. S.: Personal communication, 1969.

Handley, R. S., and Thackray, A. C.: The internal mammary lymph chain in carcinoma of the breast. Lancet, *2*:276, 1949.

Handley, R. S., and Thackray, A. C.: Invasion of internal mammary lymph nodes in carcinoma of the breast. Brit. Med. J., *1*:61, 1954.

Harrington, S. W.: Carcinoma of the breast. Results of surgical treatment when the carcinoma occurred in the course of pregnancy or lactation and when pregnancy occurred subsequent to operation (1910–1933). Ann. Surg., *106*:690, 1937.

Harrington, S. W.: Results of radical mastectomy in 5026 cases of carcinoma of the breast. Pennsylvania Med. J., *43*:413, 1940.

Harrington, S. W.: Survival rates of radical mastectomy for unilateral and bilateral carcinoma of the breast. Surgery, *19*:154, 1946.

Hartman, A. W., and Magrish, P.: Carcinoma of breast in children; case report: six-year-old boy with adenocarcinoma. Ann. Surg., *141*:792, 1955.

Hochman, A., and Schreiber, H.: Pregnancy and cancer of the breast. Obstet. & Gynec. (N.Y.), 2:268, 1953.

Holleb, A. I., and Farrow, J. H.: The relation of carcinoma of the breast and pregnancy in 283 patients. Surg., Gynec. & Obst., 115:65, 1962.

Hosbein, D. J., and Mithoefer, J.: The treatment of elderly women with cancer of the breast. Surg. Clin. N. Amer., 40:889, 1960.

Hyman, G. A.: A comparison of bone-marrow aspiration and skeletal roentgenograms in the diagnosis of metastatic carcinoma. Cancer, 8:576, 1955.

Kay, S., and Poulos, N. G.: Evaluation of the criteria of operability of carcinoma of the breast. Surg., Gynec. & Obst., 113:562, 1961.

Kennedy, C. S., Miller, E. B., and McLean, D. C.: Triple biopsy in carcinoma of the breast. J. Michigan Med. Soc., 62:389, 1963.

Kilgore, A. R.: Tumors and tumor-like lesions of the breast in association with pregnancy and lactation. Arch. Surg., 18:2079, 1929.

Kleinfeld, G., Haagensen, C. D., and Cooley, E.: Age and menstrual status as prognostic factors in carcinoma of the breast. Ann. Surg., 157:600, 1963.

Kraft, R. O., and Block, G. E.: Mammary carcinoma in the aged patient. Ann. Surg., 156:981, 1962.

Levings, A. H.: Carcinoma of the mammary gland in girl 12 years old. Amer. J. Surg., 31:29, 1917.

Lewison, E. F.: Breast cancer and pregnancy or lactation. Internat. Abstr. Surg., 99:417, 1954.

McDonald, J. J., Haagensen, C. D., and Stout, A. P.: Metastasis from mammary carcinoma to the supraclavicular and internal mammary lymph nodes. Surgery, 34:521, 1953.

McDivitt, R. W., and Stewart, F. W.: Breast carcinoma in children. J.A.M.A., 195:388, 1966.

Macdonald, I., and Wilcox, M. E.: Prognosis of mammary carcinoma in young women. Cancer, 9:281, 1956.

Mickal, A., Torres, J. E., and Mulé, J. G.: Carcinoma of the breast in pregnancy and lactation. Amer. Surg., 29:509, 1963.

Miller, E. B.: Carcinoma of the breast: Analysis according to Columbia Classification. Ann. Surg., 163:629, 1966.

Moore, S. W., and Lewis, R. J.: Carcinoma of the breast in women 30 years of age and under. Surg., Gynec. & Obst., 119:1253, 1964.

Nelson, H. M., and Howard, P. J.: Carcinoma of the breast in pregnancy and lactation. J. Michigan Med. Soc., 54:455, 1955.

Nohrman, B. A.: Cancer of the breast. Acta radiol., Supp. 77, Stockholm, 1949.

Nunn, L. L.: Cancer of the breast in the young. Northwest Med., 36:301, 1937.

Papadrianos, E., Cooley, E., and Haagensen, C. D.: Mammary carcinoma in old age. Ann. Surg., 161:189, 1965.

Parker, J. M., and Aldredge, W. M.: Carcinoma of the breast occurring during pregnancy or lactation. South. Surgeon, 15:550, 1949.

Pearson, O. H., Solaric, S., Lafferty, F. W., and Storaasli, J. P.: Calcium-47 and strontium-85 tracer studies as a guide to isotope therapy of bone metastases. Radiology, 79:446, 1962.

Peters, M. V.: Carcinoma of the breast associated with pregnancy. Radiology, 78:58, 1962.

Peters, M. V.: The effect of pregnancy on breast cancer. In Forrest, A. P. M., and Kunkler, P. B.: Prognostic Factors in Breast Carcinoma. Baltimore, Williams and Wilkins Co., 1968, p. 65.

Pirquet, C.: Allergie des Lebensalters. Leipzig, Georg Thieme, 1930.

Portmann, U. V.: Clinical and pathologic criteria as a basis for classifying cases of primary cancer of the breast. Cleveland Clin. Quart., 10:41, 1943.

Power, H. A.: Pregnancy complicating carcinoma of the breast. Pennsylvania Med. J., 45:1049, 1942.

Ratzkowski, E., and Hochman, A.: Survival of patients with "recurrent" or inoperable carcinoma of the breast with special consideration of the effect of hormonal treatment. Cancer, 14:300, 1961.

Remold, F.: Mamma-Ca und Schwangerschaft. Strahlentherapie, 87:65, 1952.

Richards, G. E.: Mammary cancer: place of surgery and of radiotherapy in its management; study of some of the factors which determine success or failure in treatment. Brit. J. Radiol., 21:109, 1948.

River, L. P., Silverstein, J., and Tope, J. W.: Breast disease in older patients. J. Amer. Geriatrics Soc., 1:854, 1953.

Rosemond, G. P.: Carcinoma of the breast during pregnancy. Clin., Obst., & Gynec., 6:994, 1963.

Rubin, P., and Ciccio, S.: Status of bone scanning for bone metastases in breast cancer. Cancer, 24:1338, 1969.

Sanger, G.: An aspect of internal mammary metastasis from carcinoma of the breast. Ann. Surg., 157:180, 1963.

Scapier, J.: Pregnancy and the development of mammary cancer. Amer. J. Med. Sci., 202:402, 1941.

Schiødt, T.: Breast Carcinoma. A Histologic and Prognostic Study of 650 Followed-up Cases. Copenhagen, Munksgaard, 1966.

Sears, J. B. and Schlesinger, M. J.: Carcinoma of the breast in 10 year old girl. New Eng. J. Med., 223:760, 1940.

Simmons, R. R.: Adenocarcinoma of the breast occurring in a boy of 13. J.A.M.A., 68:1899, 1917.

Sklaroff, D. M., and Charkes, N. D.: Diagnosis of bone metastasis by photoscanning with strontium-85. J.A.M.A., 188:1, 1964.

Smithers, D. W., Rigby-Jones, P., Galton, D. A. G., and Payne, P. M.: Cancer of the breast. Brit. J. Radiol. Supplement No., 4:45, 1952.

Spratt, J. S., and Donegan, W. L.: Cancer of the Breast. Philadelphia, W. B. Saunders Co., 1967, p. 131.

Steffen, E., and Grace, H.: Pregnancy subsequent to radical mastectomy of the breast for cancer. Amer. J. Obst. Gynec., 58:180, 1949.

Steinthal, C. F.: Zur Dauerheilung des Brustkrebses, Beitr. z. klin. Chir., 47:226, 1905.

TNM. General Rules. Geneva, Internat. Union against Cancer, 1969.

Thompson, W. H.: Case of adeno-carcinoma of the breast in a girl aged 11 years. Brit. Med. J., 2:502, 1908.

Tomlinson, W. L., and Eckert, C. T.: "Categorically inoperable" carcinoma of the breast. Ann. Surg., 130:38, 1949.

Treves, N., and Holleb, A. I.: A report of 549 cases of breast cancer in women 35 years of age or younger. Surg., Gynec. & Obst., 107:271, 1958.

Truscott, B. M.: Carcinoma of the breast. Brit. J. Cancer, 1:129, 1947.

Urban, J. A., and Baker, H. W.: Radical mastectomy in continuity with en bloc resection of the internal mammary lymph-node chain. Cancer, 5:992, 1952.

Veronesi, U.: Personal communication, 1968.

Wade, P.: Untreated carcinoma of the breast. Brit. J. Radiol., 19:272, 1946.

Weinstein, M. and Roberts, M.: Carcinoma of the breast during pregnancy. New York State J. Med., *53*:993, 1953.

Wells, D. B.: An audit of the treatment of breast carcinoma at the Hartford Hospital, 1932–1939. Connecticut Med. J., *14*:3, 1950.

Westberg, S. V.: Prognosis of breast cancer for pregnant and nursing women. Acta obst. et gynec. Scandinav., *25*(Supp. 4), 1946.

White, T. T.: Carcinoma of the breast and pregnancy; analysis of 920 cases collected from the literature and 22 new cases. Ann. Surg., *139*:9, 1954.

White, T. T.: Carcinoma of the breast in the pregnant and the nursing patient; review of 1,375 cases. Amer. J. Obst. & Gynec., *69*:1277, 1955.

White, T. T.: Prognosis of breast cancer for pregnant and nursing women; analysis of 1,413 cases. Surg., Gynec. & Obst., *100*:661, 1955.

White, T. T.: Breast cancer in women 30 years old or less. A study of 23 patients from Seattle Hospitals. Northwest Med., *59*:218, 1960.

White, T. T., and White, W. C.: Breast cancer and pregnancy. Ann. Surg., *144*:384, 1956.

Zippin, C.: Comparison of the International and American Systems for the staging of breast cancer. J. Nat. Cancer Inst., *36*:53, 1966.

Chapter Thirty-Four

The Surgical Treatment of Mammary Carcinoma

In the preceding chapter I have described the method by which we select the Halsted radical mastectomy as the treatment for the patients whose carcinomas we believe are best treated by surgery. They constitute about one-half the patients who come for treatment of primary carcinoma of the breast. The operation itself is an extensive one in which a series of related regional dissections are integrated to form an orderly comprehensive attack upon the local disease. It is an operation that cannot be improvised. Depending upon science rather than art, it is more like a carefully planned military campaign than the painting of a picture. The best introduction to the operation is a review of its evolution. Its development has followed, step by step, the advances in our knowledge of surgical pathology and the natural history of mammary carcinoma. The best historical review of the evolution of this knowledge was written by Sir D'Arcy Power. More recently, good reviews have been made by Cooper, by Craig and Holman, and by Lewison.

THE HISTORY OF THE SURGICAL ATTACK UPON BREAST CARCINOMA

Local Excision of the Tumor—Up to 1867. More than a hundred years ago, in 1863 to be exact, Sir James Paget, one of the foremost surgeons of his time, and a great

authority on breast cancer, wrote: "I am not aware of a single clear instance of recovery, that is, as that the patient should live for more than ten years free from the disease. . . . In deciding for or against the removal of a cancerous breast in any single case, we may, I think, dismiss all hope that the operation will be the final remedy for the disease." Operation for breast cancer in Paget's time was merely a palliative procedure. It was a simple local removal of the clinically obvious primary tumor in the breast, together with a margin of the surrounding mammary gland. It was crudely done, with much loss of blood, and was often followed by wound infection, and sometimes by septicemia as Dr. John Brown described so poignantly in "Rab and his Friends."

Removal of the Entire Breast and the Axillary Lymph Nodes—1867 to 1875. The second stage in the development of the surgical attack on breast cancer was the removal of the entire breast, rather than only a part of it, together with the axillary lymph nodes. Charles H. Moore, Surgeon to the Middlesex Hospital, and in charge of its cancer wards, formulated this new principle of attacking breast cancer in 1867. He maintained that recurrence of the disease after the type of operation which had previously been done was not due to the development of an entirely new tumor on the basis of a constitutional susceptibility, as was then generally considered to be the case, but to incomplete removal of the original primary carcinoma. He wrote, with wisdom far beyond his time, as follows:

It is not sufficient to remove the tumour, or any portion only of the breast in which it is situated; mammary cancer requires the careful extirpation of the entire organ.

The situation in which the operation is most likely to be incomplete is at the edge of the mamma next the sternum.

When any texture adjoining the breast is involved in or even approached by the disease, that texture should be removed with the breast. This observation relates especially to skin, to lymphatics, to much fat, and to pectoral muscle. The attempt to save skin which is in any degree unsound is of all errors perhaps the most pernicious, and whenever its condition is doubtful, that texture should be freely removed.

In the performance of the operation it is desirable to avoid, not only cutting into the tumour, but also seeing it. No actually morbid structure should be exposed lest the active microscopic elements in it should be set free and lodge in the wound. Diseased axillary glands should be taken away by the same dissection as the breast itself, without dividing the intervening lymphatics; and the practice of first roughly excising the central mass of the breast and afterwards removing successive portions which may be of doubtful soundness, should be abandoned. Only by deliberately reflecting the flaps from the whole mamma, and detaching it first at its edge, can the various undetected prolongations of the tumour and outlying nodules be included in the operation.

Moore's ideas were not generally accepted, although during the next decade two of his compatriots began to do the operation he had described. One was Joseph Lister, then at Glasgow. The other was Mitchell Banks of Liverpool. Banks deserves special credit for making a vigorous plea in 1878 and again in 1882 for the removal of the axillary lymph nodes. In the latter paper he wrote:

"In the present paper a principal object is to advocate the removal of the axillary glands as well as the breast in *all* cases, whether we can feel them enlarged or not—in fact, to make a clearing out of the axilla a necessary part of the operation for removal of the breast. I have been quietly practising this for three or four years, having been driven to the conclusion that it was the right thing to do by discovering that even in those cases where certain glands could distinctly be felt enlarged, when the axilla was opened small ones were discovered which, although most palpably affected, were quite incapable of being felt from the outside."

Removal of the Pectoral Fascia, Together With the Breast and the Axillary Lymph Nodes—1875 to 1882. The next step in the evolution of the surgical attack on breast cancer was the addition of dissection of the fascia from the pectoral muscle. Richard von Volkmann, who came home from the Franco-Prussian war to his professorship at Halle, where he introduced Lister's antiseptic methods and made it safe to operate, was perhaps the first to include removal of the pectoral fascia in the attack on breast cancer. He wrote in 1875:

I cut right down to the pectoralis muscle when I make the lower incision and clean its fibers just as I would in making a class-room dissection, carrying the knife parallel with the fibers of the muscle and penetrating the interstices. The pectoralis fascia is thus entirely removed. I was led to adopt this method because microscopical examination showed repeatedly what I had not expected that the fascia was already carcinomatous, whilst the muscle was certainly not involved.

In Philadelphia, Samuel W. Gross was performing the same operation as Volkmann. In his book *Tumors of the Mammary Gland,* published in 1880, which was certainly the best treatise on breast tumors that had been written up to that date, Gross wrote: "Within the past seven months, however, I have adopted the principles which I have just enunciated, that is to say, I removed the mamma and its coverings bodily, dissected off the pectoral fascia, and cleaned out the axilla in five cases, and all recovered."

The Modern Radical Mastectomy—1882. The final step in the evolution of the operation which we today call radical mastectomy was made by William Stewart Halsted, that heroic figure in modern surgery, at Johns Hopkins in 1882. That was the year in which, to quote his own words, "I began not only to typically clean out the axilla in all cases of cancer of the breast but also to excise in almost every case the pectoralis major muscle or at least a generous piece of it, and to give the tumor on all sides an exceedingly wide berth." Halsted's first description of his operation as he had performed it in 13 cases of carcinoma of the breast was published for the first time in 1891 in a section of a paper on "The Treatment of Wounds."

Although Halsted had received his medical education in New York, he had spent much time in Germany and was fully aware of Volkmann's surgical ideas, and of the facts concerning the lymphatic spread of carcinoma as they were emerging in several German laboratories.

Halsted was not only prepared intellectually to advance the new concept of a truly radical surgical attack upon carcinoma of the breast but he was technically prepared to carry out the concept. He was a pioneer in the development of precise meticulous surgical dissection, using small hemostats and silk ligatures. He was one of the few surgeons of his day who had mastered the technique of grafting skin, which permitted him to remove as much tissue as he wished from the chest wall and still close his wound without tension. All these features of his technique made it possible for him to carry out the extensive dissection which his concept of the treatment of breast carcinoma required, and still achieve good wound healing.

Halsted wrote four papers presenting his concept of the surgical attack on breast cancer and his results. They were published in 1894, 1898, 1907, and 1912. They should all be read by every student of breast cancer. In his first paper in 1894 Halsted reviewed the results of earlier and less radical operations in the hands of German, French, and American surgeons, and pointed out the incompleteness of these earlier operations. He then described his own operation, as it had evolved in his hands, emphasizing a cardinal principle that "the suspected tissue should be removed in one piece (1) lest the wound become infected by the division of the tissues invaded by the disease, or of lymphatic vessels containing cancer cells, and (2) because shreds or pieces of cancer tissue might readily be overlooked in a piecemeal extirpation." He included brief reports of the 50 radical mastectomies which he had performed to date without a single operative death.

During the same month of November, 1894, that Halsted's first paper appeared in print, Willy Meyer of New York read before the New York Academy of Medicine, Section on Surgery, a description of a technique for radical mastectomy which was similar to Halsted's. At the time he described his operation, Willy Meyer had performed it on six patients during the previous three years.

There is no doubt that Halsted and Willy Meyer conceived the radical mastectomy independently, but for history it must be pointed out that Halsted began to do his operation in 1882, while Willy Meyer first performed his operation in 1891.

Although the Halsted and Willy Meyer operations were similar in scope, there were important differences in the manner in which the two procedures were carried out. Halsted detached the pectoralis major muscle from the humerus, the clavicle, the sternum, and the chest wall as soon as he had dissected back his skin flaps. The operative specimen then was permitted to fall laterally, giving good access to the axilla, which was dissected last. Halsted's original illustration shows the operative specimen at the patient's side as he dissects the axilla (Fig. 34-1). In Willy Meyer's operation the axilla was dissected first. This step being completed, the operative specimen was retracted medially, the deep surface of the pectoral muscles being exposed as their attachments to the chest wall and the sternum were severed. Strong retraction was required during this step, a feature better avoided in a cancer operation. Willy Meyer's illustration (Fig. 34-2) shows this maneuver. Halsted merely divided the pectoralis minor muscle and left it in situ, while Willy Meyer removed it. Another difference between the two operations was that Halsted regularly sacrificed so much skin over the breast that it was necessary to cover the defect on the chest wall with a graft. Willy Meyer sacrificed less skin and was often able to close his wound without grafting.

An important advantage of Halsted's operation was that it was a more precise, careful dissection, carried out with meticulous hemostasis and requiring about four hours to complete. The access to the axilla, when axillary dissection was performed as a last stage with the breast out of the way at the patient's side, was excellent, and permitted gentle, accurate, sharp dissection. Willy Meyer's operation was done more rapidly, requiring only about two hours, and was bloodier and rougher. The access to the axilla, which was dissected before the breast was removed from the chest wall, was not good. The axillary dissection was done bluntly with "a scalpel handle or closed scissors or a gauze mop."

As time went by, both Halsted and Willy Meyer modified their techniques somewhat. Halsted shortly adopted excision of the pectoralis minor muscle. For many years he included a supraclavicular dissection as part of his operation, but finally gave this feature up as futile. About 1910 he made a final important technical improvement in his skin incision. He abandoned the incision extending out onto the arm, and carried his incision straight upward from his circular incision

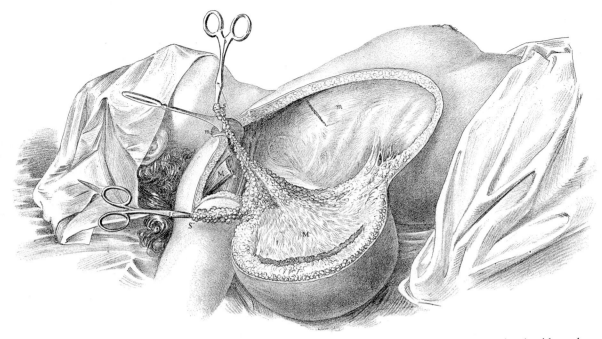

Figure 34–1. Halsted's original illustration showing the operative specimen at the patient's side as he dissects the axilla in the final step of the operation. (From Halsted, W. S.: Ann. Surg., *20*:497, 1894.)

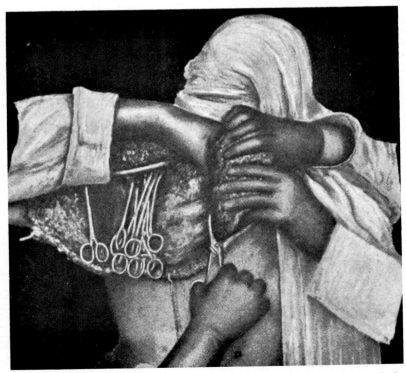

Figure 34–2. Willy Meyer's original illustration showing the operative specimen being retracted medially as the pectoral muscles and breast are detached from the chest wall in the last stage of his operation. (From Meyer, W.: Medical Record, *46*:746, 1894.)

around the breast to the strap line at the center of the shoulder. This avoided disfigurement of the axilla and upper arm by an unsightly scar.

Both of these operations were welcomed and quickly accepted in this country. Halsted's operation was performed chiefly by his pupils, however, and has never been widely practiced. Willy Meyer's operation was adopted more widely. Warren, in Boston, took it up and modified the skin incision slightly. Jackson, of Kansas City, introduced the operation in the middle west, with another modification of the skin incision. Rodman, in Philadelphia, devised still another skin incision. It was the Willy Meyer operation, not the Halsted operation, which evolved into what may be called the "standard American radical mastectomy," which is practiced throughout most of the world today. This is a quicker, less meticulous, more brutal operation than the original Halsted operation. Skin grafting is rarely done. To avoid it, less skin is sacrificed, and the wound is put together with considerable tension.

The effects of the Halsted and Willy Meyer operations upon results in carcinoma of the breast were immediate and dramatic. The results in the pre-Halsted era were unbelievably bad. For example, von Winiwarter, who published a comprehensive study of Billroth's end results in 1878, reported 82 per cent of local recurrences and only 4.7 per cent of three-year clinical cures. In 1898 Halsted reported his three-year results in 76 cases. His local recurrence rate was 10 per cent, and his clinical cure rate 41 per cent. Willy Meyer had done his operation on a total of 44 patients by 1901. His three-year clinical cure rate was 25 per cent. In interpreting these results we must remember that there was very little selection of cases for operation in these early days of the radical mastectomy. Almost all patients who came with carcinoma were operated upon. In Halsted's 1907 series, for instance, 76.4 per cent of his patients had axillary metastases.

Twenty-five years ago the Willy Meyer radical mastectomy was accepted almost everywhere as the preferred treatment for carcinoma of the breast. Then, with the end of World War II, a new generation of younger surgeons came into power. They were quite justifiably dissatisfied with the results of radical mastectomy. But they failed to realize that their basic error was the indiscriminate use of the operation. They operated upon almost all patients with breast carcinoma, including those with advanced and incurable disease. Instead of learning to classify their patients accurately on a clinical basis as to the stage of advancement of their disease, and to select for radical mastectomy only those who would benefit from it, they began to abandon radical mastectomy for a wide variety of other types of surgical attack, some less radical, some more radical, and some combined with irradiation.

I have held steadfastly to the belief that radical mastectomy is the best treatment yet devised for operable breast carcinoma, not because of blind prejudice, but because I have not seen as good results with other methods of treatment. In the present chapter I wish to describe my operation. Its performance demands much time and patience, which the rush and pressures of the modern surgeon's life do not encourage. It is my hope that the operation will become more popular when it is better known. It has given me results beyond my expectations, which I wish to present in its support.

PREPARATION OF PATIENTS FOR RADICAL MASTECTOMY

Great care is devoted to the physiological preparation of patients with breast disease for operation, which is of course important for the patient's physical welfare. But little or no attention is usually given to the mental preparation of the patient for the surgery that she is about to undergo.

The main reason why the mental preparation of patients for breast surgery is so much neglected is that it can be done only by one person—the senior surgeon in whom the patient places her trust. The physical preparation of the patient can be, and usually is, a cooperative enterprise achieved by several bright young men whom the patient need not know personally. But the detailed explanation of what is to be done at operation, and why, and the inspiring of hope and the quieting of anxiety, must come from the individual whom the patient regards as *her* surgeon. It makes no difference whether she is a ward or a private patient. The responsible attending surgeon who has the patient's confidence should sit down with her, after he has examined her, and explain her problem to her as simply and as truthfully as possible. This takes time, and many surgeons today work at such a frantic pace that they have very little time to spend preparing their patients mentally for the operations they perform on them.

As I have already emphasized in Chapter 4, fear is the most important of the factors that deter women with breast disease from seeking medical help. It has two aspects. The first is fear of mutilation. The modern woman reads a great deal about cancer, and hears a good deal about it from her friends. Her first thought when she discovers something wrong with her breast is that she has breast cancer. She assumes the worst—that she will lose her breast. It should be apparent to every physician who has had much experience with breast disease that the breasts—both breasts—are vitally important organs to every woman no matter what her age or marital status may be. This fear of breast amputation often strikes so deeply that the woman cannot bring herself to consult a physician for a long time.

A second and almost as important kind of fear that terrorizes women with breast disease is that they will not be cured of the cancer that they suspect they have. They have all known friends who were not cured, and many have had relatives who have succumbed. We must not overlook the fact that laymen do not have much confidence in our ability to cure cancer.

Many patients with breast disease get very little specific help from their surgeon to relieve these two basic fears—fear of mutilation and fear of death. Their fears are either brushed off with a hasty reassurance, or, what is worse, the surgeon attempts to calm the patient by lying to her. A common practice is to tell the patient that her breast is to be removed because her tumor *may become* malignant. Neither method is likely to succeed. Most patients have enough intelligence to see through this kind of subterfuge. They are then apt to lose confidence in their surgeon, just at the time when they most need to rely upon him.

In my experience the best weapon against these fears of breast disease is truth. The truth must of course be told patiently and sympathetically. It is important to emphasize its hopeful aspects. But the word cancer should be used openly and frankly. It has been my own practice to take as much time as is needed after I have completed my examination of the patient, to explain to her in simple terms the diagnostic problem and how we propose to solve it, and what the possibilities in store for her are. If the patient in question has a lesion that is probably benign,

I tell her so. I *always* add that my clinical diagnosis is only a guess, and explain that the microscope is the final arbiter, and that she may in fact have cancer. Plans must be made for any eventuality. When the lesion appears to me to be a carcinoma I tell the patient that there is a strong possibility that she has a cancer. I point out, however, that my clinical diagnosis may be incorrect. I emphasize the fact that the hope of cure is excellent in early breast cancer. If carcinoma is found at operation I tell the patient so without hesitation.

It has been my experience that when these truths are presented sympathetically to patients they almost always rise to the occasion and accept them with courage and dignity. Their fears are to some degree overcome by facing them. I believe that I usually succeed in gaining the confidence of my patients and in persuading them that they can trust and rely upon me. To some extent, no doubt, they transfer their burden to me.

Recently the problem of explaining the rationale of treatment for breast carcinoma to our patients has become much more complex because of our biopsy methods for sorting out those patients whose carcinomas have extended beyond the reach of surgery, and who therefore should be treated by irradiation rather than radical mastectomy. In preparing our patients mentally for what lies ahead of them, we must, therefore, tell them that even if cancer is found, the breast is not, under certain circumstances, removed. Instead, treatment with irradiation is given.

Another important advantage of telling the truth to patients with breast disease is that it makes them face the fact that they may have cancer, and that they must not delay treatment. Patients who are not made to realize this possibility are apt to delay coming into the hospital, or to go shopping around from one surgeon to another while precious weeks and months slip by, and metastasis perhaps occurs.

MY TECHNIQUE FOR THE HALSTED RADICAL MASTECTOMY

In my own surgical attack on carcinoma of the breast I have followed the fundamental principle that the disease, even in its early stage, is such a formidable enemy that it is my duty to carry out as radical an operation as the regional anatomy permits without unreasonable penalty in function and appearance. Just what this implies I will attempt to describe in the following pages. The operation that I perform is essentially the Halsted radical mastectomy, but some of the details are derived from the technique of the late Dr. George H. Semken. His carefully planned and meticulous methods of surgical attack upon several forms of cancer were my inspiration for special emphasis on this form of surgery. I am indebted to Dr. Allen O. Whipple for my apprenticeship in silk technique, which adds, I believe, to the delicacy and exactitude of radical mastectomy. It was under Dr. Whipple's sympathetic direction that I was permitted to work out the technique for radical mastectomy here presented.

Anesthesia

If radical mastectomy is to be performed safely, the surgeon must have the intelligent and sympathetic cooperation of his anesthetist. This begins with the anesthetist's preoperative visit to the patient on the night before operation. On this occasion the anesthetist not only gets acquainted with the patient and gains her confidence, but he gets an impression of her cardiorespiratory reserve. He evaluates the architecture of her airway and examines her teeth. He inquires into drug idiosyncrasy. He makes sure that her blood has been grouped and matched. He advises extra fluids and sugar during the evening preceding operation.

The anesthetist's premedication includes a barbiturate to insure a good night's sleep. Morphine, 6 to 10 mg., and scopolamine, 0.3 or 0.4 mg., is given intramuscularly one and a half hours before the patient is brought to the operating room.

For the type of radical mastectomy which I perform, we need a method of anesthesia which will maintain the patient at a relatively superficial plane of anesthesia over a period of between five and six hours. Muscle relaxation is not required. I do not mind, in fact, if the patient stirs slightly now and then. Prolonged deep anesthesia is unnecessary and is shocking and hazardous.

Our patients are usually induced with intravenous Pentothal Sodium. Anesthesia is maintained with nitrous oxide supplemented with Pentothal Sodium, or meperidine (Demerol), or morphine. If Pentothal Sodium is used the amount given should be kept judiciously small. In our average patient, with anesthesia lasting between five and six hours,

the total dose of Pentothal Sodium is usually between 0.75 and 1 gram. In patients with chronic cough resulting from sinusitis or the irritation of heavy cigarette smoking it is often desirable to use meperidine (Demerol) or morphine more freely as a supplement. In recent years a number of new anesthetic agents have been developed which are useful under certain circumstances.

During the first stage of the operation, when the skin flaps are being dissected and the electrocautery is being used, explosive anesthetic agents cannot be employed, but as soon as the cautery is disconnected, it is possible to use ethylene, cyclopropane, or ether. Cyclopropane is the preferred anesthetic for patients with extreme hypertension, and in certain other special types of cases.

Our anesthetists observe certain special precautions in these long operations. They take care to make the patient comfortable on the operating table. They remove the mask from the face every hour to make sure that the skin of the face is not damaged. They do not use airways unless they are absolutely necessary. Finally, they do not give too much fluid intravenously.

Unless my patients have a bleeding dyscrasia of some sort, very little blood is lost in the operation as I perform it. Although we have not attempted to measure the amount of blood lost in radical mastectomy, I cannot believe that I lose anywhere near the average of 821 ml. that Coller and his associates reported. The average duration of the four radical mastectomies in which Coller measured the blood loss was 179 minutes. It has been my observation that the more rapidly the operation is done, the more blood is lost, and the more often transfusion is required. We take care not to give a total of more than 1500 ml. of fluid intravenously. Blood transfusion is rarely required. If the blood pressure drops temporarily, a blood substitute usually brings it up again.

Position of the Patient upon the Operating Table

There are certain details regarding the position of the patient upon the operating table which are worth mentioning. Both of the patient's arms are stretched out at right angles upon solid metal arm boards which will not give way and permit the arm to fall backward. The brachial plexus can be injured in an unconscious patient if the arm is forced backward unreasonably. The strap over the patient's legs, fastening her to the table, should not be tight. The operating table should be one which can be tilted horizontally. Side braces padded with small pillows are placed on the side of the table opposite to the diseased breast, so that when the table is tilted, the patient will not slide off. It is desirable to incline the upper half of the operating table upward slightly so that the breast and the plane of the chest which form the operative field are inclined slightly upwards.

The skin of the arm on the tumor side is, of course, prepared down to the elbow and the whole arm enclosed in a sterile sleeve so that its position can be changed without breaking the sterility. The chest wall is prepared from the neck to the umbilicus. I do not use hexachlorophene soap for skin preparation because it seems unreasonable to me to massage a breast which may contain cancer. I have recently been preparing the skin with ether alone, and find it entirely satisfactory.

The operating table should be raised high enough so that when the operator stands erect the operative field is at elbow level. It is a common fault of tall surgeons to have the table too low, requiring them to bend over and strain their backs.

For the first stage of the operation, that is, the dissection of the lateral skin flap, it is helpful to have the operating table tilted away from the operator about 30 degrees so that the side of the breast and thorax are more accessible. After this step has been completed, the table is turned back to a level plane.

Operative Technique

The surgeon performing radical mastectomy aspires to carry out a complex maneuver so gently and precisely that every single cancer cell is removed from the operative field. The operation should be done throughout with *sharp* dissection. *Blunt* dissection should never be used. Sharp dissection is done entirely with the knife. The tissues are cleanly divided without being crushed. Blunt dissection is done with scissors, with a hemostat, or with the surgeon's finger. The tissues are scraped, torn, or pulled apart, and are badly mauled. Emboli of cancer cells may be set free by blunt dissection.

I have found it preferable to use exclusively for hemostasis the smallest size curved clamp, sometimes called the mosquito clamp. This clamp is similar to Halsted's original mosquito clamp except that the instrument he devised had a straight point and the one I prefer has a curved point. It measures about 12 cm. in length.

I tie with No. 5 black silk and use the same material for skin suture. As compared with catgut, silk is so much finer and so much more pliable that the surgeon using it develops a sense of precision and delicacy which enables him to tie small vessels more accurately.

The electrocautery is used for hemostasis only on the specimen, that is, on tissue which is to be removed.

A special effort is made to keep the operative field covered with warm, moist compresses or small towels, leaving only the small area exposed in which dissection is actually being performed. This prevents the tissues from drying out and minimizes shock and aids wound healing. It is not possible to indicate, in the accompanying drawings illustrating the steps of the operation, the extent to which I keep the operative field protected with these moist compresses or towels, but I hope the reader will understand that it is my constant care.

Since cancer cells are easily transplanted the surgeon must take care not to implant them. The fact that viable cancer cells are present on instruments used for biopsy was proved long ago by Saphir. As I indicated in describing my biopsy technique in Chapter 5, I take special precautions to avoid contamination of my mastectomy operative field by cells from the biopsy wound. It is sealed with a rubber patch, the only method that I know of which will surely keep serum and blood from escaping from it during the subsequent operative manipulations. Gowns, gloves, drapes, and all the instruments on the tray used for biopsy, are discarded before mastectomy is commenced. I suspect that a leaking biopsy wound was the source of the carcinoma cells which Brandes and White transplanted from the breast to the donor site for a skin graft on the thigh. If a surgeon *dissects* into carcinoma anywhere during the course of radical mastectomy, he will inevitably implant it in other parts of his wound, and fail to cure his patient. This course of events is often obvious in the patients of surgeons who perform radical mastectomy upon patients with advanced and inoperable carcinoma.

Step 1. Dissection of the Skin Flaps.
The skin incision is outlined with methylene
blue. The *form* of the skin incision does not
vary. It consists of an oval or circle drawn
around the breast with the tumor near its
center. Vertical extensions are then added
above and below the circle. The upper vertical extension is carried straight up to the
strap line at the middle of the shoulder. This
vertical incision must be carried up high
enough so that the axillary skin flap can be
retracted sufficiently laterally to give adequate access to the axilla. The lower vertical
extension is carried straight downward over
the hypochondrium. This skin incision (Fig.
34–3) is the one which Halsted finally came
to use. This vertical scar over the patient's
shoulder is hidden by the shoulder strap of

her brassiere and she can wear a sleeveless
dress or a bathing suit.

In the standard American radical mastectomy the skin incision is carried out onto the
arm over the anterior aspect of the pectoral
fold, as in the Willy Meyer operation. This
makes the dissection of the axillary flap a
little easier but this axillary incision is by no
means necessary. When the upper incision is
carried vertically sufficiently high in the strap
line, perfectly adequate exposure of the axilla
can be obtained with careful retraction.

It should be emphasized that the worst
mistake a surgeon can make from the point of
view of good arm function is to carry the skin
incision into the hollow of the axilla. A vertical band of scar tissue bow-stringing across
the axilla is the inevitable result, and arm

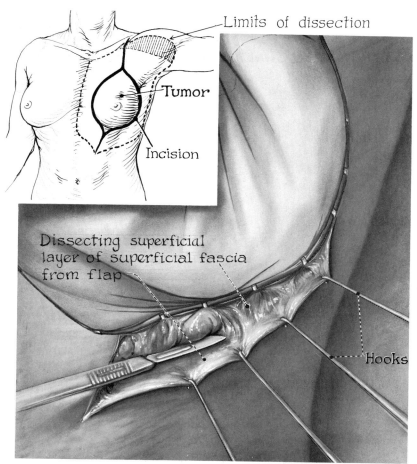

Figure 34–3. The insert shows the skin incision for a carcinoma located near the center of the breast,
the limits of the dissection of the flaps being indicated by a dotted line. The shaded area at the upper edge
of the lateral flap indicates the zone in which the flap is thicker. The drawing shows the dissection of the
lateral flap, beginning at its lower end.

motion is restricted. Willy Meyer's original incision extended into the hollow of the axilla, but he soon realized its disadvantage and placed it more cephalad so that it ran over the anterior aspect of the arm.

A large number of different skin incisions have been devised. The more complex they are, the more they are to be avoided. A transverse incision does not provide adequate access to the longitudinal extent of the operative field on the chest wall, and to the axilla.

Although I do not vary the simple basic form of my incision as a circle with upper and lower vertical extensions, I vary its position a good deal, depending upon the situation of the tumor in the breast. If the tumor is situated medially or laterally, or cephalad or caudad, the circle is correspondingly shifted so that the tumor is in its center.

All types of skin incisions which involve the shifting of flaps to cover the defect on the chest wall that remains when a wide removal of skin is carried out are impractical because they do not do away with the necessity of skin-grafting the donor area, and they further prolong an already lengthy operation.

When a breast carcinoma is situated in the axillary prolongation of the breast, and is in effect in the lower axilla, I have in several such patients been able to carry the cephalad line of my dissection several centimeters beyond the tumor and nevertheless cover the axillary structures without shifting a flap. But this is impossible when the carcinoma is situated in the center of the axilla. In these patients, who are fortunately rare, the axillary structures can be covered only by shifting a flap from the upper part of the breast, as described below.

Mrs. M. F., a 41 year old housewife, developed a small tumor beneath the skin of the central portion of her right axilla. Its true nature was missed for 10 months during which it grew slowly to reach a diameter of 1.5 cm. Biopsy then revealed it to be a mammary carcinoma.

Since it was situated beneath the skin of the axillary fold in the central axillary region, the conventional radical mastectomy could not be performed. Instead, a plastic procedure involving shifting a large flap from the upper breast skin, as shown in Figure 34-4 was used to cover the defect over the axilla. In other respects the operation was the usual radical mastectomy. A total of 26 axil-

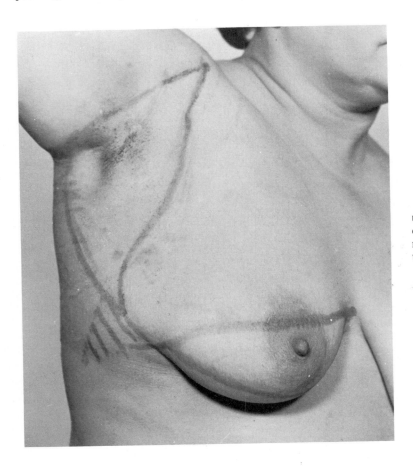

Figure 34-4. A flap from the upper half of the breast used to cover the axillary defect in carcinoma of the breast situated in the center of the axilla.

lary nodes were included in the dissection. Although they were close to the primary tumor, none of them contained metastases.

The patient developed metastases in her pelvic bones within 16 months after her operation, but there was no local recurrence of her carcinoma in the axilla or on the chest wall.

The *extent* of the skin sacrificed depends not only upon the size of the tumor but also upon the size of the breast. As a general rule I include the skin over the whole of the protuberant breast. When a tumor is eccentrically situated, an additional area of skin is necessarily included. When the tumor lies in the upper outer sector of the breast, for instance, an additional area of skin over the anterior axillary fold is sacrificed. I try to place the line of skin incision at least four finger breadths, that is, about 7 cm., beyond the edge of the palpable tumor. When the tumor is situated very high in the upper outer sector of the breast this is sometimes difficult to do. Enough of a skin flap to cover the axillary vessels must be retained. I have not seen skin recurrences in this region when this necessary compromise has been made. I see no necessity for a muscle pedicle flap utilizing the latissimus to cover the axillary structures in these cases, as advocated by Moore and Harkins. Other situations of the tumor in the breast do not limit the extent of the skin removal. Thus, for tumors of the inner sector of the breast, the area of skin removed regularly extends to the midline.

The extent of skin removal is not planned with any reference to the closing of the wound, with the exception that I have pointed out above for tumors high in the upper outer sector of the breast. Knowing that a defect of any size can be easily covered with a skin graft, I never hesitate to sacrifice as much skin as I think desirable from the viewpoint of curing the carcinoma. The result has been that in almost every patient a defect of varying size remains when the skin flaps are finally approximated. Since I know at the outset that I am going to have to do a skin graft, I never attempt to limit the amount of skin sacrificed. I will return to this question of the amount of skin sacrificed when I discuss the frequency of local recurrence later on in the present chapter.

I begin by dissecting back the lateral skin flap. The first step is to make the skin incision. Care is taken to carry the skin incision only down to the level of the superficial fascia (Fig. 34-5). The knife must not plunge through it into a deeper level. This delicate but distinct fascia is encountered just beneath the dermis. Over the lower part of the chest wall it is thicker than over the upper chest wall, but with careful hemostasis it can be identified all the way up to the clavicle. In thin patients there is only a thin film of adipose tissue, measuring not more than a millimeter or two in thickness, and the skin itself, superficial to this fascia. In obese patients the layer of subdermal fat is a little thicker. Close beneath the fascia lie relatively large thinwalled veins, which might be called the *subfascial* veins of the breast. They are accompanied by small arteries and by lymphatics.

It is a great convenience, from the viewpoint of good hemostasis, to keep the plane of dissection superficial to this fascia. In so doing the troublesome subfascial vessels, which bleed freely, are not cut, and the flap often can be dissected up without having to place a single hemostat on the flap itself. Good hemostasis makes the dissection more precise as well as less shocking.

Maintaining this level of dissection of the flap is even more important from the viewpoint of good cancer surgery. In attacking carcinoma of the breast the surgeon must remove at least all of the mammary gland. We know from our pathologic studies that carcinoma often extends widely throughout the breast tissue, and that not infrequently it is found as new and separate foci in areas of the breast remote from the dominant tumor. Mammary tissue extends far more widely over the chest wall than the protuberant breast itself. It may be found extending as a thin layer beneath the fascia which we have described to the midline of the sternum medially, to the edge of the latissimus dorsi muscle laterally, and above to the clavicle. It often extends high into the axilla. Hicken proved the wide anatomical extent of breast tissue nicely with injection studies. The surgeon who intends to remove all the breast tissue must keep his plane of dissection superficial to the superficial layer of the superficial fascia, and carry it to these peripheral limits. Unless this is done, mammary gland, as well as lymphatics accompanying the subfascial vessels, which are one of the routes along which breast carcinoma extends, will be left on the flaps.

It is convenient to begin the dissection of the lateral flap at its caudad end, and to work cephalad. The flap is retracted laterally with light, sharp, single-pronged hooks (Fig. 34-6) devised for this special purpose. These hooks injure the flaps less than the various types of

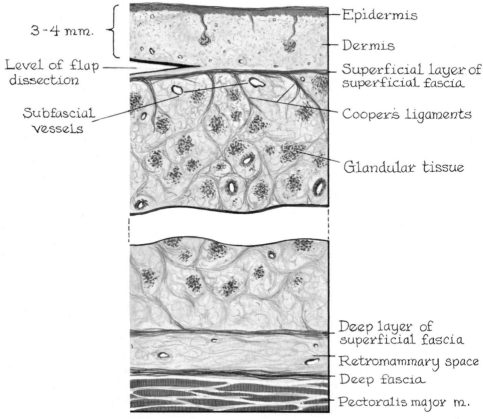

3-4 mm. {

Level of flap
dissection

Subfascial
vessels

Epidermis

Dermis

Superficial layer of
superficial fascia

Cooper's ligaments

Glandular tissue

Deep layer of
superficial fascia

Retromammary space

Deep fascia

Pectoralis major m.

Figure 34–5. Diagrammatic cross section through the breast to show the level of dissection of the skin flap.

compressive forceps or toothed hooks usually employed. In order to provide gentle countertraction from the breast side during the dissection of the flap, an ordinary surgeon's cap is clipped to the edge of the skin to be removed with the breast, using the larger size skin clips. The first assistant then grasps his side of the cap and is thus able to provide

countertraction for the surgeon dissecting up the skin flap, without having to grasp the carcinoma-containing breast itself.

As the caudad portion of the lateral flap is dissected away from the underlying tissues the line of dissection finally reaches the latissimus dorsi muscle. This marks the lateral limit of the elevation of the flap; it is unneces-

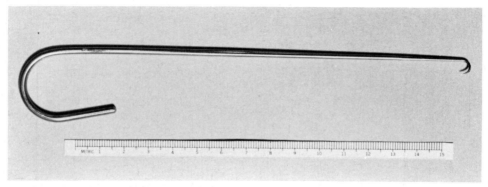

Figure 34–6. Specially designed skin hook for providing retraction in dissection of the skin flaps. (Manufactured by George Tiemann and Co., 21–28 45th Road, Long Island City, New York.)

sary to carry the dissection further posteriorly. Semken liked to call the longitudinal fibers of the outer surface of the latissimus, as they were bared at the edge of the operative field, the *red line*. He took care to develop such a red line down to muscle all around the edge of his operative field, and used it as a definitive guide as to what was to be removed. As the dissection of the lateral flap is carried cephalad the operator *must never lose sight of the latissimus*. Particularly in obese patients, it is easy to lose sight of the muscle and to dissect either too far medially into the dangerous area of carcinoma-containing axillary tissues, or to dissect needlessly far posteriorly into the tissues over the dorsum of the posterior axillary fold.

At a point about halfway upward in the dissection of the lateral flap, the skin hooks are changed to the cephalad half of the flap. I begin the dissection of this cephalad half of the lateral flap by dissecting it up along its whole length for a width of about 5 cm., thus clearly establishing my plane of dissection superficial to the superficial fascia. I then dissect up the most cephalad portion of the flap, which lies over the pectoralis major as it extends laterally over the shoulder. This portion of the flap need not be thin, because breast tissue does not extend up over this region. My level of dissection for this portion of the lateral flap is therefore just superficial to the pectoral muscle, leaving a fairly thick layer of fat on the flap (shown as a shaded zone in the drawing of the skin incision in Fig. 34–3). I next dissect the caudad portion of this upper flap, baring the latissimus dorsi muscle at the deepest point of the dissection.

I now narrow the width of my retraction upon the flap with the skin hooks, improving the definition of the structures I am about to dissect. A bridge of tissue now remains across the axilla (Fig. 34–7), with the naked fibers of the latissimus leading up to it from below and the naked fibers of the pectoralis leading down to it from above. The dissection of this axillary portion of the lateral skin flap is the final step in this phase of the operation. It must be done meticulously, for here axillary lymph nodes containing metastases may lie very close to the skin. If the surgeon scrupulously keeps his plane of dissection superficial to the superficial layer of the superficial fascia in dissecting the axillary skin flap he will lay bare the apocrine glands of the axilla on the inner surface of his flap. These are seen as small brownish nodules, interspersed

with the roots of hairs. They are an excellent guide to the operator in this region, for unless they are exposed, the flap is being cut too thick.

The final step in the dissection of the axillary flap is to identify and lay bare the axillary vein at the base of the flap. The vein lies embedded in fat upon the "white" tendinous portion of the latissimus dorsi muscle. Just caudad to the vein are several small intercostobrachial nerves and accompanying vessels, which also cross over the white tendon. The axillary vein may be identified and exposed by carrying the dissection cephalad after these nerves and small vessels have been divided. I believe, however, that it is safer and more convenient to expose and identify the axillary vein by approaching it from its cephalad side. To facilitate this I replace the retraction upon the flap with skin hooks by direct traction upon the flap held between my second assistant's fingers. In this manner better exposure is obtained at the base of the flap. The flap is then dissected away from its attachment to the fascia of the coracobrachialis muscle, and the axillary vein is finally laid bare from its cephalad side. As this part of the dissection is carried down to the axillary vein, a small and unimportant vein lying in the fascia over it and parallel to it is regularly encountered. If it is not identified and clamped before it is cut, annoying bleeding will result and may obscure the more deeply situated axillary vein. As a final step a double silk marking tie is placed on the specimen at the point where it has been dissected off the axillary vein, so that the pathologists are oriented in studying it. Figure 34–8 shows the dissection of the lateral flap completed.

The hemostasis along the entire length of the axillary flap is now carefully checked, and the flap is replaced against the chest wall so that it will not be angulated and its nutrition interfered with, and is covered with a moist towel.

The operating table is turned back to a level horizontal plane, preparatory to the dissection of the medial skin flap.

The medial skin flap is then dissected back with the same technique used for the lateral flap (Fig. 34–9). Again, it is convenient to begin at the caudad end of the flap. The dissection crosses medially over the rectus fascia to reach the midline of the sternum. I do not remove the rectus fascia except in cases in which the carcinoma is situated in the lower inner sector of the breast. Handley's patho-

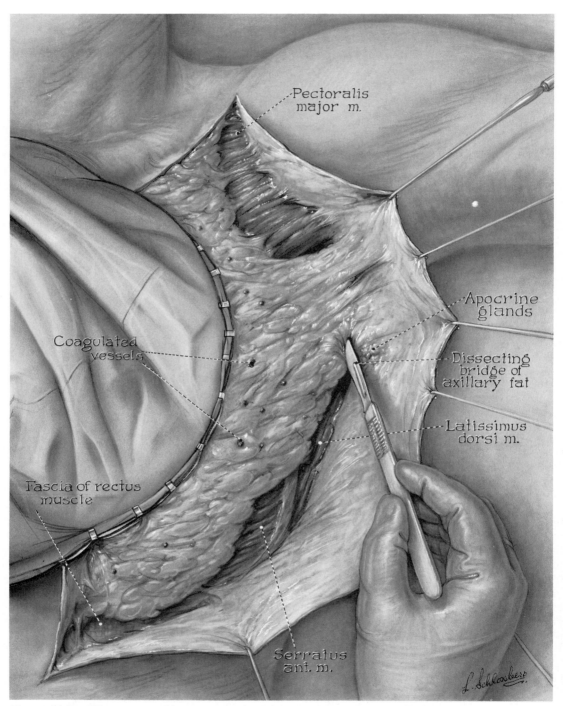

Figure 34–7. The upper and lower portions of the lateral flap dissected, leaving a bridge of tissue to be dissected from its axillary portion.

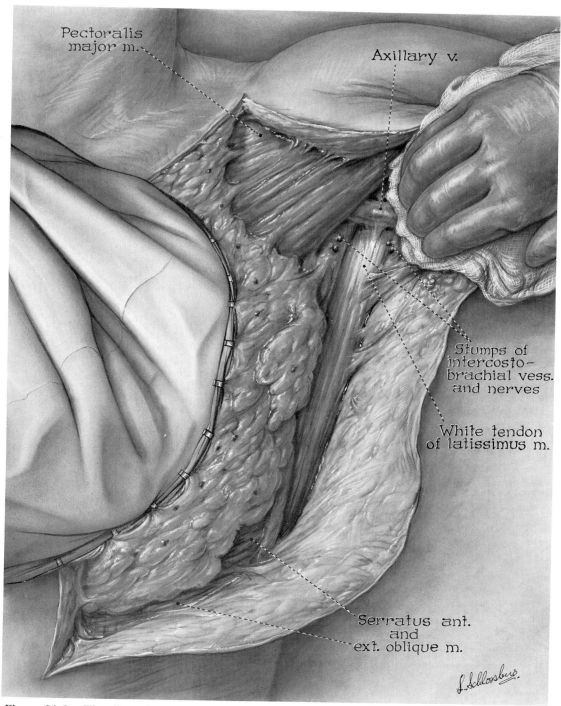

Figure 34–8. The dissection of the lateral flap completed, defining the axillary vein as it crosses the tendon of the latissimus.

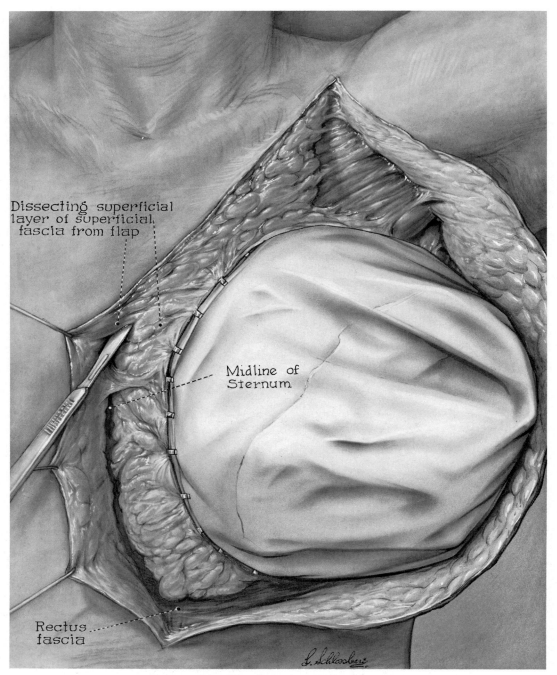

Figure 34–9. The dissection of the medial flap.

logic evidence of the permeation of this fascia with carcinoma was obtained from far advanced cases of the type which we would today classify as inoperable. In cases which we have regarded as operable we have not seen permeation of the rectus fascia, but we nevertheless sacrifice it when the tumor lies in the lower inner sector. The red line at the base of the medial flap is carried upward along the midline of the sternum to the inner end of the clavicle. The direction of the dissection then turns laterally and follows the lower edge of the clavicle. In this area fibers of the platysma coming down from the neck are encountered and severed. When the dissection of this medial flap is completed a careful check of hemostasis is made, and the flap is laid back in place so that it will not be angulated, and covered with a moist towel.

The skin flaps thus dissected up from the superficial layer of the superficial fascia and the breast tissue which lies beneath it, are thinner than the flaps that are cut in what might be called the "standard American radical mastectomy." My flaps are only 3 or 4 mm. thick and consist of the skin covered with only a delicate layer of fine fat lobules. Halsted, in his original operation, dissected this kind of flap over the axilla, for he was a good gross pathologist and realized that a thick flap in this region implied dissection perilously close to the axillary nodes. Elsewhere, however, his flaps were thicker, the incision being carried, in his own words, "through the fat." In defense of Halsted's technique it must be added that his excision was a very wide one, leaving such a large defect on the chest wall that skin grafting was regularly required.

Most present day surgeons are much less radical. Their skin excision is so limited that the edges of the flaps can be brought together and the wound closed. Moreover, the usual practice is to cut thick flaps around the whole operative field, omitting even the dissection of the thin axillary flap that Halsted empha-

sized. In Figure 34-10, reproduced from an illustration of Harrington's technique, these thick flaps are shown. The skin incision is carried directly down through the fat and mammary tissue to the muscle plane, exposing the pectoralis major medially and the serratus muscle laterally. Such thick flaps bear coarse lobules of fat and are several centimeters thick. They are easily and quickly cut. The dissection of thin flaps, such as I have described, is, however, a tedious procedure, requiring about one and one-half hours. In my technique the pectoral and serratus muscles are not laid bare except where the red line crosses them at the periphery of the operative field. These muscles remain covered with subcutaneous fat and mammary tissue after the flaps have been dissected. The difference in the extent and thickness of skin flaps in the "standard American operation" and my operation is shown diagrammatically in Figures 34-11 and 34-12.

When the skin flaps are cut as thin as I have described, the line of dissection must be exact, avoiding cuts into the corium, as well as too much tension. Otherwise necrosis will occur. It takes patience and a gentle hand to learn to cut these thin flaps and get perfect wound healing.

I believe that the dissection of thin skin

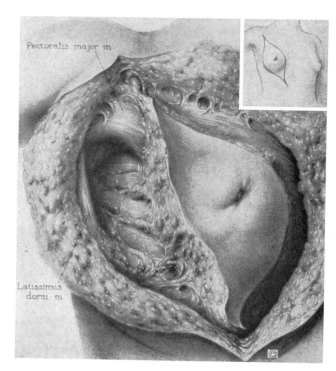

Figure 34-10. The skin flaps of a widely used technique for radical mastectomy. (From Harrington, S. W.: J.A.M.A., *92*:208, 1929.)

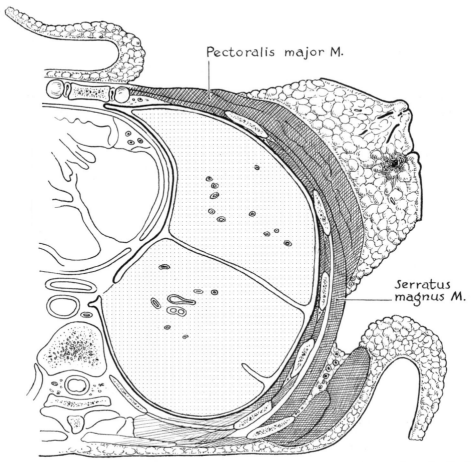

Figure 34–11. Diagrammatic cross section of breast through "Standard American Radical Mastectomy". A very limited area of skin over the breast is sacrificed. The skin flaps are long and thick, and as they are dissected the pectoralis muscle is bared medially and the serratus muscle is bared laterally.

flaps all around the operative field is a logical development of Halsted's original operative plan, and that the labor it entails is worthwhile, as indicated by the low incidence of local recurrence in my personal series of radical mastectomies.

Step 2. Dissection of the Pectoralis Major from the Arm. The dissection at a deeper plane is begun by severing the attachment of the pectoralis major to the arm. With the aid of lateral retraction at the base of the upper portion of the lateral skin flap, the surface of the pectoralis major is exposed. The dissection is then carried laterally, clearing the muscle surface until the cephalic vein, separating the pectoralis from the deltoid, is identified and exposed. The vein is followed out along the deltoid-pectoral groove until the apex of the pectoralis at its attachment of the

humerus is reached. In many patients the cephalic vein is buried in the deltoid-pectoral groove and its exact position is not apparent. Under these circumstances I do not search for it, but proceed to sever the attachment of the pectoralis to the humerus. Most operators force a finger beneath the outer tendinous edge of muscle and elevate it before severing it. This is brutal and unnecessary. Instead I grasp the lateral edge of the deeper tendinous edge of the pectoralis with a clamp, and sever it at a right angle to its fibers, 2 or 3 cm. from its attachment to the humerus (Fig. 34–13). The stump of the pectoralis which remains contains a few small vessels which should be carefully clamped and tied.

The separation of the pectoralis from the deltoid is now carried medially. The two muscles are often so fused that it is not easy to distinguish one from the other. If the cephalic vein has not been previously identified a sharp watch must be kept for it. It will soon be seen marking the line between the two muscles. It should be carefully preserved.

This dissection, freeing the pectoralis from the deltoid and retracting it cephalad, brings the deep pectoral fascia covering the deep structures of the axilla into view. Many surgeons save the clavicular portion of the pectoralis, splitting the muscle between its pectoral and clavicular divisions. This maneuver has two disadvantages. The line of cleavage is a poor one and bleeding is annoying. Also, when the clavicular portion of the pectoralis is left in place, access to the apex of the axilla is limited.

Several atypical muscles may be encountered in the pectoral region. The one most frequently found, and most likely to confuse the operator, is the so-called axillary pectoral

muscle. Paul Eisler described and illustrated it well (Fig. 34–14). As a short muscular band of varying thickness, it arches from the white tendon of the latissimus dorsi up over the axillary vessels and nerves to join the tendon of the pectoralis major at its attachment to the humerus. This muscle is well developed in the anthropoid apes and is present in about 7.7 per cent of human subjects of European stock. In the dissection that I am describing, it must, of necessity, be severed.

Step 3. Dissection of the Pectoralis Major from the Clavicle. As the dissection of the pectoralis major away from the deltoid is carried medially along the cephalic vein toward the apex of a triangle which the deltoid forms with the clavicle, this vein must not be damaged by denuding it too closely of the muscle fibers which often conceal it. In this part of the dissection, exposure is obtained and hemostasis made much easier if the opera-

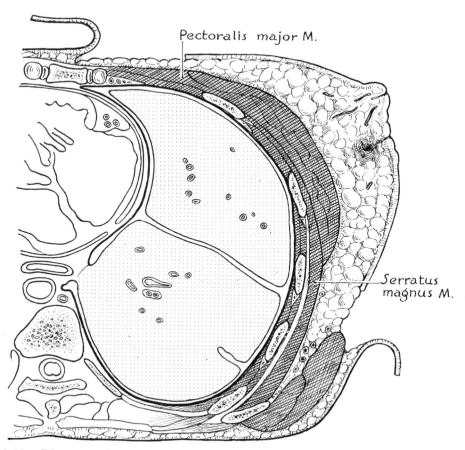

Figure 34–12. Diagrammatic cross section through radical mastectomy as I perform it. A wide area of skin over the breast is sacrificed, and short, thin skin flaps are dissected back. The pectoralis and the serratus muscles are not bared as the skin flaps are dissected.

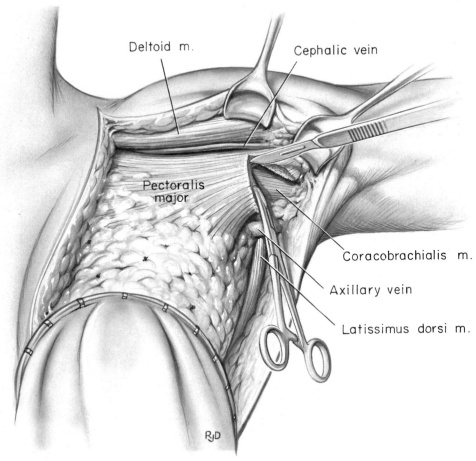

Figure 34–13. Severing the attachment of the pectoralis major to the humerus.

tor uses the fingers of his left hand holding a gauze sponge to exert firm traction in a caudad direction upon the edge of the pectoralis major which he is dissecting away from the deltoid above it. Lateral to the outer edge of the pectoralis minor, the floor of the area that comes into view in this dissection is formed by the costocoracoid fascia. English anatomists have also called this fascia the suspensory ligament of the axilla, and indeed this name is appropriate because this triangular-shaped fascia, with its apex at the coracoid process, is a broad sheet of fascia containing band-like thickenings which stretch in a caudad direction across the nerves and vessels of the axilla. German anatomists call this fascia the deep pectoral fascia. As the dissection proceeds medially, superficial to the upper portion of the pectoralis minor, a number of blood vessels crossing the operative field to enter the pectoralis major are encountered.

They are put under tension by the retraction which the operator exerts upon the pectoralis major with his left hand, making it easier to identify and clamp and cut them. At the medial edge of the pectoralis minor the thoracoacromial vessels, and the lateral anterior thoracic nerves to the pectoralis major which accompany them, come into view. The operative field at this point in the dissection is shown in Fig. 34–15. The thoracoacromial vessels are cleared from the fat in which they lie, and clamped, cut, and tied separately.

The costocoracoid fascia which forms the floor of the area being dissected in this stage of the operation is not disturbed. Beneath this fascia lie the pectoralis minor, the axillary vessels and nerves, and the lymphatics and lymph nodes in which we are particularly interested. All the dissection at this stage of the operation is carried out superficial to this fascia.

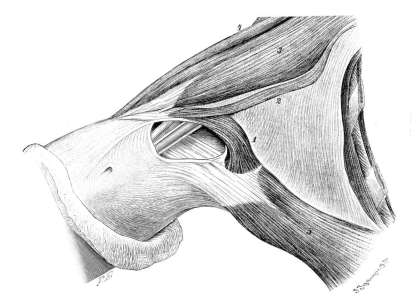

Figure 34–14. Eisler's drawing of the axillary pectoral muscle (labeled 1).

Figure 34–15. The pectoralis major has been separated from the deltoid along the cephalic vein and from the lateral half of the clavicle, and thoracoacromial vessels are defined.

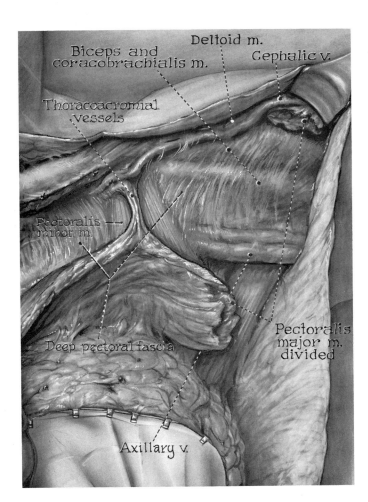

After the thoracoacromial vessels have been dealt with, the dissection is carried medially, severing the attachment of the pectoralis major to the clavicle by cutting across its fibers parallel to and about 1 cm. below the lower edge of the clavicle. Leaving a little of the muscle on the clavicle in this way makes it easier to clamp and tie the small vessels which are severed. As the muscle is cut away from its origin along the inner portion of the clavicle the first interspace is exposed.

Step 4. Dissection of the Pectoralis Major from the Chest Wall. The pectoralis major is now severed from its broad origin from the sternum, the costal cartilages and ribs, and the fascia of the rectus and external oblique muscles, allowing the whole operative specimen to fall laterally to the patient's side. This can be the bloodiest and most shocking part of the operation unless it is done with good hemostasis.

I begin this phase of the dissection by clearing the first interspace down to the intercostal muscle, at a point near the inner end of the clavicle. The thick edge of the pectoralis major muscle is retracted caudad and elevated from the second costal cartilage with a special retractor (Fig. 34–16) which I have devised. I hold it in my left hand and insert its blade between the chest wall and the free edge of the pectoral muscle. With the muscle thus elevated, as shown in Figure 34–17, detachment is begun of its origin from the inner end of the clavicle, the cartilage of the second rib, and the manubrium, at the inner end of the first interspace. Several small branches of the first perforating artery and vein will be encountered as the muscle is transected. Finally, near the deep surface of the muscle, or beneath it, the comparatively large trunks of the first perforating artery and vein will be encountered, arching up over the second costal cartilage. These vessels should be carefully isolated, and clamped before they are cut. The loss of a good deal of blood can be avoided with this technique. A little more laterally, in this same interspace, a much smaller perforating vessel usually emerges along the upper edge of the costal cartilage. It should also be clamped before it is cut. It is

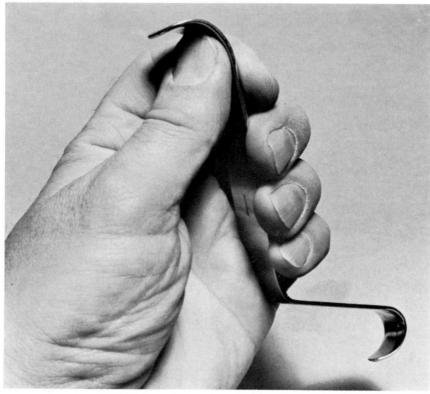

Figure 34–16. Specially designed retractor for elevating the pectoralis major muscle from the chest wall in defining the perforating vessels. (Manufactured by George Tiemann and Co., 21–28 45th Road, Long Island City, New York.)

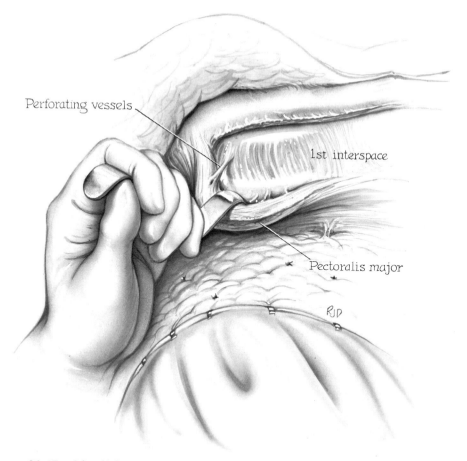

Figure 34–17. Identifying the perforating vessels at the inner end of the first interspace.

the first of a series of minor perforators which emerge in the interspaces parallel to and at a point 3 or 4 cm. lateral to the main perforators.

The dissection is then carried caudad, severing the pectoralis major from its attachment to the sternum and the costal cartilages and ribs. The perforating vessels at the sternal edge in the successive interspaces are identified as they come into view and clamped before they are cut. The position of these vessels in the lower interspaces is variable; sometimes they emerge just below and sometimes just above a costal cartilage. The intercostal spaces should be meticulously cleared of all fat and areolar tissue as the dissection proceeds. As the thoracic cage is thus denuded it should be covered with warm moist compresses or a towel in order to prevent drying of the tissues and consequent shock. The operative specimen is allowed to fall laterally and is similarly covered with a protecting towel.

When the dissection of the pectoralis major from the chest wall has been carried laterally to a point where the fan-shaped edge of the origin of the pectoralis minor comes into view, it should be discontinued. This is a convenient point at which to pause and tie the many clamped vessels, getting rid of the mass of clamps that have accumulated as the chest wall has been cleared. The pectoralis minor must now be dealt with in a separate step.

Step 5. Severing the Attachments of the Pectoralis Minor. In this step, the pectoralis minor muscle is cut across 2 or 3 cm. from its insertion on the coracoid process, and is turned back from over the axillary structures and the chest wall very much as the pectoralis major was dissected back. To free the pectoralis minor, an incision is first made through the costocoracoid fascia along the lateral edge of the muscle, near its cephalad end, where it becomes tendinous. The free edge of the muscle is then picked up with forceps and it is cut across. One or two vessels which are encountered in its substance are carefully clamped and tied. I do not find it necessary or desirable to force a finger beneath the muscle, elevating it from the underlying axillary vein, as most operators are accustomed to doing. This maneuver is apt to cause hemorrhage which obliterates the anatomic details which the operator needs for the meticulous axillary dissection which shortly follows.

A tiny branch of the thoracoacromial artery, which usually enters the pectoralis minor along its medial edge just caudad to the point where it has been transected, should be

identified and clamped and cut. Although this vessel is tiny, it bleeds freely and obscures the operative field if it is torn off as the muscle is dissected back.

The pectoralis minor is then gently retracted caudad, revealing the deep layer of the costocoracoid fascia covering the axillary structures. Since the axillary dissection is a separate and later step in the operation, I take care not to disturb these axillary structures at this stage. The operative field at this point in the dissection is shown in Figure 34–18.

As the pectoralis minor is reflected caudad, a number of vessels which emerge from the

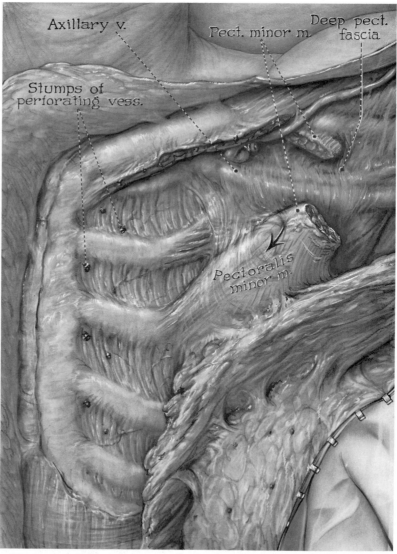

Figure 34–18. The pectoralis major has been dissected from the chest wall, and the pectoralis minor transected near its origin from the coracoid process.

deep layer of the costocoracoid fascia to enter the deep surface of the minor are encountered. They must be clamped and cut close to the muscle. This frees it so that it can be retracted caudad and laterally, giving access to its origin from the third, fourth, and fifth ribs.

The attachments of the muscle to these ribs are then severed, proceeding from the third rib downward. The muscle is friable and difficult to retract. The most convenient way to deal with it is to pick it up with thumb forceps. Along the edge of each rib several tiny vessels will be severed as the muscle fibers are cut across. The pectoralis minor interdigitates with the serratus anterior, and it requires a little special attention and practice to learn to distinguish the pectoralis minor fibers from those of the serratus digitations which lie beneath them and which should not be cut.

The pectoralis minor is allowed to fall laterally with the pectoralis major and overlying tissues already severed from the chest wall, and the dissection is continued in that portion of the operative field just caudad to the origin of the pectoralis minor. In this region the dissection of the specimen off the chest wall should include the careful removal of the fascia over the digitations of the serratus.

This dissection of the serratus fascia is carried posteriorly, the specimen being allowed to fall away to the patient's side, until the edge of the latissimus comes into view in the caudad part of the field. It is then desirable to suspend the dissection of the specimen off from the chest wall, because its detachment can be more conveniently completed after the axilla has been dissected.

Before going on to the next stage all clamped vessels on the thoracic wall should be tied, hemostasis checked, and the whole area of denuded thorax carefully covered with moist compresses.

Step 6. Dissection of the Axilla. The axilla now lies before the operator like an open book. When the arm lies beside the trunk, the axilla may be thought of as a cleft between the upper arm structures and the thoracic wall. When the arm is abducted at right angles to the trunk, however, as in radical mastectomy, the cleft becomes a tetrahedral space, with its apex at the clavicle and its base the lateral axillary wall. The three elongated triangular walls of this space are then formed by the shoulder structures cephalad, the chest wall caudad, and the pectoral muscles ventrally. In the Willy Meyer and standard American techniques for radical mas-

tectomy, in which the axilla is dissected before the pectoral muscles and the breast are removed from the chest wall, the surgeon's access to the axilla is not good because the structures forming its ventral wall (the axillary prolongation of the breast and the fat usually found in this region, and the pectoral muscles) constitute a bulky mass which tends to slide down into the field of dissection in the axilla. In the Halsted technique for radical mastectomy which I am describing, this bulky mass of tissues is out of the operator's way when he dissects the axilla, for with the dissection of the breast and pectoral muscles off the chest wall at an earlier stage in the operation they have fallen to the patient's side. Any surgeon who has compared the ease of access to the axilla with these two different techniques will at once realize the advantage, from this point of view, of the Halsted procedure. Instead of having to dissect in the depths of a deep narrow cleft, handicapped by the need for constant retraction of the overlying tissues, the surgeon can work at ease in a comparatively flat field without any retraction except that provided by the weight of the specimen itself as it lies at the patient's side.

The objection usually voiced against the technique of excising the breast and pectoral muscles from the chest wall before attacking the axilla is that it increases the chance of distant metastasis. It is true that in my operation the axillary route for metastasis remains open during the period required to dissect the breast and pectoral muscles from the chest wall, but we do this without any handling of the breast itself and with only the gentlest kind of retraction on the muscles close to the point at which they are cut from the chest wall. It should be emphasized, on the other hand, that in the final stage of the "standard American radical mastectomy" in which the breast and the pectoral muscles are retracted medially as they are severed from the chest wall, strong traction on the specimen is required and a considerable degree of pressure is often exerted upon the tumor itself. Even though this takes place after the lymphatic pathway through the axilla has been severed, I fear that it may squeeze tumor emboli into lymphatic trunks which still remain, particularly those to the internal mammary nodes.

Another objection that has been made to my technique of excising the breast and pectoral muscles from the chest wall before dissecting the axilla, has been that in so doing I cut across the pathway of lymphatic drainage from the breast to the axilla and thus risk freeing cancer cells into the wound which may be in these lymphatics. A review of the anatomy of the lymphatics of the breast will show, however, that in my technique I do not transect the main lymphatic pathway to the axilla from the breast. These lymphatic trunks run laterally and cephalad from the breast to enter the central group of axillary lymph nodes. They lie beneath the deep pectoral fascia, which remains undisturbed in my technique until I finally dissect the axilla.

Dissection of the axilla is begun by incising the costocoracoid fascia over the brachial plexus, parallel to and slightly cephalad to the axillary vein. The fascia is picked up with smooth forceps and incised with a sharp knife (Fig. 34–19). All my axillary dissection is done with smooth forceps and the knife. I never scrape the axillary contents out with a gauze sponge over the finger, as is the custom of some operators; if the nodes contain metastases this is a splendid way to implant carcinoma cells throughout the operative field and to insure local recurrence. Another disadvantage of the scraping or pawing technique in the axilla is that small vessels are torn. As they bleed and the fine details of the anat-

omy are obscured, it becomes impossible to do a meticulous dissection. Every vessel, even the most minute, must be identified and clamped before it is cut if the requisite perfect hemostasis is to be achieved. Only with this kind of technique can all of the many small lymph nodes be seen and included in the tissues removed. I use smooth rather than toothed forceps in my dissection because I fear that toothed instruments may pierce carcinomatous nodes and pick up and reimplant carcinoma cells. I try, indeed, to avoid grasping nodes even with smooth forceps. Very little traction is needed and usually it can be exerted through clamps on the specimen side of the vessels that are divided.

The costocoracoid fascia having been incised over the brachial plexus, the fascia thus released and the fat and areolar tissue attached to it are dissected caudad, bringing the wall of the vein into view. The ventral and caudad surfaces of its lateral portion are meticulously cleared to the point where the vein crosses the white tendon of the latissimus. The branches of the vein are isolated as they are encountered, and are clamped before they are cut. They vary greatly in number and arrangement. Only one thing need be kept in

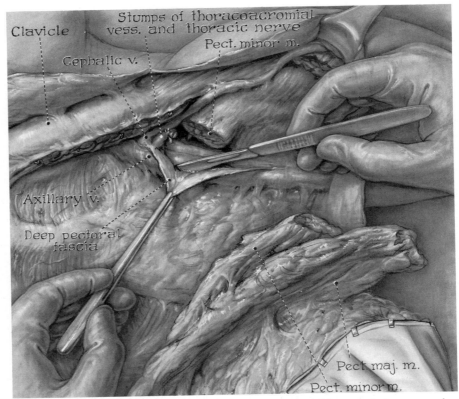

Figure 34–19. Beginning the dissection of the axillary vein with smooth forceps and scalpel.

Artery to pectoralis minor m.
Medial anterior thoracic n.

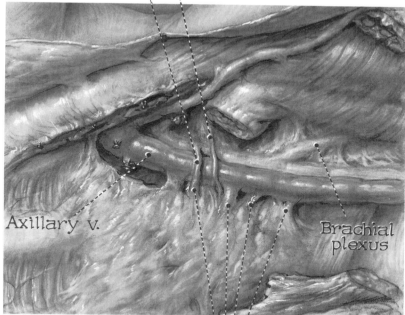

Figure 34–20. The artery to the pectoralis minor muscle and the medial anterior thoracic nerve crossing the axillary vein.

Axillary v.

Brachial plexus

Vessels to be ligated

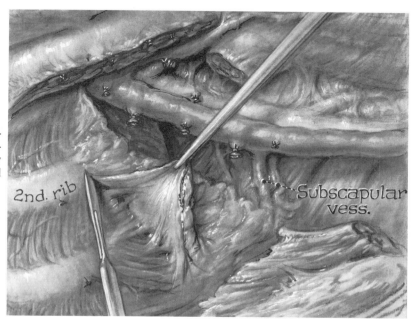

Figure 34–21. The dissection of the costocoracoid fascia and the underlying axillary tissues from the chest wall near the apex of the axilla.

2nd. rib

Subscapular vess.

mind: they should all be sacrificed. The axillary vein occasionally divides into two main trunks. These, of course, should both be preserved. I have not found it necessary to sacrifice the axillary vein on account of the extent of the axillary metastases. If our criteria of operability are followed, cases in which nodes containing metastases are adherent to the vein, and those in which the wall of the vein is involved, will not be operated upon. It may well be that the axillary vein can be excised without much penalty as Neuhof, Faugère, Lobb and Harkins, and Macdonald have maintained, but I see no excuse for the procedure. I am convinced that all cases in which the vein is involved are incurable.

It is not necessary to remove the fat and areolar tissue overlying the brachial plexus. Lymph nodes are not found lying cephalad to the axillary vein, except in the vicinity of the thoracoacromial vessels. We have occasionally found one or two nodes in this region and it is therefore our custom to clear the stumps of these vessels with care.

A small detail concerning the dissection of the axillary vein is worth mentioning. At a point from 1 to 3 cm. lateral to the origin of the thoracoacrominal vessels the axillary vein is usually crossed obliquely by a small artery and nerve (Fig. 34–20). The artery enters the deep surface of the pectoralis minor and sometimes sends a branch onto the adjacent chest wall. Its origin is hidden above and behind the vein where the surgeon does not see it, but it is from a common trunk with the thoracoacromial axis in about half the anatomical subjects I have studied, and a separate branch from the main artery, 1 or 2 cm. lateral to the thoracoacromial trunk, in the other half of the subjects. It is not described in the anatomy texts which I have consulted, so that I have had to designate it simply as the *artery to the pectoralis minor.*

The nerve which accompanies this small artery is the medial anterior thoracic nerve, which also supplies the pectoralis minor. Both the artery and the nerve are closely applied to the ventral surface of the vein in their oblique course across it, and it is from this fact that their importance to the surgeon arises. Since we strip the axillary vein clean, we necessarily identify and sever these two structures which cross over it. A small vein is usually found emptying into the axillary vein just beneath the crossing artery. In isolating, clamping, and cutting the artery and nerve, care should be taken to identify and clamp this small accompanying vein. I call these vessels the "crossing vessels." When they are out of the way the axillary vein is freed upward, and its dissection facilitated.

When the ventral and caudad aspects of the lateral portion of the axillary vein have been cleared, I turn my attention to the apex of the axilla. I dissect the fat and areolar tissue off the medial portion of the axillary vein up to the point where it passes beneath the subclavius muscle. The reflection of the costocoracoid fascia onto the chest wall opposite the upper portion of the vein is then dissected away from the chest wall to the apex of the axilla (Fig. 34–21).

The mass of fat and areolar tissue thus mobilized in the cleft between the chest wall and the most medial portion of the axillary vein contains the highest axillary lymph nodes and the lymphatic trunks that pass upward beneath the clavicle to empty into the confluence of the subclavian and internal jugular veins. A clamp is placed across the apex of the mass as high as possible and it is cut across and ligated in order to avoid backflow of lymph into the wound and to secure the small blood vessels which are usually included within the clamped tissue.

In order to help the pathologist orient the specimen it has been my custom to put a single silk marking tie on the tissue excised from the apex of the axilla. During recent years, however, I have been using a more certain method of making sure that the pathologist identifies the lymph nodes from the apex. When I have completed my dissection of the pyramidal mass of fat and lymph nodes from the apex I cut off the terminal 2 cm. of it and put it in a separate specimen bottle for the pathologist. I then put a single silk marking tie on the remaining axillary tissue at the point where I have transected it.

The next step in the operation is to continue laterally the dissection of the tissues in the cleft between the chest wall and the axillary vein. A number of small vessels spanning this cleft must be clamped and cut, and the lateral cutaneous branches of the intercostal nerves and their accompanying vessels sacrificed, as the mass of axillary tissues is dissected laterally. In the depths of this dissection the lateral thoracic artery is identified, clamped, cut, and carefully tied.

The dissection of the axillary tissues off of the chest wall is carried laterally and caudad until a lateral plane is reached corresponding approximately to that of the thoracodorsal vessels. It is then time for the operator to identify and preserve the long thoracic nerve of Bell, which will be found in the depths of the cleft between the serratus digitations and the sheet of fascia and overlying axillary contents which have been dissected away from the chest wall and retracted laterally. The nerve lies embedded in the fat just beneath the *medial* surface of this fascia. An incision is made through the fascia along the edge of the nerve and it is allowed to drop back medially against the chest wall.

This nerve need never be cut. If patients are properly selected for operation the nerve will not be found to be involved by disease, and there is no reason for sacrificing it. Cutting this nerve produces the ugly deformity of "wing scapula.'

As a final step in dealing with the long thoracic nerve, the operator must dissect it out of the small mass of fat in which it lies up behind the axillary vein in the cleft between the chest wall and the subscapularis muscle. This fat and areolar tissue may contain lymph nodes and must be dissected away from the nerve and removed in continuity with the mass of axillary tissues. To accomplish this, the axillary vein is retracted cephalad with a vein retractor, and the long thoracic nerve is put on stretch by means of gentle caudad pressure retraction with a gauze "peanut" held in a clamp. The fat surrounding the nerve at a reasonably high point behind the axillary vein is cleared with forceps and knife dissection, care being taken to clamp several small vessels which will be found in it.

The axillary dissection has now reached a point at which the thoracodorsal nerve is encountered as it arches down across the subscapular muscle from beneath the axillary vein to join the thoracordorsal vessels. A decision has to be made whether to sacrifice or to preserve it. I almost always sacrifice it. This nerve, during the last 8 or 10 cm. of its course before it enters the latissimus muscle, lies among the lymph nodes of the central and scapular group. It seems unreasonably hazardous to dissect the nerve out from among these lymph nodes, which may well contain metastases. The paralysis of the latissimus muscle which results from sacrificing the nerve, with consequent slight weakness of adduction and internal rotation of the arm, is scarcely perceptible.

The thoracordorsal vessels must now be dealt with. I always sacrifice them for the same reason that I sacrifice the thoracodorsal nerve. They are separately clamped, cut, and tied just beyond the point where the scapular circumflex branches are given off.

When the axillary vein has been cleared all the way out to the point where it crosses the outer edge of the white tendon of the latissimus dorsi muscle, and the thoracodorsal vessels and nerve have been severed, the mass of axillary tissues, now freed from all its medial and cephalad connections, is dissected in a caudad direction down over the surface of the pyramidal muscle body formed by the subscapularis medially, and the teres major and the latissimus dorsi laterally.

The final step in the axillary dissection is the excision of the specimen from along the groove between the chest wall and the latissimus dorsi, its only remaining attachment. This is carried out along a longitudinal plane, and from the chest wall toward the latissimus as shown by the arrows in Figure 34-22. When, in this final stage, the dissection reaches the level of the long thoracic nerve as it lies upon the serratus fascia, the operator must take care to dissect more superficially in order not to damage the nerve. The fascia over the serratus at this deep level is therefore not disturbed.

In this last phase of the operation a little outward traction on the specimen as it lies on the table at the patient's side enables the operator to roll, so to speak, the remaining tissues laterally over the latissimus dorsi. In this process the branches of the thoracodorsal vessels which turn medially to supply the chest wall opposite the apex of the subscapular and teres major muscle body, as well as those which enter the latissimus itself, are isolated, clamped, and ligated. These vessels are of considerable size, and the region has been aptly called the "bloody angle" of radical mastectomy. With the technique which I have described here, however, there is no need of any hemorrhage, for the surgeon's access is good and the vessels are easily identified.

It now remains only to cut the specimen free from the edge of the latissimus dorsi to complete the dissection. The specimen falls of its own weight into the basin which a nurse holds at the side of the operating table to receive it. The dissection has been completed with a minimum of traction and handling of the specimen, and a correspondingly lesser chance of the surgeon's disseminating the carcinoma. The operative field at this stage is shown in Figure 34-23.

Step 7. Closure of the Wound. The whole extent of the wound is now carefully

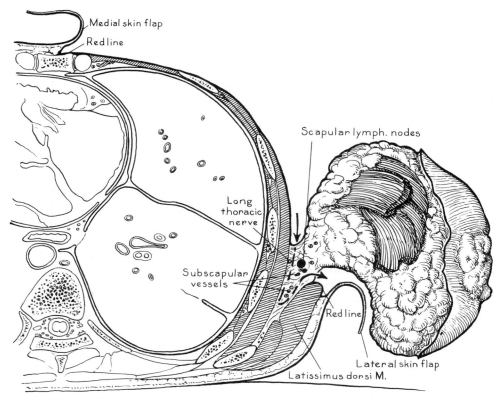

Figure 34–22. The final step in the dissection in cross section—the excision of the specimen from its attachment along the groove between the latissimus and the serrati muscles.

inspected to be sure that it is dry, for if it is to be closed without drainage, as is our custom, hemostasis must be meticulous. The surgeon must also always make sure that he has not left any sponges beneath the flaps.

The skin flaps are then replaced on the chest wall and sutured together at the upper and lower ends of the wound with interrupted sutures of No. 5 silk. The suturing is carried only as far as the flaps will come together without too much tension. A defect of varying size remains on the chest wall. This is oval in shape and usually measures at least 15 cm. in its greatest dimension. The edges of the skin flaps around the defect are sutured down to the fascia over the intercostal and serrati muscles with interrupted sutures of fine silk, their ends being left about 3 cm. long and laid out on the surface of the flaps so that they can easily be picked up when it is time to remove them (Fig. 34–24).

In suturing the flaps to the chest wall around the edges of the defect great care must be taken to avoid too much tension. By this I mean a degree of tension that will cause necrosis. My flaps are so thin that the amount

of tension required to damage them is very slight. The operator has to learn by experience how much tension is safe. Blanching of the skin of the flap beyond the suture is the best indication that too much tension has been used. I watch carefully to see if cyanosis or blanching of the skin of the flaps develops during the few minutes that it takes for me to complete the suturing of the wound. If there is any doubt about there being too much tension I remove the offending sutures and put in new ones with less tension. In teaching residents to perform radical mastectomy as I do it, this is one of the most difficult things for them to learn.

Myers has described a method of detecting portions of skin flaps with an inadequate blood supply by viewing them under ultraviolet light after the intravenous injection of fluorescin. The portions of the flaps that do not fluoresce are excised prophylactically. Myers used the method with success in a series of 52 radical mastectomies. Sanders also recommends it.

Larsen, as well as Keyes and his associates, have recommended suturing the skin

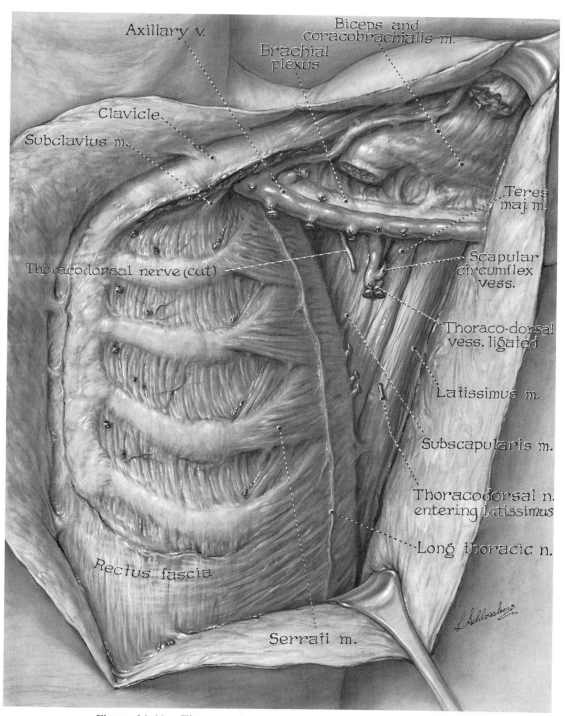

Figure 34–23. The operative field at completion of the dissection.

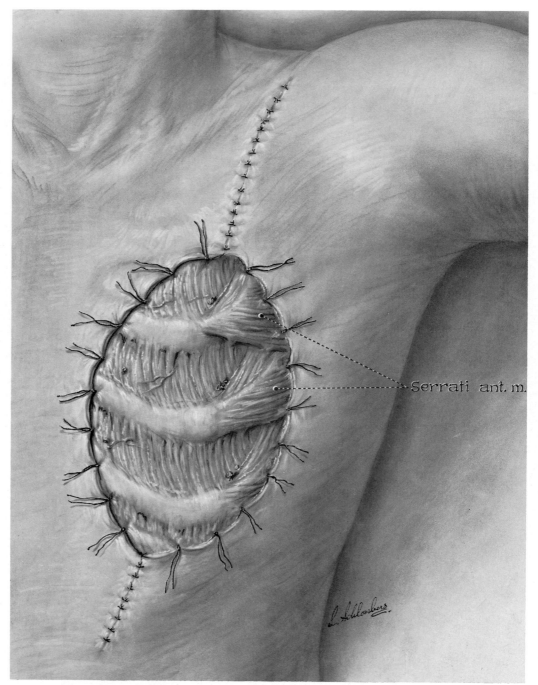

Figure 34–24. The operative wound with the skin flaps sutured in position.

flaps down to the chest wall at multiple points throughout their extent. The fact that they recommend such a procedure is an indication that their flaps are not thin. I would strongly advise against this procedure for truly thin flaps.

The defect is covered with a split-thickness or Thiersch graft (Fig. 34–25), which is usually taken from high up on the lateral aspect of the corresponding thigh. I find that the Reese dermatome is a convenient instrument with which to take the graft. I use the No. 14 shim, which gives a moderately thick graft. If this instrument is used, the graft should be removed from the adhesive tape upon which it is held upon the drum. The graft is then cut

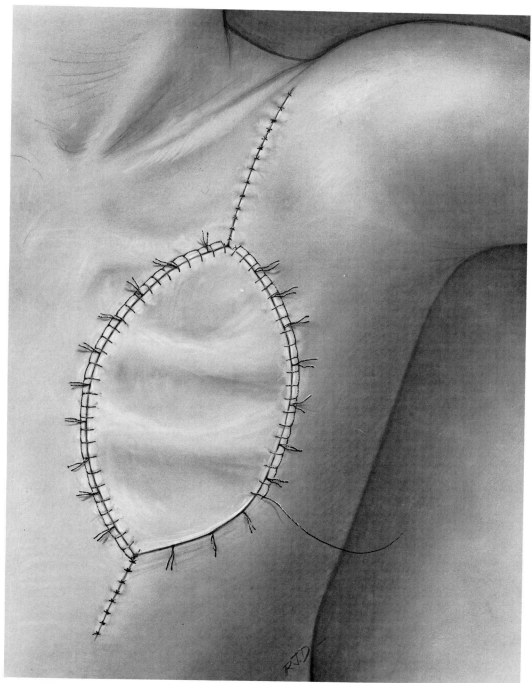

Figure 34–25. The skin graft sutured in place over the defect on the chest wall.

to fit the defect on the chest wall and sutured edge to edge with continuous locked nylon on a swedged curved needle. The graft should be perforated in several places over the inter-spaces, so that if serum or blood accumulates beneath it, it may escape. I take great care to be sure the bed for the graft is absolutely dry before applying it, but even with this precau-tion, there is occasionally some oozing be-neath it which may balloon the graft up unless it is perforated.

No drains are used. If hemostasis is meticu-lous none is required. In occasional pa-tients an accumulation of blood or serum may develop beneath the lateral flap, but this is easily dealt with by aspiration. The use of a drain favors infection in some degree at least, for it is a foreign body in the wound and it provides a channel of communication between the wound and the outside dressing. I recommend more care with hemostasis rather than elaborate arrangements for drainage such as that devised by Raffl.

Step 8. The Operative Dressing. The application of the operative dressing is an important part of the operative technique, and if good wound healing is to be achieved, the dressing must not be left to an assistant who is unfamiliar with its details. The skin graft is covered with strips of non-adhering dressing (Adaptic, Johnson & Johnson). This permits serum and blood to escape between the strips. It is necessary to apply gentle pressure to obliterate the dead space in the axilla and to hold the graft in contact with the chest wall. I use fluffed gauze to obtain this pressure, and although I have tried other materials, I have found none which is its equal for this purpose. The forearm is laid across the upper abdomen and is included within the dressing. Two eight inch ace bandages are then applied, not too tightly, around the chest and arm. The hand is left free, protruding between the folds of the ace bandage. The whole is securely fastened with safety pins and adhesive.

The donor area on the thigh is dressed with a layer of Adaptic covered with many layers of folded gauze held in place with a frame of Elastoplast.

The Prevention of Shock

An experienced operator, working steadily and rapidly, can complete this operation, including the preliminary biopsy of the tumor itself, in between five and six hours. My personal operating time has averaged 330 minutes. I take what time I need to perform the dissection that is required. I do not operate by the clock, although I do not waste time.

Unless precautions are taken to avoid it, shock will sometimes develop in patients operated upon for this length of time. The most important of these precautions are the maintenance of the anesthesia on a comparatively superficial plane, and careful hemostasis. Good hemostasis can only be achieved when the surgeon is willing to take care to identify and clamp all visible vessels before cutting them.

The gentle handling of tissues is also important. The late George Crile put it well many years ago when he classified surgeons who stretch, tear, and crush the tissues as the "carnivorous" type, and those who dissect gently as the "herbivorous" type. In radical mastectomy broad areas of tissue are exposed, and the drying of these tissues must be guarded against by keeping them covered with moist compresses if shock is to be avoided.

If, despite all these precautions to avoid shock, the blood pressure falls unreasonably, measures must be taken to bring it up again. The blood pressure must not be permitted to remain at a dangerously low level for any considerable length of time. In patients with cardiovascular disease, neglect of this precaution courts disaster. By following these general principles, and no doubt by good fortune, I am able to say that I have had no immediate operative deaths in the more than 1000 radical mastectomies for which I have been personally responsible, either as the operator or as the first assistant to my resident surgeon.

The After Care

Rest for the patient and an early resumption of fluid and food intake are the immediate objectives of the general postoperative care. With the type of anesthesia which I have described, our patients are regularly able to take fluids by mouth within a couple of hours after the completion of the operation, and they often tolerate a light meal toward the end of the day. Rest is also good for the wound, because it favors good healing. The patient is put in bed on her back and I do not permit her to be turned during the first 72 hours. Her position may be changed by gatching the head or the foot of the bed up if she desires it. This position is tedious, but since I use morphine or meperidine (Demerol) generously during this period, patients usually do not mind it.

It must be assumed that there has been a degree of bacterial contamination of all wounds in which the operation has lasted a number of hours, and in which skin grafting has been done, but I have learned that my radical mastectomy wounds nevertheless heal very well without developing infection. I therefore do not give any antibiotic prophylactically.

Patients who have had thrombophlebitis, as well as those who develop signs of it during the postoperative period, should receive anticoagulants. The only postoperative death in my personal series of radical mastectomies was the result of my failure to follow this rule. The details follow:

Mrs. F. M. began to have symptoms of cardiovascular disease in 1953 when she was 67. She was digitalized and able to continue her work in the hospital record room. In 1955 she was admitted to the hospital with a questionable diagnosis of myocardial infarct.

In May, 1962, she developed thrombophlebitis of her left leg and was again admitted to the hospital. She had developed moderately severe diabetes since her previous admission but her cardiac status had not changed much. She received anticoagulants. Her phlebitis cleared up promptly and she was discharged after two weeks.

In April, 1963, she discovered a tumor in her left breast. It was situated in the upper central region of the breast and measured 3 × 5 cm. It was clinically a carcinoma, without evidence of regional lymph node spread.

Her general condition was reviewed by her internist. Despite her cardiovascular disease, her diabetes, and her Laennec's cirrhosis, he thought she would do well, provided that she received anticoagulant therapy, since she had a history of previous attacks of thrombophlebitis.

Radical mastectomy was done on April 30, 1963. She withstood the procedure well. Unfortunately I did not follow her internist's advice and use anticoagulants. Her wound did well. She was out of bed on the seventh postoperative day, and felt generally well. She walked about during the succeeding four days and had no symptoms suggesting thrombophlebitis. Her temperature had shown a daily range of from 98 to 99.2° F. for the last five days.

At 2:45 p.m. on the eleventh postoperative day, while walking to the solarium, she felt suddenly weak, and showed signs of shock. She was cyanotic and acutely dyspnoeic but had no chest pain. Within half an hour she was unconscious. It was generally agreed that she had had massive pulmonary infarct. She died three days later without recovering consciousness. There was no autopsy.

I do all the postoperative dressings of my radical mastectomy wounds personally. I long ago learned that the care of these skin-grafted wounds is so complex that if perfect wound healing is to be achieved I cannot leave the dressings to my house staff. I must do them myself. I believe, moreover, that I myself benefit from this experience and that I still continue to learn about wound healing.

At the end of seventy-two hours, I remove the ace bandages and the fluffed gauze, and inspect the skin graft. If it has been ballooned up anywhere by accumulations of serum and blood beneath it, I evacuate them. There is no longer any need for a pressure dressing, and I cover the wound merely with several layers of gauze fastened around the periphery with a frame of Elastoplast.

The arm is now free, and I urge the patient to use it for motions of limited extent, such as holding a newspaper and eating. I caution her against abducting the arm very much from the chest wall. It is certainly very wrong to abduct the patient's arm to a right angle at this stage, as some surgeons in the past have done. This motion pulls the axillary flap out away from the chest wall, and hinders obliteration of the dead space in the axilla.

After six or seven days I take the dressing down completely for the first time, removing all the sutures around the edge of the graft except two or three of the interrupted sutures holding the axillary portion of the lateral flap down to the chest wall. It is wise to leave these few for as long as ten days to avoid the accident of the patient's abducting the arm too far and pulling the lateral flap away from the chest wall.

After 72 hours I also take down the dressing of the donor area on the thigh. The gauze will be soaked with blood and serum, and I remove it all except the final few layers which will stick to the underlying Adaptic and should not be disturbed. I again cover the area with many layers of gauze and frame it with Elastoplast. After this the donor area dressing will usually stay dry and need not be disturbed for two weeks or more. The Adaptic will then come free and leave the area healed. I do not approve of leaving the donor area exposed to the air, as is the fashion of some surgeons; it is bothersome for the patient and certainly not aesthetic.

I usually get my patients out of bed on the sixth or seventh postoperative day, and they are usually ready to go home on the twelfth to fourteenth day.

The operation which I have described does not cripple the arm. Patients are eventually able to use the arm for everything from scrubbing floors to playing tennis. Figures 34–26 and 34–27 show the absence of any constriction across the axilla in one of my patients.

By the time the patient goes home, she will be using her arm comparatively freely for limited motions. She should now be urged to begin to increase the degree of abduction and to use the arm as normally as possible. During the month that follows, a simple exercise which gains abduction gradually is that of abducting both arms together in a transverse plane, with the forearms extended. If this mo-

Fig. 34–26

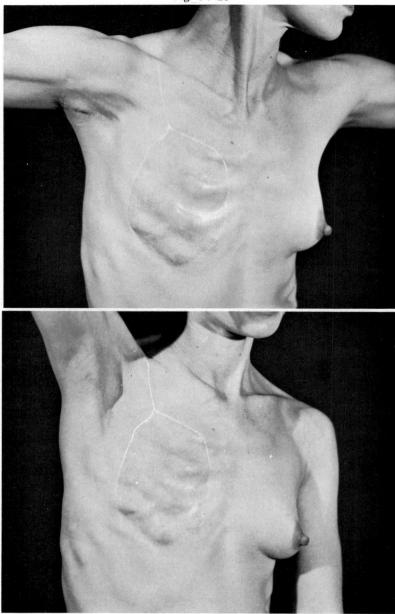

Fig. 34–27
Figures 34–26 and 34–27. Arm motion after radical mastectomy.

tion is practiced several times a day, the full range of arm motion will eventually be regained. In achieving this, patients have to bear some discomfort but this is not greater than most will tolerate. I have not referred my patients to physiotherapists for assistance in regaining arm function. I consider this a part of my duty to my patients, and I have had no difficulty in succeeding with it.

Edema of the arm has always been one of the major hazards of radical mastectomy. I will discuss it separately.

THE RESULTS OF MY METHOD OF RADICAL MASTECTOMY

The results in my personal series of radical mastectomies performed between 1935 and

1957 are presented in the following series of tables.

Table 34-1 gives a general picture of what happened to the 626 patients in my personal series during the 10 years following their operation.

In Table 34-2 I have included not only my 5- and 10-year survival rates for my patients treated by radical mastectomy, but also the survival rates for a total of 45 of my patients in whom preliminary biopsy disclosed metastases in the subclavicular lymph nodes at the apex of the axilla or the internal mammary nodes, and whose treatment was by irradiation alone. I have included in this table both 5- and 10-year survival rates to show how inadequate the 5-year data are in presenting a true picture of the results of treatment.

This table gives, in essence, complete information as to how my patients were selected for radical mastectomy. I have carefully defined elsewhere the clinical features of Clinical Stages A, B, C, and D in our Columbia Clinical Classification. Those who wish to compare my results with the results of other methods of treatment need only select their patients on the same basis that I have selected mine.

As I have explained in the preceding chapter, I have, through the years, continued to learn which patients should be treated by radical mastectomy. I now perform the operation only for patients whose disease is in Clinical Stages A and B. I have abandoned preliminary internal mammary biopsy as a criterion for selection, but continue to perform biopsy of the apical subclavicular nodes in a small proportion of patients in whom palpation of the axilla leaves me in doubt as to whether they belong in Clinical Stage B or C.

The frequency as well as the extent of axil-

Table 34-2. Five- and 10-year survival rates by clinical stage for radical mastectomy, and also for patients with metastases to subclavicular or internal mammary nodes treated only by irradiation. Personal series of cases, 1935–1957

		Radical Mastectomy			
		5 Years		10 Years	
Columbia Clinical Stage	No. of Patients	No. Survived	Per Cent Survival	No. Survived	Per Cent Survival
A	402	341	85%	280	70%
B	154	92	60%	63	41%
C	59	24	41%	14	24%
D	11	2	18%	2	18%
Totals	626				

		Positive Subclavicular or Internal Mammary Nodes Irradiation Only			
		5 Years		10 Years	
Columbia Clinical Stage	No. of Patients	No. Survived	Per Cent Survival	No. Survived	Per Cent Survival
A	14	6	43%	3	21%
B	17	5	27%	3	18%
C	14	1	7%	0	0%
D	0	0	0%	0	0%
Totals	45				

		Entire Series of Patients Treated by Primary Surgery or Irradiation			
		5 Years		10 Years	
Columbia Clinical Stage	No. of Patients	No. Survived	Per Cent Survival	No. Survived	Per Cent Survival
A	416	347	83%	283	68%
B	171	97	57%	66	39%
C	73	25	34%	14	19%
D	11	2	18%	2	18%
Totals	671				

Table 34-1. Crude 10-year survival rate for radical mastectomy. Personal series of cases, 1935–1957

1. Number of radical mastectomies		626
2. Number of operative deaths		0
3. Number of patients lost track of*		2
4. Number of patients dying of intercurrent disease within 10 years		53
5. Number of patients dying of breast carcinoma within 10 years		214
6. Number of patients surviving 10 years		359
7. Crude 10-year survival rate		57.3%

*The two patients lost to follow-up and counted as dying of breast carcinoma were both well when lost track of at 5½ and 7 years, respectively, after operation.

lary metastases in my personal series of cases is correlated with the 10-year survival rate in Table 34-3. It is clear from these data that the status of the axillary nodes is overwhelmingly important in determining the survival rate following radical mastectomy. It is also obvious that the pathologist can make a very important contribution to determining prognosis by thorough study of the axillary specimen and careful reporting of the number of axillary nodes involved and their position in the axillary lymph node filter. When only three nodes or less contain metastases in the patients whose disease is classified as Clinical Stage A the survival rate is nearly as good as when no nodes are involved. Metastasis in the subclavicular node group at the apex of the axilla is, however, an indication of incurability. All these details are of critical im-

Table 34–3. RADICAL MASTECTOMY FOR BREAST CARCINOMA. EXTENT OF AXILLARY METASTASIS CORRELATED WITH 10-YEAR SURVIVAL. PERSONAL SERIES OF CASES, 1935–1957

Columbia Clinical Classification	Number Axillary Nodes with Metastases	No. of Patients	10-year Survival
Stage A	No nodes involved	279	76%
	1 to 3 nodes involved	88	69%
	4 to 7 nodes involved	18	22%
	8 or more nodes involved	17	18%
	Total	402	70%
Stage B	No nodes involved	37	70%
	1 to 3 nodes involved	51	43%
	4 to 7 nodes involved	33	36%
	8 or more nodes involved	33	9%
	Total	154	41%
Stage C	No nodes involved	11	45%
	1 to 3 nodes involved	15	33%
	4 to 7 nodes involved	7	29%
	8 or more nodes involved	26	8%
	Total	59	24%
Stage D	No nodes involved	–	–
	1 to 3 nodes involved	2	50%
	4 to 7 nodes involved	1	–
	8 or more nodes involved	8	13%
	Total	11	18%
Total No. of Patients		626	
Per cent with Axillary Metastases		49.4%	

portance in determining further treatment in the individual patient.

As I have mentioned previously, it has been suggested by my critics that the superior results in my personal series of radical mastectomies can be explained by my selection of patients with more favorable disease. The most direct answer to this innuendo is a comparison of the frequency of axillary metastasis in other well documented series of radical mastectomies with the frequency of axillary metastasis in my own series. Table 34–4 presents these data for several carefully documented modern series of radical mastectomies. The average of axillary metastases in these case series is 51 per cent. In my personal series of radical mastectomies it was 49.4 per cent, which is not significantly different.

A feature of my personal series of cases which I should also like to emphasize is that the results were essentially as good in the series of ward patients, where I served as first assistant and the operation was performed by my pupil, the resident surgeon, as they were in my series of private patients where I operated myself. These data are shown in Table 34–5. They substantiate the point which I have repeatedly emphasized,

that the operation in itself, as we do it, is not technically difficult, and that it can be successfully performed by properly instructed surgeons who have not had a great experience with it.

LOCAL RECURRENCE FOLLOWING RADICAL MASTECTOMY

Local recurrence is a considerable threat following the usual type of radical mastectomy. It may be of three types. The first, and least frequent, type is local recurrence in the axilla. The second type is the parasternal mound-like tumor that is the outward manifestation of metastases to internal mammary nodes. They are not properly chargeable to the surgeon in the sense of his having implanted them.

The third and by far the most frequent type of local recurrence, are the nodules in the skin flaps on the chest wall. In general such nodules must result from the implantation in the wound of carcinoma emboli that have escaped from blood vessels or lymphatics cut during the operation, or the implantation of carcinoma cells by instruments or sponges from a focus of carcinoma into which

Table 34–4. THE FREQUENCY OF AXILLARY METASTASES IN RADICAL MASTECTOMY

Author	No. of Radical Mastectomies	Per cent with Axillary Metastases
Spratt and Donegan Ellis Fischel Hospital 1940-1958	704	56.7%
Lewison The Johns Hopkins Hospital 1946-1950	253	54.5%
Butcher Barnes Hospital 1950-1955	397	54.2%
Miller Grace Hospital 1951-1960	465	48.6%
Haagensen Columbia-Presbyterian Medical Center 1935-1957	626	49.4%
Dahl-Iversen and Tobiassen Rigshospitalet 1950-1955	425	41.1%
Handley Middlesex Hospital 1946-1969	804	55.4%

Table 34–5. 10-year survival of ward and private patients. Personal series of radical mastectomies, 1935–1957

Columbia Clinical Classification	Private Patients (Haagensen operator)		Ward Patients (Resident operator, Haagensen assistant)	
	No. of Patients	Per cent 10-Year Survival	No. of Patients	Per cent 10-Year Survival
Stage A	219	70.8	183	67.6
Stage B	64	40.6	90	41.1

the surgeon has unwittingly carried his dissection, or from small unrecognized foci of carcinoma in breast tissue left by the operator on his thick skin flaps.

Whatever the explanation for local recurrence on the chest wall may be, the surgeon is certainly responsible for it. Either his operative technique has been faulty, or he has erred in choosing to operate upon carcinoma so far advanced that it is impossible to get it all out. This same criticism applies when there is recurrence in the axilla.

Although most recurrent nodules on the chest wall are distressingly genuine, the pos-

sibility of pseudo-recurrence must always be kept in mind. Foreign body cysts around suture material sometimes simulate true recurrence, as described by Moschowitz. Another form of pseudo-recurrence is the bony hard, fixed nodule that develops on a rib or costal cartilage where the surgeon's knife has nicked it. These prove to be merely proliferation of periosteum or perichondrium.

The frequency and site of local recurrence within 10 years in my personal series of radical mastectomies is shown in Table 34–6. The most striking feature of these data is the infrequency of recurrence in the axilla; among a total of 299 patients with axillary metastases, only three developed axillary recurrence. I must attribute the great part of this success of our treatment for the axilla to the meticulous axillary dissection which these patients had. However, prophylactic irradiation probably played some role in preventing recurrence in the 40 patients who also received irradiation to the axilla among the 556 whose disease was classified as Clinical Stage A or B. One patient who did not receive irradiation and whose disease was classified as Clinical Stage B, developed axillary recurrence. Thirty-five other patients in the Clinical Stage A and B groups received postoper-

Table 34–6. Local recurrence within 10 years following radical mastectomy correlated with clinical stage and pathologically verified axillary metastases. Personal series of cases, 1935–1957

Columbia Clinical Classification	Status of Axillary Nodes	Parasternal Recurrence	Chest Wall Recurrence	Axillary Recurrence
Stage A	No metastases 279 cases	6	3	0
	Metastases 123 cases	7	11	0
Stage B	No metastases 37 cases	1	0	0
	Metastases 117 cases	6	18	1
Stage C	No metastases 11 cases	0	0	0
	Metastases 48 cases	4	10	2
Stage D	No metastases 0 cases	0	0	0
	Metastases 11 cases	0	7	0
Total	No metastases 327 cases	7	3	0
	Metastases 299 cases	17	46	3

ative axillary irradiation because they had extensive axillary metastasis. They had an average of 11 involved axillary nodes each. Yet not a single one developed axillary recurrence. This experience has led us to recommend postoperative prophylactic irradiation to the axilla only when a total of eight or more axillary nodes are found to be involved.

The chest wall recurrences are much the most frequent type of local recurrence following radical mastectomy. In Table 34–7 chest wall recurrence within 10 years is correlated with the extent of axillary metastasis in my personal series of cases. Chest wall recurrence was rare when there were no axillary metastases. It was distressingly frequent, however, when a total of eight or more axillary nodes were involved: thirty-five per cent of these patients whose disease was classified as Clinical Stage A, and 40 per cent of those whose disease was Clinical Stage B, developed chest wall recurrence. The 19 patients in these two groups who developed chest wall recurrence had an average of 16 axillary nodes involved by the disease.

These local recurrences on the chest wall when many axillary nodes are involved are understandable. Even the most meticulous surgeon is apt to fail to get the disease all out of the axilla under these circumstances. Since the chest wall dissection is part of the same operative field as the axillary dissection he will probably leave foci of carcinoma beneath the skin flaps.

I did not give postoperative prophylactic irradiation to the chest wall in any of my patients. I might have reduced the frequency of chest wall recurrence considerably if I had given it to the patients with extensive axillary involvement. I now recommend it for all patients who have a total of eight or more axillary nodes involved.

Local Recurrence in Relation to Skin Grafting

One of the controversial questions regarding the technique of radical mastectomy continues to be whether or not skin grafting is desirable. Halsted, in his 1912 paper describing the method of skin grafting which he had regularly employed for 16 years, concluded, "It is better to remove too much skin than

Table 34–7. RADICAL MASTECTOMY FOR BREAST CARCINOMA. EXTENT OF AXILLARY METASTASIS CORRELATED WITH FREQUENCY OF LOCAL RECURRENCE WITHIN 10 YEARS. PERSONAL SERIES OF CASES, 1935–1957

Columbia Clinical Classification	No. of Axillary Nodes with Metastases	No. of Patients	Per cent Local Recurrence in Chest Wall
Stage A	No nodes involved	279	1%
	1 to 3 nodes involved	88	5%
	4 to 7 nodes involved	18	6%
	8 or more nodes involved	17	35%
	Total	402	3.5%
Stage B	No nodes involved	37	0%
	1 to 3 nodes involved	51	4%
	4 to 7 nodes involved	33	9%
	8 or more nodes involved	33	40%
	Total	154	11.7%
Stage C	No nodes involved	11	0%
	1 to 3 nodes involved	15	13%
	4 to 7 nodes involved	7	14%
	8 or more nodes involved	26	27%
	Total	59	17%
Stage D	No nodes involved	—	—
	0 to 3 nodes involved	2	0%
	4 to 7 nodes involved	1	100%
	8 or more nodes involved	8	75%
	Total	11	64%
Total number of patients		626	

too little, for the mistake of excising an insufficient quantity is quite fatal to the patient's chance of recovery."

The opposite view was held by Sampson Handley, who wrote in 1906, "The area of skin taken away in the operation should obviously be no larger than necessary, and no healthy skin should be removed. It has already been shown that cancer does not spread in the plane of the skin. . . . The necessary conditions can usually be fulfilled by the removal of a circular area of skin 4 or 5 inches in diameter, with the growth at its center."

It is Handley's point of view that has won out in the half century that has gone by since these two distinguished students of breast carcinoma disagreed. Today the standard American radical mastectomy sacrifices so little skin that the flaps can be brought together, albeit with some tension. Skin grafting has been abandoned even by most of the pupils of Halsted's pupils. There are only a very limited number of surgeons who continue to graft skin regularly.

In a paper on the subject which he wrote in 1946, White compared the frequency of local recurrence in a number of clinics without being able to demonstate any advantage in skin grafting. He quite rightly concluded, however, that local recurrence after radical mastectomy is a distressingly common experience in most clinics.

Conway and Neumann subsequently made a detailed study of the relationship of local recurrence to skin grafting in 255 radical mastectomies performed at the New York Hospital between 1932 and 1942. Although they found that the recurrence rate was actually higher in the grafted cases, these cases had a higher incidence of axillary metastases and were therefore presumably more advanced.

Zimmerman, Montague, and Fletcher have recently presented a report of the frequency and distribution of local recurrence after radical mastectomy in their series of cases. Skin grafting was not done, but about two-thirds of the patients received preoperative or postoperative irradiation to the chest wall. The five-year incidence of local recurrence in the chest wall was approximately 8 per cent.

Donegan and his associates, in their study of local recurrence in their series of 704 patients treated by radical mastectomy, reported a 5-year cumulative local recurrence rate of 17.5 per cent. Skin grafting was done in only 289 of the 704 patients. There was no significant difference in the local recurrence rate in those whose wounds were closed primarily as compared with those whose wounds were grafted.

Unfortunately, it is a fact that skin recurrences often appear later than five years after operation. In order to provide a fair test of the value of skin grafting as regards avoidance of local recurrence we should compare the 10-year results in case series carefully classified as to clinical stage of advancement, all treated by radical mastectomy, but some series of cases grafted and the others not.

No such comparison has been available until our recent "Cooperative International Study of the Treatment of Early Breast Carcinoma" appeared. If the reader will study the data presented in this study (Table 34–8) it is evident that in my personal series of radical mastectomies the rate of local recurrence on the chest wall within 10 years is approximately 6 per cent, which is less than half that for the other methods of radical mastectomy. I attribute at least a part of this difference to my sacrifice of so much skin over the breast that I regularly close the defect with a skin graft.

A second reason why I intend to continue skin grafting is that I am convinced that it is a kindness to the patient, quite apart from the matter of local recurrence. One advantage of skin grafting is that it saves the patient discomfort. It is amazing to me how painless radical mastectomy usually is if the skin flaps are not sutured with tension. My patients often tell me they have had no pain at all postoperatively. On the other hand, I see many patients whose skin flaps have been pulled together with tension sutures, and who have had a good deal of pain as a consequence. The sensation of constriction of the chest that all patients have to some degree for a considerable time after radical mastectomy is much more marked in patients whose skin flaps have been sutured under tension.

A third reason that impels me to suture the skin flaps without tension and to graft skin is that I know that this is the easiest way to make certain of perfect wound healing and to avoid edema of the arm. Necrosis, infection, and fibrosis are the triad that lead to edema of the arm, and they are, unfortunately, frequent when the skin flaps are pulled together under tension.

Table 34–8. CARCINOMA OF THE BREAST. LOCAL RECURRENCE WITHIN 10 YEARS.
COOPERATIVE INTERNATIONAL STUDY OF THE TREATMENT OF EARLY MAMMARY CARCINOMA

Columbia Clinical Classification	Method of Treatment	Parasternal Recurrence	Chest Wall Recurrence	Axillary Recurrence	Total Patients with Local Recurrence
Stage A	Total mastectomy + ax. dissection + irradiation Williams and Stone	0%	12%	10%	22%
	Conservative radical mastectomy Handley and Thackray	5%	12%	2%	16%
	McWhirter method Kaae and Johansen	1%	10%	8%	19%
	Extended radical mastectomy Dahl-Iversen and Tobiassen	2%	10%	8%	20%
	Radical mastectomy Haagensen and Cooley	4%	3%	0%	7%
Stage B	Total mastectomy + ax. dissection + irradiation Williams and Stone	0%	12%	14%	26%
	Conservative radical mastectomy Handley and Thackray	6%	22%	0%	26%
	McWhirter method Kaae and Johansen	0%	11%	18%	29%
	Extended radical mastectomy Dahl-Iversen and Tobiassen	0%	16%	16%	32%
	Radical mastectomy Haagensen and Cooley	5%	13%	1%	18%

The Treatment of Local Recurrence

Donegan emphasized the grave prognostic significance of local recurrence after radical mastectomy. Forty-six per cent of his 146 patients who developed local recurrence died of their disease within one year after its reappearance, and only 4 per cent lived more than five years.

My experience has not been quite so unfortunate. Thirty-six per cent of the 53 patients who developed local recurrence in my personal series of 556 radical mastectomies performed for patients whose disease was classified as Clinical Stage A or B died within a year after their local recurrence. Thirteen per cent lived more than five years, and three of these still survive, 11.2, 11.5, and 19 years, respectively after diagnosis of their local recurrence.

In studying the significance of local recurrences the clinical stage of the disease as well

as the type of local recurrence should be considered. Table 34–9 shows the average length of time elapsing between operation and local recurrence, as well as the length of survival after local recurrence, in the 53 patients in my personal series of cases who developed local recurrence. These patients are classified by clinical stage, and their recurrences are classified in the three usual types—parasternal, chest wall, and axilla. It will be seen from this table that in the Clinical Stage A patients local recurrences developed later, and the patients survived somewhat longer than the Stage B cases. It will also be apparent that the patients with parasternal recurrences do a little better than those with chest wall recurrence.

Our experience has taught us that all three types of local recurrence, parasternal, axillary, and skin flap and skin graft recurrences, are better treated by irradiation than by surgery. Most surgeons have enough common

Table 34–9. Average Interval Between Radical Mastectomy and Local Recurrence and Average Length of Survival After Local Recurrence in 53 Patients in Personal Series of Cases, Clinical Stages A and B, 1935–1957

Columbia Clinical Classification	Parasternal Recurrence		Chest Wall Recurrence		Axillary Recurrence	
	Average Interval Between Operation and Recurrence	*Average Survival After Recurrence*	*Average Interval Between Operation and Recurrence*	*Average Survival After Recurrence*	*Average Interval Between Operation and Recurrence*	*Average Survival After Recurrence*
Stage A	50 months	35 months	41 months	26 months	—	—
Stage B	36 months	22 months	26 months	17 months	6 months	54 months
Total	43 months	28.5 months	33.5 months	21.5 months	6 months	54 months

sense not to attempt to excise the parasternal and axillary recurrences, but many cannot resist the temptation to excise small solitary recurrences in the skin flaps. In so doing they spread the recurrent disease around and make the radiotherapist's task of controlling it more difficult. Radiotherapy usually succeeds in controlling solitary skin recurrences, and when new ones develop in adjacent areas they too can be successfully dealt with by irradiation. This is not true of the surgical attack; the surgeon is soon hopelessly defeated in his effort to control successive local recurrences. It is therefore my practice to treat local recurrence with irradiation.

DISTANT METASTASIS FOLLOWING RADICAL MASTECTOMY

Distant metastasis is of course the sword of Damocles that hangs over the patient who has had a locally successful radical mastectomy.

In my personal series of 626 radical mastectomies, distant metastases (excluding local recurrence on the chest wall and parasternal and axillary recurrence) developed in a total of 256 patients within 10 years. The sites of first distant metastasis in these patients are shown in Table 34–10.

The striking prognostic significance of axil-

Table 34–10. Site of First Distant Metastases Within 10 Years Following Radical Mastectomy Correlated with Clinical Stage and Pathologically Verified Axillary Metastases. Personal Series of Cases, 1935–1957

Columbia Clinical Classification	Status of Axillary Nodes	Supra-clavicu-lar	Oppo-site Axilla	Oppo-site Breast	Distant Skin	Lung	Bone	Liver	Other Ab-dominal	Brain	Other	Total
Stage A	No metastasis 279 cases	4	—	—	4	20	15	5	2	5	3	58
	Metastasis 123 cases	3	3	4	2	20	22	9	5	6	2	76
Stage B	No metastasis 37 cases	—	—	—	—	5	1	—	1	—	—	7
	Metastasis 117 cases	10	3	2	2	27	39	7	7	5	1	103
Stage C	No metastasis 11 cases	—	—	—	—	—	2	1	—	1	1	5
	Metastasis 48 cases	11	4	2	3	17	16	1	3	5	3	65
Stage D	No metastasis 0 cases	—	—	—	—	—	—	—	—	—	—	—
	Metastasis 11 cases	1	—	—	—	4	4	—	2	—	—	11
Total	No metastasis 327 cases	4	—	—	4	25	18	6	3	6	4	70
	Metastasis 299 cases	25	11	8	7	68	81	17	17	16	6	256

lary metastases again emerges from these data regarding distant metastases. Distant metastases were three and one-half times more frequent in patients with axillary metastases than in those whose axillae were not involved.

Osseous and pulmonary metastases were much the most frequent types of distant metastasis to appear first in my patients.

The Time of Local Recurrence and Distant Metastasis after Radical Mastectomy

It is important to study the time of local recurrence and metastasis because it gives us a better concept of the natural history of the disease, and how its course is influenced by different types of treatment.

There have been a good many individual case reports of the very late development of local recurrence and distant metastasis. These reports have been tabulated by the Mortons, and more recently by Danckers and his associates. Pawlias, Dockerty, and Ellis reported a series of 45 cases of late local recurrence. In general it can be said that the more complete and the longer the follow-up, the more late recurrences will be found, although they are still comparatively infrequent after 10 years.

It is important to look critically into the genuineness of presumed late "recurrence." Many of the case reports are so incomplete that no definite conclusion can be drawn from them. It is more than likely that rather than being examples of true late recurrence, they represent one of three other phenomena, as follows:

1. The Persistence rather than Recurrence of Carcinoma. Patients whose carcinoma has been locked up by irradiation fibrosis until it finally begins to grow again belong in this category. Since these patients are never free from disease, it is not proper to classify them as having late recurrence.

2. Metastasis from a Different Primary Carcinoma. In patients who develop metastasis after a long period of freedom from evidence of their disease, it is often not certain that the source is the original breast carcinoma. It may be a different and occult primary carcinoma. Small primary carcinomas from the lung and pancreas are particularly likely to be missed clinically, and they may closely resemble breast carcinoma microscopically. The metastasis may be from a small

and undetected primary carcinoma in the second breast. The following is a case of this kind which only the autopsy findings saved us from mistaking for an example of late recurrence.

Miss H. M., aged 44, came to the Presbyterian Hospital in June 1940 complaining of a tumor of the left breast of one month's duration. The tumor was situated in the upper inner sector of the breast and measured 7 cm. in diameter. It was hard, irregularly nodular, and fairly well delimited. It was freely movable. There was a broad area of dimpling in the skin caudad to it, but no other skin changes. In the left axilla there were several nodes up to 1 cm. in diameter, and one of them was hard. Radical mastectomy was performed. There was no involvement of axillary nodes.

She was well for 14½ years, until January, 1955, when she developed symptoms of *right-sided* pleural effusion. X-ray examinations showed massive right pleural effusion. There was no evidence of local recurrence of her left mammary carcinoma. Careful search revealed no evidence of a new primary carcinoma anywhere else. The right breast was normal on palpation. She was treated with thoracentesis and estrogens, and survived another year, dying on February 16, 1956. Autopsy revealed an entirely unsuspected 1 cm. carcinoma situated deep in the center of the right breast, which had metastasized to the right pleural cavity, the liver, the diaphragm, the spine, the thyroid, and the right cervical lymph nodes. There was no evidence of recurrence of her original left-sided mammary carcinoma. It was assumed that the carcinoma in the right breast was a new and independent lesion.

An autopsy is always necessary to settle the question of the origin of metastases definitively. Willis described one of the best examples of late metastasis proved by autopsy. In his case signs of a brain lesion developed 14 years after radical mastectomy for carcinoma. At craniotomy, a partly calcified, partly cystic metastasis was found in the parietal area of the brain. The patient died a week later, and other metastases, seemingly from the original breast carcinoma, were found elsewhere in the brain as well as in the hilar region of both lungs, and in the mediastinal lymph nodes. No other primary carcinoma was demonstrated.

3. New Primary Mammary Carcinoma Developing from Mammary Tissue left on Thick Skin Flaps. As I have already pointed out, the skin flaps of the standard American radical mastectomy are so thick that they often include a good deal of mammary tissue. It is likely that carcinoma reappearing in the flaps a long time after operation is sometimes a new primary lesion, arising in the residual mammary tissue. Wawro has described a convincing example of this phenomenon. In his patient the new primary developed in breast tissue left on a skin flap from 2 to 4 cm. thick, 17 years after the original operation.

I have studied the time of recurrence following radical mastectomy in two different case series. The first is our Presbyterian Hospital series of 990 radical mastectomies performed between 1923 and 1938. The follow-up of these patients was not as complete as the follow-up in my own personal series of cases operated upon between 1935 and 1957. In the 1923–1938 series of cases recurrence developed more than 10 years after operation in 10, or about 1 per cent, of the patients. The details of the course of the disease in these 10 patients with late recurrence are presented in Table 34–11.

It is of interest that in nine of these 10 patients the carcinoma was microscopically well differentiated, and therefore likely to be slowly growing.

Although autopsy confirmation of the nature of the process was lacking in all but one of these cases, biopsy corroboration of the metastasis was available in the two cases with the longest latent period, Cases 6 and 7. The details of these two cases are summarized below.

CASE 6

Mrs. M. G. had been aware of a tumor in her left breast for two years. There was a transverse depression across the upper outer sector of the breast, extending around the edge of the anterior pectoral fold. The skin in the depression was reddened. Beneath it there was a firm, irregular tumor 3 cm. in diameter. It was freely movable over the underlying pectoral muscle. There were no palpable axillary nodes.

Radical mastectomy was done without skin grafting. The tumor proved to be a well differentiated Grade I carcinoma that had not metastasized to the axillary nodes.

Her first symptom of recurrent disease was pain and numbness in the left hand which began twenty years after her operation. A deep hard fullness was noted in the supraclavicular region. The arm became edematous. The pain increased in severity

Table 34–11. First recurrence of breast carcinoma more than 10 years after radical mastectomy. Presbyterian Hospital, 1923–1938

Case Number	Patient	Age	Date of Operation	Status of Axillary Nodes	Microscopic Type of Primary Tumor	First Recurrence	Interval from Operation to First Recurrence	Recurrence Elsewhere	End Result	Autopsy
1	G. DaC.*	44	Oct. 1935	1 positive in 6	Small cell	Skin graft Mar. 1954	18.5 yr.	None	Died in auto accident, Oct. 1963	0
2	E.S.	58	Feb. 1927	1 positive in 6	Grade II	Medial skin flap May 1940	12.2 yr.	Unknown	Lost track of, 1949	0
3	M.T.	50	Feb. 1934	positive	Grade I	Axilla May 1948	14.0 yr.	Unknown	Lost track of	0
4	E.I.	49	Dec. 1938	3 positive in 23	Circumscribed	Supraclavicular Jan. 1949	10.1 yr.	Pleura March 1953	Died Jan. 1959	0
5	J.R.	40	Sept. 1941	positive	Papillary	Supraclavicular + cervical March 1952	10.7 yr.	Unknown	Died Oct. 1954	0
6	M.G.	44	Nov. 1928	negative	Grade I	Supraclavicular Nov. 1948	20.0 yr.	Lung June 1951	Died Sept. 1951	0
7	R.S.	44	Nov. 1923	positive	Grade I	Lung March 1945	21.3 yr.	Unknown	Died March 1947	0
8	A.K.	50	Feb. 1937	8 positive in 8	Grade I	Ribs Sept. 1947	10.6 yr.	Unknown	Died May 1950	0
9	D.L.	38	June 1938	positive	Intraductal	Thoracic vertebrae + femur May 1953	15.0 yr.	Bone, lungs, liver	Died May 1956	+
10	E.H.	47	July 1921	positive	Small cell	Generalized skeleton Sept. 1935	14.2 yr.	Lungs Sept. 1938	Died Jan. 1939	0

*This was the only one of the 10 patients whose mastectomy wound was closed with a skin graft.

and extended up the arm into the neck. Flaccid paralysis of the arm developed. The supraclavicular area was finally explored and extensive carcinomatous involvement of the brachial plexus found. This lesion resembled the original primary breast carcinoma microscopically. She died two and one-half years later with lung metastases.

CASE 7

Mrs. R. S. noted a tumor in her right breast in November, 1922, a year before she was admitted to the Presbyterian Hospital. Examination showed a typical 2 cm. carcinoma of the upper outer sector of the breast. There were several enlarged hard axillary nodes, the largest 1 cm. in diameter. Radical mastectomy was done and the tumor proved to be a well differentiated Grade I carcinoma, largely intraductal. There were several involved axillary nodes. She was well for 21.3 years following operation. Then she began to have retrosternal pain and a hacking cough. Roentgenograms showed metastases in the right pulmonary parenchyma and pleural fluid. Thoracoscopy was done and firm yellow nodules were seen on the lung surface. Biopsy of these showed it to be a carcinoma, microscopically identical with the breast carcinoma removed many years previously. She died without any other evidence of distant metastasis two years after her first pulmonary symptom.

In studying the time of recurrence in my personal series of radical mastectomies I have focused upon the 556 patients whose disease was classified as Clinical Stages A and B because they are the ones in whom we now perform radical mastectomies. The numbers of the principal forms of recurrence are shown by year in Table 34–12. A total of 330 recurrences have been observed up to the present time in this series of cases. These data are expressed graphically in Chart 34–1.

Since patients who have recurrence of their carcinoma usually develop them in several different sites, the actual number of patients who develop recurrence is considerably smaller. I know the site and time of first recurrence of their disease in 193 of the patients in my personal series of cases. These are shown in Table 34–13, and are presented graphically in Chart 34–2.

From these data it is seen that recurrence developed with about the same frequency during each of the first five years following operation. During the next five years the frequency of recurrence steadily decreased.

At the present writing, recurrence which appeared more than 10 years after operation has developed in a total of 18, or 3 per cent, of my 556 Clinical Stage A and B patients. I have summarized the pertinent details of these 18 patients with late recurrence in Table 34–14. Their recurrences were spread over a long period of years. In two patients (Cases 7 and 4) recurrence developed more than 20 years after operation.

The details of the course of the disease in these two patients are summarized below.

CASE 7

Mrs. L. L., aged 32, discovered a small tumor in her left breast but did not consult us for a year because it did not seem to change much. When admitted in February, 1942, she had a typical 4 cm. carcinoma of the upper inner sector of the breast, without any clinically involved axillary

Table 34–12. NUMBERS OF RECURRENCES BY SITE AND YEAR FOLLOWING RADICAL MASTECTOMY IN CLINICAL STAGE A AND B CASES. PERSONAL SERIES, 1935–1957

Site of Recurrence	Postoperative Year										After 10 Years
	1	*2*	*3*	*4*	*5*	*6*	*7*	*8*	*9*	*10*	
Bone	14	13	14	7	9	6	5	2	6	1	9
Lung and pleura	9	11	17	10	11	5	4	3	2	0	7
Parasternal	1	5	2	3	3	3	0	1	1	1	2
Chest wall	5	13	4	3	3	2	2	1	0	1	4
Liver	4	6	1	4	5	0	1	0	0	0	1
Other abdominal	3	2	1	2	2	1	2	2	0	0	1
Supraclavicular	2	5	6	1	2	0	0	1	0	0	2
Contralateral axilla	2	0	0	3	0	0	1	0	0	0	0
Opposite breast	1	2	0	1	1	1	0	0	0	0	0
Distant skin	0	2	0	2	1	1	0	2	0	0	2
Brain	2	3	2	3	3	3	0	0	0	0	1
Other	0	1	0	1	1	2	0	1	0	0	3
Totals	43	63	47	40	41	24	15	13	9	3	32

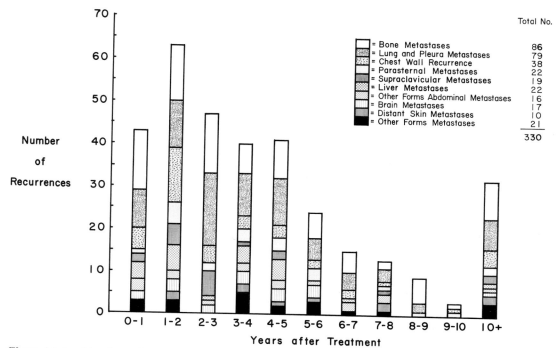

Chart 34–1. Number of recurrences by site and year following radical mastectomy in Clinical Stage A and B cases. Personal series, 1935–1957.

Table 34–13. NUMBERS OF PATIENTS WITH FIRST RECURRENCE BY SITE AND YEAR FOLLOWING RADICAL MASTECTOMY IN CLINICAL STAGE A AND B CASES. PERSONAL SERIES, 1935–1957

Site of Recurrence	Postoperative Year										After 10 Years
	1	2	3	4	5	6	7	8	9	10	
Bone	10	9	10	3	6	5	4	1	6	1	4
Lung	5	4	9	7	5	2	1	1	1	1	4
Parasternal	0	5	4	1	3	3	0	1	1	0	2
Chest wall	5	13	3	3	1	0	0	1	0	0	4
Liver	1	4	1	0	2	0	1	0	0	0	1
Other abdominal	1	1	0	0	0	1	0	1	0	0	0
Supraclavicular	2	5	3	0	0	0	0	1	0	0	1
Contralateral axilla	0	0	0	0	0	0	1	0	0	0	0
Opposite breast	0	0	0	0	0	0	0	0	0	0	0
Distant skin	0	1	0	1	1	1	0	1	0	0	1
Brain	1	2	1	0	1	1	0	0	0	0	0
Other	2	1	0	0	0	1	0	0	0	0	1
Totals	27	45	31	15	19	14	7	7	8	2	18

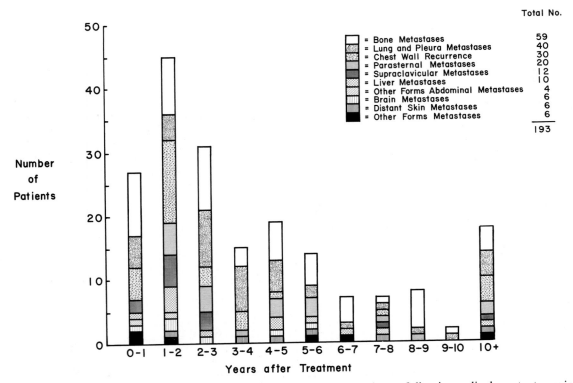

Chart 34–2. Number of patients with first recurrence by site and year following radical mastectomy in Clinical Stage A and B cases. Personal series, 1935-1957.

nodes. Her disease was classified as Clinical Stage A. Radical mastectomy was done. Eight of a total of 14 axillary nodes contained metastases. The primary tumor was a well differentiated Grade I carcinoma. No postoperative irradiation was given.

In November, 1962, 20 years and 9 months after operation, induration was noted at the base of the right side of her neck. Shortly thereafter a right Horner's syndrome developed and chest films showed slight indentation of the trachea on the right side and elevation of the right diaphragm. A biopsy of the right supraclavicular mass confirmed the diagnosis of metastases of her original breast carcinoma.

Irradiation was given to the right mediastinum and the right infraclavicular and supraclavicular regions.

Within a year the patient developed metastases to the brain, as well as to the dorsal spine, pelvic bones, and humerus. She died in August, 1964.

There was no autopsy, but it seems likely that she originally had metastases to her right internal mammary nodes, and after slowly growing over a period of many years in these nodes, her disease reached the nodes in the lymphatic terminus at the base of her right neck, and there generalized through the blood stream. Prophylactic irradiation to her internal mammary region might have saved her.

CASE 4

Miss H. B., aged 55, noticed dimpling of the skin just above the areola of her right breast and on palpation felt a lump beneath the area of skin retraction. The tumor measured 4.5 cm. in diameter and had the clinical characteristics of a carcinoma. There were no clinically involved axillary nodes and the disease was classified as a Clinical Stage A carcinoma. Radical mastectomy was performed in June, 1939. A total of 36 axillary nodes were free of metastases. The primary tumor was a well differentiated Grade I carcinoma. It is shown in Figure 34–28. The individual cells are seen to be comparatively uniform in size and shape, and are often arranged in tubules.

No postoperative irradiation was given.

In April, 1967, 27 years and 10 months later, I noted an 8 mm. erosion at the edge of the skin graft along its inner upper border. It was so characteristic of local recurrence that it was treated by irradiation. The erosion healed satisfactorily.

In October, 1969, however, the irradiated area broke down, and biopsy of the area was done. The sections showed carcinoma similar to the original breast carcinoma removed more than 30 years previously. A limited excision of the chest wall was done and the defect was closed with a flap mobilized from the opposite breast. She died in December, 1969.

Case Number	Patient	Age	Date of Operation	Clinical Stage	Size of Primary Tumor	Status of Axillary Nodes	Microscopic Type of Primary Tumor	First Recurrence	Interval from Operation to First Recurrence	Recurrence Elsewhere	End Result	Autopsy
1	H.T.	59	Oct. 1948	B	2.0 cm.	2 positive in 24	Grade I	Medial skin flap March 1959	10.4 yr.	Scalp Oct. 1961	Died May 1962	0
2	C.S.	55	April 1945	A	2.0 cm.	No metastasis in 18	Intraductal	Skin graft Feb. 1958	13.3 yr.	Liver, lungs, contra. axilla. bones, ovary	Died Aug. 1968	+
3	L.K.	65	Feb. 1941	A	2.0 cm.	No metastasis in 14	Grade I	Skin graft March 1960	19.1 yr.	Supraclavicular +pleural July 1963	Died Sept. 1968	+
4	H.B.	55	June 1939	A	4.5 cm.	No metastasis in 36	Grade I	Edge skin graft April 1967	27.8 yr.	None	Died Dec. 1969	0
5	M.H.	49	July 1945	A	4.0 cm.	1 positive in 30	Grade II	2nd interspace Feb. 1958	12.7 yr.	Bones, pleura Dec. 1959	Died July 1961	0
6	H.B.	45	Mar. 1942	B	4.5 cm.	7 positive in 14	Grade I	3rd interspace Nov. 1966	14.7 yr.	Lung, bones June 1967	Died June 1968	0
7	L.L.	32	Feb. 1942	A	4.0 cm.	8 positive in 17	Grade I	Supraclavicular nodes Nov. 1962	20.7 yr.	Brain, bones Nov. 1963	Died Aug. 1964	0
8	M.M.	47	Oct. 1949	B	3.5 cm.	4 positive in 20	Grade I	Pleura Dec. 1965	14.1 yr.		Died May 1969	+
9	A.L.B.	63	April 1950	A	3.0 cm.	2 positive in 34	Grade II	Pleura March 1964	13.9 yr.		Died Sept. 1966	0
10	H.M.	47	July 1940	B	6.5 cm.	6 positive in 19	Grade I	Pleura Feb. 1955	14.3 yr.	Spine and liver	Died Feb. 1956	+
11	N.P.	50	Jan. 1942	B	8.0 cm.	3 positive in 10	Grade I	Pleura Jan. 1954	12.0 yr.		Died Dec. 1954	0
12	L.B.	63	Sept. 1944	A	3.5 cm.	No metastasis in 18	Grade I	Bones June 1958	13.6 yr.		Died Feb. 1959	0
13	L.C.	49	Jan. 1948	B	5.0 cm.	6 positive in 14	Grade III	Bones August 1958	10.6 yr.	Lung Sept. 1958	Died Aug. 1959	0
14	L.B.	47	June 1937	B	10.0 cm.	15 positive in 18	Mucoid	Femur April 1949	11.8 yr.		Died Oct. 1953	0
15	M.V.	55	Oct. 1942	A	6.0 cm.	No metastasis in 10	Intraductal	Liver May 1956	13.5 yr.	Ovary, omentum	Died July 1956	+
16	M.T.	51	Dec. 1947	A	3.0 cm.	1 positive in 11	Small cell	Distant skin March 1959	11.6 yr.	Bones April 1959	Died Dec. 1959	+
17	M.H.	53	June 1941	A	4.0 cm.	1 positive in 18	Small cell	Subcutaneous neck Oct. 1959	18.3 yr.	Pleura Nov. 1965	Died Feb. 1966	0
18	L.C.	63	June 1947	A	2.0 cm.	3 positive in 30	Intraductal	Vertebrae August 1963	16.0 yr.	Lung August 1963	Died April 1964	+

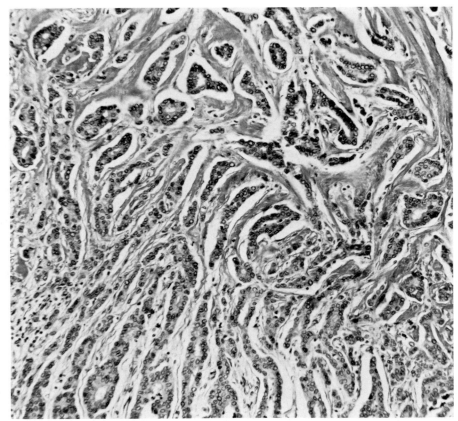

Figure 34–28. Primary carcinoma of the breast which recurred at the edge of the skin flap 27 years and 10 months after radical mastectomy.

These late skin recurrences in the skin graft and in the skin flaps in four of my patients, 10, 13, 19, and 27 years postoperatively, can be explained theoretically by the fact that my very thin flaps as well as the skin grafts provide a poorly vascularized site in which a minute focus of well differentiated carcinoma might remain locked up in scar tissue for a very long time.

The fact that these late recurrences occurred with well differentiated carcinoma is apparent in Table 34–14: 15 of my 18 patients were in this class. These lesions lack the growth vigor of undifferentiated carcinomas and grow slowly.

EDEMA OF THE ARM AFTER RADICAL MASTECTOMY

The complications of shock and infection which were formerly a hazard, to some degree, of radical mastectomy, have been solved, and edema of the arm is the only postoperative complication of any consequence. It remains, however, the greatest penalty that women have to face after the average standard American radical mastectomy.

It is necessary first of all to define what we mean by edema. A good many patients have transitory slight increase in the diameter of the arm following radical mastectomy. This kind of edema usually produces an increase of less than 3 cm. in the diameter of the arm and ordinarily disappears with the restoration of arm function. An exception must be made for the baggy enlargement of the ventral aspect of the highest part of the upper arm. This is seen in obese patients with relaxed tissues, and results from severing the axillary fascia. It cannot be avoided. The edema to which I refer as a formidable complication affects the whole of the arm or the entire upper arm. This kind of edema, which makes the patient socially unpresentable and which gives her a feeling of tension in the tissues of the arm, varies greatly in degree.

It may be defined as an increase in the

diameter of the arm by at least 3 cm. If it is not much more than that it may be classified as moderate edema. But it may become very severe and crippling, as in the patient shown in Figure 34–29. She was obese and was given postoperative irradiation to the axillary and supraclavicular regions.

Britton and Nelson, who have written one of the best papers dealing with postmastectomy lymphedema of the arm, tabulated its frequency as reported in 14 different case series. It varied between 6.7 and 62.5 per cent. Daland's experience was typical: 27.8 per cent of his patients had moderate or severe arm edema.

In tabulating the frequency of arm edema, the patients in whom edema develops as the result of local recurrence of the carcinoma in the axillary and supraclavicular regions should be set apart, or excluded. This type of edema is not directly related to the surgery that has been performed. What might be called *surgical* edema, that developing in patients who have been treated surgically but remain free of clinical evidence of axillary or supraclavicular recurrence, should be further classified into two types. *Postoperative* surgical edema is the type that occurs immediately following operation. It must be regarded as the consequence of some sort of fault in surgical technique. *Secondary* surgical edema is the type that develops many months or years after operation as the result of a new infection in the arm through a portal of entry on the hand or arm. The surgeon cannot be held responsible for secondary edema, except to the extent that he may have failed to warn his patient that any minor wound or infection on the hand or arm subsequent to radical mastectomy is a serious matter.

It is sometimes difficult to distinguish true postoperative edema from the edema develop-

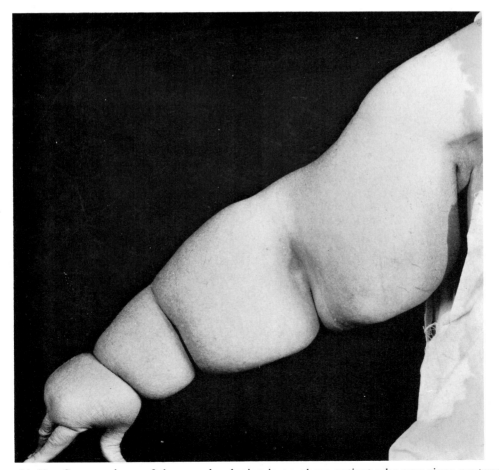

Figure 34–29. Severe edema of the arm developing in an obese patient who was given postoperative radiotherapy to the axillary and supraclavicular areas.

ing as a result of later infection. For instance, the patient may go home after operation and shortly thereafter burn her forearm while cooking, with the result that she develops edema, for which her surgeon is truly not responsible.

In my personal series of patients postoperative edema has been infrequent. Only about 5 per cent have developed it. Secondary edema, resulting from infection gaining entry through the skin of the hand or arm, has been more frequent. Approximately 8 per cent of my patients have had episodes of cellulitis of the arm which have left some degree of permanent edema.

To understand edema of the arm it is necessary to think in terms of our modern knowledge of the physiology of the lymphatics. We know that the blood carries water, electrolytes, and proteins toward the periphery of the body. The water and the electrolytes are freely diffusible from the capillaries into the extracellular spaces. Some water and electrolytes are absorbed by the lymphatics, while the remainder diffuse back into the venules. Some protein leaks from the capillaries and is also absorbed by the lymphatics.

The superficial subdermal lymphatics probably have only a minor role in the drainage of fluid from a limb. The main drainage is through the lymphatic trunks situated in the deep subcutaneous tissue, and the deep lymphatic trunks in the deep fascia and underlying muscles. When radical mastectomy is performed, these main lymphatic trunks of the subcutaneous tissue and the deep fascia are severed through a radius of at least 180° around the ventral aspect of the arm. The main lymphatic trunks from the arm drain into the axillary lymph nodes, and these are, of course, almost all extirpated. As a result, lymphatic drainage from the arm must be carried on through alternative routes. These are probably the lymphatics over the cephalad and dorsal aspects of the shoulder and those of the posterolateral chest wall.

The degree of interference with lymphatic function in the arm following radical mastectomy and in edematous arms was studied in our clinic by David Ju. He devised a lymphatic function test for this purpose, performed as follows: Three cc. of saline solution and 2 cc. of the patient's serum are added to 25 microcuries of radioactive iodinated albumin. Five cc. of this solution is then injected into the dorsal aspect of the web-space between the first and second digits. Background counts of radioactivity are taken, using the

contralateral arm. With a specially shielded Geiger counter with a long window, the edematous arm is studied in three sections — hand, forearm, and upper arm. Counts are taken immediately after injection and after 48 hours. Approximately 75 per cent of the injected dose is absorbed within a 48 hour period in a normal arm. In contrast, during the first two weeks following radical mastectomy the percentage of injected material absorbed is much lower, the average being about 45 per cent absorbed in 48 hours. After from two to four weeks the percentage absorbed increases almost to a normal level, so that the reading is approximately 65 per cent at the end of 48 hours.

These facts indicate that following the sudden extirpation of the major portion of the lymph nodes into which the arm lymphatics empty, if wound healing is normal, adequate collateral lymphatic circulation usually develops within a month. It is true that the reserve capacity of the lymphatic circulation is encroached upon. In most patients, however, no edema results. Edema, then, must be due to some other factor that causes a further encroachment upon the lymphatic drainage of the arm. The evidence indicates that this is *infection*.

Halsted, with his wonderful facility for discovering the essential truth of every problem that he put his mind to, was the first to describe the clinical picture of edema of the arm following mastectomy. He called it "elephantiasis chirurgica." He correctly described the two types which I have mentioned — that which follows shortly after operation, and that which may develop any time subsequent to operation, sometimes years later, following an episode of infection. I quote his description of the former type. "A few months ago I interviewed a patient . . . who each year for 16 years following an operation by me at The Johns Hopkins Hospital for cancer of the breast has had one or two and occasionally three or four attacks of redness and swelling of the arm on the operated side. The first symptoms, malaise and nausea, were quickly followed in the severe attacks by a chill and fever and then by slight redness and increased swelling of the arm. The arm of this patient was observed to be swollen a few days after operation. . . ."

Halsted also correctly interpreted the cause of postoperative edema as infection due to bad wound healing. He said, "Now it is within the experience of every surgeon, especially of those who employ plastic methods to cover the defect, that frequently marginal necroses of the flaps occur and occasionally sloughings of considerable dimensions, and it is usually in these cases that the swelling of the arm is most pronounced. Attendant upon the necrosis there is infection, and inflammatory reaction in varying degree, and the greater the reaction the greater in general the swelling of the arm immediate and ultimate."

Halsted found that when the axillary flap was not sutured under tension, and axillary dead space was avoided, "swollen arms of dimensions sufficient to distress or annoy the patient were no longer observed, marginal necroses rarely occurred, and the grafts took throughout with few exceptions. . . . We have been led to conclude that swelling of the arm follows the plastic operations [that is, bringing the flaps together without grafting] in greater proportion and in more pronounced form than is seen in the cases treated by skin grafting."

I have myself long been convinced that infection is the underlying cause of edema of the arm. We know that studies of the air in operating rooms often show pathogenic organisms. A considerable proportion of the personnel in operating rooms carry the same organisms in their noses and throats. Routine cultures of radical mastectomy wounds prior to closure in our hospital some time ago showed that about one-third were contaminated with pathogenic organisms, usually hemolytic *Staphylococcus aureus*.

Despite the presence of these organisms in our wounds, infection does not develop if the surgeon achieves perfect wound healing. The fact is, however, that many surgeons do not. I have so often seen edema follow bad healing of mastectomy wounds resulting from brutal surgical technique and improperly supervised wound care that I am certain that this is the usual explanation of edema. Perfect healing of radical mastectomy wounds is apt to be achieved only by experts. Other surgeons often have a varying degree of necrosis of the skin flaps because they handle them too roughly or suture them too tightly. Cultures of necrotic skin are almost always positive for hemolytic *Staphylococcus aureus*.

Another common source of infection is an imperfectly obliterated dead space in the axilla. Serum and blood accumulating in this dead space provide a perfect culture medium for the growth of the organisms often present in the wound. The infection may be of such slight degree as to escape the attention of the surgeon entirely. It is sufficient, however, to obstruct lymphatic flow beyond the critical level, and fluid begins to accumulate in the arm.

I believe that postoperative edema has not been a serious problem for me because I avoid wound infection by taking care to clamp and tie vessels precisely, using small hemostats so that I do not leave a lot of devitalized tissue in the wound, because I do not suture my thin skin flaps so tightly that I compromise their circulation, and because I dress my wounds myself. Even in the ward patients for whom I acted as a first assistant while my resident surgeon operated, I have done the postoperative dressings with the resident, supervising every detail until I felt certain that the resident had a sound knowledge of how to care for these complex wounds.

Another explanation for post-mastectomy arm edema, put forward in 1938 by Veal, was that it is due to obstruction of the axillary vein. Veal claimed that studies of venous pressure and phlebography showed that the axillary vein is often angulated and narrowed following operation. Russo and his associates confirmed Veal's studies. Smedal and Evans also reported occlusion of the axillary vein as shown by phlebography in patients with edema of the arm, and attributed it to thrombophlebitis. Deaton and Bradshaw, however, did not find increased venous pressures in patients with arm edema, and Schorr and his associates were unable to demonstrate by phlebography occlusion of the axillary vein in patients with arm edema.

The most extensive, but as yet unpublished, venographic study of post-mastectomy arms was done in our institution by Kister and his associates. They did venograms on 100 arms in 52 patients following radical mastectomy. Of these, 61 arms were on the side of the radical mastectomy and 39 were normal opposite arms serving as controls.

Their conclusions were as follows:

1. Narrowing of the axillary and cephalic veins is found in normal as well as post-mastectomy arms. In post-mastectomy arms it does not correlate with the amount of edema present in the arm.

2. Total occlusion of the axillary vein alone does not produce edema. The cephalic vein is adequate for normal venous return. In cases of total cephalic vein occlusion, the converse is true.

3. Total occlusion of both the cephalic and the axillary veins will produce acute edema. A collateral venous network then develops,

and the edge disappears within several weeks.

4. A filling defect in the major veins, which has been considered an indication of thrombophlebitis, was not found in any patient with arm edema.

5. Edema of post-mastectomy arms is not due to impairment of the venous circulation.

Postoperative irradiation to the axilla certainly increases the frequency and degree of edema of the arm. Several experienced clinicians have emphasized this relationship (Lobb and Harkins; Holman and his associates; Daland; Hollenbach).

The radiodermatitis with moist desquamation of the skin which was regularly observed following intensive 250 kilovolt radiotherapy provided an ideal portal of entry for infection. Today, with carefully supervised supervoltage therapy, this kind of radiodermatitis is not seen and the hazard of infection in the arm no longer exists. Nevertheless, my experience has convinced me that irradiation to the axillary region, no matter how skillfully

given, adds somewhat to the degree of postoperative edema of the arm, probably because it increases the amount of fibrosis in the axilla and therefore adds to the obstruction of lymphatic channels. For this reason, postoperative axillary irradiation should be avoided unless there are definite indications for it.

The patient who escapes edema of the arm immediately following radical mastectomy should be told by her surgeon that she is vulnerable to *secondary* edema for the rest of her life. She must be made to realize that any trauma to the hand or arm which provides a portal of entry for bacteria may lead to infection and edema. Burns, cuts and abrasions, and paronychia are the most frequent sources of infection. Patients should be urged to avoid manicurists, because manicurists invariably push the cuticle back and in this way induce a minor degree of infection.

Although a good many patients have such minor local infections without developing cellulitis of the arm, they should all be warned to be alert for the slightest sign of the develop-

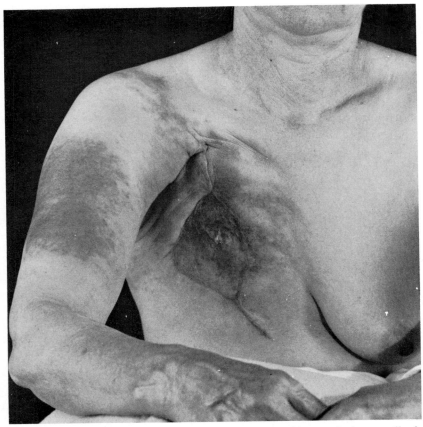

Figure 34–30. Acute "erysipeloid" cellulitis of the arm, shoulder, and chest wall, developing as a result of a paronychia.

ment of more extensive infection. This should be reported at once to the responsible surgeon and treated with a suitable antibiotic. If a positive culture can be obtained from the source of the infection and the sensitivity of the organism determined, the choice of antibiotic is easy. If the antibiotic has to be chosen empirically, it is important to keep in mind that unless there is prompt regression of the signs of arm infection within a period of three or four days it should be assumed that the organism is not sensitive to the antibiotic that is being given. Another should be tried.

Acute superficial cellulitis developing in an arm after radical mastectomy has been called erysipeloid. The name is a good one. The patient develops pain, swelling, and redness, usually involving a considerable area of the upper arm and sometimes the chest wall. She feels acutely ill with chills and a temperature which may reach 104° or 105° F. Figure 34–30 shows the zone of redness over the upper arm, the shoulder, and the skin flaps on the chest wall in a patient of mine whose infection developed from a paronychia of her right finger, which is shown in Figure 34–31. Her radical mastectomy had been done five months previously and she had had no preceding edema of the arm. She was admitted to the hospital after two days of shaking chills and malaise. Her temperature was 105° F. per rectum on admission. She was given sulfadiazine and her infection subsided within forty-eight hours. She did not develop any subsequent edema of the arm and was well 10 years later.

A patient with this erysipeloid syndrome is best treated by being admitted to the hospital and put to bed with her arm elevated while the correct antibiotic is administered. This kind of hospital care is important if subsequent permanent edema of the arm is to be avoided.

Before the development of antibiotics these patients who had developed the erysipeloid syndrome faced a dread future. Although the acute infection would subside spontaneously after a few days, the organisms apparently persisted in the tissues of the arm, because at intervals of every few months the syndrome would recur without any obvious new portal of entry for organisms. With each new bout of infection the edema of the arm would increase. Ultimately a marked degree of brawny edema would result. In this kind of edema the tissues of the arm are tense and firm, and the patient has a constant feeling of

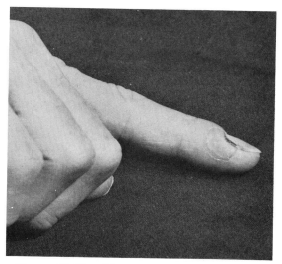

Figure 34–31. The paronychia which was the portal of entry for the infection in the patient shown in Figure 34–30.

tension in the arm. It is an exceedingly uncomfortable and crippling condition.

For the patient with well established chronic edema of the arm which has been present for some time, antibiotic treatment alone is comparatively ineffectual. In the past a number of surgical methods have been devised for treating edema of this kind. In 1912 Kondoleon proposed sleeve resection of the subcutaneous tissues and deep fascia of the arm with the aim of providing new lymphatic channels between the superficial and deep lymphatics. Although a good many of these Kondoleon operations have been done, the results have been so poor that the method has been generally abandoned.

Hutchins has proposed transplantation of the latissimus muscle across the axilla during radical mastectomy, in the hope of providing better lymphatic drainage and avoiding subsequent edema. Guthrie has treated edema by inserting celloidin strips into the subcutaneous tissues of the arm, and Treves has used laminated Gelfoam rolls in a similar way. Standard treated edema of the arm by suturing the edematous arm to the lateral chest wall. I cannot believe that any of these methods have any practical value, because they do not attack the underlying basic problem in edema of the arm, namely, the abolition of the underlying infection.

Perhaps the most important factor which limits our ability to abolish infection in a chronically edematous arm is obesity. Obese patients must reduce drastically if they are to hope to have much improvement in the condition of the arm. The arm rarely returns to a normal size, however. If the patient is having recurrent attacks of cellulitis, antibiotic therapy should be thoroughly tried. This should be done in the hospital, with the patient in bed and the arm elevated. It is important to emphasize that the arm should not be elevated in abduction, because this position is uncomfortable and constricts the axilla; the arm should be kept at the patient's side with the elbow elevated on a pillow so that it is higher than the shoulder, and the hand further elevated on an additional pillow so that it is higher than the elbow. Attempts to improve the edema by compression of the arm with an elastic bandage at this stage can only do harm.

When the signs of acute infection have subsided, and the induration of the arm has diminished, intermittent pneumatic compression of the arm is recommended by Britton. Having tried it in a considerable number of patients, I must report that although it seems to help a few of them, in general it is of so little benefit that I no longer recommend it.

Wearing a custom-made elastic sleeve extending from the wrist to the shoulder during the day, when the patient is up and about, is the most useful method of limiting and improving edema of the arm in its chronic stage. For most patients, however, even this rather bothersome method of treatment does not achieve much.

It is worthwhile trying spironolactone, the most useful of the diuretics, in moderate doses, in combination with the elastic sleeve in these patients. Used over a period of months, some improvement of the edema may be achieved.

Meanwhile, edema of the arm remains a common and crippling complication of mastectomy. It can be avoided only by a meticulous surgical technique which achieves perfect wound healing. I believe that one of the important factors in achieving perfect wound healing is skin grafting of the operative wound, because, as Halsted pointed out so long ago, it avoids the triad of tension on the skin flaps, necrosis, and infection.

OPERATIONS OTHER THAN THE HALSTED RADICAL MASTECTOMY

When radical mastectomy is used indiscriminately for cancer of the breast, and when it is performed indifferently, its results are poor. The growing awareness of modern surgeons, that their results with cancer of the breast have been poor, unfortunately has not led them to choose their patients more critically and to perform the operation more carefully. It has discouraged some surgeons, to the point that they abandon the surgical attack altogether, and hand their patients over to the radiotherapeutists. Other surgeons have given up radical mastectomy for other operations. Some of these have been less thorough, and others more comprehensive, than the conventional radical mastectomy.

The achievements of these various currently popular methods of surgical attack other than radical mastectomy must be viewed critically from three points of view. First, what is their rationale? Second, what is their morbidity and mortality? Third, what is their curative achievement?

Simple Mastectomy

There is a school of modern surgeons, exemplified by Deaton, Case, Hartmann, Fitzwilliams, and Crile, who believe that simple removal of the breast gives just as good results as radical mastectomy. They are not convinced that breast carcinoma is curable by surgery when the axillary nodes are involved. This philosophy of course goes back to Paget's time, and if these modern defeatists depended solely upon their surgical effort their results would be no better than Paget's. But patients treated today by simple surgery usually receive both irradiation and hormonal treatment in addition, with the result that life is prolonged, and the therapeutic achievement, when expressed statistically, is not much worse than the results of those surgeons who use radical mastectomy indiscriminately and unskillfully.

From the patient's point of view, the price she pays in mutilation and in morbidity is not appreciably greater for radical mastectomy than for simple mastectomy. The mortality of both operations should be nil. If she indeed has no axillary metastasis, nothing of course is gained by dissecting the axilla, but if she happens to have axillary involvement the choice between simple mastectomy and radical mastectomy is often the choice between life and death. If her axillary metastases are not excised, the only defense against them is irradiation. No one has presented solid evidence that irradiation succeeds as well with axillary metastases in operable cases as meticulous axillary dissection, which gives remarkable results. In my personal series of radical mastectomies there have been 556 patients whose disease was classified as Clinical Stage A or B and who have been followed for a minimum of 10 years. In these operable patients—according to our present criteria—there were 240 who proved to have axillary metastases. Only 35 of the 240 were given postoperative prophylactic irradiation; they were the ones who had the most axillary metastases, averaging 11 involved nodes. Among the remaining 205 patients whose axillary metastases were excised by meticulous dissection, and in whom no irradiation was given, only one developed axillary recurrence during the 10 year follow-up period (Table 34–6).

Statisticians have been of special disservice to us in the comparison of the results of simple and radical mastectomy. In 1959, Smith and Meyer studied the results of the two operations in Rockford, Illinois, and reached the conclusion that the results were similar. Two years later Shimkin, Koppel, Connelly, and Cutler of the National Cancer Institute restudied the Rockford data and reaffirmed the finding that the survival rates "were practically identical whether radical or simple mastectomy was used as the primary treatment." They reiterated the comment of Smith and Meyer that "they could demonstrate no reason for performing more than simple mastectomy." These authors from the National Cancer Institute made these statements and gave wide publicity to them, although they knew that the Rockford patients had not been accurately classified as to the clinical extent of their disease. They should have realized that under these circumstances selection might explain the similarity in results, i.e., the patients with earlier disease may have been treated by simple mastectomy and those with more advanced disease by radical mastectomy.

The best evidence regarding the efficacy of simple mastectomy has been presented by Miller in our "Cooperative International Comparison of the Treatment of Early Mammary Carcinoma." The 10-year survival rate following simple mastectomy in operable cases (Clinical Stages A and B) was 37 per cent, as compared with a 10-year survival rate of 62 per cent for radical mastectomy in my personal series of cases. To my knowledge no

one else has presented 10 year results of simple mastectomy alone for a substantial number of patients in whom the stage of advancement of the disease was defined by accurate clinical classification. Crile, who is the most vocal proponent of simple mastectomy, has not published such data, even in his most recent pronouncements (1968, 1969). I cannot understand how any conscientious surgeon can choose to treat his patients with operable breast carcinoma by simple mastectomy, which has given a 10 year survival rate of only 37 per cent.

Simple mastectomy has frequently been used as a palliative procedure to rid the patient whose carcinoma was clearly inoperable of an ulcerated tumor. As the efficacy of radiotherapy in controlling the primary tumor has improved, the need for such palliative simple mastectomy has decreased. I have personally abandoned simple mastectomy for this purpose, because I have found that radiotherapy does better.

Another use of simple mastectomy which I must strongly condemn is its use by surgeons who find themselves in a diagnostic dilemma and compromise by performing partial or simple mastectomy, with the intention of proceeding with a radical mastectomy when a definitive microscopic diagnosis becomes available. In so doing they are very apt to sacrifice their patient's only chance of cure because the initial partial dissection cuts across actual carcinoma and implants it widely. Lockhart and Ackerman reviewed a series of cases in which simple mastectomy had been done preceding radical mastectomy, and found the result disastrous.

Mastectomy Plus Axillary Dissection

A compromise between simple mastectomy and radical mastectomy consists in the removal of the breast and the performance of an axillary dissection. The pectoral muscles are left intact, being retracted medially. This kind of an operation is usually done through a transverse incision, with thick skin flaps, and primary wound closure. Techniques for this "modified" radical mastectomy have been described by Patey, by Handley, by Madden, by Auchincloss, and by others.

Patey's technique has gained wide acceptance, and is today the operation most frequently used, next to radical mastectomy, for breast carcinoma. Patey preserves the pectoralis major muscle on the assumption that it is not invaded by carcinoma except in very advanced cases. He gains access to the axilla by lifting the patient's arm so that it points toward the ceiling, and retracting the pectoralis major medially, preserving its nerve supply. The pectoralis minor is cut across close to its attachment to the carocoid process. In this way, Patey states, he is able to dissect out the contents of the axilla up to the lateral border of the first rib.

When the pectoralis major muscle is preserved, and remains to form a bridge across the axilla, the patient is, of course, less disfigured than after the Halsted mastectomy.

Among the surgeons who have championed modified radical mastectomy, Handley is the only one who has presented adequate evidence as to what can be achieved with the operation. In our "Cooperative International Comparison of the Treatment of Early Mammary Carcinoma" he reported the 10-year results in 143 patients whose disease had been carefully classified by our Columbia Clinical Classification. Study of these data will show that local recurrence is more frequent and the survival rate somewhat lower than in my personal series of patients treated by radical mastectomy.

There are perfectly good technical reasons why the results of "modified" radical mastectomy should be expected to be somewhat inferior to those of radical mastectomy.

1. When excision of the skin and subcutaneous tissues over the breast is so limited that a skin graft is not required, as in the "modified" operation, the surgeon will occasionally get too close to the carcinoma, which may extend more widely in the breast than he thinks, and local recurrence will follow. Sacrifice of all the skin over the protuberant breast and skin-grafting is followed by fewer local recurrences, as our "Cooperative International Comparison" proves.

2. When the pectoral muscles are not removed, the interpectoral nodes will not be excised, and if there are metastases in them the patient is doomed.

The following history of a patient of my own illustrates the value of including these muscles and the nodes between them in the excision.

Mrs. V. S. came to me in October, 1942, with a 3.5 cm. tumor with the clinical characteristics of a carcinoma, situated in the upper outer sector of her right breast. She also had a 3 cm. Paget's erosion of her right nipple. She had a single firm palpable 1 cm. node in each axilla, but these nodes had been present for several years and were presumed to be due to chronic dermatitis of her upper chest and neck.

Radical mastectomy was done with a large skin graft. Twenty-four axillary nodes were found. Only two, both of them interpectoral nodes situated between the two pectoral muscles, contained metastases. The carcinoma was a well differentiated intraductal one. No postoperative irradiation was given. She had had no recurrence of her breast carcinoma 28 years later.

3. The axillary dissection which is done in these "modified" radical mastectomies is less complete and more brutal than that in the Halsted radical mastectomy. In the "modified" operation, strong traction medially on the pectoralis major will expose the axillary structures for only about two-thirds of the distance from the lateral edge of the operative field where the axillary vein crosses the white tendon of the latissimus muscle, to the point at the apex of the axilla where the vein passes beneath the subclavius muscle.

Madden's illustration (Fig. 34-32) shows his limited exposure of the axillary structures, and his technique of dissection with scissors and forceps. There are a considerable number of higher lymph nodes which cannot be reached with this limited exposure, including those on the axillary vein in the vicinity of the thoracoacromial vessels, as well as the nodes which are still higher at the apex of the axilla. The axillary vein nodes in the vicinity of the thoracoacromial vessels are included in the axillary dissection that I do, and if they contain metastases the patient can be cured, but this can be accomplished only when the line of dissection is carried beyond them to include the nodes at the apex of the axilla.

A surgeon dissecting out involved lymph nodes anywhere must always carry his line of dissection at least 2 or 3 cm. beyond the site of the involved nodes, and must also dissect gently and precisely with knife and smooth forceps, if he is to succeed. Figure 34-19 shows how the axilla lies before me, like an open book, as I dissect it in this manner.

It is true that if the nodes at the very apex of the axilla contain metastases, we do not cure the patient, but if they are not involved their removal has the advantage of insuring a safer dissection of nodes situated more laterally.

The following case history illustrates very well the inadequacy of "modified" radical mastectomy.

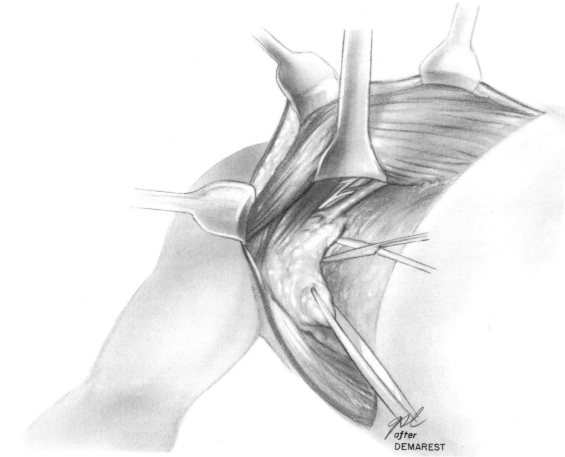

Figure 34–32. Madden's method of dissecting the axilla in his modified radical mastectomy. (From Madden, J. L.: Surg., Gynec. & Obst., *121*:1221, 1965.)

Mrs. N. D., aged 32, a housewife with two children, had a cyst excised from her left breast in another hospital. During the succeeding 10 years she had several cysts in both breasts aspirated by one of our attending surgeons. Finally, when she was 42, she developed a well delimited firm 1 cm. tumor beneath the edge of the areola of her right breast. There were no clinically involved axillary nodes. It was excised locally and proved to be the circumscribed type of carcinoma.

Six days later a "modified" radical mastectomy was performed. A transverse incision was used, the pectoral muscles were not removed, and only the lower axillary nodes were included in the dis-

section. The wound was closed *per primum* without a skin graft.

Pathologic examination of the breast revealed that in addition to the 1 cm. subareolar carcinoma there was a second 3 cm. carcinoma, intraductal in type, situated deeply in the lower portion of the breast. Three lower axillary nodes were included in the specimen; they did not contain metastases.

Five months later a 2 cm. clinically involved axillary node was noted in the axilla of the mastectomy side. An axillary dissection was then done. Many involved nodes were found and some removed. Postoperative irradiation was given to the axilla. With this degree of axillary involvement, however, the patient has very little chance of ulti-mate cure although her original carcinoma was a very favorable one.

Extended Operation Including Excision of Internal Mammary and Supraclavicular Lymph Nodes

None of the operations which I have dis-cussed above, including the Halsted mastec-tomy, attempts to remove any but the axillary lymph nodes. They are therefore all inad-equate in terms of our modern knowledge of the occurrence of metastases in other region-al lymph node groups—the internal mam-mary and the supraclavicular nodes. In an attempt to meet this challenge surgically, a variety of new operations have recently been devised which combine some type of mastec-tomy and axillary dissection with removal of either the internal mammary or the supracla-vicular nodes, or both.

1. Radical Mastectomy Combined with Supraclavicular Dissection and Internal Mammary and Mediastinal Lymph Node Dissection. Wangensteen and Lewis, at the University of Minnesota, devised the most radical surgical attack upon breast carcinoma. It included not only the conventional radical mastectomy but also supraclavicular dissec-tion as well as dissection of the internal mam-mary and mediastinal lymph nodes. To achieve this, the chest was opened widely by splitting the sternum and detaching the first rib and elevating the clavicle. The operation was done in two stages. Lewis reported a 13 per cent operative mortality in a series of 50 patients. In something over 40 per cent of the patients, no lymph node metastases were found in any of the dissected areas.

I cannot conceive of any justification for this operation. It has a high morbidity, a con-siderable mortality, and in a high percentage of the patients in whom it was done it was unnecessary. I do not believe that it is being done today by anyone who has had exper-ience with it.

2. Radical Mastectomy plus Supraclavic-ular Dissection plus Extrapleural Excision of the Internal Mammary Lymph Node Chain. Dahl-Iversen and his associates in Copenhagen began in 1948 to dissect the supraclavicular nodes as part of their radical mastectomy. In 1950 they extended their sur-gical attack to the internal mammary nodes. They evolved a conservative method of re-moving them extrapleurally, by cutting the second, third, and fourth costal cartilages 1 to 1.5 cm. from the sternal border. The costal cartilages were then raised with gauze strips so that the internal mammary vessels and nodes were exposed. The vessels and all ac-companying lymphatic and fatty tissue were removed in this way from the upper four inter-spaces.

As reported in our "Cooperative Interna-tional Study of the Treatment of Early Mam-mary Carcinoma," this operation had a con-siderable morbidity, and the results were not as good as those of the Halsted radical mas-tectomy. Dahl-Iversen and his associates abandoned their operation some time ago.

3. Radical Mastectomy Combined with en bloc Resection of the Chest Wall in the Internal Mammary Area. More radical surgical methods of combining radical mas-tectomy with *en bloc* resection of the full thickness of the chest wall in the internal mammary area have been devised by Urban and by Ariel in New York. In the Urban operation the sternum is split, and the second, third, fourth and fifth ribs are cut just lateral to their costochondral junctions. This leaves a defect of considerable size in the chest wall, which Urban closes with a *fascia lata* graft.

This operation has been more widely done than any of the other surgical procedures which include excision of the internal mam-mary nodes. The largest unselected case series are those of Veronesi and Caceres. The 10 year survival rate in these series was 13 per cent (Table 33–15). I can state again that these data do not, in my opinion, justify a continuation of surgical attempts to excise internal mammary nodes in carcinoma of the breast. I hope that prophylactic irradiation of the internal mammary nodes, following the Halsted radical mastectomy, will give us bet-ter results.

SUMMARY OF THE SURGICAL ATTACK UPON CARCINOMA OF THE BREAST

The current confusion among surgeons themselves as to which operation is the prefer-able one for carcinoma of the breast will only be resolved when better standards are used for the comparison of the results of these different methods of treatment in care-fully studied case series.

I have emphasized in Chapter 33 that these

Table 34–15. RESULTS OF TREATMENT IN MAMMARY CARCINOMA – 10-YEAR SURVIVAL, COLUMBIA CLINICAL CLASSIFICATION*

Columbia Clinical Classification	Miller Simple Mastectomy		Handley and Thackray Conservative Radical Mastectomy		Butcher Radical Mastectomy		Haagensen and Cooley Radical Mastectomy		Dahl-Iversen and Tobiassen Extended Mastectomy		Williams and Stone Total Mastectomy +Axillary Dissec.+Irrad.		Kaae and Johansen, McWhirter Method	
	No. of Patients	10-Year Survival	No. of Patients	10-Year Survival	No. of Patients	10-Year Survival	No. of Patients	10-Year Survival	No. of Patients	10-Year Survival	No. of Patients	10-Year Survival	No. of Patients	10-Year Survival
A	105	40%	77	61%	216	56%	344	70%	352	57%	68	59%	159	50%
B	34	26%	58	25%	135	30%	138	40%	75	24%	57	46%	28	32%
C	18	22%	8	14%	48	31%	63	27%	34	35%	16	19%	9	0%
D	45	9%	0		26	0%	11	18%	15	7%	1	0%	3	0%
Totals	202		143		425		556		476		142		199	

*From Haagensen, C. D., et al.: Treatment of early mammary carcinoma: Cooperative International Study. Ann. Surg., *170*:875, 1969.

standards must include accurate case histories from which the clinical extent of the disease in each patient can be determined on the basis of a practical clinical classification such as our Columbia Clinical Classification. These data define how the patients were selected for treatment, and make it possible to compare the results of treatment in different series of patients whose disease is at the same stage of advancement. A complete 10 year follow-up is equally essential for any comparison of results.

Our recently published "Cooperative International Study of the Treatment of Early Mammary Carcinoma" is the only comparison of the results of different methods of treatment which meets these standards. Table 34–15 presents the 10-year survival rates in the seven different case series included in the study. I invite the reader to study our comparison carefully. The differences in the results of the different methods of treatment are of course much more apparent in the earlier and operable Clinical Stage A and B cases. In the more advanced Stage C and D cases all methods of treatment give poor results.

It is fashionable today to suggest for this kind of therapeutic problem so-called random studies, in which alternate and unselected patients are treated by different methods and the results compared. Fisher has recently been quoted in the columns of the Wall Street Journal in an appeal for such a random study comparing the results of simple mastectomy alone, simple mastectomy followed by irradiation, and radical mastectomy. There are several reasons why his suggestion is not a practical one. Accurate clinical staging of the disease in all patients included in such a study is essential if the results of the different methods of treatment are to be compared in alternate patients whose disease is at the same stage of advancement. It would be very difficult to organize, in a considerable number of different hospitals, the collection of the clinical data which permits this kind of clinical staging of breast carcinoma. And as one who has spent a lifetime studying the disease I must emphasize that it would take a very long time, perhaps 25 years, to carry out such a random study. In each hospital cooperating in the study it would take some years to collect the substantial numbers of cases treated by each of the different methods: after that a minimum of 10 years of follow-up is necessary.

Another serious objection to the random study that Fisher proposes is a moral one. Will surgeons who are asked to take part in the study be willing to condemn a proportion of their patients to treatment by simple mastectomy? The majority of surgeons with adequate experience in the pathology, natural history and treatment of breast carcinoma certainly believe, on the basis of data now available, that simple mastectomy is inferior to radical mastectomy. I hope that conscience will prevent them from treating patients whom they have come to know as human beings in desperate peril, with what they believe to be an inferior method. That is my own stand.

REFERENCES

Andreassen, M., Dahl-Iversen, E., and Soerensen, B.: Glandular metastases in carcinoma of the breast. Lancet, *1*:176, 1954.

Ariel, I. M.: A conservative method of resecting the internal mammary lymph nodes en bloc with radical mastectomy. Surg., Gynec. & Obst., *100*:623, 1955.

Auchincloss, H.: Significance of location and number of axillary metastases in carcinoma of the breast; a justification for a conservative operation. Ann. Surg., *158*:37, 1963.

Banks, W. M.: A plea for the more free removal of cancerous growths. Liverpool and Manchester M. & S. Rep., 5:192, 1878.

Banks, W. M.: Some Results of the Operative Treatment of Cancer of the Breast. Edinburgh, Neill & Co., 1882, p. 16.

Berg, J. W., and Robbins, G. F.: Factors influencing short and long term survival of breast cancer patients. Surg., Gynec. & Obst., *122*:1311, 1966.

Boyd, A. K., Enterline, H. T., and Donald, J. G.: Carcinoma of the breast. Surg., Gynec. & Obst., 99:9, 1954.

Brandes, W. W., White, W. C., and Sutton, J. B.: Accidental transplantation of cancer in the operating room. Surg., Gynec. & Obst., *82*:212, 1946.

Brenier, J. L.: La chirurgie élargie du cancer du sein. Rev. de chir. (Paris), *72*:72, 1953.

Britton, R. C., and Nelson, P. A.: Causes and treatment of postmastectomy lymphedema of the arm. J.A.M.A., *180*:95, 1962.

Butcher, H. R., Jr.: Effectiveness of radical mastectomy for mammary cancer; analysis of mortalities by methods of probits. Ann. Surg., *154*:383, 1961.

Case, T. C.: Extended simple mastectomy for carcinoma of the breast. J. Internat. Coll. Surgeons, *18*:26, 1952.

Chilko, A. J., and Quastler, H.: Delayed metastases in cancer of the breast. Am. J. Surg., *55*:75, 1942.

Cogswell, H. D.: Excision of the skin in radical mastectomy. Arch. Surg., *61*:305, 1950.

Coller, F. A., Crook, C. E., and Iob, V.: Blood loss in surgical operations. J.A.M.A., *126*:1, 1944.

Conway, H., and Neumann, C. G.: Evaluation of skin grafting in the technique of radical mastectomy in relation to local recurrence of carcinoma. Surg. Gynec. & Obst., *88*:45, 1949.

Cooper, W. A.: The history of the radical mastectomy. Ann. M. Hist., *3*:36, 1941.

Craig, C., and Holman, W. P.: The development of the surgical treatment of carcinoma of the breast. Med. J. Australia, 2:201, 1944.

Crile, G., Jr.: Simplified treatment of cancer of the breast; early results of a clinical study. Ann. Surg., *153*:745, 1961.

Crile, G., Jr.: Results of simple mastectomy without irradiation in the treatment of operative stage I cancer of the breast. Ann. Surg., *168*:330, 1968.

Crile, G., Jr.: Possible role of uninvolved regional nodes in preventing metastasis from breast cancer. Cancer, *24*:1283, 1969.

Dahl-Iversen, E.: Carcinoma of the Breast. Copenhagen, Official Tr. Northern Surg. A., 1951, p. 150.

Dahl-Iversen, E., and Tobiassen, T.: Radical mastectomy with parasternal and supraclavicular dissection for mammary carcinoma. Ann. Surg., *157*:170, 1963.

Daland, E. M.: Some unusual aspects of cancer of the breast. New Eng. J. Med., *233*:515, 1945.

Daland, E. M.: The incidence of swollen arms after radical mastectomy and suggestions for prevention. New Eng. J. Med., *242*:497, 1950.

Daland, E. M., and Greenough, R. B.: Cancer of the breast. New Eng. J. Med., *201*:1240, 1929.

Danckers, U. F., Hamann, A., and Savage, J. L.: Postoperative recurrence of breast cancer after 32 years. Surgery, *47*:656, 1960.

Deaton, W. R., Jr.: Simple mastectomy for carcinoma of the breast. Surgery, *37*:720, 1955.

Deaton, W. R., Jr., and Bradshaw, H. H.: Postmastectomy edema of the arm. Arch. Surg., *66*:641, 1953.

Demaree, E. W.: Local recurrence following surgery for cancer of the breast. Ann. Surg., *134*:863, 1951.

Devenish, E. A., and Jessop, W. H. G.: The nature and cause of swelling of the upper limb after radical mastectomy. Brit. J. Surg., *28*:222, 1940.

Dieulafé, R., and Grimoud, M.: Les "gros bras" consécutifs au traitement du cancer du sein. Rev. de chir. (Paris), *77*:161, 1939.

Donegan, W. L., Perez-Mesa, C. M., and Watson, F. R.: A biostatistical study of locally recurrent breast carcinoma. Surg., Gynec. & Obst., *122*:529, 1966.

Donegan, W. L., and Spratt, J. S., Jr.: Cancer of the second breast. In Spratt, J. S., Jr., and Donegan, W. L.: Cancer of the Breast. Philadelphia, W. B. Saunders Co., 1967, page 179.

Eisler, P.: Die Muskeln des Stammes. In Bardeleben: Handbuch der Anatomie des Menschen, Jena, Gustav Fischer, 1912, vol. 2, part 2, section 1.

Endler, F.: Prognose und Heilungsergebnisse des Brustdrüsenkrebses an der I. Chirurg. Universitätsklinik in Wien. Wien. Med. Wchnschr., *103*:568, 1953.

Faugère, G., and Prat-Rousseau, C.: Résection de la veine axillaire au cours de l'opération radicale du cancer du sein. Bordeaux chir., *3*:131, 1942.

Finney, G. G., Merkel, W. C., and Miller, D. B.: Carcinoma of the breast; study of 298 consecutive cases. Ann. Surg., *125*:673, 1947.

Fitts, W. T., Jr., Keuhnelian, J. G., Ravdin, I. S., and Schor, S.: Swelling of the arm after radical mastectomy. Surgery, *35*:460, 1954.

Fitzwilliams, D. C. L.: A plea for a more local operation in really early breast carcinoma. Brit. Med. J., 2:405, 1940.

Ginsburg, S.: Osteoplastic skeletal metastases from carcinoma of the breast. Arch. Surg. *11*:219, 1925.

Glover, D. M.: Rationale of internal mammary lymph node dissection for carcinoma of the breast. Arch. Surg., *69*:393, 1954.

Gray, E. B., Jr., and Anglem, T. J.: Radical mastectomy for carcinoma of the breast. New Eng. J. Med., *261*:1310, 1959.

Greenough, R. B.: Carcinoma of the breast; results of treatment 1918–1919–1920. Am. J. Roentgenol., *16*:439, 1926.

Greenough, R. B., and Simmons, C. C.: End-results in cancer cases; cancer of the breast (1911–1914). Boston M. & S. J., *185*:253, 1921.

Greenough, R. B., and Taylor, G. W.: Cancer of the breast; end results, Massachusetts General Hospital 1921, 1922, and 1923. New England J. Med., *210*:831, 1934.

Gross, S. W.: Tumors of the Mammary Gland. New York, D. Appleton & Co., 1880.

Gumrich, H.: Beitrag zur Klärung der Genese der Elephantiasis nach Mammaamputation. Arch. f. klin. Chir., *279*:129, 1954.

Guthrie, D., and Gagnon, G.: The prevention and treatment of post-operative lymphedema of the arm. Ann. Surg., *123*:925, 1946.

Haagensen, C. D.: A technique for radical mastectomy. Surgery, *19*:100, 1946.

Haagensen, C. D.: The treatment and results in cancer of the breast at the Presbyterian Hospital, New York, Am. J. Roentgenol., *62*:328, 1949.

Haagensen, C. D., and Stout, A. P.: Carcinoma of the breast. I. Results of treatment, 1915–1934. Ann. Surg., *116*:801, 1942.

Haagensen, C. D., and Stout, A. P.: Carcinoma of the breast. Criteria of operability. Ann. Surg., *118*:1032, 1943.

Haagensen, C. D., and Stout, A. P.: Carcinoma of the breast. III. Results of treatment, 1935–1942. Ann. Surg., *134*:151, 1951.

Haagensen, C. D., et al.: Treatment of early mammary carcinoma: a cooperative international study. Ann. Surg., *170*:875, 1969.

Halsted, W. S.: The treatment of wounds with especial reference to the value of the blood clot in the management of dead spaces. John Hopkins Hosp. Rep., *2*:255, 1890–91.

Halsted, W. S.: The results of operations for the cure of cancer of the breast performed at the Johns Hopkins Hospital from June, 1889 to January, 1894, Johns Hopkins Hosp. Rep. *4*:297, 1894–95.

Halsted, W. S.: A clinical and histological study of certain adenocarcinomata of the breast; and a brief consideration of the supraclavicular operation and of the results of the operations for cancer of the breast from 1889–1898 at the Johns Hopkins Hospital. Tr. Am. S.A., *16*:144, 1898.

Halsted, W. S.: The results of radical operations for the cure of carcinoma of the breast. Tr. Am. S. A., *25*:61, 1907.

Halsted, W. S.: Developments in the skin-grafting operation for mammary cancer. Tr. Am. S. A., *30*:287, 1912.

Halsted, W. S.: The swelling of the arm after operations for cancer of the breast—*elephantiasis chirurgica*—its cause and prevention. Bull. Johns Hopkins Hosp., *32*:309, 1921.

Handley, R. S.: Some observations and reflections on breast cancer. J. Roy. Coll. Surgeons, Edinburgh, *6*:1, 1960.

Handley, R. S.: Indications and contraindications for mastectomy. J.A.M.A., *200*:610, 1967.

Handley, R. S.: Personal communication, 1969.

Handley, R. S., Patey, D. H., and Hand, B. H.: Excision of the internal mammary chain in radical mastectomy. Lancet, *1*:457, 1956.

Handley, W. S.: Cancer of the Breast. London, John Murray, 1906, p. 182.

Harrington, S. W.: Survival rates of radical mastectomy for unilateral and bilateral carcinoma of the breast. Surgery, *19*:154, 1946.

Harrington, S. W.: Results of surgical treatment of unilateral carcinoma of the breast in women. J.A.M.A., *148*:1007, 1952.

Harrington, S. W.: Fifteen-year to forty-year survival rates following radical mastectomy for cancer of the breast. Ann. Surg., *137*:843, 1953.

Hartmann, H.: Quelques cas de récidives tardives de cancers. Bull. Acad de méd., Paris, *113*:281, 1935.

Hartmann, H.: Résultats des opérations limitées dans le cancer du sein. Internat. Union Against Cancer, *8*:161, 1952.

Hicken, N. F.: Mastectomy; a clinical pathologic study demonstrating why most mastectomies result in incomplete removal of the mammary gland. Arch. Surg., *40*:6, 1940.

Hollenbach, F.: Vermeidung des Armödems nach Mamma-Amputation. Chirurg, *20*:374, 1949.

Holman, C. C.: Cancer of the breast: The principles of surgical treatment. Lancet, *1*:174, 1954.

Holman, C., McSwain, B., and Beal, J. M.: Swelling of the upper extremity following radical mastectomy. Surgery, *15*:757, 1944.

Hoopes, B. F., and McGraw, A. B.: The Halsted radical mastectomy. Surgery, *12*:892, 1942.

Hutchins, E. H.: A method for the prevention of elephantiasis chirurgica. Surg., Gynec. & Obst., *69*:795, 1939.

Ju, D. M. C., Blakemore, A., and Stevenson, T. W.: A lymphatic function test. Clin. Congress of Am. Coll. of Surgeons, 1954, Surgical Forum, p. 607.

Keyes, E. L., Hawk, B. O., and Sherwin, C. S.: Basting the axillary flap for wounds of radical mastectomy. Arch. Surg., *66*:446, 1953.

Kinmonth, J. B., and Taylor, G. W.: The lymphatic circulation in lymphedema. Ann. Surg., *139*:129, 1954.

Kister, S.: Personal communication, 1970.

Kondoleon, E.: Die operative Behandlung der elephantiastischen Oedeme. Zentralbl. f. Chir. *39*:1022, 1912.

Larsen, B. B.: Fixation of skin flaps by subcutaneous sutures in radical mastectomy. J.A.M.A., *159*:24, 1955.

Lewis, D., and Rienhoff, W. F., Jr.: A study of the results of operations for the cure of cancer of the breast, performed at The Johns Hopkins Hospital from 1889 to 1931. Ann. Surg., *95*:336, 1932.

Lewis, F. J.: Extended or super-radical mastectomy for cancer of the breast. Minnesota Med., *36*:763, 1953.

Lewison, E. F.: The surgical treatment of breast cancer. Surgery, 34:904, 1953.

Lewison, E. F.: Breast Cancer. Baltimore, Williams and Wilkins Co., 1955.

Lewison, E. F.: An appraisal of long-term results in the treatment of breast cancer. Internat. Union Against Cancer, *19*:1547, 1963.

Lewison, E. F., Trimble, F. H., and Griffith, P. C.: Results of surgical treatment of breast cancer at Johns Hopkins Hospital, 1935–1940, J.A.M.A., *153*:905, 1953.

Lobb, A. W., and Harkins, H. N.: Postmastectomy swelling of the arm. West. J. Surg., *57*:550, 1949.

Lockhart, C. E., and Ackerman, L. V.: The implications of local excision or simple mastectomy prior to radical mastectomy for carcinoma of the breast. Surgery, *26*:577, 1949.

Macdonald, I.: Resection of the axillary vein in radical mastectomy. Cancer, *1*:618, 1948.

McDonald, J. J., Haagensen, C. D., and Stout, A. P.: Metastasis from mammary carcinoma to the supraclavicular and internal mammary lymph nodes. Surgery, *34*:521, 1953.

Madden, J. L.: Modified radical mastectomy. Surg., Gynec. & Obst., *121*:1221, 1965.

McWhirter, R.: Cancer of the breast. Am. J. Roentgenol., *62*:335, 1949.

McWhirter, R.: Should more radical treatment be attempted in breast cancer? Am. J. Roentgenol., *92*:3, 1964.

Margottini, M., and Bucalossi, P.: Le metastasi linfoghiandolari mammarie interne nel cancro della mammella. Oncologia, *23*:70, 1949.

Mathews, F. S.: The ten-year survivors of radical mastectomy. Ann. Surg., *98*:635, 1933.

Meyer, W.: An improved method of the radical operation for carcinoma of the breast. M. Rec., *46*:746, 1894.

Meyer, W.: Carcinoma of the breast; ten years' experience with my method of radical operation. J.A.M.A., *45*:297, 1905.

Miller, E. B.: Five-year review of carcinoma of the breast. Ann. Surg., *163*:629, 1966.

Miller, E. B., and Kennedy, C. S.: Some factors in the choice of treatment of carcinoma of the breast. Ann. Surg., *150*:993, 1959.

Moore, C. H.: On the influence of inadequate operations on the theory of cancer. Roy. Med. & Chir. Soc., London, *1*:245, 1867.

Moore, H. G., Jr., and Harkins, H. N.: The use of a latissimus dorsi pedicle flap graft in radical mastectomy. Surg., Gynec. & Obst., 96:430, 1953.

Morton, J. J., Jr., and Morton, J. H.: Cancer as a chronic disease. Ann. Surg., 137:683, 1953.

Moschcowitz, A. V.: Pseudo recurrences after radical amputation of the breast for carcinoma. Ann. Surg., 81:81, 1925.

Myers, M. B.: Wound tension and vascularity in the etiology and prevention of skin sloughs. Surgery, 56:945, 1964.

Neuhof, H.: Excision of the axillary vein in the radical operation for carcinoma of the breast. Ann. Surg., 108:15, 1938.

Neumann, C. G., and Conway, H.: Evaluation of skin grafting in the technique of radical mastectomy in relation to function of the arm. Surgery, 23:584, 1948.

Nohrman, B. A.: Cancer of the breast; a clinical study of 1042 cases treated at the Radium-hemmet, 1936–41. Acta Radiol. Supp., 77, 1949.

Paget, Sir J.: Lectures on Surgical Pathology. London, Longman, Green, Longman, Roberts and Green, 1863, p. 630.

Parker, J. M., Russo, P. E., and Oesterreicher, D. L.: Investigation of cause of lymphedema of the upper extremity after radical mastectomy. Radiology, 59:538, 1952.

Patey, D. H.: Carcinoma of the female breast: Correspondence. Brit. Med. J., 2:1046, 1953.

Patey, D. H., and Dyson, W. H.: The prognosis of carcinoma of the breast in relation to the type of operation performed. Brit. J. Cancer, 2:7, 1948.

Pawlias, K. T., Dockerty, M. B., and Ellis, F. H. Jr.: Late local recurrent carcinoma of the breast. Ann. Surg., 148:192, 1958.

Pendergrass, E. P., and Hodes, P. J.: Some observations on carcinoma of the breast. Am. J. Roentgenol., 39:397, 1938.

Pendergrass, E. P., and Hodes, P. J.: Further observations on carcinoma of the breast. Am. J. Roentgenol., 42:393, 1939.

Plenk, A.: Ueber ein Mammakarzinom mit vielen Lokalrezidiven, welches bisher durch 26 Jahr beherrscht wurde. Krebsarzt, Wien, 13:554, 1958.

Power, Sir D.: The history of the amputation of the breast to 1904. Liverpool Med.-Chir. J., 42:29, 1934.

Prudente, A.: L'amputation inter-scapulo-mammo-thoracique. J. de chir., 65:729, 1949.

Raffl, A. B.: The use of negative pressure under skin flaps after radical mastectomy. Ann. Surg., 136:1048, 1952.

Redon, H., and Lacour, J.: Technique d'amputation large du sein avec ablation des muscles pectoraux et triple curage mammaire interne, sus-claviculaire, et axillaire. J. de chir., 69:197, 1953.

Redon, H., and Lacour, J.: Constatations fournies par le curage mammaire interne dans le cancer du sein. Mém. Acad. Chir., 80:568, 1954.

Rigby-Jones, P.: The influence of various factors on metastases in carcinoma of the breast. Brit. J. Cancer, 7:431, 1953.

Robnett, A. H., Jones, T. E., and Hazard, J. B.: Carcinoma of the breast. Cancer, 3:757, 1950.

Rodman, J. S.: Skin removal in radical breast amputation. Ann. Surg., 118:694, 1943.

Russo, P. E., Parker, J. M., and Mathews, H. H.: Changes of the axillary vein after radical mastectomy. South. Med. J., 47:430, 1954.

Sanders, G.: Personal communication, 1969.

Saphir, O.: The transfer of tumor cells by the surgical knife. Surg., Gynec. & Obst., 63:775, 1936.

Schorr, S., Hochmann, A., and Fraenkel, M.: Phlebographic study of the swollen arm following radical mastectomy. J. Fac. Radiol., London, 6:104, 1954.

Shimkin, M. B., Koppel, M., Connelly, R. R., and Cutler, S. J.: Simple and radical mastectomy for breast cancer; A re-analysis of Smith and Meyer's report from Rockford, Ill. J. Nat. Cancer Inst., 27:1197, 1961.

Simmons, C. C.: Cancer of the breast; ten year end-results. Surg., Gynec. & Obst., 74:763, 1942.

Smedal, M. I., and Evans, J. A.: The cause and treatment of edema of the arm after mastectomy. Surg., Gynec. & Obst., 111:29, 1960.

Smith, S. S., and Meyer, A. C.: Cancer of the breast in Rockford, Illinois. Am. J. Surg., 98:653, 1959.

Smithers, D. W., Rigby-Jones, P., Galton, D. A. G., and Payne, P. M.: Cancer of the Breast. Brit. J. Radiol. Supp. No. 4, 1952.

Spratt, J. S., and Donegan, W. L.: Cancer of the Breast. Philadelphia, W. B. Saunders Co., 1967.

Standard, S.: Lymphedema of the arm following radical mastectomy for carcinoma of the breast. Ann. Surg., 116:816, 1942.

Stocks, P.: Methods of measuring results in the treatment of cancer, J. Fac. Radiol., 1:187, 1950.

Taylor, G. W.: Carcinoma of the breast in young women. New Eng. J. Med., 215:1276, 1936.

Taylor, G. W.: Treatment and results in cancer of the breast. Am. J. Roentgenol., 62:341, 1949.

Taylor, G. W., and Bruce, N. H.: Prognostic factors in carcinoma of the breast. New Eng. J. Med., 222:790, 1940.

Taylor, G. W., and Daland, E. M.: The Greenough technique of radical mastectomy. Surg., Gynec. & Obst., 65:807, 1937.

Taylor, G. W., and Wallace, R. H.: Carcinoma of the breast. Surg. Clin. N. Amer., 27:1151, 1947.

Taylor, G. W., and Wallace, R. H.: Carcinoma of the breast; end-results, Massachusetts General Hospital 1933–1935. New Eng. J. Med., 237:475, 1947.

Taylor, G. W., and Wallace, R. H.: Carcinoma of the breast; fifty years' experience at the Massachusetts General Hospital. Ann. Surg., 132:833, 1950.

Treves, N.: Prophylaxis of postmammectomy lymphedema by the use of gelfoam laminated rolls. Cancer, 5:73, 1952.

Trout, H. H.: Carcinoma of the breast. Ann. Surg., 107:733, 1938.

Trout, H. H., Jr.: Five-year follow-up carcinoma of the breast treated with radical mastectomy and postoperative irradiation. Tr. South. S.A., 62:231, 1950.

Truscott, B. M.: Carcinoma of the breast; an analysis of the symptoms, factors affecting prognosis, results of treatment, and recurrences in 1211 cases treated at the Middlesex Hospital. Brit. J. Cancer, 1:129, 1947.

Urban, J. A.: Radical excision of the chest wall for mammary cancer. Cancer, 4:1263, 1951.

Veal, J. R.: The pathologic basis for swelling of the arm following radical amputation of the breast. Surg., Gynec. & Obst., 67:752, 1938.

Veronesi, U., and Zingo, L.: Extended mastectomy for cancer of the breast. Cancer, 20:677, 1967.

Villasor, R. P., and Lewison, E. F.: Postmastectomy lymphedema. Surg., Gynec. & Obst., 100:743, 1955.

von Volkmann, R.: Beiträge zur Chirurgie. Leipzig, Breitkoff und Härtel, 1875, p. 329.

Wangensteen, O. H.: In discussion: Bell, H. G.: Cancer of the breast. Ann. Surg., 130:315, 1949.

Wawro, N. W.: The case for de novo origin of late recurrence of cancer of the female breast. Surgery, 35:470, 1954.

Webster, J. H. D.: The periodicity of recurrences in cancer of the breast. Internat. Union against Cancer, 8:161, 1952.

White, W. C.: Late results of operation for carcinoma of the breast. Ann. Surg., 86:695, 1927.

White, W. C.: Skin removal in radical mastectomy. Ann. Surg., 115:1182, 1942.

White, W. C.: The problem of local recurrence after radical mastectomy for carcinoma. Surgery, 19:149, 1946.

White, W. C.: Radical breast surgery and local recurrence. Am. Surg., 17:237, 1951.

Williams, I. G., Murley, R. S., and Curwen, M. P.: Carcinoma of the female breast; conservative and radical surgery. Brit. Med. J., 2:787, 1953.

Willis, R. A.: The Spread of Tumors in the Human Body. London, J. & A. Churchill, 1934, p. 112, Case 42.

Willis, R. A.: Pathology of Tumours, St. Louis, C. V. Mosby Co., 1948, p. 244.

von Winiwarter, A.: Beiträge zur Statistik der Carcinome mit besonderer Rücksicht auf die dauernde Heilbarkeit durch operative Behandlung. Stuttgart, Ferdinand Enke, 1878.

Zimmerman, K. W., Montague, E. D., and Fletcher, G. H.: Frequency, anatomical distribution, and management of local recurrences after definitive therapy for breast cancer. Cancer, 19:67, 1966.

Chapter Thirty-Five

The Radiotherapy of Breast Carcinoma

The irradiation treatment of carcinoma of the breast is a subject of great importance, because more than one-half of our patients require it. I cannot attempt, as a surgeon, to present the technical details of radiotherapy. These must be sought for in books on radiotherapy. I wish, however, to present certain basic facts and principles concerning the use of irradiation in breast carcinoma.

Irradiation is used in carcinoma of the breast in three ways: (1) as a primary method of treatment attempting to cure the disease; (2) as an auxiliary form of therapy supplementing radical mastectomy, again with the intention of cure; (3) as a palliative method of therapy. These three usages are best discussed separately. They all depend, however, upon the same biological effect of irradiation upon mammary carcinoma, and it is helpful to consider this fundamental matter before discussing the special usages of irradiation.

THE BIOLOGICAL EFFECTS OF IRRADIATION UPON MAMMARY CARCINOMA

Although we do not know the precise mechanism by which irradiation damages cells, we know from clinical and microscopic observations that its effects are profound. Tumor masses shrink and disappear. The carcinoma cells themselves show marked morpho-logical changes and finally disintegrate and disappear. The degree of cell destruction depends not only upon the amount of irradiation reaching them but upon the relative sensitivity of the tumor cells to irradiation in comparison with the cells of the surrounding tissues. Irradiation of sufficient intensity can destroy any tissue, but from a practical aspect the aim of the radiotherapeutist has to be to deliver a sufficient dosage to the carcinoma to destroy it without irreparably damaging the surrounding normal tissues.

It is important to review the microscopic evidence as to what success has been achieved in the effort to destroy breast carcinoma. The studies that are pertinent are recent, because it is only recently that sufficiently fractionated irradiation, capable of delivering a high dosage to the carcinoma, has been employed. To be of value, such studies must not only include accurate data as to the dosage of irradiation delivered to the tumor, but after the completion of irradiation, the breast and axillary contents must have been removed and detailed microscopic studies carried out. Studies providing information of this kind are summarized in Table 35–1.

One of the first such studies was that carried out by Lenz in our own clinic in the Presbyterian Hospital. Between 1933 and 1937 a total of 38 patients with breast carcinoma, most of them with comparatively advanced disease, were treated intensively

Table 35-1. Microscopic Effects of Roentgen Therapy

Year	Author	No. of Cases Treated	Tumor Dosage	Persisting Cancer in Breast		Persisting Cancer in Axillary Nodes
				No.	Per cent	Number
1947	Lenz	38	up to 4500 rads	38	100	31 of 38
1950	Lumb	60	2000 to 4500 rads	53	88.4	not reported
1951	Williams	36	3000 to 3500 rads	35	97.1	14 of 24
1953	Peters	135	4000 rads	111	82	not reported
1962	Baclesse	101	4500 to 9500 rads	86	85.9	54 of 61

with roentgen rays. The breast and the axilla each received a tumor dose of up to 4500 rads during a total period of six to eight weeks.

After a varying interval of time radical mastectomy was performed. The surgical specimens were meticulously studied by Stout. The microscopic changes in some of these cases were described by Beach. They illustrate the effects of irradiation on mammary carcinoma cells very well. The earliest change is perhaps suppression of mitosis. The nuclei then become pyknotic, the cytoplasms vacuolated. Abnormal cell division occurs with the formation of bizarre and gigantic cells. Changes of this kind are shown in Figure 35-1. The tumor cells finally disintegrate and disappear. Meanwhile, fibrosis of the stroma develops and the remaining carcinoma cells are imprisoned in dense collagen. Figure 35-2 shows residual carcinoma cells in a dense fibrous stroma of this kind. Figure 35-3 shows a biopsy of the same carcinoma before irradiation. The radiation effect may be so marked that only scattered individual carcinoma cells can be identified, as in Figure 35-4. Ultimately calcification may develop in the areas of fibrosis as shown in Figure 35-5. Despite these marked microscopic effects of radiation seen in Lenz's series of cases, Stout

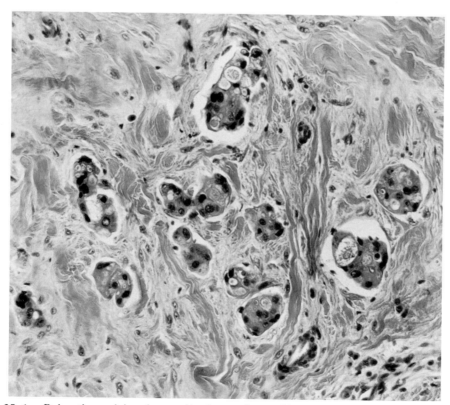

Figure 35-1. Pyknotic nuclei and vacuolated cytoplasm of irradiated mammary carcinoma cells.

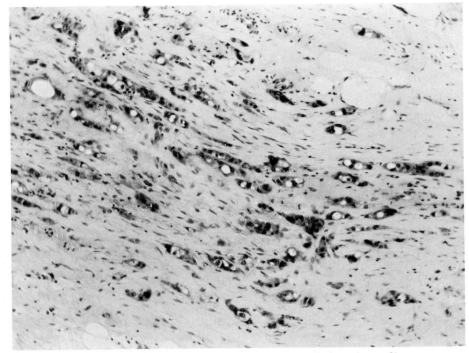

Figure 35–2.   Atypical residual mammary carcinoma cells in a dense fibrous stroma.

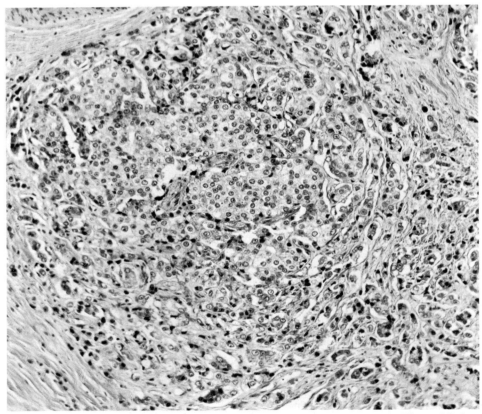

Figure 35–3.   Pre-irradiation biopsy of mammary carcinoma shown in Figure 35–2.

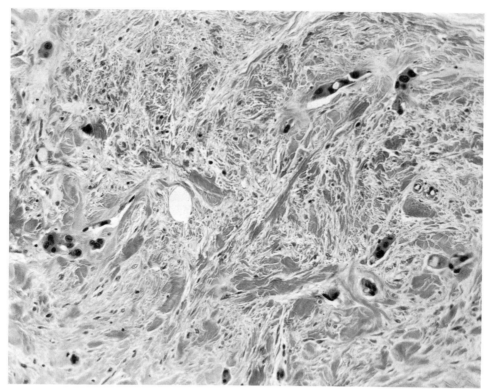

Figure 35–4. Isolated atypical mammary carcinoma cells persisting in dense fibrotic stroma after irradiation.

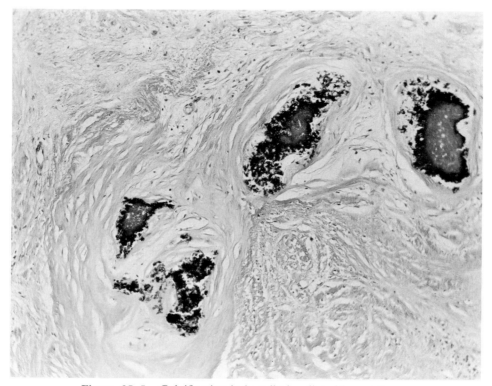

Figure 35–5. Calcification in heavily irradiated breast tissue.

was able to find persisting carcinoma cells in
every case, although in some cases only a very
few remaining cells could be identified, and
they were so distorted that their viability
might be questioned.

Lumb studied the microscopic changes in a
series of 60 cases of carcinoma of the breast
treated by radiation at the Westminster Hospital, London. In his cases the tumor dose
ranged from 2000 to 4000 rads, administered
during a period of between 20 and 40 days.
Lumb found no remaining carcinoma in seven
of the 60 cases. Four of these were among
the 11 cases in which a dose of 3500 to 4000
rads had been given. In the other seven cases
in this group only small numbers of isolated
cells showing gross degenerative changes
were found. The changes produced by dosages of 2500 rads or less were slight. Lumb
concluded that a dose of between 3500 and
4000 rads is required to destroy the majority
of breast carcinomas.

Williams described his findings in 36 cases
treated by fractionated x-rays. In 32 cases
the dosage varied from 3000 to 3500 rads.,
delivered in from 21 to 28 days. In four other
cases, the only ones which have been reported treated by supervoltage x-rays, the
dose was 4500 rads delivered in 30 days.
Williams' supervoltage was given with a 1000
kilovolt unit, using a half layer value of 9.2
mm. of copper. Residual carcinoma was
found in the breast of 35 of the 36 cases. The
only case in which the tumor had been completely destroyed was one of the four treated
by supervoltage x-rays. In the 24 cases in
which the axillary lymph nodes were removed and studied microscopically, viable
carcinoma was found in 14.

Peters reported the microscopic findings in
135 cases in which a tumor dose of 4000 rads
was administered over a period of two weeks,
and radical mastectomy subsequently performed. Residual carcinoma was found in
111, or 82 per cent of the cases. Peters did
not state how many lymph nodes were found
to contain residual tumor.

Baclesse was one of the foremost students
of irradiation in the treatment of breast carcinoma. In 1962 he reported his findings in a
series of 101 patients treated with x-rays between the years 1935 and 1955 with subsequent radical mastectomy. No Stage I cases
were included. The approximate tumor dose
varied between 4500 and 9500 rads. At least
two months, and sometimes much longer,
were required to deliver this amount of radiation. In 86 of the 101 patients residual carci-

noma was found in the breast. In 54 of 61
patients with clinically involved axillary
nodes, persisting axillary metastases were
found.

The apparent conclusion from these facts
about the microscopic evidence of irradiation
effect upon mammary carcinoma is that a tumor dose of 5000 to 6000 rads is desirable,
and that even with the highest dosages yet
employed, carcinoma persists in about four-
fifths of the cases. The carcinoma cells are
locked up in a dense fibrous stroma but they
are apparently viable. The threat that they
may break free and begin to grow again remains one of the basic disadvantages of irradiation treatment.

NEW TECHNIQUES AND FORMS OF IRRADIATION

As a deeply interested observer watching
from the sidelines, so to speak, the struggle
for the control of breast carcinoma with
irradiation, I have seen important basic advances during my 45 years experience with
the disease. My early mentor in radiotherapy,
Maurice Lenz, has summarized them in a
recent paper.

The first of these important basic advances
was the development of highly fractionated
irradiation. It evolved at the Curie Institute
in Paris in the 1920's. Regaud, in his famous
experiment studying the sterilization of the
testicle in rams and rabbits, proved the importance of the distribution of the dose of
irradiation in time. Coutard then carried out
a series of clinical experiments in which the
time required to give the desired dose varied
from one to 12 weeks. Baclesse analyzed
Coutard's data, and carried fractionation
much farther. These experiments clearly
showed that lengthening of the time required
to give the irradiation, and giving it daily,
made it possible to give a much larger total
dose and yet spare the normal tissues.

The result of these studies has been a
general agreement among the best modern
radiotherapists that five or six weeks is an
optimum period in which to administer a total
dose of 5000 or 6000 rads.

With this increased dosage radiotherapists
have learned to be more precise about defining the fields they treat. The best ones set
their patients up personally for each treatment instead of leaving it to a technician.
They assume the same kind of personal re-

sponsibility for each treatment that a good surgeon assumes. There is no doubt whatever in my mind that this kind of irradiation achieves a good deal more. I have seen the difference.

Most of the fractionated irradiation to the breast of the past generation was done with orthovoltage of from 200 to 280 kilovolts. Some nausea and malaise frequently resulted. The skin often suffered severely with this plan of treatment. Moist desquamation was the rule, as shown in Figure 35–6. Late telangiectasia and fibrosis usually followed.

The second basic advance in radiotherapy in recent times has been the development of higher voltage x-rays (above 1000 kilovolts) and cobalt-60 beam therapy. This kind of irradiation spares the skin so that only a mild tanning results, as shown in Figure 35–7. There is much less late fibrosis. Systemic symptoms are minimal. Both Baclesse and Guttmann have described the advantages of this type of irradiation. The patient is penalized less by it, although the survival rate may not be any better than with orthovoltage irradiation.

The newest form of irradiation is the high energy electron beam produced by the betatron. This type of irradiation has the special advantage of a limited penetration, thus sparing deeper tissues. Chu and her associates have reported their results in treating 549 patients with breast carcinoma with their betatron. They state that the electron beam is particularly effective in delivering a satisfactory tumor dose without injuring the underlying normal tissues. They conclude, "We have found electron beam therapy indispensible in our treatment of breast cancer." Tapley and Fletcher have also discussed the use of the betatron in breast carcinoma.

Irradiation Injuries. It is to be expected that the modern intensive irradiation which destroys breast carcinoma will damage normal tissues. These injuries are of several types.

Much the most frequent type of injury is that sustained by the pleura and lung. Pleurisy and pneumonitis, producing chest pain, cough, and dyspnea, occur in a significant proportion of patients even when the irradiation is directed tangentially to the chest wall in an effort to spare the lung. Bate and Guttmann wrote a good description of these changes occurring in patients treated by supervoltage irradiation in our Francis Delafield Hospital. Our radiologists, Bachman and Macken, discussed the diagnosis and significance of pleural effusions in these patients.

The symptoms of pleural and pulmonary damage develop within a month or two after irradiation is completed, and subside within four to six months. The fibrosis of the underlying lung is seen in x-ray films as a broad

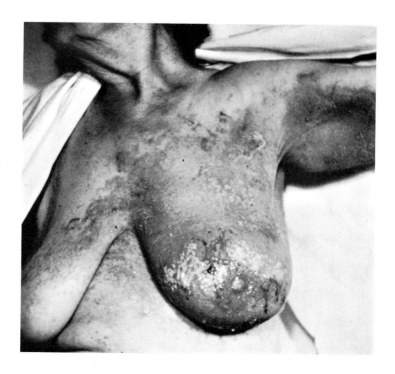

Figure 35–6. The severe skin reaction which develops following intensive irradiation with 250 kilovolts.

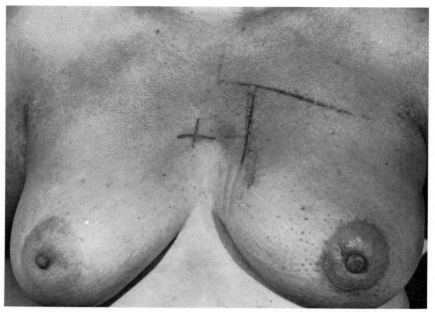

Figure 35–7. The mild skin reaction following intensive irradiation with higher voltage x-rays or cobalt beam therapy.

zone of increased density which eventually clears.

The frequency of these changes has been variously reported as from 7 per cent to 90 per cent. (Chu et at.; Ross; Rouquès; Lougheed and Maguire; Fleming et al.; Smith; O'Neill; Greenberg and Jacobs). These pulmonary changes are usually not severe. They must not be confused with pulmonary metastases.

Damage to the heart by irradiation given for breast carcinoma has been reported but this is certainly infrequent (Whitfield and Kunkler; Jones and Wedgwood, Rubin et al.).

A number of instances of irradiation necrosis of ribs, clavicle, scapula, and humerus have been reported (Kolar and Vrabec; Baudisch; Kikuchi et al.). Ribs thus damaged sometimes fracture. I have myself observed two such cases.

The extent to which irradiation can damage the bones of the shoulder girdle is illustrated in the roentgenogram reproduced in Figure 35-8. This patient consulted me 11 years after intensive prophylactic irradiation to the supraclavicular and axillary regions. She had no clinical evidence of recurrence of her breast carcinoma, but the upper humerus, scapula, and clavicle showed many areas of necrosis. These changes had been interpreted as metastasis, and she was about to be given additional irradiation when we recognized their true nature.

Primary Treatment with Irradiation

Reliance upon roentgen rays as a primary method of treating carcinoma of the breast, even when it is in the so-called operable stage, is a comparatively recent development which has been carried on only in a few centers. The use of x-rays for this purpose has evolved with the modern development of fractionated intensive treatment which has made it possible to deliver sufficiently large tumor doses to profoundly affect breast carcinoma. This type of primary radiologic treatment has evolved chiefly under Baclesse. Between 1936 and 1951 he treated a total of 431 patients with irradiation alone. Their carcinomas were classified by the Columbia Clinical Classification. In 136 the disease was classified as Clinical Stage A or B. Baclesse did not himself choose to treat these patients with operable breast carcinoma by irradiation alone. Most of them were patients who refused radical mastectomy; others were sent to him by surgeons who requested this form of treatment. In all, the tumor had been excised for biopsy. The patients with Clinical Stage C and D carcinoma were treated by irradiation because their disease was inoperable.

X-rays of 200 kilovolts were used. The approximate minimal dosage, through 6 or 7 portals, was 6500 rads to the breast, and 6000 rads to the axillary, supraclavicular, and internal mammary regions.

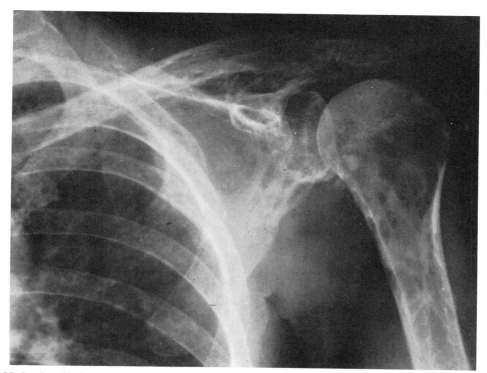

Figure 35–8. Irradiation necrosis of the bones of the shoulder girdle resulting from radiotherapy given prophylactically to the axilla and supraclavicular region for carcinoma of the breast.

Baclesse's 5 and 10 year results are shown in Table 35–2. He has expressed them as "apparent clinical cure" rates. The ten year "clinical cure rate" for the Clinical Stage A and B patients was 34 per cent. This 10 year rate would, of course, be somewhat higher if it were presented as a 10 year survival rate, as is the usual custom.

Baclesse did not advise irradiation alone as a general method of treatment for operable breast carcinoma, but he believed that it provided an alternative method of treatment for patients who refused mastectomy.

His data are of great value from several points of view. They show that the results of irradiation alone in the early operable Clinical Stage A and B cases are greatly inferior to those of radical mastectomy. His data are equally valuable in showing that irradiation alone does almost as well as radical mastectomy in the advanced inoperable Clinical Stage C and D cases. In these patients with advanced disease, the results of all methods of treatment are very poor; the kindest method of treatment is to be preferred, and in this sense irradiation is surely preferable.

Papillon has repeated Baclesse's experiment, treating early breast carcinoma with irradiation alone following excisional biopsy of the tumor. Between 1946 and 1956 he treated a total of 73 patients, most of whom were classified as Clinical Stage I (T.N.M.

Table 35–2. IRRADIATION ONLY FOR BREAST CARCINOMA. BACLESSE, 1936–1951

Columbia Clinical Classification	5 Year Results		10 Year Results	
	No. of Patients	Per cent Apparent Clinical Cure	No. of Patients	Per cent Apparent Clinical Cure
Stage A	50	54%	33	30.3%
Stage B	86	61%	64	35.9%
Stage C	95	34.7%	75	14.7%
Stage D	200	10%	137	4.4%
Total	431	—	309	—

Classification). At five years the disease was "stabilized" in 67 per cent of the patients. In 46 per cent of the 30 patients treated more than 10 years previously "stabilization" was achieved.

Peters has also treated a series of patients with radiotherapy alone following excisional biopsy of the primary tumor. Most of the 124 patients in her series of cases had refused radical mastectomy. In all the disease was classified as Clinical Stage I or II (T.N.M. Classification). They were treated between 1935 and 1960. Peters used 400 kilovolt x-ray irradiation, and since 1953 cobalt beam therapy, to give a total of 4500 rads in four weeks.

The five year survival rate for Peters' 124 patients was 76 per cent. Forty-five per cent of the 62 patients treated more than 10 years ago have survived.

In considering Peters' results it should be kept in mind that the Clinical Stage I and II patients in the T.N.M. Classification have carcinoma in an earlier clinical stage than the Clinical Stage A and B patients staged by our Columbia Clinical Classification. Yet Peters' 10 year survival rates with her method of treatment are much inferior to the 10 year survival rate of 62 per cent for Clinical Stages A and B in my personal series of radical mastectomies.

At our Frances Delafield Hospital the careful clinical classification of our patients as to the stage of advancement of their disease, and the further refinement of classification by the performance, in some patients, of preliminary biopsy of the lymph nodes at the periphery of the regional lymph node filter, has provided us with a number of patients whose disease was clinically operable, yet incurable by surgery because of proven metastases in the apex of the axilla or internal mammary lymph nodes. Guttmann has treated these patients with irradiation alone.

She used 2,000 kilovolt x-rays to deliver a dose of 5000 to 6000 rads in five or six weeks. The filtration was 7 mm. of lead and the target skin distance 100 cm. The irradiation was given through four portals as shown in Figure 35–9. The two breast fields were directed tangentially as shown in Figure 35–10.

Patients tolerate this treatment very well. The skin reaction which occurs develops somewhat later than with orthovoltage irradiation, and is much less marked. Patients treated with 2000 kilovolts also have less malaise and nausea. Their blood picture must

of course be followed with the customary care necessary when high doses of irradiation are given.

The 5 and 10 year results in Guttmann's series of 63 patients treated in this manner are shown in Table 35–3. In all, the stage of advancement of their disease was classified by our Columbia Clinical Classification.

The 10 year survival rate of 33.3 per cent for these patients with metastases at the periphery of the regional lymph node filter, for whom even the extended surgical attack has given very poor results, is a tribute to Guttmann's skill as a radiotherapist.

From autopsy studies of several of these patients she has irrefutable evidence that the type of irradiation she gives to the internal mammary region can destroy metastatic carcinoma in the internal mammary nodes. The following case history illustrates this point.

Mrs. J. W., aged 64, was admitted to the Frances Delafield Hospital in January 1954 with a 3.5 cm. carcinoma in the upper outer sector of the right breast. Her disease was classified as Clinical Stage A. A preliminary internal mammary biopsy showed metastases in the first interspace. She was treated by irradiation to the breast, the axilla and supraclavicular region, and the internal mammary region. The latter received 5000 rads of 2 millivolt irradiation.

The patient died of cardiovascular disease in January 1965, 11 years later. Autopsy study showed no persisting carcinoma in the internal mammary region.

The most discouraging handicap of primary irradiation for breast carcinoma is the fact that although the initial response to irradiation is often excellent, the disease is apt to break free of the fibrous bonds in which it has been imprisoned and grow again after a number of years. This is much less true of the surgical attack. Thus the survival rate following primary irradiation treatment falls by almost 50 per cent between 5 and 10 years, but it decreases by only about 20 per cent between 5 and 10 years following radical mastectomy.

Very late recurrence is also seen following primary irradiation treatment, as illustrated in the following cases.

CASE 1

Mrs. G. P., aged 48, came to Presbyterian Hospital in February, 1939, with a tumor of the right breast which she said she had had for three weeks. She had a 10 cm. carcinoma filling the central area

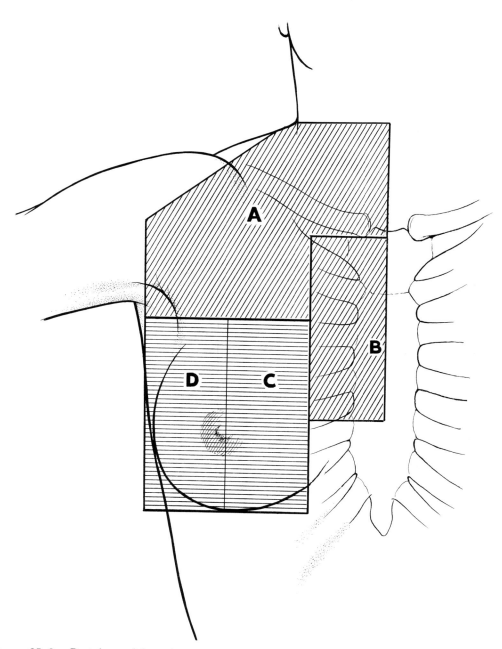

Figure 35–9. Portals used for primary treatment of breast carcinoma with 2000 kilovolt x-rays.

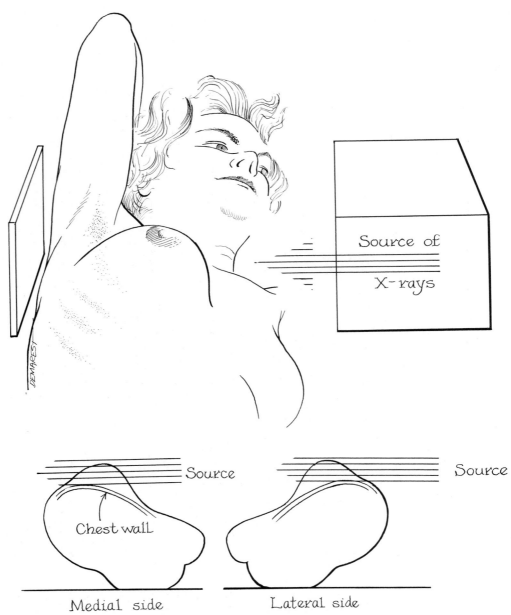

Figure 35–10. Tangential irradiation to the breast through two fields, with 2000 kilovolt x-rays.

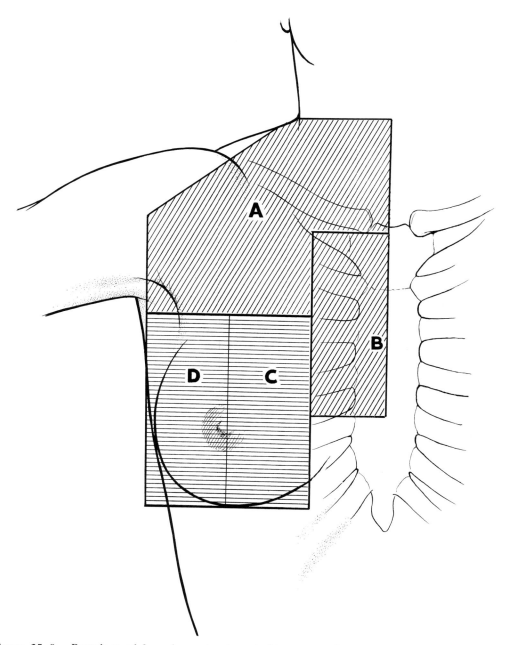

Figure 35–9. Portals used for primary treatment of breast carcinoma with 2000 kilovolt x-rays.

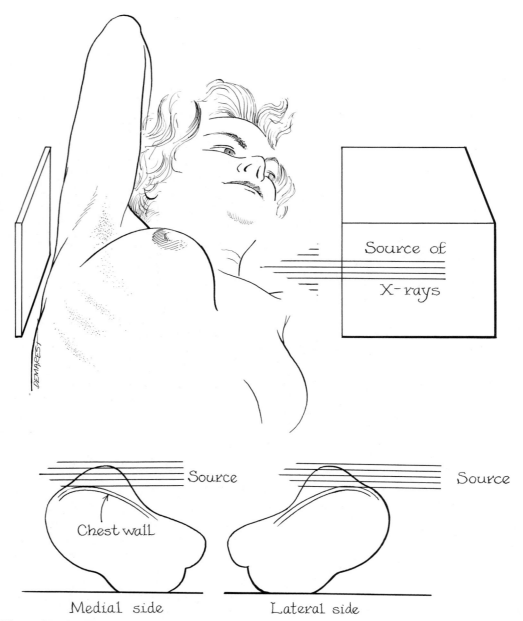

Figure 35–10. Tangential irradiation to the breast through two fields, with 2000 kilovolt x-rays.

Table 35-3. IRRADIATION ONLY FOR BREAST CARCINOMA WITH BIOPSY-PROVEN INTERNAL MAMMARY OR APEX OF AXILLA NODES. GUTTMANN, FRANCES DELAFIELD HOSPITAL, 1955–1960

Columbia Clinical Classification	Internal Mammary Node Metastases			Apex of Axilla Node Metastases			Metastases to Internal Mammary and Apex of Axilla Nodes			All Patients with Internal Mammary or Apex of Axilla Node Metastases		
		Number Survived			Number Survived			Number Survived			Number Survived	
	Number Patients	5 Years	10 Years	Number Patients	5 Years	10 Years	Number Patients	5 Years	10 Years	Number Patients	5 Years	10 Years
Stage A	12	9	7	1		0	—		—	13	9	7
Stage B	17	10	4	4	3	2	5		1	26	15	7
Stage C	16	9	7	3		0	5		0	24	9	7
Totals	45	28	18	8	3	2	10		1	63	33	21

of the right breast. There was edema of the skin over the central portion of the breast. There was a clinically involved node in the right axilla.

It was decided that the carcinoma was inoperable, although there was no evidence of distant metastasis, and she was treated with irradiation given through four fields to the breast and three fields to the axilla, each field receiving approximately 2000 rads over a period of three months. The tumor dose to the breast lesion was 5600 rads. Both the primary tumor and the axillary metastasis disappeared.

The patient had no further evidence of her carcinoma until August, 1951, twelve years and three months after radiation had been completed, when a number of small recurrent nodules were found in the skin along the lower portion of the right edge of the sternum. These were treated successfully with radiation, but during the following year new skin nodules continued to appear in the skin over the right chest. Carcinoma finally appeared in the opposite breast, and bone metastasis developed. The patient died in December, 1955, 16 years after her irradiation treatment was begun.

CASE 2

In this case the primary tumor in the breast was controlled by irradiation but the axillary metastasis began to grow after being held in check for many years.

Mrs. M. M., aged 52, came to the Presbyterian Hospital in February, 1940, with a tumor of the central portion of the left breast which she had had for seven months. The tumor measured 5 cm. in diameter. It was freely movable over the chest wall. There was a very small area of edema of the skin just caudad to the areola. The nipple was markedly retracted. There was a small satellite nodule in the skin just lateral to the areola. In the lower left axilla there was a firm 1 cm. node. There were no evidences of distant metastasis.

It was decided that her carcinoma was locally inoperable and her breast was treated through four portals and the axilla through three portals. Each

of these received 2000 rads except the superior and inferior breast portals which received 1500 rads. This treatment was given over a period of four months. The breast tumor regressed, leaving only an area of thickening. The axillary node also disappeared.

There was no reactivation of her breast disease until 14½ years later, in November, 1954. On a follow-up examination on that date I noted that at the site of the original node in the lower axilla there was a recurrent tumor measuring 2 cm. in diameter. There was a small ulcer in the overlying skin. The breast itself showed no change, although the skin showed marked telangiectasia and atrophy. During the following year the area of recurrent carcinoma in the axillary region slowly increased in size. Her arm became edematous and began to pain her a good deal. The axillary recurrence was given additional irradiation which held it in check until she died in a nursing home of other causes in October, 1959, 19 years and 8 months after her initial irradiation treatment.

Radiation Supplementing Radical Mastectomy

Fifty years ago it was the general practice to supplement radical mastectomy with radiation given either preoperatively or postoperatively. Postoperative radiation was the most popular, and it was usually given in small doses repeated at intervals of weeks or months, on the basis of the theory that this kind of treatment would restrain the growth of residual carcinoma. Critical evaluation of the results of radical mastectomy supplemented by this kind of radiation, by such able students of the disease as Harrington (1935) and Greenough (1929), failed to show any advantage of this combined treatment over radical mastectomy alone. When Stout and I published our study of end results at the Presbyterian Hospital for the period of 1915 to 1934 inclusive, we were likewise unable to demonstrate any advantage of either preoperative or postoperative irradiation. German radiotherapeutists, such as Hintze and Anschütz, were the chief proponents of supplementary prophylactic irradiation, but it gradually fell into disfavor in American clinics when it was realized that this kind of feeble interrupted irradiation was not sufficient to have much effect on carcinoma.

In several important European clinics, such as the Radiumhemmet (Berven) and the Radium Center in Copenhagen (Nielsen), supplementary prophylactic irradiation continued to be given. With the development of modern radiotherapy techniques which provide a far larger tumor dose, prophylactic irradiation supplementing radical mastectomy has had a revival in American clinics. Today it is widely used, often, I believe, when there is no justification whatever for giving it. It is of two types, preoperative and postoperative. I will discuss them separately.

Irradiation Preceding Radical Mastectomy

Although irradiation preceding radical mastectomy has the handicap of delaying operation at least six or eight weeks, arguments in its favor have come from several clinics during the last decade. These reports are listed in Table 35–4.

Baclesse carried out a careful study of the value of preoperative irradiation in a series of 101 patients treated between 1935 and 1951. He emphasized that all of the patients were treated with *high doses* of *fractionated* irra-

diation of 200 kilovolts. In 96 of the patients, radical mastectomy followed; in five, simple mastectomy was done.

The extent of the disease in this series of patients was classified by the T.N.M. Clinical Classification. There were no Stage I cases, 47 Stage II cases, 63 Stage III cases, and one Stage IV case.

The 5 year "apparent cure" rate for the 101 patients was 41.5 per cent. Eighty-six of the patients had been treated more than 10 years previously; 35 per cent of them were "apparently well."

Baclesse believed that his results indicated that this method gives superior results in the more advanced stages of breast carcinoma.

Delarue and his associates advise preoperative irradiation for locally advanced breast carcinoma (Clinical Stage III, T.N.M. Classification) on the basis of their experience with 266 such patients.

Fletcher has made a plea for preoperative irradiation, based on a comparison of the frequency of local recurrence and the 5 year survival rates in a series of 254 patients given preoperative irradiation, and another series of 301 patients given postoperative irradiation. Local recurrence was much less frequent, and the five year survival rate 10 per cent better, in the group treated by preoperative irradiation. In evaluating Fletcher's data, it must be kept in mind that the clinical stage of advancement of the disease in the patients making up his two case series is not precisely stated. There is, therefore, no way of knowing what part selection played in determining the results.

Lindgren and his associates treated a series of 166 patients with preoperative irradiation. The cases were carefully staged both clinically and microscopically. The frequency of local recurrence and the five and 10 year survival rates in these patients were compared with the corresponding results in another series of 148 patients whose disease was clinically and microscopically similar, and who were treated by radical mastectomy alone. No statistically significant differences in results were demonstrated.

Prophylactic Postoperative Irradiation Following Radical Mastectomy

It has become the general custom to give postoperative prophylactic irradiation following radical mastectomy. The expense and the morbidity of this kind of irradiation in

Table 35–4. IRRADIATION PRECEDING RADICAL MASTECTOMY

Author	Years of Treatment	Number of Patients Treated Pre- operatively	Number of Patients Having Radical Mastectomy Only
Baclesse, 1962	1935–1955	101	no comparable group
Delarue et al., 1965	1938–1956	266	no comparable group
Fletcher, 1967	1949–1962	254	301
Lindgren et al., 1968	1952–1961	166	148

terms of increased edema of the arm are considerable.

Fortunately, surgeons who perform a good radical mastectomy with a skin graft need not fear to irradiate their skin graft if postoperative prophylactic irradiation to the chest wall is indicated. Cram and his associates have found that skin grafts will tolerate a dose of 4500 rads if it is given over a 5 week period.

Whether or not postoperative prophylactic irradiation improves the survival rate continues to be debated. Several reports published during the past decade, however, have begun to clarify the question (Table 35–5).

Lewison and Smith compared the 5 and 10 year survival rates in 153 patients given postoperative prophylactic irradiation with the results in 100 patients who did not receive it. They concluded that the survival rate was "somewhat" better in the irradiated group. Since the clinical stage of advancement of the disease in their patients was not stated, selection may well have been responsible for the difference.

Archambault and his associates reported a 5 year survival rate of 54.3 per cent in a series of 168 patients to whom they gave postoperative prophylactic irradiation consisting of 6000 rads over a period of 11 to 14 weeks. Because the clinical stage of advancement of the disease in his patients was not classified in terms of a modern clinical classification, it is difficult to evaluate his results.

Butcher and his associates compared survival in 129 patients treated by radical mastectomy alone with survival in 78 patients who were, in addition, given postoperative prophylactic irradiation to the supraclavicular and internal mammary regions. There was no difference in survival rate in the two case series.

Robbins and his associates reported the five year survival rates for 386 patients treated by radical mastectomy alone, and for 349 patients who were given postoperative prophylactic irradiation to the supraclavicular and internal mammary regions. A dose of 4000 rads was given over a four week period. There was "no significant difference in the five year cure rates." Unfortunately, their patients were not classified as to the clinical stage of advancement of their disease.

Fletcher, Montague, and White have reviewed their experience with postoperative prophylactic irradiation between 1948 and 1964. They state that it was given to all patients except those with microscopically negative axillary nodes and those whose lesions were situated in the outer sectors of the breast. Supraclavicular and internal mammary portals were used to deliver a tumor dose of 3500 to 5000 rads.

A total of 281 patients were treated by radical mastectomy alone, and 363 others were given postoperative prophylactic irradiation in addition. Although their report does not include a statement of the comparative clinical stage of advancement of the disease in these two groups of patients, the authors conclude that "the judiciously planned use of irradiation in conjunction with radical mastectomy . . . has considerably diminished the incidence of local recurrence in all categories." This statement may be correct, but I do not believe that the data which Fletcher and his associates present justify it.

The most convincing study of the value of postoperative prophylactic irradiation in breast carcinoma is the one which was begun at the Christie Hospital in Manchester in 1949. This is a true random study carried out upon patients whose disease was operable, and who had a standard radical mastectomy.

The 10 year results of this study have recently been presented by Easson. This series included 707 patients who were given postoperative prophylactic irradiation, and 750 pa-

Table 35–5. PROPHYLACTIC IRRADIATION FOLLOWING RADICAL MASTECTOMY

Author	Years of Treatment	Number of Patients Irradiated Prophylactically Postoperatively	Number of Patients Having Radical Mastectomy only
Lewison and Smith, 1963	1946–1950	153	100
Archambault, 1964	1952–1959	168	no comparable group
Butcher et al., 1964	1952–1958	78	129
Robbins et al., 1966	1954–1955	349	386
Fletcher, Montague & White, 1968	1948–1964	363	281
Easson, 1968	1948–1955	707	750

Table 35–6. INCIDENCE OF LOCAL RECURRENCE
TO TENTH YEAR: IRRADIATED VERSUS
WATCHED GROUPS. EASSON,
CHRISTIE HOSPITAL, 1968

| Clinical Stage | Number of Cases | Incidence of Local Recurrence Within 10 Years | |
		Prophylactic Irradiation	Watched
1	527	9.5%	16.0%
2	934	25.0%	41.5%
Total		19.0%	32.0%

tients who were "watched" but not irradiated. The prophylactic irradiation reduced the incidence of local recurrence considerably, as shown in Easson's table (Table 35–6). But there was no significant difference between the survival curves for the "watched" and treated groups of patients. I reproduce Easson's chart illustrating this fact (Chart 35–1). Thirty-five per cent of the "watched" patients died of metastases without ever having developed local recurrence; they were spared the disadvantages of prophylactic irradiation. The local recurrences

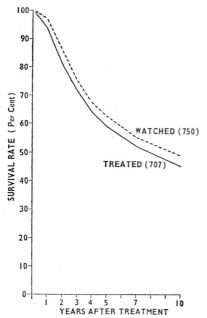

Chart 35–1. Survival curves for patients "watched," and for those given postoperative prophylactic irradiation. From Easson, E. C., in: Forrest, A. P. M., and Kunkler, P. B.: Prognostic Factors in Breast Cancer. Baltimore, Williams and Wilkins, 1968, p. 118, reproduced with permission.

which developed in the surviving "watched" patients were treated by irradiation as the need arose. The local recurrences responded so well that at death the incidence of persisting local recurrence was almost the same in the "watched" patients as it was in the patients who had been given prophylactic irradiation.

Easson drew the following conclusions from this important study: (1) X-ray therapy following Halsted mastectomy does not prevent death from metastases. (2) Locally recurrent disease can be usefully controlled when the need arises. (3) There is advantage to the patient in avoiding prophylactic radiation therapy.

Simple Mastectomy Plus Postoperative Irradiation — the McWhirter Method

In 1941 Robert McWhirter, radiotherapist to the Royal Infirmary in Edinburgh, being dissatisfied with the results of radical mastectomy, conceived a plan for treating breast carcinoma by combining limited removal of the breast with a single course of postoperative irradiation. The method achieved great popularity in Great Britain where today — 30 years later — almost half of the patients with breast cancer are treated with some version of McWhirter's method, according to Handley. It has also been widely used in the United States.

Neither the surgery nor the irradiation which follows it in McWhirter's technique can be regarded as very aggressive. The operation, as described by McWhirter in 1949, removes the bulk of the mammary tissue, but since the extent of skin removal is very limited, the flaps are cut thick, and very little undermining of them is done, some breast tissue is certainly not removed. The axilla is not dissected. Strictly speaking, this procedure should be called a partial mastectomy. It is very much like the mastectomy of 100 years ago: by itself it cannot be expected to give any better results than it did then.

The irradiation which McWhirter gives to the chest wall, the axilla, and the supraclavicular region following this operation consists of 3750 rads administered to each of four fields over a period of three weeks. This is rather limited irradiation as compared with the 5000 to 6000 rads administered over a period of 6 to 8 weeks which the followers

Table 35–7. RESULTS OF SIMPLE MASTECTOMY AND X-RAY THERAPY IN PATIENTS UNDER 65 YEARS OF AGE. McWHIRTER, 1966*

International T N M Classification	Number of Patients	10 Year Survival
Stage I	600	54%
Stage II	491	43%
Stage III	690	24%
Total	1781	

*McWhirter, R.: J. de Radiol., 48:768, 1967.

of the French school of radiotherapy administer when it is indicated for breast carcinoma.

In 1964 McWhirter presented the 10 year survival rates for 1429 patients with "operable" breast carcinoma treated by his method. He defined as "operable" those patients whose disease is classified as Stage I and II by the Manchester clinical classification. However, McWhirter excluded his results in patients over the age of 65 from his report: this makes his case series a particularly favorable one because these older patients are more apt to succumb to intercurrent disease during the follow-up period, and thus worsen the end results. McWhirter's 10 year survival rate as thus determined was 46 per cent.

In 1966 McWhirter reported his results in terms of the International TNM clinical classification. Again, he excluded his patients over the age of 65. These results are shown in Table 35–7.

Fortunately, the Danes Kaae and Johansen have classified a series of their patients according to our Columbia Clinical Classification and treated them with the McWhirter method. This has made it possible to compare the results obtained with this method with the results of radical mastectomy and five other methods of treating breast carcinoma as reported in our Cooperative International Study. Kaae and Johansen's 10 year survival rates for the McWhirter technique are shown in Table 35–8.

These data of McWhirter and of Kaae and Johansen clearly indicate that in the earlier stages of breast carcinoma our radical mastectomy gives much better results than the McWhirter method. In patients whose disease was classified as Stages A and B of the Columbia Clinical Classification the 10 year survival rate in my personal series of radical mastectomies was 62 per cent, as compared with 42 per cent for Kaae's and

Johansen's series of patients treated by the McWhirter method. In patients whose disease has advanced to Clinical Stage C and for whom radical mastectomy should not be done, McWhirter's method may be considered as an alternative to irradiation alone. Better data are needed to settle this special question.

The Palliative Use of Roentgen Therapy

It was formerly my custom to do palliative simple mastectomy for fungating tumors which were so objectionable locally that something had to be done about them. As the years have gone by and my appreciation of the ability of modern, intensive, fractionated roentgen therapy to produce regression of breast carcinoma has grown, I have abandoned surgery and rely entirely upon radiation for this purpose. What can be achieved with irradiation in the local control of inoperable breast carcinoma is illustrated by the following cases.

CASE 1

Mrs. M. L., age 75, came to the Delafield Hospital with a large, fungating carcinoma, shown in Figure 35–11. She had first noticed the tumor two years previously. She had a chain of clinically involved axillary nodes. She was also in congestive heart failure.

The lesion was treated with 2 millivolt x-rays. Through tangential fields a total tumor dose of 4400 rads was delivered during five weeks. During 20 succeeding days an additional tumor dose of 1800 rads was given with 250 kilovolt x-rays through a single portal directly over the tumor.

The tumor regressed as shown in Figure 35–12. Six months later osteoblastic metastases developed in the lumbar spine. The patient died with generalized metastases 10 months later, but her primary breast lesion remained controlled.

Table 35–8. RESULTS OF SIMPLE MASTECTOMY PLUS POSTOPERATIVE IRRADIATION BY THE METHOD OF McWHIRTER. KAAE AND JOHANSEN, 1969*

Columbia Clinical Classification	Number of Patients	10 Year Survival
Stage A	159	50%
Stage B	28	32%
Stage C	9	–
Stage D	3	–
Total	199	

*Haagensen, C. D. et al.: Ann. Surg., 170:875, 1969.

CASE 2

C. B., a 77 year old housewife, came to the Presbyterian Hospital with a 9 cm. fungating carcinoma of the upper outer sector of her right breast. Its appearance is shown in Figure 35–13. There was a chain of firm clinically involved axillary nodes extending high into the axilla.

The lesion was treated with 2000 kilovolt x-rays through four portals, three being directed to the breast and one to the axilla, each averaging 2300 rads delivered during a period of 8 weeks.

The primary tumor and the axillary nodes regressed very satisfactorily, leaving only a shallow 1 cm. ulcer at the site of the tumor (Fig. 35–14). The patient died of arteriosclerotic heart disease, without any further evidence of her breast carcinoma, six years after it was irradiated.

Roentgen therapy is much the preferred weapon in dealing with metastasis to the skin and local skin recurrence. The fact that the skin nodules are small makes it possible to treat them through a very small field and to deliver to them comparatively large amounts of irradiation—so large that they are almost invariably controlled. Guttmann prefers to treat skin metastases with 100 or 120 kilovoltage, using 3 mm. of aluminum as a filter with a target skin distance of 30 cm. A field of sufficient size to surround the lesion with a generous margin is used. A skin dose of 350 to 450 rads is given at each treatment, a total of 3000 rads being administered during a three week treatment period.

It is, in my opinion, an error to excise skin nodules surgically. Surgical excision is not only much less successful than irradiation, but excision carries a risk of producing further embolism and metastasis of the carcinoma.

One of the most valuable uses of irradiation is in the treatment of metastasis to bone. Treatment should be begun at once when pain suggests the likelihood of bone metastases, even though they cannot be seen roentgenographically. In this way the patient is spared unnecessary pain. If the involvement of bone is generalized it is of course impossible, from a practical point of view, to use roentgen therapy, but in most patients the bone metastases are few and isolated, at least at an earlier stage in the metastatic process. For such le-

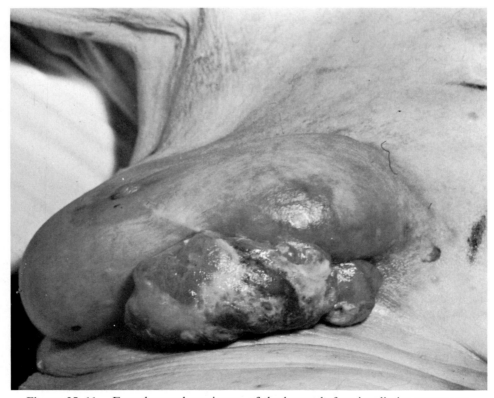

Figure 35–11. Far advanced carcinoma of the breast before irradiation treatment.

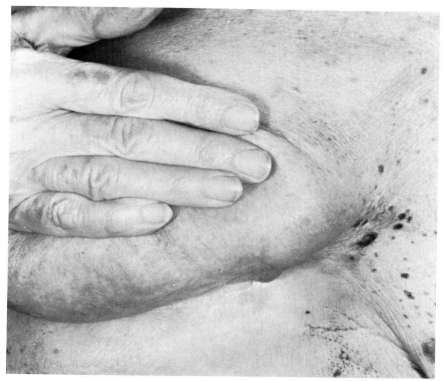

Figure 35–12. The result of irradiation treatment of the carcinoma shown in Figure 35–11.

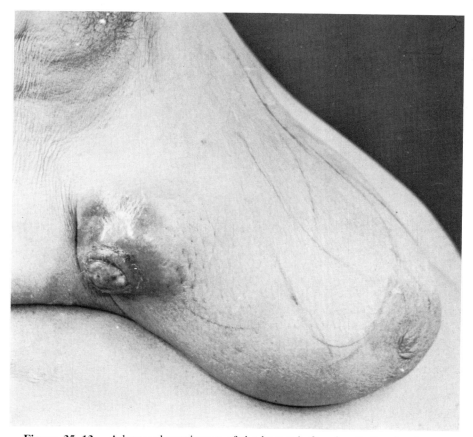

Figure 35–13. Advanced carcinoma of the breast before irradiation treatment.

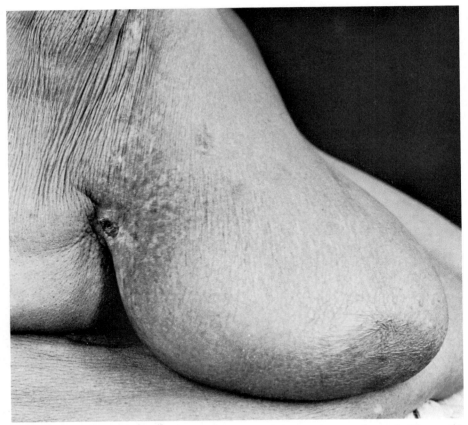

Figure 35–14.   The result of irradiation treatment of the carcinoma shown in Figure 35–13.

sions no other therapy is as successful as ir-radiation.

Irradiation is occasionally indicated to pre-vent fracture of a large silent bone metastasis.

For the treatment of bone metastases, Gutt-mann prefers to use 250 kilovoltage, with a filter of 2 mm. of copper, and a target skin distance of 50 cm. Deep-seated bone lesions are usually treated through opposing fields. When this method cannot be employed oblique fields may be used to avoid a moist skin reac-tion. A daily tumor dose of 200 rads is given. A total tumor dose of 2000 to 2500 rads is delivered over a period of from two to three weeks.

Approximately three-quarters of the pa-tients with bone metastasis who are treated with irradiation will get fairly satisfactory pain relief. Table 35–9 shows the percentage of successful pain relief reported by several authors, and also the average survival time following the development of bone metasta-sis. It will be seen that this was about one year. Occasional patients will survive much

longer following the successful treatment of bone metastasis, and live several years in comfort. Nohrman reported that 33.3 per cent of the patients from the Radiumhemmet treated for bone metastasis lived more than one year, 15.8 per cent more than two years, 7.6 per cent more than three years, 5.3 per cent more than four years, 3.5 per cent more than five years, and 0.9 per cent more than eight years.

More than 90 per cent of bone metastases are osteolytic in type. Even when irradiation successfully relieves pain, it often fails to produce restoration of the bony architecture. Garland reported that this occurred in only 26.3 per cent of his cases treated with irra-diation.

Irradiation is much superior to hormonal treatment of bone metastasis. It gives pain relief more quickly and more surely, and it does not have the unpleasant side effects of hormonal therapy.

Irradiation is useful for pulmonary paren-chymal metastases only if they are of limited

Table 35–9. Results of Roentgen Therapy of Bone Metastases from Cancer of the Breast *

Author	Number of Cases	Percentage of Pain Relief	Average Survival Period (Months after Discovery of Bone Metastasis)
Lenz and Freid	31	71	11
Burch	41	70.6	15.5
Pohle and Benson	18	65	?
Copeland	74	?	18
Deucher	145	78	13
Leddy and Desjardins	106	80	?
Wulff	44	46	14.3
Bouchard	23	65	13.6
Garland et al.	79	68.4	12
Guttmann	52	75	15

*After Garland, 1950.

extent and unilateral. Bilateral metastases and pleural metastases should not be irradiated. For patients whose pleural effusion accumulates so rapidly that they have to be tapped every few days, the intrapleural administration of radioactive gold is worthwhile. It will produce a significant diminution in the effusion in at least 50 per cent of cases (Hansen and Haug; Lambrethsen and Sell; Karras and Moss; Botsford).

Irradiation is of only temporary help in controlling metastases to the brain and spinal cord. These types of metastases usually occur late in the course of the disease, and the patients are not likely to survive long. Irradiation must be given very carefully when the intracranial pressure is elevated, because the edema resulting from it may produce a further rise in intracranial pressure.

A SUMMARY OF THE ROLE OF IRRADIATION IN BREAST CARCINOMA

The radiotherapist is an essential member of the team dealing with breast carcinoma, and should examine all new patients and be a party to all decisions made regarding choice of treatment. My colleagues and I, working together in the breast clinics in our institution, have reached the following conclusions regarding the place of irradiation in the treatment of breast carcinoma.

1. Patients whose disease is classified as Clinical Stage C or D, as well as the occasional patients whose disease is classified as Clinical Stage A or B but who are shown by preliminary biopsy to have metastases in the nodes at the apex of the axilla, should be treated exclusively by irradiation.

2. Preoperative prophylactic irradiation has no place in our plan of therapy.

3. Postoperative prophylactic irradiation to the internal mammary area only will be given to all patients except those whose primary carcinoma is in the outer half of the breast and measures less than 3 cm. in diameter. The internal mammary area will of course be irradiated postoperatively in all patients who are found to have axillary metastases.

In patients in whom eight or more axillary nodes are found to be involved, postoperative prophylactic irradiation will also be given to the supraclavicular and axillary regions, and to the operative field on the chest wall. We appreciate the fact, established by the Christie Hospital random experiment, that in this group of patients the prophylactic irradiation will probably not prolong survival, but it spares these patients, who are very likely to get local recurrence, the distress associated with such recurrence.

4. Local recurrence, when it does develop, is always treated by irradiation.

5. Metastases to bones are treated initially by irradiation provided they are not so widespread that it is impossible to encompass them. Hormonal methods of control are used when irradiation has failed, or is inapplicable.

REFERENCES

Anschütz, W., and Hellmann, J.: Ueber die Erfolge der Nachbestrahlung radikal operierter Mammakarzinome. Deutsche Ztschr. f. Chir., 197:47, 1926.

Archambault, M., Griem, M. L., and Lochman, D. J.: Results of ultrafractionation radiation therapy in breast carcinoma. Am. J. Roentgenol., 91:62, 1964.

Bachman, A. L., and Macken, K.: Pleural effusions following supervoltage radiation for breast carcinoma. Radiology, 72:699, 1959.

Baclesse, F.: Le pronostic éloigné des cancers du sein (stades II, III, IV, a l'exclusion du stade I) traités par roentgentherapie seule d'après le siège de la lésion primaire. Bull. Assoc. franç. p. l'étude du cancer, 46:594, 1959.

Baclesse, F.: Roentgentherapy alone in the cancer of the breast. Internat. Union against Cancer, 15:1023, 1959.

Baclesse, F.: Les irradiations préopératoires à dose élevée et fractionée dans le traitement du cancer du sein. J. de radiol., et d'électrol., 43:826, 1962.

Baclesse, F.: Hyperfractionation. Am. J. Roentgenol., 91:32, 1964.

Baclesse, F.: Conventional radiation vs. cobalt-60 therapy. J.A.M.A., 200:613, 1967.

Baclesse, F.: Personal communication, 1968.

Baclesse, F., Ennuyer, A., and Cheguillaume, J.: Est-on autorisé à pratiquer une tumorectomie simple, suivie de radiothérapie en cas de tumeur mammaire? J. de radiol. et d'électrol., 41:137, 1960.

Bate, D., and Guttmann, R. J.: Changes in lung and pleura following two-million-volt therapy for carcinoma of the breast. Radiology, 69:372, 1957.

Baudisch, E.: Beitrag zu den Strahlenschaden der Rippen und Schlusselbeine bei Brustkrebs-Patienten. Strahlentherapie, 113:312, 1960.

Beach, A.: The effects of roentgen-ray dosage in breast carcinoma. Am. J. Roentgenol., 46:89, 1941.

Berven, E.: Treatment and results in cancer of the breast. Am. J. Roentgenol., 62:320, 1949.

Botsford, T. W.: Experiences with radioactive colloidal gold in the treatment of pleural effusion caused by metastatic cancer of the breast. Tr. New England S. Soc., 44:106, 1964.

Bouchard, J.: Skeletal metastases in cancer of the breast; study of character, incidence and response to roentgen therapy. Am. J. Roentgenol., 54:156, 1945.

Burch, H. A.: Osseous metastases from graded cancers of the breast, with particular reference to roentgen treatment. Am. J. Roentgenol., 52:1, 1954.

Butcher, H. R., Jr., Seaman, W. B., Eckert, C., and Saltzstein, S.: An assessment of radical mastectomy and postoperative irradiation therapy in the treatment of mammary cancer. Cancer, 17:480, 1964.

Chu, F. C. H., et al.: Electron beam therapy of cancer of the breast. Radiology, 89:216, 1967.

Chu, F. C. H., Phillips, R., Nickson, J. J., and McPhee, J. G.: Pneumonitis following radiation therapy of cancer of the breast by tangential technic. Radiology, 64:642, 1955.

Cole, M. P.: The value of post-operative radiotherapy in the management of breast cancer. Internat. Union against Cancer, 18:976, 1962.

Cram, R. W., Weder, C., and Watson, T. A.: Tolerance of skin grafts to radiation; a study of post-mastectomy irradiated grafts. Ann. Surg., 149:65, 1959.

Delarue, N. C., Ash, C. L., Peters, V., and Fielden, R.: Preoperative irradiation in management of locally advanced breast cancer. Arch. Surg., 91:136, 1965.

Deucher, W. G.: Results of roentgen therapy for metastatic neoplasms. Am. J. Roentgenol., 50:197, 1943.

Easson, E. C.: Post-operative radiotherapy in breast cancer. In Forrest, A. P. M. and Kunkler, P. B.: Prognostic Factors in Breast Cancer. Baltimore, Williams and Wilkins Co., 1968, p. 118.

Fleming, J. A. C., Filbee, J. F., and Wiernik, G.: Sequelae to radical irradiation in carcinoma of the breast. An inquiry into the incidence of certain radiation injuries. Brit. J. Radiol., 34:713, 1961.

Fletcher, G. H.: Textbook of Radiotherapy. Philadelphia, Lea and Febiger, 1966.

Fletcher, G. H.: The advantages of preoperative irradiation. J.A.M.A., 200:140, 1967.

Fletcher, G. H., Montague, E. D., and White, E. C.: Evaluation of irradiation of the peripheral lymphatics in conjunction with radical mastectomy for cancer of the breast. Cancer, 21:791, 1968.

Freid, J. R., and Goldberg, H.: Treatment of metastases from cancer of the breast. Am. J. Roentgenol., 63:312, 1950.

Garland, L. H., Baker, M., Picard, W. H., and Sisson, M. A.: Roentgen and steroid hormone therapy in mammary cancer metastatic to bone. J.A.M.A., 144:997, 1950.

Greenberg, H. B., and Jacobs, S.: Incidence of radiation fibrosis after use of a standardized technique of radiotherapy for breast cancer. Cancer, 19:1289, 1966.

Greenough, R. B.: Treatment of malignant diseases with radium and x-ray. Report No. 3. Cancer of the breast. Surg., Gynec. & Obst., 49:253, 1929.

Griscom, N. I., and Wang, C. C.: Radiation therapy of inoperable breast carcinoma. Radiology, 79:18, 1962.

Guttmann, R. J.: The treatment of inoperable carcinoma of the breast with conventional 250-kv irradiation as compared with 2-mv irradiation. Radiology, 67:497, 1956.

Guttmann, R. J.: Radiotherapy in the treatment of primary operable carcinoma of the breast with proved lymph node metastases. Am. J. Roentgenol., 89:58, 1963.

Guttmann, R. J.: Role of supervoltage irradiation of regional lymph node bearing areas in breast cancer. Am. J. Roentgenol., 96:560, 1966.

Guttmann, R. J.: Radiotherapy in locally advanced cancer of the breast. Cancer, 20:1046, 1967.

Guttmann, R. J.: Personal communication, 1970.

Haagensen, C. D., et al.: Treatment of early mammary carcinoma: A cooperative international study. Ann. Surg., 170:875, 1969.

Hamperl, V. H., Huhn, F. O., Kaufman, C., and Ober, K.-G.: Histologische Untersuchungen präoperativ bestrahlter Mammakarzinome. Deutsche med. Wchnschr., 88:616, 1963.

Hansen, P. B., and Haug, A.: Treatment of pleural and peritoneal carcinomatous effusions with radioactive gold. (1956-1959). Acta radiol., 53:321, 1960.

Harrington, S. W.: Unilateral carcinoma of the breast treated by surgical operation and radiation. Surg., Gynec. & Obst., 60:499, 1935.

Hintze, A.: Unsere Fortschritte bei der Behandlung des Brustkrebses durch Nachbestrahlung. Strahlentherapie, 41:601, 1931.

Hochman, A., and Robinson, E.: Eighty-two cases of mammary cancer treated exclusively with roentgen therapy. Cancer, 13:670, 1960.

Jones, A., and Wedgwood, J.: Effects of radiations on the heart. Brit. J. Radiol., 33:138, 1960.

Karras, B. G., and Moss, W. T.: Radioactive gold in the control of malignant serous effusions. Quart. Bull., Northwestern Univ. M. School, 36:57, 1962.

Kikuchi, A., et al.: Five cases of rib fractures following postoperative roentgen treatment of the breast cancer. Nippon Acta Radiol., 23:264, 1963.

Lambrethsen, E., and Sell, A.: Palliative treatment of carcinomatous effusions in the pleural and peritoneal cavities with radioactive gold. Acta radiol., 56:33, 1961.

Leddy, E. T.: Roentgen treatment of metastases to vertebrae and bones of pelvis from carcinoma of the breast. Am. J. Roentgenol., 24:657, 1930.

Lenz, M.: Tumor dosage and results in roentgen therapy of cancer of the breast. Am. J. Roentgenol., 56:67, 1946.

Lenz, M.: Tissue dosage in roentgenotherapy of mammary cancer. Acta Radiol., 28:583, 1947.

Lenz, M.: Radiocurability of cancer. Am. J. Roentgenol., 67:428, 1952.

Lenz, M.: Radiotherapy of mammary cancer. In Progress in Radiation Therapy. New York, Grune and Stratton, 1965, p. 118.

Lewison, E. F., and Smith, R. I.: Results of breast cancer treatment at Johns Hopkins Hospital, 1946–1950. Surgery, 53:644, 1963.

Lindgren, M., Borgstrom, S., and Landberg, T.: Pre-operative radiotherapy in operable breast cancer. *In* Forrest, A. P. M., and Kunkler, P. B.: Prognostic Factors in Breast Cancer. Baltimore, Williams and Wilkins, 1968, p. 103.

Lougheed, M. N., and Maguire, G. H.: Irradiation pneumonitis in the treatment of carcinoma of the breast. J. Canad. Assoc. Radiol., *11*:1, 1960.

Lumb, G.: Changes in carcinoma of the breast following irradiation. Brit. J. Surg., *38*:82, 1950.

McIntosh, H. C.: Changes in the lungs and pleura following roentgen treatment of cancer of the breast by prolonged fractional method. Radiology, *23*:558, 1934.

McWhirter, R.: Cancer of the breast. Am. J. Roentgenol., *62*:335, 1949.

McWhirter, R.: Should more radical treatment be attempted in breast cancer? Am. J. Roentgenol., *92*:3, 1964.

McWhirter, R.: Cancer of the breast. J. de Radiol., *48*:768, 1967.

Miller, M. W., and Pendergrass, E. P.: Some observations concerned with carcinoma of the breast; part I. Am. J. Roentgenol., *72*:263, 1954.

Miller, M. W., and Pendergrass, E. P.: Some observations concerned with carcinoma of the breast; part 2. Am. J. Roentgenol., *72*:462, 1954.

Nielsen, J.: Carcinoma of the Breast, Copenhagen, Official Tr. Northern Surg., A., 1951, p. 211.

Nohrman, B. A.: Cancer of the Breast; a clinical study of 1042 cases treated at the Radiumhemmet, 1936–41. Acta Radiol. Supp. 77, 1949.

O'Neill, A., Cunningham, R. M., and Cudkowicz, L.: The effects of mediastinal irradiation upon respiratory function in patients with mastectomy for carcinoma of the breast. Canad. M. A. J., *90*:484, 1964.

Papillon, J., et al.: Résultats du traitement du cancer du sein par l'association tumorectomie-radiothérapie à doses élevées. Semaine d. hôp. Paris, Ann. de radiol., *5*:485, 1962.

Peters, M. V.: Wedge resection and irradiation. J.A.M.A., *200*:134, 1967.

Robbins, G. F., et al.: An evaluation of postoperative prophylactic radiation therapy in breast cancer. Surg., Gynec. & Obst., *122*:979, 1966.

Ross, W. M.: Radiotherapeutic and radiological aspects of radiation fibrosis of the lungs. Thorax, *11*:241, 1956.

Rouquès, L.: Les épanchements pleuraux chez les malades atteintes de cancer du sein et traitées par les irradiations sous très haut voltage. Presse Méd., *67*:1614, 1959.

Rubin, E., et al.: Radiation-induced cardiac fibrosis, Am. J. Med., *34*:71, 1963.

Smith, J. C.: Radiation pneumonitis. Am. Rev. Resp. Dis., *87*:647, 1963.

Tapley, N. D., and Fletcher, G. H.: Patterns of use of 6-18 MEV electron beam radiation therapy. Am. J. Roentgenol., *99*:924, 1967.

Veronesi, U., and Zingo, L.: Extended mastectomy for cancer of the breast. Cancer, *20*.677, 1967.

Whitfield, A. G. W., and Kunkler, P. B.: Radiation reactions in the heart. Brit. Heart J., *19*:53, 1957.

Williams, I. G., and Cunningham, G. J.: Histological changes in irradiated carcinoma of the breast. Brit. J. Radiol., *24*:123, 1951.

Chapter Thirty-Six

The Hormonal Treatment of Mammary Carcinoma

Hormonal treatment is an important weapon against breast cancer. Even though it is only palliative it adds to the quality, as well as the length, of life of those in whom surgery and irradiation have failed. Since most hormonal methods penalize the patient to some degree, they should not be given in conjunction with surgery or irradiation; the superiority of combined treatment of this kind has not been proved. Hormonal treatment should be given only to those whose disease is incurable by surgery, and to those in whom irradiation has either failed or cannot be used because the disease is too widespread.

Whatever I write today about hormonal treatment will be somewhat out of date tomorrow because of the rapid evolution of knowledge in this special field of investigation. Treatment has so far been empirical and is based either upon the administration of some one of the various estrogenic or androgenic hormones, upon the suppression of ovarian, adrenal, or pituitary function by irradiation, or upon the destruction or removal of these glands. This therapy cannot in any way be regarded as scientific in the sense that it is dependent upon an understanding of the relationship of the origin and growth of mammary carcinoma to any of these hormones.

All that I shall attempt to do in the present chapter is to present a review of what has been achieved by these various hormonal methods of treatment, and to state our plan for the hormonal treatment of carcinoma of the breast.

The effects of hormonal treatment have been discussed in many individual reports, some of which I will refer to. Two cooperative American study groups have made important contributions. The first was the Therapeutic Trials Committee of the Council on Pharmacy and Chemistry of the American Medical Association, organized in 1947. In 1960, a re-analysis of the data collected by the committee concerning the treatment of 1983 patients was presented by Edwards. His report contains much useful information. More recently, the Cooperative Breast Cancer Group sponsored by the National Institutes of Health has reported extensive studies of hormonal methods of treating breast carcinoma.

HORMONE ADMINISTRATION

In 1939 Ulrich reported that testosterone had favorably influenced breast carcinoma in two patients. By 1946 Adair and Herrmann were able to document its value in 11 patients.

Haddow and his associates reported in 1944 that estrogen also had a favorable effect upon advanced breast carcinoma.

Androgen

Testosterone propionate was the original androgen widely used in the palliation of advanced breast carcinoma. In 580 patients treated with it and reported by the American Medical Association committee in 1960, the rate of objective regression was 21.4 per cent. In 564 such cases reported by the Cooperative Breast Cancer Group in 1964 the regression rate was 21 per cent. Subjective benefits of testosterone are relief of pain, a feeling of well-being, and a gain in weight.

The chief unfavorable effect is virilization, manifested by hoarseness, hirsutism, acne, the development of a ruddy complexion, and increased libido.

The degree of masculinization increases over a period of months as the treatment is continued. In a sensitive feminine woman it is sometimes so distressing that she finally refuses to continue taking the hormone, even though it has relieved her pain. To such a patient the treatment is worse than the disease. I am entirely in sympathy with this point of view and I am glad to note that Gordan agrees with me.

The masculinization that testosterone propionate produces is so unpleasant that this hormone should never be given prophylactically, as some have suggested.

Estrogen

Stilbestrol has been the estrogen most widely used. The side effects are less distressing than those of testosterone, but they can occasionally be severe. The usual dose is 15 mg. daily. If the full dose is given to begin with, anorexia, nausea, and vomiting are common; but if a lesser dose is given at first, tolerance is acquired after a week or two. The deep pigmentation of the nipple and areola is the most obvious outward sign that a full estrogen effect has been obtained. The breasts may become somewhat engorged. Uterine bleeding is the most troublesome phenomenon produced by estrogen. It is usually easily controlled by stopping the estrogen temporarily and then continuing with a smaller dosage.

While hypercalcemia may develop in any patient with extensive bone metastases, this complication is sometimes precipitated by the administration of estrogen. It can be very serious and lead to anuria and death unless recognized and treated promptly. The administration of estrogen as a provocative test of estrogen dependence is dangerous and should be condemned.

The objective regression rate for 364 patients treated by estrogen reported by the Therapeutic Trials Committee of the American Medical Association in 1960 was 36.8 per cent. One of the most extensive individual studies of the efficacy of estrogen administration was that reported by Douglas in 1952. She treated 322 patients. Her results, shown in Table 36-1, illustrate the fact that the effects of estrogen upon carcinoma of the breast are closely correlated with the age of the patient; the older the patient, the better the palliative effect. This same age relationship was apparent in the American Medical Association committee's (1960) data.

The objective regression rate for 283 patients treated by stilbestrol reported in 1964 by the Cooperative Breast Cancer Group was 18 per cent.

The efficacy of testosterone propionate and stilbestrol have been compared by the American Medical Association committee (1960) and also by the Cooperative Breast Cancer Group (1964). The objective regression rates for the two hormones were similar, and increased with the patient's age. Both testosterone propionate and stilbestrol gave a somewhat higher regression rate for local breast and lymph node disease. The poorest results were in patients with visceral lesions. In the American Medical Association committee's 1960 study, the estrogen-treated patients in whom regression occurred lived significantly longer than the corresponding group treated with androgen—the average times of survival being 27 and 20 months, respectively. Those who did not respond to androgen or to estro-

Table 36-1. RESULTS FOLLOWING TREATMENT WITH STILBESTROL DIPROPIONATE — DOUGLAS — 1952

Response	No. of Cases	Average Survival Time (Months)	Average Age (Years)	Per cent Premeno-pausal
Good	33	30.5	66.3	0
Fair	65	19.9	62.9	9.2
None	183	9.1	57.9	17.5
Adverse	33	6.3	54.7	33.3
Withdrawal	8	27.3	58.1	12.5

gen survived almost the same length of time — 10 and 11 months, respectively.

New Hormones Related to Androgen and Estrogen

A whole new series of hormones related to androgens and estrogens have been tested by the Cooperative Breast Cancer Group during recent years. Several new androgens are clearly better than testosterone propionate because they penalize the patients less. Some compounds may give higher regression rates than any previously known hormones. I will review the most promising.

1. Fluoxymesterone (Halotestin, Upjohn), developed in 1958, is effective when given by mouth, and has little masculinizing effect. It has enjoyed great popularity, but Lowe and his associates found the objective regression rate obtained with it to be only 13 per cent. The Cooperative Breast Cancer Group (1964) reported that fluoxymesterone gave only 15 per cent of objective remissions. The response of breast, osseous, and visceral lesions was similar.

2. 1-Delta Testolactone (Teslac, Squibb), developed in 1953, is a compound that has neither androgenic or estrogenic effects, and can be given by mouth or intramuscularly. It is nontoxic, even when given in massive doses (Cantino and Gordan). Bisel reported an objective regression rate of 20 per cent, approximately the same as for testosterone propionate. The regression rate for osseous metastases was slightly better than for breast and visceral lesions.

3. 2-Alpha Methyldihydrotestosterone Propionate (Drolban, Lilly) is an androgen which is much less masculinizing than testosterone propionate. It is given intramuscularly.

The objective regression rate achieved with this hormone in studies conducted by Thomas et al., by Goldenberg and Hayes, and by Blackburn, was 25.5 per cent — approximately the same as the regression rate for testosterone propionate.

4. 7-Beta, 17-Alpha Dimethyltestosterone. Gordan has recently made a preliminary report of his results with this new non-virilizing, nontoxic compound. In a series of 15 patients with advanced breast carcinoma who had not responded to the administration of other hormones, objective regression occurred in 14. In five patients, soft tissue lesions regressed; in ten, bone metastases regressed; and in two, pulmonary lesions regressed.

Progesterone

A third group of steroid sex hormones, the progestins, have also been used in advanced breast carcinoma. In 1951, Taylor and Morris as well as Gordan and his associates treated small series of patients with progesterone. The results were not impressive.

In 1965, Crowley and Macdonald reported better results when they combined estrogen with 17-Alpha hydroxyprogesterone caproate (Delantin). Objective regression occurred in six of 27 patients, all of whom had been refractory to previous treatment with estrogen.

The progestins have nevertheless found little favor in treating advanced breast carcinoma.

Corticosteroids

The corticosteroids have been widely used for advanced breast cancer and have produced striking palliation. The mechanism of their action is presumably the suppression of estrogen production by the adrenals, as indicated by adrenal atrophy (Jantet et al.) and by decrease in urinary estrogenic metabolites (Smith and Emerson), in postmenopausal women following treatment with corticosteroids.

The earlier efforts to palliate breast carcinoma with cortisone were not encouraging, but when more potent corticoid derivatives such as prednisone became available the usefulness of this method of adrenal suppression in postmenopausal patients became evident. Lemon deserves credit for emphasizing the value of prednisone. In his 1959 report he described objective benefit in 48 per cent of his series of 31 patients treated with it.

Gardner, Thomas, and Gordan in 1962 obtained objective remission in 24 per cent of a series of 46 postmenopausal patients treated with prednisone. Regressions were more frequent in older women, but the presence of ovaries did not reduce the chance of regression.

The most extensive series of patients treated with corticosteroids has been reported by Moore and his associates. In a total of 223 patients treated for recurrent breast carcinoma a positive response was obtained in from 41 to 57 per cent.

Moore has emphasized that, unlike some other hormones, corticosteroids can be given without fear of stimulating breast carcinoma. Hypercalcemia, a very real hazard with estrogen and androgen therapy, does not occur with prednisone. Indeed, prednisone is of great value in the treatment of hypercalcemia. It is also the best hormonal treatment for brain metastases.

Prednisone does, however, produce bothersome complications. It regularly induces some degree of Cushing's syndrome, of which fullness of the face is the most obvious sign. Gain in body weight and edema of the lower extremities are common. Exacerbation of latent diabetes and duodenal ulcer are less frequent complications.

A great advantage of prednisone is that the patient very quickly feels better, even though her disease is not objectively checked. Her appetite is improved, and she often regains her long-lost feeling of well-being.

Large doses of prednisone are not required. Thirty milligrams daily are usually adequate.

It has been emphasized by several authors that the remissions produced by prednisone are shorter than those obtained with other hormonal methods. Moore states that the usual duration of remission is 6 months. My own impression is that it is often longer. We have had a few patients in whom remission lasted several years. The following case history is an example:

Miss T. G., aged 44, came to the Francis Delafield Hospital in April, 1955, with a 4 cm., well delimited, movable tumor of the left breast. Her only sister had a breast carcinoma. Biopsy revealed the tumor to be a simple cyst.

Seven years later, in January 1962, when she was 51, she was found to have a firm 4 cm. tumor of the upper outer sector of her right breast. There was a 1.5 cm. clinically involved axillary node. Biopsy of the breast tumor showed it to be a carcinoma, and biopsy of the apex of the axilla revealed metastases in one of seven subclavicular nodes. Her disease was therefore classified as inoperable and she was treated with irradiation alone.

One year after the completion of her irradiation her breast tumor was obviously growing, and measured 10 cm. in diameter. Bilateral oophorectomy was done in March, 1963.

Three months later, in June, 1963, her disease was clearly progressing. She was put on prednisone, 30 mg. daily. She had a remarkable regression of her supraclavicular, axillary, and chest wall disease. Seven years later, in June, 1970, her carcinoma was still controlled by the prednisone.

Rebound Regression

One of the basic facts of hormone administration is that the objective regression rates for a number of androgens and estrogens are similar. This suggests that it is not a specific hormonal effect which produces the regression, but rather the abrupt change in the patient's hormonal physiology. If this is true, merely stopping the administration of an androgen or estrogen which has been given for a long time might be expected to produce a new regression. This kind of rebound regression has occasionally been observed. Kaufman and Escher have described it well. In their series of 674 patients to whom hormones had been administered, rebound regression occurred in 3.5 per cent of those who had been treated with androgen and in 9 per cent of those who had been given estrogen. The mean duration of the rebound regression for both groups was 9 to 10 months. The mean survival time following rebound regression was approximately 25 months in both groups.

OOPHORECTOMY AND OVARIAN IRRADIATION FOR BREAST CARCINOMA

The fact that the ovaries influence mammary physiology in both animals and human beings led Beatson to remove the ovaries in women with breast cancer in 1896. He obtained striking palliation with the operation in a few cases. The procedure was taken up by several English surgeons, and during the following decade they did about a hundred of these operations. Lett, in 1905, reported that temporary improvement was observed in about one third of the cases. But contemporary surgeons were not impressed by these results, and the operation lost favor.

A few among the next generation of surgeons continued to perform prophylactic oophorectomy, and reports of its results in small series of cases began to appear (Raven, Horsley and Horsley, Miller and Pendergrass, Smith and Smith). These studies did not, however, answer the question of the value of prophylactic oophorectomy. The numbers of cases were too small, and the data did not always include such basic information as the age of the patients and the clinical stage of advancement of their carcinomas. Only 5 year survival rates were reported.

In the 1920's, radiotherapists introduced suppression of ovarian function by irradiation. This added a new impetus to the study of the role of the ovaries in breast carcinoma. Taylor reported that in a series of 47 younger patients with carcinoma of the breast given prophylactic ovarian irradiation there was no demonstrable benefit. He concluded, however, that artificial menopause induced by irradiation in patients with inoperable and recurrent carcinoma of the breast had a definite palliative effect in about one third. The most striking benefit was observed in patients with bone metastases. Ahlbom was not able to prove that ovarian irradiation given therapeutically to 163 patients with recurrent or metastatic mammary carcinoma had any definite favorable effect. Miller and Pendergrass reported their results in 71 patients who had therapeutic ovarian radiation. They were not able to show that life was prolonged for these irradiated patients in comparison with patients in their series whose ovaries were not treated. Douglas, however, reported that in a series of 175 patients given ovarian irradiation therapeutically, a good response was obtained in 9.7 per cent and a fair response in 10.9 per cent. Most of the patients who were benefited were premenopausal.

It is apparent that irradiation given to the ovaries does not entirely suppress estrogen formation in them. Evidence to this effect in terms of a smaller rise in urinary gonadotrophin, and a smaller decrease in urinary estrogens, following irradiation of the ovaries as compared with surgical castration, was presented by Nathanson, Rice, and Meigs.

Another type of evidence concerning the relationship of ovarian function to breast carcinoma comes from pathological study of ovaries removed therapeutically from patients with breast cancer and ovaries removed at autopsy of patients dying of breast carcinoma. Sommers and Teloh reported that a large majority of the ovaries from such patients showed hyperplasia of the cortical ovarian stroma. They found no difference in the length of life in autopsied patients whose ovaries showed cortical hyperplasia as compared with the length of life in patients whose ovaries were atrophic. Studying the length of life, however, in patients whose ovaries were removed therapeutically, they reported that the mean duration of life was 47 months for those with ovarian stroma hyperplasia and only 27 months for those with atrophic ovaries. But the number of cases in their series was so small that these

differences were not statistically significant. Moreover, they did not state the ages of their patients, data which are certainly of basic importance. In a more recent study of the significance of ovarian cortical stroma hyperplasia, Osborne and Pitts found no difference in the length of survival of patients whose ovaries showed this phenomenon.

With the general recognition of the importance of all hormonal methods of treating breast carcinoma which has come about during the last 20 years, there has been wide acceptance of the fact that ovarian function influences the natural history of the disease. Although proof of the value of prophylactic oophorectomy and irradiation suppression of ovarian function has been lacking, these procedures have been very widely done. It is high time that their usefulness should be critically reviewed. In considering their value it is essential to distinguish the results of prophylactic oophorectomy or ovarian irradiation done in conjunction with radical mastectomy, from the therapeutic ovarian procedures done for inoperable or recurrent disease.

Fortunately, several studies have recently appeared which provide much more comprehensive information concerning these questions. The most interesting of these reports are listed in Table 36–2.

Siegert compared the recurrence-free period in 347 premenopausal patients given prophylactic postoperative ovarian irradiation, with the recurrence-free period in 260 patients who were not irradiated. The recurrence-free period was 16 months longer in the irradiated group. Very few details of this study are included in the report—for example, the clinical stage of advancement of the disease in the two groups of patients is lacking.

McWhirter gave prophylactic ovarian irradiation to a series of 275 patients with breast carcinoma whose disease was Stage I or II in terms of the Manchester Clinical Classification, and who were treated by his method of simple mastectomy and irradiation to the chest wall and regional lymph node areas. The five year survival rate for these patients was identical with the survival rate for a series of 493 patients who did not get prophylactic ovarian irradiation.

Rosenberg and Uhlmann reported that the five year survival rate in a total of 78 patients in whom prophylactic castration was done following radical mastectomy was 59 per cent. In a control series of 122 patients in whom no ovarian treatment was given, the

Table 36–2. RECENT REPORTS OF RESULTS OF OOPHORECTOMY AND OF OVARIAN IRRADIATION FOR BREAST CARCINOMA

Author	Year	Prophy-lactic	Procedure	No. of Patients	No. of Controls	Thera-peutic	Procedure	No. of Patients
Siegert	1952	+	Ovarian irradiation	347	260	—	—	—
McWhirter	1956	+	Ovarian irradiation	275	493	—	—	—
Rosenberg and Uhlmann	1959	+	Oophorectomy,	12		—	—	—
			Ovarian irradiation	66	122			
Horsley and Horsley	1962	+	Oophorectomy	72	None	—	—	—
Taylor	1962	—	—	—	—	+	Oophorectomy	409
Kennedy et al.	1964	+	Oophorectomy,	34		+	Oophorectomy,	54
			Ovarian irradiation	85			Ovarian irradiation	123
Fracchia et al.	1969	+	Oophorectomy	100	—	+	Oophorectomy	101
Nissen-Meyer	1965	+	Oophorectomy,	74	255	—	—	—
			Ovarian irradiation	590				
Fracchia et al.	1969	—	—	—	—	+	Oophorectomy,	466
							Ovarian irradiation	61
Cole	1968	+	Ovarian irradiation	369	375	—	—	—

five year survival rate was 36 per cent. This study has two defects—no clinical staging, and a follow-up period of only five years.

The Horsleys reported their results with prophylactic oophorectomy following radical mastectomy in a total of 72 women between the ages of 28 and 54. There was no clinical staging, and only 27 patients had been followed for 10 years.

Taylor summarized the data regarding the results of oophorectomy in a total of 381 premenopausal and 28 postmenopausal patients with disseminated mammary carcinoma. These data had been collected by a Joint Committee of the American College of Physicians and the American College of Surgeons. Regression occurred in only 16.3 per cent of the patients 34 years or younger, while it occurred in 31.6 per cent of the patients between 35 years and up to one year after the menopause. Regression occurred in only one of 28 patients more than one year past the menopause.

There were several other basic lessons concerning oophorectomy derived from Taylor's data. The longer the "free interval" following the primary treatment, the higher the incidence of regression resulting from oophorectomy for recurrent disease. Soft tissue, pleural, and skeletal metastases responded best—approximately 39 per cent. Only 22.6 per cent of visceral metastases responded. The average survival after oophorectomy in all responders was 31.2 months.

Kennedy and his associates were the first to compare the efficacy of prophylactic suppression of ovarian function with that of therapeutic suppression of ovarian function. There were 119 patients in the prophylactic group and 177 patients in the therapeutic group. Almost all were premenopausal. Unfortunately, the two groups were not strictly comparable, the disease being more advanced in the therapeutic group. The authors conclude that the total survival time from initial breast cancer therapy to death was not significantly different in the prophylactic and therapeutic groups.

Fracchia and his associates also compared the results of prophylactic oophorectomy with those obtained by therapeutic oophorectomy done for recurrent disease. They chose to make this comparison in a selected group of premenopausal patients who had all been treated initially by radical mastectomy, and who had all died of their disease. Since the initial surgery had failed in all, it was to some degree eliminated as a disturbing factor in the comparison of results. It is obvious, however, that differences in the initial stage of advancement of the disease in the prophylactic group as compared with the therapeutic group might have influenced the results. This factor could have been eliminated by selecting groups of patients in whom the clinical stage of advancement was the same, but Fracchia and his associates did not stage their patients.

They found that the overall survival time in the two series was not significantly different—it was 43.8 months for the prophylactic series and 48 months for the therapeutic series. They therefore favor waiting and performing oophorectomy therapeutically when it is indicated for recurrence in premenopausal patients.

Nissen-Meyer described a prospective randomized study of prophylactic suppression of ovarian function in a large number of patients. In 590 ovarian irradiation was given and in 74 oophorectomy was done. Both premenopausal and postmenopausal patients were included. A series of 255 patients treated initially by operation alone was used as a control group. His patients were not staged clinically.

Nissen-Meyer expressed his results in a series of graphs showing five year free of disease rates as well as survival rates. He calculated that patients in whom prophylactic sterilization was done had an increased recurrence free time of about one year and survived about one year longer. He recommended prophylactic ovarian irradiation for all patients with breast carcinoma between the ages of 45 and 70, and for all patients under 45 who have axillary metastases.

Fracchia and his associates reported the results of therapeutic oophorectomy and ovarian irradiation in a total of 527 patients who had primary inoperable or recurrent breast carcinoma. Four hundred and forty-three were premenopausal. Ovarian metastases were found in 24.2 per cent of the patients in whom oophorectomy was done.

Objective regression or arrest of the disease of at least six months' duration occurred in 27 per cent of the premenopausal patients. Three of the 42 patients who had had their menopause within one year had objective regression, but none of the 43 patients who were more than one year postmenopausal responded.

Lesions of the breast, skin, lymph nodes, and other soft tissue responded best. Bone and lung metastases responded almost as well. Liver metastases responded poorly, and brain metastases did not respond at all.

The duration of remission in the premenopausal patients was 6 months—31.6 per cent, 12 months—24.4 per cent, 18 months—16.7 per cent, and 24 months—10.4 per cent. Seventeen patients had remissions that lasted five years or more, and two were still in remission after 10 years.

Much the most interesting study of the value of postoperative prophylactic suppression of ovarian function was begun at the Christie Hospital in Manchester in 1948. All patients who were premenopausal or within two years of the menopause were included in the study. They were allocated in two groups by their dates of birth. In one group, prophylactic ovarian irradiation was given. The other group served as a control. Cole has recently reported the 10 year results in the two groups. The crude 10 year survival rate for the irradiated group was 46.6 per cent; for the control group it was 41.6 per cent. The increased survival in the irradiated group was greater in the patients who did not have axillary metastases; in them it was statistically significant.

Although Cole concludes that the crude survival time can be somewhat increased by prophylactic ovarian irradiation, she points out that the difference in survival between irradiated and control groups can be narrowed by the use of other modern hormonal procedures.

Cole also reports interesting findings regarding the effect of prophylactic ovarian irradiation upon recurrence. The incidence of local recurrence in the breast area and in regional lymph node areas at 10 years was reduced: it was 23.9 per cent in the irradiated group as compared with 29.7 per cent in the control group. The frequency of distant metastases at 10 years was also less in the irradiated group—46.1 per cent as compared with 54.5 per cent in the control group.

ADRENALECTOMY

Bilateral total adrenalectomy for advanced, disseminated carcinoma was first employed by Huggins and Scott for prostatic cancer patients in 1945. The surgical procedure, as well as postoperative maintenance of their early patients, was very difficult, because the patients were operated upon before the advent of cortisone therapy and, with it, easy substitution therapy. In 1951 Huggins and Bergenstal described bilateral total adrenalectomy for metastatic breast cancer. In breast carcinoma, as in prostatic carcinoma, the theoretical basis for the operation was the fact of the common embryonic origin of the gonads and adrenal cortex, plus the belief that these are the only structures having the capacity to synthesize endogenous steroid hormonal substances.

By 1957 Dao and Huggins were able to report their results with adrenalectomy in 52 consecutive patients with disseminated mammary carcinoma. Objective remission occurred in 37.5 per cent of the patients treated by adrenalectomy alone and in 44 per cent of those treated by adrenalectomy plus oophorectomy. Seven patients survived longer than 36 months. One patient continued in good health after 12 years.

By 1962, Daicoff, Harmon, and Van Prohaska, Huggins' colleagues at the University of Chicago, were able to report their results in a total of 455 adrenalectomized breast cancer patients and compare the course of the disease in them with the course of the disease in a total of 415 patients who did not have adrenalectomy.

Twenty-eight per cent of the adrenalectomized patients had objective remission of their metastases. The frequency of response was much lower in patients under the age of 40. Brain and liver metastases responded much less often than other types of metastases.

The data concerning survival in Daicoff's two groups of patients suggests that adrenalectomy added appreciably to the length of life. The actual survival times were as follows:

	Patients Adrenal-ectomized	Patients Not Adrenal-ectomized
50 per cent survived:	20 months	8.5 months
25 per cent survived:	36 months	17 months
12.5 per cent survived:	60 months	31 months

The operation was adopted in many clinics in this country and abroad. I will review the larger case series.

Cade championed adrenalectomy in Britain. By 1957 he was able to report his results in 136 patients. Objective improvement occured in 39 per cent. Cade's series of cases included a large proportion of patients with very advanced disease. He presented the details of some of the remarkable examples of regression of disease—including liver metastases—in his series.

Byron and his associates in 1962 evaluated their results in a series of 215 patients who survived six months or more following adrenalectomy. There was objective improvement in 37.7 per cent. There was no significant difference in the results in premenopausal and postmenopausal patients. The frequency of objective improvement was greater in the

Table 36–3. Results of Adrenalectomy and of Hypophysectomy, Macdonald, 1962

	Adrenalectomy	Hypophysectomy
Number of patients	690	340
Per cent patients with inoperable primary lesion	10.6%	10.6%
Mean age at mastectomy	44.6	43.8
Mean free interval (months)	32.8	33.6
Mean interval, metastasis to ablation (months)	15.2	18.8
Per cent objective remission	28.4%	32.6%
Soft tissue metastases	34.6%	31.1%
Bone metastases	37.5%	37.8%
Visceral metastases	16.4%	23.2%
Survival ablation to death in responders (months) Soft tissue and bone metastases	25	21.8
Visceral metastases	22.8	25.2
Mean interval mastectomy to death in responders (months)	79.2	82.9
Mean interval mastectomy to death in nonresponders (months)	52.4	54.6

patients who had had a longer interval free of disease between the original treatment and the development of metastases.

Macdonald, in 1962, summarized the data concerning adrenalectomy and hypophysectomy collected by the Joint Committee of the American College of Physicians and the American College of Surgeons, and compared the results of the two procedures in breast carcinoma.

The basic features of the disease in the two case series were very similar. I have reproduced these data in Table 36–3.

The conclusions from these data are that, when performed for recurrent or inoperable breast carcinoma, adrenalectomy and hypophysectomy have almost identical beneficial results. Objective remission occurs in approximately one third of the patients, and they live from 20 to 25 months longer than those who do not respond. The results of previous therapeutic oophorectomy are an important guide to the probable success of subsequent adrenalectomy or hypophysectomy. Patients who had not responded to oophorectomy had less than a 1 in 3 chance of benefit from adrenalectomy or hypophysectomy, while those who had responded to oophorectomy had an even chance of benefit.

Dao and Nemoto in 1965 reported their results with primary adrenalectomy in 86 patients with advanced breast cancer, and of secondary adrenalectomy in another series of 72 patients who had been receiving androgen therapy. Primary adrenalectomy produced objective remission in 45 per cent, while secondary adrenalectomy gave objective remission in 35 per cent.

Mye and Neal in 1965 described their results with adrenalectomy in 83 patients with advanced mammary carcinoma. Objective improvement occurred in 36 per cent. The average survival in those who responded was 12.2 months. One patient survived 54 months. The longer the interval that the patient was free of disease following her primary treatment, the longer she survived following adrenalectomy. No patient under 40 responded.

Moore and his associates reviewed their results with adrenalectomy in 1967. Objective remission occurred in 51 per cent of their 86 patients.

In 1967 Fracchia and his associates published their results with adrenalectomy in a series of 500 patients with advanced breast carcinoma. Objective improvement lasting six months or longer resulted in 31 per cent of the 245 patients treated by adrenalectomy alone, and in 33.7 per cent of the 255 patients in which the ovaries as well as the adrenals were removed.

There were 75 patients with inflammatory carcinoma in the series. Fracchia and his colleagues report that 34 per cent were "improved" by adrenalectomy.

The patients who had remission following adrenalectomy lived longer than those who did not respond to the operation. The length of the free interval between the primary treatment and the first appearance of metastases correlated closely with the response to adrenalectomy; the longer the free interval the greater the likelihood of remission.

In 1969 Harris and Spratt reported their results in 64 patients treated by adrenalectomy. Thirty-three per cent had objective regression of their disease. Soft tissue and bone lesions responded in 35 per cent, pulmonary lesions in 15 per cent and liver lesions not at all. There were 10 women under 40 in the series and only one of them responded.

HYPOPHYSECTOMY AND OTHER METHODS OF SUPPRESSING THE FUNCTION OF THE HYPOPHYSIS

With the palliative value of the removal of the ovaries and the adrenals in breast cancer firmly established, it was inevitable that attempts to influence the disease by removing or destroying the hypophysis would follow. Luft and Olivecrona began to do transfrontal hypophysectomy for breast carcinoma in 1951, and by 1955 they were able to report their results in 37 patients. Evaluation of the results was possible in 30 patients: 13 "improved markedly."

The operation was taken up in a number of clinics and by 1962 Macdonald was able to present the summary of the results of hypophysectomy in a total of 340 patients which I have referred to above.

Ray has the largest series of transfrontal hypophysectomies. They totalled 630 in 1966. The most recent evaluation of results was published by Ray and Pearson in 1962. Forty-two per cent of those who survived the operation had remission for more than six months. The average duration of remission was more than 17 months. The average survival after hypophysectomy in the group who had remissions was more than 24.5 months. This is about five times the average survival of the patients who did not have remission after hypophysectomy. About 30 per cent of Ray's patients lost their sense of smell, and in 20 per cent diabetes insipidus was a continuing problem.

Ray emphasizes that the best indication as to whether or not hypophysectomy will be of benefit is the response to a previous therapeutic oophorectomy. If oophorectomy produced a remission, a new remission will follow hypophysectomy in 85 per cent of the patients.

Hamberger introduced transantrosphenoidal hypophysectomy in 1961 and obtained results similar to those when the skull is opened in the classical manner. Hamberger's technique is more tedious, and has not achieved much popularity. In our breast clinic at the Columbia-Presbyterian Hospital it has been done with good results by Baker and Bridges.

The destruction of the pituitary by irradiation has been attempted with several different techniques.

Evans and his associates in 1954 began to implant yttrium[90] into the pituitary through a right frontal trephine opening. In eight of 31 patients with breast carcinoma, arrest followed, and lasted 12 months or more. It was soon found that the implantation could be more simply performed via the nasal and sphenoidal route. Yttrium implantation was taken up in Britain by Forrest and his associates, and by Greening and his associates. Juret and his associates at the Institut Gustav Roussy began to use yttrium implantation in 1958, and by 1964 they were able to report their results in 150 patients with advanced breast cancer. Objective regression resulted in 37 per cent. In 84 per cent of the patients who had an initial remission it lasted more than one year.

Scheer and Klar in 1961 reported their results with the transethmoidal implantation of radioactive gold seeds into the pituitary in 387 patients with breast carcinoma. Objective improvement occurred in 23 per cent.

Ray points out that the implantation of yttrium has not given as high a percentage of remission as hypophysectomy, and that rhinorrhea is a frequent complication.

A PLAN FOR HORMONAL THERAPY

In my review of hormonal methods of treatment the wide divergence of opinion regarding many aspects of this form of treatment is obvious. The question is not only which method promises the longest survival. The quality of life during the period of survival is, in my personal opinion, more important than the length of survival. It is unreasonable to prolong life which promises only misery.

Premenopausal Patients

For the premenopausal patient who has had radical mastectomy, there are two reasons why I do not advise prophylactic oophorectomy, even if she is found to have more axillary metastases than I expected.

1. Although I recognize that immediate oophorectomy may reduce the frequency of both local and regional lymph node recurrence, I know that such recurrences can usually be treated effectively with irradiation if and when they develop. The penalty of precipitate menopausal symptoms which prophylactic oophorectomy inflicts on the entire group of patients who have it outweighs the possible gain in recurrence-free time of a few.

2. If prophylactic oophorectomy is performed I will not have the help of the response to therapeutic oophorectomy performed for recurrence in planning subsequent hormone therapy. Many authors have emphasized the value of the response to therapeutic oophorectomy as a guide to subsequent treatment. Hall and his associates studied this question in a series of 282 patients who had had therapeutic oophorectomy. Of those who had responded to oophorectomy 23 per cent had a favorable response to subsequent hormonal treatment. Of those who had not responded to oophorectomy only 7 per cent had a favorable response to subsequent hormonal treatment. Obviously it is not worthwhile performing hypophysectomy or adrenalectomy when only 7 per cent of patients respond.

Returning to my premenopausal patient treated by radical mastectomy alone, who develops recurrence of her carcinoma, I do not at once remove her ovaries. If her recurrent disease is sufficiently limited in extent to be treated by irradiation, I much prefer it. The probability of irradiation controlling local or regional lymph node recurrence, or bone metastases of limited extent, is much greater than the likelihood of control by oophorectomy. When irradiation finally fails I of course advise oophorectomy. And I usually prefer to remove the ovaries rather than to irradiate them, because at this stage of the evolution of my patient's disease I want as prompt a response as possible.

When the remission obtained by therapeutic oophorectomy ends, adrenalectomy or hypophysectomy will achieve a second remission in a considerable proportion of patients. The choice between adrenalectomy and hypophysectomy depends upon the availability of experts in these techniques; the results are very similar. The following case history illustrates the fact that successive long recessions can sometimes be obtained with this sequential ablative hormone therapy.

Mrs. M. P. had a left radical mastectomy when she was 36. There were no metastases in 22 axillary lymph nodes. Three and one-half years later she was found to have generalized osteoblastic skeletal metastases. Oophorectomy was done. Almost all x-ray evidence of these metastases disappeared during the following year.

She was perfectly well for the following 6½ years. A small local recurrence then appeared in the skin just above the upper end of the medial flap of her mastectomy. It was excised for biopsy and the area irradiated.

Twenty months later skeletal films showed reappearance and progression of her generalized bone metastases. They were both osteolytic and osteoblastic. Since she had had such a good response to oophorectomy, transantrosphenoidal hypophysectomy was performed.

Her bone metastases showed no change following hypophysectomy. Her general condition continued to be fairly good during the next 27 months. She then became weaker, began to have epigastric distress, and her abdomen enlarged. She was found to have massive ascites with marked bone marrow depression. Her spleen was greatly enlarged. Despite supportive measures, her condition deteriorated and she is near death 14 years after her radical mastectomy, 10½ years after her oophorectomy, and 3 years and 4 months after her hypophysectomy.

For the premenopausal patient with recurrent disease which does not respond to oophorectomy, I advise one of the non-virilizing androgens. Testolactone, at the moment, appears to be the best one, but I hope that 7-beta, 17-alpha-dimethyltestosterone will prove to be better.

Postmenopausal Patients

When irradiation is no longer useful for recurrence in postmenopausal patients, I do not advise oophorectomy — it is futile in them. Adrenalectomy and hypophysectomy are formidable procedures compared with the administration of hormones. It usually seems reasonable to try this simpler type of hormonal treatment first. From the viewpoint of the usefulness of androgen and estrogen, the postmenopausal patients should be divided into two groups — those less than five years postmenopausal and those more than five years postmenopausal. Careful study of the detailed reports of the Cooperative Breast Cancer Group (1964) shows that the frequency of objective regression in patients less than five years postmenopausal treated with androgen or estrogen was only about 6 per cent. In patients between five and 10 years past the menopause the regression rate rose to 17 per cent, and in patients more than 10 years past the menopause it was 23 per cent.

Age particularly restricts the use of estrogen. We know all too well that in premenopausal patients it sets breast cancer on fire, so to speak. In my own experience I have seen a number of patients in the decade following the menopause in whom the disease was aggravated by estrogen. I am fearful of giving it to patients under the age of 65.

In view of these limitations of androgen and estrogen in the decade following the menopause I have usually advised prednisone. It gives subjective improvement very quickly; and objective remissions are at least as frequent as with androgen or estrogen.

In aged women, estrogen gives the best palliation. I use stilbestrol for all patients beyond the age of 65 who have recurrent disease which is not amenable to irradiation. The dosage needs to be adjusted to individual needs.

There is general agreement that the local disease in the breast and on the chest wall, and in the regional lymph nodes, responds best to hormonal treatment. Bone metastases respond less well. Metastases to the viscera — lungs, intestinal tract, brain, and liver — are the least responsive. Nemoto and Dao have emphasized that all hormonal methods fail in patients with extensive liver involvement.

In considering the length of survival following hormonal treatment it should be kept in mind that the better differentiated and more slowly growing breast carcinomas usually recur later; the free interval between the primary treatment and recurrence is longer. As might be expected, when these late recurring tumors respond to hormonal treatment, the regression lasts longer.

I do not mean to suggest that the plan which I have outlined for the use of hormonal methods can be rigidly followed. I often make exceptions to it. But it provides general guidelines which, experience has convinced me, are sound.

REFERENCES

Adair, F. E., and Herrmann, J. B.: The use of testosterone propionate in the treatment of advanced carcinoma of the breast. Ann. Surg., *123*:1023, 1946.

Adair, F. E., et al.: Use of estrogens and androgens in advanced mammary cancer: Clinical and laboratory study of 105 female patients. J.A.M.A., *140*:1193, 1949.

Ahlbom, H.: Castration by roentgen rays as an auxiliary treatment in the radiotherapy of cancer mammae at Radiumhemmet, Stockholm. Acta radiol., *11*:614, 1930.

A.M.A. Therapeutic Trials Committee: Current status of hormone therapy of advanced mammary cancer. J.A.M.A., *146*:471, 1951.

A.M.A. Therapeutic Trials Committee: Androgens and estrogens in the treatment of disseminated mammary carcinoma — Retrospective study of 944 patients, J.A.M.A., *172*:1271, 1960.

Baker, D. C., Jr., and Bridges, T. J.: Transantrosphenoidal hypophysectomy. Tr. Am. Acad. Ophth., *68*:60, 1964.

Beatson, G. T.: On the treatment of inoperable cases of carcinoma of the mamma; suggestions for a new method of treatment. Lancet, 2:104 and 162, 1896.

Bisel, H. F.: Treatment of advanced breast carcinoma with delta-I testolactone. Internat. Union against Cancer, 20:429, 1964.

Blackburn, C. M.: Use of 2α-methyldihydrotestosterone propionate in treatment of advanced cancer of the breast. Cancer Chemother. Rep., 16:279, 1962.

Boyd, S.: On oöphorectomy in cancer of breast. Brit. M. J., 2:1161, 1900.

Byron, R. L., Jr., et al.: Bilateral adrenalectomy in advanced breast cancer. Surgery, 52:725, 1962.

Cade, S.: The role of adrenalectomy in cancer of the breast. Cancer, 10:777, 1957.

Cantino, T. J., and Gordan, G. S.: High-dosage delta-I testolactone therapy of disseminated carcinoma of the breast. Cancer, 20:458, 1967.

Cole, M. P.: Suppression of ovarian function in primary breast cancer. In Forrest, A. P. M., and Kunkler, P. B.: Prognostic Factors in Breast Cancer. Baltimore, Williams and Wilkins Co., 1968, p. 146.

Cooperative Breast Cancer Group: Testosterone propionate therapy in breast cancer. J.A.M.A., 188:1069, 1964.

Cooperative Breast Cancer Group: Results of Studies of the Cooperative Breast Cancer Group—1961-1963. Suppl. Cancer Chemotherapy Reports, 41:1, 1964.

Crowley, L. G., and Macdonald, I.: Delantin and estrogens for the treatment of advanced mammary carcinoma in postmenopausal women. Cancer, 18:436, 1965.

Daicoff, G. R., Harmon, R., and Van Prohaska, J.: Effect of adrenalectomy on mammary carcinoma. Arch. Surg., 85:800, 1962.

Dao, T. L-Y., and Huggins, C.: Bilateral adrenalectomy in the treatment of cancer of the breast. Arch. Surg., 71:645, 1955.

Dao, T. L-Y., and Huggins, C.: Metastatic cancer of the breast treated by adrenalectomy; evaluation and 5-year results. J.A.M.A., 165:1793, 1957.

Dao, T. L-Y., and Nemoto, T.: An evaluation of adrenalectomy and androgen in disseminated mammary carcinoma. Surg., Gynec. & Obst., 121:1257, 1965.

Douglas, M.: Treatment of advanced breast cancer by hormone therapy. Brit. J. Cancer, 6:32, 1952.

Dragstedt, L. R., Humphreys, E. M., and Dragstedt, L. R., II: Prophylactic bilateral adrenalectomy and oophorectomy for advanced cancer of the breast. Surgery, 47:885, 1960.

Evans, J. P., Fenge, W., Kelly, W. A., and Harper, P. V.: Transcranial yttrium⁹⁰ hypophysectomy. Surg., Gynec. & Obst., 108:393, 1959.

Fairgrieve, J.: Selective criteria for surgical removal of endocrine glands in advanced breast cancer. Surg., Gynec. & Obst., 120:371, 1965.

Forrest, A. P. M., et al.: Radio-active implantation of the pituitary. Brit. J. Surg., 47:61, 1959.

Fracchia, A. A., et al.: The results of adrenalectomy in advanced breast cancer in 500 consecutive patients. Surg., Gynec. & Obst., 125:747, 1967.

Fracchia, A. A., et al.: Castration for primary inoperable or recurrent breast carcinoma. Surg., Gynec. & Obst., 128:1226, 1969.

Fracchia, A. A., Murray, D. R., Farrow, J. H., and Balachandra, V. K.: Comparison of prophylactic and therapeutic castration in breast carcinoma. Surg., Gynec. & Obst., 129:270, 1969.

Gardner, B., Thomas, A. N., and Gordan, G. S.: Antitumor efficacy of prednisone and sodium liothyronine in advanced breast cancer. Cancer, 15:334, 1962.

Gardner, B., et al.: Calcium and phosphate metabolism in patients with disseminated breast cancer; effect of androgens and of prednisone. J. Clin. Endocrinol., 23:1115, 1963.

Goldenberg, I. S., and Hayes, M. A.: Hormonal therapy of metastatic female breast carcinoma. II. 2-α-methyl dihydrotestosterone propionate. Cancer, 14:705, 1961.

Gordan, G. S.: Progress in the treatment of advanced breast cancer. California Med., 111:38, 1969.

Gordon, D., et al.: Hormonal therapy in cancer of the breast. III. The effect of progesterone on clinical course and hormonal excretion. Cancer, 5:275, 1952.

Greening, W. P., et al.: Results in the treatment of the breast by interstitial irradiation of the pituitary. Brit. J. Cancer, 14:627, 1960.

Haddow, A., Watkinson, J. M., and Paterson, E.: Influence of synthetic oestrogens upon advanced malignant disease. Brit. M. J., 2:393, 1944.

Hall, T. C., et al.: Prognostic value of response of patients with breast cancer to therapeutic castration. Cancer Chemother. Rep., 31:47, 1963.

Hamberger, C. A., Hammer, G., Norlen, G., and Sjögren, B.: Transantrosphenoidal hypophysectomy. Arch. Otolaryng., 74:2, 1961.

Harris, H. S., and Spratt, J. S.: Bilateral adrenalectomy in metastatic mammary cancer. Cancer, 23:145, 1969.

Horsley, J. S., and Horsley, G. W.: Twenty years' experience with prophylactic bilateral oophorectomy in the treatment of carcinoma of the breast. Ann. Surg., 155:935, 1962.

Huggins, C., and Bergenstal, D. M.: Surgery of the adrenals. J.A.M.A., 147:101, 1951.

Huggins, C., and Dao, T. L-Y.: Adrenalectomy for mammary cancer; surgical technic of bilateral one-stage adrenalectomy in man. Ann. Surg., 136:595, 1952.

Huggins, C., and Scott, W. W.: Bilateral adrenalectomy in prostatic cancer; clinical features and urinary excretion of 17-ketosteroids and estrogen. Ann. Surg., 122:1031, 1945.

Jantet, G., Crocker, D. W., Shiraki, M., and Moore, F. D.: Adrenal suppression in disseminated carcinoma of the breast. I. The effect on adrenal morphology of hypophysectomy and corticosteroid treatment. New England J. Med., 269:1, 1963.

Juret, P., Hayem, M., and Faisler, A.: A propos 150 implantations intra-hypophysaires dans le traitement du cancer du sein à une stade avancée. J. Chir., 87:409, 1964.

Kaufman, R. J., and Escher, G. C.: Rebound regression in advanced mammary carcinoma. Surg., Gynec. & Obst., 113:635, 1961.

Kennedy, B. J.: Fluoxymesterone therapy in advanced breast cancer. New England J. Med., 259:673, 1958.

Kennedy, B. J., and Fortuny, I. E.: Therapeutic castration in the treatment of advanced breast cancer. Cancer, 17:1197, 1964.

Kennedy, B. J., Mielke, P. W. Jr., and Fortuny, I. E.: Therapeutic castration versus prophylactic castration in breast cancer. Surg., Gynec. & Obst., 118:524, 1964.

Kennedy, B. J., and Nathanson, I. T.: Effects of intensive sex steroid hormone therapy in advanced breast cancer. J.A.M.A., 152:1135, 1953.

Kofman, S., Garvin, J. S., Nagamani, D., and Taylor, S. G., III: Treatment of cerebral metastases from breast carcinoma with prednisolone. J.A.M.A., 163:147, 1957.

Lemon, H. M.: Prednisone therapy of advanced mammary cancer. Cancer, *12*:93, 1959.

Lett, H.: Analysis of 99 cases of inoperable carcinoma of breast treated by oophorectomy. Lancet, *1*:227, 1905.

Lowe, R., DeLorimier, A. A., Jr., Gordan, G. S., and Goldman, L.: Antitumor efficacy of Fluoxymesterone; use in advanced breast cancer. Arch. Int. Med., *107*:241, 1961.

Luft, R., and Olivecrona, H.: Hypophysectomy in man. Experiences in metastatic cancer of the breast. Cancer, *8*:261, 1955.

Macdonald, I.: Endocrine ablation in disseminated mammary carcinoma. Surg., Gynec. & Obst., *115*:215, 1962.

McWhirter, R.: Some factors influencing prognosis in breast cancer. J. Fac. Radiol., London, *8*:220, 1956.

Miller, M. W., and Pendergrass, E. P.: Some observations concerned with carcinoma of the breast; part 3. Am. J. Roentgenol., *72*:942, 1954.

Moore, F. D., Woodrow, S. I., Aliapoulios, M. A., and Wilson, R. E.: Carcinoma of the breast (concluded). New England J. Med., *277*:460, 1967.

Mye, G. L., and Neal, W.: Bilateral adrenalectomy for advanced mammary cancer—9 year review of 84 cases. Amer. Surg., *31*:621, 1965.

Nathanson, I. T.: Sex hormones and castration in advanced breast cancer. Radiology, *56*:535, 1951.

Nathanson, I. T., Rice, C., and Meigs, J. V.: Hormonal studies in artifical menopause produced by roentgen rays. Am. J. Obst. & Gynec., *40*:936, 1940.

Nemoto, T., and Dao, T. L-Y.: Significance of liver metastases in women with disseminated breast cancer undergoing endocrine ablative surgery. Cancer, *19*:421, 1966.

Nissen-Meyer, R.: Castration as part of the primary treatment for operable female breast cancer. Acta Radiol. Supp. 249, 1965.

Osborne, M. P., and Pitts, R. M.: Therapeutic oophorectomy for advanced breast cancer. Cancer, *114*:126, 1961.

Raven, R. W.: Cancer of the breast treated by oophorectomy. Brit. M. J., *1*:1343, 1950.

Ray, B. S.: Current cancer concepts: Hypophysectomy as palliative treatment. J.A.M.A., *200*:974, 1967.

Ray, B. S., and Pearson, O. H.: Hypophysectomy in the treatment of disseminated breast cancer. Surg. Clin. N. Amer., *42*:419, 1962.

Rosenberg, M. F., and Uhlmann, E. M.: Prophylactic castration in carcinoma of the breast. Arch. Surg., *78*:376, 1959.

Scheer, K. E., and Klar, E.: Pituitary implantation with Au^{198}. A report of 500 cases. Nuclearmedizin, *2*:143, 1961.

Segaloff, A., et al.: Hormonal therapy in cancer of the breast. XVI. The effect of delta-1-testolactone on clinical course and hormonal excretion. Cancer, *13*:1017, 1960.

Segaloff, A., et al.: Hormonal therapy in cancer of the breast. XIX. Effect of oral administration of delta-1-testolactone on clinical course and hormonal excretion. Cancer, *15*:633, 1962.

Segaloff, A.: Hormones and breast cancer. Recent Prog. in Hormonal Research, *22*:351, 1966.

Siegert, A.: Kastration und Mamma-Ca. Strahlentherapie, *87*:62, 1952.

Smith, G. V., and Smith, O. W.: Carcinoma of the breast; results, evaluation of x-radiation and relation of age and surgical castration to length of survival. Surg., Gynec. & Obst., *97*:508, 1953.

Smith, O. W., and Emerson, K., Jr.: Urinary estrogens and related compounds in postmenopausal women with mammary cancer; effect of cortisone treatment. Proc. Soc. Exper. Biol. Med., *85*:264, 1954.

Sommers, S. C., Teloh, H. A., and Goldman, G.: Ovarian influence upon survival in breast cancer. Arch. Surg., *67*:916, 1953.

Taylor, G. W.: Evaluation of ovarian sterilization for breast cancer. Surg., Gynec. & Obst., *68*:452, 1939.

Taylor, S. G., III: Endocrine ablation in disseminated mammary carcinoma. Surg., Gynec. & Obst., *115*:443, 1962.

Taylor, S. G., III, and Morris, R. S., Jr.: Hormones in breast metastasis therapy. Med. Clin. N. Amer. *35*:51, 1951.

Thomas, A. N., Gordan, G. S., Goldman, L., and Lowe, R.: Antitumor efficacy of 2-α-methyl dihydrotestosterone propionate in advanced breast cancer. Cancer, *15*:176, 1962.

Ulrich, P.: Testosterone (hormone male) et son role possible dans le traitement de certains cancers du sein. Internat. Union against Cancer, *4*:377, 1939.

Witt, J. A., et al.: Secondary hormonal therapy of disseminated breast cancer—comparison of hypophysectomy replacement therapy, estrogens, and androgens. Arch. Int. Med., *111*:557, 1963.

Chapter Thirty-Seven

The Chemotherapy of Breast Cancer

by SVEN J. KISTER, M.D.

Hormonal chemotherapy has been discussed in the preceding chapter. Therefore, this chapter will describe the present status of non-hormonal chemotherapy in the treatment of disseminated breast cancer. Chemotherapy, like hormone therapy, is merely palliative; no chemical compound is capable of curing breast cancer. In comparison to hormonal therapy, chemotherapy is even less effective and of greater potential harm to the patient.

THE HISTORY OF CHEMOTHERAPY

The use of chemicals in the treatment of cancer spans from antiquity to the present time. Acids, alkalies, and salts of various metals, particularly those of arsenic, have found application as anticancer agents in the past. Their use was commonly limited to local treatment by topical application to either ulcerated tumors or skin cancers. Apparently, the first systemic use of a chemical agent in the treatment of cancer was carried out more than a century ago by Lissauer, who described the beneficial effects of potassium arsenite solution in two patients with leukemia. A few years later, Billroth used the same agent with repeated success in a case of lymphoma. Although Ehrlich first investigated the biological effects of an alkylating agent at the turn of the century, it was not until the investigation of war gases during World War II that a compound capable of marked white blood cell depression, and its possible application in the treatment of leukemia, was discovered (Gilman and Philips). This report of the therapeutic application of nitrogen mustard in the treatment of a malignant disease in 1946 was the beginning of the modern era of cancer chemotherapy.

In 1948, Farber and associates first used aminopterin in the treatment of acute leukemia in children, introducing a new group of chemicals, known as antimetabolites, into cancer chemotherapy. Another antimetabolite, a fluorinated pyrimidine, 5-fluorouracil, was developed by Heidelberger and his associates in 1957, and is possibly the most effective chemical against breast cancer. The number of new chemotherapeutic agents continues to proliferate. A host of antibiotics, the Vinca alkaloids, and other C-mitotic arrestors, and most recently the precious metals, particularly some platinum compounds (Rosenberg et al.; Talley), have taken their place in the long list of anticancer drugs. The number of chemicals developed and considered potentially useful against cancer is in the thousands. More than 2000 nitrogen mustards alone were known by the mid-1960's (Bratzel et al.). Of all those drugs developed, relatively few have been considered useful in man, and only about 30 chemotherapeutic agents are presently in clinical use.

Paralleling this extensive search for newer

and more effective chemicals against cancer has been the effort in evaluating their clinical usefulness. Since no single institution has a large enough cancer patient population of a given kind in the relatively short period of time necessary for drug evaluation, the concept of cooperative clinical study groups emerged under the auspices of the National Cancer Institute. During the past 15 years, more than 30 cooperative study groups have dealt with various cancer treatments, of which chemotherapy has constituted a major proportion.

THE CHEMOTHERAPEUTIC AGENTS AND THEIR EFFECT

The literature concerning the efficacy of various chemotherapeutic agents has been mushrooming. In order to accommodate the many reports, the National Cancer Institute has sponsored the publication of two new journals, *Cancer Chemotherapy Reports* and *Cancer Chemotherapy Abstracts*. Even today there is no certainty regarding the site of action of the various chemotherapeutic agents upon the cancer cell; anticancer drugs are, nevertheless, grouped according to their most likely site of action into three broad categories: (1) biological alkylating agents, (2) antimetabolites, and (3) others, which include the antibiotics, the Vinca alkaloids and, most recently, some precious metals.

It is not the intent of this brief discussion to review all chemotherapeutic agents used in the clinical treatment of breast cancer—nor to discuss the supposed mechanisms of their action in any detail. Suffice it to say that many of the cytotoxic agents have been used in the treatment of human mammary carcinoma. The most commonly used alkylating agents, antimetabolites, and "other substances" are listed in Table 37–1.

The alkylating agents, although dissimilar in their structure and chemical reactivity, seem to affect the cancer cells in a similar manner. The majority of them are bifunctional or trifunctional. They react at body temperature under neutral aqueous conditions, and are, therefore, described as biological. They react with many cellular constituents, but most importantly with the proteins and nucleic acids. There is increasing evidence that DNA is the biologic site of action (Ochoa and Hirschberg; Ross; Warwick). In their reaction, the alkylating agents exchange alkyl groups of their own with hydrogens of the reacting substance (Kihlman; Ochoa and Hirschberg; Ross; Warwick).

Antimetabolic substances are compounds designed to interfere with the synthesis of deoxyribonucleic and ribonucleic acid and in this fashion inhibit cellular growth and replication of the tumor cells. They are accepted into the metabolic pathways of the tumor cell by virtue of their close similarity to the "true" metabolite. Once in the cell, they exert their effect because of their dissimilarity from the normal (Kihlman).

Table 37–1. CHEMOTHERAPEUTIC AGENTS MOST COMMONLY USED IN THE TREATMENT OF BREAST CANCER

	Brand Name	Generic Name	Route of Administration	Dosage	Toxicity
Alkylating agents	Thiotepa	Triethylenethiophosporamide	I.V.	0.2 mg./kg./day for 4 days	Bone marrow depression
	Cytoxan	Cyclophosphamide	P.O.	50–200 mg./day	Bone marrow depression, alopecia, cystitis, jaundice
	Melphalan	Phenylalanine mustard	P.O.	2–6 mg./day initially 2–4 mg./day maintenance	Bone marrow depression
Antimetabolites	Fluorouracil, 5-FU	5-Fluorouracil	I.V.	10–15 mg./kg./day 3–5 days 5–7.5 mg./kg./for 3–5 alternate days	Gastrointestinal, bone marrow depression, alopecia
	Methotrexate	Methtrexate	P.O.	0.5 mg./kg./day	Gastrointestinal, liver damage, bone marrow depression
Others	Oncovin	Vincristine	I.V.	0.02–0.05 mg./kg./weekly	Gastrointestinal, peripheral neuritis, bone marrow depression
	Velban	Vinblastine	I.V.	0.1–0.15 mg./kg./weekly	Gastrointestinal, bone marrow depression, alopecia

The vinca alkaloids, vinblastine and vincristine, are derived from the plant, periwinkle. They act at a specific point of the cycle to destroy the spindle or the C-stage (metaphase) mitosis to produce mitotic arrest. They also have other biological effects, including interference with nucleic acid synthesis (Kihlman; Sartorelli and Creasey).

Essentially, the action of all present day anticancer drugs is in essence the inhibition of growth, whatever the site or mode of action of each agent. All the drugs lack selectivity of action and act equally upon both tumor and normal cells. Their effect is greatest on tissues with rapidly dividing cells, such as some tumor cells and cells of the bone marrow and intestinal mucosa. Therefore, at least theoretically, we may be able to destroy all cells of a breast cancer without destroying the normal breast, but in so doing, we may severely harm the bone marrow or some other normal tissues.

There are two other problems inherent in chemotherapy that also plague cancer chemotherapy: the development of drug-resistant tumors and the inability of the drug to reach the tumor cells. An attempt at resolving the first problem has been made through the use of multiple agents in combination or sequentially. At this time, there is no practical solution to the second problem. One can only state that blood supply to tumors varies considerably, and, therefore, certain anatomic sites provide "tumor sanctuaries."

With the increased interest in the immunologic aspects of malignant growths, another dimension has been introduced into the problem of cancer chemotherapy. The remarkable control, if not cure, that chemotherapeutic agents offer in the treatment of Burkitt's lymphoma, trophoblastic tumors, and acute leukemias in childhood can undoubtedly be attributed to the strong immunologic component of these tumors (Bagshawe; Hertz). Furthermore, there is increasing evidence that many of the anticancer agents suppress delayed immunity in man (Al-Sarraf et al.; Mitchell and DiConti), a supposed antitumor mechanism of the host.

CLINICAL RESULTS OF CHEMOTHERAPY

Most of the clinically available chemotherapeutic agents have also been used for the treatment of metastatic breast carcinoma. Their efficacy has been described in many clinical studies. Reported response rates range from 0 to 85 per cent of patients so treated (Cooper; Nadler and Moore). These remarkably variable results were obtained, irrespective of whether single drugs (Ahmenn et al.; Ansfield and Curreri, 1959, 1963, Ansfield et al.; Brennan, 1966; Dao and Grinberg; Donegan; Edelstyn; Freckman et al.; Goldenberg; Gordon and MacArthur; Greening; Greenspan, 1965, 1966, 1968; Grinberg et al.; Hadfield; Mackman et al.; Ravdin and Eisman; Samp and Ansfield; Sedgwick and Vernon; Stoll and Matar; Talley et al.; Talley, 1970), combinations of cytotoxic drugs (Ahmenn et al.; Bateman and Carlton; Brennan, 1966; Dobson; Eastern Cooperative Group; Grady; Greenspan, 1964, 1965, 1966, 1968), or cytotoxic drugs in combination with hormonal treatment (Brennan, 1967, 1968; Freckman et al.; Mackman et al.; Wilson and Moore; Wright et al.) were used.

At least a partial explanation for these widely differing results can be found in the lack of uniformity among the various studies in the following criteria: selection of patients for chemotherapy, definition of disseminated disease, the timing of initiation of treatment, response to treatment, duration of response and quality of life prolonged.

Selection of Patients. The general condition of the patient at initiation of chemotherapy is all important. Adequate tumor dose often means mild to moderate systemic toxicity. Advanced age, poor nutritional status, and the presence of metabolic disturbances, or infection, all increase the patient's vulnerability to these cytotoxic agents and make the administration of an adequate tumor dose hazardous, if not impossible. It is obviously for this reason that some investigators exclude certain poor risk patients as candidates for chemotherapy. Sears defines two such categories. In the first category, increased risk for chemotherapy is present in patients with advanced breast cancer who are in poor nutrition, are over 65 years of age, have a falling hemoglobin, white cell count, and platelet count, have renal or hepatic insufficiency, have extensive bone metastases, and, finally, have had prior antitumor therapy, either in the form of radiotherapy, chemotherapy, surgical therapy, or adrenal ablation. The second category defines patients with breast cancer ineligible for chemotherapy when expected survival is less than two months, when they have myelophthisic anemia with greater than 10 to 15 per cent immature red blood cells, when the white blood cell count is below 3000, when platelets are below 50 per cent of normal, and when severe renal insufficiency exists. Moore et al. also exclude patients from chemotherapy when they have "too far advanced disease." On the other hand, chemotherapy is often used only when other palliative measures have been exhausted or have failed.

Definition of Disseminated Breast Cancer. The precise assessment of dissemination of breast cancer prior to initiation of chemotherapy is difficult, but most important (Rall). Without a precise starting line for all patients receiving a given treatment, comparisons of survival between responders and nonresponders are of little value. The Subcommittee on Breast and Genital Cancer, in its report to the American Medical Association Council, defines dissemination as follows: "unequivocal evidence of distant dissemination of the disease was present, which was unsuitable for radiotherapy or surgical palliation. Specifically, it was required that spread beyond the regional (axillary) nodes be demonstrable in multiple foci or be of such extent in dominant areas that irradiation was impractical, or both. Each patient represented genuine distant dissemination so advanced as to require a systemic approach in treatment." Although specifying dissemination, these criteria leave the degree of dissemination poorly defined. The determination of unsuitability and impracticality of radiotherapy of certain metastases is frequently a reflection of the skill of the radiotherapist, rather than of uniform criteria within acceptable dose ranges. The Cooperative Breast Cancer Group (1961) has categorized metastases according to the dominant lesion into three groups: (1) visceral, which includes liver, lung, and brain; (2) osseous; and (3) breast, which includes lymph nodes, skin, and subcutaneous tissues. Many authors, however, state that metastases were present, without attempting any kind of localization or measurement of the extent of the disseminated disease.

The Timing of Initiation of Treatment of Disseminated Disease. No chemical compound is capable of curing breast cancer. The usefulness of chemotherapy is, therefore, only in palliation. Palliation in turn implies that there has to be something to alleviate. Should patients with definite but asymptomatic disseminated breast cancer be treated with chemotherapy? The answer would seem to be quite simple and answerable through the meaning of the word palliation; only symptoms can and should be palliated. Asymptomatic

patients exhibiting abnormal chemical tests and x-rays should usually not be treated. There is no evidence, to date, that life is prolonged or that the quality of the prolonged life improved with the earlier use of the available chemotherapeutic agents. Most reports fail to describe precisely when, in the course of dissemination, chemotherapy was introduced.

Thus, an additional variable, the timing of initiation of chemotherapy in disseminated breast cancer, is introduced in the evaluation of the efficacy of chemotherapeutic agents.

Even more important is the choice of type of treatment for disseminated breast cancer. As previously mentioned, chemotherapy may be used as the first form of treatment, or after palliation by hormonal manipulation has failed or has become ineffectual. These choices of timing during the course of breast cancer may strongly influence the apparent duration of the effect of the chemotherapeutic agent.

Criteria for Response to Chemotherapeutic Treatment. What is improvement? At the present time, the most commonly utilized criteria of improvement in response to chemotherapy of disseminated breast cancer are those defined by Ansfield and Curreri. These criteria include, (1) at least a 50 per cent reduction in size of tumors with no lesions showing progression, (2) subjective improvement, (3) leveling off, or reversal, of the downward weight curve, (4) improvement in performance status, and (5) the existence of all of these criteria for at least two months.

The reduction in size of a measurable metastatic lesion in man does not correlate well with survival. Furthermore, tumor size often reflects also stromal response of the host to the tumor cells (Brennan, 1965). Subjective improvement, such as decrease in pain, decrease in dyspnea, decrease in cough, and increase in well-being, are most difficult to evaluate unless it is accompanied by corroborative objective improvement, e.g., some improvement of findings on chest x-ray or skeletal films.

Implicit in the term "improvement" are two qualifications, duration or prolongation of survival and the quality of such survival.

DURATION OF RESPONSE. Duration of survival is most commonly expressed in terms of average survival in months, and according to the aforementioned definition, two months qualifies as regression. The duration of survival is sometimes expressed in terms of prolonged survival of responders over nonresponders in a group of patients with disseminated breast cancer receiving the same drug (Ansfield et al.). This type of comparison is dependent particularly upon the definition of "disseminated breast cancer" and the timing of the institution of chemotherapy. Differences in survival time between responders and nonresponders may merely reflect two different populations of breast cancer behavior. Shorter survival in nonresponders may also reflect drug toxicity.

The information required to identify various populations of breast cancer behavior at the time of dissemination can only derive from the knowledge of the given breast cancer behavior before its dissemination, i.e., from the time of the initial diagnosis of breast cancer. It must include precise clinical staging of the cancer at the time of first diagnosis, pathologic diagnosis, primary treatment, axillary lymph node status if surgery was performed, and all subsequent additive or prophylactic treatment administered prior to the disease becoming systemic. Frequent follow-up at 3 to 4 month intervals after primary treatment is extremely important for the precise assessment of the time and extent of dissemination. The disease-free interval, i.e., the time interval between primary treatment and the appearance of recurrent or metastatic disease, is influenced primarily by the initial stage and the type of the treatment of the breast cancer. If these two factors are known and are constant, then the disease-free interval may reflect the basic biologic behavior of a given breast cancer.

Data of this kind are sorely lacking in most of the aforementioned reports, and may not even be available, since most cancer chemotherapy is administered in larger centers to which patients have been referred. These referrals frequently lack information pertaining to the primary diagnosis, staging, and subsequent treatment of the breast cancer. Statistical allowances cannot compensate for the lack of basic information, nor should complex methodology lend it respectability. This situation is reflected by the great diversity of reported regression rates. Brennan (1968) recognizes the dilemma and states, "How can we express the results of chemotherapeutic treatment of disseminated breast cancer without making arbitrary decisions, creating artificial categories or inflating the significance of our efforts in the minds of our colleagues?"

THE QUALITY OF LIFE PROLONGED. Probably the most poorly defined criterion of improvement is the quality of life prolonged. The sole measure of improvement is an increase in performance status, according to the criteria described by Ansfield and Curreri (1959, 1963). Yet, the most important aspect of survival is its quality. A patient who shows a 50 per cent decrease in her osseous lesions, still has severe bone pain, is bedridden, and lives for more than two months with a performance status that has improved from "moribund" to "very sick" or "severely disabled status requiring hospitalization," would qualify as a responder according to the above criteria. If performance status is to reflect quality of life, it must be given a numerical value according to criteria originally described by Karnovsky and associates.

SEQUENCE OF PALLIATIVE MEASURES

There is no evidence that chemotherapy is superior to radiotherapy or hormonal treatment in prolonging useful life when used as the first palliative measure at the time of breast cancer dissemination. Weighing the positive and negative effects derived from any palliative measure in the treatment of breast cancer, a certain logical order emerges. Symptomatic metastases should be treated. The first treatment of soft tissue and osseous metastases should be radiotherapy. Visceral metastases and radio-resistant osseous and soft tissue metastases are managed with hormonal treatment. Only when the metastases are not responsive to, or have escaped, the palliative effects of radiotherapy and hormonal therapy should chemotherapy be instituted.

The choice of chemotherapeutic agents often depends on such variables as route, and ease and cost of administration, as well as on personal preference of the physician, rather than on relative effectiveness of the drug.

ALTERNATIVE CRITERIA FOR THE USEFULNESS OF CHEMOTHERAPY

The presently utilized criteria for response to chemotherapy are inadequate to measure the true efficacy of these agents. In the selection of candidates for chemotherapy, patients with evidence of bone marrow depression (white cell count below 3500 per cu. mm. and platelet count below 120,000) and significant renal failure (blood urea nitrogen over 30 mg.

per ml.) should be excluded. All other patients are eligible, irrespective of age or extent of disseminated disease. The timing of initiation of chemotherapy should follow the order outlined under "sequence of palliative measures." If the two factors indicated above are kept constant, a beneficial response to chemotherapy can be defined as prolongation of quality of life for the minimum duration of six months. During this time, all evident metastases at the time of onset of treatment should remain stationary or regress. No new lesions should become apparent. The quality of life is defined as improvement in performance status to 80 per cent, according to the criteria originally described by Karnovsky et al. Any improvement to less than 70 per cent performance status should not be considered a satisfactory response.

CHOICE OF CHEMOTHERAPEUTIC AGENT

5-Fluorouracil. Although conclusive evidence is presently not available, 5-fluorouracil seems to be the chemotherapeutic agent offering the greatest potential for remission in the treatment of disseminated mammary carcinoma (Donegan, Kennedy, The Medical Letter).

Reported results following treatment with 5-fluorouracil differ widely. Regression rates range from 0 to 42 per cent in reported studies over the past five years. Silva et al. (1965) report a regression rate of 38 per cent in 108 patients for a minimum of one month; Kennedy and Theologides (1966), a regression rate of 42 per cent in 43 women for a minimum duration of two months, the Eastern Cooperative Group (1967) a regression rate of 27 per cent in 30 patients for a duration of two weeks, Ravdin and Eisman (1967) a regression rate of 30 per cent in 63 patients, Sears a regression rate of 33 per cent in 108 patients, Moore et al. a regression rate of 32 per cent in 389 women for two months, Nadler and Moore no regression in seven patients, Ansfield et al. (1969) a regression rate of 21 per cent in 535 patients for a minimum of two months and Fracchia et al. (1970) a regression rate of 9 per cent in 347 women for the duration of two months, Nemoto and Dao a regression rate of 13 per cent in 133 patients for a minimum of one month.

In addition, the Eastern Cooperative Group reports no difference in duration of survival between responders and non-responders, while Ravdin and Eisman report a shorter survival for the responders compared with the non-responders.

The above reported regression rates are difficult to evaluate and compare because of variation in the selection of patients for chemotherapy, timing of initiation of treatment and sequence of palliative measures. For example, Moore et al. excluded 187 patients because of "too far advanced disease." Ansfield et al. used 5-fluorouracil as the first mode of treatment in all postmenopausal patients, whereas Fracchia et al. instituted chemotherapy only after other palliative measures such as radiotherapy and hormonal treatment had either proven ineffective or their efficacy had been exhausted.

Our own rather limited experience with 5-fluorouracil thus far includes 17 patients. Ten of them initially had a clinically operable carcinoma of the breast, Columbia Clinical Classification Stages A or B and were treated with a Halsted radical mastectomy. One was inoperable at time of initial diagnosis, Columbia Clinical Classification Stage D. She received radiotherapy as the first treatment. Six patients had their operative treatment elsewhere and the stage of the disease at initial diagnosis is not known.

At the time of dissemination, 9 patients were postmenopausal, and 8 premenopausal. All 17 patients received radiation and hormonal manipulations prior to initiation of chemotherapy. Ten patients had failed to respond to previous treatment. All patients had received steroids as part of their hormonal treatment and continued to do so during 5-fluorouracil administration.

Our dosage schedule of 5-fluorouracil is 15 mg. per kg. for four consecutive days, followed by 7.5 mg. per kg. on days 6, 8, 10, and 12, administered intravenously. Maintenance dose is 500 mg. weekly. At the sign of the least toxicity, treatment is interrupted. Toxic effects of 5-fluorouracil are shown in Table 37-2.

According to the criteria for improvement outlined by Ansfield and Curreri we had no responders. In one patient, pulmonary and pleural metastases regressed completely while the soft tissue lesions remained stationery. Her performance status, however, increased from 40 to 80 per cent for the duration of ten months.

Quintuple Chemotherapy. Multiple drug therapy with chemotherapeutic agents was developed in order to prevent the development of drug-resistance of the tumor. At the

Table 37–2. TOXIC EFFECTS OF 5-FLUOROURACIL

Source	No. of Cases	Symptoms			
		Nausea and Vomiting	Bone Marrow Depression	Diarrhea	Stomatitis
Ansfield et al. (1969)*	535	25%	39%	61%	30%
Fracchia et al. (1970)	347	43%	26%	37%	26%
Nadler and Moore (1968)	389	48%	46%	38%	28%

*Ansfield reported that 4 per cent of his patients also developed alopecia.

same time, it was hoped that lowering the dosage of each individual drug would result in decreased total toxicity. Cooper reported his results with quintuple chemotherapy at the American Association for Cancer Research meeting in San Francisco in early 1969. Sixty unselected patients with far-advanced metastatic breast cancer were given vincristine, 0.035 mg. per kg. intravenously weekly; cyclophosphamide, 2.5 mg. per kg. by mouth daily; prednisone, 0.75 mg. per kg. daily by mouth; 5-fluorouracil, 12 mg. per kg. intravenously for four days followed by 500 mg. once a week; methotrexate, 25 to 50 mg. intramuscularly weekly. The initial course was 8 weeks. Smaller dosages were suggested for maintenance. Cooper reported complete remission in 53 of 60 patients for an average of 10 months. The results were unrelated to age of the patient or previous treatment of the metastatic breast cancer. This amazing remission was seen in 8 of 9 patients

with pulmonary metastases, in 19 of 22 patients with metastases to the liver, in 14 of 16 with bone metastases, in 7 of 8 with brain metastases, and in all 5 with skin lesions. The attendant toxicity was as follows: alopecia occurred in 67 per cent, significant bone marrow depression as manifested by a low white blood cell count was present in 45 per cent, and gastrointestinal symptoms were present in 10 per cent. Two patients died of drug toxicity.

Our experience with quintuple chemotherapy includes 11 patients. Five of them had operable lesions at first diagnosis of breast cancer (Columbia Clinical Classification, Stage A and B). The remaining six patients had more advanced disease and received radiotherapy as the primary mode of treatment. All patients received repeated courses of palliative treatment in the form of radiation or hormonal measures prior to the initiation of chemotherapy. Quintuple chemotherapy was

Table 37–3. QUINTUPLE CHEMOTHERAPY FOR METASTATIC CARCINOMA OF BREAST FOR PATIENTS NOT RESPONSIVE TO RADIOTHERAPEUTIC OR HORMONAL MANAGEMENT

Treatment   For 6 weeks then maintenance with drugs 1, 2, and 3.
1. Prednisone... 0.5 mg./kg. P.O. daily
2. Cyclophosphamide (Cytoxan)........................... 50.0 mg. P.O. daily
3. Fluorouracil.. 12.0 mg./kg. IV weekly
4. Methotrexate... 0.25 mg./kg. IV weekly, maximum dose 15 mg.
5. Vinblastine... 0.1 mg./kg. IV weekly

If BUN more than 30 mg. per 100 ml., omit methotrexate.
WBC above 5000, give full dose of drugs 2, 3, 4, and 5.
WBC below 5000, give ½ *dose of four drugs* (2, 3, 4, 5) and continue prednisone full dose.

WBC below 3500 or platelets below 120,000, *omit four drugs* for one week.

WBC below 3000 or platelets below 100,000, *discontinue four drugs.*

If diarrhea or stomatitis develops, stop fluorouracil and methotrexate. Omit prednisone with history of previous or current peptic ulcer, congestive failure, or emotional disturbance.

Maintenance with three drugs.
1. Fluorouracil .... 7.5   mg./kg. IV weekly
2. Cyclophosphamide .... 50.0   mg. P.O. o.d.
3. Prednisone.. 0.375 mg./kg. O.D. P.O.

attempted when or after all other modalities had failed.

None of our patients was able to tolerate the regime in the dosages recommended by Cooper. Three changes in protocol were carried out during the 12 months to reduce toxicity. Our present dosage schedule is shown in Table 37–3. We have no responders among 11 patients. Our series is too small to allow any statistical analysis. It is difficult to reconcile Cooper's regression rate of 88 per cent with our own results, but a larger number of patients is necessary for valid comparison. Such an attempt is presently in progress.

SUMMARY

Chemical treatment of mammary carcinoma has been in use for 20 years. During this time, a host of agents have been tried singly or in combination with various hormonal treatments. Different ways of administration and dosages of these drugs have come and gone. As the decades have passed, the overall results have been disappointing. The benefits of chemotherapy in terms of frequency are in the order of 10 to 20 per cent for the duration of two months, while the life prolonged is of questionable quality. Toxicity, difficulty and expense of administration, particularly with multiple drug therapy, have not infrequently outweighed the transient benefits gained from the drugs. The not yet understood, but possibly significant effects of these chemicals upon the patient's own antitumor mechanisms are an additional factor to be considered.

In view of the occasional real success in prolonging useful life and the attendant psychological benefits of active treatment, it would seem that chemotherapy may be used in selected cases: in early menopausal patients with visceral metastases who respond poorly to hormonal therapy or for whom hormonal methods have failed. If chemotherapy is used, great care must be exercised not to harm the patient. The drugs should be used in doses that do not produce toxicity. The choice and administration of these drugs should be carried out by a physician well versed in the intricacies of this type of treatment.

Perhaps the greatest value of the cancer chemotherapeutic agents and their clinical use has been the contribution they have made to the understanding of cancer mechanisms.

REFERENCES

Ahmenn, D. L., Bisel, H. F., and Hahn, R. G.: An evaluation of 5-fluorouracil in the treatment of advanced breast cancer. Proc. Mayo Clin., 42:193–199, 1967.

Al-Sarraf, M., Wong, P., Sardesai, S., and Vaitkevicius, V. K.: Clinical immunologic responsiveness in malignant disease. I. Delayed hypersensitivity reaction and the effect of cytotoxic drugs. Cancer, 26:262, 1970.

Ansfield, F. J., and Curreri, A. R.: Further clinical comparison between 5-fluorouracil (5-FU) and 5-fluoro -2- deoxyuridine (5-FUDR). Cancer Chemother. Rep., 32:101, 1963.

Ansfield, F. J., and Curreri, A. R.: Further clinical studies with 5-fluorouracil. J. Nat. Cancer Inst., 22:497–507, 1959.

Ansfield, F. J., Ramirez, G., Mackman, S., Bryan, G., and Curreri, A. R.: A ten-year study of 5-fluorouracil in disseminated breast cancer with clinical results and survival times. Cancer Res., 29:1062–1066, 1969.

Bagshawe, K. D.: Choriocarcinoma: The Clinical Biology of the Trophoblast and Its Tumours. London, Edward Arnold, 1969.

Bagshawe, K. D.: Some immunological aspects of choriocarcinoma. In Maxwell Anderson, J., ed.: The Biology and Surgery of Tissue Transplantation. Oxford and Edinburgh, Blackwell, 1970, Chap. 13.

Bateman, J. C., and Carlton, H. N.: Palliation of mammary carcinoma with phosphoramide drugs. J.A.M.A., 162:8, 701–706, 1956.

Bratzel, R. P., Ross, R. B., Goodridge, T. H., Huntress, W. T., Flather, M. T., and Johnson, D. E.: Survey of nitrogen mustards. Cancer Chemother. Rep., 26:1, 1963.

Brennan, M. J.: Indices of response to breast cancer therapy. In Hayward, J. H., and Bulbrook, R. D., eds.: Clinical Evaluation in Breast Cancer. New York, Academic Press, 1965.

Brennan, M. J.: Chemotherapy of Solid Tumors in Modern Treatment. New York, Harper and Row, 1966, Vol. 3, p. 791.

Brennan, M. J.: Comparison of cumulative functions for breast cancer series differing in treatment plan. In Segaloff, A., Myer, K., and Debakey, S., eds.: Current Concepts of Breast Cancer. Baltimore, Williams and Wilkins, 1967, p. 228.

Brennan, M. J.: The value of hormonal and chemotherapeutic treatment in disseminated breast cancer. In Forrest, A. P. M., and Kunkler, P. V., eds.: Prognostic Factors in Breast Cancer. Proceedings of First Tenovus Symposium, Cardiff, April 12–14, 1967. Edinburg and London, E. and S. Livingstone, Ltd., 1968.

Cooper, R. G.: Breast cancer remission achieved with five drugs. Combination therapy in hormone resistant breast cancer. Proc. Amer. Assoc. Cancer Res., 10:15, 1969.

Cooperative Breast Cancer Group. Progress Report: Results of studies by the cooperative breast cancer group, 1956–1960. Cancer Chemother. Rep., 11:109–141, 1961.

Dao, T. L., and Grinberg, R.: Fluorinated pyrimidines in treatment of breast cancer patients with liver metastasis. Cancer Chemother. Rep., 27:71–77, 1963.

Dobson, L.: The treatment of recurrent or metastatic breast cancer with emphasis of the use of 5-fluorouracil. Amer. J. Surg., 104:143, 1962.

Donegan, W. L.: Chemotherapy. *In* Spratt, J. S., Jr., and Donegan, W. L., eds.: Cancer of the Breast. Philadelphia and London, W. B. Saunders Co., 1967, Chap. 11, p. 231.

Eastern Cooperative Group in Solid Tumor Chemotherapy. Comparison of antimetabolites in the treatment of breast and colon cancer. J.A.M.A., *200*:110–118, 1967.

Edelstyn, A. G.: Cyclophosphamide in treatment of locally recurrent breast cancer. Lancet, *1*:237, 1965.

Ehrlich, P.: *In* Himmelweit, ed.: The Collected Papers of Paul Ehrlich. London, Pergamon, 1956, vol. 1, p. 612.

Farber, S., Diamond, L. K., Mercer, R. D., Sylvester, R. F., and Wolff, J. A.: Temporary remission in acute leukemia in children produced by folic acid antagonist, 4-aminopteroyl-glutamic acid (aminopterin). New Eng. J. Med., *238*:787, 1948.

Fracchia, A. A., Farrow, J. H., Adam, Y. G., Monroy, J., and Knapper, W. H.: Systemic chemotherapy for advanced breast cancer. Cancer, *26*:642, 1970.

Freckman, A. H., Fry, H. L., Mendez, F. L., and Maurer, E. R.: Chlorambucil-prednisolone therapy for disseminated breast carcinoma. J.A.M.A., *189*:23, 1964.

Gilman, A., and Philips, F. S.: The biological actions and therapeutic application of the B-chloroethyl amines and sulfides. Science, *103*:409, 1946.

Goldenberg, I.: Vincristine: Therapy of women with advanced breast cancer. Cancer Chemother. Rep., *41*:7–9, 1964.

Gordon, I., and MacArthur, J.: Thio-tepa and cyclophosphamide in the treatment of advanced mammary cancer. Scot. Med. J., *10*:27, 1965 (also Victoria Informary Glasgow Excerpta Medica, *14*:222, 1966).

Grady, E. D.: The treatment of advanced cancer with a combination of 5-fluorouracil, cytoxan and methotrexate. J. Med. Assoc. Georgia, *53*:285, 1964.

Greening, W. P.: Methotrexate in the treatment of advanced cancer of the breast. *In* Porter, R., and Wiltshaw, E., eds.: Methotrexate in the Treatment of Cancer. Briston, England. John Wright and Sons, Ltd., 1962.

Greenspan, E. M.: Regression of metastatic hepatomegaly from mammary carcinoma. New York State J. Med., *64*:2442–2449, 1964.

Greenspan, E. M.: Results of four drugs sequential combination chemotherapy of breast carcinoma in relation to predominant organ metastases. Proc. Amer. Assoc. Cancer Res., *6*:24, 1965.

Greenspan, E. M.: Combination of cytotoxic chemotherapy in advanced disseminated breast cancer. J. Mount Sinai Hosp., *33*:1–27, 1966.

Greenspan, E. M.: Combination antimetabolite and alkylating agent chemotherapy in advanced breast carcinoma. New York State J. Med., *68*:780, 1968.

Grinberg, P., Nemoto, T., and Dao, T. L.: Vincristine (NSC-67574): Dosage and response in advanced breast cancer. Cancer Chemother. Rep., *45*:57–61, 1965.

Hadfield, J.: The place of chemotherapy in management of disseminated mammary cancer. J.A.M.A., *200*: 168, 1967.

Heidelberger, C., Chandhuri, N. K., Dannberg, P., Mooren, D., and Griesbach, L.: Fluorinated pyrimidines, a new class of tumor inhibitory compounds. Nature, *179*:663, 1957.

Heidelberger, C., and Ansfield, F. J.: Experimental and clinical use of fluorinated pyrimidines in cancer chemotherapy. Cancer Res., *23*:1226, 1963.

Hertz, R.: Eight years' experience with chemotherapy of choriocarcinoma and related trophoblasic tumors in women. *In* Holland, J. F., and Hreschchyshyn, M. M., eds.: Choriocarcinoma: Transactions of a Conference of the International Union Against Cancer. Berlin, Springer-Verlag, 1967, pp. 66–71.

Ivy. H. C.: Treatment of breast cancer with 5-fluorouracil. Ann. Int. Med., *57*:598–605, 1962.

Karnofsky, D. A., Ellison, R. R., and Golbey, R. D.: Selection of patients for evaluation of chemotherapeutic procedures in advanced cancer. J. Chronic. Dis., *15*:243, 1962.

Kennedy, B. J., and Theologides, A.: The role of 5-fluorouracil in malignant disease. Ann. Int. Med., *55*:719, 1961.

Kennedy, B. J.: Chemotherapy for Cancer in Modern Treatment. New York, Hoeber Med. Div., Harper and Row, 1966, vol. 3, pp. 683.

Kihlman, B. A.: Actions of Chemicals on Dividing Cells. Englewood Cliffs, New Jersey, Prentice-Hall, 1966.

Lissauer: Zwei Falle von Leucaemia, Berl. Klin. Wschr., *2*:403, 1865.

Mackman, S., Ramirez, G., and Ansfield, F. J.: Results of 5-fluorouracil (NSC-19893) given by the multiple daily dose method in disseminated breast cancer. Cancer Chemother. Rep., *51*:483–489, 1967.

Mitchell, M. S., and DeConti, R. C.: Immunosuppression by 5-fluorouracil. Cancer, *26*:884, 1970.

Moore, G. E., Bross, I. D. J., Ausman, R., Nadler, S., Jones, R., Jr., Slack, N., and Rinum, A. A.: Effects of 5-fluorouracil in 389 patients with cancer. Eastern Clinical Drug Evaluation Program, CCR, *52*:641, 1968.

Nadler, S. H., and Moore, G. S.: A Clinical Study of fluorouracil. Surg., Gynec. & Obst., *127*:1210, 1968.

Nemoto, T., and Dao, T. L.: 5-Fluorouracil and cyclophosphamide in disseminated breast cancer. N.Y. State J. Med., *7*:554, 1971.

Nichol, C. A.: The application of new knowledge to the effective administration of anticancer agents. Cancer Res., *29*:2469, 1969.

Ochoa, N., and Hirschberg, E.: *In* Schnitzer, R. J., and Hawking, F., eds.: Experimental Chemotherapy. New York, Academic Press, 1967.

Rall, D. P.: New approaches in administration of anticancer drugs. Cancer Res., *29*:2471, 1969.

Ravdin, R. G., and Eisman, S. H.: Disseminated breast cancer: relationship of response to endocrine manipulation, cytoxan and fluorouracil. *In* Segaloff, A., Myer, K., and Debakey, S., eds.: Current Concepts in Breast Cancer. Baltimore, Williams and Wilkins, 1967, p. 203.

Rosenberg, B., Vancamp, L., Trosko, J. E., and Mansour, V. H.: Platinum compounds: A new class of potent antitumor agents. Nature (London), *222*:385, 1969.

Ross, W. C. J.: Biological Alkylating Agents. London, Butterworths, 1962.

Samp, R. J., and Ansfield, F. J.: Breast cancer treated with fluorouracil. J.A.M.A., *198*:148, 1966.

Sartorelli, A. C., and Creasey, W. A.: Cancer Chemotherapy. Rev. Pharm. Ann., *9*:51, 1969.

Sears, M. E.: Chemotherapy for advanced breast cancer. In Breast Cancer, Early and Late. Conference of Cancer, 1968, at the University of Texas, M. D. Anderson Hospital and Tumor Institute at Houston, Texas, Chicago, Year Book Medical Publishers, p. 387.

Sedgwick, C. E., and Vernon, J. K.: Management of carcinoma of the breast. Surg. Clin. N. Amer., *47*:707, 1967.

Silva, A. R., Smart, C. R., and Rochlin, D. N.: Chemotherapy of breast cancer. Surg., Gynec. & Obstet., *121*:494, 1965.

Stoll, B. A., and Matar, J. H.: Cyclophosphamide in advanced breast cancer. Brit. Med. J., *2*:283–286, 1961.

Subcommittee on Breast and Genital Cancer. Androgens and Estrogens in the Treatment of Disseminated Mammary Carcinoma. J.A.M.A., *172*:1271–1283, 1960.

Symposium on vincristine. Cancer Chemother. Rep., 1968, p. 52.

Talley, R. W., Vaitkevicius, V. K., and Leighton, G. A.: Comparison of cyclophosphamide and 5-fluorouracil in the treatment of patients with metastatic breast cancer. Clin. Pharmacol. Ther., *6*:740, 1965.

Talley, R. W.: Systemic chemotherapy of human malignant neoplasms, *In* Cole, W. H., ed.: Philadelphia, Chemotherapy of Cancer. Lea and Febiger, 1970, p. 148.

Talley, R. W.: Chemotherapy of a mouse reticulum cell sarcoma with platinum salts. Proc. Amer. Assoc. Cancer Res., *11*:310, 1970.

The choice of therapy in the treatment of cancer. The Medical Letter, *12* :16, 1970.

Wilson, R. E., and Moore, F. D.: Biochemical and clinical factors in the selection of patients for endocrine surgery. *In* Forrest, A. P. M., and Kunkler, P. V., eds.: Prognostic Factors in Breast Cancer. Proceedings of First Tenovus Symposium, Cardiff, April, 1967, Edinburgh and London, E. and S. Livingstone, Ltd., 1968.

Warwick, G. P.: The mechanisms of action of alkylating agents. Cancer Res., *23*:1315, 1963.

Wright, J. C., Cobb, J. P., Golomb, F. M., Gumport, S. L., Lyall, D., and Safadi, D.: Chemotherapy of disseminated carcinoma of the breast. Ann. Surg., *150*:221, 1959.

Chapter Thirty-Eight

Carcinoma of the Male Breast

Carcinoma of the breast occurs so infrequently in men that it is not at all well known either to patients or physicians; and it is therefore apt to be missed or diagnosed late. When the disease is advanced the results of treatment are very poor. Education is needed to the effect that breast cancer occurs in males, that it has the same general characteristics as in females, and that the surgical attack on it can be successful when the diagnosis is made early.

Epidemiology

Several interesting features of the epidemiology of male breast carcinoma have been emphasized by Schottenfeld and Lilienfeld. The age-specific mortality rates for the disease in the United States increase exponentially during life, with a greater rate of increase before 40 to 50 years of age. They are higher for non-whites.

The Connecticut data show that the incidence rates for the disease in this country declined sharply between 1941 and 1951. The mortality rates for this disease in Japan and Finland are strikingly lower than in other countries where these data are available.

The infrequency of breast cancer in males has led several American students of the disease to collect the published cases (Wainwright, 401; Sachs, 178). More precise data are to be found in several reports of original case series which have been published during recent years. The largest of these original case series from a single clinic, that reported by Treves and Holleb, included 146 patients. These case series are listed in Table 38-1. Included is our Columbia-Presbyterian series of 49 cases observed over a 37 year period, 1933 to 1970. During this time some 6000 primary breast carcinomas were observed in our clinic. Male breast carcinoma therefore constituted 0.8 per cent of all breast carcinomas in our clinic. In other clinics the proportion of male breast carcinomas has been slightly higher—averaging about 1 per cent.

Carcinoma of the male breast occurs at a later age than carcinoma of the female breast. The average age of males with the disease—as listed in the original case series in Table 38-1—approximates 60 years. Females develop breast carcinoma at an average age of about 50 years.

In males, as in females, breast carcinoma is infrequent below the age of 30. There were three patients under 30 in Treves' series of 146 cases; the youngest was 24. In Norris and Taylor's series of 113 patients, there was only one patient under 30; he was 21.

Etiology

There is a lamentable lack of data as to familial history in the published reports of carcinoma of the male breast. Wainwright, Sachs, Huggins and Taylor, Treves, and Norris and Taylor, present no information as to family history of their patients.

In our own series of male patients with

779

Table 38–1.   FREQUENCY AND AGE INCIDENCE OF CARCINOMA OF THE BREAST IN MALES

Year	Author	Number of Cases	Average Age	Proportion of All Breast Carcinomas
		Collected Case Series		
1927	Wainwright	401	52.6 years	
1941	Sachs	178	57.2 years	
		Original Case Series		
1933	Neal	50	57.7 years	1.2%
1955	Huggins and Taylor	75	63.0 years	
1955	Treves and Holleb	146	52.1 years	< 1.0%
1961	Sinner	27	60.4 years	1.1%
1964	Moss	507		1.1%
1967	Liechty et al.	40	67 years	
1969	Norris and Taylor	113	59 years	
1970	Haagensen	49	62 years	0.8%

breast carcinoma I regret to state that the case histories have not in general included reliable data as to family history of the disease. In my small personal series of 12 patients I have this information but their number is so small that it has, of course, no significance.

It is important to point out, however, that in my history-taking in female patients with breast carcinoma I have found a number of families in which there were many women who developed the disease. In such families it is the rule to find one or more males with breast carcinoma. Chart 21–1 presents two of these families. In Family V, consisting of 23 individuals, nine females and one male have developed the disease. In Family Z, including 29 individuals, five females and two males have had it. It is therefore important to be alert for the disease in both sexes in such a family.

There is strong evidence, which has been summed up by El-Gazayerli and Abdel-Aziz, that bilharziasis is an indirect etiological factor. The disease damages the liver and causes hyperestrogenism in males. In Egypt, where as much as 70 per cent of subjects have bilharziasis, carcinoma of the male breast constitutes about 6 per cent of all breast cancer as compared with 1 per cent in other countries.

There have been several reports in the German medical literature (Gleichmann, Meyer-Laack, Ritschel and Schultze-Jena, Botsztejn and Schinz) which suggest that the increased frequency of gynecomastia in European countries, where starvation conditions existed during the last war, can be correlated with a subsequent increase in carcinoma of the male breast, the assumption being that starvation causes liver damage which leads to hyperestrogenism. There is also some clinical evidence that gynecomastia predisposes to breast cancer. Seven of Liechty's 40 patients with breast carcinoma had clinically evident gynecomastia. Five per cent of Norris and Taylor's 113 patients had clinical gynecomastia. In Chapter 3, in discussing the senescent type of hypertrophy of the male breast I described a patient of my own in which this form of gynecomastia was followed seven years later by carcinoma.

More direct evidence of the role of estrogen in the etiology of breast carcinoma in males is found in the reports of the disease developing in men with carcinoma of the prostate who have been treated with estrogen. I have discussed this question in Chapter 21. Some of these cases are no doubt examples of metastasis of prostatic carcinoma to the breast. In others, however, the evidence is strongly suggestive that the estrogen has actually caused primary breast carcinoma. The most convincing case of this kind has recently been reported by O'Grady and McDivitt. The patient was a man aged 77 with prostatic carcinoma who had taken diethylstilbestrol for 6 years. He soon developed marked bilateral gynecomastia, and after four years, erosion of the epithelium of the right nipple. Radical mastectomy was done. Extensive intraductal mammary carcinoma with characteristic Paget's involvement of the nipple epithelium was found.

I will discuss Paget's carcinoma of the breast in males later on in the present chapter, but at this point, I should emphasize that it is a very rare lesion. In view of this fact I am convinced that O'Grady's and McDivitt's case is a genuine example of estrogen inducing mammary carcinoma in a male. If this has occurred in one patient it has probably occurred in others.

Dodge and his associates have found that there is a high incidence of breast carcinoma in males with Kleinfelter's syndrome. They have described four such lesions in a series of 22 patients with Kleinfelter's syndrome—an estimated incidence 66.5 times that expected. In this syndrome there are complex hormone abnormalities that are not as yet well understood.

It is not infrequent for men with carcinoma of the breast to give a history of antecedent trauma. Treves reports that 12 per cent of his patients gave such a history. He was unable to trace any definite correlation between the trauma and the carcinomas, however.

Symptoms

Treves' data regarding symptomatology are so much more extensive than any other, that I reproduce his table (Table 38–2) listing the symptoms in his patients.

Nipple discharge not associated with ulceration of the nipple—particularly a bloody discharge—occurs more frequently in males with carcinoma of the breast than in females with the disease. Treves and his associates wrote a good discussion of this phenomenon.

Martin, in 1930, emphasized that a bloody nipple discharge in a male suggests carcinoma. In Sachs' collected series of 178 patients with verified breast carcinoma, 14.6 per cent had a bloody nipple discharge. In Treves' series of 131 patients, 13.7 per cent had a nipple discharge; the discharge was serous in three and bloody in 15. Only two of Liechty's 40 patients had a nipple discharge. In our Columbia-Presbyterian Hospital series of 49 patients five, or 10 per cent, gave a history of a nipple discharge not associated with ulceration. In contrast with this considerable frequency of a nipple discharge in males with breast cancer, only 3.3 per cent of my personal series of 1669 women with mammary carcinoma had a nipple discharge.

The circumstances of the nipple discharge in three of our male patients are worth reporting. In one the first sign of disease was a slight amount of bloody discharge, which stained his pajamas, occurring seven years pre-

Table 38–2. INITIAL SYMPTOM IN 146 CASES OF CANCER OF THE MALE BREAST—TREVES—1955

Symptom	No. of Cases
Breast mass only	89 (67.4%)
Breast mass plus	
Retracted nipple	7
Discharging nipple	4
Discharging nipple, pain	1
Encrusted nipple	3
Encrusted nipple, pain	1
Nipple discharge only	8
Nipple encrustation only	5
Nipple retraction only	4
Nipple encrustation, retraction	0
Ulceration	7
Axillary swelling	3
Pain only	0
Pain, breast mass	0
Total	132
Uncertain	14
Total	146

viously. Examining his breast, the patient found a small mass beneath the nipple which, when he pressed it, produced the nipple discharge. He consulted a physician who told him "it was only a pimple." The mass persisted and grew very slowly in size. The nipple became retracted. Six months before admission a few small nodules were noticed around the retracted nipple. The breast finally began to pain him, and he decided to consult a surgeon. In two other patients an intermittent serous and bloody nipple discharge was the only sign of breast disease; in one it had been present for four years and in the other for seven months. There was no palpable tumor in either of these two patients.

There are three other conditions in males in which a nipple discharge may occur. The most frequent is in men with gynecomastia induced by estrogen given for prostatic carcinoma; a slight serous discharge occasionally develops. It is also true that men given large doses of androgen may develop a slight serous nipple discharge.

Benign solitary intraductal papilloma is very rare in males, but when it does occur it may be accompanied by a serous or bloody nipple discharge.

It is obvious from these facts that a nipple discharge in a male who has not been taking any hormone is a clear indication for biopsy.

Duration of Symptoms. There is no doubt but that men with breast carcinoma come for treatment considerably later than women who develop the disease. The average duration of the breast tumor on admission in

Wainwright's series of cases was 2.4 years. Every series of cases of carcinoma of the male breast contains a number of cases in which it would appear that the lesion had been present for many years. One of Huggins and Taylor's patients had had an ulcerated tumor for 30 years. Thirteen per cent of Treves' series of patients had had symptoms for four or more years before consulting a physician. The average duration of symptoms in Liechty's series of patients was 17 months.

In our Columbia-Presbyterian series of patients, five, or 10 per cent, had had symptoms for four years or more; the duration in them was four, five, seven, eight, and ten years, respectively. The average duration of symptoms in our male patients was 19 months. This can be compared with an average duration of symptoms of 5.5 months in my personal series of 1669 women with breast carcinoma.

Three of our male patients with breast carcinoma did not find the breast tumor which indicated that they had breast disease; it was found in the course of a routine physical examination.

Physical Characteristics

Carcinoma developing in the male breast forms a hard, poorly delimited tumor, usually situated beneath the nipple or areola. All but one of our patients had a palpable tumor. In the one who had no tumor the only sign of disease was a bloody nipple discharge.

Since the carcinoma develops so close to the nipple, changes in it are apparent in many of the patients. The nipple was retracted in 15, or about one third, of our patients. As the disease progresses it also narrows and distorts the areola, and finally appears on the surface of the areola and the skin immediately surrounding it in the form of small nodules. Figure 38–1 shows the typical appearance of the disease at this stage.

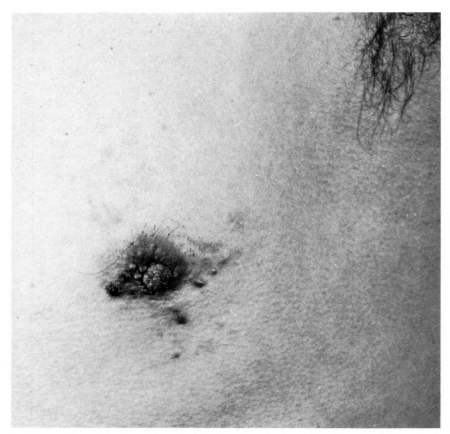

Figure 38–1.   The typical appearance of a locally advanced carcinoma of the male breast.

These carcinomas of the male breast are often fixed to the underlying pectoral fascia, since they lie very close to it.

Most of these breast carcinomas in the male are small. Not including two bulky tumors in our series of cases, their average size was 3.1 cm. The two bulky tumors measured 8 and 16 cm. in diameter, respectively. The larger of these is shown in Figure 38–2. It had begun as a small tumor beneath the nipple eight years previously, and had grown slowly during the intervening years. It was a well differentiated intraductal carcinoma.

One of the noteworthy features of these breast carcinomas in the male is that they may metastasize extensively to the axillary nodes even though the primary tumor is very small. Figure 38–3 shows a well differentiated carcinoma which formed a 5 mm. elevated nodule near the base of the nipple. It was covered with intact epithelium. On biopsy, it proved to be a carcinoma, and radical mastectomy was performed. No other evidence of carcinoma was found in the breast,

yet there were metastases in 16 of 33 axillary nodes.

In the later stages of breast carcinoma in the male ulceration often occurs. None of our six patients with an ulcerated tumor was cured.

Paget's Disease of the Male Breast

A few examples of Paget's carcinoma occurring in males have been reported. The first comprehensive discussion of this lesion with a review of previously reported cases and detailed descriptions of two cases was published by Treves in 1954. Treves emphasized that this lesion in males sometimes progresses exceedingly slowly, as we know it occasionally does in females. He referred to a patient in whom Paget's erosion had slowly extended during a period of 14 years to cover the entire left thoracic wall. Yet when radical mastectomy was finally performed, there were no axillary metastases.

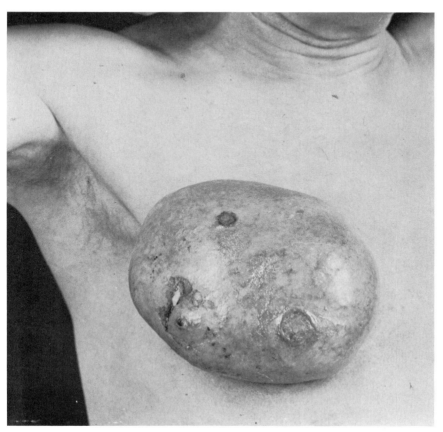

Figure 38–2. A bulky carcinoma of the male breast of eight years' duration.

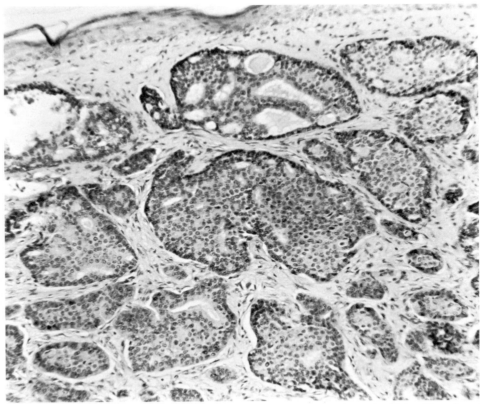

Figure 38–3.   A 5 mm. carcinoma of the male breast that metastasized to 16 of 33 axillary lymph nodes.

In recent years there have been three reviews of the reported cases of Paget's disease in males. Hutchin and Houlihan found reports of 12 cases and added one of their own. O'Grady and McDivitt collected reports of 14 cases and added the remarkable case, referred to above, which appears to have been induced by estrogen. Crichlow and Czernobilsky in their review accepted only 11 previously reported cases as genuine, and added two cases from their own clinic.

Study of the cases included in these reviews suggests that Paget's carcinoma of the male breast has the same clinical and pathological features as its counterpart in females. The results of treatment of the disease in the male appear to have been disastrous. There appear to be no reports of 10 year cures.

I am able to present a hitherto unreported case of my own in which the outcome has been happier. The patient was an engineer aged 43 years who came to me in 1957 with the story that five months previously he had developed a crusted, slightly raised lesion at the edge of his left nipple. The lesion finally extended onto the areola. A small biopsy excision suggested Paget's carcinoma, and the patient was referred to me.

When I examined him, the nipple and areola appeared to be normal except for the recent biopsy scar. There was no tumor in the underlying breast.

In order to make certain of the nature of the lesion I excised the nipple, areola, and breast tissue immediately beneath, through an elliptical incision. The epidermis of both the nipple and areola was extensively infiltrated by typical Paget's cells, arranged singly and in clusters (Figure 38–4). In the underlying nipple ducts and breast tissue, however, we did not find any carcinoma, although we blocked all the tissue and cut it in serial sections.

In view of these facts, I performed only a simple mastectomy with an axillary dissection. In this surgical specimen, including 28 axillary lymph nodes, no carcinoma was found.

The patient has no evidence of recurrence 12 years later. I have not found any other 10

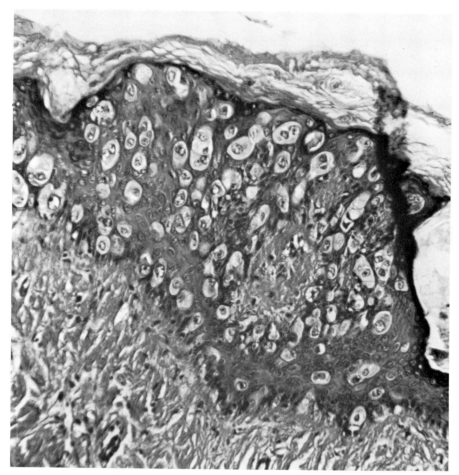

Figure 38–4.   Paget's carcinoma of the male breast.

year clinical cure of Paget's carcinoma of the male breast reported.

Differential Diagnosis

Carcinoma of the male breast is a rare disease which has to be distinguished from several much more frequent and entirely harmless lesions which also form tumors in the male breast. The most frequent of these is the adolescent type of benign hypertrophy of the breast. This occurs with puberty, or sometimes a year or so later, and forms a discoid mass beneath the areola. The youth of the patient, and the well delimited character of the tumor and its lack of fixation, serve to distinguish it. True gynecomastia, occurring in the late teens or early twenties, is usually apparent from the larger and softer nature of the tumor, which mimics the character of the

female breast on a small scale. Hypertrophy of the male breast, due to liver disease or of idiopathic origin, may form a discoid, movable, somewhat tender tumor beneath the areola. Carcinoma of the male breast is so rare before the age of 30 that there is no justification for biopsying tumors in these younger patients. Their benign nature is apparent, moreover, from their physical character.

In older patients, beyond the age of 50, carcinoma of the breast has to be distinguished from the senile type of benign hypertrophy of the breast. I have described this rather frequent but not very well known condition in Chapter 3. This form of hypertrophy has two characteristics which almost always make it possible to distinguish it from carcinoma. It begins as a tender small discoid tumor situated beneath the areola. Its tenderness is out of all proportion to its size. Small carcinomas are not ordinarily tender. More important is the well delimited, rounded, movable character of hypertrophy. Carcinomas are usually poorly delimited and somewhat fixed. I see a good many older patients with the senile type of hypertrophy and I rarely find it necessary to biopsy their lesions. In the typical case of hypertrophy the tenderness will begin to diminish after two or three months, and within six months the tumor itself will disappear. If it persists much longer, or if it is in any way atypical, I perform a biopsy.

Pathology

Microscopic study of our series of carcinomas of the male breast has convinced us that this disease differs microscopically from its counterpart in females. The same microscopic types are found in both males and females, but the carcinomas in the males are more often well differentiated. The distribu-tion of microscopic types in our series of 47 cases in which microscopical sections were available for study is as follows:

Papillary carcinoma	7
Intraductal carcinoma	11
Mucoid carcinoma	1
Paget's carcinoma	1
Small cell carcinoma	1
Apocrine carcinoma	1
No special type	
Grade I — well differentiated	5
Grade II — moderately differentiated	5
Grade III — undifferentiated	15
Total	47

Figure 38–5 shows a typical papillary carcinoma of the male breast. Figures 38–6 and 38–7 illustrate two forms of intraductal carcinoma in males. Figure 38–8 shows the one example of the small cell type of breast carcinoma in our series of carcinomas in males. The patient with this lesion was one of our eight patients surviving 10 years, although the tumor is seen in Figure 38–9 infiltrating the sheath of a small nerve in the breast. In discussing the small cell type of breast carcinoma as it occurs in females, I have

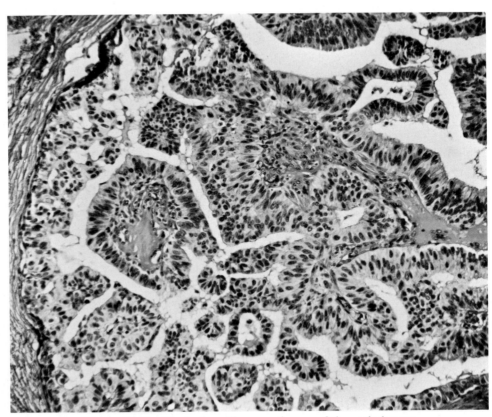

Figure 38–5. Typical papillary carcinoma of the male breast.

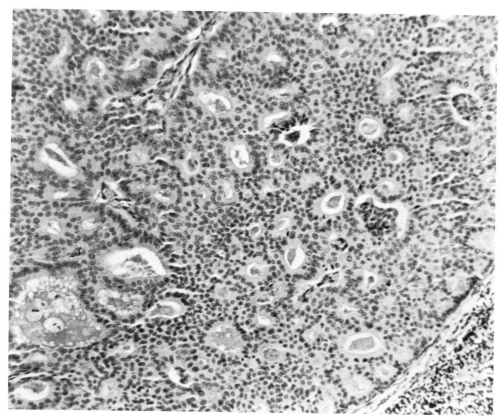

Figure 38–6. The en rognon form of intraductal carcinoma of the male breast.

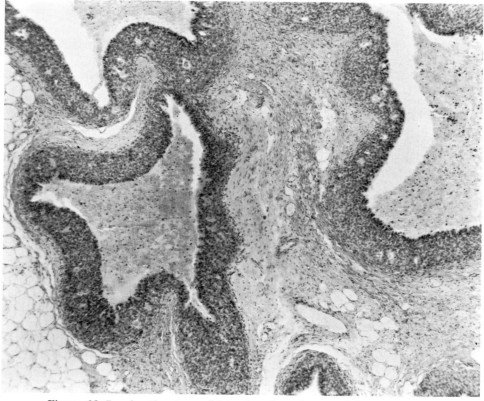

Figure 38–7. Another type of intraductal carcinoma of the male breast.

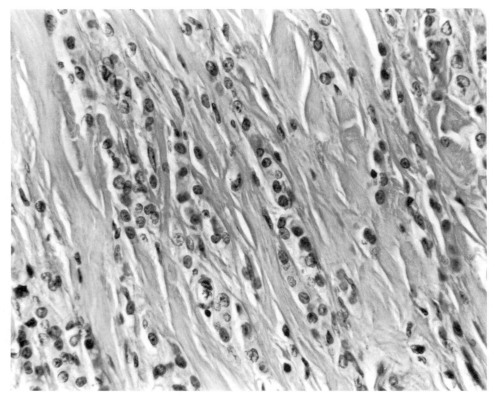

Figure 38–8. The small cell type of carcinoma of the male breast.

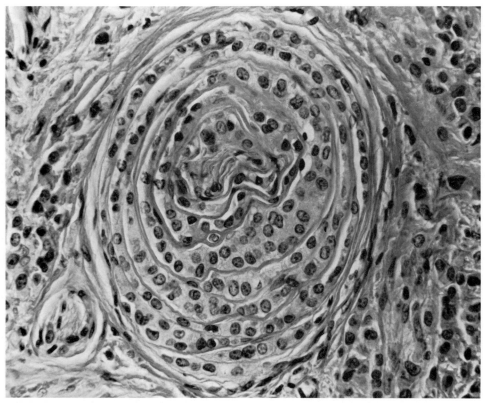

Figure 38–9. The small cell type of carcinoma of the male breast infiltrating the sheath of a small nerve.

emphasized that it is a favorable type of carcinoma.

The papillary and the intraductal carcinomas, in particular, seem to occur with unusual frequency in males. They constituted 39 per cent of the carcinomas of the breast in males in our case series. In contrast, these two types of breast carcinoma have formed only about 6 per cent of the breast carcinomas in females studied in our laboratory.

Treatment

Carcinoma of the breast in males has the reputation of being very difficult to cure. I believe this is due to two factors. In the first place the disease is often not recognized until it is comparatively far advanced. I have classified the stage of advancement of the disease in our 49 patients in terms of our Columbia Clinical Classification, as follows:

Columbia Clinical Classification	Number of Patients
Stage A	25
Stage B	4
Stage C	3
Stage D	17
Total	49

Our experience with breast carcinoma in both males and females has led us to believe that only Clinical Stage A and B disease should be treated by radical mastectomy. On this basis only 29, or 59 per cent, of our 49 male patients with breast carcinoma have come to us in a stage in which their disease was operable.

The second reason why carcinoma of the male breast has a bad reputation is that it presents a special technical challenge to the surgeon who attempts radical mastectomy for it. Although I believe that wide sacrifice of skin over the breast and a skin graft to cover the defect are important features of radical mastectomy for carcinoma of the breast in the female, these features are absolutely essential in operating upon the disease in the male. If the surgeon sacrifices skin widely enough in males, he cannot possibly close his wound without using skin graft. The great majority of males with breast carcinoma have not had skin grafts, and local recurrence has been very frequent.

As with breast carcinoma in the female the end results with the disease in males should be expressed in terms of 10 year survival. Five year results mean very little in this comparatively slowly growing disease, as I will illustrate in several of our patients. Unfortunately, the only 10 year results which have been reported are those of Liechty and his associates: three, or 9 per cent, of their 33 patients who had been treated more than 10 years previously survived.

The 10 year survival rates for the radical mastectomies performed in our Columbia-Presbyterian series of carcinomas of the male breast are shown in Table 38–3. With the exception of my patient with Paget's disease who had only a simple mastectomy and axillary dissection, these results were obtained

Table 38–3. 10 YEAR SURVIVAL FOLLOWING RADICAL MASTECTOMY FOR CARCINOMA OF THE MALE BREAST BY CLINICAL STAGE. COLUMBIA-PRESBYTERIAN MEDICAL CENTER, 1933–1961

Columbia Clinical Classification	No. of Patients	No Axillary Metastases		Axillary Metastases		All Patients, 10 Year Survival	
		No. of Patients	No. of 10 Year Survivors	No. of Patients	No. of 10 Year Survivors	No. of Patients	Per cent
Stage A*	14	10	6	4	1	7	50%
Stage B**	3	2	1	1	—	1	33%
Total	17	12	7	5	1	8	47%
Stage C	1	—	—	1	—	—	—
Stage D	3	—	—	3	—	—	—
Total	21	12	7	9	—	8	38%

*One of these patients, who had papillary carcinoma, died of coronary disease two years postoperatively. Autopsy revealed no evidence of his breast carcinoma, but his case is included.

**One of these patients, who had the apocrine type of carcinoma, died of coronary disease eight years postoperatively. Autopsy showed no evidence of his breast carcinoma, but his case is included.

with our usual radical mastectomy in which a wide area of skin is sacrificed and the defect closed with a skin graft. Both pectoral muscles are sacrificed, and a meticulous and thorough axillary dissection is performed. An average of 26 axillary nodes were found in the surgical specimen in this series of cases.

There are several aspects of these results which merit comment. The 10 year survival rate of 47 per cent in these male patients with operable Clinical Stage A and B carcinoma is much inferior to the 10 year survival rate of 62 per cent for females with Clinical Stage A and B carcinoma in my personal case series.

Only one of five males with axillary metastases survived 10 years.

None of the four males who were treated by radical mastectomy even though their disease was classified as Clinical Stage C or D, and was therefore inoperable, survived 10 years.

The microscopic type of the carcinoma plays a very important role in prognosis. Six of our eight patients who survived for 10 years had favorable microscopic types—two had papillary carcinoma, two intraductal carcinoma, one small cell carcinoma, and the other Paget's carcinoma.

Unfortunately, I must report that survival for even 10 years is no guarantee of cure of these well differentiated carcinomas occurring in the breast in males. Two of my own patients, one with a papillary carcinoma and the other with an intraductal carcinoma, succumbed 14½ and 13½ years, respectively, after operation. Both had had wide local excision of their primary lesion before being referred to me. In both I did a particularly extensive sacrifice of tissues on the chest wall and a large skin graft as part of my radical mastectomy. The patient with the papillary carcinoma had no axillary metastases. The one with the intraductal carcinoma had one of 23 axillary nodes involved.

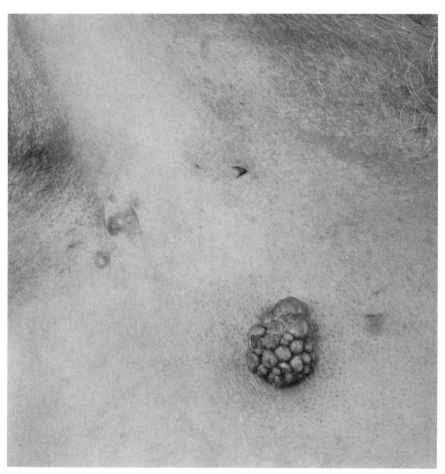

Figure 38–10.   Advanced carcinoma of the male breast on admission.

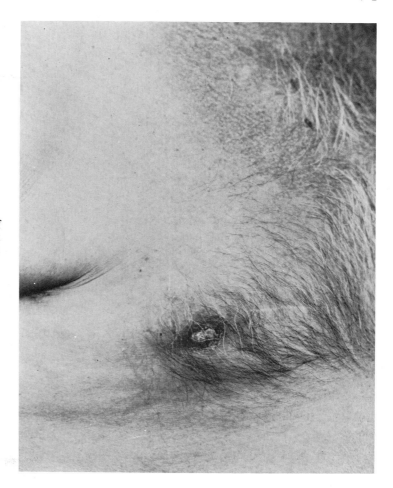

Figure 38–11. The appearance of the local disease in the patient shown in Figure 38–10 two years after orchiectomy.

Neither patient had local recurrence, but the one with the papillary lesion developed pulmonary metastases 7½ years after operation. Its nature was proved by thoracotomy and biopsy. The pulmonary metastases regressed almost completely with stilbestrol treatment. Cerebral metastases developed, however, while the hormone treatment was continuing, 12½ years postoperatively. He succumbed to this last manifestation of his disease 14½ years after radical mastectomy.

The other patient, whose carcinoma was an intraductal one, developed pleural and pulmonary metastases eight years after his operation. Prednisone held his disease in check for some time but he finally developed generalized metastases and died 13½ years after radical mastectomy.

Hormonal Treatment of Breast Carcinoma in Males. Treves discovered the striking palliation which orchiectomy provides in carcinoma of the male breast. His first report was published in 1944, his latest in 1959. The latter report described the results of the operation in 41 patients. At the time of this report 5 patients were living and without evidence of carcinoma from 9 to 60 months after orchiectomy. Seven had died without evidence of carcinoma from 7 to 136 months post-orchiectomy. Twenty-eight of Treves' 41 orchiectomized patients had showed objective improvement for an average of 29.6 months.

In our series of carcinomas of the breast in males we have also seen these dramatic results of orchiectomy. One of our 8 patients who had the operation survived 5½ years afterwards. His case history follows:

Mr. F. A., aged 70, was admitted to the Presbyterian Hospital in October, 1947, with an advanced carcinoma of the right breast. The primary tumor formed a protruding mass in the nipple region that measured 3 cm. in diameter (Fig. 38–10). There were metastatic nodules in the skin over the anterior pectoral fold, and large fixed axillary nodes. There was also a supraclavicular metastasis and a retroperitoneal mass.

Orchiectomy was performed with remarkable local and general palliative benefits. His general health improved strikingly and the breast tumor and its regional metastases regressed remarkably. His appearance two years after orchiectomy is shown in Figure 38-11. He ultimately succumbed to his disease in May, 1953, 5½ years after operation.

The average survival time for our eight patients with advanced or recurrent disease treated by orchiectomy has been 36.8 months.

Understandably, men with breast carcinoma are usually reluctant to submit to orchiectomy. It must be kept in mind that irradiation is a useful alternative method of treatment as long as the disease is sufficiently limited.

The administration of estrogen also produces palliation in this disease, and deserves consideration as an alternative method of treatment. In one of my patients it held pulmonary metastases in check for seven years, although it did not prevent the development of brain metastases. There are not enough reports of the results with estrogen in carcinoma of the breast in males to provide any estimate of how often it will provide palliation.

Treves reported that estrogen given for relapse after orchiectomy in 18 patients was of very little value.

The number of reports of the results of adrenalectomy and of hypophysectomy for carcinoma of the breast in males is too small to permit any conclusions as to their value.

REFERENCES

Botsztejn, C., and Schinz, H. R.: Der Brustkrebs beim Manne. Oncologia, *1*:110, 1948.
Crichlow, R. W., and Czernobilsky, B.: Paget's disease of the male breast. Cancer, *24*:1033, 1969.
Dodge, O. G., Jackson, A. W., and Muldal, S.: Breast cancer and interstitial-cell tumor in a patient with Kleinfelter's syndrome. Cancer, *24*:1027, 1969.
El-Gazayerli, M. M., and Abdel-Aziz, A. S.: On bilharziasis and male breast cancer in Egypt. Brit. J. Cancer, *17*:566, 1963.
Gleichmann, H. G.: Die Beziehungen zwischen Gynäkomastie und Karzinom der Mamma. Ztschr. f. ges. inn. Med., *8*:567, 1953.
Greene, W. W., and Howard, N. J.: Relation of trauma to lesions of the male breast. Am. J. Surg., *85*:431, 1953.
Huggins, C., Jr., and Taylor, G. W.: Carcinoma of the male breast. Arch. Surg., *70*:303, 1955.
Hutchin, P., and Houlihan, R. K.: Paget's disease of the male breast: a case report and a review of the literature. Ann. Surg., *159*:305, 1964.
Liechty, R. D., Davis, J., and Gleysteen, J.: Cancer of the male breast: forty cases. Cancer, *20*:1617, 1967.
Martin, B.: Blutende Mamma beim Manne. Zentralbl. f. Chir., *57*:130, 1930.
Meyer-Laack, H.: Männliche Mammakarzinome und ihre Beziehungen zur Gynaekomastie. Strahlentherapie, *87*:67, 1952.
Moss, N. H.: Cancer of the male breast. Ann. New York Acad. Sci., *114*:937, 1964.
Norris, H. J., and Taylor, H. B.: Carcinoma of the male breast. Cancer, *23*:1428, 1969.
O'Grady, W. P., and McDivitt, R. W.: Breast cancer in a man treated with Diethylstilbestrol. Arch. Path., *88*:162, 1969.
Ritschel, E., and Schultze-Jena, B. S.: Increase of fibrosis mammae virilis (gynaecomastia) after the war. Frankfurt. Ztschr. f. Path., *61*:476, 1950.
Sachs, M. D.: Carcinoma of the male breast. Radiology, *37*:458, 1941.
Schottenfeld, D., Lilienfeld, A. M., and Diamond, H.: Some observations on the epidemiology of breast cancer among males. Am. J. Pub. Health, *53*:890, 1963.
Schottenfeld, D., and Lilienfeld, A. M.: Some epidemiological features of breast cancer among males. J. Chronic Dis., *16*:71, 1963.
Schreiner, B. F.: Tumors of the male breast; based on a study of 31 cases. Radiology, *18*:90, 1932.
Sinner, W.: Karzinome der mannlicher Brustdruse. Strahlentherapie, *115*:522, 1961.
Smith, V. G., and Painter, R. W.: Carcinoma of the male breast: experience at Hartford Hospital, 1930–1950. Amer. Surg., *29*:133, 1963.
Treves, N.: Castration as a therapeutic measure in cancer of the male breast. Cancer, *2*:191, 1949.
Treves, N.: Paget's disease of the male mamma: a report on two cases. Cancer, *7*:325, 1954.
Treves, N.: The treatment of cancer, especially inoperable cancer, of the male breast by ablative surgery (orchiectomy, adrenalectomy, and hypophysectomy) and hormone therapy (estrogens and corticosteroids). Cancer, *12*:820, 1959.
Treves, N., Abels, J. C., Woodard, H. Q., and Farrow, J. H.: The effects of orchiectomy on primary and metastatic carcinoma of the breast. Surg., Gynec. & Obst., *79*:589, 1944.
Treves, N., and Holleb, A. I.: Cancer of the male breast, a report of 146 cases. Cancer, *8*:1239, 1955.
Treves, N., Robbins, G. F., and Amoroso, W. L.: Serous and serosanguineous discharge from the male nipple. Arch. Surg., *73*:319, 1956.
Wainwright, J. M.: Carcinoma of the male breast. Arch. Surg., *14*:836, 1927.
Williams, I. G.: Carcinoma of the male breast. Lancet, *1*:701, 1942.

Chapter Thirty-Nine

The Problem of Breast Carcinoma in Profile

In this concluding chapter I wish to review the challenge which breast carcinoma presents to us today.

Etiology. During the last 100 years much has been learned concerning breast cancer; but we have not found a key to its control as we have for two other common forms of cancer. We know today, for example, that cancer of the lung is, in general, due to cigarette smoking, and that if we could abolish cigarettes the disease would again become a rarity. For cancer of the cervix of the uterus we have a diagnostic method in the cervical smear, which, if generally applied, would reveal the disease at such an early stage that it would regularly be cured. With breast carcinoma, however, our best hope still lies in early diagnosis and a good operation. We often fail to achieve either.

Many facts which have been learned from cancer registries during the past 25 years concerning the occurrence of breast carcinoma provide strong suggestions as to its etiology. In our country the disease has doubled in frequency during the last 35 years, as indicated by the data from the Connecticut Registry. During the same period of time, the most striking change that has occurred in the United States in terms of breast physiology is the abandonment of breast-feeding. In some highly evolved societies, such as that of Japan, in which almost all the children are nursed for a long time, breast cancer is much less frequent than in our American society; and in primitive societies, in which women are usually either pregnant or nursing children, breast cancer is a rarity. Women should be informed of these data and encouraged to breast-feed their children.

Diagnosis. The detection of breast cancer at an earlier stage, in which surgery is more successful, should be one of our basic aims. I do not believe that mammography contributes substantially to earlier diagnosis. We still have to rely upon the education of women to alert them to the possibility of finding their own breast tumors at an early stage by self-examination, and upon careful examination of the breasts by physicians.

In this effort to find breast carcinoma at an earlier stage, it is important to keep in mind that we have five groups of women who are predisposed to develop the disease. They are:

1. Women who have had breast cancer occur in their families;

2. Women who have had gross cystic disease of their breasts;

3. Women who have had carcinoma in one breast;

4. Women who have been found to have lobular neoplasia (lobular carcinoma in situ) in either breast;

5. Women who have had multiple papilloma in either breast.

The women in these five groups should be alerted to their predisposition. Their breasts should be examined by a physician more often than those of other women, preferably every three months.

To achieve earlier detection of breast carcinoma, a carefully planned educational effort will be required. Education of laymen regarding cancer is a two-edged sword and will do more harm than good if it frightens them. We know beyond question that it is fear more than ignorance that makes women with a breast tumor delay so long in consulting a physician. The average duration of symptoms in my most recent personal series of cases is about 5 months. This is, to be sure, an improvement over my figures of 15 years ago; the average delay was then 7.5 months. The challenge to educators is to shorten this period of delay by overcoming fear.

When the patient with breast carcinoma finally consults her physician, he not infrequently misses the diagnosis and causes further delay. This is a distressing fact for medical educators to face, and necessitates improvement in clinical teaching regarding breast cancer.

We have not had much success as yet in meeting this challenge, either as regards lay or professional education. We must hope that better progress will be made and that our modern communications media will be used more effectively.

Our provisions for medical care for those who need financial help, as well as for those who are insured, should make breast examination (as well as other diagnostic examinations) available without cost. Many underprivileged women today are deterred from having these examinations because of such obstacles as the $50 deductible clause for the initial medical expense every year, and the fact that Blue Shield insurance does not pay for check-up examinations.

Another obstacle to the prompt treatment of carcinoma of the breast is our present shortage of hospital beds. In the Columbia-Presbyterian Medical Center for example, our attack on this disease has been seriously handicapped during the past year or so by the fact that it takes about a month to get the patient into the hospital. Priority in admission should be given to patients with probable malignant disease.

Treatment. No new curative methods of treatment for breast carcinoma have been found during the present century. Surgery and irradiation, the latter being a very poor second, remain our only curative weapons. But we have not succeeded in using either of them as skillfully as they should be used.

The surgical attack has recently been seriously weakened by the substitution of a variety of inadequate operations for the classical Halsted radical mastectomy. We surgeons are, of course, to blame. We have not until very recently developed accurate methods of comparing the results of different surgical techniques, and it is tempting for less critical and less conscientious surgeons to abandon the tedious Halsted radical mastectomy. Halsted himself characterized his operation as a "very great labor."

I have described the three basic requirements for the kind of comparison of these different techniques which will lead us to the truth.

1. Detailed and accurate clinical case records;
2. Reliable clinical classification of the stage of advancement of the disease in the patients constituting the case series being compared. (our Columbia Clinical Classification is the only practical classification);
3. Ten-year survival data for the entire number of patients originally treated by the methods being compaired.

This kind of comparison of different surgical methods of treating breast carcinoma was published for the first time in 1969 by our international group. It shows that the classical Halsted radical mastectomy as exemplified by the operation which I and a number of my associates at Columbia perform, yields a lower local recurrence rate and a higher 10-year survival rate than any other surgical method of treatment.

This is only what might be expected in terms of the facts of the natural history of breast carcinoma and its pathology. Simple mastectomy, as well as many of the "limited" and "modified" radical mastectomies now so much in vogue, do not remove all of the mammary gland, although we know that carcinoma may be multicentric or may infiltrate much more widely than the clinician suspects. Moreover, many of these limited operations do not remove all of the axillary lymph nodes which may contain metastases even in the early stages of the disease.

Irradiation alone for breast carcinoma in its operable stages has been tried by several skillful radiotherapists. The five-year survival rates are inferior—although not greatly inferior—to radical mastectomy; but between 5 and 10 years the survival rate falls off so tragically that irradiation cannot be seriously considered as a substitute for the Halsted radical mastectomy.

Although irradiation has, I believe, proved to be inferior as the sole method of treatment for operable carcinoma of the breast, it has great value when judiciously used as an auxiliary prophylactic form of treatment supplementing radical mastectomy. There are two situations in which we at Columbia advise its use following radical mastectomy:

1. *Internal mammary irradiation.* Probably the most challenging therapeutic problem we face today in dealing with operable breast carcinoma (Clinical Stages A and B in our Columbia Clinical Classification) is how best to deal with occult internal mammary metastases. I have described recent studies which show that from 20 to 25 per cent of all patients with operable breast carcinoma have occult internal mammary metastases, and I have documented the failure of the extended radical mastectomy which includes removal of these nodes. Our own method of treatment, which has been to remove these nodes for biopsy and to rely upon irradiation alone for the treatment of the disease if these nodes are found to be involved has also failed. We have recently abandoned this method and turned to the one remaining alternative, namely, to perform radical mastectomy on all our operable patients and to give postoperative prophylactic irradiation to the internal mammary region to all except those who have very small carcinomas of the outer half of the breast. This limited kind of irradiation does not penalize the patient and we hope it will improve our results.

2. Analysis of our end-results with the Halsted radical mastectomy indicates that postoperative irradiation should be given prophylactically to the chest wall, axillary, supraclavicular, and internal mammary regions, in all patients who are found to have a total of eight or more axillary nodes involved. We believe that the postoperative irradiation so often given to these regions in patients who have less extensive axillary metastases does more harm than good.

Hormones in Breast Carcinoma. The hormonal methods of treatment for breast carcinoma which have evolved during the last 50 years have important palliative value, and this form of treatment is perhaps our best hope for the future. It is the chemists who must find the keys to the precise roles of the various hormones in the etiology and control of breast carcinoma. We need quantitative analytic methods which will make it possible to study ovarian, adrenal, and pituitary hormones in the bloodstream.

Chemotherapy. The recent chemotherapeutic attack upon breast carcinoma has been very disappointing. A great deal of money has been spent, and probably more harm than good has come of it.

The experience with chemotherapy has been a good example of the fact that in exceedingly complex biological problems such as cancer, large amounts of money and bureaucratic organization of research on a large scale are not necessarily successful. It is more reasonable to concentrate our effort in highly trained and devoted teams of research workers, surgeons, internists, radiotherapists, and educators—all cooperating to make the best use of the weapons which modern science has given us—and to emphasize quality rather than quantity in research. The courage which our patients display should inspire us to put aside prejudice, and in all humility to intensify our effort to conquer the disease.

Author Index

Note: Page numbers in *italics* refer to bibliographic references.

Subject Index

Note: Page numbers in *italics* refer to illustrations.